ICD-10

International Statistical Classification of Diseases and Related Health Problems

10th Revision

Volume 3
Alphabetical index

2010 Edition

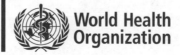
World Health Organization

WHO Library Cataloguing-in-Publication Data

International statistical classification of diseases and related health problems. - 10th revision, edition 2010.

3 v.

Contents: v. 1. Tabular list – v. 2. Instruction manual – v. 3. Alphabetical index.

1.Diseases - classification. 2.Classification. 3.Manuals. I.World Health Organization. II.ICD-10.

ISBN 978 92 4 154834 2   (NLM classification: WB 15)

The 43rd World Health Assembly in 1990 approved the Tenth Revision of the International Classification of Diseases (WHA 43,24) and endorsed the recommendation of the International Conference for the Tenth Revision of the ICD held in Geneva from 26 September to 2 October 1989 concerning the establishment of an updating process within the 10-year revision cycle. This recommendation was put into motion at the annual meeting of WHO Collaborating Centres for the Family of International Classifications in Tokyo, Japan in 1996 and later a formal mechanism to guide the updating process was established. According to this updating mechanism minor updates are made each year while major updates are made, if required, every three years.

For more information regarding the updating process and a cumulative list of the updates please see http://www.who.int/classifications. Future updates will also be posted on this site.

The 2010 edition of ICD-10 can also be referred to as the 4th edition of ICD-10. It includes updates that came into effect between 1998 and 2010, as well as the corrigenda to Volume 1, which appeared as an addendum to Volume 3 of the first edition.

Printed in Malta

Contents

Introduction   1

   General arrangement of the Index   1
   Conventions used in the Index   5

Alphabetical index to diseases and nature of injury   11

External causes of injury   663

Table of drugs and chemicals   717

Introduction

Volume 3 of the *International Statistical Classification of Diseases and Related Health Problems* is an alphabetical index to the Tabular List of Volume 1. Although the Index reflects the provisions of the Tabular List in regard to the notes varying the assignment of a diagnostic term when it is reported with other conditions, or under particular circumstances (e.g. certain conditions complicating pregnancy), it is not possible to express all such variations in the index terms. Volume 1 should therefore be regarded as the primary coding tool. The Alphabetical Index is, however, an essential adjunct to the Tabular List, since it contains a great number of diagnostic terms that do not appear in Volume 1. The two volumes must therefore be used together.

The terms included in a category of the Tabular List are not exhaustive; they serve as examples of the content of the category or as indicators of its extent and limits. The Index, on the other hand, is intended to include most of the diagnostic terms currently in use. Nevertheless, reference should always be made back to the Tabular List and its notes, as well as to the guidelines provided in Volume 2, to ensure that the code given by the Index fits with the information provided by a particular record.

Because of its exhaustive nature, the Index inevitably includes many imprecise and undesirable terms. Since these terms are still occasionally encountered on medical records, coders need an indication of their assignment in the classification, even if this is to a rubric for residual or ill-defined conditions. The presence of a term in this volume, therefore, should not be taken as implying approval of its usage.

General arrangement of the Index

Main sections

The Alphabetical Index consists of the three sections, as follows:

Section I is the index of diseases, syndromes, pathological conditions, injuries, signs, symptoms, problems and other reasons for contact with health services, i.e. the type of information that would be recorded by a physician. It includes all terms classifiable to categories A00–T98 and Z00–Z99 except drugs and other chemical substances giving rise to poisoning or other adverse effects (these are included in Section III).

Section II is the index of external causes of injury. The terms included here are not medical diagnoses but descriptions of the circumstances in which the violence occurred (e.g. fire, explosion, fall, assault, collision, submersion). It includes all terms classifiable to V01–Y98, except drugs and chemicals.

Section III is the index of drugs and other chemical substances giving rise to poisoning or other adverse effects (referred to in Sections I and II as the Table of drugs and chemicals). For each substance the Table gives the Chapter XIX code for poisoning (T36–T65) and the external cause (Chapter XX) codes for accidental poisoning by and exposure to noxious substances (X40–X49), intentional self-harm (X60–X69), and poisoning, undetermined whether accidental or intentional (Y10–Y19). For drugs, medicaments and biological substances, it also gives the code for these substances causing adverse effects in therapeutic use (Y40–Y59).

Structure

To avoid unnecessary repetition, the Index is organized in the form of lead terms, which start at the extreme left of a column, and various levels of indentation, which start progressively further right. A complete index term, therefore, may be composed of several lines, sometimes quite widely separated. For example, in the entry:

> Erythroblastosis (fetalis) (newborn) P55.9
> – due to
> – – ABO (antibodies) (incompatibility) (isoimmunization) P55.1
> – – Rh (antibodies) (incompatibility) (isoimmunization) P55.0

the last line stands for "Erythroblastosis due to Rh antibodies, incompatibility or isoimmunization".

Usually, the lead term is the name of a disease or pathological condition, while the terms indented beneath it (the "modifiers") refer either to varieties of the condition, to the anatomical sites affected by it, or to circumstances that affect its coding. The coder should therefore look up the disease or condition as a lead term and then find the variety, anatomical site, etc., indented beneath it. Thus "tuberculosis of hip" is under the letter T and not under H, and stomach ulcer is under U, not under S. Only occasionally are anatomical sites indexed as the lead term. Usually, after the name of the anatomical site there will be a cross-reference to the disease, e.g. Ankle – *see condition*.[1]

---

[1] The name of an anatomical site appears as a lead term when it is part of the name of the disease, e.g. "abdomen, acute R10.0". This does not occur frequently in English, and in the English-language version applies mainly to Latin expressions for some conditions, e.g. "Cor biloculare".

In some diagnostic statements, the disease condition is expressed in adjectival form. Sometimes, the index lists both forms but often only the noun form will be found and the coder must make the necessary transformation.

Among the indented modifiers, it is always feasible to include a complete listing of the various combinations of modifiers that could apply to a given term. In such circumstances, some types of modifier tend to have priority in assignment over others. For instance, under the lead term "Abscess" are indented a large number of anatomical sites and their appropriate codes. However, tuberculous abscesses are not classified to these codes but to the codes for tuberculosis of these sites. Instead of inserting an indent "tuberculous" under each anatomical site, the index uses one single indent "tuberculous – see Tuberculosis, abscess" under the lead term "Abscess". In general, the types of modifiers that tend to have priority in Section I are those indicating that a disease or condition is infectious or parasitic, malignant, neoplastic, psychogenic, hysterical, congenital, traumatic, complicating or affecting the management of pregnancy, childbirth or the puerperium, or affecting the fetus or newborn, or that the disease was reported in circumstances where the patient was looking for health advice but was not necessarily sick (cases in Chapter XXI). In Section II, the priority modifiers are those indicating transport accidents, complications of medical and surgical procedures, intentional self-harm, assault, legal intervention, or war operations.

Section I incorporates an index of the categories to be used with Chapter XXI[1] for terms relating to problems or circumstances rather than diseases or injuries. Some special lead terms, or "key" words, are used for these, indicating the type of problem or circumstances. The main key words are "Counseling", "Examination", "History", "Observation", "Pregnancy", "Problem", "Screening", "Status", and "Vaccination".

In both Sections I and II, this key word form of lead term is also used instead of, or in addition to, the standard method for certain conditions or circumstances where terminology is diverse and reported descriptions might not easily be found in the Index, or where the normal method of indexing might be misleading. Some obstetric complications, especially the more common ones, can be found under the specific condition, e.g. Hemorrhage, complicating delivery. More often, however, the complication will be listed under "Labor", "Pregnancy", "Puerperal", or "Maternal condition affecting fetus or newborn". In Section II, key words are "Complication" (for medical or surgical procedures), "Sequelae", "Suicide", "Assault", "Legal intervention" and "War operations". Coders should remember the presence of

---

[1] Formerly the supplementary "V" code.

the special lists whenever they have difficulty locating index entries for the relevant conditions, problems or circumstances; by scrutinizing the indented terms, guidance can be found as to the code numbers of all the relevant categories even if not reported in precisely the same words.

Code numbers

The code numbers that follow the terms in the Index are those of the three- or four-character categories to which the terms are classified. In some cases, the fourth character is replaced by a dash, e.g. Burn, ankle (and foot) T25.–. This indicates that a fourth character exists and should be used, and that it will be found either in a note in the Index (e.g. the fourth-character subdivisions common to many sites of burns are given in a note under the lead term "Burn") or by reference to Volume 1.

When a set of fourth characters is applicable to a group of categories, the common fourth characters may be presented in a note or, in the case of pregnancies with abortive outcome, in a table in order to facilitate their application to different types of complete or incomplete abortion and to molar pregnancies. In other cases, the complication or main manifestation is listed in the Index with a cross-reference to the entire group of categories, with specification of the fourth character, e.g. Coma, diabetic – *code to* E10–E14 with fourth character .0.

Where an index term is one of the diagnostic statements for which there is a dual classification according to etiology and manifestation (see Volume 2), both codes are given, the first followed by a dagger (†) and the second by an asterisk (*), e.g. Pott's disease A18.0† M49.0*.

Multiple diagnoses

The Tabular List includes a number of categories for the classification of two or more conditions jointly reported, e.g. "Influenza with pneumonia" (J11.0), "Acute appendicitis with generalized peritonitis" (K35.0). Such combinations of conditions, which are specifically classified in the Tabular List, also appear in the Index. Classification rules for certain other combinations appear in Volume 2 in the section "Mortality: guidelines for certification and rules for coding" under the heading "Notes for use in underlying cause mortality coding", e.g. "Atherosclerosis" should not be coded when it is reported with conditions in I60–I69 (cerebrovascular diseases). These provisions, since they are not inherent in the classification itself, are not indexed.

Spelling

In order to avoid repetitions caused by the differences between American and British spelling, the American form has been used in the Index. Users familiar with the British form should remember that the first letter of the vowel combinations ae and oe and the u in words ending in -our have been dropped, and the "re" reversed to "er" in words ending thus. It is only when the initial letters are affected that any great displacement in alphabetical order is caused, and in this case, the word is usually also listed with the British spelling and a reference given to the American spelling, thus: "Oedema, oedematous – *see* Edema".

Conventions used in the Index

Parentheses

In the Index, as in the Tabular List, parentheses have a special meaning which the coder must bear in mind. A term that is followed by other terms in parentheses is classified to the given code number whether any of the terms in parentheses are reported or not. For example:

> Abscess (embolic) (infective) (metastatic) (multiple) (pyogenic) (septic)
> – brain (any part) G06.0

Brain abscess is classified to G06.0 regardless of the part of the organ affected and whether or not the abscess is described as embolic, infective, metastatic, multiple, pyogenic, or septic.

Cross-references

Some categories, particularly those subject to notes linking them with other categories, require rather complex indexing arrangements. To avoid repeating this arrangement for each of the inclusion terms involved, a cross-reference is used. This may take a number of forms, as in the following examples:

> Inflammation
> – bone – *see* Osteomyelitis

This indicates that the term "Inflammation, bone" is to be coded in the same way as the term "Osteomyelitis". On looking up the latter term, the coder will find listed various forms of osteomyelitis: acute, acute hematogenous, chronic, etc.

When a term has a number of modifiers which might be listed beneath more than one term, the cross-reference (*see also...*) is used.

> Paralysis
> – shaking (*see also* Parkinsonism) G20

The coder is told that if the term "shaking paralysis" is the only term on the medical record, the code number is G20, but that if any other information is present which is not found indented below, he or she should look up "Parkinsonism". There alternative codes will be found for the condition if further or otherwise qualified as, for example, due to drugs or syphilitic.

> Enlargement, enlarged – *see also* Hypertrophy

If the coder does not find the site of the enlargement among the indentations beneath "Enlargement", he or she should look among the indentations beneath "Hypertrophy" where a more complete list of sites is given.

> Bladder – *see* condition

> Hereditary – *see* condition

As stated previously, anatomical sites and very general adjectival modifiers are not usually used as lead terms in the Index and the coder is instructed to look up the disease or injury reported on the medical record and under that term to find the site or adjectival modifier.

> Abdomen, abdominal – *see also* condition
> – acute R10.0
> – convulsive equivalent G40.8
> – muscle deficiency syndrome Q79.4

The term "acute abdomen" is coded to R10.0; "abdominal convulsive equivalent" is coded to G40.8; and "abdominal muscle deficiency syndrome" is coded to Q79.4. For other abdominal conditions, the coder should look up the disease or injury reported.

Abbreviation NEC

The letters NEC stand for "not elsewhere classified". They are added after terms classified to residual or unspecific categories and to terms in themselves ill defined as a warning that specified forms of the conditions are classified differently. If the medical record includes more precise information the coding should be modified accordingly, e.g.

> Anomaly, anomalous (congenital) (unspecified type) Q89.9
> – aorta (arch) NEC Q25.9

The term "anomaly of aorta" is classified to Q25.4 only if no more precise description appears on the medical record. If a more precise term, e.g. atresia of aorta, is recorded, this term should be looked up for the appropriate code.

Special signs

The following special signs will be found attached to certain code numbers or index terms:

† / * Used to designate the etiology code and the manifestation code respectively, for terms subject to dual classification. See above under "Code numbers".

/ ◇ Attached to certain terms in the list of sites under "Neoplasm" to refer the coder to Notes 2 and 3, respectively, at the start of that list.

Section I

Alphabetical index to diseases and nature of injury

Primary Diagnosis

1. The main condition treated or investigated during the relevant episode of healthcare

2. where there is no definitive diagnosis, The main symptom, abnormal findings or problem should be selected as the main condition

Con Code: 'Probable'; 'Presumed'; or 'Treat As'

Cant code: 'likely'; 'Possible'

(cc. Jan 2000)

A

Aarskog's syndrome Q87.1
Abandonment T74.0
Abasia(-astasia) (hysterical) F44.4
Abdomen, abdominal – *see also condition*
– acute R10.0
– convulsive equivalent G40.8
– muscle deficiency syndrome Q79.4
Abdominalgia R10.4
Abduction contracture, hip or other joint – *see* Contraction, joint
Aberrant (congenital) – *see also* Malposition, congenital
– adrenal gland Q89.1
– artery (peripheral) NEC Q27.8
– breast Q83.8
– endocrine gland NEC Q89.2
– hepatic duct Q44.5
– pancreas Q45.3
– parathyroid gland Q89.2
– pituitary gland Q89.2
– sebaceous glands, mucous membrane, mouth, congenital Q38.6
– spleen Q89.0
– subclavian artery Q27.8
– thymus (gland) Q89.2
– thyroid gland Q89.2
– vein (peripheral) NEC Q27.8
Aberration, mental F99
Abetalipoproteinemia E78.6
Abiotrophy R68.8
Ablatio, ablation
– placentae (*see also* Abruptio placentae) O45.9
– – affecting fetus or newborn P02.1
– retinae (*see also* Detachment, retina) H33.2
– uterus Z90.7
Ablepharia, ablepharon Q10.3
Abnormal, abnormality, abnormalities – *see also* Anomaly
– acid-base balance (mixed) E87.4
– – fetus – *see* Distress, fetal
– albumin R77.0
– alphafetoprotein R77.2
– amnion, amniotic fluid O41.9
– – affecting fetus or newborn P02.9
– apertures, congenital, diaphragm Q79.1
– auditory perception NEC H93.2
– autosomes NEC Q99.9

Abnormal, abnormality—*continued*
– autosomes NEC—*continued*
– – fragile site Q95.5
– basal metabolic rate R94.8
– biosynthesis, testicular androgen E29.1
– blood level (of)
– – cobalt R79.0
– – copper R79.0
– – iron R79.0
– – lithium R78.8
– – magnesium R79.0
– – mineral NEC R79.0
– – zinc R79.0
– blood-gas level R79.8
– bowel sounds R19.1
– breathing NEC R06.8
– caloric test R94.1
– cervix NEC (acquired) (congenital), in pregnancy or childbirth O34.4
– – causing obstructed labor O65.5
– – – affecting fetus or newborn P03.1
– chemistry, blood R79.9
– – specified NEC R79.8
– chest sounds (friction) (rales) R09.8
– chorion O41.9
– – affecting fetus or newborn P02.9
– chromosome, chromosomal Q99.9
– – analysis result R89.8
– – dicentric replacement Q93.2
– – female with more than three X chromosomes Q97.1
– – fetal (suspected), affecting management of pregnancy O35.1
– – ring replacement Q93.2
– – sex Q99.8
– – – female phenotype Q97.9
– – – – specified NEC Q97.8
– – – male phenotype Q98.9
– – – – specified NEC Q98.8
– – – structural, male Q98.6
– – specified NEC Q99.8
– clinical findings NEC R68.8
– coagulation D68.9
– – newborn, transient P61.6
– communication – *see* Fistula
– course, eustachian tube Q16.4
– diagnostic imaging
– – abdomen, abdominal region NEC R93.5

11

Abnormal, abnormality—*continued*
- diagnostic imaging—*continued*
- – biliary tract R93.2
- – breast R92
- – central nervous system NEC R90.8
- – coronary circulation R93.1
- – digestive tract NEC R93.3
- – gastrointestinal (tract) R93.3
- – genitourinary organs R93.8
- – head R93.0
- – heart R93.1
- – intrathoracic organs NEC R93.8
- – limbs R93.6
- – liver R93.2
- – lung (field) R91
- – musculoskeletal system NEC R93.7
- – retroperitoneum R93.5
- – sites specified NEC R93.8
- – skin and subcutaneous tissue R93.8
- – skull R93.0
- – urinary organs R93.4
- ear ossicles, acquired NEC H74.3
- echocardiogram R93.1
- echoencephalogram R90.8
- echogram – *see* Abnormal, diagnostic imaging
- electrocardiogram (ECG) (EKG) R94.3
- electroencephalogram (EEG) R94.0
- electrolyte (*see also* Imbalance, electrolyte) E87.8
- electromyogram (EMG) R94.1
- electro-oculogram (EOG) R94.1
- electrophysiological intracardiac studies R94.3
- electroretinogram (ERG) R94.1
- feces (color) (contents) (mucus) R19.5
- fetus, fetal
- – acid-base balance, complicating labor and delivery O68.3
- – affecting management of pregnancy O35.9
- – causing disproportion O33.7
- – – with obstructed labor O66.3
- – – affecting fetus or newborn P03.1
- – heart rate – *see* Distress, fetal
- finding
- – antenatal screening, mother O28.9
- – – biochemical NEC O28.1
- – – chromosomal NEC O28.5
- – – cytological NEC O28.2
- – – genetic NEC O28.5
- – – hematological NEC O28.0
- – – radiological NEC O28.4
- – – specified NEC O28.8

Abnormal, abnormality—*continued*
- finding—*continued*
- – antenatal screening, mother—*continued*
- – – ultrasonic O28.3
- – specimen – *see* Abnormal, specimen
- fluid
- – amniotic R89.-
- – cerebrospinal R83.-
- – peritoneal R85.-
- – pleural R84.-
- – respiratory organs (bronchial washings) (nasal secretions) (pleural fluid) (sputum) (throat scrapings) R84.-
- – synovial R89.-
- – thorax (bronchial washings) (pleural fluid) R84.-
- – vaginal R87.-
- forces of labor O62.9
- – affecting fetus or newborn P03.6
- – specified type NEC O62.8
- form
- – teeth K00.2
- – uterus – *see* Anomaly, uterus
- function studies
- – bladder R94.8
- – brain R94.0
- – cardiovascular R94.3
- – endocrine NEC R94.7
- – kidney R94.4
- – liver R94.5
- – nervous system
- – – central R94.0
- – – peripheral R94.1
- – pulmonary R94.2
- – special senses R94.1
- – spleen R94.8
- – thyroid R94.6
- gait (*see also* Gait) R26.8
- – hysterical F44.4
- globulin R77.1
- – cortisol-binding E27.8
- – thyroid-binding E07.8
- glomerular, minor – *code to* N00-N07 with fourth character .0
- glucose tolerance (test) R73.0
- – in pregnancy, childbirth or puerperium O99.8
- gravitational (G) forces or states (effect of) T75.8
- hair (color) (shaft) L67.9
- – specified NEC L67.8
- hard tissue formation in pulp (dental) K04.3
- head movement R25.0

Abnormal, abnormality—*continued*
- heart
- – rate NEC R00.8
- – – fetus – *see* Distress, fetal
- – shadow R93.1
- – sounds NEC R01.2
- hematological NEC, resulting from HIV disease B23.2
- hemoglobin (disease) (*see also* Disease, hemoglobin) D58.2
- – trait – *see* Trait, hemoglobin, abnormal
- histology NEC R89.7
- immunological findings R89.4
- – in serum R76.9
- – – specified NEC R76.8
- – resulting from HIV disease B23.2
- involuntary movement R25.8
- jaw closure K07.5
- karyotype R89.8
- kidney function test R94.4
- labor NEC O75.8
- – affecting fetus or newborn P03.6
- leukocyte (cell) (differential) NEC R72
- loss of weight R63.4
- Mantoux test R76.1
- membranes (fetal)
- – affecting fetus or newborn P02.9
- – complicating pregnancy O41.9
- – specified type NEC, affecting fetus or newborn P02.8
- movement (disorder) (*see also* Disorder, movement) G25.9
- – head R25.0
- – involuntary R25.8
- myoglobin (Aberdeen) (Annapolis) R89.-
- organs or tissues of pelvis NEC
- – in pregnancy or childbirth O34.9
- – – affecting fetus or newborn P03.8
- – – causing obstructed labor O65.5
- – – – affecting fetus or newborn P03.1
- – – specified NEC O34.8
- palmar creases Q82.8
- Papanicolaou (smear)
- – cervix R87.6
- – sites NEC R89.6
- parturition
- – affecting fetus or newborn P03.9
- – mother – *see* Delivery, complicated
- pelvis (bony) – *see* Deformity, pelvis
- percussion, chest (tympany) R09.8
- periods (grossly) (*see also* Menstruation) N92.6
- phonocardiogram R94.3

Abnormal, abnormality—*continued*
- placenta NEC (*see also* Placenta, abnormal) O43.1
- plasma
- – protein R77.9
- – – specified NEC R77.8
- – viscosity R70.1
- pleural (folds) Q34.0
- position – *see* Malposition
- posture R29.3
- presentation (fetus) (*see also* Presentation, fetal, abnormal) O32.9
- – before labor, affecting fetus or newborn P01.7
- product of conception O02.9
- – specified type NEC O02.8
- pulmonary
- – artery, congenital Q25.7
- – function, newborn P28.8
- – test results R94.2
- – ventilation, newborn P28.8
- pupillary function (reaction) (reflex) H57.0
- radiological examination – *see* Abnormal, diagnostic imaging
- red blood cell(s) (morphology) (volume) R71
- reflex NEC (*see also* Reflex) R29.2
- renal function test R94.4
- response to nerve stimulation R94.1
- retinal correspondence H53.3
- rhythm, heart (*see also* Arrhythmia) I49.9
- – fetus – *see* Distress, fetal
- saliva R85.-
- secretion
- – gastrin E16.4
- – glucagon E16.3
- semen, seminal fluid R86.-
- serum level (of)
- – acid phosphatase R74.8
- – alkaline phosphatase R74.8
- – amylase R74.8
- – enzymes R74.9
- – – specified NEC R74.8
- – lipase R74.8
- – triacylglycerol lipase R74.8
- shape, gravid uterus – *see* Anomaly, uterus
- sinus venosus Q21.1
- size, tooth, teeth K00.2
- spacing, tooth, teeth K07.3
- specimen
- – cervix uteri R87.-

Abnormal, abnormality—*continued*
- specimen—*continued*
-   – digestive organs (peritoneal fluid) (saliva) R85.-
-   – female genital organs (secretions) (smears) R87.-
-   – male genital organs (prostatic secretions) (semen) R86.-
-   – nipple discharge R89.-
-   – respiratory organs (bronchial washings) (nasal secretions) (pleural fluid) (sputum) (throat scrapings) R84.-
-   – specified organ, system or tissue NEC R89.-
-   – synovial fluid R89.-
-   – thorax (bronchial washings) (pleural fluids) R84.-
-   – vagina (secretion) (smear) R87.-
-   – vulva (secretion) (smear) R87.-
-   – wound secretion R89.-
- spermatozoa R86.-
- sputum (amount) (color) (odor) R09.3
- stool (color) (contents) (mucus) R19.5
- synchondrosis Q78.8
- thermography – *see* Abnormal, diagnostic imaging
- thyroid-binding globulin E07.8
- tooth, teeth (form) (size) K00.2
- toxicology (findings) R78.9
- transport protein E88.0
- ultrasound results – *see* Abnormal, diagnostic imaging
- umbilical cord
-   – affecting fetus or newborn P02.6
-   – complicating delivery O69.9
- urination NEC R39.1
- urine (constituents) NEC R82.9
-   – cytological examination R82.8
-   – heavy metals R82.6

Abnormal, abnormality—*continued*
- urine—*continued*
-   – histological examination R82.8
-   – microbiological examination (culture) R82.7
-   – positive culture R82.7
-   – specified NEC R82.9
-   – substances nonmedical R82.6
- vagina (acquired) (congenital), in pregnancy or childbirth O34.6
-   – causing obstructed labor O65.5
-   – – affecting fetus or newborn P03.1
- vectorcardiogram R94.3
- visually evoked potential (VEP) R94.1
- vulva and perineum (acquired) (congenital), in pregnancy or childbirth O34.7

Abnormal, abnormality—*continued*
- vulva and perineum—*continued*
-   – causing obstructed labor O65.5
-   – – affecting fetus or newborn P03.1
- white blood cells NEC R72
- X-ray examination – *see* Abnormal, diagnostic imaging

Abnormity (any organ or part) – *see* Anomaly

ABO hemolytic disease (fetus or newborn) P55.1

Abolition, language R48.8

Aborter, habitual or recurrent NEC
- care in current pregnancy O26.2
- current abortion – *see* categories O03-O06
-   – affecting fetus or newborn P01.8
- without current pregnancy N96

Abortion (complete) (incomplete) O06.-
- accidental O03.-
- attempted (failed) (induced) (nonmedical) O07.9

Note: The following fourth-character list is provided to be used with categories O03-O06 and O08. A distinction is made between an episode of care at which a disease or injury and resulting complications or manifestations are treated together - "current episode" - and an episode of care for complications or manifestations of diseases or injuries treated previously - "subsequent episode".

	Complication of abortion, current episode (O03-O06)		Complication of pregnancy with abortive outcome, subsequent episode (O08)
	complete or unspecified	incomplete	
Abortion			
– complicated (by)	.8	.3	.9
– – afibrinogenemia	.6	.1	.1
– – cardiac arrest	.8	.3	.8
– – chemical damage			
– – – bladder	.8	.3	.6
– – – bowel	.8	.3	.6
– – – broad ligament	.8	.3	.6
– – – cervix	.8	.3	.6
– – – periurethral tissue	.8	.3	.6
– – – uterus	.8	.3	.6
– – circulatory collapse	.8	.3	.3
– – condition specified NEC	.8	.3	.8
– – damage to pelvic organs or tissues NEC	.8	.3	.6
– – defibrination syndrome	.6	.1	.1
– – electrolyte imbalance	.8	.3	.5
– – embolism	.7	.2	.2
– – – air	.7	.2	.2
– – – amniotic fluid	.7	.2	.2
– – – blood clot	.7	.2	.2
– – – pulmonary	.7	.2	.2
– – – pyemic	.7	.2	.2
– – – septic	.7	.2	.2
– – – septicopyemic	.7	.2	.2
– – – soap	.7	.2	.2
– – endometritis	.5	.0	.0
– – hemorrhage (delayed) (excessive)	.6	.1	.1
– – infection			
– – – genital	.5	.0	.0
– – – pelvic	.5	.0	.0
– – – urinary tract	.8	.3	.8
– – intravascular coagulation	.6	.1	.1
– – laceration			
– – – bladder	.8	.3	.6
– – – bowel	.8	.3	.6
– – – broad ligament	.8	.3	.6
– – – cervix	.8	.3	.6
– – – periurethral tissue	.8	.3	.6
– – – uterus	.8	.3	.6
– – metabolic disorder	.8	.3	.5
– – oliguria	.8	.3	.4
– – oophoritis	.5	.0	.0
– – parametritis	.5	.0	.0
– – pelvic peritonitis	.5	.0	.0

[handwritten annotation: New Consult episode or Readmission]

15

	Complication of abortion, current episode (O03-O06)		Complication of pregnancy with abortive outcome, subsequent episode (O08)
	complete or unspecified	incomplete	
Abortion—*continued*			
– complicated (by) —*continued*	.8	.3	.9
– – perforation			
– – – bladder	.8	.3	.6
– – – bowel	.8	.3	.6
– – – cervix	.8	.3	.6
– – – uterus	.8	.3	.6
– – renal failure (acut)	.8	.3	.4
– – renal shutdown	.8	.3	.4
– – salpingitis	.5	.0	.0
– – salpingo-oophoritis	.5	.0	.0
– – sepsis	.5	.0	.0
– – septic shock	.5	.0	.0
– – shock (postoperative)	.8	.3	.3
– – tear			
– – – bladder	.8	.3	.6
– – – bowel	.8	.3	.6
– – – broad ligament	.8	.3	.6
– – – cervix	.8	.3	.6
– – – periurethral tissue	.8	.3	.6
– – – uterus	.8	.3	.6
– – tubular necrosis (renal)	.8	.3	.4
– – uremia	.8	.3	.4
– – urinary infection	.8	.3	.8

Abortion—*continued*
– attempted—*continued*
– – complicated by
– – – afibrinogenemia O07.6
– – – cardiac arrest O07.8
– – – chemical damage of pelvic organ(s) O07.8
– – – circulatory collapse O07.8
– – – defibrination syndrome O07.6
– – – electrolyte imbalance O07.8
– – – embolism (amniotic fluid) (blood clot) (pulmonary) (septic) (soap) O07.7
– – – endometritis O07.5
– – – hemorrhage (delayed) (excessive) O07.6
– – – infection, genital tract or pelvic O07.5
– – – intravascular coagulation O07.6
– – – laceration of pelvic organ(s) O07.8
– – – oliguria O07.8
– – – oophoritis O07.5
– – – parametritis O07.5
– – – pelvic peritonitis O07.5

Abortion—*continued*
– attempted—*continued*
– – complicated by—*continued*
– – – perforation of pelvic organ(s) O07.8
– – – renal failure or shutdown O07.8
– – – salpingitis or salpingo-oophoritis O07.5
– – – sepsis O07.5
– – – septic shock O07.5
– – – shock O07.8
– – – – septic O07.5
– – – specified condition NEC O07.8
– – – tubular necrosis (renal) O07.8
– – – urinary infection O07.8
– – illegal O07.-
– – medical O07.4
– – – complicated by
– – – – afibrinogenemia O07.1
– – – – cardiac arrest O07.3
– – – – chemical damage of pelvic organ(s) O07.3
– – – – circulatory collapse O07.3
– – – – defibrination syndrome O07.1
– – – – electrolyte imbalance O07.3

Abortion—*continued*
- attempted—*continued*
- - medical—*continued*
- - - complicated by—*continued*
- - - - embolism (amniotic fluid) (blood clot) (pulmonary) (septic) (soap) O07.2
- - - - endometritis O07.0
- - - - hemorrhage (delayed) (excessive) O07.1
- - - - infection, genital tract or pelvic O07.0
- - - - intravascular coagulation O07.1
- - - - laceration of pelvic organ(s) O07.3
- - - - oliguria O07.3
- - - - oophoritis O07.0
- - - - parametritis O07.0
- - - - pelvic peritonitis O07.0
- - - - perforation of pelvic organ(s) O07.3
- - - - renal failure or shutdown O07.3
- - - - salpingitis or salpingo-oophoritis O07.0
- - - - sepsis O07.0
- - - - septic shock O07.0
- - - - shock O07.3
- - - - - septic O07.0
- - - - specified condition NEC O07.3
- - - - tubular necrosis (renal) O07.3
- - - - urinary infection O07.3
- failed – *see* Abortion, attempted
- fetus or newborn P96.4
- following threatened abortion O03.-
- - with current abortion – *see* categories O03-O06
- - - fetus P01.8
- - care in current pregnancy O26.2
- - without current pregnancy N96
- illegal O05.-
- induced O06.-
- - for
- - - legal indications O04.-
- - - medical indications O04.-
- - - psychiatric indications O04.-
- - nonmedical O05.-
- legal (induced) O04.-
- - fetus P96.4
- medical O04.-
- - fetus P96.4
- missed O02.1
- operative – *see* Abortion, medical
- spontaneous O03.-
- - fetus P01.8

Abortion—*continued*
- spontaneous—*continued*
- - threatened O20.0
- - - affecting fetus or newborn P01.8
- therapeutic O04.-
- - fetus P96.4
- threatened (spontaneous) O20.0
- - affecting fetus or newborn P01.8
- tubal O00.1
Abrami's disease D59.8
Abrasion (*see also* Injury, superficial) T14.0
- tooth, teeth (dentifrice) (habitual) (hard tissues) (occupational) (ritual) (traditional) (wedge defect) K03.1
Abruptio placentae O45.9
- with coagulation defect O45.0
- affecting fetus or newborn P02.1
Abruption, placenta – *see* Abruptio placentae
Abscess (embolic) (infective) (metastatic) (multiple) (pyogenic) (septic) L02.9
- with
- - diverticular disease (intestine) K57.8
- - - large K57.2
- - - - and small K57.4
- - - small K57.0
- - lymphangitis – code site under Abscess
- abdomen, abdominal
- - cavity K65.0
- - wall L02.2
- abdominopelvic K65.0
- accessory sinus (chronic) (*see also* Sinusitis) J32.9
- - acute (*see also* Sinusitis, acute) J01.9
- alveolar K04.7
- amebic A06.4
- - brain (and liver or lung abscess) A06.6† G07*
- - liver (without mention of brain or lung abscess) A06.4† K77.0*
- - lung (and liver) (without mention of brain abscess) A06.5† J99.8*
- - specified site NEC A06.8
- - spleen A06.8† D77*
- ankle L02.4
- anorectal K61.2
- antecubital space L02.4
- antrum (chronic) (Highmore) (*see also* Sinusitis, maxillary) J32.0
- anus K61.0
- apical (tooth) K04.7
- - with sinus (alveolar) K04.6
- appendix K35.3

17

Abscess—*continued*
- areola (acute) (chronic) (nonpuerperal) N61
- – puerperal, postpartum or gestational O91.0
- arm (any part) L02.4
- artery (wall) I77.8
- auricle, ear H60.0
- axilla (region) L02.4
- – lymph gland or node L04.2
- back (any part, except buttock) L02.2
- Bartholin's gland N75.1
- Bezold's H70.0
- bladder (wall) N30.8
- bone (subperiosteal) M86.9
- – accessory sinus (chronic) (*see also* Sinusitis) J32.9
- – chronic M86.6
- – jaw (lower) (upper) K10.2
- – mastoid H70.0
- – petrous H70.2
- – spinal (tuberculous) A18.0† M49.0*
- – – nontuberculous M46.2
- bowel K63.0
- brain (any part) G06.0
- – amebic (with abscess of any other site) A06.6† G07*
- – cystic G06.0
- – gonococcal A54.8† G07*
- – otogenic G06.0
- – pheomycotic (chromomycotic) B43.1† G07*
- – tuberculous A17.8† G07*
- breast (acute) (chronic) (nonpuerperal) N61
- – gestational O91.1
- – newborn P39.0
- – puerperal, postpartum O91.1
- broad ligament (*see also* Disease, pelvis, inflammatory) N73.2
- Brodie's (chronic) (localized) M86.8
- bronchi J98.0
- buccal cavity K12.2
- bulbourethral gland N34.0
- bursa M71.0
- – pharyngeal J39.1
- buttock L02.3
- canthus H10.5
- cartilage M94.8
- cerebellum, cerebellar G06.0
- cerebral (embolic) G06.0
- cervical (meaning neck) L02.1
- – lymph gland or node L04.0
- cervix (uteri) (*see also* Cervicitis) N72
- cheek (external) L02.0

Abscess—*continued*
- chest J86.9
- – with fistula J86.0
- – wall L02.2
- chin L02.0
- choroid H30.0
- ciliary body H20.8
- cold (lung) (tuberculous) (*see also* Tuberculosis, abscess, lung) A16.2
- – articular – *see* Tuberculosis, joint
- colon (wall) K63.0
- colostomy or enterostomy K91.4
- conjunctiva H10.0
- connective tissue NEC L02.9
- cornea H16.3
- corpus
- – cavernosum N48.2
- – luteum (*see also* Salpingo-oophoritis) N70.9
- Cowper's gland N34.0
- cranium G06.0
- Crohn's disease K50.9
- – large intestine K50.1
- – – and small intestine K50.8
- – small intestine (duodenum, ileum or jejunum) K50.0
- cul-de-sac (Douglas') (posterior) (*see also* Peritonitis, pelvic, female) N73.5
- cutaneous (*see also* Abscess, by site) L02.9
- dental K04.7
- – with sinus (alveolar) K04.6
- dentoalveolar K04.7
- – with sinus K04.6
- diaphragm, diaphragmatic K65.0
- Douglas' cul-de-sac or pouch (*see also* Peritonitis, pelvic, female) N73.5
- ear (middle) H66.4
- – acute H66.0
- – external H60.0
- entamebic – *see* Abscess, amebic
- epididymis N45.0
- epidural G06.2
- – brain G06.0
- – spinal cord G06.1
- epiglottis J38.7
- epiploon, epiploic K65.0
- erysipelatous (*see also* Erysipelas) A46
- esophagus K20
- ethmoid (bone) (chronic) (sinus) J32.2
- external auditory canal H60.0
- extradural G06.2
- – brain G06.0
- – spinal cord G06.1
- extraperitoneal K65.0

Abscess—*continued*
- eye H44.0
- eyelid H00.0
- face (any part, except ear, eye and nose) L02.0
- fallopian tube (*see also* Salpingo-oophoritis) N70.9
- fascia M72.8
- fauces J39.1
- femoral (region) L02.4
- filaria, filarial (*see also* Infestation, filarial) B74.9
- finger (any) L02.4
- − − nail L03.0
- fistulous NEC L02.9
- foot (any part) L02.4
- forehead L02.0
- frontal sinus (chronic) J32.1
- gallbladder K81.0
- genital organ or tract NEC
- − female (external) N76.4
- − − following
- − − − abortion (subsequent episode) O08.0
- − − − ectopic or molar pregnancy O08.0
- − male N49.9
- − − multiple sites N49.8
- − − specified NEC N49.8
- gingival K05.2
- gland, glandular (lymph) (acute) (*see also* Lymphadenitis, acute) L04.9
- gluteal (region) L02.3
- gonorrheal NEC (*see also* Gonococcus) A54.1
- groin L02.2
- gum K05.2
- hand L02.4
- head NEC L02.8
- heart (*see also* Carditis) I51.8
- heel L02.4
- hepatic (cholangitic) (hematogenic) (lymphogenic) (pylephlebitic) K75.0
- hip (region) L02.4
- ileocecal K35.3
- ileostomy (bud) K91.4
- iliac (region) L02.2
- infraclavicular (fossa) L02.4
- inguinal (region) L02.2
- − lymph gland or node L04.1
- intestine, intestinal NEC K63.0
- − rectal K61.1
- intra-abdominal (*see also* Abscess, peritoneum) K65.0
- intracranial G06.0
- intramammary – *see* Abscess, breast

Abscess—*continued*
- intraorbital H05.0
- intraperitoneal K65.0
- intrasphincteric (anus) K61.4
- intraspinal G06.1
- intratonsillar J36
- iris H20.8
- ischiorectal (fossa) K61.3
- jaw (bone) (lower) (upper) K10.2
- joint M00.9
- − − spine (tuberculous) A18.0† M49.0*
- − − − nontuberculous M46.5
- kidney N15.1
- − − with calculus N20.0
- − − − with hydronephrosis N13.6
- − − complicating pregnancy O23.0
- − − − affecting fetus or newborn P00.1
- − − puerperal, postpartum O86.2
- knee L02.4
- − joint M00.9
- labium (majus) (minus) N76.4
- − complicating pregnancy O23.5
- − puerperal, postpartum O86.1
- lacrimal
- − caruncle H04.3
- − gland H04.0
- − passages (duct) (sac) H04.3
- larynx J38.7
- leg (any part) L02.4
- lens H27.8
- limb (lower) (upper) L02.4
- lingual K14.0
- lip K13.0
- Littré's gland N34.0
- liver (cholangitic) (hematogenic) (lymphogenic) (pylephlebitic) K75.0
- − − amebic A06.4
- − − − with
- − − − − brain abscess (and lung abscess) A06.6† G07*
- − − − − lung abscess A06.5† J99.8*
- − − due to Entamoeba histolytica (*see also* Abscess, liver, amebic) A06.4
- loin (region) L02.2
- lumbar (tuberculous) A18.0† M49.0*
- − − nontuberculous L02.2
- lung (miliary) (putrid) J85.2
- − − with pneumonia J85.1
- − − − due to specified organism – *see* Pneumonia, in (due to)
- − − amebic (with liver abscess) A06.5† J99.8*
- − − − with
- − − − − brain abscess A06.6† G07*
- − − − − pneumonia A06.5† J17.0*

Abscess—*continued*
- lymph, lymphatic, gland or node (acute) (*see also* Lymphadenitis, acute) L04.9
- – mesentery I88.0
- mammary gland – *see* Abscess, breast
- marginal, anus K61.0
- mastoid H70.0
- maxilla, maxillary K10.2
- – sinus (chronic) J32.0
- mediastinum J85.3
  meibomian gland H00.0
- meninges G06.2
- mesentery, mesenteric K65.0
- mesosalpinx (*see also* Salpingo-oophoritis) N70.9
- mons pubis L02.2
- mouth (floor) K12.2
- muscle M60.0
- myocardium I40.0
- nabothian (follicle) (*see also* Cervicitis) N72
- nail (chronic) (with lymphangitis) L03.0
- nasopharyngeal J39.1
- navel L02.2
- – newborn P38
- neck (region) L02.1
- – lymph gland or node L04.0
- nephritic (*see also* Abscess, kidney) N15.1
- nipple N61
- – puerperal, postpartum or gestational O91.0
- nose (external) (fossa) (septum) J34.0
- – sinus (chronic) (*see also* Sinusitis) J32.9
- omentum K65.0
- operative wound T81.4
- orbit, orbital H05.0
- ovary, ovarian (corpus luteum) (*see also* Salpingo-oophoritis) N70.9
- oviduct (*see also* Salpingo-oophoritis) N70.9
- palate (soft) K12.2
- – hard K10.2
- palmar (space) L02.4
- pancreas (duct) K85.-
- paradontal K05.2
- parametric, parametrium (*see also* Disease, pelvis, inflammatory) N73.2
- parapharyngeal J39.0
- pararectal K61.1
- parasinus (*see also* Sinusitis) J32.9
- parauterine (*see also* Disease, pelvis, inflammatory) N73.2

Abscess—*continued*
- paravaginal N76.0
- parietal region (scalp) L02.8
- parotid (duct) (gland) K11.3
- pectoral (region) L02.2
- pelvis, pelvic
    female (*see also* Disease, pelvis, inflammatory) N73.9
- – male, peritoneal K65.0
- penis N48.2
- – gonococcal (accessory gland) (periurethral) A54.1
- perianal K61.0
- periapical K04.7
- – with sinus (alveolar) K04.6
- periappendicular K35.3
- pericardial I30.1
- pericemental K05.2
- pericoronal K05.2
- peridental K05.2
- perimetric (*see also* Disease, pelvis, inflammatory) N73.2
- perinephric, perinephritic (*see also* Abscess, kidney) N15.1
- perineum, perineal (superficial) L02.2
- – urethra N34.0
- periodontal (parietal) K05.2
- periosteum, periosteal M86.8
- – with osteomyelitis M86.8
- – – acute M86.1
- – – chronic M86.6
- peripharyngeal J39.0
- periprostatic N41.2
- perirectal K61.1
- perirenal (tissue) (*see also* Abscess, kidney) N15.1
- peritoneum, peritoneal (perforated) (ruptured) K65.0
- – with appendicitis K35.3
- – following
- – – abortion (subsequent episode) O08.0
- – – ectopic or molar pregnancy O08.0
- – pelvic
- – – female (*see also* Peritonitis, pelvic, female) N73.5
- – – male K65.0
- – postoperative T81.4
- – puerperal, postpartum, childbirth O85
- – tuberculous A18.3† K67.3*
- peritonsillar J36
- periureteral N28.8
- periurethral N34.0
- – gonococcal (accessory gland) (periurethral) A54.1

Abscess—*continued*
- periuterine (*see also* Disease, pelvis, inflammatory) N73.2
- perivesical N30.8
- pernicious NEC L02.9
- petrous bone H70.2
- phagedenic NEC L02.9
- – chancroid A57
- pharynx, pharyngeal (lateral) J39.1
- pilonidal L05.0
- pituitary (gland) E23.6
- pleura J86.9
- – with fistula J86.0
- popliteal L02.4
- postlaryngeal J38.7
- postnasal J34.0
- postoperative (any site) T81.4
- postpharyngeal J39.0
- post-typhoid A01.0
- pouch of Douglas (*see also* Peritonitis, pelvic, female) N73.5
- premammary – *see* Abscess, breast
- prepatellar L02.4
- prostate N41.2
- – gonococcal (acute) (chronic) A54.2† N51.0*
- psoas, nontuberculous M60.0
- puerperal – code site under Puerperal, abscess
- pulmonary – *see* Abscess, lung
- pulp, pulpal (dental) K04.0
- rectovesical N30.8
- rectum K61.1
- regional NEC L02.8
- renal (*see also* Abscess, kidney) N15.1
- respiratory, upper J39.8
- retina H30.0
- retrobulbar H05.0
- retrocecal K65.0
- retrolaryngeal J38.7
- retromammary – *see* Abscess, breast
- retroperitoneal K65.0
- retropharyngeal J39.0
- retrouterine (*see also* Peritonitis, pelvic, female) N73.5
- retrovesical N30.8
- round ligament (*see also* Disease, pelvis, inflammatory) N73.2
- rupture (spontaneous) NEC L02.9
- sacrum (tuberculous) A18.0† M49.0*
- – nontuberculous M46.2
- salivary (duct) (gland) K11.3
- scalp (any part) L02.8
- scapular M86.8
- sclera H15.0

Abscess—*continued*
- scrofulous (tuberculous) A18.2
- scrotum N49.2
- seminal vesicle N49.0
- shoulder (region) L02.4
- sigmoid K63.0
- sinus (accessory) (chronic) (nasal) (*see also* Sinusitis) J32.9
- – intracranial venous (any) G06.0
- Skene's duct or gland N34.0
- skin (*see also* Abscess, by site) L02.9
- sloughing NEC L02.9
- specified site NEC L02.8
- spermatic cord N49.1
- sphenoidal (sinus) (chronic) J32.3
- spinal cord (any part) (staphylococcal) G06.1
- – tuberculous A17.8† G07*
- spine (column) (tuberculous) A18.0† M49.0*
- – nontuberculous M46.2
- spleen D73.3
- – amebic A06.8† D77*
- stitch T81.4
- subarachnoid G06.2
- – brain G06.0
- – spinal cord G06.1
- subareolar (*see also* Abscess, breast) N61
- – puerperal, postpartum O91.1
- subcutaneous (*see also* Abscess, by site) L02.9
- – pheomycotic (chromomycotic) B43.2† L99.8*
- subdiaphragmatic K65.0
- subdural G06.2
- – brain G06.0
- – spinal cord G06.1
- subgaleal L02.8
- subhepatic K65.0
- sublingual K12.2
- – gland K11.3
- submammary – *see* Abscess, breast
- submandibular (region) (space) (triangle) K12.2
- – gland K11.3
- submaxillary (region) L02.0
- submental L02.0
- subperiosteal – *see* Abscess, bone
- subphrenic K65.0
- – postoperative T81.4
- suburethral N34.0
- sudoriparous L75.8
- suppurative NEC L02.9
- supraclavicular (fossa) L02.4
- sweat gland L74.8

Abscess—*continued*
- tear duct H04.3
- temple L02.0
- temporal region L02.0
- temporosphenoidal G06.0
- tendon (sheath) M65.0
- testis N45.0
- thigh L02.4
- thorax J86.9
- – with fistula J86.0
- throat J39.1
- thumb L02.4
- – nail L03.0
- thymus (gland) E32.1
- thyroid (gland) E06.0
- toe (any) L02.4
- – nail L03.0
- tongue (staphylococcal) K14.0
- tonsil(s) J36
- tonsillopharyngeal J36
- tooth, teeth (root) K04.7
- – with sinus (alveolar) K04.6
- – supporting structures NEC K05.2
- trachea J39.8
- trunk L02.2
- tubal (*see also* Salpingo-oophoritis) N70.9
- tuberculous – *see* Tuberculosis, abscess
- tubo-ovarian (*see also* Salpingo-oophoritis) N70.9
- tunica vaginalis N49.1
- umbilicus L02.2
- – newborn P38
- urethral (gland) N34.0
- uterus, uterine (wall) (*see also* Endometritis) N71.9
- – ligament (*see also* Disease, pelvis, inflammatory) N73.2
- – neck (*see also* Cervicitis) N72
- vagina (wall) (*see also* Vaginitis) N76.0
- vaginorectal (*see also* Vaginitis) N76.0
- vas deferens N49.1
- vermiform appendix K35.3
- vertebra (column) (tuberculous) A18.0† M49.0*
- – nontuberculous M46.2
- vesical N30.8
- vesico-uterine pouch (*see also* Peritonitis, pelvic, female) N73.5
- vitreous (humor) H44.0
- vocal cord J38.3
- von Bezold's H70.0
- vulva N76.4
- – complicating pregnancy O23.5
- – puerperal, postpartum O86.1

Abscess—*continued*
- vulvovaginal gland N75.1
- web space L02.4
- wound T81.4
- wrist L02.4

Absence (organ or part) (complete or partial)
- adrenal (gland) (congenital) Q89.1
- – acquired E89.6
- albumin in blood E88.0
- alimentary tract (congenital) Q45.8
- – upper Q40.8
- ankle (acquired) – *see* Absence, foot and ankle
- anus (congenital) Q42.3
- – with fistula Q42.2
- aorta (congenital) Q25.4
- appendix, congenital Q42.8
- arm (acquired) (unilateral) Z89.2
- – with leg (any level) Z89.8
- – bilateral (any level) Z89.3
- – – with leg(s) (any level) Z89.8
- – congenital Q71.9
- artery (congenital) (peripheral) Q27.8
- – brain Q28.3
- – coronary Q24.5
- – pulmonary Q25.7
- atrial septum (congenital) Q21.1
- auditory canal (congenital) (external) Q16.1
- auricle (ear), congenital Q16.0
- bile, biliary duct, congenital Q44.5
- bladder (acquired) Z90.6
- – congenital Q64.5
- bowel sounds R19.1
- brain Q00.0
- – part of Q04.3
- breast(s) (acquired) Z90.1
- – congenital Q83.8
- broad ligament Q50.6
- bronchus (congenital) Q32.4
- canaliculus lacrimalis, congenital Q10.4
- cerebellum (vermis) Q04.3
- cervix (acquired) Z90.7
- – congenital Q51.5
- chin (congenital) Q18.8
- cilia (congenital) Q10.3
- – acquired H02.7
- clitoris (congenital) Q52.6
- coccyx (congenital) Q76.4
- cold sense R20.8
- congenital
- – lumen – *see* Atresia
- – organ or site NEC – *see* Agenesis
- – septum – *see* Imperfect, closure

Absence—*continued*
- corpus callosum Q04.0
- cricoid cartilage, congenital Q31.8
- diaphragm (with hernia), congenital Q79.1
- digestive organ(s) or tract (acquired) Z90.4
- – congenital Q45.8
- duodenum (acquired) Z90.4
- – congenital Q41.0
- ear (acquired) Z90.0
- – congenital Q16.9
- – – auricle Q16.0
- – – lobe, lobule Q17.8
- ejaculatory duct (congenital) Q55.4
- endocrine gland (congenital) NEC Q89.2
- – acquired E89.9
- epididymis (congenital) Q55.4
- – acquired Z90.7
- epiglottis, congenital Q31.8
- epileptic NEC G40.7
- – status G41.1
- esophagus (congenital) Q39.8
- – acquired (partial) Z90.4
- eustachian tube (congenital) Q16.2
- extremity (acquired) Z89.9
- – congenital Q73.0
- – lower (above knee) (unilateral) Z89.6
- – – with upper extremity (any level) Z89.8
- – – below knee (unilateral) Z89.5
- – – bilateral (any level) Z89.7
- – – – with upper extremity (any level) Z89.8
- – upper (unilateral) Z89.2
- – – with lower extremity (any level) Z89.8
- – – bilateral (any level) Z89.3
- eye (acquired) Z90.0
- – congenital Q11.1
- – muscle (congenital) Q10.3
- eyeball (acquired) Z90.0
- eyelid (fold) (congenital) Q10.3
- – acquired Z90.0
- fallopian tube(s) (acquired) Z90.7
- – congenital Q50.6
- family member (causing problem in home) Z63.3
- femur, congenital Q72.4
- finger(s) (acquired) (unilateral) Z89.0
- – bilateral Z89.3
- – congenital Q71.3
- foot and ankle (acquired) (unilateral) Z89.4
- – with upper limb (any level) Z89.8

Absence—*continued*
- foot and ankle—*continued*
- – bilateral Z89.7
- – – with upper limb (any level) Z89.8
- – congenital Q72.3
- forearm (acquired) (unilateral) (*see also* Absence, arm) Z89.2
- – congenital Q71.1
- – – and hand Q71.2
- gallbladder (acquired) Z90.4
- – congenital Q44.0
- gamma globulin in blood D80.1
- – hereditary D80.0
- genital organs
- – acquired (female) (male) Z90.7
- – female, congenital Q52.8
- – – external Q52.7
- – – internal NEC Q52.8
- – male, congenital Q55.8
- genitourinary organs, congenital NEC
- – female Q52.8
- – male Q55.8
- globe (acquired) Z90.0
- – congenital Q11.1
- glottis, congenital Q31.8
- hand and wrist (acquired) (unilateral) Z89.1
- – with lower limb (any level) Z89.8
- – bilateral Z89.3
- – – with lower limb (any level) Z89.8
- – congenital Q71.3
- head, part (acquired) NEC Z90.0
- heat sense R20.8
- hymen (congenital) Q52.4
- ileum (acquired) Z90.4
- – congenital Q41.2
- incus (acquired) H74.3
- – congenital Q16.3
- inner ear, congenital Q16.5
- intestine (acquired) (small) Z90.4
- – congenital Q41.9
- – – specified NEC Q41.8
- – large Z90.4
- – – congenital Q42.9
- – – – specified NEC Q42.8
- iris, congenital Q13.1
- jejunum (acquired) Z90.4
- – congenital Q41.1
- joint, congenital NEC Q74.8
- kidney(s) (acquired) Z90.5
- – congenital Q60.2
- – – bilateral Q60.1
- – – unilateral Q60.0
- larynx (congenital) Q31.8
- – acquired Z90.0

Absence—*continued*
- leg (acquired) (above knee) (unilateral) Z89.6
- – with arm(s) (any level) Z89.8
- – below knee Z89.5
- – bilateral (any level) Z89.7
- – – with arm(s) (any level) Z89.8
- – congenital Q72.8
- lens (acquired) H27.0
- – congenital Q12.3
- limb (acquired) – *see* Absence, extremity
- liver (congenital) Q44.7
- lung (fissure) (lobe) (bilateral) (unilateral) (congenital) Q33.3
- – acquired (any part) Z90.2
- menstruation (*see also* Amenorrhea) N91.2
- muscle (congenital) (pectoral) Q79.8
- – ocular Q10.3
- neutrophil D70
- nipple, congenital Q83.2
- nose (congenital) Q30.1
- – acquired Z90.0
- organ
- – acquired Z90.8
- – congenital Q89.8
- – of Corti, congenital Q16.5
- ovary (acquired) Z90.7
- – congenital Q50.0
- oviduct (acquired) Z90.7
- – congenital Q50.6
- pancreas (congenital) Q45.0
- – acquired Z90.4
- parathyroid gland (acquired) E89.2
- – congenital Q89.2
- patella, congenital Q74.1
- penis (congenital) Q55.5
- – acquired Z90.7
- pericardium (congenital) Q24.8
- pituitary gland (congenital) Q89.2
- – acquired E89.3
- prostate (acquired) Z90.7
- – congenital Q55.4
- punctum lacrimale (congenital) Q10.4
- radius, congenital Q71.4
- rectum (congenital) Q42.1
- – with fistula Q42.0
- – acquired Z90.4
- rib (acquired) Z90.8
- – congenital Q76.6
- sacrum, congenital Q76.4
- salivary gland(s), congenital Q38.4
- scrotum, congenital Q55.2
- seminal vesicles (congenital) Q55.4
- – acquired Z90.7

Absence—*continued*
- septum
- – atrial (congenital) Q21.1
- – between aorta and pulmonary artery Q21.4
- – ventricular (congenital) Q20.4
- sex chromosome
-   female phenotype Q97.8
- – male phenotype Q98.8
- skull bone Q75.8
- – with
- – – anencephaly Q00.0
- – – encephalocele (*see also* Encephalocele) Q01.9
- – – hydrocephalus Q03.9
- – – – with spina bifida (*see also* Spina bifida, with hydrocephalus) Q05.4
- – – microcephaly Q02
- spermatic cord, congenital Q55.4
- spine, congenital Q76.4
- spleen (congenital) Q89.0
- – acquired D73.0
- sternum, congenital Q76.7
- stomach (acquired) (partial) Z90.3
- – congenital Q40.2
- superior vena cava, congenital Q26.8
- tendon (congenital) Q79.8
- testis (congenital) Q55.0
- – acquired Z90.7
- thumb (acquired) (unilateral) Z89.0
- – bilateral Z89.3
- – congenital Q71.3
- thyroid (gland) (acquired) E89.0
- – cartilage, congenital Q31.8
- – congenital E03.1
- toe(s) (acquired) (unilateral) (bilateral) Z89.4
- – with foot – *see* Absence, foot and ankle
- – congenital Q72.3
- tongue, congenital Q38.3
- tooth, teeth (congenital) K00.0
- – acquired K08.1
- – – with malocclusion K07.3
- trachea (cartilage), congenital Q32.1
- transverse aortic arch, congenital Q25.4
- umbilical artery, congenital Q27.0
- upper arm and forearm with hand present, congenital Q71.1
- ureter (congenital) Q62.4
- – acquired Z90.6
- urethra, congenital Q64.5
- uterus (acquired) Z90.7
- – congenital Q51.0
- uvula, congenital Q38.5
- vagina, congenital Q52.0

Absence—*continued*
- vas deferens (congenital) Q55.4
- – acquired Z90.7
- vein (peripheral), congenital Q27.8
- – brain Q28.3
- – great Q26.8
- – portal Q26.5
- – specified NEC Q27.8
- vena cava (inferior) (superior), congenital Q26.8
- vertebra, congenital Q76.4
- vulva, congenital Q52.7
- wrist (acquired) (*see also* Absence, hand and wrist) Z89.1

Absorption
- carbohydrate, disturbance K90.4
- chemical T65.9
- – specified chemical or substance – *see* Table of drugs and chemicals
- – through placenta (fetus or newborn) P04.9
- – – environmental substance P04.6
- – – nutritional substance P04.5
- – – obstetric anesthetic or analgesic drug P04.0
- – – suspected, affecting management of pregnancy O35.8
- drug NEC (*see also* Reaction, drug) T88.7
- – addictive
- – – through placenta (fetus or newborn) P04.4
- – – – suspected, affecting management of pregnancy O35.5
- – through placenta (fetus or newborn) P04.1
- – – obstetric anesthetic or analgesic medication P04.0
- fat, disturbance K90.4
- – pancreatic K90.3
- maternal medication NEC through placenta (fetus or newborn) P04.1
- noxious substance – *see* Absorption, chemical
- protein, disturbance K90.4
- starch, disturbance K90.4
- toxic substance – *see* Absorption, chemical
- uremic – *see* Uremia

Abstinence symptoms, syndrome
- alcohol F10.3
- drug – *see* F11-F19 with fourth character .3

Abulia R68.8

Abuse
- alcohol (non-dependent) F10.1
- – counseling and surveillance Z71.4
- – personal history of (no longer current) Z86.4
- – rehabilitation measures Z50.2
- amfetamine (or related substance) F15.1
- antacids F55
- anxiolytic F13.1
- cannabis, cannabinoids F12.1
- child T74.9
- – physical, alleged Z61.6
- – sexual, alleged (by)
- – – family member Z61.4
- – – person outside family Z61.5
- – specified NEC T74.8
- cocaine F14.1
- drugs
- – anxiolytics F13.1
- – counseling and surveillance Z71.5
- – hypnotics F13.1
- – non-dependent (psychoactive) F19.1
- – – amfetamine-type F15.1
- – – analgesics (non-prescribed) F55
- – – antacids F55
- – – antidepressants F55
- – – barbiturates F13.1
- – – caffeine F15.1
- – – cannabis F12.1
- – – cocaine-type F14.1
- – – hallucinogens F16.1
- – – hashish F12.1
- – – herbal or folk remedies F55
- – – hormones F55
- – – laxatives F55
- – – LSD F16.1
- – – marihuana F12.1
- – – mixed F19.1
- – – morphine-type (opioids) F11.1
- – – sedatives F13.1
- – – specified NEC F19.1
- – – steroids F55
- – – stimulants NEC F15.1
- – – tranquilizers F13.1
- – – vitamins F55
- – personal history of (no longer current) Z86.4
- – rehabilitation measures Z50.3
- – sedatives F13.1
- – stimulants NEC F15.1
- hallucinogens F16.1
- herbal or folk remedies F55
- hormones F55
- hypnotics F13.1
- inhalants F18.1

Abuse—*continued*
- laxatives F55
- opioids F11.1
- PCP (phencyclidine) (or related substance) F19.1
- physical (adult) (child) T74.1
- psychoactive substance (specified NEC) F19.1
- psychological (adult) (child) T74.3
- sedative F13.1
- sexual T74.2
- – child, alleged (by) family member Z61.4
- – – person outside family Z61.5
- solvent F18.1
- steroids F55
- tobacco F17.1
- – counseling and surveillance Z71.6
- – personal history of (no longer current) Z86.4
- vitamins F55

Acalculia R48.8
- developmental F81.2

Acanthamebiasis (with) B60.1
- conjunctiva B60.1† H13.1*
- keratoconjunctivitis B60.1† H19.2*

Acanthocephaliasis B83.8

Acanthocheilonemiasis B74.4

Acanthocytosis E78.6

Acantholysis L11.9

Acanthosis (acquired) (nigricans) L83
- benign Q82.8
- congenital Q82.8
- seborrheic L82
- tongue K14.3

Acardia, acardius Q89.8

Acardiacus amorphus Q89.8

Acariasis B88.0
- scabies B86

Acarodermatitis (urticarioides) B88.0†
L99.8*

Acarophobia F40.2

Acatalasemia, acatalasia E80.3

Accelerated atrioventricular conduction I45.6

Accentuation of personality traits (type A) Z73.1

Accessory (congenital)
- adrenal gland Q89.1
- anus Q43.4
- appendix Q43.4
- atrioventricular conduction I45.6
- auditory ossicles Q16.3
- auricle (ear) Q17.0
- biliary duct or passage Q44.5

Accessory—*continued*
- bladder Q64.7
- blood vessels NEC Q27.9
- bone NEC Q79.8
- breast tissue, axilla Q83.1
- carpal bones Q74.0
- cecum Q43.4
- chromosome(s) NEC (non-sex) Q92.9
- – with complex rearrangements NEC Q92.5
- – – seen only at prometaphase Q92.4
- – partial Q92.9
- – sex
- – – female phenotype Q97.8
- – – male phenotype Q98.8
- – 13 – *see* Trisomy, 13
- – 18 – *see* Trisomy, 18
- – 21 – *see* Trisomy, 21
- coronary artery Q24.5
- cusp(s), heart valve NEC Q24.8
- – pulmonary Q22.3
- cystic duct Q44.5
- digit(s) Q69.9
- ear (auricle) (lobe) Q17.0
- endocrine gland NEC Q89.2
- eye muscle Q10.3
- eyelid Q10.3
- face bone(s) Q75.8
- fallopian tube (fimbria) (ostium) Q50.6
- finger(s) Q69.0
- foreskin N47
- frontonasal process Q75.8
- gallbladder Q44.1
- genital organ(s)
- – female Q52.8
- – – external Q52.7
- – – internal NEC Q52.8
- – male Q55.8
- hallux Q69.2
- heart Q24.8
- – valve NEC Q24.8
- – – pulmonary Q22.3
- hepatic ducts Q44.5
- hymen Q52.4
- intestine (large) (small) Q43.4
- kidney Q63.0
- lacrimal canal Q10.6
- leaflet, heart valve NEC Q24.8
- liver Q44.7
- – duct Q44.5
- lobule (ear) Q17.0
- lung (lobe) Q33.1
- muscle Q79.8
- navicular of carpus Q74.0
- nervous system, part NEC Q07.8

Accessory—*continued*
- nipple Q83.3
- nose Q30.8
- organ or site not listed – *see* Anomaly, by site
- ovary Q50.3
- oviduct Q50.6
- pancreas Q45.3
- parathyroid gland Q89.2
- parotid gland (and duct) Q38.4
- pituitary gland Q89.2
- preauricular appendage Q17.0
- prepuce N47
- renal arteries (multiple) Q27.2
- rib Q76.6
- - cervical Q76.5
- roots (teeth) K00.2
- salivary gland Q38.4
- sesamoid bones Q74.8
- - foot Q74.2
- - hand Q74.0
- skin tags Q82.8
- spleen Q89.0
- sternum Q76.7
- submaxillary gland Q38.4
- tarsal bones Q74.2
- tendon Q79.8
- thumb Q69.1
- thymus gland Q89.2
- thyroid gland Q89.2
- toes Q69.2
- tongue Q38.3
- tooth, teeth K00.1
- - causing crowding K07.3
- tragus Q17.0
- ureter Q62.5
- urethra Q64.7
- urinary organ or tract NEC Q64.8
- uterus Q51.2
- vagina Q52.1
- valve, heart NEC Q24.8
- vertebra Q76.4
- vocal cords Q31.8
- vulva Q52.7

Accident
- birth – *see* Birth, injury
- cardiac (*see also* Infarct, myocardium) I21.9
- cardiovascular (*see also* Disease, cardiovascular) I51.6
- cerebral I64
- cerebrovascular I64
- - hemorrhagic I61.9
- - old I69.4

Accident—*continued*
- coronary (*see also* Infarct, myocardium) I21.9
- craniovascular I64
- during pregnancy, to mother
- - affecting fetus or newborn P00.5
- vascular, brain I64

Accidental – *see* condition

Accommodation (disorder) (paresis) (spasm) (*see also* condition) H52.5
- hysterical paralysis of F44.8

Accouchement – *see* Delivery

Accreta placenta
- complication during delivery (with hemorrhage) O72.0
- - without hemorrhage O73.0
- maternal care O43.2

Accretio cordis I31.0

Accretions, tooth, teeth K03.6

Acculturation difficulty Z60.3

Accumulation secretion, prostate N42.8

Acephalia, acephalism, acephalus, acephaly Q00.0

Acephalobrachia monster Q89.8

Acephalochirus monster Q89.8

Acephalogaster Q89.8

Acephalostomus monster Q89.8

Acephalothorax Q89.8

Acetonemia R79.8
- diabetic – *see* E10-E14 with fourth character .1

Acetonuria R82.4

Achalasia (cardia) (esophagus) K22.0
- congenital Q39.5
- pylorus Q40.0

Ache(s) – *see* Pain

Achilloburitis M76.6

Achillodynia M76.6

Achlorhydria, achlorhydric (neurogenic) K31.8
- anemia D50.8
- diarrhea K31.8
- psychogenic F45.3
- secondary to vagotomy K91.1

Acholuric jaundice (familial) (splenomegalic) (*see also* Spherocytosis) D58.0
- acquired D59.8

Achondrogenesis Q77.0

Achondroplasia (osteosclerosis congenita) Q77.4

Achromatism, achromatopsia (acquired) (congenital) H53.5

Achylia gastrica K31.8
- psychogenic F45.3

Acid
- burn – *see* Corrosion
- deficiency
- – amide nicotinic E52
- – ascorbic E54
- – folic E53.8
- – nicotinic E52
- – pantothenic E53.8
- intoxication E87.2
- phosphatase deficiency E83.3
- stomach K31.8
- – psychogenic F45.3
Acidemia E87.2
- argininosuccinic E72.2
- fetal – *see* Distress, fetal
- isovaleric E71.1
- methylmalonic E71.1
- pipecolic E72.3
- propionic E71.1
Acidity, gastric (high) (low) K31.8
- psychogenic F45.3
Acidosis (lactic) (respiratory) E87.2
- diabetic – *see* E10-E14 with fourth character .1
- fetal – *see* Distress, fetal
- intrauterine – *see* Distress, fetal
- kidney, tubular N25.8
- metabolic NEC E87.2
- – late, of newborn P74.0
- renal (hyperchloremic) (tubular) N25.8
Aciduria
- argininosuccinic E72.2
- glutaric E72.3
- orotic (congenital) (hereditary) (pyrimidine deficiency) E79.8
- – anemia D53.0
Aclasis, diaphyseal Q78.6
Acne L70.9
- artificialis L70.8
- atrophica L70.2
- cachecticorum (Hebra) L70.8
- conglobata L70.1
- cystic L70.0
- decalvans L66.2
- excoriée des jeunes filles L70.5
- frontalis L70.2
- indurata L70.0
- infantile L70.4
- keloid L73.0
- necrotic, necrotica (miliaris) L70.2
- nodular L70.0
- occupational L70.8
- pustular L70.0
- rosacea L71.9
- specified NEC L70.8

Acne—*continued*
- tropica L70.3
- varioliformis L70.2
- vulgaris L70.0
Acnitis (primary) A18.4
Acosta's disease T70.2
Acoustic – *see condition*
Acquired – *see also condition*
- immunodeficiency syndrome (AIDS) (*see also* Human, immunodeficiency virus (HIV) disease) B24
- – complicating pregnancy, childbirth or the puerperium O98.7
Acrania Q00.0
Acroasphyxia, chronic I73.8
Acrocephalopolysyndactyly Q87.0
Acrocephalosyndactyly Q87.0
Acrocephaly Q75.0
Acrocyanosis I73.8
- newborn P28.2
Acrodermatitis L30.8
- atrophicans (chronica) L90.4
- continua (Hallopeau) L40.2
- enteropathica (hereditary) E83.2
- Hallopeau's L40.2
- infantile papular L44.4
- perstans L40.2
- pustulosa continua L40.2
- recalcitrant pustular L40.2
Acrodynia T56.1
Acromegaly, acromegalia E22.0
Acromicria, acromikria Q79.8
Acroparesthesia (simple) (vasomotor) I73.8
Acrophobia F40.2
Acroscleriasis, acroscleroderma, acrosclerosis (*see also* Scleroderma) M34.8
Acrospiroma, eccrine (M8402/0) – *see* Neoplasm, skin, benign
ACTH ectopic syndrome E24.3
Actinic – *see condition*
Actinobacillosis, actinobacillus A28.8
Actinomyces israelii (infection) – *see* Actinomycosis
Actinomycetoma (foot) B47.1
Actinomycosis, actinomycotic A42.9
- with pneumonia A42.0† J17.0*
- abdominal A42.1
- cervicofacial A42.2
- cutaneous A42.8
- gastrointestinal A42.1
- pulmonary A42.0
- septicemia A42.7

Actinomycosis, actinomycotic—*continued*
- specified site NEC A42.8
Actinoneuritis G62.8
Action, heart
- disorder I49.9
- irregular I49.9
- - psychogenic F45.3
Active – *see condition*
Acute – *see also condition*
- abdomen NEC R10.0
Acyanotic heart disease (congenital)
Q24.9
Acystia Q64.5
Adamantinoblastoma (M9310/0) – *see*
Adamantinoma
Adamantinoma (M9310/0) D16.5
- jaw (bone) (lower) D16.5
- - upper D16.4
- long bones (M9261/3) C40.9
- malignant (M9310/3) C41.1
- - jaw (bone) (lower) C41.1
- - - upper C41.0
- mandible D16.5
- tibial (M9261/3) C40.2
Adamantoblastoma (M9310/0) – *see*
Adamantinoma
Adams-Stokes(-Morgagni) disease or
syndrome I45.9
Adaptation reaction F43.2
Addiction (*see also* Dependence) – *code to*
F10-F19 with fourth character .2
- alcohol, alcoholic (ethyl) (methyl) (wood)
F10.2
- - complicating pregnancy, childbirth or
puerperium O99.3
- - - affecting fetus or newborn P04.3
- - suspected damage to fetus affecting
management of pregnancy O35.4
- drug F19.2
- ethyl alcohol F10.2
- heroin F11.2
- methyl alcohol F10.2
- methylated spirit F10.2
- morphine(-like substances) F11.2
- nicotine F17.2
- opium and opioids F11.2
- tobacco F17.2
Addisonian crisis E27.2
Addison's
- anemia D51.0
- disease (bronze) or syndrome E27.1
- - tuberculous A18.7† E35.1*
- keloid L94.0
Addison-Schilder complex E71.3
Additional – *see* Accessory

Adduction contracture, hip or other
joint – *see* Contraction, joint
Adenitis (*see also* Lymphadenitis) I88.9
- acute, unspecified site L04.9
- axillary I88.9
- - acute L04.2
- - chronic or subacute I88.1
- Bartholin's gland N75.8
- bulbourethral gland (*see also* Urethritis)
N34.2
- cervical I88.9
- - acute L04.0
- - chronic or subacute I88.1
- chancroid (Haemophilus ducreyi) A57
- chronic, unspecified site I88.1
- Cowper's gland (*see also* Urethritis)
N34.2
- epidemic, acute B27.0
- gangrenous L04.9
- gonorrheal NEC A54.8
- groin I88.9
- - acute L04.1
- - chronic or subacute I88.1
- infectious (acute) (epidemic) B27.0
- inguinal I88.9
- - acute L04.1
- - chronic or subacute I88.1
- lymph gland or node, except mesenteric
I88.9
- - acute (*see also* Lymphadenitis, acute)
L04.9
- - chronic or subacute I88.1
- mesenteric (acute) (chronic) (nonspecific)
(subacute) I88.0
- parotid gland (suppurative) K11.2
- salivary gland (any) (recurring)
(suppurative) K11.2
- scrofulous (tuberculous) A18.2
- Skene's duct or gland (*see also* Urethritis)
N34.2
- strumous, tuberculous A18.2
- subacute, unspecified site I88.1
- sublingual gland (suppurative) K11.2
- submandibular gland (suppurative) K11.2
- tuberculous (*see also* Tuberculosis, lymph
gland) A18.2
- urethral gland (*see also* Urethritis) N34.2
Adenoacanthoma (M8570/3) – *see*
Neoplasm, malignant
Adenoameloblastoma (lower jaw)
(M9300/0) D16.5
- upper jaw (bone) D16.4
Adenocarcinoid (tumor) (M8245/3) – *see*
Neoplasm, malignant

Adenocarcinoma (M8140/3) – *see also*
Neoplasm, malignant

Note: The list of adjectival modifiers below is not exhaustive. A description of adenocarcinoma that does not appear in this list should be coded in the same manner as carcinoma with that description. Thus, "mixed acidophil-basophil adenocarcinoma" should be coded in the same manner as "mixed acidophil-basophil carcinoma", which apperas in the list under "Carcinoma".

- with
- – apocrine metaplasia (M8573/3)
- – cartilaginous (and osseous) metaplasia (M8571/3)
- – osseous (and cartilaginous) metaplasia (M8571/3)
- – spindle cell metaplasia (M8572/3)
- – squamous metaplasia (M8570/3)
- acidophil (M8280/3)
- – specified site – *see* Neoplasm, malignant
- – unspecified site C75.1
- acinar (M8550/3)
- acinic cell (M8550/3)
- adrenal cortical (M8370/3) C74.0
- alveolar (M8251/3) – *see* Neoplasm, lung, malignant
- and
- – carcinoid, combined (M8244/3)
- – epidermoid carcinoma, mixed (M8560/3)
- – squamous cell carcinoma, mixed (M8560/3)
- apocrine (M8401/3)
- – breast – *see* Neoplasm, breast, malignant
- – in situ (M8401/2)
- – – breast D05.7
- – – specified site NEC – *see* Neoplasm, skin, in situ
- – – unspecified site D04.9
- – specified site NEC – *see* Neoplasm, skin, malignant
- – unspecified site C44.9
- basal cell (M8147/3)
- – specified site – *see* Neoplasm, malignant
- – unspecified site C08.9
- basophil (M8300/3)
- – specified site – *see* Neoplasm, malignant
- – unspecified site C75.1
- bile duct type (M8160/3) C22.1

Adenocarcinoma—*continued*
- bile duct type—*continued*
- – liver C22.1
- – specified site NEC – *see* Neoplasm, malignant
- – unspecified site C22.1
- bronchiolar (M8250/3) – *see* Neoplasm, lung, malignant
- bronchioloalveolar (M8250/3) – *see* Neoplasm, lung, malignant
- ceruminous (M8420/3) C44.2
- chromophobe (M8270/3)
- – specified site – *see* Neoplasm, malignant
- – unspecified site C75.1
- clear cell (mesonephroid) (M8310/3)
- colloid (M8480/3)
- cylindroid (M8200/3)
- diffuse type (M8145/3)
- – specified site – *see* Neoplasm, malignant
- – unspecified site C16.9
- duct (M8500/3)
- – infiltrating (M8500/3)
- – – with Paget's disease (M8541/3) – *see* Neoplasm, breast, malignant
- – – specified site – *see* Neoplasm, malignant
- – – unspecified site (female) C50.9
- embryonal (M9070/3)
- endometrioid (M8380/3)
- – specified site – *see* Neoplasm, malignant
- – unspecified site
- – – female C56
- – – male C61
- eosinophil (M8280/3)
- – specified site – *see* Neoplasm, malignant
- – unspecified site C75.1
- follicular (M8330/3)
- – with papillary (M8340/3) C73
- – moderately differentiated (M8332/3) C73
- – specified site – *see* Neoplasm, malignant
- – trabecular (M8332/3) C73
- – unspecified site C73
- – well differentiated (M8331/3) C73
- gelatinous (M8480/3)
- granular cell (M8320/3)
- Hurthle cell (M8290/3) C73
- in
- – adenomatous
- – – polyp (M8210/3)

Adenocarcinoma—*continued*
− in—*continued*
− − adenomatous—*continued*
− − − polyp—*continued*
− − − − multiple (M8221/3)
− − − polyposis coli (M8220/3) C18.9
− − polyp (adenomatous) (M8210/3)
− − − multiple (M8221/3)
− − polypoid adenoma (M8210/3)
− − tubular adenoma (M8210/3)
− − tubulovillous adenoma (M8263/3)
− − villous adenoma (M8261/3)
− infiltrating duct (M8500/3)
− − with Paget's disease (M8541/3) – *see*
    Neoplasm, breast, malignant
− − specified site – *see* Neoplasm,
    malignant
− − unspecified site C50.9
− inflammatory (M8530/3)
− − specified site – *see* Neoplasm,
    malignant
− − unspecified site C50.9
− intestinal type (M8144/3)
− − specified site – *see* Neoplasm,
    malignant
− − unspecified site C16.9
− intracystic papillary (M8504/3)
− intraductal (M8500/2)
− − breast D05.1
− − noninfiltrating (M8500/2)
− − − breast D05.1
− − − papillary (M8503/2)
− − − − with invasion (M8503/3)
− − − − − specified site – *see* Neoplasm,
        malignant
− − − − − unspecified site C50.9
− − − − breast D05.1
− − − − specified site NEC – *see*
        Neoplasm, in situ
− − − − unspecified site D05.1
− − − specified site NEC – *see* Neoplasm,
    in situ
− − − unspecified site D05.1
− − papillary (M8503/2)
− − − with invasion (M8503/3)
− − − − specified site – *see* Neoplasm,
        malignant
− − − − unspecified site C50.9
− − − breast D05.1
− − − specified site – *see* Neoplasm, in situ
− − − unspecified site D05.1
− − specified site NEC – *see* Neoplasm, in
    situ
− − unspecified site D05.1
− islet cell (M8150/3)

Adenocarcinoma—*continued*
− islet cell—*continued*
− − with exocrine, mixed (M8154/3)
− − − specified site – *see* Neoplasm,
    malignant
− − − unspecified site C25.9
− − pancreas C25.4
− − specified site NEC – *see* Neoplasm,
    malignant
− − unspecified site C25.4
− lobular (M8520/3)
− − in situ (M8520/2)
− − − breast D05.0
− − − specified site NEC – *see* Neoplasm,
    in situ
− − − unspecified site D05.0
− − specified site – *see* Neoplasm,
    malignant
− − unspecified site C50.9
− medullary (M8510/3)
− mesonephric (M9110/3)
− mixed cell (M8323/3)
− mucinous (M8480/3)
− − metastatic (M8480/6) – *see* Neoplasm,
    secondary
− mucin-producing (M8481/3)
− mucin-secreting (M8481/3)
− mucoid (M8480/3) – *see also* Neoplasm,
    malignant
− − cell (M8300/3)
− − − specified site – *see* Neoplasm,
    malignant
− − − unspecified site C75.1
− mucous (M8480/3)
− nonencapsulated sclerosing (M8350/3)
    C73
− oncocytic (M8290/3)
− oxyphilic (M8290/3)
− papillary (M8260/3)
− − with follicular (M8340/3) C73
− − follicular variant (M8340/3) C73
− − intraductal (noninfiltrating) (M8503/2)
− − − with invasion (M8503/3)
− − − − specified site – *see* Neoplasm,
        malignant
− − − − unspecified site C50.9
− − − breast D05.1
− − − specified site NEC – *see* Neoplasm,
    in situ
− − − unspecified site D05.1
− − serous (M8460/3)
− − − specified site – *see* Neoplasm,
    malignant
− − − unspecified site C56
− papillocystic (M8450/3)

Adenocarcinoma—*continued*
- papillocystic—*continued*
- – specified site – *see* Neoplasm, malignant
- – unspecified site C56
- pseudomucinous (M8470/3)
- – specified site – *see* Neoplasm, malignant
- – unspecified site C56
- renal cell (M8312/3) C64
- scirrhous (M8141/3)
- sebaceous (M8410/3) – *see* Neoplasm, skin, malignant
- serous (M8441/3) – *see also* Neoplasm, malignant
- – papillary (M8460/3)
- – – specified site – *see* Neoplasm, malignant
- – – unspecified site C56
- signet ring cell (M8490/3)
- superficial spreading (M8143/3)
- sweat gland (M8400/3) – *see* Neoplasm, skin, malignant
- trabecular (M8190/3)
- tubular (M8211/3)
- villous (M8262/3)
- water-clear cell (M8322/3) C75.0

Adenocarcinoma in situ (M8140/2) –
  see also Neoplasm, in situ
- breast D05.9
- in
- – adenoma (polypoid) (tubular) (M8210/2)
- – – tubulovillous (M8263/2)
- – – villous (M8261/2)
- – polyp, adenomatous (M8210/2)

Adenofibroma (M9013/0)
- clear cell (M8313/0) – *see* Neoplasm, benign
- endometrioid (M8381/0) D27
- – borderline malignancy (M8381/1) D39.1
- – malignant (M8381/3) C56
- mucinous (M9015/0)
- – specified site – *see* Neoplasm, benign
- – unspecified site D27
- papillary (M9013/0)
- – specified site – *see* Neoplasm, benign
- – unspecified site D27
- prostate D29.1
- serous (M9014/0)
- – specified site – *see* Neoplasm, benign
- – unspecified site D27
- specified site – *see* Neoplasm, benign
- unspecified site D27

Adenofibrosis, breast N60.2
Adenoiditis (chronic) J35.0
- acute J03.9
Adenoids – *see condition*
Adenolipoma (M8324/0) – *see* Neoplasm, benign
Adenolipomatosis, Launois-Bensaude E88.8
Adenolymphoma (M8561/0)
- specified site – *see* Neoplasm, benign
- unspecified site D11.9
Adenoma (M8140/0) – *see also* Neoplasm, benign

Note: Except where otherwise indicated, the morphological varieties of adenoma in the list below should be coded by site as for "Neoplasm, benign".

- acidophil (M8280/0)
- – specified site – *see* Neoplasm, benign
- – unspecified site D35.2
- acidophil-basophil, mixed (M8281/0)
- – specified site – *see* Neoplasm, benign
- – unspecified site D35.2
- acinar (cell) (M8550/0)
- acinic cell (M8550/0)
- adrenal (cortical) (M8370/0) D35.0
- – clear cell (M8373/0) D35.0
- – compact cell (M8371/0) D35.0
- – glomerulosa cell (M8374/0) D35.0
- – heavily pigmented variant (M8372/0) D35.0
- – mixed cell (M8375/0) D35.0
- alpha-cell (M8152/0)
- – pancreas D13.7
- – specified site NEC – *see* Neoplasm, benign
- – unspecified site D13.7
- alveolar (M8251/0) D14.3
- apocrine (M8401/0)
- – breast D24
- – specified site NEC – *see* Neoplasm, skin, benign
- – unspecified site D23.9
- basal cell (M8147/0) D11.9
- basophil (M8300/0)
- – specified site – *see* Neoplasm, benign
- – unspecified site D35.2
- basophil-acidophil, mixed (M8281/0)
- – specified site – *see* Neoplasm, benign
- – unspecified site D35.2
- beta-cell (M8151/0)
- – pancreas D13.7
- – specified site NEC – *see* Neoplasm, benign

Adenoma—*continued*
- beta-cell—*continued*
- – unspecified site D13.7
- bile duct (M8160/0) D13.4
- – common D13.5
- – extrahepatic D13.5
- – intrahepatic D13.4
- – specified site NEC – *see* Neoplasm,
  benign
- – unspecified site D13.4
- black (M8372/0) D35.0
- bronchial (M8140/1) D38.1
- – carcinoid type (M8240/3) – *see*
  Neoplasm, lung, malignant
- – cylindroid type (M8200/3) – *see*
  Neoplasm, lung, malignant
- ceruminous (M8420/0) D23.2
- chief cell (M8321/0) D35.1
- chromophobe (M8270/0)
- – specified site – *see* Neoplasm, benign
- – unspecified site D35.2
- clear cell (M8310/0)
- colloid (M8334/0)
- – specified site – *see* Neoplasm, benign
- – unspecified site D34
- duct (M8503/0)
- eccrine, papillary (M8408/0) – *see*
  Neoplasm, skin, benign
- embryonal (M8191/0)
- endocrine, multiple (M8360/1)
- – single specified site – *see* Neoplasm,
  uncertain behavior
- – two or more specified sites D44.8
- – unspecified site D44.8
- endometrioid (M8380/0) – *see also*
  Neoplasm, benign
- – borderline malignancy (M8380/1) – *see*
  Neoplasm, uncertain behavior
- eosinophil (M8280/0)
- – specified site – *see* Neoplasm, benign
- – unspecified site D35.2
- fetal (M8333/0)
- – specified site – *see* Neoplasm, benign
- – unspecified site D34
- follicular (M8330/0)
- – specified site – *see* Neoplasm, benign
- – unspecified site D34
- hepatocellular (M8170/0) D13.4
- Hurthle cell (M8290/0) D34
- intracystic papillary (M8504/0)
- islet cell (M8150/0)
- – pancreas D13.7
- – specified site NEC – *see* Neoplasm,
  benign
- – unspecified site D13.7

Adenoma—*continued*
- liver cell (M8170/0) D13.4
- macrofollicular (M8334/0)
- – specified site – *see* Neoplasm, benign
- – unspecified site D34
- malignant (M8140/3) – *see* Neoplasm,
  malignant
- mesonephric (M9110/0)
- microcystic (M8202/0)
- – pancreas D13.7
- – specified site NEC – *see* Neoplasm,
  benign
- – unspecified site D13.7
- microfollicular (M8333/0)
- – specified site – *see* Neoplasm, benign
- – unspecified site D34
- mixed cell (M8323/0)
- monomorphic (M8146/0)
- mucinous (M8480/0)
- mucoid cell (M8300/0)
- – specified site – *see* Neoplasm, benign
- – unspecified site D35.2
- multiple endocrine (M8360/1)
- – single specified site – *see* Neoplasm,
  uncertain behavior
- – two or more specified sites D44.8
- – unspecified site D44.8
- nipple (M8506/0) D24
- oncocytic (M8290/0)
- oxyphilic (M8290/0)
- papillary (M8260/0) – *see also* Neoplasm,
  benign
- – eccrine (M8408/0) – *see* Neoplasm,
  skin, benign
- – intracystic (M8504/0)
- papillotubular (M8263/0)
- Pick's tubular (M8640/0)
- – specified site – *see* Neoplasm, benign
- – unspecified site
- – – female D27
- – – male D29.2
- pleomorphic (M8940/0)
- – carcinoma in (M8941/3) – *see*
  Neoplasm, salivary gland, malignant
- – – specified site – *see* Neoplasm,
  malignant
- – – unspecified site C08.9
- polypoid (M8210/0) – *see also* Neoplasm,
  benign
- – adenocarcinoma in (M8210/3) – *see*
  Neoplasm, malignant
- – adenocarcinoma in situ (M8210/2) –
  see Neoplasm, in situ
- prostate D29.1

Adenoma—*continued*
- sebaceous (M8410/0) – *see* Neoplasm, skin, benign
- Sertoli cell (M8640/0)
- – specified site – *see* Neoplasm, benign
- – unspecified site
- – – female D27
- – – male D29.2
  skin appendage (M8390/0) – *see* Neoplasm, skin, benign
- sudoriferous gland (M8400/0) – *see* Neoplasm, skin, benign
  sweat gland (M8400/0) *see* Neoplasm, skin, benign
- testicular (M8640/0)
- – specified site – *see* Neoplasm, benign
- – unspecified site
- – – female D27
- – – male D29.2
- trabecular (M8190/0)
- tubular (M8211/0) – *see also* Neoplasm, benign
- – adenocarcinoma in (M8210/3) – *see* Neoplasm, malignant
- – adenocarcinoma in situ (M8210/2) – *see* Neoplasm, in situ
- – Pick's (M8640/0)
- – – specified site – *see* Neoplasm, benign
- – – unspecified site
- – – – female D27
- – – – male D29.2
- tubulovillous (M8263/0) – *see also* Neoplasm, benign
- – adenocarcinoma in (M8263/3) – *see* Neoplasm, malignant
- – adenocarcinoma in situ (M8263/2) – *see* Neoplasm, in situ
- villoglandular (M8263/0)
- villous (M8261/1) – *see* Neoplasm, uncertain behavior
- – adenocarcinoma in (M8261/3) – *see* Neoplasm, malignant
- – adenocarcinoma in situ (M8261/2) – *see* Neoplasm, in situ
- water-clear cell (M8322/0) D35.1
- wolffian duct (M9110/0)

Adenomatosis (M8220/0)
- endocrine (multiple) (M8360/1)
- – single specified site – *see* Neoplasm, uncertain behavior
- – two or more specified sites D44.8
- – unspecified site D44.8
- erosive of nipple (M8506/0) D24
- pluriendocrine (M8360/1) – *see* Adenomatosis, endocrine (multiple)

Adenomatosis—*continued*
- pulmonary (M8250/1) D38.1
- – – malignant (M8250/3) – *see* Neoplasm, lung, malignant
- specified site – *see* Neoplasm, benign
- unspecified site D12.6
Adenomatous
- goiter (nontoxic) E04.9
- – – with hyperthyroidism E05.2
- – – toxic E05.2
Adenomyoma (M8932/0) – *see also* Neoplasm, benign
- prostate D29.1
Adenomyosis N80.0
Adenopathy (lymph gland) R59.9
- generalized R59.1
- inguinal R59.0
- localized R59.0
- mediastinal R59.0
- mesentery R59.0
- syphilitic (secondary) A51.4
- tracheobronchial R59.0
- – tuberculous A16.3
- – – primary (progressive) A16.7
- – – – with bacteriological and histological confirmation A15.7
- tuberculous (*see also* Tuberculosis, lymph gland) A18.2
- – tracheobronchial A16.3
- – – primary (progressive) A16.7
- – – – with bacteriological and histological confirmation A15.7
Adenosarcoma (M8933/3) – *see* Neoplasm, malignant
Adenosclerosis I88.8
Adenosis (sclerosing) breast N60.2
Adenovirus, as cause of disease classified elsewhere B97.0
Adherent – *see also* Adhesions
- labia (minora) N90.8
- pericardium I31.0
- – rheumatic I09.2
- placenta (morbidly) O43.2
- prepuce N47
- scar (skin) L90.5
Adhesions, adhesive (postinfective) K66.0
- with intestinal obstruction K56.5
- abdominal (wall) (*see also* Adhesions, peritoneum) K66.0
- amnion to fetus O41.8
- – affecting fetus or newborn P02.8
- appendix K38.8
- bile duct (common) (hepatic) K83.8
- bladder (sphincter) N32.8

Adhesions, adhesive—*continued*
- bowel (*see also* Adhesions, peritoneum) K66.0
- cardiac I31.0
- – rheumatic I09.2
- cecum (*see also* Adhesions, peritoneum) K66.0
- cervicovaginal N88.1
- – congenital Q52.8
- – postpartal O90.8
- – – old N88.1
- cervix N88.1
- ciliary body NEC H21.5
- clitoris N90.8
- colon (*see also* Adhesions, peritoneum) K66.0
- common duct K83.8
- congenital (*see also* Anomaly, by site)
- – fingers Q70.0
- – omental, anomalous Q43.3
- – peritoneal Q43.3
- – toes Q70.2
- – tongue (to gum or roof of mouth) Q38.3
- conjunctiva (acquired) H11.2
- – congenital Q15.8
- cystic duct K82.8
- diaphragm (*see also* Adhesions, peritoneum) K66.0
- due to foreign body – *see* Foreign body
- duodenum (*see also* Adhesions, peritoneum) K66.0
- epididymis N50.8
- epidural – *see* Adhesions, meninges
- epiglottis J38.7
- eyelid H02.5
- female pelvis N73.6
- gallbladder K82.8
- globe H44.8
- heart I31.0
- – rheumatic I09.2
- ileocecal (coil) (*see also* Adhesions, peritoneum) K66.0
- ileum (*see also* Adhesions, peritoneum) K66.0
- intestine (*see also* Adhesions, peritoneum) K66.0
- – with obstruction K56.5
- intra-abdominal (*see also* Adhesions, peritoneum) K66.0
- iris NEC H21.5
- – to corneal graft T85.8
- joint M24.8
- – knee M23.8
- labium (majus) (minus), congenital Q52.5

Adhesions, adhesive—*continued*
- liver (*see also* Adhesions, peritoneum) K66.0
- lung J98.4
- mediastinum J98.5
- meninges
- – cerebral G96.1
- – – congenital Q04.8
- – congenital Q07.8
- – spinal G96.1
- – – congenital Q06.8
- – tuberculous (cerebral) (spinal) A17.0† G01*
- mesenteric (*see also* Adhesions, peritoneum) K66.0
- nasal (septum) (to turbinates) J34.8
- ocular muscle H50.6
- omentum (*see also* Adhesions, peritoneum) K66.0
- ovary N73.6
- – congenital (to cecum, kidney or omentum) Q50.3
- paraovarian N73.6
- pelvic (peritoneal)
- – female N73.6
- – – postprocedural N99.4
- – male (*see also* Adhesions, peritoneum) K66.0
- – postpartal (old) N73.6
- – tuberculous A18.1† N74.1*
- penis to scrotum (congenital) Q55.8
- periappendiceal (*see also* Adhesions, peritoneum) K66.0
- pericardium I31.0
- – focal I31.8
- – rheumatic I09.2
- – tuberculous A18.8† I32.0*
- perigastric (*see also* Adhesions, peritoneum) K66.0
- periovarian N73.6
- periprostatic N42.8
- perirenal N28.8
- peritoneum, peritoneal K66.0
- – with obstruction (intestinal) K56.5
- – congenital Q43.3
- – pelvic, female N73.6
- – – postprocedural N99.4
- – postpartal, pelvic N73.6
- – to uterus N73.6
- peritubal N73.6
- periureteral N28.8
- periuterine N73.6
- perivesical N32.8
- perivesicular (seminal vesicle) N50.8
- pleura, pleuritic J94.8

Adhesions, adhesive—*continued*
- pleura, pleuritic—*continued*
- - tuberculous NEC A16.5
- pleuropericardial J94.8
- postoperative
- - with obstruction K91.3
- - due to foreign body accidentally left in wound T81.5
- - pelvic peritoneal N99.4
- - vagina N99.2
- postpartal, old (vulva or perineum) N90.8
- preputial, prepuce N47
- pulmonary J98.4
- pylorus (*see also* Adhesions, peritoneum) K66.0
- sciatic nerve G57.0
- seminal vesicle N50.8
- shoulder (joint) M75.0
- sigmoid flexure (*see also* Adhesions, peritoneum) K66.0
- spermatic cord (acquired) N50.8
- - congenital Q55.4
- spinal canal G96.1
- stomach (*see also* Adhesions, peritoneum) K66.0
- subscapular M75.0
- tendinitis M65.8
- - shoulder M75.0
- testis N50.8
- tongue, congenital (to gum or roof of mouth) Q38.3
- trachea J39.8
- tubo-ovarian N73.6
- tunica vaginalis N50.8
- uterus N73.6
- - internal N85.6
- - to abdominal wall N73.6
- vagina (chronic) N89.5
- - postoperative N99.2
- vitreous H43.8
- vulva N90.8
Adiaspiromycosis B48.8
Adie(-Holmes) pupil or syndrome H57.0
Adiponecrosis neonatorum P83.8
Adiposis E66.9
- cerebralis E23.6
- dolorosa E88.2
Adiposity E66.9
- heart (*see also* Degeneration, myocardial) I51.5
- localized E65
Adiposogenital dystrophy E23.6
Adjustment
- disorder F43.2
- implanted device – *see* Management

Adjustment—*continued*
- prosthesis, external – *see* Fitting
- reaction F43.2
Administration, prophylactic
- antibiotics Z29.2
- chemotherapeutic agents NEC Z29.2
- gamma globulin Z29.1
- immunoglobulin Z29.1
Admission (for)
- in vitro fertilization Z31.2
- observation – *see* Observation
- ovum harvesting or implantation Z31.2
- prophylactic organ removal Z40.0
Adnexitis (suppurative) (*see also* Salpingo-oophoritis) N70.9
Adrenal (gland) – *see* condition
Adrenalism, tuberculous A18.7† E35.1*
Adrenalitis, adrenitis E27.8
- autoimmune E27.1
- meningococcal, hemorrhagic A39.1† E35.1*
Adrenocortical syndrome – *see* Cushing's syndrome
Adrenogenital syndrome E25.9
- acquired E25.8
- congenital E25.0
- salt loss E25.0
Adrenogenitalism, congenital E25.0
Adrenoleukodystrophy E71.3
Adventitious bursa M71.8
Advice – *see* Counseling
Adynamia episodica hereditaria G72.3
Aeration lung imperfect, newborn P28.1
Aerobullosis T70.3
Aerocele – *see* Embolism, air
Aerodontalgia T70.2
Aeroembolism T70.3
Aero-otitis media T70.0
Aerophagy, aerophagia (psychogenic) F45.3
Aerosinusitis T70.1
Aerotitis T70.0
Affection – *see* Disease
Afibrinogenemia (*see also* Defect, coagulation) D68.8
- acquired D65
- congenital D68.2
Aftercare (*see also* Care) Z51.9
- following surgery Z48.9
- - specified NEC Z48.8
- involving dialysis
- - extracorporeal Z49.1
- - peritoneal Z49.2
- - renal Z49.1
- orthodontics Z51.8

Aftercare—*continued*
- orthopedic (*see also* Removal) Z47.9
- - specified NEC Z47.8
- specified type NEC Z51.8
After-cataract H26.4
Agalactia (primary) O92.3
- elective, secondary or therapeutic O92.5
Agammaglobulinemia D80.1
- with
- - immunoglobulin-bearing B-
  lymphocytes D80.1
- - lymphopenia D81.9
- acquired (secondary) D80.1
- autosomal recessive (Swiss type) D80.0
- Bruton's X-linked D80.0
- common variable (CVAgamma) D80.1
- congenital sex-linked D80.0
- hereditary D80.0
- lymphopenic D81.9
- nonfamilial D80.1
- Swiss type (autosomal recessive) D80.0
- X-linked (with growth hormone
  deficiency) (Bruton) D80.0
Aganglionosis (bowel) (colon) Q43.1
Age (old) (*see also* Senile, senility) R54
Agenesis
- adrenal (gland) Q89.1
- alimentary tract (complete) (partial) NEC
  Q45.8
- - upper Q40.8
- anus, anal (canal) Q42.3
- - with fistula Q42.2
- aorta Q25.4
- appendix Q42.8
- arm (complete) Q71.0
- artery (peripheral) Q27.9
- - brain Q28.3
- - coronary Q24.5
- - pulmonary Q25.7
- - specified NEC Q27.8
- - umbilical Q27.0
- auditory (canal) (external) Q16.1
- auricle (ear) Q16.0
- bile duct or passage Q44.5
- bladder Q64.5
- bone NEC Q79.9
- brain Q00.0
- - part of Q04.3
- breast (with nipple present) Q83.8
- - with absent nipple Q83.0
- bronchus Q32.4
- canaliculus lacrimalis Q10.4
- carpus Q71.3
- cartilage Q79.9
- cecum Q42.8

Agenesis—*continued*
- cerebellum Q04.3
- cervix Q51.5
- chin Q18.8
- cilia Q10.3
- circulatory system, part NEC Q28.9
- clavicle Q74.0
- clitoris Q52.6
- coccyx Q76.4
- colon Q42.9
- - specified NEC Q42.8
- corpus callosum Q04.0
- cricoid cartilage Q31.8
- diaphragm (with hernia) Q79.1
- digestive organ(s) or tract (complete)
  (partial) NEC Q45.8
- - upper Q40.8
- duodenum Q41.0
- ear Q16.9
- - auricle Q16.0
- - lobe Q17.8
- ejaculatory duct Q55.4
- endocrine (gland) NEC Q89.2
- epiglottis Q31.8
- esophagus Q39.8
- eustachian tube Q16.2
- eye Q11.1
- - adnexa Q15.8
- eyelid (fold) Q10.3
- face
- - bones NEC Q75.8
- - specified part NEC Q18.8
- fallopian tube Q50.6
- femur Q72.4
- fibula Q72.6
- finger (complete) (partial) Q71.3
- foot (and toes) (complete) (partial) Q72.3
- gallbladder Q44.0
- gastric Q40.2
- genitalia, genital (organ(s))
- - female Q52.8
- - - external Q52.7
- - - internal NEC Q52.8
- - male Q55.8
- glottis Q31.8
- hair Q84.0
- hand (and fingers) (complete) (partial)
  Q71.3
- heart Q24.8
- - valve NEC Q24.8
- hepatic Q44.7
- humerus Q71.8
- hymen Q52.4
- ileum Q41.2
- incus Q16.3

Agenesis—*continued*
- intestine (small) Q41.9
- – large Q42.9
- – – specified NEC Q42.8
- iris (dilator fibers) Q13.1
- jaw K07.0
- jejunum Q41.1
- kidney(s) (partial) Q60.2
- – bilateral Q60.1
- – unilateral Q60.0
- labium (majus) (minus) Q52.7
- labyrinth, membranous Q16.5
- lacrimal apparatus Q10.4
- larynx Q31.8
- leg
- – lower Q72.8
- – – and foot Q72.2
- – meaning lower limb Q72.0
- lens Q12.3
- limb (complete) Q73.0
- – lower Q72.0
- – upper Q71.0
- lip Q38.0
- liver Q44.7
- lung (fissure) (lobe) (bilateral) (unilateral) Q33.3
- mandible, maxilla K07.0
- metacarpus Q71.3
- metatarsus Q72.3
- muscle Q79.8
- – eyelid Q10.3
- – ocular Q15.8
- musculoskeletal system NEC Q79.8
- nail(s) Q84.3
- neck, part Q18.8
- nerve Q07.8
- nervous system, part NEC Q07.8
- nipple Q83.2
- nose Q30.1
- nuclear Q07.8
- oesophagus Q39.8
- organ
- – of Corti Q16.5
- – or site not listed – *see* Anomaly, by site
- osseous meatus (ear) Q16.1
- ovary Q50.0
- oviduct Q50.6
- pancreas Q45.0
- parathyroid (gland) Q89.2
- parotid gland(s) Q38.4
- patella Q74.1
- pelvic girdle (complete) (partial) Q74.2
- penis Q55.5
- pericardium Q24.8
- pituitary (gland) Q89.2

Agenesis—*continued*
- prostate Q55.4
- punctum lacrimale Q10.4
- radioulnar Q71.8
- radius Q71.4
- rectum Q42.1
- – with fistula Q42.0
- renal Q60.2
- – bilateral Q60.1
- – unilateral Q60.0
- respiratory organ NEC Q34.8
- rib Q76.6
- roof of orbit Q75.8
- round ligament Q52.8
- sacrum Q76.4
- salivary gland Q38.4
- scapula Q74.0
- scrotum Q55.2
- seminal vesicles Q55.4
- septum
- – atrial Q21.1
- – between aorta and pulmonary artery Q21.4
- – ventricular Q20.4
- shoulder girdle (complete) (partial) Q74.0
- skull (bone) Q75.8
- – with
- – – anencephaly Q00.0
- – – encephalocele (*see also* Encephalocele) Q01.9
- – – hydrocephalus Q03.9
- – – – with spina bifida (*see also* Spina bifida, with hydrocephalus) Q05.4
- – – microcephaly Q02
- spermatic cord Q55.4
- spinal cord Q06.0
- spine Q76.4
- spleen Q89.0
- sternum Q76.7
- stomach Q40.2
- submaxillary gland(s) (congenital) Q38.4
- tarsus Q72.3
- tendon Q79.8
- testicle Q55.0
- thymus (gland) Q89.2
- thyroid (gland) E03.1
- – cartilage Q31.8
- tibia Q72.5
- tibiofibular Q72.8
- toe (and foot) (complete) (partial) Q72.3
- tongue Q38.3
- trachea (cartilage) Q32.1
- ulna Q71.5
- upper limb Q71.0
- – with hand present Q71.1

Agenesis—*continued*
- ureter Q62.4
- urethra Q64.5
- urinary tract NEC Q64.8
- uterus Q51.0
- uvula Q38.5
- vagina Q52.0
- vas deferens Q55.4
- vein(s) (peripheral) Q27.9
- – brain Q28.3
- – great NEC Q26.8
- – portal Q26.5
- vena cava (inferior) (superior) Q26.8
- vermis of cerebellum Q04.3
- vertebra Q76.4
- vulva Q52.7

Ageusia R43.2
Agitated – *see condition*
Agitation R45.1
Aglossia (congenital) Q38.3
Aglossia-adactylia syndrome Q87.0
Agnosia (body image) (tactile) (other senses) R48.1
- developmental F88
- verbal R48.1
- – auditory R48.1
- – – developmental F80.2
- – developmental F80.2
- – visual R48.1

Agoraphobia (with history of panic disorder) F40.0
Agrammatism R48.8
Agranulocytosis (angina) (chronic) (cyclical) (genetic) (infantile) (periodic) (pernicious) D70
Agraphia (absolute) R48.8
- developmental F81.8

Ague – *see* Malaria
Agyria Q04.3
Ahumada-del Castillo syndrome E23.0
AIDS (related complex) (*see also* Human, immunodeficiency virus (HIV) disease) B24
- complicating pregnancy, childbirth or the puerperium O98.7

Ailment, heart – *see* Disease, heart
Ainhum (disease) L94.6
Air
- anterior mediastinum J98.2
- conditioner lung or pneumonitis J67.7
- embolism (artery) (cerebral) (any site) T79.0
- – due to implanted device NEC – *see* Complications, by site and type, specified NEC

Air—*continued*
- embolism—*continued*
- – following infusion, therapeutic injection or transfusion T80.0
- – in pregnancy, childbirth or puerperium O88.0
- – traumatic T79.0
- hunger, psychogenic F45.3
- pollution Z58.1
- – occupational NEC Z57.3
- rarefied, effects of – *see* Effect, adverse, high altitude
- sickness T75.3

Akathisia, treatment-induced G21.1
Akinesia R29.8
Akinetic mutism R41.8
Akureyri's disease G93.3
Alactasia, congenital E73.0
Alagille's syndrome Q44.7
Alalia R47.0
- developmental F80.0

Alastrim B03
Albers-Schönberg syndrome Q78.2
Albert's syndrome M76.6
Albinism, albino (cutaneous) (generalized) (isolated) (partial) E70.3
- ocular, oculocutaneous E70.3

Albinismus E70.3
Albright (-McCune) (-Sternberg) syndrome Q78.1
Albuminous – *see condition*
Albuminuria, albuminuric (acute) (chronic) (subacute) (*see also* Proteinuria) R80
- complicating pregnancy, childbirth or puerperium O12.1
- – with
- – – gestational hypertension (*see also* Pre-eclampsia) O14.9
- – – pre-existing hypertensive disorder O11
- gestational O12.1
- – with
- – – gestational hypertension (*see also* Pre-eclampsia) O14.9
- – – pre-existing hypertensive disorder O11
- orthostatic N39.2
- postural N39.2
- pre-eclamptic (*see also* Pre-eclampsia) O14.9
- – affecting fetus or newborn P00.0
- – severe O14.1
- – – affecting fetus or newborn P00.0

Alcaptonuria E70.2

39

Alcohol, alcoholic, alcohol-induced
- addiction F10.2
- brain syndrome, chronic F10.7
- counseling and surveillance Z71.4
- delirium (acute) (tremens) (withdrawal) F10.4
- - chronic F10.6
- dependence F10.2
- dementia F10.7
- detoxification therapy Z50.2
- hallucinosis (acute) F10.5
- intoxication (acute) F10.0
- - with delirium F10.0
- jealousy F10.5
- liver K70.9
- paranoia, paranoid (type) psychosis F10.5
- pellagra E52
- poisoning, accidental (acute) NEC T51.9
- - specified type of alcohol – see Table of drugs and chemicals
- psychosis – see Psychosis, alcoholic
- rehabilitation measures Z50.2
- use NEC Z72.1
- withdrawal F10.3
- - with delirium F10.4
Alcoholism (chronic) F10.2
- with psychosis (see also Psychosis, alcoholic) F10.5
- complicating pregnancy, childbirth or puerperium O99.3
- - affecting fetus or newborn P04.3
- Korsakov's F10.6
- suspected damage to fetus affecting management of pregnancy O35.4
Alder's anomaly or syndrome D72.0
Aldosteronism (see also Hyperaldosteronism) E26.9
Aldrich(-Wiskott) syndrome D82.0
Aleppo boil B55.1
Aleukemic – see condition
Aleukia hemorrhagica D61.9
Alexia R48.0
- developmental F81.0
Algoneurodystrophy M89.0
Alienation, mental (see also Psychosis) F29
Alkalemia E87.3
Alkalosis (metabolic) (respiratory) E87.3
Alkaptonuria E70.2
Allen-Masters syndrome N83.8
Allergy, allergic (reaction) T78.4
- airborne substance NEC (rhinitis) J30.3
- animal (dander) (epidermal) (hair) (rhinitis) J30.3

Allergy, allergic—continued
- biological – see Allergy, drug, medicament and biological
- colitis K52.2
- dander (animal) (rhinitis) J30.3
- dandruff (rhinitis) J30.3
- dermatitis (see also Dermatitis, due to) L23.9
- drug, medicament and biological (any) (correct medicinal substance properly administered) (external) (internal) T88.7
- - wrong substance given or taken NEC T50.9
- - - specified drug or substance – see Table of drugs and chemicals
- dust (house) (stock) (rhinitis) J30.3
- - with asthma J45.0
- eczema (see also Dermatitis, due to) L23.9
- epidermal (animal) (rhinitis) J30.3
- feathers (rhinitis) J30.3
- food (any) (ingested) NEC T78.1
- - anaphylactic shock T78.0
- - dietary counseling and surveillance Z71.3
- - in contact with skin L23.6
- gastrointestinal K52.2
- grass (hay fever) (pollen) J30.1
- - asthma J45.0
- hair (animal) (rhinitis) J30.3
- horse serum – see Allergy, serum
- inhalant (rhinitis) J30.3
- kapok (rhinitis) J30.3
- medicine – see Allergy, drug, medicament and biological
- nasal, seasonal due to pollen J30.1
- pollen (any) (hay fever) J30.1
- - asthma J45.0
- ragweed (hay fever) (pollen) J30.1
- - asthma J45.0
- rose (pollen) J30.1
- Senecio jacobae (pollen) J30.1
- serum (prophylactic) (therapeutic) T80.6
- - anaphylactic shock T80.5
- shock (anaphylactic) T78.2
- - due to
- - - adverse effect of correct medicinal substance properly administered T88.6
- - - serum or immunization T80.5
- tree (any) (hay fever) (pollen) J30.1
- - asthma J45.0
- upper respiratory J30.4
- vaccine – see Allergy, serum
Allescheriasis B48.2

Alligator skin disease Q80.9
Allocheiria, allochiria R20.8
Almeida's disease (*see also*
Paracoccidioidomycosis) B41.9
Alopecia (hereditaria) (seborrheica)
L65.9
– androgenic L64.9
– – drug-induced L64.0
– – specified NEC L64.8
– areata L63.9
– – specified NEC L63.8
– cicatricial L66.9
– – specified NEC L66.8
– circumscripta L63.9
– congenital, congenitalis Q84.0
– due to cytotoxic drugs NEC L65.8
– mucinosa L65.2
– postinfective NEC L65.8
– postpartum L65.0
– premature L64.8
– specific (syphilitic) A51.3† L99.8∗
– specified NEC L65.8
– syphilitic (secondary) A51.3† L99.8∗
– totalis (capitis) L63.0
– universalis (entire body) L63.1
– X-ray L58.1
Alpers' disease G31.8
Alpine sickness T70.2
Alport's syndrome Q87.8
**Altered pattern of family relationships
affecting child** Z61.2
Alternating – *see condition*
Altitude, high (effects) – *see* Effect,
adverse, high'altitude
Aluminosis (of lung) J63.0
Alveolitis
– allergic (extrinsic) J67.9
– – due to
– – – inhaled organic dusts NEC J67.8
– – – organisms (fungal, thermophilic
actinomycetes, other) growing in
ventilation (air conditioning) systems
J67.7
– due to
– – Aspergillus clavatus J67.4
– – Cryptostroma corticale J67.6
– fibrosing (cryptogenic) (idiopathic) J84.1
– jaw K10.3
Alveolus, alveolar – *see condition*
Alymphocytosis D72.8
– thymic (with immunodeficiency) D82.1
Alymphoplasia, thymic D82.1
Alzheimer's disease or sclerosis G30.9
– dementia in G30.9† F00.9∗
– – atypical or mixed G30.8† F00.2∗

Alzheimer's disease or sclerosis—
continued
– dementia in—*continued*
– – early onset (presenile) G30.0† F00.0∗
– – late onset (senile) G30.1† F00.1∗
– early onset (presenile) G30.0
– late onset (senile) G30.1
– specified NEC G30.8
Amastia (with nipple present) Q83.8
– with absent nipple Q83.0
**Amaurosis (acquired)
(congenital)** (*see also* Blindness) H54.0
– fugax G45.3
– hysterical F44.6
– Leber's congenital H35.5
– uremic – *see* Uremia
**Amaurotic idiocy (infantile) (juvenile)
(late)** E75.4
Ambiguous genitalia Q56.4
**Amblyopia (congenital) (deprivation)
(partial) (strabismic) (suppression)**
H53.0
– anisometropic H53.0
– ex anopsia H53.0
– hysterical F44.6
– nocturnal H53.6
– – vitamin A deficiency E50.5† H58.1∗
– tobacco H53.8
– toxic NEC H53.8
– uremic – *see* Uremia
Ameba, amebic – *see* Amebiasis
Amebiasis A06.9
– with abscess – *see* Abscess, amebic
– acute A06.0
– chronic (intestine) A06.1
– – with abscess – *see* Abscess, amebic
– cutaneous A06.7
– hepatic (*see also* Abscess, liver, amebic)
A06.4
– intestine A06.0
– nondysenteric colitis A06.2
– skin A06.7
– specified site NEC A06.8
Ameboma (of intestine) A06.3
Amelia Q73.0
– lower limb Q72.0
– upper limb Q71.0
Ameloblastoma (M9310/0) D16.5
– jaw (bone) (lower) D16.5
– – upper D16.4
– long bones (M9261/3) C40.9
– malignant (M9310/3) C41.1
– – jaw (bone) (lower) C41.1
– – – upper C41.0
– mandible D16.5

Ameloblastoma—*continued*
– tibial (M9261/3) C40.2
Amelogenesis imperfecta K00.5
– nonhereditaria (segmentalis) K00.4
Amenorrhea N91.2
– hyperhormonal E28.8
– primary N91.0
– secondary N91.1
Amentia (*see also* Retardation, mental)
F79.-
Ametropia H52.7
Amianthosis J61
Amimia R48.8
Amino-acid disorder E72.9
– anemia D53.0
Aminoacidopathy E72.9
Aminoaciduria E72.9
Amnes(t)ic syndrome
– alcohol-induced F10.6
– drug-induced – *see* F11-F19 with fourth
character .6
Amnesia R41.3
– anterograde R41.1
– auditory R48.8
– dissociative F44.0
– hysterical F44.0
– postictal in epilepsy G40.9
– psychogenic F44.0
– retrograde R41.2
– transient global G45.4
Amniocentesis screening (for) Z36.2
– alphafetoprotein level, raised Z36.1
– chromosomal anomalies Z36.0
Amnion, amniotic – *see* condition
Amnionitis
– affecting fetus or newborn P02.7
– complicating pregnancy O41.1
Amok F68.8
Amoral traits F61
Ampulla
– lower esophagus K22.8
– phrenic K22.8
Amputation – *see also* Absence, by limb or
organ, acquired
– any part of fetus, to facilitate delivery
P03.8
– cervix (uteri) Z90.7
– – in pregnancy or childbirth O34.4
– neuroma T87.3
– stump (surgical)
– – abnormal, painful, or with complication
(late) T87.6
– – healed or old NEC Z89.9
– traumatic (complete) (partial) T14.7

Amputation—*continued*
– traumatic—*continued*
– – abdomen, lower back and pelvis NEC
S38.3
– – arm
– – – meaning upper limb – *see*
Amputation, traumatic, limb, upper
– – – upper S48.9
– – – – at shoulder joint S48.0
– – – – between shoulder and elbow
S48.1
– – ear S08.1
– – finger
– – – one (except thumb) S68.1
– – – – with other parts of wrist and hand
S68.3
– – – two or more (except thumb) S68.2
– – – – with other parts of wrist and hand
S68.3
– – foot S98.4
– – – and other lower limb(s) (leg) (any
level, except foot) T05.4
– – – at ankle level S98.0
– – – both T05.3
– – – one toe S98.1
– – – other parts S98.3
– – – parts of foot and toe(s) S98.3
– – two or more toes S98.2
– – forearm S58.9
– – – at elbow level S58.0
– – – between elbow and wrist S58.1
– – genital organ(s) (external) S38.2
– – hand S68.9
– – – and other upper limb(s) (arm) (any
level, except hand) T05.1
– – – and wrist S68.9
– – – – parts NEC S68.8
– – – at wrist level S68.4
– – – both T05.0
– – – parts NEC S68.8
– – head
– – – decapitation (at neck level) S18
– – – ear S08.1
– – – nose S08.8
– – – part S08.9
– – – – scalp S08.0
– – – – specified NEC S08.8
– – hip (and thigh) S78.9
– – – at hip joint S78.0
– – labium (majus) (minus) S38.2
– – leg
– – – lower S88.9
– – – – and other foot T05.4
– – – – at knee level S88.0
– – – – between knee and ankle S88.1

Amputation—*continued*
- traumatic—*continued*
- – leg—*continued*
- – – lower—*continued*
- – – – both (any level) T05.5
- – – meaning lower limb – *see*
    Amputation, traumatic, limb, lower
- – limb T14.7
- – – lower T13.6
- – – – and other foot T05.4
- – – – both T05.5
- – – upper T11.6
- – – – and other hand T05.1
- – – – both T05.2
- – lower limb(s) except toe(s) T13.6
- – multiple T05.9
- – – specified site NEC T05.8
- – nose S08.8
- – pelvis S38.3
- – penis S38.2
- – scrotum S38.2
- – shoulder S48.9
- – – at shoulder joint S48.0
- – testis S38.2
- – thigh S78.9
- – – at hip joint S78.0
- – – between hip and knee S78.1
- – thorax, part of S28.1
- – thumb S68.0
- – toe
- – – one S98.1
- – – – with other parts of foot S98.3
- – – two or more S98.2
- – – – with other parts of foot S98.3
- – trunk NEC T09.6
- – upper limb(s) T11.6
- – – with lower limb(s), any level(s)
    T05.6
- – – both T05.2
- – vulva S38.2
- – wrist S68.9
- – – parts NEC S68.8
Amputee (bilateral) (old) Z89.9
Amsterdam dwarfism Q87.1
Amusia R48.8
- developmental F80.8
Amyelencephalus, amyelencephaly Q00.0
Amyelia Q06.0
Amygdalitis – *see* Tonsillitis
Amygdalolith J35.8
Amyloid heart (disease) E85.4† I43.1*
Amyloidosis (generalized) (primary)
    E85.9
- with lung involvement E85.4† J99.8*
- familial E85.2

Amyloidosis—*continued*
- genetic E85.2
- heart E85.4† I43.1*
- hemodialysis-associated E85.3
- heredofamilial E85.2
- – neuropathic E85.1
- – non-neuropathic E85.0
- liver E85.4† K77.8*
- localized E85.4
- neuropathic heredofamilial E85.1
- non-neuropathic heredofamilial E85.0
- organ-limited E85.4
- Portuguese E85.1
- pulmonary E85.4† J99.8*
- skin (lichen) (macular) E85.4† L99.0*
- specified NEC E85.8
- subglottic E85.4† J99.8*
- systemic, secondary E85.3
Amylopectinosis (brancher enzyme
    deficiency) E74.0
Amyoplasia congenita Q79.8
Amyotonia M62.8
- congenita G70.2
Amyotrophia, amyotrophy, amyotrophic
    G71.8
- congenita Q79.8
- diabetic (*see also* E10-E14 with fourth
    character .4) E14.4† G73.0*
- lateral sclerosis G12.2
- neuralgic G54.5
- spinal progressive G12.2
Anacidity, gastric K31.8
- psychogenic F45.3
Anaerosis of newborn P28.8
Analbuminemia E88.0
Analgesia (*see also* Anesthesia) R20.0
Analphalipoproteinemia E78.6
Anaphylactic shock or reaction – *see*
    Shock, anaphylactic
Anaphylactoid syndrome of pregnancy
    O88.1
Anaphylactoid shock or reaction – *see*
    Shock, anaphylactic
Anaphylaxis T78.2
Anaplasia cervix (*see also* Dysplasia,
    cervix) N87.9
Anarthria R47.1
Anasarca R60.1
- cardiac (*see also* Failure, heart,
    congestive) I50.0
- fetus or newborn P83.2
Anastomosis
- aneurysmal – *see* Aneurysm
- arteriovenous, ruptured, brain I60.8
- intestinal Z98.0

Anastomosis—*continued*
– intestinal—*continued*
– – complicated NEC K91.8
– – – involving urinary tract N99.8
– retinal and choroidal vessels (congenital)
  Q14.8
Anatomical narrow angle H40.0
**Ancylostoma, ancylostomiasis
  (braziliense) (caninum) (ceylanicum)
  (duodenale) (infection) (infestation)**
  B76.0
Andersen's disease (glycogen storage)
  E74.0
Anderson-Fabry disease E75.2
Andes disease T70.2
Androblastoma (M8630/1)
– benign (M8630/0)
– – specified site – *see* Neoplasm, benign
– – unspecified site
– – – female D27
– – – male D29.2
– malignant (M8630/3)
– – specified site – *see* Neoplasm,
  malignant
– – unspecified site
– – – female C56
– – – male C62.9
– specified site – *see* Neoplasm, uncertain
  behavior
– tubular (M8640/0)
– – with lipid storage (M8641/0)
– – – specified site – *see* Neoplasm, benign
– – – unspecified site
– – – – female D27
– – – – male D29.2
– – specified site – *see* Neoplasm, benign
– – unspecified site
– – – female D27
– – – male D29.2
– unspecified site
– – female D39.1
– – male D40.1
Androgen resistance syndrome E34.5
Android pelvis Q74.2
– with disproportion (fetopelvic) O33.3
– – affecting fetus or newborn P03.1
– – causing obstructed labor O65.3
Anemia D64.9
– with disorder of
– – anaerobic glycolysis D55.2
– – pentose phosphate pathway D55.1
– achlorhydric D50.8
– achrestic D53.1
– Addison(-Biermer) D51.0
– amino-acid-deficiency D53.0

Anemia—*continued*
– aplastic D61.9
– – congenital D61.0
– – constitutional D61.0
– – drug-induced D61.1
– – due to
– – – drugs D61.1
– – – external agents NEC D61.2
– – – infection D61.2
– – – radiation D61.2
– – idiopathic D61.3
– – red cell (pure) D60.9
– – – chronic D60.0
– – – congenital D61.0
– – – specified type NEC D60.8
– – – transient D60.1
– – specified type NEC D61.8
– – toxic D61.2
– asiderotic D50.9
– atypical (primary) D64.9
– Baghdad spring D55.0
– Balantidium coli A07.0
– Biermer's D51.0
– brickmaker's B76.9† D63.8*
– cerebral I67.8
– childhood D64.9
– chlorotic D50.8
– chronic simple D53.9
– combined system disease NEC D51.0†
  G32.0*
– – due to dietary vitamin B_{12} deficiency
  D51.3† G32.0*
– complicating pregnancy, childbirth or
  puerperium O99.0
– congenital P61.4
– – due to isoimmunization NEC P55.9
– – dyserythropoietic, dyshematopoietic
  D64.4
– – following fetal blood loss P61.3
– – Heinz body D58.2
– – hereditary hemolytic NEC D58.9
– Cooley's (erythroblastic) D56.1
– deficiency D53.9
– – amino-acid D53.0
– – 2,3-diphosphoglycerate mutase (2,3-
  PG) D55.2
– – enzyme D55.9
– – – drug-induced (hemolytic) D59.2
– – – glucose-6-phosphate dehydrogenase
  (G6PD) D55.0
– – – glycolytic D55.2
– – – nucleotide metabolism D55.3
– – – related to hexose monophosphate
  (HMP) shunt pathway NEC D55.1
– – – specified type NEC D55.8

Anemia—*continued*
- deficiency—*continued*
- - erythrocytic glutathione D55.1
- - folate D52.9
- - - dietary D52.0
- - - drug-induced D52.1
- - folic acid D52.9
- - - dietary D52.0
- - - drug-induced D52.1
- - GSH D55.1
- - GGS-R D55.1
- - glucose-6-phosphate dehydrogenase (G6PD) D55.0
- - glutathione reductase (GGS-R) D55.1
- - glyceraldehyde phosphate dehydrogenase D55.2
- - G6PD D55.0
- - hexokinase D55.2
- - iron D50.9
- - - secondary to blood loss (chronic) D50.0
- - nutritional D53.9
- - - with
- - - - poor iron absorption D50.8
- - - - specified deficiency NEC D53.8
- - 2,3-PG D55.2
- - 6-PGD D55.1
- - phosphofructo-aldolase D55.2
- - 6-phosphogluconate dehydrogenase (6-PGD) D55.1
- - phosphoglycerate kinase (PK) D55.2
- - PK D55.2
- - protein D53.0
- - pyruvate kinase D55.2
- - transcobalamin II D51.2
- - triose-phosphate isomerase D55.2
- - vitamin B_{12} D51.9
- - - dietary D51.3
- - - due to
- - - - intrinsic factor deficiency D51.0
- - - - selective vitamin B_{12} malabsorption with proteinuria D51.1
- - - specified type NEC D51.8
- Diamond-Blackfan D61.0
- dimorphic D53.1
- diphasic D53.1
- Diphyllobothrium (Dibothriocephalus) B70.0† D63.8*
- drepanocytic (*see also* Disease, sickle-cell) D57.1
- due to
- - deficiency
- - - amino-acid D53.0
- - - copper D53.8

Anemia—*continued*
- due to—*continued*
- - deficiency—*continued*
- - - folate (folic acid) D52.9
- - - - dietary D52.0
- - - - drug-induced D52.1
- - - molybdenum D53.8
- - - protein D53.0
- - - zinc D53.8
- - dietary vitamin B_{12} deficiency D51.3
- - disorder of
- - - glutathione metabolism D55.1
- - - nucleotide metabolism D55.3
- - enzyme disorder D55.9
- - fetal blood loss P61.3
- - hemorrhage (chronic) D50.0
- - - acute D62
- - loss of blood (chronic) D50.0
- - - acute D62
- - myxedema E03.9† D63.8*
- - prematurity P61.2
- - selective vitamin B_{12} malabsorption with proteinuria D51.1
- - transcobalamin II deficiency D51.2
- Dyke-Young type (secondary) (symptomatic) D59.1
- dyserythropoietic (congenital) D64.4
- dyshematopoietic (congenital) D64.4
- Egyptian B76.9† D63.8*
- elliptocytosis (*see also* Elliptocytosis) D58.1
- enzyme-deficiency, drug-induced D59.2
- erythroblastic
- - familial D56.1
- - fetus or newborn (*see also* Disease, hemolytic) P55.9
- - of childhood D56.1
- erythrocytic glutathione deficiency D55.1
- essential D64.9
- familial erythroblastic D56.1
- Fanconi's D61.0
- favism D55.0
- fetus or newborn P61.4
- - due to
- - - ABO (antibodies) (isoimmunization) (maternal/fetal incompatibility) P55.1
- - - Rh (antibodies) (isoimmunization) (maternal/fetal incompatibility) P55.0
- - following fetal blood loss P61.3
- folate (folic acid) deficiency D52.9
- general D64.9
- glucose-6-phosphate dehydrogenase (G6PD) deficiency D55.0

Anemia—*continued*
- glutathione-reductase deficiency D55.1
- goat's milk D52.0
- Heinz body, congenital D58.2
- hemoglobin deficiency D64.9
- hemolytic D58.9
- - acquired D59.9
- - - with hemoglobinuria NEC D59.6
- - - autoimmune NEC D59.1
- - - infectious D59.4
- - - non-autoimmune NEC D59.4
- - drug-induced D59.2
- - - specified type NEC D59.8
- - - toxic D59.4
- - acute D59.9
- - - due to enzyme deficiency specified type NEC D55.8
- - - fetus or newborn (*see also* Disease, hemolytic) P55.9
- - - Lederer's D59.1
- - autoimmune D59.1
- - - drug-induced D59.0
- - chronic D58.9
- - - idiopathic D59.9
- - cold type (secondary) (symptomatic) D59.1
- - congenital (spherocytic) (*see also* Spherocytosis) D58.0
- - due to
- - - cardiac conditions D59.4
- - - drugs (nonautoimmune) D59.2
- - - - autoimmune D59.0
- - - enzyme disorder D55.9
- - - - drug-induced D59.2
- - - presence of shunt or other internal prosthetic device D59.4
- - familial D58.9
- - hereditary D58.9
- - - due to enzyme disorder D55.9
- - - - specified type NEC D55.8
- - - specified type NEC D58.8
- - idiopathic (chronic) D59.9
- - mechanical D59.4
- - microangiopathic D59.4
- - nonautoimmune D59.4
- - - drug-induced D59.2
- - nonspherocytic
- - - congenital or hereditary NEC D55.8
- - - - glucose-6-phosphate dehydrogenase deficiency D55.0
- - - - pyruvate kinase deficiency D55.2
- - - - type I D55.1
- - - - type II D55.2
- - - type I D55.1
- - - type II D55.2

Anemia—*continued*
- hemolytic—*continued*
- - secondary D59.4
- - - autoimmune D59.1
- - - - drug-induced D59.0
- - specified (hereditary) type NEC D58.8
- - Stransky-Regala type (*see also* Hemoglobinopathy) D58.2
- - symptomatic D59.4
- - - autoimmune D59.1
- - toxic NEC D59.4
- - warm type (secondary) (symptomatic) D59.1
- hemorrhagic (chronic) D50.0
- - acute D62
- Herrick's (*see also* Disease, sickle-cell) D57.1
- hexokinase deficiency D55.2
- hookworm B76.9† D63.8*
- hypochromic D50.9
- - familial sex-linked D64.0
- - microcytic D50.8
- - normoblastic D50.8
- - pyridoxine-responsive D64.3
- - sideroblastic, sex-linked D64.0
- hypoplasia, red blood cells D61.9
- - congenital or familial D61.0
- hypoplastic D61.9
- - congenital or familial D61.0
- hypoproliferative (refractive) D61.9
- idiopathic D64.9
- - aplastic D61.3
- - hemolytic, chronic D59.9
- in
- - chronic kidney disease
- - - stage 3 N18.3† D63.8*
- - - stage 4 N18.4† D63.8*
- - - stage 5 N18.5† D63.8*
- - - unspecified N18.9† D63.8*
- - neoplastic disease NEC (M8000/1) (*see also* Neoplasm) D48.9† D63.0* [handwritten: Ｐ – Any neoplasm]
- infantile D64.9
- iron deficiency D50.9
- - secondary to blood loss (chronic) D50.0
- - specified type NEC D50.8
- Lederer's (hemolytic) D59.1
- leukoerythroblastic D64.8
- macrocytic D52.9
- - nutritional D52.0
- - of or complicating pregnancy O99.0
- - tropical D52.8
- malarial (*see also* Malaria) B54† D63.8*
- malignant D51.0

Anemia—*continued*
- malnutrition D53.9
- marsh (*see also* Malaria) B54† D63.8∗
- Mediterranean D56.9
- megaloblastic D53.1
- − hereditary D51.1
- − nutritional D52.0
- − of or complicating pregnancy O99.0
- − orotic aciduria D53.0
- − refractory D53.1
- − specified type NEC D53.1
- megalocytic D53.1
- microcytic D50.8
- − due to blood loss (chronic) D50.0
- − − acute D62
- − familial D56.8
- − hypochromic D50.8
- microelliptopoikilocytic (Rietti-Greppi-Micheli) D56.9
- miner's B76.9† D63.8∗
- myelodysplastic (related to alkylating agent) (related to Epipodophyllotoxin) (related to therapy) D46.9
- myelofibrosis D47.1† D63.0∗
- myelogenous D64.8
- myelopathic D64.8
- myelophthisic D61.9
- myeloproliferative D47.1
- newborn P61.4
- − posthemorrhagic (fetal) P61.3
- nonspherocytic hemolytic – *see* Anemia, hemolytic, nonspherocytic
- normocytic (infection) D64.9
- − due to blood loss (chronic) D50.0
- − − acute D62
- − myelophthisic D61.9
- nutritional (deficiency) D53.9
- − with poor iron absorption D50.8
- − megaloblastic D52.0
- − specified NEC D53.8
- of or complicating pregnancy O99.0
- − affecting fetus or newborn P00.8
- of prematurity P61.2
- orotaciduric D53.0
- osteosclerotic D64.8
- paludal (*see also* Malaria) B54† D63.8∗
- pernicious (congenital) (malignant) (progressive) D51.0
- − of or complicating pregnancy O99.0
- pleochromic D64.8
- − of sprue D52.8
- posthemorrhagic (chronic) D50.0
- − acute D62
- − newborn P61.3
- pressure D64.8

Anemia—*continued*
- primary D64.9
- profound D64.9
- progressive D64.9
- protein-deficiency D53.0
- pseudoleukemica infantum D64.8
- puerperal O99.0
- pure red cell D60.9
- − congenital D61.0
- pyridoxine-responsive D64.3
- pyruvate kinase deficiency D55.2
- refractory (related to alkylating agent) (related to Epipodophyllotoxin) (related to therapy) NEC D46.4
- − with
- − − dysplasia, multi lineage D46.5
- − − excess
- − − − blasts in transformation C92.0
- − − − of blasts (RAEB I) (RAEB II) D46.2
- − − hemochromatosis D46.1
- − − sideroblasts, ring D46.1
- − sideroblastic D46.1
- − sideropenic D50.8
- − without sideroblasts, ring D46.0
- Rietti-Greppi-Micheli D56.9
- scorbutic D53.2
- secondary to
- − blood loss (chronic) D50.0
- − − acute D62
- − hemorrhage (chronic) D50.0
- − − acute D62
- semiplastic D61.8
- septic D64.8
- sickle-cell D57.1
- − with crisis D57.0
- sideroblastic D64.3
- − hereditary D64.0
- − hypochromic, sex-linked D64.0
- − pyridoxine-responsive NEC D64.3
- − secondary (due to)
- − − disease D64.1
- − − drugs and toxins D64.2
- − specified type NEC D64.3
- sideropenic (refractory) D50.9
- simple chronic D53.9
- specified type NEC D64.8
- spherocytic (hereditary) (*see also* Spherocytosis) D58.0
- splenic D64.8
- splenomegalic D64.8
- syphilitic (acquired) (late) A52.7† D63.8∗
- target cell D64.8
- thalassemia D56.9

Anemia—*continued*
- thrombocytopenic (*see also*
  Thrombocytopenia) D69.6
- toxic D61.2
- tropical B76.9† D63.8*
- – macrocytic D52.8
  tuberculous A18.8† D63.8*
- vegan D51.3
- vitamin B₆-responsive D64.3
- von Jaksch's D64.8
- Witts' D50.8

Anencephalus, anencephaly Q00.0
- fetus (suspected), affecting management
  of pregnancy O35.0

Anesthesia, anesthetic (*see also* Effect,
adverse, anesthesia) R20.0
- complication or reaction NEC (*see also*
  Complications, anesthesia) T88.5
- – due to
- – – correct substance properly
  administered T88.5
- – – overdose or wrong substance given
  T41.-
- – – – specified anesthetic – *see* Table of
  drugs and chemicals
- cornea H18.8
- death from
- – correct substance properly administered
  T88.2
- – during delivery O74.8
- – in pregnancy O29.9
- – overdose or wrong substance given
  T41.-
- – – specified anesthetic – *see* Table of
  drugs and chemicals
- – postpartum, puerperal O89.8
- dissociative F44.6
- functional (hysterical) F44.6
- hysterical F44.6
- local skin lesion R20.0
- sexual (psychogenic) F52.1
- shock T88.2
- – correct substance properly administered
  T88.2
- – overdose or wrong substance given
  T41.-
- – – specified anesthetic – *see* Table of
  drugs and chemicals
- skin R20.0

Anetoderma (maculosum) (of) L90.8
- Jadassohn-Pellizzari L90.2
- Schweniger-Buzzi L90.1

Aneurin deficiency E51.9

**Aneurysm (anastomotic) (artery) (cirsoid)
(diffuse) (false) (fusiform) (multiple)
(saccular)** I72.9
- abdominal (aorta) I71.4
- – dissecting (ruptured) I71.0
- – ruptured I71.3
- – syphilitic A52.0† I79.0*
- aorta, aortic (nonsyphilitic) I71.9
- – abdominal I71.4
- – – ruptured I71.3
- – arch I71.2
- – – ruptured I71.1
- – arteriosclerotic NEC I71.9
- – – ruptured I71.8
- – ascending I71.2
- – – ruptured I71.1
- – congenital Q25.4
- – descending I71.9
- – – abdominal I71.4
- – – – ruptured I71.3
- – – ruptured I71.8
- – – thoracic I71.2
- – – – ruptured I71.1
- – dissecting (any part) (ruptured) I71.0
- – ruptured I71.8
- – sinus, congenital Q25.4
- – syphilitic A52.0† I79.0*
- – thoracoabdominal I71.6
- – – ruptured I71.5
- – thorax, thoracic (arch) I71.2
- – – ruptured I71.1
- – transverse I71.2
- – – ruptured I71.1
- – valve (heart) (*see also* Endocarditis,
  aortic) I35.8
- arteriosclerotic I72.9
- cerebral I67.1
- – – ruptured (*see also* Hemorrhage,
  subarachnoid) I60.9
- arteriovenous (congenital) (peripheral)
  Q27.3
- – acquired I77.0
- – brain I67.1
- – – pulmonary I28.0
- – brain Q28.2
- – – ruptured I60.8
- – precerebral vessels (nonruptured)
  Q28.0
- – – ruptured I72.5
- – specified site NEC Q27.3
- – – acquired I77.0
- – traumatic (complication) (early) T14.5
- basal – *see* Aneurysm, brain
- brain I67.1
- – arteriosclerotic I67.1

Aneurysm—*continued*
- brain—*continued*
- − − arteriosclerotic—*continued*
- − − − ruptured (*see also* Hemorrhage,
    subarachnoid) I60.9
- − − arteriovenous (congenital)
    (nonruptured) Q28.2
- − − − acquired I67.1
- − − − − ruptured I60.8
- − − − ruptured I60.8
- − − berry (nonruptured) I67.1
- − − − ruptured (*see also* Hemorrhage,
    subarachnoid) I60.7
- − − congenital Q28.3
- − − − berry (nonruptured) Q28.3
- − − − − ruptured I60.7
- − − − ruptured I60.9
- − − meninges I67.1
- − − − ruptured I60.8
- − − ruptured NEC (*see also* Hemorrhage,
    subarachnoid) I60.9
- − − syphilitic (hemorrhage) A52.0† I68.8∗
- cardiac (false) (*see also* Aneurysm, heart)
    I25.3
- carotid (internal) I72.0
- − − ruptured into brain I60.0
- − − syphilitic A52.0† I79.8∗
- − − − intracranial A52.0† I68.8∗
- cavernous sinus I67.1
- − − arteriovenous (congenital)
    (nonruptured) Q28.3
- − − − ruptured I60.8
- central nervous system, syphilitic A52.0†
    I68.8∗
- cerebral – *see* Aneurysm, brain
- chest – *see* Aneurysm, thorax
- circle of Willis I67.1
- − − congenital Q28.3
- − − − ruptured I60.6
- − − ruptured I60.6
- congenital (peripheral) Q27.8
- − − brain Q28.3
- − − − ruptured (*see also* Hemorrhage,
    subarachnoid) I60.9
- − − coronary Q24.5
- − − pulmonary Q25.7
- − − retina Q14.1
- conjunctiva H11.4
- conus arteriosus (*see also* Aneurysm,
    heart) I25.3
- coronary (arteriosclerotic) (artery) I25.4
- − − arteriovenous, congenital Q24.5
- − − congenital Q24.5
- − − ruptured (*see also* Infarct, myocardium)
    I21.9

Aneurysm—*continued*
- coronary—*continued*
- − − syphilitic A52.0† I52.0∗
- − − vein I25.8
- cylindroid (aorta) I71.9
- − − ruptured I71.8
- − − syphilitic A52.0† I79.0∗
- dissecting (*see also* Dissection, artery)
    I72.9
- − − aorta (any part) (ruptured) I71.0
- − − syphilitic A52.0† I79.0∗
- femoral (artery) (ruptured) I72.4
- heart (wall) (chronic or with a stated
    duration of over 4 weeks) I25.3
- − − acute or with a stated duration of 4
    weeks or less I21.9
- − − valve – *see* Endocarditis
- iliac (common) (artery) (ruptured) I72.3
- infective I72.9
- innominate (nonsyphilitic) I72.8
- − − syphilitic A52.0† I79.8∗
- interauricular septum (*see also* Aneurysm,
    heart) I25.3
- interventricular septum (*see also*
    Aneurysm, heart) I25.3
- intrathoracic (nonsyphilitic) I71.2
- − − ruptured I71.1
- − − syphilitic A52.0† I79.0∗
- jugular vein I86.8
- lower limb I72.4
- mediastinal (nonsyphilitic) I72.8
- − − syphilitic A52.0† I79.8∗
- miliary I67.1
- − − ruptured (*see also* Hemorrhage,
    subarachnoid) I60.7
- mitral (heart) (valve) I34.8
- mural (*see also* Aneurysm, heart) I25.3
- mycotic I72.9
- − − ruptured, brain (*see also* Hemorrhage,
    subarachnoid) I60.9
- myocardium (*see also* Aneurysm, heart)
    I25.3
- peripheral NEC I72.8
- − − congenital Q27.8
- popliteal (artery) (ruptured) I72.4
- precerebralNEC I72.5
- − − acquired (ruptured) I72.5
- − − − carotid (internal) I72.0
- − − − vertebral I72.5
- − − congenital (nonruptured) Q28.1
- pulmonary I28.1
- − − arteriovenous Q25.7
- − − − acquired I28.0
- − − syphilitic A52.0† I79.8∗

Aneurysm—*continued*
- pulmonary—*continued*
- – valve (heart) (*see also* Endocarditis, pulmonary) I37.8
- racemose (peripheral) I72.9
- – congenital Q27.8
- Rasmussen's NEC A16.2
- renal (artery) I72.2
- retina H35.0
- – congenital Q14.1
- – diabetic (*see also* E10-E14 with fourth character .3) E14.3† H36.0*
- spinal (cord) I72.8
- – syphilitic (hemorrhage) A52.0† I79.8*
- splenic I72.8
- subclavian (artery) (ruptured) I72.8
- – syphilitic A52.0† I79.8*
- syphilitic (aorta) A52.0† I79.0*
- – central nervous system A52.0† I68.8*
- – congenital (late) A50.5† I79.0*
- – spine, spinal A52.0† I79.8*
- thoracoabdominal (aorta) I71.6
- – ruptured I71.5
- thorax, thoracic (aorta) (arch) (nonsyphilitic) I71.2
- – dissecting (ruptured) I71.0
- – ruptured I71.1
- – syphilitic A52.0† I79.0*
- traumatic (complication) (early), specified site – *see* Injury, blood vessel
- tricuspid (heart) (valve) I07.8
- upper limb (ruptured) I72.1
- valve, valvular – *see* Endocarditis
- venous (*see also* Varix) I86.8
- – congenital Q27.8
- ventricle (*see also* Aneurysm, heart) I25.3
Angelman syndrome Q93.5
Anger R45.4
Angiectasis, angiectopia I99
Angiitis I77.6
- allergic granulomatous M30.1
- hypersensitivity M31.0
- necrotizing M31.9
- – specified NEC M31.8
Angina (attack) (cardiac) (chest) (heart) (pectoris) (syndrome) (vasomotor) I20.9
- with documented spasm I20.1
- agranulocytic D70
- angiospastic I20.1
- aphthous B08.5
- crescendo I20.0
- cruris I73.9
- de novo effort I20.0
- decubitus I20.0

Angina—*continued*
- diphtheritic, membranous A36.0
- Ludwig's K12.2
- membranous J31.2
- – diphtheritic A36.0
- – Vincent's A69.1
- monocytic (*see also* Mononucleosis, infectious) B27.9
- of effort I20.8
- pre-infarctional I20.0
- Prinzmetal I20.1
- pseudomembranous A69.1
- septic J02.0
- spasm-induced I20.1
- specified NEC I20.8
- unstable I20.0
- variant I20.1
- Vincent's A69.1
- worsening effort I20.0
Angioblastoma (M9161/1) – *see* Neoplasm, connective tissue, uncertain behavior
Angiocholecystitis (*see also* Cholecystitis, acute) K81.0
Angiodysplasia (cecum) (colon) K55.2
Angioedema (allergic) (any site) (with urticaria) T78.3
- hereditary D84.1
Angioendothelioma (M9130/1) – *see also* Neoplasm, uncertain behavior
- benign (M9130/0) D18.0
- bone (M9130/3) – *see* Neoplasm, bone, malignant
- Ewing's (M9260/3) – *see* Neoplasm, bone, malignant
- nervous system (M9130/0) D18.0
Angioendotheliomatosis C85.9
Angiofibroma (M9160/0) – *see also* Neoplasm, benign
- juvenile (M9160/0)
- – specified site – *see* Neoplasm, benign
- – unspecified site D10.6
Angiohemophilia (A) (B) D68.0
Angioid streaks (choroid) (macula) (retina) H35.3
Angiokeratoma (M9141/0) – *see* Neoplasm, skin, benign
- corporis diffusum E75.2
Angioleiomyoma (M8894/0) – *see* Neoplasm, connective tissue, benign
Angiolipoma (M8861/0) (*see also* Lipoma) D17.9
- infiltrating (M8856/0) – *see* Lipoma
Angioma (M9120/0) D18.0
- malignant (M9120/3) – *see* Neoplasm, connective tissue, malignant

Angioma—*continued*
– placenta O43.1
– plexiform (M9131/0) D18.0
– senile I78.1
– serpiginosum L81.7
– spider I78.1
– stellate I78.1
Angiomatosis Q82.8
– encephalotrigeminal Q85.8
– liver K76.4
Angiomyolipoma (M8860/0) – *see* Lipoma
Angiomyoliposarcoma (M8860/3) – *see*
Neoplasm, connective tissue, malignant
Angiomyoma (M8894/0) – *see* Neoplasm,
connective tissue, benign
Angiomyosarcoma (M8894/3) – *see*
Neoplasm, connective tissue, malignant
Angiomyxoma (M8841/1) – *see* Neoplasm,
connective tissue, uncertain behavior
Angioneurosis F45.3
**Angioneurotic edema (allergic) (any site)
(with urticaria)** T78.3
– hereditary D84.1
Angiopathia, angiopathy I99
– cerebral I67.9
– – amyloid E85.4† I68.0∗
– diabetic (peripheral) (*see also* E10-E14
with fourth character .5) E14.5† I79.2∗
– peripheral I73.9
– – diabetic (*see also* E10-E14 with fourth
character .5) E14.5† I79.2∗
– retinae syphilitica A52.0† H36.8∗
Angiosarcoma (M9120/3) – *see also*
Neoplasm, connective tissue, malignant
– liver C22.3
Angiosclerosis – *see* Arteriosclerosis
Angiospasm I73.9
– cerebral G45.9
– peripheral NEC I73.9
– traumatic (foot) (leg) I73.9
– vessel (peripheral) I73.9
Angiostrongyliasis
– due to
– – Angiostrongylus
– – – cantonensis B83.2
– – – costaricensis B81.3
– – Parastrongylus
– – – cantonensis B83.2
– – – costaricensis B81.3
– intestinal B81.3
Anguillulosis (*see also* Strongyloidiasis)
B78.9
Angulation
– cecum (*see also* Obstruction, intestine)
K56.6

Angulation—*continued*
– coccyx (acquired) M43.8
– – congenital NEC Q76.4
– femur (acquired) M21.8
– – congenital Q74.2
– intestine (large) (small) (*see also*
Obstruction, intestine) K56.6
– sacrum (acquired) M43.8
– – congenital NEC Q76.4
– sigmoid (flexure) (*see also* Obstruction,
intestine) K56.6
– spine (*see also* Curvature, spine) M43.8
– tibia (acquired) M21.8
– – congenital Q74.2
– ureter N13.5
– – with infection N13.6
– wrist (acquired) M21.8
– – congenital Q74.0
Angulus infectiosus (lips) K13.0
Anhedonia (sexual) F52.1
Anhidrosis L74.4
Anhydration, anhydremia E86
Anidrosis L74.4
Aniridia (congenital) Q13.1
Anisakiasis (infection) (infestation) B81.0
Anisakis larvae infestation B81.0
Aniseikonia H52.3
Anisocoria (pupil) H57.0
– congenital Q13.2
Anisocytosis R71
Anisometropia (congenital) H52.3
Ankle – *see condition*
Ankyloblepharon (eyelid) (acquired)
H02.5
– filiforme (adnatum) (congenital) Q10.3
– total Q10.3
Ankyloglossia Q38.1
Ankylosis (fibrous) (osseous) (joint)
M24.6
– ankle M24.6
– arthrodesis status Z98.1
– cricoarytenoid (cartilage) (larynx) J38.7
– dental K03.5
– ear ossicles H74.3
– elbow M24.6
– finger M24.6
– hip M24.6
– incudostapedial (infectional) H74.3
– knee M24.6
– lumbosacral M43.2
– multiple sites, except spine M24.6
– postoperative (status) Z98.1
– produced by surgical fusion, status Z98.1
– sacro-iliac M43.2
– shoulder M24.6

Ankylosis—*continued*
- specified site NEC M24.6
- spine M43.2
- surgical M24.6
- tooth, teeth (hard tissues) K03.5
- wrist M24.6

Ankylostoma – *see* Ancylostoma

Ankylostomiasis – *see* Ancylostoma

Ankylurethria (*see also* Stricture, urethra)
N35.9

Annular – *see also* condition
- organ or site, congenital NEC – *see*
Distortion
- pancreas (congenital) Q45.1

Anodontia (complete) (partial) (vera)
K00.0
- acquired K08.1

Anomaly, anomalous (congenital)
(unspecified type) Q89.9
- abdominal wall NEC Q79.5
- acoustic nerve Q07.8
- adrenal (gland) Q89.1
- Alder's D72.0
- alimentary tract Q45.9
- – upper Q40.9
- ankle (joint) Q74.2
- anus Q43.9
- aorta (arch) NEC Q25.4
- – coarctation (preductal) (postductal)
Q25.1
- aortic cusp or valve NEC Q23.9
- appendix Q43.8
- apple peel syndrome Q41.1
- aqueduct of Sylvius Q03.0
- – with spina bifida (*see also* Spina bifida,
with hydrocephalus) Q05.4
- arm Q74.0
- artery (peripheral) Q27.9
- – basilar NEC Q28.1
- – cerebral Q28.3
- – coronary Q24.5
- – eye Q15.8
- – great Q25.9
- – – specified NEC Q25.8
- – peripheral Q27.9
- – – specified NEC Q27.8
- – pulmonary NEC Q25.7
- – retina Q14.1
- – vertebral NEC Q28.1
- aryteno-epiglottic folds Q31.8
- atrial
- – bands or folds Q20.8
- – septa Q21.1
- atrioventricular excitation I45.6
- auditory canal Q17.8

Anomaly, anomalous—*continued*
- auricle
- – ear Q17.8
- – – causing impairment of hearing
Q16.9
- – heart Q20.8
- Axenfeld's Q15.0
- band
- – atrial Q20.8
- – heart Q24.8
- – ventricular Q24.8
- Bartholin's duct Q38.4
- biliary duct or passage Q44.5
- bladder (neck) Q64.7
- bone NEC Q79.9
- – arm Q74.0
- – face Q75.9
- – leg Q74.2
- – pelvic girdle Q74.2
- – shoulder girdle Q74.0
- – skull Q75.9
- – – with
- – – – anencephaly Q00.0
- – – – encephalocele (*see also*
Encephalocele) Q01.9
- – – – hydrocephalus Q03.9
- – – – – with spina bifida (*see also* Spina
bifida, with hydrocephalus)
Q05.4
- – – – microcephaly Q02
- brain (multiple) Q04.9
- – vessel Q28.3
- breast Q83.9
- broad ligament Q50.6
- bronchus Q32.4
- bursa Q79.9
- canal of Nuck Q52.4
- canthus Q10.3
- capillary Q27.9
- cardiac Q24.9
- – chambers Q20.9
- – – specified NEC Q20.8
- – septal closure Q21.9
- – – specified NEC Q21.8
- – valve NEC Q24.8
- – – pulmonary Q22.3
- cardiovascular system Q28.8
- carpus Q74.0
- caruncle, lacrimal Q10.6
- cauda equina Q06.3
- cecum Q43.9
- cerebral Q04.9
- – vessels Q28.3
- cervix Q51.9
- – in pregnancy or childbirth O34.4

Anomaly, anomalous—*continued*
- cervix—*continued*
- − − in pregnancy or childbirth—*continued*
- − − − affecting fetus or newborn P03.8
- − − − causing obstructed labor O65.5
- − − − − affecting fetus or newborn P03.1
- Chediak-Higashi(-Steinbrinck) E70.3
- cheek Q18.9
- chest wall Q67.8
- − − bones Q76.9
- chin Q18.9
- chordae tendineae Q24.8
- choroid Q14.3
- − plexus Q07.8
- chromosomes, chromosomal Q99.9
- − − D(1) – *see* condition, chromosome 13
- − − E(3) – *see* condition, chromosome 18
- − − G – *see* condition, chromosome 21
- − − sex
- − − − female phenotype Q97.9
- − − − − specified NEC Q97.8
- − − − gonadal dysgenesis (pure) Q99.1
- − − − Klinefelter's Q98.4
- − − − male phenotype Q98.9
- − − − − specified NEC Q98.8
- − − − Turner's Q96.9
- − − − − specified NEC Q96.8
- − − specified NEC Q99.8
- cilia Q10.3
- circulatory system NEC Q28.9
- clavicle Q74.0
- clitoris Q52.6
- coccyx Q76.4
- colon Q43.9
- common duct Q44.5
- concha (ear) Q17.3
- connection
- − portal vein Q26.5
- − pulmonary venous Q26.4
- − − partial Q26.3
- − − total Q26.2
- − renal artery with kidney Q27.2
- cornea (shape) Q13.4
- coronary artery or vein Q24.5
- cranium – *see* Anomaly, skull
- cricoid cartilage Q31.8
- cystic duct Q44.5
- dental arch relationship K07.2
- dentofacial K07.9
- − functional K07.5
- − specified NEC K07.8
- dermatoglyphic Q82.8
- diaphragm (apertures) NEC Q79.1
- digestive organ(s) or tract NEC Q45.9
- − lower Q43.9

Anomaly, anomalous—*continued*
- digestive organ(s) or tract NEC— *continued*
- − upper Q40.9
- ductus
- − arteriosus Q25.0
- − botalli Q25.0
- duodenum Q43.9
- dura (brain) Q04.9
- − − spinal cord Q06.9
- ear Q17.9
- − − causing impairment of hearing Q16.9
- − − inner Q16.5
- − − middle (causing impairment of hearing) Q16.4
- − − ossicles Q16.3
- Ebstein's Q22.5
- ectodermal Q82.9
- ejaculatory duct Q55.4
- elbow Q74.0
- endocrine gland NEC Q89.2
- epididymis Q55.4
- epiglottis Q31.8
- esophagus Q39.9
- eustachian tube Q16.4
- eye Q15.9
- − − anterior segment Q13.9
- − − posterior segment Q14.9
- − − specified NEC Q15.8
- eyelid Q10.3
- face Q18.9
- − − bone(s) Q75.9
- fallopian tube Q50.6
- fascia Q79.9
- femur NEC Q74.2
- fibula NEC Q74.2
- finger Q74.0
- fixation, intestine Q43.3
- flexion (joint) NEC Q74.9
- − − hip or thigh Q65.8
- foot NEC Q74.2
- − − varus (congenital) Q66.3
- forearm Q74.0
- forehead (*see also* Anomaly, skull) Q75.8
- fovea centralis Q14.1
- frontal bone (*see also* Anomaly, skull) Q75.9
- gallbladder (position) (shape) (size) Q44.1
- Gartner's duct Q50.6
- gastrointestinal tract NEC Q45.9
- genitalia, genital organ(s) or system
- − − female Q52.9
- − − − external Q52.7
- − − − internal NEC Q52.9

Anomaly, anomalous—*continued*
- genitalia, genital organ(s) or system—*continued*
- - male Q55.9
- - - specified NEC Q55.8
- genitourinary NEC
- - female Q52.9
- - male Q55.9
- glottis Q31.8
- granulation or granulocyte, genetic D72.0
- gum Q38.6
- hair Q84.2
- hand Q74.0
- head (*see also* Anomaly, skull) Q75.9
- heart Q24.9
- - auricle Q20.8
- - bands or folds Q24.8
- - septum Q21.9
- - - auricular Q21.1
- - - specified NEC Q21.8
- - - ventricular Q21.0
- - valve NEC Q24.8
- - - pulmonary Q22.3
- - ventricle Q20.8
- heel NEC Q74.2
- Hegglin's D72.0
- hepatic duct Q44.5
- hip NEC Q74.2
- humerus Q74.0
- hydatid of Morgagni
- - female Q50.5
- - male (epididymal) Q55.4
- - - testicular Q55.2
- hymen Q52.4
- hypophyseal Q89.2
- ileocecal (coil) (valve) Q43.9
- ileum Q43.9
- ilium NEC Q74.2
- integument Q84.9
- - specified NEC Q84.8
- intervertebral cartilage or disk Q76.4
- intestine (large) (small) Q43.9
- - with anomalous adhesions, fixation or malrotation Q43.3
- iris Q13.2
- ischium NEC Q74.2
- jaw K07.9
- - size (major) K07.0
- - specified NEC K07.8
- jaw-cranial base relationship K07.1
- jejunum Q43.8
- joint NEC Q74.9
- - specified NEC Q74.8
- kidney(s) (calyx) (pelvis) Q63.9
- - artery Q27.2

Anomaly, anomalous—*continued*
- kidney(s)—*continued*
- - specified NEC Q63.8
- knee Q74.1
- labium (majus) (minus) Q52.7
- labyrinth, membranous Q16.5
- lacrimal apparatus or duct Q10.6
- larynx, laryngeal (muscle) Q31.9
- - web(bed) Q31.0
- lens Q12.9
- leukocytes, genetic D72.0
- lid (fold) Q10.3
- ligament Q79.9
- - broad Q50.6
- - round Q52.8
- limb Q74.9
- - lower NEC Q74.2
- - - reduction deformity Q72.8
- - upper Q74.0
- lip Q38.0
- liver Q44.7
- - duct Q44.5
- lower limb NEC Q74.2
- lumbosacral (joint) (region) Q76.4
- lung (fissure) (lobe) Q33.9
- May-Hegglin D72.0
- meatus urinarius NEC Q64.7
- meningeal bands or folds Q07.9
- - constriction of Q07.8
- - spinal Q06.9
- meninges Q07.9
- - cerebral Q04.8
- - spinal Q06.9
- mesentery Q45.9
- metacarpus Q74.0
- metatarsus NEC Q74.2
- middle ear Q16.4
- mitral (leaflets) (valve) Q23.9
- - specified NEC Q23.8
- mouth Q38.6
- multiple NEC Q89.7
- muscle Q79.9
- - eyelid Q10.3
- musculoskeletal system, except limbs Q79.9
- myocardium Q24.8
- nail Q84.6
- narrowness, eyelid Q10.3
- nasal sinus (wall) Q30.9
- neck (any part) Q18.9
- nerve Q07.9
- - acoustic Q07.8
- - optic Q07.8
- nervous system (central) NEC Q07.9
- nipple Q83.9

Anomaly, anomalous—*continued*
- nose, nasal (bones) (cartilage) (septum) (sinus) Q30.9
- − − specified NEC Q30.8
- ocular muscle Q15.8
- oesophagus Q39.9
- opening, pulmonary veins Q26.4
- optic
- − − disk Q14.2
- − − nerve Q07.8
- opticociliary vessels Q13.2
- orbit (eye) Q10.7
- organ NEC Q89.9
- − − of Corti Q16.5
- origin
- − artery
- − − − innominate Q25.8
- − − − pulmonary Q25.7
- − − − renal Q27.2
- − − − subclavian Q25.8
- osseous meatus (ear) Q16.1
- ovary NEC Q50.3
- oviduct Q50.6
- palate (hard) (soft) NEC Q38.5
- pancreas or pancreatic duct Q45.3
- papillary muscles Q24.8
- parathyroid gland Q89.2
- paraurethral ducts Q64.7
- parotid (gland) Q38.4
- patella Q74.1
- Pelger-Huet D72.0
- pelvic girdle NEC Q74.2
- pelvis (bony) NEC Q74.2
- penis (glans) Q55.6
- pericardium Q24.8
- peripheral vascular system Q27.9
- Peter's Q13.4
- pharynx Q38.8
- pigmentation L81.9
- pituitary (gland) Q89.2
- pleural (folds) Q34.0
- portal vein Q26.5
- − − connection Q26.5
- position, tooth, teeth K07.3
- precerebral vessel Q28.1
- prepuce Q55.6
- prostate Q55.4
- pulmonary Q33.9
- − − artery NEC Q25.7
- − − valve Q22.3
- − − venous connection Q26.4
- − − − partial Q26.3
- − − − total Q26.2
- pupil Q13.2
- − − function H57.0

Anomaly, anomalous—*continued*
- pylorus Q40.3
- radius Q74.0
- rectum Q43.9
- reduction (extremity) (limb)
- − − femur (longitudinal) Q72.4
- − − fibula (longitudinal) Q72.6
- − − lower limb Q72.9
- − − − specified NEC Q72.8
- − − radius (longitudinal) Q71.4
- − − tibia (longitudinal) Q72.5
- − − ulna (longitudinal) Q71.5
- − − upper limb Q71.9
- − − − specified NEC Q71.8
- refraction H52.7
- renal Q63.9
- − − artery Q27.2
- − − pelvis Q63.9
- − − − specified NEC Q63.8
- respiratory system Q34.9
- − − specified NEC Q34.8
- retina Q14.1
- rib Q76.6
- − − cervical Q76.5
- Rieger's Q13.8
- rotation − *see also* Malrotation Q43.3
- − − hip or thigh Q65.8
- round ligament Q52.8
- sacroiliac (joint) NEC Q74.2
- sacrum NEC Q76.4
- salivary duct or gland Q38.4
- scapula Q74.0
- scrotum Q55.2
- sebaceous gland Q82.9
- seminal vesicles Q55.4
- sense organs NEC Q07.8
- sex chromosomes NEC − *see* Anomaly, chromosomes, sex
- shoulder (girdle) (joint) Q74.0
- sigmoid (flexure) Q43.9
- simian crease Q82.8
- sinus of Valsalva Q25.4
- skeleton generalized NEC Q78.9
- skin (appendage) Q82.9
- skull Q75.9
- − − with
- − − − anencephaly Q00.0
- − − − encephalocele (*see also* Encephalocele) Q01.9
- − − − hydrocephalus Q03.9
- − − − − with spina bifida (*see also* Spina bifida, with hydrocephalus) Q05.4
- − − − microcephaly Q02
- specified organ or site NEC Q89.8
- spermatic cord Q55.4

Anomaly, anomalous—*continued*
- spine, spinal NEC Q76.4
- – column NEC Q76.4
- – cord Q06.9
- – nerve root Q07.8
- spleen Q89.0
- stenonian duct Q38.4
- sternum NEC Q76.7
- stomach Q40.3
- submaxillary gland Q38.4
- tarsus NEC Q74.2
- tendon Q79.9
- testis Q55.2
- thigh NEC Q74.2
- thorax (wall) Q67.8
- – bony Q76.9
- throat Q38.8
- thumb Q74.0
- thymus gland Q89.2
- thyroid (gland) Q89.2
- – cartilage Q31.8
- tibia NEC Q74.2
- toe Q74.2
- tongue Q38.3
- tooth, teeth NEC K00.9
- – eruption K00.6
- – position K07.3
- – spacing K07.3
- trachea (cartilage) Q32.1
- trichromata, trichromatopsia H53.5
- tricuspid (leaflet) (valve) Q22.9
- – atresia or stenosis Q22.4
- – Ebstein's Q22.5
- Uhl's (hypoplasia of myocardium, right ventricle) Q24.8
- ulna Q74.0
- union
- – cricoid cartilage and thyroid cartilage Q31.8
- – thyroid cartilage and hyoid bone Q31.8
- – trachea with larynx Q31.8
- upper limb Q74.0
- urachus Q64.4
- ureter Q62.8
- – obstructive NEC Q62.3
- urethra NEC Q64.7
- – obstructive Q64.3
- urinary tract Q64.9
- uterus Q51.9
- – with only one functioning horn Q51.8
- – in pregnancy or childbirth NEC O34.0
- – – affecting fetus or newborn P03.8
- – – causing obstructed labor O65.5
- – – – affecting fetus or newborn P03.1
- uvula Q38.5

Anomaly, anomalous—*continued*
- vagina Q52.4
- valleculae Q31.8
- valve (heart) NEC Q24.8
- – coronary sinus Q24.5
- – inferior vena cava Q24.8
- – pulmonary Q22.3
- – sinus coronario Q24.5
- – venae cavae inferioris Q24.8
- vas deferens Q55.4
- vascular NEC Q27.9
- – brain Q28.3
- – ring Q25.4
- vein(s) (peripheral) Q27.9
- – brain Q28.3
- – cerebral Q28.3
- – coronary Q24.5
- – great Q26.9
- – – specified NEC Q26.8
- vena cava (inferior) (superior) Q26.9
- venous return Q26.8
- ventricular
- – bands or folds Q24.8
- – septa Q21.0
- vertebra Q76.4
- vesicourethral orifice NEC Q64.7
- vessel(s) Q27.9
- – optic papilla Q14.2
- – precerebral Q28.1
- vitreous body or humor Q14.0
- vulva Q52.7
- wrist (joint) Q74.0

Anomia R48.8
Anonychia (congenital) Q84.3
- acquired L60.8
Anophthalmos, anophthalmus (congenital) (globe) Q11.1
- acquired Z90.0
Anopsia, quadrant H53.4
Anorchia, anorchism, anorchidism Q55.0
Anorexia R63.0
- hysterical F44.8
- nervosa F50.0
- – atypical F50.1
- – binge-eating type F50.2
Anorgasmy (psychogenic) F52.3
Anosmia (*see also* Disturbance, sensation) R43.0
- hysterical F44.6
Anosognosia R41.8
Anovulatory cycle N97.0
Anoxemia R09.0
- newborn (*see also* Asphyxia, newborn) P21.9

Anoxia R09.0
– altitude T70.2
– cerebral G93.1
– – complicating
– – – anesthesia (general) (local) or other
   sedation
– – – – in labor and delivery O74.3
– – – – in pregnancy O29.2
– – – – postpartum, puerperal O89.2
– – – delivery (cesarean) (instrumental)
   O75.4
– – during or resulting from a procedure
   G97.8
– – newborn (*see also* Asphyxia, newborn)
   P21.9
– due to drowning T75.1
– heart – *see* Insufficiency, coronary
– high altitude T70.2
– intrauterine – *see* Hypoxia, intrauterine
– myocardial – *see* Insufficiency, coronary
– newborn (*see also* Asphyxia, newborn)
   P21.9
– pathological R09.0
Anteflexion – *see* Anteversion
Antenatal
– care, normal pregnancy Z34.9
– – first Z34.0
– – specified NEC Z34.8
– screening (for) Z36.9
– – abnormal findings – *see* Abnormal,
   finding, antenatal screening, mother
– – based on amniocentesis Z36.2
– – chromosomal anomalies Z36.0
– – fetal growth retardation using
   ultrasound and other physical methods
   Z36.4
– – hemoglobinopathy Z36.8
– – isoimmunization Z36.5
– – malformations using ultrasound and
   other physical methods Z36.3
– – raised alphafetoprotein levels in
   amniotic fluid Z36.1
– – specified NEC Z36.8
Antepartum – *see* condition
Anterior – *see* condition
Anteversion
– cervix (*see also* Anteversion, uterus)
   N85.4
– femur (neck), congenital Q65.8
– uterus, uterine (cervix) (postinfectional)
   (postpartal, old) N85.4
– – congenital Q51.8
– – in pregnancy or childbirth O34.5
– – – affecting fetus or newborn P03.8
– – – causing obstructed labor O65.5

Anteversion—*continued*
– uterus, uterine—*continued*
– – in pregnancy or childbirth—*continued*
– – – causing obstructed labor—*continued*
– – – – affecting fetus or newborn P03.1
Anthracosilicosis J60
Anthracosis (lung) J60
Anthrax A22.9
– with pneumonia A22.1† J17.0*
– cerebral A22.8† G01*
– cutaneous A22.0
– gastrointestinal A22.2† K93.8*
– inhalation A22.1† J17.0*
– meningitis A22.8† G01*
– pulmonary A22.1† J17.0*
– respiratory A22.1† J17.0*
– sepsis A22.7
– specified manifestation NEC A22.8
Anthropoid pelvis Q74.2
– with disproportion (fetopelvic) O33.0
– – affecting fetus or newborn P03.1
Anthropophobia F40.1
**Antibodies, maternal (blood
   group)** (*see also* Incompatibility) O36.1
– anti-D O36.0
– – fetus or newborn P55.0
Anticardiolipin syndrome D68.6
Antidiuretic hormone syndrome E22.2
Antimonial cholera T56.8
Antiphospholipid syndrome D68.6
Antisocial personality F60.2
Antithrombinemia (*see also* Circulating
   anticoagulants) D68.5
Antithromboplastinemia (*see also*
   Circulating anticoagulants) D68.3
Antithromboplastinogenemia (*see also*
   Circulating anticoagulants) D68.3
Antitoxin complication or reaction – *see*
   Complications, vaccination
Antritis (chronic) J32.0
– acute J01.0
Antrum, antral – *see* condition
Anuria R34
– calculous (impacted) (recurrent) (*see also*
   Calculus, urinary) N20.9
– following
– – abortion (subsequent episode) O08.4
– – – current episode – *see* Abortion
– – ectopic or molar pregnancy O08.4
– newborn P96.0
– postprocedural N99.0
– sulfonamide
– – correct substance properly administered
   R34

Anuria—*continued*
- sulfonamide—*continued*
- - overdose or wrong substance given or taken T37.0
- traumatic (following crushing) T79.5
Anus, anal – *see condition*
Anusitis K62.8
Anxiety F41.9
- depression F41.2
- episodic paroxysmal F41.0
- generalized F41.1
- hysteria F41.8
- neurosis F41.1
- reaction F41.1
- separation, abnormal (of childhood) F93.0
- specified NEC F41.8
- state F41.1
Aorta, aortic – *see condition*
Aortitis (nonsyphilitic) (calcific) I77.6
- arteriosclerotic I70.0
- Doehle-Heller A52.0† I79.1*
- luetic A52.0† I79.1*
- rheumatic (*see also* Endocarditis, acute, rheumatic) I01.1
- specific (syphilitic) A52.0† I79.1*
- syphilitic A52.0† I79.1*
- - congenital A50.5† I79.1*
Apathy R45.3
Apepsia K31.8
- psychogenic F45.3
Apert's syndrome Q87.0
Apgar (score)
- low NEC, with asphyxia P21.9
- 0-3 at 1 minute, with asphyxia P21.0
- 4-7 at 1 minute, with asphyxia P21.1
Aphagia R63.0
- psychogenic F50.1
Aphakia (acquired) H27.0
- congenital Q12.3
Aphasia (amnestic) (global) (nominal) (semantic) (syntactic) R47.0
- acquired, with epilepsy (Landau-Kleffner syndrome) F80.3
- auditory (developmental) F80.2
- developmental (receptive type) F80.2
- - expressive type F80.1
- - Wernicke's F80.2
- progressive isolated G31.0
- sensory F80.2
- syphilis, tertiary A52.1† G94.8*
- uremic N19
- Wernicke's (developmental) F80.2
Aphemia R47.0

Aphonia R49.1
- hysterical F44.4
- organic R49.1
- psychogenic F44.4
Aphthae, aphthous – *see also condition*
- Bednar's K12.0
- epizootic B08.8
- fever B08.8
- oral (recurrent) K12.0
- stomatitis (major) (minor) K12.0
- thrush B37.0
- ulcer (oral) (recurrent) K12.0
- - genital organ(s) NEC
- - - female N76.6
- - - male N50.8
- - larynx J38.7
Apical – *see condition*
Aplasia – *see also* Agenesis
- abdominal muscle syndrome Q79.4
- alveolar process (acquired) K08.8
- - congenital Q38.6
- aorta (congenital) Q25.4
- axialis extracorticalis (congenita) E75.2
- bone marrow (myeloid) D61.9
- brain Q00.0
- - part of Q04.3
- bronchus Q32.4
- cementum K00.4
- cerebellum Q04.3
- cervix (congenital) Q51.5
- corpus callosum Q04.0
- cutis congenita Q84.8
- extracortical axial E75.2
- eye Q11.1
- fovea centralis (congenital) Q14.1
- gallbladder, congenital Q44.0
- labyrinth, membranous Q16.5
- limb (congenital) Q73.0
- - lower Q72.0
- - upper Q71.0
- lung, congenital (bilateral) (unilateral) Q33.3
- pancreas Q45.0
- parathyroid-thymic D82.1
- Pelizaeus-Merzbacher E75.2
- penis Q55.5
- prostate Q55.4
- red cell (pure) (with thymoma) D60.9
- - chronic D60.0
- - congenital D61.0
- - of infants D61.0
- - primary D61.0
- - specified type NEC D60.8
- - transient D60.1
- round ligament Q52.8

Aplasia—*continued*
– skin Q84.8
– spermatic cord Q55.4
– testicle Q55.0
– thymic, with immunodeficiency D82.1
– thyroid (congenital) (with myxedema) E03.1
– uterus Q51.0
– ventral horn cell Q06.1
Apnea, apneic (spells) R06.8
– newborn NEC P28.4
– – sleep (primary) P28.3
– sleep (central) (obstructive) G47.3
Apocrine metaplasia (breast) N60.8
Apophysitis (bone) (*see also* Osteochondrosis) M93.9
– calcaneus M92.8
– juvenile M92.9
Apoplectiform convulsions (cerebral ischemia) I67.8
Apoplexia, apoplexy, apoplectic I64
– attack I64
– basilar I64
– brain I64
– bulbar I64
– capillary I64
– cerebral I64
– chorea I64
– congestive I64
– embolic I63.4
– fit I64
– heart (auricle) (ventricle) (*see also* Infarct, myocardium) I21.9
– heat T67.0
– hemorrhagic (stroke) (*see also* Hemorrhage, intracerebral) I61.9
– meninges, hemorrhagic (*see also* Hemorrhage, subarachnoid) I60.9
– progressive I64
– seizure I64
– stroke I64
– thrombotic I63.3
– uremic N18.5† I68.8*
Appearance
– bizarre R46.1
– specified NEC R46.8
– very low level of personal hygiene R46.0
Appendage
– epididymal (organ of Morgagni) Q55.4
– intestine (epiploic) Q43.8
– preauricular Q17.0
– testicular (organ of Morgagni) Q55.2
Appendicitis K37
– with
– – peritoneal abscess K35.3

Appendicitis—*continued*
– with—*continued*
– – peritonitis, generalized K35.2
– – – with mention of perforation or rupture K35.2
– – peritonitis, localized K35.3
– – – with mention of perforation or rupture K35.3
– acute (catarrhal) (fulminating) (gangrenous) (obstructive) (retrocecal) (suppurative) K35.8
– – with
– – – peritoneal abscess K35.3
– – – peritonitis, generalized K35.2
– – – – with mention of perforation or rupture K35.2
– – – peritonitis, localized K35.3
– – – – with mention of perforation or rupture K35.3
– amebic A06.8
– chronic (recurrent) K36
– exacerbation – *see* Appendicitis, acute
– gangrenous – *see* Appendicitis, acute
– healed (obliterative) K36
– interval K36
– obstructive K36
– pneumococcal K37
– recurrent K36
– retrocecal K37
– subacute (adhesive) K36
– suppurative – *see* Appendicitis, acute
– tuberculous A18.3† K93.0*
Appendix, appendicular – *see also* condition
– epididymis Q55.4
– Morgagni
– – female Q50.5
– – male (epididymal) Q55.4
– – – testicular Q55.2
– testis Q55.2
Appetite
– depraved F50.8
– – in childhood F98.3
– excessive R63.2
– lack or loss (*see also* Anorexia) R63.0
– – nonorganic origin F50.8
– – psychogenic F50.8
– perverted (hysterical) F50.8
Apple peel syndrome Q41.1
Apprehension state F41.1
Apprehensiveness, abnormal F41.9
Apraxia (classic) (ideational) (ideokinetic) (ideomotor) (motor) (verbal) R48.2
– oculomotor, congenital H51.8
Aptyalism K11.7

Apudoma (M8248/1) – *see* Neoplasm, uncertain behavior
Arachnidism T63.3
Arachnitis – *see* Meningitis
Arachnodactyly Q87.4
Arachnoiditis (acute) (adhesive) (basal) (cerebrospinal) (*see also* Mcningitis) G03.9
– meningococcal (chronic) A39.0† G01*
– syphilitic (late) (tertiary) A52.1† G01*
– tuberculous A17.0† G01*
Arachnophobia F40.2
Araneism T63.3
Arboencephalitis, Australian A83.4
Arborization block (heart) I45.5
ARC (AIDS-related complex) (*see also* Human, immunodeficiency virus (HIV) disease) B24
– complicating pregnancy, childbirth or the puerperium O98.7
Arches – *see condition*
Arcuatus uterus Q51.8
Arcus senilis (cornea) H18.4
Arc-welder's lung J63.4
Areola – *see condition*
Argentaffinoma (M8241/1) – *see also* Neoplasm, uncertain behavior
– malignant (M8241/3) – *see* Neoplasm, malignant
Argininemia E72.2
Argyll Robertson phenomenon, pupil or syndrome (syphilitic) A52.1† H58.0*
– atypical H57.0
– nonsyphilitic H57.0
Argyria, argyriasis, argyrosis NEC T56.8
– conjunctival H11.1
– from drug or medicament
– – correct substance properly administered L81.8
– – overdose or wrong substance given or taken T37.8
Arhinencephaly Q04.1
Ariboflavinosis E53.0
Arm – *see condition*
Arnold-Chiari obstruction or syndrome Q07.0
Aromatic amino-acid metabolism disorder E70.9
– specified NEC E70.8
Arrest, arrested
– active phase of labor O62.1
– – affecting fetus or newborn P03.6
– any plane in pelvis
– – complicating delivery O66.9
– cardiac I46.9

Arrest, arrested—*continued*
– cardiac—*continued*
– – with successful resuscitation I46.0
– – complicating
– – – anesthesia (general) (local) or other sedation
– – – – correct substance properly administered I46.9
– – – – in labor and delivery O74.2
– – – – in pregnancy O29.1
– – – – overdose or wrong substance given T41.-
– – – – – specified anesthetic – *see* Table of drugs and chemicals
– – – – postpartum, puerperal O89.1
– – – delivery (cesarean) (instrumental) O75.4
– – – surgery T81.8
– – newborn P29.1
– – postoperative I97.8
– – – long-term effect of cardiac surgery I97.1
– cardiorespiratory (*see also* Arrest, cardiac) I46.9
– circulatory (*see also* Arrest, cardiac) I46.9
– deep transverse O64.0
– – affecting fetus or newborn P03.1
– development or growth
– – bone M89.2
– – child R62.8
– – fetus P05.9
– – – affecting management of pregnancy O36.5
– – tracheal rings Q32.1
– epiphyseal M89.1
– heart – *see* Arrest, cardiac
– legal, anxiety concerning Z65.3
– respiratory R09.2
– – newborn P28.5
– sinus I45.5
– spermatogenesis (complete) (incomplete) N46
– transverse (deep) O64.0
Arrhenoblastoma (M8630/1)
– benign (M8630/0)
– – specified site – *see* Neoplasm, benign
– – unspecified site
– – – female D27
– – – male D29.2
– malignant (M8630/3)
– – specified site – *see* Neoplasm, malignant
– – unspecified site
– – – female C56

Arrhenoblastoma—*continued*
- malignant—*continued*
- – unspecified site—*continued*
- – – male C62.9
- specified site – *see* Neoplasm, uncertain behavior
- unspecified site
- – female D39.1
- – male D40.1

Arrhythmia (cardiac) I49.9
- extrasystolic I49.4
- newborn P29.1
- psychogenic F45.3
- specified NEC I49.8
- ventricular re-entry I47.0

Arsenical pigmentation L81.8
- from drug or medicament – *see* Table of drugs and chemicals

Arterial – *see condition*

Arteriofibrosis – *see* Arteriosclerosis

Arteriolar sclerosis – *see* Arteriosclerosis

Arteriolith – *see* Arteriosclerosis

Arteriolitis I77.6
- renal – *see* Hypertension, kidney

Arteriolosclerosis – *see* Arteriosclerosis

Arterionephrosclerosis (*see also* Hypertension, kidney) I12.9

Arteriopathy I77.9

Arteriosclerosis, arteriosclerotic (diffuse) (disease) (general) (obliterans) (senile) (with calcification) I70.9
- aorta I70.0
- arteries of extremities I70.2
- brain I67.2
- cardiac I25.1
- cardiopathy I25.1
- cardiorenal (*see also* Hypertension, cardiorenal) I13.9
- cardiovascular I25.0
- carotid artery I65.2
- central nervous system I67.2
- cerebral I67.2
- cerebrovascular I67.2
- coronary (artery) I25.1
- extremities I70.2
- heart (disease) I25.1
- kidney (*see also* Hypertension, kidney) I12.9
- medial I70.2
- mesenteric (chronic) K55.1
- Mönckeberg's I70.2
- peripheral (of extremities) I70.2
- pulmonary I27.0
- renal (arterioles) (*see also* Hypertension, kidney) I12.9

Arteriosclerosis, arteriosclerotic—*continued*
- renal—*continued*
- – artery I70.1
- retina (vascular) I70.8
- specified artery NEC I70.8
- spinal (cord) G95.1
- vertebral (artery) I67.2

Arteriospasm I73.9

Arteriovenous – *see condition*

Arteritis I77.6
- allergic M31.0
- aorta (nonsyphilitic) I77.6
- – syphilitic A52.0† I79.1∗
- aortic arch M31.4
- brachiocephalic M31.4
- brain I67.7
- – syphilitic A52.0† I68.1∗
- cerebral I67.7
- – in systemic lupus erythematosus M32.1† I68.2∗
- – listerial A32.8† I68.1∗
- – syphilitic A52.0† I68.1∗
- – tuberculous A18.8† I68.1∗
- coronary (artery) I25.8
- – rheumatic I01.8
- – – chronic I09.8
- – syphilitic A52.0† I52.0∗
- cranial (left) (right), giant cell M31.6
- deformans – *see* Arteriosclerosis
- giant cell NEC M31.6
- – with polymyalgia rheumatica M31.5
- necrosing or necrotizing M31.9
- – specified NEC M31.8
- nodosa M30.0
- obliterans – *see* Arteriosclerosis
- rheumatic – *see* Fever, rheumatic
- senile – *see* Arteriosclerosis
- suppurative I77.2
- syphilitic (general) A52.0† I79.8∗
- – brain A52.0† I68.1∗
- – coronary A52.0† I52.0∗
- – spinal A52.0† I79.8∗
- temporal, giant cell M31.6
- young female aortic arch syndrome M31.4

Artery, arterial – *see also condition* –abscess I77.8
- single umbilical Q27.0

Arthralgia (allergic) M25.5
- psychogenic F45.4

Arthritis, arthritic (acute) (chronic) (subacute) M13.9
- allergic M13.8
- ankylosing (crippling) (spine) M45
- – sites other than spine M13.8

Arthritis, arthritic—*continued*
- atrophic M19.9
- – spine M45
- back (*see also* Arthritis, spine) M46.9
- blennorrhagic (gonococcal) A54.4†
  M01.3*
- Charcot's (tabetic) A52.1† M14.6*
- – diabetic (*see also* E10-E14 with fourth
  character .6) E14.6† M14.6*
- – nonsyphilitic NEC G98† M14.6*
- – syringomyelic G95.0† M49.4*
- chylous (filarial) B74.9† M01.8*
- climacteric (any site) NEC M13.8
- crystal(-induced) M11.9
- deformans M19.9
- epidemic erythema A25.1
- febrile – *see* Fever, rheumatic
- gonococcal A54.4† M01.3*
- gouty (acute) M10.0
- in (due to)
- – acromegaly E22.0† M14.5*
- – amyloidosis E85.4† M14.4*
- – bacterial disease A49.9† M01.3*
- – – specified NEC A48.8† M01.3*
- – Behçet's disease M35.2
- – caisson disease T70.3† M14.8*
- – coliform bacilli (Escherichia coli)
  M00.8
- – colitis, ulcerative K51.-† M07.5*
- – Crohn's disease K50.-† M07.4*
- – crystals M11.9
- – – dicalcium phosphate M11.8
- – – hydroxyapatite M11.0
- – – pyrophosphate M11.8
- – – specified NEC M11.8
- – dermatoarthritis, lipoid E78.8† M14.3*
- – dracontiasis (dracunculiasis) B72†
  M01.8*
- – endocrine disorder NEC E34.9†
  M14.5*
- – enteritis NEC A09.9† M03.-*
- – – infectious NEC A09.0† M03.-*
- – – regional K50.-† M07.4*
- – – specified organism NEC A08.5†
  M01.8*
- – erythema
- – – multiforme L51.-† M14.8*
- – – nodosum L52† M14.8*
- – gastrointestinal condition NEC K63.9†
  M03.6*
- – gout M10.0
- – Haemophilus influenzae M00.8
- – helminthiasis NEC B83.9† M01.8*
- – hematological disorder NEC D75.9†
  M36.3*

Arthritis, arthritic—*continued*
- in—*continued*
- – hemochromatosis E83.1† M14.5*
- – hemoglobinopathy NEC D58.2†
  M36.3*
- – hemophilia NEC D66† M36.2*
- – Henoch(-Schönlein) purpura D69.0†
  M36.4*
- – hyperparathyroidism NEC E21.3†
  M14.1*
- – hypersensitivity reaction NEC T78.4†
  M36.4*
- – hypogammaglobulinemia D80.1†
  M14.8*
- – hypothyroidism NEC E03.9† M14.5*
- – infection M00.9
- – – spine M46.5
- – infectious disease NEC B99† M01.8*
- – leprosy A30.-† M01.3*
- – leukemia NEC C95.9† M36.1*
- – lipoid dermatoarthritis E78.8† M14.3*
- – Lyme disease A69.2† M01.2*
- – Mediterranean fever, familial E85.0†
  M14.4*
- – meningococcus A39.8† M01.0*
- – metabolic disorder NEC E88.9†
  M14.5*
- – multiple myeloma C90.0† M36.1*
- – mumps B26.8† M01.5*
- – mycosis NEC B49† M01.6*
- – myelomatosis (multiple) C90.0†
  M36.1*
- – neurological disorder NEC G98†
  M14.6*
- – ochronosis E70.2† M14.5*
- – O'nyong-nyong A92.1† M01.5*
- – parasitic disease NEC B89† M01.8*
- – paratyphoid fever A01.-† M01.3*
- – Pseudomonas M00.8
- – psoriasis L40.5† M07.3*
- – pyogenic organism NEC M00.8
- – regional enteritis K50.-† M07.4*
- – Reiter's disease M02.3
- – respiratory disorder NEC J98.9†
  M14.8*
- – reticulosis, malignant C86.0† M14.8*
- – rubella B06.8† M01.4*
- – Salmonella (arizonae) (cholerae-suis)
  (enteritidis) (typhimurium) A02.2†
  M01.3*
- – sarcoidosis D86.8† M14.8*
- – sporotrichosis B42.8† M01.6*
- – syringomyelia G95.0† M49.4*
- – thalassemia NEC D56.9† M36.3*

Post traumatic arthritis — See arthrosis

Arthritis, arthritic—*continued*
- in—*continued*
- - tuberculosis – *see* Tuberculosis, arthritis
- - typhoid fever A01.0† M01.3∗
- - ulcerative colitis K51.-† M07.5∗
- - urethritis, Reiter's M02.3
- - viral disease NEC B34.9† M01.5∗
- infectious or infective (*see also* Arthritis, in) M00.9
- - spine M46.5
- juvenile M08.9
- - with systemic onset M08.2
- - in (due to)
- - - Crohn's disease K50.-† M09.1∗
- - - psoriasis L40.5† M09.0∗
- - - regional enteritis K50.-† M09.1∗
- - - ulcerative colitis K51.-† M09.2∗
- - pauciarticular M08.4
- - rheumatoid M08.0
- - specified NEC M08.8
- meningococcal A39.8† M01.0∗
- menopausal (any site) NEC M13.8
- mutilans (psoriatic) L40.5† M07.1∗
- mycotic NEC B49† M01.6∗
- neuropathic (Charcot) (tabetic) A52.1† M14.6∗
- - diabetic (*see also* E10-E14 with fourth character .6) E14.6† M14.6∗
- - nonsyphilitic NEC G98† M14.6∗
- - syringomyelic G95.0† M49.4∗
- nonpyogenic NEC M13.9
- ochronotic E70.2† M14.5∗
- palindromic (any site) M12.3
- pneumococcal (any site) M00.1
- postdysenteric M02.1
- postmeningococcal A39.8† M03.0∗
- postrheumatic, chronic M12.0
- primary progressive M13.8
- - spine M45
- psoriatic L40.5† M07.3∗
- purulent (any site except spine) M00.9
- - spine M46.5
- pyogenic or pyemic (any site except spine) M00.9
- - spine M46.5
- rheumatic, acute or subacute – *see* Fever, rheumatic
- rheumatoid M06.9
- - with
- - - carditis M05.3† I52.8∗
- - - endocarditis M05.3† I39.8∗
- - - heart involvement NEC M05.3† I52.8∗
- - - lung involvement M05.1† J99.0∗

Arthritis, arthritic—*continued*
- rheumatoid—*continued*
- - with—*continued*
- - - myocarditis M05.3† I41.8∗
- - - myopathy M05.3† G73.7∗
- - - pericarditis M05.3† I32.8∗
- - - polyneuropathy M05.3† G63.6∗
- - - splenoadenomegaly and leukopenia M05.0
- - - systemic involvement NEC M05.3
- - - torticollis M06.8
- - - vasculitis M05.2
- - - visceral involvement NEC M05.3
- - juvenile (with or without rheumatoid factor) M08.0
- - seronegative M06.0
- - seropositive M05.9
- - - specified NEC M05.8
- - specified NEC M06.8
- - spine M45
- rubella B06.8† M01.4∗
- scorbutic E54† M14.5∗
- senile or senescent (*see also* Arthrosis) M19.9
- septic (any site except spine) M00.9
- - spine M46.5
- serum (nontherapeutic) (therapeutic) M02.2
- specified form NEC M13.8
- spine M46.9
- - infectious or infective NEC M46.5
- - Marie-Strümpell M45
- - pyogenic M46.5
- - rheumatoid M45
- - traumatic (old) M48.3
- - tuberculous A18.0† M49.0∗
- staphylococcal (any site) M00.0
- streptococcal NEC (any site) M00.2
- suppurative (any site) M00.9
- syphilitic (late) A52.1† M01.3∗
- - congenital A50.5† M03.1∗
- syphilitica deformans (Charcot) A52.1† M14.6∗
- temporomandibular K07.6
- toxic of menopause (any site) M13.8
- transient M12.8
- traumatic (chronic) M12.5
- tuberculous A18.0† M01.1∗
- - spine A18.0† M49.0∗
- uratic M10.0
- urethritica, Reiter's M02.3
- vertebral (*see also* Arthritis, spine) M46.9
- villous (any site) M12.8
Arthrocele M25.4
Arthrodesis status Z98.1

Arthrodynia M25.5
– psychogenic F45.4
Arthrofibrosis, joint M24.6
Arthrogryposis (congenital) Q68.8
– multiplex congenita Q74.3
Arthrokatadysis M24.7
Arthropathy (*see also* Arthritis) M13.9
– Charcot's (tabetic) A52.1† M14.6*
– – diabetic (*see also* E10-E14 with fourth
  character .6) E14.6† M14.6*
– – nonsyphilitic NEC G98† M14.6*
– – syringomyelic G95.0† M49.4*
– cryoarytenoid I38.7
– crystal(-induced) M11.9
– diabetic NEC (*see also* E10-E14 with
  fourth character .6) E14.6† M14.2*
– – neuropathic E14.6† M14.6*
– distal interphalangeal, psoriatic L40.5†
  M07.0*
– following intestinal bypass M02.0
– gouty M10.0
– – in (due to)
– – – Lesch-Nyhan syndrome E79.1†
  M14.0*
– – – sickle-cell disorders D57.-† M14.0*
– hemophilic NEC D66† M36.2*
– – in (due to)
– – – hyperparathyroidism NEC E21.3†
  M14.1*
– – – metabolic disease NEC E88.9†
  M14.1*
– in (due to)
– – acromegaly E22.0† M14.5*
– – amyloidosis E85.-† M14.4*
– – blood disorder NEC D75.9† M36.3*
– – Crohn's disease K50.-† M07.4*
– – diabetes (*see also* E10-E14 with fourth
  character .6) E14.6† M14.2*
– – endocrine disorder NEC E34.9†
  M14.5*
– – enteritis NEC A09.9† M03.-*
– – – infectious NEC A09.9† M03.-*
– – enteropathic NEC A09.9† M07.6*
– – – infectious A09.9† M03.-*
– – erythema
– – – multiforme L51.-† M14.8*
– – – nodosum L52† M14.8*
– – hematologic disorders NEC (*see also*
  categories D50-D77) D75.9† M36.3*
– – hemochromatosis E83.1† M14.5*
– – hemoglobinopathy NEC D58.2†
  M36.3*
– – hemophilia NEC D66† M36.2*
– – Henoch-Schönlein purpura D69.0†
  M36.4*

Arthropathy—*continued*
– in—*continued*
– – hepatitis viral (*see also* categories B15-
  B19) B19.9† M03.2*
– – hyperthyroidism E05.-† M14.5*
– – hypothyroidism E03.9† M14.5*
– – infective endocarditis I33.0† M03.6*
– – leukemia NEC (*see also* categories
  C91-C95) C95.9† M36.1*
– – malignant histiocytosis C96.8† M36.1*
– – metabolic disorder NEC E88.9†
  M14.5*
– – multiple myeloma (M9732/3) C90.0†
  M36.1*
– – mycosis NEC (*see also* categories B35-
  B49) B49† M01.6*
– – neoplastic disease NEC
  (M8000/1) (*see also* Neoplasm)
  D48.9† M36.1*
– – nutritional deficiency E63.9† M14.5*
– – psoriasis NEC L40.5† M07.3*
– – regional enteritis K50.-† M07.4*
– – sarcoidosis D86.8† M14.8*
– – syphilis (late) A52.7† M01.3*
– – – congenital A50.5† M03.1*
– – thyrotoxicosis E05.-† M14.5*
– – ulcerative colitis K51.-† M07.5*
– – viral hepatitis (postinfectious)
  NEC (*see also* categories B15-B19))
  B19.9† M03.2*
– – Whipple's disease K90.8† M14.8*
– Jaccoud M12.0
– juvenile – *see* Arthritis, juvenile
– neurogenic, neuropathic (Charcot)
  (tabetic) A52.1† M14.6*
– – diabetic (*see also* E10-E14 with fourth
  character .6) E14.6† M14.6*
– – nonsyphilitic NEC G98† M14.6*
– – syringomyelic G95.0† M49.4*
– osteopulmonary M89.4
– postdysenteric M02.1
– postimmunization M02.2
– postinfectious NEC B99† M03.2*
– – in (due to)
– – – enteritis due to Yersinia
  enterocolitica A04.6† M03.2*
– – – syphilis A52.7† M03.1*
– – – viral hepatitis NEC B19.9† M03.2*
– postrheumatic, chronic (Jaccoud) M12.0
– psoriatic NEC L40.5† M07.3*
– – interphalangeal, distal L40.5† M07.0*
– reactive M02.9
– – in infective endocarditis I33.0†
  M03.6*
– – specified NEC M02.8

Arthropathy—*continued*
- specified NEC M12.8
- syringomyelic G95.0† M49.4∗
- tabes dorsalis A52.1† M14.6∗
- tabetic A52.1† M14.6∗
- traumatic M12.5

Arthropyosis M00.9

Arthrosis (deformans) (degenerative)
  M19.9
- erosive M15.4
- first carpometacarpal joint M18.9
- - post-traumatic (unilateral) M18.3
- - - bilateral M18.2
- - primary (unilateral) M18.1
- - - bilateral M18.0
- - secondary NEC (unilateral) M18.5
- - - bilateral M18.4
- generalized, primary M15.0
- hip – *see* Coxarthrosis
- joint NEC
- - post-traumatic M19.1
- - primary M19.0
- - secondary NEC M19.2
- knee – *see* Gonarthrosis
- localized M19.9
- polyarticular M15.9
- post-traumatic NEC M19.1
- primary NEC M19.0
- secondary NEC M19.2
- - multiple M15.3
- specified NEC M19.8
- spine M47.9

Arthus' phenomenon or reaction T78.4
- due to
- - correct substance properly administered
  T88.7
- - overdose or wrong substance given or
  taken T50.9
- - - specified drug – *see* Table of drugs
  and chemicals
- - serum T80.6

Articular – *see condition*

Artificial
- insemination Z31.1
- - complication (*see also* Complications,
  artificial, fertilization or insemination)
  N98.9
- vagina status Z93.8

Arytenoid – *see condition*

Asbestosis J61

Ascariasis, ascaridosis, ascaridiasis B77.9
- with
- - complications NEC B77.8
- - intestinal complications B77.0†
  K93.8∗

Ascariasis, ascaridosis—*continued*
- with—*continued*
- - pneumonia, pneumonitis B77.8†
  J17.3∗

Ascaris (infection) (infestation)
  (lumbricoides) (*see also* Ascariasis)
  B77.9

Ascending – *see condition*

Aschoff's bodies (*see also* Myocarditis,
  rheumatic) I09.0

Ascites (abdominal) R18
- chylous (nonfilarial) I89.8
- - filarial (*see also* Filaria) B74.9
- fetal, causing obstructed labor (mother)
  O66.3
- malignant C78.6
- syphilitic A52.7
- tuberculous A18.3

Aseptic – *see condition*

Asialia K11.7

Askin's tumor (M8803/3) – *see* Neoplasm,
  connective tissue, malignant

Asocial personality F60.2

Aspartylglucosaminuria E77.1

Asperger's disease or syndrome F84.5

Aspergillosis, aspergilloma B44.9
- with pneumonia B44.-† J17.2∗
- disseminated B44.7
- generalized B44.7
- pulmonary NEC B44.1† J99.8∗
- - invasive B44.0† J99.8∗
- specified NEC B44.8
- tonsillar B44.2† J99.8∗

Aspergillus (flavus) (fumigatus)
  (infection) (terreus) (*see also*
  Aspergillosis) B44.9

Aspermatogenesis N46

Aspermia (testis) N46

Asphyxia, asphyxiation (by) R09.0
- antenatal (*see also* Distress, fetal) P20.9
- bedclothes T71
- birth (*see also* Asphyxia, newborn) P21.9
- carbon monoxide T58
- cave-in T71
- - crushing S28.0
- constriction T71
- crushing S28.0
- drowning T75.1
- fetal (*see also* Distress, fetal) P20.9
- food or foreign body (in) T17.9
- - bronchioles T17.8
- - bronchus (main) T17.5
- - larynx T17.3
- - lung T17.8
- - nasal sinus T17.0

Asphyxia, asphyxiation—*continued*
- food or foreign body—*continued*
- – – nasopharynx T17.2
- – – newborn P24.3
- – – nose, nostril T17.1
- – – pharynx T17.2
- – – respiratory tract T17.9
- – – – specified part NEC T17.8
- – – throat T17.2
- – – trachea T17.4
- gas, fumes, or vapor T59.9
- – specified – *see* Table of drugs and chemicals
- gravitational changes T71
- hanging T71
- inhalation – *see* Inhalation
- intrauterine (*see also* Distress, fetal) P20.9
- local I73.0
- mechanical T71
- mucus (in) T17.9
- – bronchioles T17.8
- – bronchus (main) T17.5
- – larynx T17.3
- – lung T17.8
- – nasal sinus T17.0
- – nasopharynx T17.2
- – newborn P24.1
- – nose, nostril T17.1
- – pharynx T17.2
- – respiratory tract T17.9
- – – specified part NEC T17.8
- – throat T17.2
- – trachea T17.4
- newborn P21.9
- – with 1-minute Apgar score
- – – low NEC P21.9
- – – – 0-3 P21.0
- – – – 4-7 P21.1
- – blue P21.1
- – livida P21.1
- – mild or moderate P21.1
- – pallida P21.0
- – severe P21.0
- – white P21.0
- pathological R09.0
- postnatal (*see also* Asphyxia, newborn) P21.9
- – mechanical T71
- prenatal (*see also* Distress, fetal) P20.9
- pressure T71
- reticularis R23.1
- strangulation T71
- submersion T75.1
- traumatic NEC T71

Asphyxia, asphyxiation—*continued*
- traumatic NEC—*continued*
- – – due to crushed chest S28.0
- vomiting, vomitus – *see* Asphyxia, food or foreign body

Aspiration
- amniotic fluid (newborn) P24.1
- blood, newborn P24.2
- food or foreign body (with asphyxiation) – *see* Asphyxia, food or foreign body
- liquor (amnii) (newborn) P24.1
- meconium (newborn) P24.0
- milk (newborn) P24.3
- mucus T17.9
- – into
- – – bronchioles T17.8
- – – bronchus (main) T17.5
- – – larynx T17.3
- – – lung T17.8
- – – nasal sinus T17.0
- – – nose, nostril T17.1
- – – pharynx T17.2
- – – respiratory tract T17.9
- – – – specified part NEC T17.8
- – – throat T17.2
- – – trachea T17.4
- – newborn P24.1
- syndrome of newborn (massive) P24.9
- – meconium P24.0
- vernix caseosa (newborn) P24.8

Asplenia (congenital) Q89.0
- postsurgical D73.0

Assam fever B55.0

Assmann's focus NEC A16.2

Astasia(-abasia) (hysterical) F44.4

Asteatosis cutis L85.3

Astereognosis R48.1

Asterixis R27.8

Asthenia, asthenic R53
- cardiac (*see also* Failure, heart) I50.9
- – psychogenic F45.3
- cardiovascular (*see also* Failure, heart) I50.9
- – psychogenic F45.3
- heart (*see also* Failure, heart) I50.9
- – psychogenic F45.3
- hysterical F44.4
- myocardial (*see also* Failure, heart) I50.9
- – psychogenic F45.3
- nervous F48.0
- neurocirculatory F45.3
- neurotic F48.0
- psychogenic F48.0
- psychoneurotic F48.0
- psychophysiologic F48.0

Asthenia, asthenic—*continued*
- reaction (psychophysiologic) F48.0
- senile R54

Asthenopia H53.1
- accommodative H52.5
- hysterical F44.6
- psychogenic F44.6

Asthenospermia R86.9

Asthma, asthmatic (bronchial) (catarrh) (spasmodic) J45.9
- with
- - hay fever J45.0
- - rhinitis, allergic J45.0
- acute, severe J46
- allergic extrinsic J45.0
- atopic J45.0
- cardiac (*see also* Failure, ventricular, left) I50.1
- childhood J45.0
- collier's J60
- croup J45.9
- due to detergent J69.8
- eosinophilic J82
- extrinsic, allergic J45.0
- grinder's J62.8
- heart I50.1
- idiosyncratic J45.1
- intrinsic, nonallergic J45.1
- late-onset J45.9
- Millar's J38.5
- miner's J60
- mixed J45.8
- nervous J45.1
- nonallergic J45.1
- platinum J45.0
- pneumoconiotic NEC J64
- potter's J62.8
- predominantly allergic J45.0
- pulmonary eosinophilic J82
- Rostan's I50.1
- sandblaster's J62.8
- severe, acute J46
- status J46
- stonemason's J62.8
- tuberculous (*see also* Tuberculosis, pulmonary) A16.2

Astigmatism (compound) (congenital) (any type) H52.2

Astroblastoma (M9430/3)
- specified site – *see* Neoplasm, malignant
- unspecified site C71.9

Astrocytoma (cystic) (M9400/3)
- anaplastic (M9401/3)
- - specified site – *see* Neoplasm, malignant

Astrocytoma—*continued*
- anaplastic—*continued*
- - unspecified site C71.9
- fibrillary (M9420/3)
- - specified site – *see* Neoplasm, malignant
- - unspecified site C71.9
- fibrous (M9420/3)
- - specified site – *see* Neoplasm, malignant
- - unspecified site C71.9
- gemistocytic (M9411/3)
- - specified site – *see* Neoplasm, malignant
- - unspecified site C71.9
- juvenile (M9421/3)
- - specified site – *see* Neoplasm, malignant
- - unspecified site C71.9
- pilocytic (M9421/3)
- - specified site – *see* Neoplasm, malignant
- - unspecified site C71.9
- piloid (M9421/3)
- - specified site – *see* Neoplasm, malignant
- - unspecified site C71.9
- protoplasmic (M9410/3)
- - specified site – *see* Neoplasm, malignant
- - unspecified site C71.9
- specified site NEC – *see* Neoplasm, malignant
- subependymal (M9383/1) D43.2
- - giant cell (M9384/1)
- - - specified site – *see* Neoplasm, uncertain behavior
- - - unspecified site D43.2
- - specified site – *see* Neoplasm, uncertain behavior
- - unspecified site D43.2
- unspecified site C71.9

Astroglioma (M9400/3)
- specified site – *see* Neoplasm, malignant
- unspecified site C71.9

Asymbolia R48.8

Asymmetry – *see also* Distortion
- face Q67.0
- jaw K07.1
- pelvis with disproportion (fetopelvic) O33.0
- - affecting fetus or newborn P03.1
- - causing obstructed labor O65.0

Asynergia, asynergy R27.8

Asystole (heart) (*see also* Arrest, cardiac)
 I46.9
Ataxia, ataxy, ataxic R27.0
– brain (hereditary) G11.9
– cerebellar (hereditary) G11.9
– – with defective DNA repair G11.3
– – alcoholic G31.2
– – early-onset G11.1
– – in
– – – alcoholism G31.2
– – – myxedema E03.9† G13.2*
– – – neoplastic disease NEC
  (M8000/1) (*see also* Neoplasm)
  D48.9† G13.1*
– – late-onset (Marie's) G11.2
– cerebral (hereditary) G11.9
– congenital nonprogressive G11.0
– family, familial – *see* Ataxia, hereditary
– Friedreich's (cerebellar) (heredofamilial)
  (spinal) G11.1
– gait R26.0
– – hysterical F44.4
– general R27.8
– hereditary G11.9
– – with neuropathy G60.2
– – cerebellar – *see* Ataxia, cerebellar
– – spastic G11.4
– – specified NEC G11.8
– – spinal (Friedreich's) G11.1
– heredofamilial – *see* Ataxia, hereditary
– Hunt's G11.1
– hysterical F44.4
– locomotor (partial) (progressive) (spastic)
  (syphilitic) A52.1
– Marie's (cerebellar) (heredofamilial) (late-
  onset) G11.2
– nonorganic origin F44.4
– nonprogressive, congenital G11.0
– psychogenic F44.4
– Roussy-Lévy G60.0
– Sanger-Brown's (hereditary) G11.2
– spinal
– – hereditary (Friedreich's) G11.1
– – progressive (syphilitic) A52.1
– spinocerebellar, X-linked recessive G11.1
– telangiectasia (Louis-Bar) G11.3
Ataxia-telangiectasia (Louis-Bar) G11.3
Atelectasis (massive) (partial) (pressure)
  (pulmonary) J98.1
– fetus or newborn (secondary) P28.1
– – due to resorption P28.1
– – partial P28.1
– – primary P28.0
– primary (newborn) P28.0

Atelectasis—*continued*
– tuberculous (*see also* Tuberculosis,
  pulmonary) A16.2
Atelocardia Q24.9
Atelomyelia Q06.1
Atheroma, atheromatous (*see also*
  Arteriosclerosis) I70.9
– aorta, aortic I70.0
– – valve (*see also* Endocarditis, aortic)
  I35.8
– aorto-iliac I70.0
– artery – *see* Arteriosclerosis
– basilar (artery) I67.2
– carotid (artery) (common) (internal) I67.2
– cerebral (arteries) I67.2
– coronary (artery) I25.1
– degeneration – *see* Arteriosclerosis
– heart, cardiac I25.1
– mitral (valve) I34.8
– myocardium, myocardial I25.1
– pulmonary valve (heart) (*see also*
  Endocarditis, pulmonary) I37.8
– tricuspid (heart) (valve) I36.8
– valve, valvular – *see* Endocarditis
– vertebral (artery) I67.2
Atheromatosis – *see* Arteriosclerosis
Atherosclerosis – *see* Arteriosclerosis
Athetosis (acquired) R25.8
– bilateral (congenital) G80.3
– congenital (bilateral) (double) G80.3
  double (congenital) G80.3
– unilateral R25.8
Athlete's
– foot B35.3
– heart I51.7
Athyrea (acquired) – *see* Hypothyroidism
Atonia, atony, atonic
– bladder (sphincter) (neurogenic) N31.2
– capillary I78.8
– cecum K59.8
– – psychogenic F45.3
– colon – *see* Atonia, intestine
– congenital P94.2
– esophagus K22.8
– intestine K59.8
– – psychogenic F45.3
– stomach K31.8
– – neurotic or psychogenic F45.3
– uterus, during labor O62.2
– – affecting fetus or newborn P03.6
Atopy – *see* Hypersensitive, hypersensitivity
Atransferrinemia, congenital E88.0
Atresia, atretic
– alimentary organ or tract NEC Q45.8
– – upper Q40.8

Atresia, atretic—*continued*
- ani, anus, anal (canal) Q42.3
- – with fistula Q42.2
- aorta (arch) (ring) Q25.2
- aortic (orifice) (valve) Q23.0
- – arch Q25.2
- – congenital with hypoplasia of ascending aorta and defective development of left ventricle (with mitral stenosis) Q23.4
- – in hypoplastic left heart syndrome Q23.4
- aqueduct of Sylvius Q03.0
- – with spina bifida (*see also* Spina bifida, with hydrocephalus) Q05.4
- artery NEC Q27.8
- – cerebral Q28.3
- – coronary Q24.5
- – eye Q15.8
- – pulmonary Q25.5
- – umbilical Q27.0
- auditory canal (external) Q16.1
- bile duct (common) (congenital) (hepatic) Q44.2
- – acquired (*see also* Obstruction, bile duct) K83.1
- bladder (neck) Q64.3
- bronchus Q32.4
- cecum Q42.8
- cervix (acquired) N88.2
- – congenital Q51.8
- – in pregnancy or childbirth O34.4
- – – causing obstructed labor O65.5
- – – – affecting fetus or newborn P03.1
- choana Q30.0
- colon Q42.9
- – specified NEC Q42.8
- common duct Q44.2
- cystic duct Q44.2
- – acquired (*see also* Obstruction, gallbladder) K82.0
- digestive organs NEC Q45.8
- duodenum Q41.0
- ear canal Q16.1
- ejaculatory duct Q55.4
- esophagus Q39.0
- – with tracheoesophageal fistula Q39.1
- eustachian tube Q16.4
- fallopian tube (congenital) Q50.6
- – acquired N97.1
- foramen of
- – Luschka Q03.1
- – – with spina bifida (*see also* Spina bifida, with hydrocephalus) Q05.4
- – Magendie Q03.1

Atresia, atretic—*continued*
- foramen of—*continued*
- – Magendie—*continued*
- – – with spina bifida (*see also* Spina bifida, with hydrocephalus) Q05.4
- gallbladder Q44.1
- genital organ
- – external
- – – female Q52.7
- – – male Q55.8
- – internal
- – – female Q52.8
- – – male Q55.8
- gullet Q39.0
- – with tracheoesophageal fistula Q39.1
- heart valve NEC Q24.8
- – pulmonary Q22.0
- – tricuspid Q22.4
- hymen Q52.3
- – acquired (postinfective) N89.6
- ileum Q41.2
- intestine (small) Q41.9
- – large Q42.9
- – – specified NEC Q42.8
- iris, filtration angle Q15.0
- jejunum Q41.1
- lacrimal apparatus Q10.4
- larynx Q31.8
- meatus urinarius Q64.3
- mitral valve Q23.2
- – in hypoplastic left heart syndrome Q23.4
- nares (anterior) (posterior) Q30.0
- nasopharynx Q34.8
- nose, nostril Q30.0
- – acquired J34.8
- oesophagus Q39.0
- – with tracheoesophageal fistula Q39.1
- organ or site NEC Q89.8
- osseous meatus (ear) Q16.1
- oviduct (congenital) Q50.6
- – acquired N97.1
- parotid duct Q38.4
- – acquired K11.8
- pulmonary (artery) Q25.5
- – valve Q22.0
- pupil Q13.2
- rectum Q42.1
- – with fistula Q42.0
- salivary duct Q38.4
- – acquired K11.8
- sublingual duct Q38.4
- – acquired K11.8
- submandibular duct Q38.4
- – acquired K11.8

Atresia, atretic—*continued*
- trachea Q32.1
- tricuspid valve Q22.4
- ureter Q62.1
- ureteropelvic junction Q62.1
- ureterovesical orifice Q62.1
- urethra (valvular) Q64.3
- urinary tract NEC Q64.8
- uterus Q51.8
- – acquired N85.8
- vagina (congenital) Q52.4
- – acquired (postinfectional) (senile) N89.5
- vas deferens Q55.3
- vascular NEC Q27.8
- – cerebral Q28.3
- vein NEC Q27.8
- – great Q26.8
- – portal Q26.5
- – pulmonary Q26.3
- vena cava (inferior) (superior) Q26.8
- vesicourethral orifice Q64.3
- vulva Q52.7
- – acquired N90.5
Atrichia, atrichosis (*see also* Alopecia) L65.9
- congenital (universal) Q84.0
Atrophia – *see also* Atrophy
- cutis senilis L90.8
- – due to radiation L57.8
- gyrata of choroid and retina H31.2
- senilis R54
- – dermatological L90.8
- – – due to radiation (nonionizing) (solar) L57.8
- unguium L60.3
- – congenita Q84.6
Atrophie blanche (en plaque) (de Milian) L95.0
Atrophoderma, atrophodermia (of) L90.9
- diffusum (idiopathic) L90.4
- maculatum L90.8
- – et striatum L90.8
- – – due to syphilis A52.7† L99.8*
- – syphilitic A51.3† L99.8*
- neuriticum L90.8
- Pasini and Pierini L90.3
- pigmentosum Q82.1
- reticulatum symmetricum faciei L66.4
- senile L90.8
- – due to radiation (nonionizing) (solar) L57.8
- vermiculata (cheeks) L66.4
Atrophy, atrophic
- adrenal (capsule) (gland) E27.4

Atrophy, atrophic—*continued*
- adrenal—*continued*
- – primary E27.1
- alveolar process or ridge (edentulous) K08.2
- appendix K38.8
- arteriosclerotic – *see* Arteriosclerosis
- bile duct (common) (hepatic) K83.8
- bladder N32.8
- – neurogenic N31.8
- blanche (en plaque) (of Milian) L95.0
- bone (senile) NEC M89.8
- – due to
- – – tabes dorsalis (neurogenic) A52.1† M90.2*
- brain (cortex) (progressive) (*see also* Degeneration, brain) G31.9
- – circumscribed G31.0
- – – dementia in G31.0† F02.0*
- – presenile NEC G31.8
- – – dementia in G31.8† F02.8*
- – senile NEC G31.1
- breast N64.2
- – puerperal, postpartum O92.2
- buccal cavity K13.7
- cardiac (*see also* Degeneration, myocardial) I51.5
- cartilage (infectional) (joint) M94.8
- cerebellar – *see* Atrophy, brain
- cerebral – *see* Atrophy, brain
- cervix (mucosa) (senile) (uteri) N88.8
- – menopausal N95.8
- Charcot-Marie-Tooth G60.0
- choroid (central) (macular) (myopic) (retina) (senile) H31.1
- – gyrate H31.2
- ciliary body H21.2
- conjunctiva (senile) H11.8
- corpus cavernosum N48.8
- cortical (*see also* Atrophy, brain) G31.9
- cystic duct K82.8
- Déjerine-Thomas G23.8
- disuse NEC M62.5
- Duchenne-Aran G12.2
- ear H93.8
- edentulous alveolar ridge K08.2
- endometrium (senile) N85.8
- – cervix N88.8
- enteric K63.8
- epididymis N50.8
- eyeball H44.5
- eyelid (senile) H02.7
- facial (skin) L90.9
- facioscapulohumeral G71.0
- fallopian tube (senile) N83.3

Atrophy, atrophic—*continued*
- fatty, thymus (gland) E32.8
- gallbladder K82.8
- gastric K29.4
- gastrointestinal K63.8
- glandular I89.8
- globe H44.5
- gum K06.0
- hair L67.8
- hemifacial Q67.4
- – Romberg G51.8
- infantile paralysis, acute (*see also* Poliomyelitis, paralytic) A80.3
- intestine K63.8
- iris (essential) (progressive) H21.2
- kidney (senile) (terminal) (*see also* Sclerosis, renal) N26
- – with hypertension (*see also* Hypertension, kidney) I12.9
- – congenital or infantile Q60.5
- – – bilateral Q60.4
- – – unilateral Q60.3
- – hydronephrotic N13.3
- – – with infection N13.6
- lacrimal gland H04.1
- Landouzy-Déjerine G71.0
- laryngitis, infective J37.0
- larynx J38.7
- Leber's optic (hereditary) H47.2
- lip K13.0
- liver (yellow) K72.9
- – acute, subacute K72.0
- – chronic K72.1
- lung (senile) J98.4
- macular (dermatological) L90.8
- – syphilitic, skin A51.3† L99.8*
- – – striated A52.7† L99.8*
- multiple system (brain) (CNS) G90.3
- muscle, muscular M62.5
- – diffuse M62.5
- – Duchenne-Aran G12.2
- – general M62.5
- – limb (lower) (upper) M62.5
- – myelopathic – *see* Atrophy, muscle, spinal
- – neuritic G58.9
- – neuropathic (peroneal) (progressive) G60.0
- – peroneal G60.0
- – primary (idiopathic) M62.5
- – progressive (bulbar) (spinal) G12.2
- – pseudohypertrophic G71.0
- – spinal G12.9
- – – adult form G12.1
- – – childhood form, type II G12.1

Atrophy, atrophic—*continued*
- muscle, muscular—*continued*
- – spinal—*continued*
- – – distal G12.1
- – – hereditary NEC G12.1
- – – infantile, type I (Werdnig-Hoffmann) G12.0
- – – juvenile form, type III (Kugelberg-Welander) G12.1
- – – progressive G12.2
- – – scapuloperoneal form G12.1
- – – specified NEC G12.8
- – syphilitic A52.7† M63.8*
- myocardium (*see also* Degeneration, myocardial) I51.5
- myometrium (senile) N85.8
- – cervix N88.8
- myopathic NEC M62.5
- nail L60.3
- nasopharynx J31.1
- nerve – *see also* Disorder, nerve
- – abducens H49.2
- – cranial
- – – fourth (trochlear) H49.1
- – – second (optic) H47.2
- – – sixth (abducens) H49.2
- – – third (oculomotor) H49.0
- – oculomotor H49.0
- – optic (papillomacular bundle) H47.2
- – – syphilitic (late) A52.1† H48.0*
- – – – congenital A50.4† H48.0*
- – trochlear H49.1
- neurogenic, bone, tabetic A52.1† M90.2*
- old age R54
- olivopontocerebellar G23.8
- orbit H05.3
- ovary (senile) N83.3
- oviduct (senile) N83.3
- palsy, diffuse (progressive) G12.2
- pancreas (duct) (senile) K86.8
- parotid gland K11.0
- penis N48.8
- pharynx J39.2
- pluriglandular E31.8
- – autoimmune E31.0
- polyarthritis M15.9
- prostate N42.2
- pseudohypertrophic (muscle) G71.0
- renal (*see also* Sclerosis, renal) N26
- retina, retinal (postinfectional) H35.8
- salivary gland K11.0
- scar L90.5
- sclerosis, lobar (of brain) G31.0
- – dementia in G31.0† F02.0*
- scrotum N50.8

Atrophy, atrophic—*continued*
- seminal vesicle N50.8
- senile R54
- – due to radiation (nonionizing) (solar) L57.8
- skin (patches) (spots) L90.9
- – degenerative (senile) L90.8
- – due to radiation (nonionizing) (solar) L57.8
- – senile L90.8
- spermatic cord N50.8
- spinal (cord) G95.8
- – muscular (*see also* Atrophy, muscle, spinal) G12.9
- – paralysis G12.2
- – – infantile (*see also* Poliomyelitis, paralytic) A80.3
- – – meaning progressive muscular atrophy G12.2
- spine (column) M48.8
- spleen (senile) D73.0
- stomach K29.4
- striate (skin) L90.6
- – syphilitic A52.7† L99.8*
- subcutaneous L90.9
- sublingual gland K11.0
- submandibular gland K11.0
- Sudeck's M89.0
- suprarenal (capsule) (gland) E27.4
- – primary E27.1
- systemic, affecting central nervous system
- – in
- – – myxedema E03.9† G13.2*
- – – neoplastic disease NEC (M8000/1) (*see also* Neoplasm) D48.9† G13.1*
- tarso-orbital fascia, congenital Q10.3
- testis N50.0
- thymus (fatty) E32.8
- thyroid (gland) (acquired) E03.4
- – with cretinism E03.1
- – congenital (with myxedema) E03.1
- tongue (senile) K14.8
- – papillae K14.4
- trachea J39.8
- tunica vaginalis N50.8
- turbinate J34.8
- upper respiratory tract J39.8
- uterus, uterine (senile) N85.8
- – cervix N88.8
- – due to radiation (intended effect) N85.8
- – – adverse effect or misadventure N99.8
- vagina (senile) N95.2

Atrophy, atrophic—*continued*
- vas deferens N50.8
- vascular I99
- vertebra (senile) M48.8
- vulva (senile) N90.5
- yellow (*see also* Failure, hepatic) K72.9

Attack
- Adams-Stokes I45.9
- akinetic – *see* Epilepsy
- angina – *see* Angina
- atonic G40.3
- cardiovascular I51.6
- cataleptic – *see* Catalepsy
- cerebral I64
- coronary – *see* Infarct, myocardium
- cyanotic, newborn P28.2
- epileptic – *see* Epilepsy
- epileptiform R56.8
- hysterical F44.9
- jacksonian G40.1
- myoclonic G40.3
- panic F41.0
- paroxysmal – *see* Convulsions
- psychomotor (*see also* Epilepsy) G40.2
- salaam G40.4
- schizophreniform, brief F23.2
- sensory and motor – *see* Convulsions
- Stokes-Adams I45.9
- syncope R55
  transient ischemic (TIA) G45.9
- – specified NEC G45.8
- unconsciousness R55
- – hysterical F44.8
- vasomotor R55
- vasovagal (paroxysmal) (idiopathic) R55

Attention (to)
- artificial
- – opening (of) Z43.9
- – – digestive tract NEC Z43.4
- – – specified NEC Z43.8
- – – urinary tract NEC Z43.6
- – vagina Z43.7
- colostomy Z43.3
- cystostomy Z43.5
- deficit disorder or syndrome F98.8
- – with hyperactivity F90.0
- gastrostomy Z43.1
- ileostomy Z43.2
- nephrostomy Z43.6
- surgical dressings Z48.0
- sutures Z48.0
- tracheostomy Z43.0
- ureterostomy Z43.6
- urethrostomy Z43.6

Attrition, tooth, teeth (excessive) (hard tissues) K03.0
Atypical, atypism – *see also condition*
– endometrium N85.9
– – hyperplasia (adenomatous) N85.1
– parenting situation Z60.1
Auditory – *see condition*
Aujeszky's disease B33.8
Aura, jacksonian G40.1
Aurantiasis, cutis E67.1
Auricle, auricular – *see also condition*
– cervical Q18.2
Austin Flint murmur (aortic insufficiency) I35.1
Australian
– Q fever A78
– X disease A83.4
Autism, autistic (childhood) (infantile) F84.0
– atypical F84.1
Autodigestion R68.8
Autoerythrocyte sensitization (syndrome) D69.2
Autographism L50.3
Autoimmune disease (systemic) NEC M35.9
Autointoxication R68.8
Automatism
– epileptic G40.2
– paroxysmal, idiopathic G40.2
Autonomic, autonomous
– bladder (neurogenic) N31.2
– hysteria seizure F44.5
Autosensitivity, erythrocyte D69.2
Autosensitization, cutaneous L30.2
Autosome – *see* condition by chromosome involved
Autotopagnosia R48.1
Autotoxemia R68.8
Autumn – *see condition*
Avellis' syndrome I65.0† G46.8*
Aversion, sexual F52.1
Aviator's
– disease or sickness (*see also* Effects, adverse, high altitude) T70.2
– ear T70.0

Avitaminosis (multiple NEC) (*see also* Deficiency, vitamin) E56.9
Avulsion (traumatic) T14.7
– blood vessel – *see* Injury, blood vessel
– bone – *see* Fracture, by site
– cartilage (*see also* Dislocation, by site) T14.3
– – symphyseal (inner), complicating delivery O71.6
– external site other than limb – *see* Wound, open, by site
– eye S05.7
– head NEC (intracranial) S08.9
– – complete S18
– – external site NEC S08.8
– – scalp S08.0
– internal organ or site – *see* Injury, by site
– joint (*see also* Dislocation, by site) T14.3
– – capsule – *see* Sprain, by site
– ligament – *see* Sprain, by site
– limb – *see also* Amputation, traumatic, by site
– – skin and subcutaneous tissue – *see* Wound, open, by site
– muscle – *see* Injury, muscle
– nerve (root) – *see* Injury, nerve
– scalp S08.0
– skin and subcutaneous tissue – *see* Wound, open, by site
– symphyseal cartilage (inner), complicating delivery O71.6
– tendon – *see* Injury, muscle
– tooth S03.2
Awareness of heart beat R00.2
Axenfeld's
– anomaly or syndrome Q15.0
– degeneration (calcareous) Q13.4
Axilla, axillary – *see also condition*
– breast Q83.1
Axonotmesis – *see* Injury, nerve
Ayerza's disease or syndrome I27.0
Azoospermia N46
Azotemia R79.8
Aztec ear Q17.3
Azygos
– continuation inferior vena cava Q26.8
– lobe (lung) Q33.1

B

Baastrup's disease M48.2
Babesiosis B60.0
Babinski's syndrome A52.7
Baby
– crying constantly R68.1
  floppy (syndrome) P94.2
Bacillary – *see condition*
Bacilluria N39.0
Bacillus – *see also* Infection, bacillus
– fragilis, as cause of disease classified
  elsewhere B96.6
Back – *see condition*
Backache (postural) M54.9
– psychogenic F45.4
– sacroiliac M53.3
– specified NEC M54.8
Backflow – *see* Reflux
Backward reading (dyslexia) F81.0
Bacteremia A49.9
– with sepsis – *see* Sepsis
– meningococcal (*see also*
  Meningococcemia) A39.4
Bacterid, bacteride (pustular) L40.3
Bacterium, bacteria, bacterial – *see also*
  condition
– agent NEC, as cause of disease classified
  elsewhere B96.8
– in blood – *see* Bacteremia
– infection NEC, resulting from HIV
  disease B20.1
– in urine – *see* Bacteriuria
Bacteriuria, bacteruria N39.0
– asymptomatic N39.0
– – in pregnancy O23.4
– – puerperal, postpartum O86.2
Bad
– heart – *see* Disease, heart
– trip – *see* F11-F19 with fourth character .0
Baelz's disease K13.0
Bagasse disease or pneumonitis J67.1
Bagassosis J67.1
Baker's cyst M71.2
– tuberculous A18.0† M01.1*
**Balanitis (circinata) (erosiva)
  (gangrenosa) (infectional)
  (nongonococcal) (phagedenic) (vulgaris)**
  N48.1
– amebic A06.8† N51.2*
– candidal B37.4† N51.2*

Balanitis—*continued*
– due to Haemophilus ducreyi A57
– gonococcal (acute) (chronic) A54.0
– venereal NEC A64† N51.2*
– xerotica obliterans N48.0
Balanoposthitis N48.1
– gonococcal (acute) (chronic) A54.0
– ulcerative (specific) A63.8† N51.2*
Balanorrhagia – *see* Balanitis
Balantidiasis, balantidiosis A07.0
Baldness (*see also* Alopecia) L65.9
– male-pattern (*see also* Alopecia,
  androgenic) L64.9
Balkan grippe A78
Balloon disease (*see also* Effect, adverse,
  high altitude) T70.2
Balo's disease (concentric sclerosis) G37.5
Bamberger-Marie disease M89.4
Bancroft's filariasis B74.0
Band(s)
– adhesive (*see also* Adhesions,
  peritoneum) K66.0
– anomalous or congenital – *see also*
  Anomaly, by site
– – heart (atrial) (ventricular) Q24.8
– – omentum Q43.3
– cervix N88.1
– constricting, congenital Q79.8
– gallbladder (congenital) Q44.1
– intestinal (adhesive) (*see also* Adhesions,
  peritoneum) K66.0
– obstructive
– – intestine K56.5
– – peritoneum K56.5
– periappendiceal, congenital Q43.3
– peritoneal (adhesive) (*see also* Adhesions,
  peritoneum) K66.0
– uterus N73.6
– – internal N85.6
– vagina N89.5
**Bandl's ring (contraction), complicating
  delivery** O62.4
– affecting fetus or newborn P03.6
Bankruptcy, anxiety concerning Z59.8
Bannister's disease T78.3
– hereditary D84.1
**Banti's disease or syndrome (with
  cirrhosis) (with portal hypertension)**
  K76.6

Bar, median, prostate N40
Barcoo disease or rot (*see also* Ulcer, skin)
  L98.4
Barlow's disease E54
Barodontalgia T70.2
Baron Münchhausen syndrome F68.1
Barosinusitis T70.1
Barotitis T70.0
Barotrauma T70.2
– odontalgia T70.2
– otitic T70.0
– sinus T70.1
Barraquer(-Simons) disease or syndrome
  E88.1
Barré-Guillain disease or syndrome
  G61.0
Barrel chest M95.4
Barrett's
– disease K22.7
– esophagus K22.7
– – malignant – *see* Neoplasm, esophagus,
  malignant
– syndrome K22.7
– ulcer K22.1
Bartholinitis (suppurating) N75.8
– gonococcal (acute) (chronic) (with
  abscess) A54.1
Bartonellosis A44.9
– cutaneous A44.1
– mucocutaneous A44.1
– specified NEC A44.8
– systemic A44.0
Bartter's syndrome E26.8
Basal – *see condition*
Baseball finger S63.1
Basedow's disease E05.0
Basic – *see condition*
Basilar – *see condition*
Basophilia D75.8
Basophilism (cortico-adrenal) (Cushing's)
  (pituitary) E24.0
Bassen-Kornzweig disease or syndrome
  E78.6
Bat ear Q17.5
Bateman's disease B08.1
Bathing cramp T75.1
Bathophobia F40.2
Batten(-Mayou) disease E75.4
– retina E75.4† H36.8*
Battered
– baby or child (syndrome) NEC T74.1
– spouse syndrome T74.1
Battey mycobacterium infection A31.0
Battle exhaustion F43.0

Battledore placenta – *see* Placenta,
  abnormal
Baumgarten-Cruveilhier cirrhosis, disease
  or syndrome K74.6
Bauxite fibrosis (of lung) J63.1
Bayle's disease (general paresis) A52.1
Bazin's disease (primary) (tuberculous)
  A18.4
Beach ear H60.3
Beaded hair (congenital) Q84.1
Béal conjunctivitis or syndrome B30.2†
  H13.1*
Beard's disease F48.0
Beat(s)
– atrial, premature I49.1
– ectopic I49.4
– elbow M70.3
– escaped, heart I49.4
– hand M70.1
– knee M70.5
– premature I49.4
– – atrial I49.1
Beau's lines L60.4
Bechterev's syndrome M45
Becker's
– cardiomyopathy I42.8
– dystrophy G71.0
– pigmented hairy nevus (M8720/0) D22.5
Beckwith-Wiedemann syndrome Q87.3
Bedclothes, asphyxiation or suffocation by
  T71
Bedfast NEC R26.3
– requiring health care provider Z74.0
Bednar('s)
– aphthae K12.0
– tumor (M8833/3) – *see* Neoplasm, skin,
  malignant
Bedsore L89.-
– stage
– – I L89.0
– – II L89.1
– – III L89.2
– – IV L89.3
Bedwetting (*see also* Enuresis) R32
Bee sting (with allergic or anaphylactic
  shock) T63.4
Beer drinker's heart (disease) I42.6
Behavior
– antisocial, child or adolescent Z72.8
– disorder, disturbance – *see* Disorder,
  conduct
– disruptive (*see also* Disorder, conduct)
  F91.8
– inexplicable R46.2

Behavior—*continued*
– marked evasiveness R46.5
– overactivity R46.3
– poor responsiveness R46.4
– self-damaging (lifestyle) Z72.8
– slowness R46.4
– specified NEC R46.8
– strange (and inexplicable) R46.2
– suspiciousness R46.5
– type A pattern Z73.1
  undue concern or preoccupation with
  stressful events R46.6
– verbosity and circumstantial detail
  obscuring reason for contact R46.7
Behçet's disease or syndrome M35.2
Behr's disease H35.5
Beigel's disease B36.8
Bejel A65
Bekhterev's syndrome M45
Belching (*see also* Eructation) R14
Bell's
– mania F30.8
– palsy, paralysis G51.0
– spasm G51.3
**Bence Jones albuminuria or proteinuria
  NEC** R80
Bends T70.3
Benedikt's paralysis or syndrome I67.9†
  G46.3*
Bennett's fracture S62.2
Benson's disease H43.2
Bent
– back (hysterical) F44.4
– nose M95.0
– – congenital Q67.4
Bereavement (uncomplicated) Z63.4
Bergeron's disease (hysterical chorea)
  F44.4
Berger's disease – *see* Nephropathy, IgA
Beriberi (dry) E51.1
– wet E51.1
– – involving circulatory system E51.1†
  I98.8*
– – polyneuropathy E51.1† G63.4*
Berlin's disease or edema (traumatic)
  S05.8
Berlock (berloque) dermatitis L56.2
Bernard-Horner syndrome G90.2
**Bernard-Soulier disease or
  thrombopathia** D69.1
Bernhardt(-Roth) disease or paresthesia
  G57.1
Bernheim's syndrome (*see also* Failure,
  heart, congestive) I50.0

Bertielliasis B71.8
Berylliosis (lung) J63.2
**Besnier-Boeck(-Schaumann)
  disease** (*see also* Sarcoidosis) D86.9
Besnier's
– lupus pernio D86.3
– prurigo L20.0
Bestiality F65.8
Best's disease H35.5
Betalipoproteinemia, broad or floating
  E78.2
Betting and gambling Z72.6
– pathological (compulsive) F63.0
Bezoar T18.9
– intestine T18.3
– stomach T18.2
Bezold's abscess H70.0
Bianchi's syndrome R48.8
Bicornate or bicornis uterus Q51.3
– in pregnancy or childbirth O34.0
– – affecting fetus or newborn P03.8
– – causing obstructed labor O65.5
Bicuspid aortic valve Q23.1
Biedl-Bardet syndrome Q87.8
Bielschowsky(-Jansky) disease E75.4
Biermer's anemia or disease D51.0
Biett's disease L93.0
Bifid (congenital)
– apex, heart Q24.8
– clitoris Q52.6
– kidney Q63.8
– nose Q30.2
– patella Q74.1
– scrotum Q55.2
– toe NEC Q74.2
– tongue Q38.3
– ureter Q62.8
– uterus Q51.3
– uvula Q35.7
Biforis uterus (suprasimplex) Q51.3
Bifurcation (congenital)
– gallbladder Q44.1
– kidney pelvis Q63.8
– renal pelvis Q63.8
– rib Q76.6
– tongue Q38.3
– trachea Q32.1
– ureter Q62.8
– urethra Q64.7
– vertebra Q76.4
Bigeminal pulse R00.8
Bilateral – *see condition*
Bile
– duct – *see condition*

Bile—*continued*
- pigments in urine R82.2
Bilharziasis (*see also* Schistosomiasis)
  B65.9
- chyluria B65.0
- galacturia B65.0
- hematochyluria B65.0
- intestinal B65.1
- lipuria B65.0
- oriental B65.2
- pulmonary NEC B65.-† J99.8∗
- - pneumonia B65.-† J17.3∗
- tropical hematuria B65.0
- vesical B65.0
Biliary – *see condition*
Bilious (attack) (*see also* Vomiting) R11
Bilirubin metabolism disorder E80.7
- specified NEC E80.6
Bilirubinemia, familial nonhemolytic
  E80.4
Biliuria R82.2
Bilocular stomach K31.2
Binswanger's disease I67.3
Biparta, bipartite
- carpal scaphoid Q74.0
- patella Q74.1
- vagina Q52.1
Bird
- face Q75.8
- fancier's disease or lung J67.2
Birth
- abnormal NEC, affecting fetus or newborn
  P03.9
- complications in mother – *see* Delivery,
  complicated
- defect – *see* Anomaly
- delayed, fetus P03.8
- difficult NEC, affecting fetus or newborn
  P03.9
- forced NEC, affecting fetus or newborn
  P03.8
- forceps, affecting fetus or newborn P03.2
- immature (between 28 and 37 completed
  weeks) P07.3
- - extremely (less than 28 completed
  weeks) P07.2
- inattention, at or after T74.0
- induced, affecting fetus or newborn P03.8
- injury P15.9
- - basal ganglia P11.1
- - brachial plexus NEC P14.3
- - brain (compression) (pressure) P11.2
- - central nervous system NEC P11.9
- - cerebellum P11.1

Birth—*continued*
- injury—*continued*
- - cerebral hemorrhage P10.1
- - external genitalia P15.5
- - eye P15.3
- - face P15.4
- - fracture
- - - bone P13.9
- - - - specified NEC P13.8
- - - clavicle P13.4
- - - femur P13.2
- - - humerus P13.3
- - - long bone, except femur P13.3
- - - radius and ulna P13.3
- - - skull P13.0
- - - spine P11.5
- - - tibia and fibula P13.3
- - intracranial P11.2
- - - laceration or hemorrhage P10.9
- - - - specified NEC P10.8
- - intraventricular hemorrhage P10.2
- - laceration
- - - brain P10.1
- - - - by scalpel P15.8
- - - peripheral nerve P14.9
- - liver P15.0
- - meninges
- - - brain P11.1
- - - spinal cord P11.5
- - nerve
- - - brachial plexus P14.3
- - - cranial NEC (except facial) P11.4
- - - facial P11.3
- - - peripheral P14.9
- - - phrenic (paralysis) P14.2
- - penis P15.5
- - scalp P12.9
- - scalpel wound P15.8
- - scrotum P15.5
- - skull NEC P13.1
- - - fracture P13.0
- - specified type NEC P15.8
- - spinal cord P11.5
- - spine P11.5
- - spleen P15.1
- - sternomastoid (hematoma) P15.2
- - subarachnoid hemorrhage P10.3
- - subcutaneous fat necrosis P15.6
- - subdural hemorrhage P10.0
- - tentorial tear P10.4
- - testes P15.5
- - vulva P15.5
- instrumental NEC, affecting fetus or
  newborn P03.8

77

Birth—*continued*
- lack of care, at or after T74.0
- multiple, affecting fetus or newborn
  P01.5
- neglect, at or after T74.0
- palsy or paralysis, newborn, NEC (birth
  injury) P14.9
- post-term (42 weeks or more) P08.2
- precipitate, affecting fetus or newborn
  P03.5
- premature (infant) P07.3
- prolonged, affecting fetus or newborn
  P03.8
- retarded, affecting fetus or newborn
  P03.8
- shock, newborn P96.8
- trauma – *see* Birth, injury
- twin, affecting fetus or newborn P01.5
- vacuum extractor, affecting fetus or
  newborn P03.3
- ventouse, affecting fetus or newborn
  P03.3
- weight
- – low (between 1000 and 2499 grams)
  P07.1
- – – extremely (999 grams or less) P07.0
- – 4500 grams or more P08.0
Birthmark Q82.5
Bisalbuminemia E88.0
Biskra's button B55.1
Bite(s)
- amphibian (venomous) T63.8
- animal (*see also* Wound, open) T14.1
- – multiple T01.9
- – venomous T63.9
- – – specified NEC T63.8
- arthropod NEC T63.4
- centipede T63.4
- chigger B88.0
- flea – *see* Injury, superficial
- human (open wound) (*see also* Wound,
  open) T14.1
- insect (nonvenomous) (*see also* Injury,
  superficial) T14.0
- – venomous T63.4
- lizard (venomous) T63.1
- marine animal (venomous) NEC T63.6
- poisonous (*see also* Bite(s), venomous)
  T63.9
- reptile NEC T63.1
- – nonvenomous – *see* Wound, open
- scorpion T63.2
- sea-snake (venomous) T63.0
- snake T63.0

Bite(s)—*continued*
- snake—*continued*
- – nonvenomous – *see* Wound, open
- spider (venomous) T63.3
- – nonvenomous (*see also* Injury,
  superficial) T14.0
- venomous T63.9
- – specified NEC T63.8
Biting, cheek or lip K13.1
Biventricular failure (heart) I50.0
Black
- eye S00.1
- hairy tongue K14.3
- lung J60
Blackfan-Diamond anemia or syndrome
  D61.0
Blackhead L70.0
Blackout R55
Bladder – *see* condition
Blast (air) (hydraulic) (immersion)
  (underwater)
- blindness S05.8
- injury T14.8
- – abdomen or thorax – *see* Injury, by site
- – syndrome NEC T70.8
Blastoma (M8000/3) – *see* Neoplasm,
  malignant
- pulmonary (M8972/3) – *see* Neoplasm,
  lung, malignant
Blastomycosis, blastomycotic B40.9
- Brazilian (*see also*
  Paracoccidioidomycosis) B41.9
- cutaneous B40.3† L99.8*
- disseminated B40.7
- European (*see also* Cryptococcosis)
  B45.9
- generalized B40.7
- keloidal B48.0
- North American B40.9
- primary pulmonary B40.0† J99.8*
- pulmonary B40.2† J99.8*
- – acute B40.0† J99.8*
- – chronic B40.1† J99.8*
- skin B40.3† L99.8*
- South American (*see also*
  Paracoccidioidomycosis) B41.9
- specified NEC B40.8
Bleb(s) R23.8
- emphysematous (lung) J43.9
- endophthalmitis H59.8
- inflamed (infected), postprocedural
  H59.8
- lung (ruptured) J43.9
- – fetus or newborn P25.8

Blebitis, postprocedural H59.8
Bleeder (familial) (hereditary) (*see also*
Defect, coagulation) D68.9
Bleeding (*see also* Hemorrhage) R58
– atonic, following delivery O72.1
– capillary I78.8
– – puerperal O72.2
– contact (postcoital) N93.0
– familial (*see also* Defect, coagulation)
D68.9
– following intercourse N93.0
– hemorrhoids NEC I84.8
– intermenstrual (regular) N92.3
– – irregular N92.1
– irregular N92.6
– ovulation N92.3
– postclimacteric N95.0
– postcoital N93.0
– postmenopausal N95.0
– postoperative T81.0
– puberty (excessive, with onset of
menstrual periods) N92.2
– rectum, rectal K62.5
– – newborn P54.2
– tendencies (*see also* Defect, coagulation)
D68.9
– tooth socket (post-extraction) T81.0
– umbilical stump P51.9
– uterus, uterine NEC N93.9
– – climacteric N92.4
– – dysfunctional or functional N93.8
– – menopausal N92.4
– – preclimacteric or premenopausal N92.4
– – unrelated to menstrual cycle N93.9
– vagina, vaginal (abnormal) N93.9
– – dysfunctional or functional N93.8
– – newborn P54.6
– vicarious N94.8
Blennorrhagia, blennorrhagic – *see*
Gonorrhea
Blennorrhea (acute) (chronic) (*see also*
Gonorrhea) A54.9
– lower genitourinary tract (gonococcal)
A54.0
– neonatorum (gonococcal ophthalmia)
A54.3† H13.1*
Blepharelosis H02.0
**Blepharitis (angularis) (ciliaris) (eyelid)
(marginal) (nonulcerative) (squamous)
(ulcerative)** H01.0
– zoster (herpes) B02.3† H03.1*
Blepharochalasis H02.3
– congenital Q10.0
Blepharoclonus H02.5

Blepharoconjunctivitis H10.5
Blepharophimosis (eyelid) H02.5
– congenital Q10.3
Blepharoptosis H02.4
– congenital Q10.0
Blepharopyorrhea, gonococcal A54.3†
H03.1*
Blepharospasm G24.5
Blighted ovum O02.0
Blind – *see also* Blindness
– bronchus (congenital) Q32.4
– loop syndrome K90.2
– – congenital Q43.8
– sac, fallopian tube (congenital) Q50.6
– spot, enlarged H53.4
– tract or tube, congenital NEC – *see*
Atresia, by site
**Blindness (acquired) (binocular)
(congenital) (both eyes)** H54.0
– blast S05.8
– color H53.5
– concussion S05.8
– day H53.1
– due to injury (current episode) S05.9
– – sequelae T90.4
– eclipse (total) H31.0
– emotional (hysterical) F44.6
– hysterical F44.6
– mind R48.8
– monocular H54.4
– night H53.6
– – vitamin A deficiency E50.5
– one eye (other eye normal) H54.4
– – low vision, other eye H54.4
– psychic F44.6
– river B73† H45.1*
– snow H16.1
– sun, solar H31.0
– transient H53.1
– traumatic (current episode) S05.9
– uremic N19
– word (developmental) F81.0
Blister – *see also* Injury, superficial
– beetle dermatitis L24.8
– due to burn – *see* Burn, by site, second
degree
– fever B00.1
– multiple, skin, nontraumatic R23.8
Bloating R14
Bloch-Sulzberger disease or syndrome
Q82.3
Block
– alveolocapillary J84.1
– arborization (heart) I45.5

Block—*continued*
- arrhythmic I45.9
- atrioventricular (incomplete) (partial) I44.3
- - complete I44.2
- - first degree I44.0
- - second degree (types I and II) I44.1
- - specified NEC I44.3
- - types I and II I44.1
- auriculoventricular – *see* Block, atrioventricular
- bifascicular I45.2
- bundle-branch (complete) (false) (incomplete) I45.4
- - left I44.7
- - - hemiblock I44.6
- - - - anterior I44.4
- - - - posterior I44.5
- - right I45.1
- - Wilson's type I45.1
- cardiac I45.9
- conduction I45.9
- fascicular (left) I44.6
- - anterior I44.4
- - posterior I44.5
- - right I45.0
- foramen Magendie (acquired) G91.1
- - congenital Q03.1
- - - with spina bifida (*see also* Spina bifida, with hydrocephalus) Q05.4
- heart I45.9
- - complete (atrioventricular) I44.2
- - congenital Q24.6
- - first degree (atrioventricular) I44.0
- - second degree (atrioventricular) I44.1
- - specified type NEC I45.5
- - third degree (atrioventricular) I44.2
- hepatic vein I82.0
- intraventricular (nonspecific) I45.4
- kidney (*see also* Failure, kidney) N19
- - postcystoscopic or postprocedural N99.0
- Möbitz (types I and II) I44.1
- myocardial (*see also* Block, heart) I45.9
- nodal I45.5
- organ or site, congenital NEC – *see* Atresia, by site
- portal (vein) I81
- sinoatrial I45.5
- sinoauricular I45.5
- trifascicular I45.3
- tubal N97.1
- vein NEC I82.9
- Wenckebach (types I and II) I44.1

Blockage – *see* Obstruction
Blocq's disease F44.4
Blood
- constituents, abnormal R78.9
- disease D75.9
- dyscrasia D75.9
- - fetus or newborn P61.9
- - puerperal, postpartum O72.3
- flukes NEC (*see also* Schistosomiasis) B65.9
- in
- - feces (*see also* Melena) K92.1
- - - occult R19.5
- - urine (*see also* Hematuria) R31
- mole O02.0
- pressure
- - decreased, due to shock following injury T79.4
- - examination only Z01.3
- - fluctuating I99
- - high (*see also* Hypertension) I10
- - - incidental reading, without diagnosis of hypertension R03.0
- - low (*see also* Hypotension) I95.9
- - - incidental reading, without diagnosis of hypotension R03.1
- spitting (*see also* Hemoptysis) R04.2
- staining cornea H18.0
- tranfusion (session) Z51.3
- - reaction or complication – *see* Complications, transfusion
- - without reported diagnosis Z51.3
- vessel rupture – *see* Hemorrhage
- vomiting (*see also* Hematemesis) K92.0
Blood-forming organs, disease D75.9
Bloodgood's disease N60.1
Bloom (-Machacek) (-Torre) syndrome Q82.8
Blount's disease or osteochondrosis M92.5
Blue
- baby Q24.9
- dome cyst (breast) N60.0
- dot cataract Q12.0
- nevus (M8780/0) D22.9
- sclera Q13.5
- - with fragility of bone and deafness Q78.0
Blueness – *see* Cyanosis
Blushing (abnormal) (excessive) R23.2
Boarder, hospital NEC Z76.4
- accompanying sick person Z76.3
Bockhart's impetigo L01.0

Bodechtel-Guttman disease (subacute sclerosing panencephalitis) A81.1
Body, bodies
- Aschoff's (*see also* Myocarditis, rheumatic) I09.0
- cytoid (retina) H34.2
- drusen (degenerative) (macula) (retinal) H35.3
- − optic disk H47.3
- foreign − *see* Foreign body
- loose
- − − joint, except knee M24.0
- − − − knee M23.4
- − − sheath, tendon M67.8
- Mallory's R89.7
- Mooser's A75.2
- rice M24.0
- − − knee M23.4
Boeck's
- disease or sarcoid (*see also* Sarcoidosis) D86.9
- lupoid (miliary) D86.3
Boggy
- cervix N88.8
- uterus N85.8
Boil (*see also* Abscess, by site) L02.9
- Aleppo B55.1
- Baghdad B55.1
- corpus cavernosum N48.2
- Delhi B55.1
- eyelid H00.0
- lacrimal
- − gland H04.0
- − − passages (duct) (sac) H04.3
- Natal B55.1
- orbit, orbital H05.0
- penis N48.2
- tropical B55.1
Bombé, iris H21.4
Bone − *see condition*
Bonnevie-Ullrich syndrome Q87.1
Bonnier's syndrome H81.8
Bonvale dam fever T73.3
Bony block of joint M24.6
Bornholm disease B33.0
Boston exanthem A88.0
Botulism (foodborne intoxication) A05.1
- infant A05.1
- wound A05.1
Bouba (*see also* Yaws) A66.9
Bouchard's nodes (with arthropathy) M15.2

Bouffée délirante (without symptoms of schizophrenia) F23.0
- with symptoms of schizophrenia F23.1
Bouillaud's disease or syndrome I01.8
Bourneville's disease Q85.1
Boutonnière deformity (finger) M20.0
Bouveret(-Hoffmann) syndrome I47.9
Bovine heart − *see* Hypertrophy, cardiac
Bowel − *see condition*
Bowen's
- dermatosis (precancerous) (M8081/2) − *see* Neoplasm, skin, in situ
- disease (M8081/2) − *see* Neoplasm, skin, in situ
- epithelioma (M8081/2) − *see* Neoplasm, skin, in situ
- type
- − epidermoid carcinoma in situ (M8081/2) − *see* Neoplasm, skin, in situ
- − intraepidermal squamous cell carcinoma (M8081/2) − *see* Neoplasm, skin, in situ
Bowing
- femur M21.8
- − congenital Q68.3
- fibula M21.8
- − congenital Q68.4
- forearm M21.8
- leg(s), long bones, congenital Q68.5
- radius M21.8
- tibia M21.8
- − congenital Q68.4
Bowleg(s) (acquired) M21.1
- congenital Q68.5
- rachitic E64.3
Boyd's dysentery A03.2
Brachial − *see condition*
Brachycardia R00.1
Brachycephaly Q75.0
Bradley's disease A08.1
Bradyarrhythmia, cardiac I49.8
Bradycardia (sinoatrial) (sinus) (vagal) R00.1
- fetal − *see* Distress, fetal
Bradypnea R06.8
Bradytachycardia I49.5
Brailsford's disease or osteochondrosis M92.1
Brain − *see also condition*
- syndrome − *see* Syndrome, brain
Branched-chain amino-acid disorder E71.2
Branchial − *see condition*
- cartilage, congenital Q18.2

Branchiogenic remnant (in neck) Q18.0
Brash (water) R12
Brass-founders' ague T56.8
Bravais-jacksonian epilepsy G40.1
Braziers' disease T56.8
Break, retina (without detachment) H33.3
– with retinal detachment H33.0
Breakdown
– device, graft or implant (*see also*
  Complications, by site and type,
  mechanical) T85.8
– – arterial graft NEC T82.3
– – – coronary (bypass) T82.2
– – breast T85.4
– – catheter NEC T85.6
– – – dialysis (renal) T82.4
– – – – intraperitoneal T85.6
– – – infusion NEC T82.5
– – – – spinal (epidural) (subdural) T85.6
– – – urinary (indwelling) T83.0
– – corneal T85.3
– – electronic (electrode) (pulse generator)
  (stimulator)
– – – bone T84.3
– – – cardiac T82.1
– – – nervous system (brain) (peripheral
    nerve) (spinal) T85.1
– – – urinary T83.1
– – fixation, internal (orthopedic) NEC
  T84.2
– – – bones of limb T84.1
– – gastrointestinal (bile duct) (esophagus)
  T85.5
– – genital NEC T83.4
– – – intrauterine contraceptive device
    T83.3
– – heart NEC T82.5
– – – valve (prosthesis) T82.0
– – – – graft T82.2
– – joint prosthesis T84.0
– – ocular (corneal graft) (orbital implant)
  NEC T85.3
– – – intraocular lens T85.2
– – orthopedic NEC T84.4
– – – bone graft T84.3
– – specified NEC T85.6
– – urinary NEC T83.1
– – – graft T83.2
– – vascular NEC T82.5
– – ventricular intracranial shunt T85.0
– nervous F48.8
– perineum (obstetric) O90.1
Breast – *see condition*

Breath
– foul R19.6
– holder, child R06.8
– holding spells R06.8
– shortness R06.0
Breathing
– exercises Z50.1
– labored (*see also* Hyperventilation) R06.4
– mouth R06.5
– periodic R06.3
Breathlessness R06.8
Breda's disease (*see also* Yaws) A66.9
Breech
– delivery NEC O83.1
– – affecting fetus or newborn P03.0
– – assisted NEC O83.1
– extraction O83.0
– – affecting fetus or newborn P03.0
– presentation (mother) O32.1
– – before labor, affecting fetus or newborn
    P01.7
– – causing obstructed labor O64.1
– – during labor, affecting fetus or newborn
    P03.0
Breisky's disease N90.4
Brennemann's syndrome I88.0
Brenner
– tumor (benign) (M9000/0) D27
– – borderline malignancy (M9000/1)
    D39.1
– – malignant (M9000/3) C56
– – proliferating (M9000/1) D39.1
Bretonneau's disease or angina A36.0
Breus' mole O02.0
Brevicollis Q76.4
Bright's
– disease (*see also* Nephritis) N05.-
– – arteriosclerotic (*see also* Hypertension,
    kidney) I12.9
Brill(-Zinsser) disease A75.1
Brill-Symmers' disease C82.9
Briquet's disorder or syndrome F45.0
Brissaud's infantilism or dwarfism E23.0
Brittle
– bones disease Q78.0
– nails L60.3
– – congenital Q84.6
Broad ligament – *see also condition*
– laceration syndrome N83.8
Broad- or floating-betalipoproteinemia
  E78.2
Brock's syndrome J98.1
Brodie's abscess or disease M86.8

Broken
- arches M21.4
- – – congenital Q66.5
- – arm T10
- – – meaning upper limb – *see* Fracture, limb, upper
- – – upper – *see* Fracture, arm, upper
- – back – *see* Fracture, vertebra
- – bone – *see* Fracture
- – implant or internal device – *see* Complications, by site and type, mechanical
- – leg T12
- – – lower – *see* Fracture, leg, lower
- – – meaning lower limb – *see* Fracture, limb, lower
- – nose S02.2
- – tooth, teeth S02.5

Bromhidrosis, bromidrosis L75.0
Bromidism, bromism
- acute, overdose or wrong substance given or taken T42.6
- chronic (dependence) F13.2
- correct substance properly administered G92

Bromidrosiphobia F40.2
Bronchi, bronchial – *see condition*
Bronchiectasis (cylindrical) (diffuse) (fusiform) (localized) (saccular) J47
- congenital Q33.4
- tuberculous NEC (*see also* Tuberculosis, pulmonary) A16.2

Bronchiolectasis – *see* Bronchiectasis
Bronchiolitis (acute) (infective) (subacute) J21.9
- with
- – bronchospasm or obstruction J21.9
- – influenza, flu or grippe (*see also* Influenza, with, respiratory manifestations) J11.1
- chemical (chronic) J68.4
- chronic (fibrosing) (obliterative) J44.8
- due to
- – external agent – *see* Bronchitis, acute or subacute, due to
- – human metapneumovirus J21.1
- – respiratory syncytial virus J21.0
- – specified organism NEC J21.8
- fibrosa obliterans J44.8
- influenzal (*see also* Influenza, with, respiratory manifestations) J11.1
- obliterative (chronic) (subacute) J44.8
- – due to chemicals, gases, fumes or vapors (inhalation) J68.4

Bronchitis (diffuse) (fibrinous) (hypostatic) (infective) (membranous) (with tracheitis) (15 years of age and above) J40
- with
- – influenza, flu or grippe (*see also* Influenza, with, respiratory manifestations) J11.1
- – obstruction (airway) (lung) J44.8
- acute or subacute (with bronchospasm or obstruction) J20.9
- – chemical (due to gases, fumes or vapors) J68.0
- – due to
- – – coxsackievirus J20.3
- – – echovirus J20.7
- – – Haemophilus influenzae J20.1
- – – human metapneumovirus J20.8
- – – Mycoplasma pneumoniae J20.0
- – – parainfluenza virus J20.4
- – – radiation J70.0
- – – respiratory syncytial virus J20.5
- – – rhinovirus J20.6
- – – specified organism NEC J20.8
- – – streptococcus J20.2
- – viral NEC J20.8
- allergic (acute) – *see* Asthma
- arachidic T17.5
- asthmatic – *see* Asthma
- capillary (*see also* Pneumonia, broncho) J21.9
- caseous (tuberculous) A16.4
- catarrhal (15 years of age and above) J40
- – acute – *see* Bronchitis, acute or subacute
- – chronic J41.0
- – under 15 years of age J20.9
- chemical (acute) (subacute) J68.0
- – chronic J68.4
- chronic J42
- – with
- – – airways obstruction J44.8
- – – tracheitis (chronic) J42
- – asthmatic (obstructive) J44.8
- – chemical (due to fumes or vapors) J68.4
- – due to
- – – chemicals, gases, fumes or vapors (inhalation) J68.4
- – – radiation J70.1
- – emphysematous J44.8
- – mucopurulent J41.1
- – obliterans J44.8
- – obstructive J44.8

Bronchitis—*continued*
- chronic—*continued*
- - purulent J41.1
- - simple J41.0
- croupous (*see also* Bronchitis, acute or subacute) J20.9
  due to gases, fumes or vapors (chemical) J68.0
- emphysematous (obstructive) J44.8
- exudative (*see also* Bronchitis, acute or subacute) J20.9
- fetid J41.1
- grippal (*see also* Influenza, with, respiratory manifestations) J11.1
- in those under 15 years of age – *see also* Bronchitis, acute or subacute
- - chronic – *see* Bronchitis, chronic
- influenzal (*see also* Influenza, with, respiratory manifestations) J11.1
- membranous, acute or subacute (*see also* Bronchitis, acute or subacute) J20.-
- mixed simple and mucopurulent J41.8
- mucopurulent (chronic) (recurrent) J41.1
- - acute or subacute J20.9
- - and simple (mixed) J41.8
- obliterans (chronic) J44.8
- obstructive (chronic) (diffuse) J44.8
- pneumococcal, acute or subacute J20.2
- purulent (chronic) (recurrent) J41.1
- - acute or subacute (*see also* Bronchitis, acute or subacute) J20.9
- senile (chronic) J42
- septic, acute or subacute (*see also* Bronchitis, acute or subacute) J20.9
- simple and mucopurulent (mixed) J41.8
- smokers' J41.0
- spirochetal NEC A69.8† J99.8*
- subacute – *see* Bronchitis, acute or subacute
- suppurative (chronic) J41.1
- - acute or subacute (*see also* Bronchitis, acute or subacute) J20.-
- tuberculous A16.4
- - with bacteriological and histological confirmation A15.5
- under 15 years of age – *see also* Bronchitis, acute or subacute
- - chronic – *see* Bronchitis, chronic
- viral NEC, acute or subacute (*see also* Bronchitis, acute or subacute) J20.8
Bronchoaspergillosis B44.1† J99.8*
Broncholithiasis J98.0
- tuberculous NEC A16.4

Broncholithiasis—*continued*
- tuberculous NEC—*continued*
- - with bacteriological and histological confirmation A15.5
Bronchomalacia J98.0
- congenital Q32.2
Bronchomycosis NEC B49† J99.8*
- candidal B37.8† J99.8*
Bronchopleuropneumonia – *see* Pneumonia, broncho
Bronchopneumonia (*see also* Pneumonia, broncho) J18.0
Bronchopneumonitis – *see* Pneumonia, broncho
Bronchopulmonary – *see condition*
Bronchopulmonitis – *see* Pneumonia, broncho
Bronchorrhagia – *see* Hemoptysis
Bronchorrhea J98.0
- chronic (infective) (purulent) J42
Bronchospasm J98.0
- with
- - bronchiolitis, acute J21.9
- - bronchitis, acute (conditions in J20.-) (*see also* Bronchitis, acute or subacute) J20.9
Bronchospirochetosis A69.8
- Castellani A69.8
Bronchostenosis J98.0
Bronchus – *see condition*
Bronze baby syndrome P83.8
Brooke's tumor (M8100/0) – *see* Neoplasm, skin, benign
Brown's sheath syndrome H50.6
Brown-Séquard disease, paralysis or syndrome G83.8
Bruce septicemia A23.0
Brucella, brucellosis (infection) A23.9
- abortus A23.1
- canis A23.3
- melitensis A23.0
- mixed A23.8
- sepsis A23.9
- - melitensis A23.0
- - specified NEC A23.8
- suis A23.2
Bruck-de Lange disease Q87.1
Bruck's disease M21.8
Brugsch's syndrome Q82.8
Bruise (skin surface intact) (*see also* Contusion) T14.0
- with open wound – *see* Wound, open
- fetus or newborn P54.5
- internal organ – *see* Injury, by site

Bruise—*continued*
- scalp, due to birth injury, newborn P12.3
- umbilical cord O69.5
- – affecting fetus or newborn P02.6
Bruit (arterial) R09.8
- cardiac R01.1
Brushburn – *see* Burn, by site
Bruton's X-linked agammaglobulinemia
D80.0
Bruxism F45.8
Bubbly lung syndrome P27.0
Bubo I88.8
- blennorrhagic (gonococcal) A54.8
- chancroidal A57
- climatic A55
- due to
- – Haemophilus ducreyi A57
- – Yersinia pestis A20.0
- gonococcal A54.8
- inguinal (nonspecific) I88.8
- – chancroidal A57
- – climatic A55
- – due to Haemophilus ducreyi A57
- – infective I88.8
- – venereal A64
- scrofulous (tuberculous) A18.2
- soft chancre A57
- suppurating (*see also* Lymphadenitis, acute) L04.9
- syphilitic (primary) A51.0
- – congenital A50.0
- tropical A55
- venereal A64
- virulent (chancroidal) A57
Bubonocele – *see* Hernia, inguinal
Buccal – *see condition*
Buchanan's disease or osteochondrosis
M91.0
Bucket-handle fracture or tear (semilunar cartilage) (*see also* Tear, meniscus)
S83.2
Budd-Chiari syndrome I82.0
Budgerigar fancier's disease or lung J67.2
Buerger's disease I73.1
Bulbar – *see condition*
Bulbus cordis (left ventricle) (persistent)
Q21.8
Bulimia (nervosa) F50.2
- atypical F50.3
- normal weight F50.3
Bulky
- stools R19.5
- uterus N85.2

Bulla(e) R23.8
- lung J43.9
- – fetus or newborn P25.8
Bullet wound – *see also* Wound, open
- fracture – *code as* Fracture, by site
- internal organ – *see* Injury, by site
Bundle
- branch block (complete) (false) (incomplete) – *see* Block, bundle-branch
- of His – *see condition*
Bunion M20.1
Buphthalmia, buphthalmos (congenital)
Q15.0
Burdwan fever B55.0
Bürger-Grütz disease or syndrome E78.3
Buried roots K08.3
Burkholderia NEC A49.8 – *Cepacia*
- mallei A24.0
- – as the cause of disease classified elsewhere B96.8
- pseudomallei (*see also* Melioidosis) A24.4
- – as the cause of disease classified elsewhere B96.8
Burkitt
- cell leukemia C91.8
- lymphoma (malignant) C83.7
- – resulting from HIV disease B21.1
- – small noncleaved, diffuse C83.7
- – undifferentiated C83.7
- tumor C83.7
- type
- – acute lymphoblastic leukemia (M9826/3) C91.8
- – undifferentiated (M9687/3) C83.7
Burn (electricity) (flame) (hot gas, liquid or object) (radiation) (steam) (thermal)
T30.0

Note: The following fourth-character subdivisions are for use with categories T20-T25, T29 and T30: *multiple burns code to highest deg.*
  - .0 Unspecified degree
  - .1 First degree [Erythema] *Superficial*
  - .2 Second degree [Blisters, epidermal loss] *Partial thickness*
  - .3 Third degree [Deep necrosis of underlying tissue][Full-thickness skin loss] *Full thickness*
- abdomen, abdominal (muscle) (wall) T21.-
- acid (caustic) (external) (internal) – *see* Corrosion, by site
- alimentary tract NEC T28.2

Burn—*continued*
- alkaline (caustic) (external) (internal) – *see* Corrosion, by site
- ankle (and foot) T25.-
- – with leg T29.-
- anus T21.-
- arm (lower) (upper) – *see* Burn, limb, upper
- axilla T22.-
- back (lower) T21.-
- blisters – *code as* Burn, by site, with fourth character .2
- breast(s) T21.-
- buttock(s) T21.-
- caustic acid or alkaline – *see* Corrosion, by site
- cervix T28.3
- chemical (acids) (alkalines) (caustics) (external) (internal) – *see* Corrosion, by site
- chest wall T21.-
- colon T28.2
- conjunctiva (and cornea) T26.1
- – chemical T26.6
- cornea (and conjunctiva) T26.1
- – chemical T26.6
- corrosion (external) (internal) – *see* Corrosion, by site
- deep necrosis of underlying tissue – *code as* Burn, by site, with fourth character .3
- due to ingested chemical agent – *see* Corrosion, by site
- ear (auricle) (canal) (drum) (external) T20.-
- entire body T29.-
- epidermal loss – *code as* Burn, by site, with fourth character .2
- erythema, erythematous – *code as* Burn, by site, with fourth character .1
- esophagus T28.1
- extremity – *see* Burn, limb
- eye(s) and adnexa T26.4
- – with resulting rupture and destruction of eyeball T26.2
- – specified part (*see also* Burn, by site) T26.3
- eyeball – *see* Burn, eye(s) and adnexa
- eyelid(s) T26.0
- – chemical T26.5
- face T20.-
- finger(s) (nail) (subungual) T23.-
- first degree – *code as* Burn, by site, with fourth character .1
- flank T21.-

Burn—*continued*
- foot (and ankle) (phalanges) T25.-
- – with leg T29.-
- fourth degree – *code as* Burn, by site, with fourth character .3
- friction – *see* Burn, by site
- from swallowing caustic or corrosive substance NEC – *see* Corrosion, by site
- full-thickness skin loss – *code as* Burn, by site, with fourth character .3
- gastrointestinal tract NEC T28.2
- – from swallowing caustic or corrosive substance T28.7
- genitourinary organs
- – external T21.-
- – internal T28.3
- – – from caustic or corrosive substance T28.8
- groin T21.-
- hand(s) (phalanges) (and wrist) T23.-
- – with arm T29.-
- head (and face) (and neck) T20.-
- – eye(s) only – *see* Burn, eye(s) and adnexa
- – – specified part – *see* Burn, by site
- hip(s) T24.-
- inhalation NEC (*see also* Burn, by site) T27.3
- – caustic or corrosive substance (fumes) – *see* Corrosion, by site
- internal organs NEC (*see also* Burn, by site) T28.4
- – from caustic or corrosive substance (swallowing) NEC (*see also* Corrosion, by site) T28.9
- interscapular region T21.-
- intestine (large) (small) T28.2
- knee T24.-
- labium (majus) (minus) T21.-
- lacrimal apparatus, duct, gland or sac T26.3
- – – chemical T26.8
- larynx T27.0
- – with lung T27.1
- leg(s) (lower) (upper) – *see* Burn, limb(s), lower
- lightning – *see* Burn, by site
- limb(s)
- – lower (except ankle or foot alone) T24.-
- – – with ankle and foot T29.-
- – upper (except wrist and hand alone) T22.-
- – – with wrist and hand T29.-

Burn—*continued*
- lip(s) T20.-
- lower back T21.-
- lung (with larynx and trachea) T27.1
- mouth T28.0
- multiple body regions (sites classifiable to more than one category in T20-T28) T29.0
- – first degree (only, without second or third degree) T29.1
- – second degree (with first degree) T29.2
- – third degree (with first and second degree) T29.3
- neck T20.-
- nose (septum) T20.-
- ocular adnexa T26.4
- palm(s) T23.-
- partial thickness skin damage – *code as* Burn, by site, with fourth character .2
- pelvis T21.-
- penis T21.-
- perineum T21.-
- periocular area T26.0
- – chemical T26.5
- pharynx T28.0
- rectum T28.2
- respiratory tract T27.3
- – specified part NEC T27.2
- scalp T20.-
- scapular region T22.-
- sclera T26.3
- scrotum T21.-
- second degree – *code as* Burn, by site, with fourth character .2
- shoulder(s) T22.-
- skin NEC T30.0
- stomach T28.2
- temple T20.-
- testis T21.-
- thigh(s) T24.-
- third degree – *code as* Burn, by site, with fourth character .3
- thorax (external) T21.-
- throat (meaning pharynx) T28.0
- thumb(s) T23.-
- toe(nail) (subungual) T25.-
- tongue T28.0
- tonsil(s) T28.0
- total body T29.-
- trachea T27.0
- – with lung T27.1
- trunk T21.-

Burn—*continued*
- unspecified site with extent of body surface involved specified
- – less than 10 per cent T31.0
- – 10-19 per cent T31.1
- – 20-29 per cent T31.2
- – 30-39 per cent T31.3
- – 40-49 per cent T31.4
- – 50-59 per cent T31.5
- – 60-69 per cent T31.6
- – 70-79 per cent T31.7
- – 80-89 per cent T31.8
- – 90 per cent or more T31.9
- uterus T28.3
- vagina T28.3
- vulva T21.-
- wrist (and hand) T23.-
- – with arm T29.-

Burnett's syndrome E83.5
Burning
- feet syndrome E53.9
- sensation R20.8
- tongue K14.6
Burn-out (state) Z73.0
Burns' disease or osteochondrosis M92.1
Bursa – *see condition*
Bursitis M71.9
- Achilles M76.6
- adhesive M71.5
- ankle M76.8
- calcaneal M77.5
- due to use, overuse or pressure M70.9
- – specified NEC M70.8
- Duplay's M75.0
- elbow NEC M70.3
- finger M70.8
- foot M77.5
- gonococcal A54.4† M73.0*
- gouty M10.0
- hand M70.1
- hip NEC M70.7
- infective NEC M71.1
- ischial M70.7
- knee NEC M70.5
- occupational NEC M70.9
- olecranon M70.2
- pharyngeal J39.1
- popliteal M70.5
- prepatellar M70.4
- radiohumeral M77.8
- rheumatoid M06.2
- scapulohumeral M75.5
- semimembranous muscle (knee) M70.5
- shoulder M75.5

Bursitis—*continued*
- specified NEC M71.5
- subacromial M75.5
- subcoracoid M75.5
- subdeltoid M75.5
- syphilitic A52.7† M73.1*
- Thornwaldt, Tornwaldt J39.2
- tibial collateral M76.4
- toe M77.5
- trochanteric (area) M70.6
- wrist M70.1

Bursopathy (*see also* Bursitis) M71.9
- specified NEC M71.8

Burst stitches or sutures (complication of surgery) T81.3

Buruli ulcer A31.1
Bury's disease L95.1
Buschke's
- disease B45.3† M90.2*
- scleredema M34.8
Busse-Buschke disease B45.3† M90.2*
Buttock – *see condition*
Button
- Biskra B55.1
- Delhi B55.1
- oriental B55.1
Buttonhole deformity (finger) M20.0
Bwamba fever A92.8
Byssinosis J66.0
Bywaters' syndrome T79.5

C

Cachexia R64
- cancerous (M8000/3) C80.-
- cardiac – *see* Disease, heart
- due to malnutrition E41
- heart – *see* Disease, heart
- hypophyseal E23.0
- hypopituitary E23.0
- lead T56.0
- malignant (M8000/3) C80.-
- marsh (*see also* Malaria) B54
- nervous F48.0
- old age R54
- paludal (*see also* Malaria) B54
- pituitary E23.0
- saturnine T56.0
- senile R54
- Simmonds' E23.0
- splenica D73.0
- strumipriva E03.4
- tuberculous NEC (*see also* Tuberculosis) A16.9
Café au lait spots L81.3
Caffey's syndrome M89.8
Caisson disease T70.3
Cake kidney Q63.1
Caked breast (postpartum) (puerperal) O92.2
Calabar swelling B74.3
Calcaneo-apophysitis M92.8
Calcareous – *see* condition
Calcicosis J62.8
Calcification
- adrenal (capsule) (gland) E27.4
- – tuberculous B90.8† E35.1*
- aorta I70.0
- artery (annular) – *see* Arteriosclerosis
- auricle (ear) H61.1
- basal ganglia G23.8
- bladder N32.8
- brain (cortex) – *see* Calcification, cerebral
- bronchus J98.0
- bursa NEC M71.4
- – shoulder M75.3
- cerebral (cortex) G93.8
- – artery I67.2
- cervix (uteri) N88.8
- choroid plexus G93.8
- conjunctiva H11.1
- corpus cavernosum (penis) N48.8

Calcification—*continued*
- cortex (brain) – *see* Calcification, cerebral
- dental pulp (nodular) K04.2
- dentinal papilla K00.4
- falx cerebri G96.1
- gallbladder K82.8
- general E83.5
- heart (*see also* Degeneration, myocardial) I51.5
- – valve – *see* Endocarditis
- intervertebral cartilage or disk (postinfective) M51.8
- intracranial – *see* Calcification, cerebral
- joint M25.8
- kidney N28.8
- – tuberculous B90.1† N29.1*
- larynx (senile) J38.7
- lens H26.8
- lung (active) (postinfectional) J98.4
- – tuberculous B90.9
- lymph gland or node (postinfectional) I89.8
- – tuberculous B90.8
- massive (paraplegic) M61.2
- meninges (cerebral) (spinal) G96.1
- metastatic E83.5
- Mönckeberg's I70.2
- muscle M61.9
- – due to burns M61.3
- – paralytic M61.2
- – specified NEC M61.4
- myocardium, myocardial (*see also* Degeneration, myocardial) I51.5
- ovary N83.8
- pancreas K86.8
- penis N48.8
- periarticular M25.8
- pericardium (*see also* Pericarditis) I31.1
- pineal gland E34.8
- pleura J94.8
- – postinfectional J94.8
- – tuberculous NEC B90.9
- – – with bacteriological and histological confirmation A15.6
- pulpal (dental) (nodular) K04.2
- sclera H15.8
- spleen D73.8
- subcutaneous L94.2
- suprarenal (capsule) (gland) E27.4

Calcification—*continued*
- tendon (sheath) M65.8
- – with bursitis, synovitis or tenosynovitis M65.2
- trachea J39.8
- ureter N28.8
- uterus N85.8
- vitreous H43.2

Calcified – *see* Calcification

Calcinosis (interstitial) (tumoral) (universalis) E83.5
- with Raynaud's phenomenon, esophageal dysfunction, sclerodactyly, telangiectasia (CREST syndrome) M34.1
- circumscripta (skin) L94.2
- cutis L94.2

Calcium
- deposits – *see* Calcification, by site
- metabolism disorder E83.5
- salts or soaps in vitreous (body) H43.2

Calciuria R82.9

Calculi – *see* Calculus

Calculosis, intrahepatic (*see also* Choledocholithiasis) K80.5

Calculus, calculi, calculous
- ampulla of Vater (*see also* Choledocholithiasis) K80.5
- appendix K38.1
- bile duct (common) (hepatic) K80.5
- – with cholangitis K80.3
- biliary K80.2
- – specified NEC K80.8
- bilirubin, multiple (*see also* Cholelithiasis) K80.2
- bladder (diverticulum) (encysted) (impacted) (urinary) N21.0
- bronchus J98.0
- calyx (kidney) (renal) (*see also* Calculus, kidney) N20.0
- – congenital Q63.8
- cholesterol (pure) (solitary) (*see also* Cholelithiasis) K80.2
- common duct (bile) K80.5
- conjunctiva H11.1
- cystic N21.0
- – duct (*see also* Cholelithiasis) K80.2
- dental (subgingival) (supragingival) K03.6
- diverticulum
- – bladder N21.0
- – kidney N20.0
- epididymis N50.8
- gallbladder K80.2
- – with cholecystitis (chronic) K80.1

Calculus, calculi—*continued*
- gallbladder—*continued*
- – with cholecystitis—*continued*
- – – acute K80.0
- hepatic (duct) K80.5
- intestinal (impaction) (obstruction) K56.4
- kidney (impacted) (multiple) (pelvis) (recurrent) (staghorn) N20.0
- – with calculus, ureter – *see* Calculus, ureter, with calculus, kidney
- – congenital Q63.8
- lacrimal passages H04.5
- liver (impacted) K80.5
- lung J98.4
- nephritic (impacted) (recurrent) (*see also* Calculus, kidney) N20.0
- nose J34.8
- pancreas (duct) K86.8
- parotid duct or gland K11.5
- pelvis, encysted (*see also* Calculus, kidney) N20.0
- prostate N42.0
- pulmonary J98.4
- pyelitis (impacted) (recurrent) N20.9
- – with hydronephrosis N13.2
- pyelonephritis (impacted) (recurrent) N20.9
- – with hydronephrosis N13.2
- renal (impacted) (recurrent) (*see also* Calculus, kidney) N20.0
- – congenital Q63.8
- salivary (duct) (gland) K11.5
- seminal vesicle N50.8
- staghorn (*see also* Calculus, kidney) N20.0
- Stensen's duct K11.5
- stomach K31.8
- sublingual duct or gland K11.5
- – congenital Q38.4
- submandibular duct, gland or region K11.5
- suburethral N21.8
- tonsil J35.8
- tooth, teeth (subgingival) (supragingival) K03.6
- tunica vaginalis N50.8
- ureter (impacted) (recurrent) N20.1
- – with
- – – calculus, kidney N20.2
- – – – with hydronephrosis N13.2
- – – – – with infection N13.6
- – – hydronephrosis N13.2
- – – – with infection N13.6
- urethra (impacted) N21.1

Calculus, calculi—*continued*
- urinary (duct) (impacted) (passage) (tract) N20.9
- − − with hydronephrosis N13.2
- − − − with infection N13.6
- − − lower NEC N21.9
- − − − specified NEC N21.8
- vagina N89.8
- vesical (impacted) N21.0
- Wharton's duct K11.5
- xanthine E79.8† N22.8∗
Calicectasis N28.8
California disease B38.9
Callositas, callosity (infected) L84
Callus (infected) L84
- excessive, following fracture – *see* Sequelae, fracture
Calorie deficiency (*see also* Malnutrition) E46
Calvé-Perthes disease M91.1
Calvé's disease M42.0
Calvities (*see also* Alopecia, androgenic) L64.9
Cameroon fever (*see also* Malaria) B54
Camptocormia (hysterical) F44.4
Camurati-Engelmann syndrome Q78.3
Canal – *see also condition*
- atrioventricular common Q21.2
Canaliculitis (acute) (lacrimal) (subacute) H04.3
- Actinomyces A42.8
- chronic H04.4
Canavan's disease E75.2
Cancelled procedure (surgical) Z53.9
- because of
- − − contraindication Z53.0
- − − patient's decision NEC Z53.2
- − − − for reasons of belief or group pressure Z53.1
- − − specified reason NEC Z53.8
- vaccination Z28.9
- − − because of
- − − − contraindication Z28.0
- − − − patient's decision NEC Z28.2
- − − − − for reasons of belief or group pressure Z28.1
- − − − specified reason NEC Z28.8
Cancer (M8000/3) – *see also* Neoplasm, malignant

Note: The term "cancer", when modified by an adjective or adjectival phrase indicating a morphological type, should be coded in the same manner as "carcinoma" with that adjective or phrase. Thus, "squamous cell cancer" should be coded in the same manner as "squamous cell carcinoma", which appears in the list under "Carcinoma".

Cancer(o)phobia F45.2
Cancerous (M8000/3) – *see* Neoplasm, malignant
Cancrum oris A69.0
Candidiasis, candidal B37.9
- balanitis B37.4† N51.2∗
- congenital P37.5
- disseminated B37.8
- endocarditis B37.6† I39.8∗
- intertrigo B37.2
- lung B37.1† J99.8∗
- meningitis B37.5† G02.1∗
- mouth B37.0
- nails B37.2
- neonatal P37.5
- onychia B37.2
- paronychia B37.2
- pneumonia B37.1† J17.2∗
- resulting from HIV disease B20.4
- sepsis B37.7
- skin B37.2
- specified site NEC B37.8
- systemic B37.8
- urethritis B37.4† N37.0∗
- urogenital site NEC B37.4
- vagina B37.3† N77.1∗
- vulva B37.3† N77.1∗
- vulvovaginitis B37.3† N77.1∗
Candidid L30.2
Candidosis – *see* Candidiasis
Candiru infection or infestation B88.8
Canities (premature) L67.1
- congenital Q84.2
Canker (sore) (mouth) K12.0
Cannabinosis J66.2
Cantrell's syndrome Q87.8
Capillariasis (intestinal) B81.1
- hepatic B83.8
Capillary – *see condition*
Caplan's syndrome M05.1† J99.0∗
Capsule – *see condition*
Capsulitis (joint) M77.9
- adhesive M77.9
- − − shoulder M75.0
- hepatic K65.8
Caput
- crepitus Q75.8
- medusae I86.8
- succedaneum P12.8
Car sickness T75.3
Carapata (disease) A68.0

Carate – *see* Pinta
Carbon lung J60
Carboxyhemoglobinemia T58
Carbuncle (*see also* Abscess, by site)
L02.9
– auricle, ear H60.0
– corpus cavernosum N48.2
– ear (external) (middle) H60.0
– external auditory canal H60.0
– eyelid II00.0
– kidney (*see also* Abscess, kidney) N15.1
– labium (majus) (minus) N76.4
– lacrimal
– – gland H04.0
– – passages (duct) (sac) H04.3
– malignant A22.0
– nose J34.0
– orbit, orbital H05.0
– penis N48.2
– urethra N34.0
– vulva N76.4
Carcinoid (tumor) (M8240/3) – *see also*
Neoplasm, malignant
– with struma ovarii (M9091/1) D39.1
– appendix (M8240/1) D37.3
– argentaffin (M8241/1) – *see* Neoplasm,
uncertain behavior
– – malignant (M8241/3) – *see* Neoplasm,
malignant
– composite (M8244/3) – *see* Neoplasm,
malignant
– goblet cell (M8243/3) C80.-
– – specified site – *see* Neoplasm,
malignant
– – unspecified site C18.1
– malignant (M8240/3) – *see* Neoplasm,
malignant
– mucinous (M8243/3)
– – specified site – *see* Neoplasm,
malignant
– – unspecified site C18.1
– strumal (M9091/1) D39.1
– syndrome E34.0
– type bronchial adenoma (M8240/3) – *see*
Neoplasm, lung, malignant
Carcinoma (M8010/3) – *see also* Neoplasm,
malignant

Note: Except where otherwise indicated, the
morphological varieties of carcinoma in the
list below should be coded by site as for
Neoplasm, malignant.

– with
– – apocrine metaplasia (M8573/3)

Carcinoma—*continued*
– with—*continued*
– – cartilaginous (and osseous) metaplasia
(M8571/3)
– – osseous (and cartilaginous) metaplasia
(M8571/3)
– – productive fibrosis (M8141/3)
– – spindle cell metaplasia (M8572/3)
– – squamous metaplasia (M8570/3)
– acidophil (M8280/3)
– – specified site – *see* Neoplasm,
malignant
– – unspecified site C75.1
– acidophil-basophil, mixed (M8281/3)
– – specified site – *see* Neoplasm,
malignant
– – unspecified site C75.1
– acinar (cell) (M8550/3)
– acinic cell (M8550/3)
– adenocystic (M8200/3)
– adenoid
– – cystic (M8200/3)
– – squamous cell (M8075/3)
– adenosquamous (M8560/3)
– adnexal (skin) (M8390/3) – *see* Neoplasm,
skin, malignant
– adrenal cortical (M8370/3) C74.0
– alveolar (M8251/3) – *see* Neoplasm, lung,
malignant
– – cell (M8250/3) – *see* Neoplasm, lung,
malignant
– ameloblastic (M9270/3) C41.1
– – upper jaw (bone) C41.0
– anaplastic type (M8021/3)
– apocrine (M8401/3)
– – breast – *see* Neoplasm, breast,
malignant
– – specified site NEC – *see* Neoplasm,
skin, malignant
– – unspecified site C44.9
– basal cell (pigmented) (M8090/3) –
see also Neoplasm, skin, malignant
– – fibro-epithelial (M8093/3) – *see*
Neoplasm, skin, malignant
– – morphea (M8092/3) – *see* Neoplasm,
skin, malignant
– – multicentric (M8091/3) – *see*
Neoplasm, skin, malignant
– basaloid (M8123/3)
– basal-squamous cell, mixed (M8094/3) –
see Neoplasm, skin, malignant
– basophil (M8300/3)
– – specified site – *see* Neoplasm,
malignant

Carcinoma—*continued*
- basophil—*continued*
- – unspecified site C75.1
- basophil-acidophil, mixed (M8281/3)
- – specified site – *see* Neoplasm,
  malignant
- – unspecified site C75.1
- basosquamous (M8094/3) – *see*
  Neoplasm, skin, malignant
- bile duct (M8160/3)
- – with hepatocellular, mixed (M8180/3)
  C22.0
- – liver C22.1
- – specified site NEC – *see* Neoplasm,
  malignant
- – unspecified site C22.1
- branchial or branchiogenic C10.4
- bronchial or bronchogenic – *see*
  Neoplasm, lung, malignant
- bronchiolar (M8250/3) – *see* Neoplasm,
  lung, malignant
- bronchioloalveolar (M8250/3) – *see*
  Neoplasm, lung, malignant
- C cell (M8510/3)
- – specified site – *see* Neoplasm,
  malignant
- – unspecified site C73
- ceruminous (M8420/3) C44.2
- chorionic (M9100/3)
- – specified site – *see* Neoplasm,
  malignant
- – unspecified site
- – – female C58
- – – male C62.9
- chromophobe (M8270/3)
- – specified site – *see* Neoplasm,
  malignant
- – unspecified site C75.1
- clear cell (mesonephroid) (M8310/3)
- cloacogenic (M8124/3)
- – specified site – *see* Neoplasm,
  malignant
- – unspecified site C21.2
- colloid (M8480/3)
- cribriform (M8201/3)
- cylindroid (M8200/3)
- diffuse type (M8145/3)
- – specified site – *see* Neoplasm,
  malignant
- – unspecified site C16.9
- duct (cell) (M8500/3)
- – with Paget's disease (M8541/3) – *see*
  Neoplasm, breast, malignant
- – infiltrating (M8500/3)

Carcinoma—*continued*
- duct—*continued*
- – infiltrating—*continued*
- – – with lobular carcinoma (in situ)
    (M8522/3)
- – – – specified site – *see* Neoplasm,
      malignant
- – – – unspecified site C50.9
- – – specified site – *see* Neoplasm,
    malignant
- – – unspecified site (female) C50.9
- ductal (M8500/3)
- – with lobular (M8522/3)
- – – specified site – *see* Neoplasm,
    malignant
- – – unspecified site C50.9
- ductular, infiltrating (M8521/3)
- – specified site – *see* Neoplasm,
  malignant
- – unspecified site C50.9
- embryonal (M9070/3)
- – with teratoma, mixed (M9081/3)
- – combined with choriocarcinoma
    (M9101/3)
- – infantile type (M9071/3)
- – liver C22.7
- – polyembryonal type (M9072/3)
- endometrioid (M8380/3)
- – specified site – *see* Neoplasm,
  malignant
- – unspecified site
- – – female C56
- – – male C61
- eosinophil (M8280/3)
- – specified site – *see* Neoplasm,
  malignant
- – unspecified site C75.1
- epidermoid (M8070/3) – *see also*
  Carcinoma, squamous cell
- – with adenocarcinoma, mixed
    (M8560/3)
- – in situ, Bowen's type (M8081/2) – *see*
  Neoplasm, skin, in situ
- – keratinizing (M8071/3)
- – large cell, nonkeratinizing (M8072/3)
- – small cell, nonkeratinizing (M8073/3)
- – spindle cell (M8074/3)
- – verrucous (M8051/3)
- epithelial-myoepithelial (M8562/3)
- fibroepithelial, basal cell (M8093/3) – *see*
  Neoplasm, skin, malignant
- follicular (M8330/3)
- – with papillary (mixed) (M8340/3) C73

Carcinoma—*continued*
- follicular—*continued*
- – – moderately differentiated (M8332/3) C73
- – – pure follicle (M8331/3) C73
- – – specified site – *see* Neoplasm, malignant
- – – trabecular (M8332/3) C73
- – – unspecified site C73
- – – well differentiated (M8331/3) C73
- – gelatinous (M8480/3)
- – giant cell (M8031/3)
- – – with spindle cell (M8030/3)
- – glycogen-rich (M8315/3) – *see* Neoplasm, breast, malignant
- – granular cell (M8320/3)
- – granulosa cell (M8620/3) C56
- – hepatic cell (M8170/3) C22.0
- – hepatocellular (M8170/3) C22.0
- – – with bile duct, mixed (M8180/3) C22.0
- – – fibrolamellar (M8171/3) C22.0
- – hepatocholangiolitic (M8180/3) C22.0
- – Hurthle cell (M8290/3) C73
- – in
- – – adenomatous
- – – – polyp (M8210/3)
- – – – polyposis coli (M8220/3) C18.9
- – – pleomorphic adenoma (M8941/3) – *see* Neoplasm, salivary gland, malignant
- – – polyp (M8210/3)
- – – polypoid adenoma (M8210/3)
- – – situ (M8010/2) – *see* Carcinoma in situ
- – – tubular adenoma (M8210/3)
- – – villous adenoma (M8261/3)
- – infiltrating
- – – duct (M8500/3)
- – – – with lobular (M8522/3)
- – – – – specified site – *see* Neoplasm, malignant
- – – – – unspecified site C50.9
- – – – with Paget's disease (M8541/3) – *see* Neoplasm, breast, malignant
- – – – specified site – *see* Neoplasm, malignant
- – – – unspecified site (female) C50.9
- – – ductular (M8521/3)
- – – – specified site – *see* Neoplasm, malignant
- – – – unspecified site C50.9
- – – lobular (M8520/3)
- – – – specified site – *see* Neoplasm, malignant
- – – – unspecified site C50.9
- – inflammatory (M8530/3)

Carcinoma—*continued*
- inflammatory—*continued*
- – – specified site – *see* Neoplasm, malignant
- – – unspecified site (female) C50.9
- – intestinal type (M8144/3)
- – – specified site – *see* Neoplasm, malignant
- – – unspecified site C16.9
- – intracystic (M8504/3)
- – – noninfiltrating (M8504/2) – *see* Neoplasm, in situ
- – intraductal (noninfiltrating) (M8500/2)
- – – with Paget's disease (M8543/3) – *see* Neoplasm, breast, malignant
- – – breast D05.1
- – – papillary (M8503/2)
- – – – with invasion (M8503/3)
- – – – – specified site – *see* Neoplasm, malignant
- – – – – unspecified site C50.9
- – – – breast D05.1
- – – – specified site NEC – *see* Neoplasm, in situ
- – – – unspecified site D05.1
- – – specified site NEC – *see* Neoplasm, in situ
- – – unspecified site D05.1
- – intraepidermal (M8070/2) – *see* Neoplasm, in situ
- – – squamous cell, Bowen's type (M8081/2) – *see* Neoplasm, skin, in situ
- – intraepithelial (M8010/2) – *see* Neoplasm, in situ
- – – squamous cell (M8070/2) – *see* Neoplasm, in situ
- – intraosseous (M9270/3) C41.1
- – – upper jaw (bone) C41.0
- – islet cell (M8150/3)
- – – with exocrine, mixed (M8154/3)
- – – – specified site – *see* Neoplasm, malignant
- – – – unspecified site C25.9
- – – pancreas C25.4
- – – specified site NEC – *see* Neoplasm, malignant
- – – unspecified site C25.4
- – juvenile, breast (M8502/3) – *see* Neoplasm, breast, malignant
- – large cell (M8012/3)
- – – small cell (M8045/3)
- – – – specified site – *see* Neoplasm, malignant
- – – – unspecified site C34.9

Carcinoma—*continued*
– large cell—*continued*
– – squamous cell (M8070/3)
– – – keratinizing (M8071/3)
– – – nonkeratinizing (M8072/3)
– Leydig cell (testis) (M8650/3)
– – specified site – *see* Neoplasm,
  malignant
– – unspecified site
– – – female C56
– – – male C62.9
– lipid-rich (M8314/3) C50.9
– liver cell (M8170/3) C22.0
– lobular (infiltrating) (M8520/3)
– – with intraductal (M8522/3)
– – – specified site – *see* Neoplasm,
  malignant
– – – unspecified site C50.9
– – noninfiltrating (M8520/2)
– – – breast D05.0
– – – specified site NEC – *see* Neoplasm,
  in situ
– – – unspecified site D05.0
  specified site – *see* Neoplasm,
  malignant
– – unspecified site (female) C50.9
– lymphoepithelial (M8082/3)
– medullary (M8510/3)
– – with
– – – amyloid stroma (M8511/3)
– – – – specified site – *see* Neoplasm,
  malignant
– – – – unspecified site C73
– – – lymphoid stroma (M8512/3)
– – – – specified site – *see* Neoplasm,
  malignant
– – – – unspecified site (female) C50.9
– Merkel cell (M8247/3) – *see* Neoplasm,
  skin, malignant
– mesometanephric (M9110/3)
– mesonephric (M9110/3)
– metastatic (M8010/6) – *see* Neoplasm,
  secondary
– metatypical (M8095/3) – *see* Neoplasm,
  skin, malignant
– morphea, basal cell (M8092/3) – *see*
  Neoplasm, skin, malignant
– mucinous (M8480/3)
– mucin-producing (M8481/3)
– mucin-secreting (M8481/3)
– mucoepidermoid (M8430/3)
– mucoid (M8480/3)
– – cell (M8300/3)

Carcinoma—*continued*
– mucoid—*continued*
– – cell—*continued*
– – – specified site – *see* Neoplasm,
  malignant
– – – unspecified site C75.1
– mucous (M8480/3)
– myoepithelial-epithelial (M8562/3)
– neuroendocrine (M8246/3)
– – specified site – *see* Neoplasm,
  malignant
– nonencapsulated sclerosing (M8350/3)
  C73
– noninfiltrating (M8010/2)
– – intracystic (M8504/2) – *see* Neoplasm,
  in situ
– – intraductal (M8500/2)
– – – breast D05.1
– – – papillary (M8503/2)
– – – – breast D05.1
– – – – specified site NEC – *see*
  Neoplasm, in situ
– – – – unspecified site D05.1
– – – specified site – *see* Neoplasm, in situ
– – – unspecified site D05.1
– – lobular (M8520/2)
– – – breast D05.0
– – – specified site NEC – *see* Neoplasm,
  in situ
– – – unspecified site D05.0
– oat cell (M8042/3)
– – specified site – *see* Neoplasm,
  malignant
– – unspecified site C34.9
– odontogenic (M9270/3) C41.1
– – upper jaw (bone) C41.0
– oncocytic (M8290/3)
– oxyphilic (M8290/3)
– papillary (M8050/3)
– – with follicular (mixed) (M8340/3) C73
– – epidermoid (M8052/3)
– – follicular variant (M8340/3) C73
– – intraductal (noninfiltrating) (M8503/2)
– – – with invasion (M8503/3)
– – – – specified site – *see* Neoplasm,
  malignant
– – – – unspecified site C50.9
– – – breast D05.1
– – – specified site NEC – *see* Neoplasm,
  in situ
– – – unspecified site D05.1
– – serous (M8460/3)
– – – specified site – *see* Neoplasm,
  malignant

95

Carcinoma—*continued*
- papillary—*continued*
- – serous—*continued*
- – – surface (M8461/3)
- – – – specified site – *see* Neoplasm, malignant
- – – – unspecified site C56
- – – unspecified site C56
- – – squamous cell (M8052/3)
- – – transitional cell (M8130/3)
- papillocystic (M8450/3)
- – specified site – *see* Neoplasm, malignant
- – – unspecified site C56
- parafollicular cell (M8510/3)
- – specified site – *see* Neoplasm, malignant
- – – unspecified site C73
- pilomatrix (M8110/3) – *see* Neoplasm, skin, malignant
- pleomorphic (M8022/3)
- polygonal cell (M8034/3)
- pseudoglandular, squamous cell (M8075/3)
- pseudomucinous (M8470/3)
- – specified site – *see* Neoplasm, malignant
- – – unspecified site C56
- pseudosarcomatous (M8033/3)
- renal cell (M8312/3) C64
- reserve cell (M8041/3)
- round cell (M8041/3)
- Schmincke (M8082/3) – *see* Neoplasm, nasopharynx, malignant
- Schneiderian (M8121/3)
- – specified site – *see* Neoplasm, malignant
- – – unspecified site C30.0
- scirrhous (M8141/3)
- sebaceous (M8410/3) – *see* Neoplasm, skin, malignant
- secondary (M8010/6) – *see* Neoplasm, secondary
- secretory, breast (M8502/3) – *see* Neoplasm, breast, malignant
- serous (M8441/3)
- – papillary (M8460/3)
- – – specified site – *see* Neoplasm, malignant
- – – unspecified site C56
- – surface, papillary (M8461/3)
- – – specified site – *see* Neoplasm, malignant
- – – unspecified site C56

Carcinoma—*continued*
- Sertoli cell (M8640/3)
- – specified site – *see* Neoplasm, malignant
- – unspecified site C62.9
- – – female C56
- – – male C62.9
- signet ring cell (M8490/3)
- – metastatic (M8490/6) – *see* Neoplasm, secondary
- simplex (M8231/3)
- skin appendage (M8390/3) – *see* Neoplasm, skin, malignant
- small cell (M8041/3)
- – fusiform cell (M8043/3)
- – – specified site – *see* Neoplasm, malignant
- – – unspecified site C34.9
- – intermediate cell (M8044/3)
- – – specified site – *see* Neoplasm, malignant
- – – unspecified site C34.9
- – large cell (M8045/3)
- – – specified site – *see* Neoplasm, malignant
- – – unspecified site C34.9
- – squamous cell, nonkeratinizing (M8073/3)
- solid (M8230/3)
- spheroidal cell (M8010/3)
- spindle cell (M8032/3)
- – with giant cell (M8030/3)
- spinous cell (M8070/3)
- squamous (cell) (M8070/3)
- – with adenocarcinoma, mixed (M8560/3)
- – adenoid (M8075/3)
- – keratinizing, large cell (M8071/3)
- – large cell, nonkeratinizing (M8072/3)
- – metastatic (M8070/6) – *see* Neoplasm, secondary
- – microinvasive (M8076/3)
- – – specified site – *see* Neoplasm, malignant
- – – unspecified site C53.9
- – nonkeratinizing (large cell) (M8072/3)
- – papillary (M8052/3)
- – pseudoglandular (M8075/3)
- – small cell, nonkeratinizing (M8073/3)
- – spindle cell (M8074/3)
- – verrucous (M8051/3)
- superficial spreading (M8143/3)
- sweat gland (M8400/3) – *see* Neoplasm, skin, malignant

Carcinoma—*continued*
- theca cell (M8600/3) C56
- thymic (M8580/3) C37
- trabecular (M8190/3)
- transitional (cell) (M8120/3)
- – papillary (M8130/3)
- – spindle cell (M8122/3)
- tubular (M8211/3)
- undifferentiated (M8020/3)
- urothelial (M8120/3)
- verrucous (epidermoid) (squamous cell) (M8051/3)
- villous (M8262/3)
- water-clear cell (M8322/3) C75.0
- wolffian duct (M9110/3)

Carcinoma in situ (M8010/2) – *see also* Neoplasm, in situ   *with microinvasia – malignant*
- breast NEC D05.9
- epidermoid (M8070/2) – *see also* Neoplasm, in situ
- – with questionable stromal invasion (M8076/2)
- – – cervix D06.9
- – – specified site NEC – *see* Neoplasm, in situ
- – – unspecified site D06.9
- – Bowen's type (M8081/2) – *see* Neoplasm, skin, in situ
- in
- – adenomatous polyp (M8210/2)
- – polyp NEC (M8210/2)
- intraductal (M8500/2)
- – breast D05.1
- – specified site NEC – *see* Neoplasm, in situ
- – unspecified site D05.1
- lobular (M8520/2)
- – with
- – – infiltrating duct (M8522/3)
- – – – breast C50.9
- – – – specified site NEC – *see* Neoplasm, malignant
- – – – unspecified site C50.9
- – – intraductal (M8522/2)
- – – – breast D05.7
- – – – specified site NEC – *see* Neoplasm, in situ
- – – – unspecified site D05.7
- – breast D05.0
- – specified site NEC – *see* Neoplasm, in situ
- – unspecified site D05.0
- papillary (M8050/2) – *see* Neoplasm, in situ

Carcinoma in situ—*continued*
- squamous cell (M8070/2) – *see also* Neoplasm, in situ
- – with questionable stromal invasion (M8076/2)
- – – cervix D06.9
- – – specified site NEC – *see* Neoplasm, in situ
- – – unspecified site D06.9
- transitional cell (M8120/2) – *see* Neoplasm, in situ

Carcinomaphobia F45.2
Carcinomatosis
- peritonei (M8010/6) C78.6
- specified site NEC (M8010/3) – *see* Neoplasm, malignant
- unspecified site (M8010/6) C79.9
- – primary site not indicated C80.9
- – primary site unknown, so stated C80.0

Carcinosarcoma (M8980/3) – *see* Neoplasm, malignant
- embryonal (M8981/3) – *see* Neoplasm, malignant

Cardia, cardial – *see condition*
Cardiac – *see also condition*
- death, sudden I46.1
- pacemaker
- – in situ Z95.0
- – management or adjustment Z45.0
- tamponade I31.9
Cardialgia (*see also* Pain, precordial) R07.2
Cardiectasis – *see* Hypertrophy, cardiac
Cardiochalasia K21.9
Cardiomegalia glycogenica diffusa E74.0† I43.1*
Cardiomegaly (*see also* Hypertrophy, cardiac) I51.7
- congenital Q24.8
- glycogen E74.0† I43.1*
- idiopathic I51.7
Cardiomyopathy (familial) (idiopathic) I42.9
- alcoholic I42.6
- amyloid E85.4† I43.1*
- arteriosclerotic I25.1
- beriberi E51.1† I43.2*
- complicating pregnancy O99.4
- congenital I42.4
- congestive I42.0
- constrictive NEC I42.5
- dilated I42.0
- due to
- – alcohol I42.6

Cardiomyopathy—*continued*
- due to—*continued*
- – drugs I42.7
- – external agents NEC I42.7
- hypertensive (*see also* Hypertension, heart) I11.9
- hypertrophic (nonobstructive) I42.2
- – obstructive I42.1
- – – congenital Q24.8
- in
- – Chagas' disease (chronic) B57.2† I41.2*
- – – acute B57.0† I41.2*
- – – sarcoidosis D86.8† I43.8*
- ischemic I25.5
- metabolic E88.9† I43.1*
- nutritional E63.9† I43.2*
- obscure of Africa I42.8
- postpartum O90.3
- restrictive NEC I42.5
- rheumatic I09.0
- secondary I42.9
- thyrotoxic E05.9† I43.8*
- tuberculous A18.8† I43.0*
- viral B33.2† I43.0*
Cardionephritis (*see also* Hypertension, cardiorenal) I13.9
Cardionephropathy (*see also* Hypertension, cardiorenal) I13.9
Cardionephrosis (*see also* Hypertension, cardiorenal) I13.9
Cardiopathy (*see also* Disease, heart) I51.9
- idiopathic I42.9
- mucopolysaccharidosis E76.3† I52.8*
Cardiopericarditis (*see also* Pericarditis) I31.9
Cardiophobia F45.2
Cardiorenal – *see condition*
Cardiorrhexis (*see also* Infarct, myocardium) I21.9
Cardiosclerosis I25.1
Cardiosis – *see* Disease, heart
Cardiospasm (esophagus) (reflex) (stomach) K22.0
- congenital (without mention of megaesophagus) Q40.2
- – with megaesophagus Q39.5
Cardiostenosis – *see* Disease, heart
Cardiovascular – *see condition*
Carditis (acute) (chronic) (subacute) I51.8
- meningococcal A39.5† I52.0*
- rheumatic – *see* Disease, heart, rheumatic
- rheumatoid M05.3† I52.8*
- viral B33.2† I52.1*

Care (of) (for) (following)
- child (routine) Z76.2
- family member (handicapped) (sick) Z63.6
- foundling Z76.1
- holiday relief Z75.5
- improper T74.0
- lack of (at or after birth) (infant) T74.0
- lactating mother Z39.1
- orthodontic Z51.8
- palliative Z51.5
- postpartum
- – immediately after delivery Z39.0
- – routine follow-up Z39.2
- pregnancy – *see* Maternal care
- preparatory, for subsequent treatment Z51.4
- – for dialysis Z49.0
- respite Z75.5
- unavailable, due to
- – absence of person rendering care Z74.2
- – inability (any reason) of person rendering care Z74.2
- well-baby Z76.2
Caries
- bone NEC A18.0† M90.0*
- cementum K02.2
- – arrested K02.3
- – specified NEC K02.8
- dental K02.9
- dentin (acute) (chronic) K02.1
- enamel (acute) (chronic, incipient) K02.0
- external meatus H61.8
- hip (tuberculous) A18.0† M01.1*
- initial K02.0
- knee (tuberculous) A18.0† M01.1*
- labyrinth H83.8
- limb NEC (tuberculous) A18.0† M90.0*
- mastoid process (chronic) H70.1
- – tuberculous A18.0† H75.0*
- middle ear H74.8
- nose (tuberculous) A18.0† M90.0*
- orbit (tuberculous) A18.0† M90.0*
- ossicles, ear H74.3
- petrous bone H70.2
- sacrum (tuberculous) A18.0† M49.0*
- spine, spinal (column) (tuberculous) A18.0† M49.0*
- syphilitic A52.7† M90.2*
- – congenital (early) A50.0† M90.2*
- tooth, teeth K02.9
- tuberculous A18.0† M90.0*
- vertebra (column) (tuberculous) A18.0† M49.0*

Carious teeth K02.9
Carneous mole O02.0
Carotid body or sinus syndrome G90.0
Carotinosis (cutis) (skin) E67.1
Carpal tunnel syndrome G56.0
Carpenter's syndrome Q87.0
Carpopedal spasm (*see also* Tetany) R29.0
Carr-Barr-Plunkett syndrome Q97.1
Carrier (suspected) of
– amebiasis Z22.1
– bacterial disease NEC Z22.3
– cholera Z22.1
– diphtheria Z22.2
– gastrointestinal pathogens NEC Z22.1
– gonorrhea Z22.4
– HB(c) (s)Ag Z22.5
– hepatitis
– – Australia antigen (HAA) Z22.5
– – B surface antigen (HBAg) Z22.5
– – – with acute delta-(super)infection
    B17.0
– – viral Z22.5
– human T-cell lymphotropic virus type 1
  (HTLV-1) infection Z22.6
– infectious organism Z22.9
– – specified NEC Z22.8
– meningococci Z22.3
– staphylococci Z22.3
– streptococci Z22.3
– syphilis Z22.4
– typhoid Z22.0
– venereal disease NEC Z22.4
Carrion's disease A44.0
Carter's relapsing fever (Asiatic) A68.1
Cartilage – *see condition*
Caruncle (inflamed)
– labium (majus) (minus) N90.8
– lacrimal H04.3
– myrtiform N89.8
– urethral (benign) N36.2
Caseation lymphatic gland (tuberculous)
  A18.2
Castellani's disease A69.8
Castration, traumatic, male S38.2
Casts in urine R82.9
Cat
– cry syndrome Q93.4
– ear Q17.3
Catabolism, senile R54
Catalepsy (hysterical) F44.2
– schizophrenic F20.2
Cataplexy (idiopathic) G47.4

Cataract (cortical) (immature)
  (incipient) (*see also* Cataracta) H26.9
– anterior
– – and posterior axial embryonal Q12.0
– – pyramidal Q12.0
– blue Q12.0
– central Q12.0
– cerulean Q12.0
– complicated H26.2
– congenital Q12.0
– coralliform Q12.0
– coronary Q12.0
– crystalline Q12.0
– diabetic (*see also* E10-E14 with fourth
  character .3) E14.3† H28.0∗
– drug-induced H26.3
– due to radiation H26.8
– electric H26.8
– glass-blower's H26.8
– heat ray H26.8
– heterochromic H26.2
– in (due to)
– – chronic iridocyclitis H26.2
– – diabetes (*see also* E10-E14 with fourth
    character .3) E14.3† H28.0∗
– – endocrine disease NEC E34.9† H28.1∗
– – eye disease H26.2
– – hypoparathyroidism E20.-† H28.1∗
– – malnutrition-dehydration E46† H28.1∗
– – metabolic disease NEC E88.9† H28.1∗
– – myotonic disorders G71.1† H28.2∗
– – nutritional disease NEC E63.9†
    H28.1∗
– infantile H26.0
– irrradiational H26.8
– juvenile H26.0
– malnutrition-dehydration E46† H28.1∗
– morgagnian H25.2
– myotonic G71.1† H28.2∗
– myxedema E03.9† H28.1∗
– nuclear
– – embryonal Q12.0
– – sclerosis H25.1
– presenile H26.0
– secondary H26.4
– – to eye disease H26.2
– senile H25.9
– – brunescens H25.1
– – combined forms H25.8
– – coronary H25.0
– – cortical H25.0
– – hypermature H25.2
– – incipient H25.0
– – morgagnian type H25.2

Cataract—*continued*
- senile—*continued*
- - nuclear (sclerosis) H25.1
- - polar subcapsular (anterior) (posterior) H25.0
- - punctate H25.0
- - specified NEC H25.8
- - subcapsular polar (anterior) (posterior) H25.0
- toxic H26.3
- traumatic H26.1
- zonular (perinuclear) Q12.0

Cataracta (*see also* Cataract) H26.9
- brunescens H25.1
- centralis pulverulenta Q12.0
- cerulea Q12.0
- complicata H26.2
- congenita Q12.0
- coralliformis Q12.0
- coronaria Q12.0
- membranacea
- - accreta H26.4
- - congenita Q12.0
- sunflower H26.2

Catarrh, catarrhal (inflammation) (*see also condition*) J00
- acute J00
- bronchial – *see* Bronchitis
- chronic J31.0
- enteric – *see* Enteritis
- eustachian H68.0
- eye (acute) H10.2
- fauces (*see also* Pharyngitis) J02.9
- febrile J00
- gastrointestinal – *see* Enteritis
- hay fever J30.1
- - with asthma J45.0
- infectious J00
- intestinal – *see* Enteritis
- larynx, chronic J37.0
- middle ear, chronic H65.2
- nasal (chronic) (*see also* Rhinitis) J31.0
- - acute J00
- nasopharyngeal (chronic) J31.1
- - acute J00
- spring (eye) (vernal) H10.1
- summer (hay) (*see also* Fever, hay) J30.1
- throat J31.2
- tubotympanal H65.9
- - chronic H65.2

Catatonia (schizophrenic) F20.2

Catscratch (*see also* Injury, superficial) T14.0
- disease or fever A28.1

Cauda equina – *see condition*

Caul over face (causing asphyxia) P21.9

Cauliflower ear M95.1

Causalgia G56.4

Cause
- external, general effects T75.8
- not stated (morbidity) R69
- - mortality R99
- unknown (morbidity) R69
- - mortality R99

Caustic burn – *see* Corrosion, by site

Cavare's disease G72.3

Cave-in, injury
- crushing (severe) T14.7
- suffocation T71

Cavernitis (penis) N48.2

Cavernositis N48.2

Cavernous – *see condition*

Cavitation of lung (*see also* Tuberculosis, pulmonary) A16.2
- nontuberculous J98.4

Cavity
- lung – *see* Cavitation of lung
- optic papilla Q14.2
- pulmonary – *see* Cavitation of lung

Cavus foot (congenital) Q66.7
- acquired M21.6

Cazenave's disease L10.2

Cecitis K52.9
- with perforation, peritonitis, or rupture K65.8

Cecum – *see condition*

Cell(s), cellular – *see also condition*
- anterior chamber (eye) H20.0
- in urine R82.9

Cellulitis (diffuse) (with lymphangitis) L03.9
- abdominal wall L03.3
- anaerobic A48.0
- ankle L03.1
- anus K61.0
- arm (any part, except finger or thumb) L03.1
- auricle (ear) H60.1
- axilla L03.1
- back (any part) L03.3
- buttock L03.3
- cervical (meaning neck) L03.8
- cervix (uteri) (*see also* Cervicitis) N72
- chest wall L03.3
- chronic NEC L03.9
- clostridial A48.0
- corpus cavernosum N48.2
- drainage site (following operation) T81.4

Cellulitis—*continued*
- ear (external) H60.1
- eosinophilic (granulomatous) L98.3
- erysipelatous (*see also* Erysipelas) A46
- external auditory canal H60.1
- eyelid H00.0
- face (any part, except ear, eye and nose) L03.2
- finger (intrathecal) (periostcal) (subcutaneous) (subcuticular) L03.0
- foot, except toe(s) L03.1
- gangrenous (*see also* Gangrene) R02
- genital organ NEC
- – female (external) N76.4
- – male N49.9
- – – multiple sites N49.8
- – – specified NEC N49.8
- gluteal (region) L03.3
- gonococcal NEC A54.8
- groin L03.3
- hand, except finger or thumb L03.1
- head NEC L03.8
- heel L03.1
- hip L03.1
- jaw (region) L03.2
- knee L03.1
- labium (majus) (minus) (*see also* Vulvitis) N76.4
- lacrimal apparatus H04.3
- larynx J38.7
- leg, except toe(s) L03.1
- mouth (floor) K12.2
- multiple sites, so stated L03.8
- nasopharynx J39.1
- navel L03.3
- – newborn P38
- neck (region) L03.8
- nose (external) (septum) J34.0
- orbit, orbital H05.0
- pectoral (region) L03.3
- pelvis, pelvic (chronic)
- – female (*see also* Disease, pelvis, inflammatory) N73.2
- – following
- – – abortion (subsequent episode) O08.0
- – – – current episode – *see* Abortion
- – – ectopic or molar pregnancy O08.0
- – male K65.0
- penis N48.2
- perineal, perineum L03.3
- perirectal K61.1
- peritonsillar J36
- periurethral N34.0

Cellulitis—*continued*
- periuterine (*see also* Disease, pelvis, inflammatory) N73.2
- pharynx J39.1
- rectum K61.1
- retroperitoneal K65.0
- scalp (any part) L03.8
- scrotum N49.2
- septic NEC L03.9
- shoulder L03.1
- specified site NEC L03.8
- suppurative NEC L03.9
- thigh L03.1
- thumb (intrathecal) (periosteal) (subcutaneous) (subcuticular) L03.0
- toe (intrathecal) (periosteal) (subcutaneous) (subcuticular) L03.0
- tonsil J36
- trunk L03.3
- tuberculous (primary) A18.4
- umbilicus L03.3
- – newborn P38
- vaccinal T88.0
- vocal cord J38.3
- vulva (*see also* Vulvitis) N76.2
- wrist L03.1

Cementoblastoma, benign (M9273/0) D16.5
- upper jaw (bone) D16.4

Cementoma (M9272/0) D16.5
- gigantiform (M9275/0) D16.5
- – upper jaw (bone) D16.4
- upper jaw (bone) D16.4

Cementosis K03.4

Cephalematocele, cephal(o)hematocele
- fetus or newborn P52.8
- – birth injury P10.8
- traumatic S09.8

Cephalematoma, cephalhematoma (calcified)
- fetus or newborn (birth injury) P12.0
- traumatic S09.8

Cephalgia, cephalalgia (*see also* Headache) R51
- nonorganic origin F45.4

Cephalic – *see condition*

Cephalitis – *see* Encephalitis

Cephalocele (*see also* Encephalocele) Q01.9

Cephalomenia N94.8

Cephalopelvic – *see condition*

Cerclage (with cervical incompetence) in pregnancy O34.3

Cerebellitis – *see* Encephalitis

Cerebellum, cerebellar – *see condition*
Cerebral – *see condition*
Cerebritis – *see* Encephalitis
Cerebrohepatorenal syndrome Q87.8
Cerebromalacia (*see also* Softening, brain)
G93.8
Cerebroside lipidosis E75.2
Cerebrospasticity (congenital) G80.1
Cerebrospinal – *see condition*
Cerebrum – *see condition*
Ceroid-lipofuscinosis, neuronal E75.4
Cerumen (accumulation) (impacted)
H61.2
Cervical – *see also condition*
– auricle Q18.2
– dysplasia in pregnancy O34.4
– erosion in pregnancy O34.4
– fibrosis in pregnancy O34.4
– fusion syndrome Q76.1
– rib Q76.5
Cervicalgia M54.2
Cervicitis (acute) (chronic) (nonvenereal)
(subacute) (with ulceration) N72
– chlamydial A56.0
– complicating pregnancy O23.5
– – affecting fetus or newborn P00.8
– gonococcal A54.0
– herpesviral A60.0† N74.8*
– puerperal, postpartum O86.1
– senile (atrophic) N72
– syphilitic A52.7† N74.2*
– trichomonal A59.0† N74.8*
– tuberculous A18.1† N74.0*
Cervicocolpitis (emphysematosa) (*see also*
Cervicitis) N72
Cervix – *see condition*
Cesarean
– emergency O82.1
– operation or section NEC (*see also*
Delivery, cesarean) O82.9
– – with hysterectomy O82.2
– – affecting fetus or newborn P03.4
– – post mortem, affecting fetus or newborn
P01.6
– – preterm NEC O60.1
– – – with spontaneous labor O60.1
– – – without spontaneous labor O60.3
– – previous, affecting management of
pregnancy O34.2
Cestan(-Chenais) paralysis or syndrome
I63.0† G46.3*
Cestode infection or infestation B71.9
– specified type NEC B71.8
Cestodiasis B71.9

Chafing L30.4
Chagas'(-Mazza) disease (chronic) B57.2
– with
– – cardiovascular involvement NEC
B57.2† I98.1*
– – digestive system involvement NEC
B57.3† K93.8*
– – megacolon B57.3† K93.1*
– – megaesophagus B57.3† K23.1*
– – myocarditis B57.2† I41.2*
– – nervous system involvement B57.4†
G99.8*
– – other organ involvement B57.5
– acute (with) B57.1
– – cardiovascular NEC B57.0† I98.1*
– – myocarditis B57.0† I41.2*
Chagres fever B50.9
Chairfast NEC R26.3
– requiring health care provider Z74.0
Chalasia (cardiac sphincter) K21.9
Chalazion H00.1
Chalcosis H44.3
– cornea H18.0
– crystalline lens H26.2
– retina H35.8
Chalicosis J62.8
Chancre (genital) (hard) (primary)
(seronegative) (seropositive) (syphilitic)
A51.0
– conjunctiva A51.2
– Ducrey's A57
– extragenital A51.2
– eyelid A51.2
– hunterian A51.0
– lip A51.2
– mixed A51.0
– nipple A51.2
– of
– – carate A67.0
– – pinta A67.0
– – yaws A66.0
– simple A57
– soft A57
– – bubo A57
– – palate A51.2
– urethra A51.0
Chancroid (anus) (genital) (rectum) A57
Change(s) (of) – *see also* Removal
– arteriosclerotic – *see* Arteriosclerosis
– bone M89.9
– – diabetic E14.6† M90.8*
– bowel habit R19.4
– cardiorenal (vascular) (*see also*
Hypertension, cardiorenal) I13.9

Change(s)—*continued*
- cardiovascular – *see* Disease, cardiovascular
- circulatory I99
- cognitive (mild) (organic) due to or secondary to general medical condition F06.7
- color, tooth, teeth
- – during formation K00.8
- – posteruptive K03.7
- contraceptive device Z30.5
- corneal membrane H18.3
- degenerative, spine or vertebra M47.9
- dressing Z48.0
- fixation device (internal) Z47.0
- – external Z47.8
- heart – *see* Disease, heart
- hyperplastic larynx J38.7
- hypertrophic
- – nasal sinus J34.8
- – upper respiratory tract J39.8
- indwelling catheter Z46.6
- inflammatory – *see also* Inflammation
- – sacroiliac M46.1
- job, anxiety concerning Z56.1
- Kirschner wire Z47.0
- malignant (M8000/3) – *code as* primary malignant neoplasm of the site of the lesion

Note: For malignant change occurring in a neoplasm, use the appropriate M code with behavior code /3, e.g. malignant change in uterine fibroid, M8890/3. For malignant change occuring in a non-neoplastic condition (e.g. gastric ulcer) use the M code M8000/3.

- mental NEC F99
- minimal (glomerular) – *code to* N00-N07, with fourth character .0
- myocardium, myocardial – *see* Degeneration, myocardial
- of life (*see also* Menopause) N95.1
- pacemaker Z45.0
- personality (enduring) (*see also* Personality, change) F62.9
- – due to (secondary to) general medical condition F07.0
- – secondary (nonspecific) F61
- plaster cast Z47.8
- renal (*see also* Disease, renal) N28.9
- retina, myopic H44.2
- sacroiliac joint M53.3
- senile (*see also* condition) R54

Change(s)—*continued*
- sensory R20.8
- skin R23.8
- – acute, due to ultraviolet radiation L56.9
- – – specified NEC L56.8
- – chronic, due to nonionizing radiation L57.9
- – – specified NEC L57.8
- – texture R23.4
- splint, external Z47.8
- suture Z48.0
- traction device Z47.8
- vascular I99
- vasomotor I73.9
- voice R49.8
- – psychogenic F44.4
Chapping skin T69.8
Charcot-Marie-Tooth disease, paralysis or syndrome G60.0
Charcot's
- arthropathy (tabetic) A52.1† M14.6*
- – diabetic (*see also* E10-E14 with fourth character.6) E14.6† M14.6*
- – nonsyphilitic NEC G98† M14.6*
- – syringomyelic G95.0† M49.4*
- cirrhosis K74.3
- disease (tabetic arthropathy) – *see* Charcot's arthropathy
- joint (disease) (tabetic) – *see* Charcot's arthropathy
- syndrome I73.9
Charley-horse (quadriceps) S76.1
- muscle, except quadriceps
- – traumatic – *see* Injury, muscle
- – non traumatic – *see* Cramp(s)
Cheadle's disease E54
Checking (of)
- cardiac pacemaker (battery) (electrode(s)) (pulse generator) Z45.0
- device
- – contraceptive Z30.5
- – fixation (internal) Z47.0
- – – external Z47.8
- – traction Z47.8
- Kirschner wire Z47.0
- plaster cast Z47.8
- splint, external Z47.8
Check-up, health (routine) Z00.0
- infant (not sick) Z00.1
- occupational Z10.0
Chediak-Higashi(-Steinbrinck) anomaly, disease or syndrome E70.3
Cheek – *see* condition
Cheese itch B88.0

Cheese-washer's lung J67.8
Cheese-worker's lung J67.8
Cheilitis (angular) (exfoliative)
   (glandular) K13.0
– actinic (due to sun) L56.8
– – other than from sun L59.8
– candidal B37.8
Cheilodynia K13.0
Cheiloschisis (*see also* Cleft, lip) Q36.9
Cheilosis (angular) K13.0
– with pellagra E52† K93.8*
– due to vitamin B₂ (riboflavin) deficiency
   E53.0† K93.8*
Cheiromegaly M79.8
Cheiropompholyx L30.1
Cheloid (*see also* Keloid) L91.0
Chemical burn – *see also* Corrosion, by site
– following induced abortion O08.6
Chemodectoma (M8693/1) – *see*
   Paraganglioma, nonchromaffin
Chemoprophylaxis Z29.2
Chemosis, conjunctiva H11.4
Chemotherapy (session) (for) Z51.2
– cancer Z51.1
– – maternal, affecting fetus or newborn
   P04.1
– maintenance NEC Z51.2
– – neoplasm Z51.1
– neoplasm Z51.1
– prophylactic NEC Z29.2
Cherubism K10.8
Chest – *see condition*
Cheyne-Stokes breathing (respiration)
   R06.3
Chiari's
– disease (Budd) I82.0
– net Q24.8
Chicago disease B40.9
Chickenpox (*see also* Varicella) B01.9
– congenital P35.8
Chiclero ulcer or sore B55.1
Chigger (infestation) B88.0
Chignon (disease) B36.8
– fetus or newborn (birth injury) (from
   vacuum extraction) P12.1
Chilblain(s) T69.1
Child behavior causing concern Z63.8
Childbirth (mother) (*see also* Delivery)
   O80.9
Chill(s) R68.8
– with fever R50.8
– septic – *see* Sepsis
Chilomastigiasis A07.8
Chimera 46,XX/46,XY Q99.0

See Arnold Chiari P60 for Congenital brain

Chin – *see condition*
Chlamydia, chlamydial A74.9
– cervicitis A56.0
– conjunctivitis A74.0† H13.1*
– cystitis A56.0
– endometritis A56.1† N74.4*
– epididymitis A56.1† N51.1*
– female
– – pelvic inflammatory disease A56.1†
   N74.4*
– – pelviperitonitis A56.1† N74.4*
– orchitis A56.1† N51.1*
– peritonitis A74.8† K67.0*
– pharyngitis A56.4
– proctitis A56.3
– psittaci (infection) A70
– salpingitis A56.1† N74.4*
– sexually transmitted infection NEC A56.8
– specified NEC A74.8
– urethritis A56.0
– vulvovaginitis A56.0
Chlamydiosis (*see also* Chlamydia) A74.9
Chloasma (idiopathic) (symptomatic)
   L81.1
– eyelid H02.7
– – hyperthyroid E05.9† H03.8*
Chloroma C92.3
Chlorosis D50.8
– Egyptian B76.9† D63.8*
– miner's B76.9† D63.8*
Chocolate cyst (ovary) N80.1
Choked
– disk H47.1
– on food, phlegm, or vomitus
   NEC (*see also* Asphyxia, food or foreign
   body) T17.9
– while vomiting NEC (*see also* Asphyxia,
   food or foreign body) T17.9
Chokes (resulting from bends) T70.3
Choking sensation R06.8
Cholangiectasis K83.8
Cholangiocarcinoma (M8160/3)
– with hepatocellular carcinoma, combined
   (M8180/3) C22.0
– liver C22.1
– specified site NEC – *see* Neoplasm,
   malignant
– unspecified site C22.1
Cholangiohepatoma (M8180/3) C22.0
Cholangiolitis (acute) (chronic)
   (extrahepatic) (gangrenous)
   (intrahepatic) K83.0

Cholangioma (M8160/0) D13.4
- malignant (M8160/3) – *see*
Cholangiocarcinoma
**Cholangitis (primary) (recurrent)
(sclerosing) (secondary) (stenosing)
(suppurative)** K83.0
- with calculus, bile duct K80.3
- – and cholecystitis K80.4
- chronic nonsuppurative destructive K74.3
Cholecystectasia K82.8
Cholecystitis K81.9
- with
- – calculus, stones in
- – – bile duct (common) (hepatic) K80.4
- – – cystic duct K80.1
- – – gallbladder K80.1
- – choledocholithiasis K80.4
- – cholelithiasis K80.1
- acute K81.0
- – with
- – – calculus, stones in
- – – – cystic duct K80.0
- – – – gallbladder K80.0
- – – choledocholithiasis K80.4
- – – cholelithiasis K80.0
- chronic K81.1
- emphysematous (acute) K81.0
- gangrenous K81.0
- specified NEC K81.8
- suppurative K81.0
Cholecystolithiasis K80.2
Choledochitis (suppurative) K83.0
Choledocholith K80.5
Choledocholithiasis (common duct) K80.5
- with
- – cholangitis K80.3
- – cholecystitis (and cholangitis) K80.4
- cystic K80.2
**Cholelithiasis (cystic duct) (gallbladder)
(impacted) (multiple)** K80.2
- with cholecystitis (chronic) K80.1
- – acute K80.0
- bile duct (common) (hepatic) K80.5
- common duct K80.5
- hepatic duct K80.5
- specified NEC K80.8
Cholemia (*see also* Jaundice) R17
- familial (simple) (congenital) E80.4
- Gilbert's E80.4
Choleperitoneum, choleperitonitis K65.8
Cholera (Asiatic) (epidemic) (malignant)
A00.9
- antimonial T56.8
- classical A00.0

Cholera—*continued*
- due to Vibrio cholerae 01 A00.9
- – biovar cholerae A00.0
- – biovar eltor A00.1
Cholestasis NEC K83.1
- with hepatocyte injury K71.0
- complicating pregnancy, childbirth or the
puerperium (intrahepatic) O26.6
- pure K71.0
**Cholesteatoma (ear) (middle) (mastoid)
(with reaction)** H71
- external ear (canal) H60.4
- postmastoidectomy cavity (recurrent)
H95.0
- tympani H71
Cholesterin in vitreous (body) H43.2
Cholesterol deposit
- retina H35.8
- vitreous (body) H43.2
**Cholesterolemia (essential) (familial)
(hereditary) (pure)** E78.0
**Cholesterolosis, cholesterosis
(gallbladder)** K82.4
- cerebrotendinous E75.5
Choluria R82.2
Chondritis M94.8
- costal M94.0
- – Tietze's M94.0
- purulent M94.8
- tuberculous NEC A18.0† M01.1*
- – intervertebral A18.0† M49.0*
Chondroblastoma (M9230/0) – *see also*
Neoplasm, bone, benign
- malignant (M9230/3) – *see* Neoplasm,
bone, malignant
Chondrocalcinosis M11.2
- familial M11.1
- specified NEC M11.2
**Chondrodermatitis nodularis chronica
helicis or anthelicis** H61.0
Chondrodysplasia Q78.9
- with hemangioma Q78.4
- calcificans congenita Q77.3
- fetalis Q77.4
- metaphyseal (Jansen's) (McKusick's)
(Schmid's) Q78.5
- punctata Q77.3
**Chondrodystrophy, chondrodystrophia
(familial) (fetalis) (hypoplastic)** Q78.9
- calcificans congenita Q77.3
- punctata Q77.3
Chondroectodermal dysplasia Q77.6
Chondrogenesis imperfecta Q77.4
Chondrolysis M94.3

Chondroma (M9220/0) – *see also*
Neoplasm, cartilage, benign
– juxtacortical (M9221/0) – *see* Neoplasm,
bone, benign
– periosteal (M9221/0) – *see* Neoplasm,
bone, benign
Chondromalacia M94.2
– patella, patellae M22.4
– systemic M94.2
Chondromatosis (M9220/1) – *see also*
Neoplasm, cartilage, uncertain behavior
– internal Q78.4
Chondromyxosarcoma (M9220/3) – *see*
Neoplasm, cartilage, malignant
**Chondro-osteodysplasia (Morquio-
Brailsford type)** E76.2
Chondro-osteodystrophy E76.2
Chondro-osteoma (M9210/0) – *see*
Neoplasm, bone, benign
Chondropathia tuberosa M94.0
Chondrosarcoma (M9220/3) – *see also*
Neoplasm, cartilage, malignant
– juxtacortical (M9221/3) – *see* Neoplasm,
bone, malignant
– mesenchymal (M9240/3) – *see* Neoplasm,
connective tissue, malignant
– myxoid (M9231/3) – *see* Neoplasm,
cartilage, malignant
Chordee (nonvenereal) N48.8
– congenital Q54.4
– gonococcal A54.0
Chorditis (fibrinous) (nodosa) (tuberosa)
J38.2
Chordoma (M9370/3) – *see* Neoplasm,
malignant
Chorea (gravis) (spasmodic) G25.5
– with
– – heart involvement I02.0
– – – active or acute (conditions in I01.-)
I02.0
– – rheumatic heart disease (chronic)
(inactive) (quiescent) – *code to*
rheumatic heart condition involved
– apoplectic I64
– chronic G25.5
– drug-induced G25.4
– habit F95.8
– hereditary G10
– Huntington's G10
– hysterical F44.4
– minor I02.9
– – with heart involvement I02.0
– posthemiplegic G25.5
– progressive G25.5

Chorea—*continued*
– progressive—*continued*
– – hereditary G10
– rheumatic (chronic) I02.9
– – with heart involvement I02.0
– senile G25.5
– Sydenham's I02.9
– – with heart involvement I02.0
Choreoathetosis (paroxysmal) G25.5
Chorioadenoma (destruens) (M9100/1)
D39.2
Chorioamnionitis O41.1
– fetus or newborn P02.7
Chorioangioma O02.8
Choriocarcinoma (female) (M9100/3) C58
– combined with
– – embryonal carcinoma (M9101/3) – *see*
Neoplasm, malignant
– – other germ cell elements (M9101/3) –
see Neoplasm, malignant
– – teratoma (M9101/3) – *see* Neoplasm,
malignant
– male C62.9
– specified site – *see* Neoplasm, malignant
– unspecified site
– – female C58
– – male C62.9
**Chorioencephalitis (acute) (lymphocytic)
(serous)** A87.2† G05.1*
Chorioepithelioma (M9100/3) – *see*
Choriocarcinoma
**Choriomeningitis (acute) (lymphocytic)
(serous)** A87.2† G02.0*
Chorionepithelioma (M9100/3) – *see*
Choriocarcinoma
Chorioretinitis H30.9
– disseminated H30.1
– – in neurosyphilis A52.1† H32.0*
– focal (acute) (chronic) (central)
(exudative) (Jensen's) H30.0
– histoplasmic B39.9† H32.0*
– in (due to)
– – histoplasmosis B39.9† H32.0*
– – syphilis (secondary) – *see*
Chorioretinitis, syphilitic
– – toxoplasmosis (acquired) B58.0†
H32.0*
– – – congenital (active) P37.1† H32.0*
– – tuberculosis A18.5† H32.0*
– juxtapapillary, juxtapapillaris H30.0
– progressive myopia (degeneration) H44.2
– specified NEC H30.8
– syphilitic (secondary) A51.4† H32.0*
– – congenital (early) A50.0† H32.0*

Chorioretinitis—*continued*
- syphilitic—*continued*
- - congenital—*continued*
- - - late A50.3† H32.0*
- - late A52.7† H32.0*
- tuberculous A18.5† H32.0*

Chorioretinopathy, central serous H35.7
Choroid – *see condition*
Choroideremia H31.2
Choroiditis (*see also* Chorioretinitis) H30.9
- leprous A30.-† H32.0*
- syphilitic (secondary) A51.4† H32.0*
- - congenital (early) A50.0† H32.0*
- - - late A50.3† H32.0*
- - late A52.7† H32.0*
- tuberculous A18.5† H32.0*

Choroidopathy H31.9
- degenerative H31.1
- hereditary H31.2

Choroidoretinitis – *see* Chorioretinitis
Choroidoretinopathy, central serous H35.7
Christian-Weber disease M35.6
Christmas disease D67
Chromaffinoma (M8700/0) – *see also* Neoplasm, benign
- malignant (M8700/3) – *see* Neoplasm, malignant

Chromatopsia H53.1
Chromhidrosis, chromidrosis L75.1
Chromoblastomycosis (*see also* Chromomycosis) B43.9
Chromomycosis B43.9
- brain abscess B43.1† G07*
- cerebral B43.1† G07*
- cutaneous B43.0† L99.8*
- skin B43.0† L99.8*
- specified NEC B43.8
- subcutaneous abscess or cyst B43.2† L99.8*

Chromophytosis B36.0
Chromosome – *see* condition by chromosome involved
- D(1) – *see* condition, chromosome 13
- E(3) – *see* condition, chromosome 18
- G – *see* condition, chromosome 21
- long arm 18 or 21 syndrome Q93.5

Chronic – *see condition*
Churg-Strauss syndrome M30.1
Chyle cyst, mesentery I89.8
Chylocele (nonfilarial) I89.8
- filarial (*see also* Filaria) B74.-† N51.8*
- tunica vaginalis N50.8
- - filarial (*see also* Filaria) B74.-† N51.8*

Chylopericardium I31.3
Chylothorax (nonfilarial) I89.8
- filarial (*see also* Filaria) B74.9† J91*
Chylous – *see condition*
Chyluria R82.0
- due to
- - Brugia (malayi) B74.1
- - - timori B74.2
- - schistosomiasis (bilharziasis) B65.0
- - Wuchereria (bancrofti) B74.0
- filarial (*see also* Filaria) B74.9
- nonfilarial R82.0

Cicatricial (deformity) – *see* Cicatrix
Cicatrix (adherent) (contracted) (painful) (vicious) (*see also* Scar) L90.5
- adenoid (and tonsil) J35.8
- anus K62.8
- auricle H61.1
- bile duct (common) (hepatic) K83.8
- bladder N32.8
- bone M89.8
- brain G93.8
- cervix (postoperative) (postpartal) N88.1
- common duct K83.8
- cornea H17.9
- - tuberculous A18.5† H19.8*
- duodenum (bulb), obstructive K31.5
- eyelid H02.5
- hypopharynx J39.2
- lacrimal passages H04.5
- larynx J38.7
- lung J98.4
- middle ear H74.8
- mouth K13.7
- muscle M62.8
- - with contracture M62.4
- nasopharynx J39.2
- palate (soft) K13.7
- penis N48.8
- pharynx J39.2
- prostate N42.8
- rectum K62.8
- retina H31.0
- semilunar cartilage – *see* Derangement, meniscus
- seminal vesicle N50.8
- skin L90.5
- - infected L08.8
- - postinfective L90.5
- - tuberculous B90.8
- throat J39.2
- tongue K14.8
- tonsil (and adenoid) J35.8
- trachea J39.2

Cicatrix—*continued*
- tuberculous NEC B90.9
- urethra N36.8
- uterus N85.8
- vagina N89.8
- – postoperative N99.2
- vocal cord J38.3

CIN – *see* Neoplasia, intraepithelial, cervix

Cinchonism
- correct substance properly administered H91.0
- overdose or wrong substance given or taken T37.2

Circle of Willis – *see condition*

Circular – *see condition*

Circulating anticoagulants D68.3
- following childbirth O72.3

Circulation
- collateral, any site I99
- defective I99
- – congenital Q28.9
- failure (peripheral) R57.9
- – fetus or newborn P29.8
- fetal, persistent P29.3
- heart, incomplete Q28.9

Circulatory system – *see condition*

Circulus senilis (cornea) H18.4

Circumcision (in absence of medical indication) (ritual) (routine) Z41.2

Circumscribed – *see condition*

Circumvallate placenta (*see also* Placenta, abnormal) O43.1

Cirrhosis, cirrhotic (hepatic) K74.6
- alcoholic K70.3
- atrophic – *see* Cirrhosis, liver
- Baumgarten-Cruveilhier K74.6
- biliary (cholangiolitic) (cholangitic) (hypertrophic) (obstructive) (pericholangiolitic) K74.5
- – primary K74.3
- – secondary K74.4
- cardiac (of liver) K76.1
- Charcot's K74.3
- cholangiolitic, cholangitic, cholostatic (primary) K74.3
- congestive K76.1
- Cruveilhier-Baumgarten K74.6
- cryptogenic – *see* Cirrhosis, liver
- dietary K74.6
- Hanot's (hypertrophic) K74.3
- hypertrophic K74.3
- Indian childhood K74.6
- kidney – *see* Sclerosis, renal
- Laennec's K70.3

Cirrhosis, cirrhotic—*continued*
- Laennec's—*continued*
- – non-alcoholic K74.6
- liver (chronic) (hepatolienal) (hypertrophic) (nodular) (splenomegalic) K74.6
- – alcoholic K70.3
- congenital P78.8
- – syphilitic A52.7† K77.0*
- lung (chronic) – *see* Fibrosis, lung
- macronodular K74.6
- – alcoholic K70.3
- micronodular K74.6
- – alcoholic K70.3
- mixed type K74.6
- monolobular K74.3
- nodular K74.6
- nutritional K74.6
- – alcoholic K70.3
- obstructive (intrahepatic) (secondary) – *see* Cirrhosis, biliary
- pancreas (duct) K86.8
- periportal K74.6
- portal K74.6
- – alcoholic K70.3
- posthepatitic K74.6
- postnecrotic K74.6
- – alcoholic K70.3
- pulmonary – *see* Fibrosis, lung
- septal K74.6
- stasis K76.1
- Todd's K74.3
- trabecular K74.6
- unilobar K74.3

Citrullinemia E72.2

Citrullinuria E72.2

Civatte's disease or poikiloderma L57.3

Clammy skin R23.1

Clap – *see* Gonorrhea

Clastothrix L67.8

Claude Bernard-Horner syndrome G90.2
- traumatic S14.5

Claude's disease or syndrome I66.8† G46.3*

Claudication, intermittent I73.9
- cerebral (artery) G45.9
- spinal cord (arteriosclerotic) G95.1
- syphilitic A52.0† I79.8*
- venous I87.8

Claustrophobia F40.2

Clavus (infected) L84

Clawfoot (congenital) Q66.8
- acquired M21.5

Clawhand (acquired) M21.5
– congenital Q68.1
Clawtoe (congenital) Q66.8
– acquired M20.5
Cleansing of artificial opening – *see*
Attention, artificial, opening
Cleft (congenital) – *see also* Imperfect,
closure
– alveolar process K08.8
– branchial (cyst) (persistent) Q18.2
– cricoid cartilage, posterior Q31.8
– lip (unilateral) Q36.9
– – median Q36.1
– – with cleft palate Q37.9
– – – hard Q37.1
– – – – and soft Q37.5
– – – soft Q37.3
– – bilateral Q36.0
– – – with cleft palate Q37.8
– – – – hard Q37.0
– – – – – and soft Q37.4
– – – – soft Q37.2
– nose Q30.2
– palate Q35.9
– – with cleft lip (unilateral) Q37.9
– – – bilateral Q37.8
– – hard Q35.1
– – – with cleft
– – – – lip (unilateral) Q37.1
– – – – – bilateral Q37.0
– – – – soft palate Q35.5
– – – – – with cleft lip (unilateral) Q37.5
– – – – – – bilateral Q37.4
– – medial Q35.5
– – soft Q35.3
– – – with cleft
– – – – hard palate Q35.5
– – – – – with cleft lip (unilateral) Q37.5
– – – – – – bilateral Q37.4
– – – – lip (unilateral) Q37.3
– – – – – bilateral Q37.2
– penis Q55.6
– scrotum Q55.2
– thyroid cartilage Q31.8
– uvula Q35.7
Cleidocranial dysostosis Q74.0
Cleidotomy, fetus or newborn P03.8
– to facilitate delivery O83.4
Clicking hip (newborn) R29.4
Climacteric (*see also* Menopause) N95.1
– arthritis (any site) NEC M13.8
– depression (single episode) F32.8
– disease (female) N95.1
– male (symptoms) (syndrome) NEC N50.8

Climacteric—*continued*
– paranoid state F22.8
– polyarthritis NEC M13.8
– symptoms (female) N95.1
**Clinical research investigation (control
subject)** Z00.6
Clitoris – *see condition*
Cloaca (persistent) Q43.7
Clonorchiasis, clonorchis infection B66.1
– liver B66.1† K77.0*
Clonus R25.8
**Clostridium perfringens, as cause of
disease classified elsewhere** B96.7
Closure
– cranial sutures, premature Q75.0
– defective or imperfect NEC – *see*
Imperfect, closure
– fistula, delayed – *see* Fistula
– foramen ovale, imperfect Q21.1
– hymen N89.6
– interauricular septum, defective Q21.1
– interventricular septum, defective Q21.0
– lacrimal duct H04.5
– – congenital Q10.5
– nose, congenital Q30.0
– of artificial opening – *see* Attention,
artificial, opening
– vagina N89.5
– valve – *see* Endocarditis
– vulva N90.5
Clot (blood) – *see also* Embolism
– artery (obstruction) (occlusion) (*see also*
Embolism) I74.9
– bladder N32.8
– brain (intradural or extradural) (*see also*
Occlusion, artery, cerebral) I66.9
– circulation I74.9
– coronary (*see also* Infarct, myocardium)
I21.9
– – not resulting in infarction I24.0
– vein (*see also* Thrombosis) I82.9
Clouded state R40.1
– epileptic G40.8
– paroxysmal G40.8
Cloudy antrum, antra J32.0
Clouston's (hidrotic) ectodermal dysplasia
Q82.8
Clubbed nail pachydermoperiostosis
M89.4† L62.0*
Clubbing of finger(s) (nails) R68.3
Clubfinger R68.3
– congenital Q68.1
Clubfoot (congenital) Q66.8
– acquired M21.5

Clubfoot—*continued*
− paralytic M21.5
Clubhand (congenital) (radial) Q71.4
− acquired M21.5
Clubnail R68.3
− congenital Q84.6
Clump, kidney Q63.1
Clumsiness, clumsy child syndrome F82
Cluttering F98.6
Clutton's joints A50.5† M03.1*
Coagulation, intravascular (diffuse) (disseminated) (*see also* Defibrination) D65
− fetus or newborn P60
Coagulopathy (*see also* Defect, coagulation) D68.9
− consumption D65
− − newborn P60
Coalminer's
− elbow M70.2
− lung or pneumoconiosis J60
Coalition
− calcaneo-scaphoid Q66.8
− tarsal Q66.8
Coalworker's lung or pneumoconiosis J60
Coarctation of aorta (preductal) (postductal) Q25.1
Coated tongue K14.3
Coats' disease (exudative retinopathy) H35.0
Cocainism F14.2
Coccidioidomycosis, coccidioidosis B38.9
− cutaneous B38.3† L99.8*
− disseminated B38.7
− generalized B38.7
− meninges B38.4† G02.1*
− prostate B38.8† N51.0*
− pulmonary B38.2† J17.2*
− − acute B38.0† J17.2*
− − chronic B38.1† J17.2*
− skin B38.3† L99.8*
− specified NEC B38.8
Coccidiosis (intestinal) A07.3
Coccydynia, coccygodynia M53.3
Coccyx − *see condition*
Cockayne's syndrome Q87.1
Cocked up toe M20.5
Cock's peculiar tumor L72.1
Codman's tumor (M9230/0) − *see* Neoplasm, bone, benign
Coenurosis B71.8
Coffee-worker's lung J67.8
Cogan's syndrome H16.3
− oculomotor apraxia H51.8

Coitus, painful (female) N94.1
− male N48.8
− psychogenic F52.6
Cold J00
− with influenza, flu, or grippe (*see also* Influenza, with, respiratory manifestations) J11.1
− agglutinin disease or hemoglobinuria D59.1
− bronchial or chest − *see* Bronchitis
− common (head) J00
− effects of T69.9
− − specified NEC T69.8
− excessive, effects of T69.9
− − specified NEC T69.8
− exhaustion from T69.8
− exposure to T69.9
− − specified effect NEC T69.8
− injury syndrome (newborn) P80.0
− sensitivity, auto-immune D59.1
− virus J00
Coldsore B00.1
Colibacillosis NEC A49.8
− generalized A41.5
Colic (recurrent) R10.4
− abdomen R10.4
− − psychogenic F45.3
− appendix, appendicular K38.8
− bile duct (*see also* Choledocholithiasis) K80.5
− biliary K80.5
− bilious R10.4
− common duct K80.5
− cystic duct (*see also* Cholelithiasis) K80.2
− Devonshire NEC T56.0
− flatulent R14
− gallbladder K80.2
− gallstone K80.2
− − gallbladder or cystic duct (*see also* Cholelithiasis) K80.2
− hepatic (duct) (*see also* Choledocholithiasis) K80.5
− hysterical F45.3
− infantile R10.4
− intestinal R10.4
− kidney N23
− lead NEC T56.0
− nephritic N23
− painter's NEC T56.0
− psychogenic F45.3
− renal N23
− saturnine NEC T56.0
− spasmodic R10.4

Colic—*continued*
- ureter N23
- urethral N36.8
- - due to calculus N21.1
- uterus NEC N94.8
- - menstrual (*see also* Dysmenorrhea) N94.6

Colicystitis (*see also* Cystitis) N30.8
Colitis (acute) (catarrhal) (hemorrhagic) (*see also* Enteritis) A09.9
- allergic K52.2
- amebic (acute) (*see also* Amebiasis) A06.0
- - nondysenteric A06.2
- anthrax A22.2
- bacillary (*see also* Infection, Shigella) A03.9
- balantidial A07.0
- chronic (noninfectious) K52.9
- coccidial A07.3
- collagenous K52.8
- cystica superficialis K52.8
- dietary counseling and surveillance (for)) Z71.3
- dietetic K52.2
- due to radiation K52.0
- food hypersensitivity K52.2
- giardial A07.1
- granulomatous K50.1
- hemi-, left K51.5
- indeterminate K52.3
- infectious (*see also* Enteritis, infectious) A09.0
- ischemic K55.9
- - acute (fulminant) (subacute) K55.0
- - chronic K55.1
- - fulminant (acute) K55.0
- left sided K51.5
- lymphocytic K52.8
- microscopic K52.8
- noninfectious K52.9
- - specified NEC K52.8
- pan-, ulcerative (chronic) K51.0
- polyposa K51.4
- protozoal A07.9
- pseudomembranous A04.7
- regional K50.1
- septic (*see also* Enteritis, infectious) A09.0
- spastic K58.9
- - with diarrhea K58.0
- toxic K52.1
- trichomonal A07.8
- tuberculous (ulcerative) A18.3† K93.0*

Colitis—*continued*
- ulcerative (chronic) K51.9
- - specified NEC K51.8
Collagenosis, collagen disease (nonvascular) (vascular) M35.9
- cardiovascular I42.8
- reactive perforating L87.1
- specified NEC M35.8
Collapse R55
- adrenal E27.2
- cardiorenal I13.2
- cardiorespiratory R57.0
- cardiovascular R57.9
- - newborn P29.8
- circulatory (peripheral) R57.9
- - during or after labor and delivery O75.1
- - fetus or newborn P29.8
- - following
- - - abortion (subsequent episode) O08.3
- - - - current episode – *see* Abortion
- - - ectopic or molar pregnancy O08.3
- during or after labor and delivery O75.1
- external ear canal H61.3
- general R55
- heart I50.9
- heat T67.1
- hysterical F44.8
- labyrinth, membranous (congenital) Q16.5
- lung (massive) (*see also* Atelectasis) J98.1
- - pressure due to anesthesia (general) (local) or other sedation T88.2
- - - during labor and delivery O74.1
- - - in pregnancy O29.0
- - - postpartum, puerperal O89.0
- myocardial – *see* Disease, heart
- nervous F48.8
- neurocirculatory F45.3
- nose M95.0
- postoperative (cardiovascular) T81.1
- pulmonary (*see also* Atelectasis) J98.1
- trachea J39.8
- tracheobronchial J98.0
- valvular – *see* Endocarditis
- vascular (peripheral) R57.9
- - cerebral I64
- - during or after labor and delivery O75.1
- - - affecting fetus or newborn P03.8
- - fetus or newborn P29.8
- vertebra NEC M48.5

Collapse—*continued*
- vertebra NEC—*continued*
- – in (due to)
- – – metastasis (M8000/6) C79.5†
  M49.5*
- – – osteoporosis (*see also* Osteoporosis)
  M80.9
Colles' fracture S52.5
Collet(-Sicard) syndrome G52.7
Collier's asthma or lung J60
Collodion baby Q80.2
Colloid nodule (cystic) (of thyroid) E04.1
Coloboma Q13.0
- eyelid Q10.3
- fundus Q14.8
- iris Q13.0
- lens Q12.2
- optic disk Q14.2
Coloenteritis – *see* Enteritis
Colon – *see condition*
Coloptosis K63.4
Color blindness H53.5
Colostomy
- attention to Z43.3
- fitting or adjustment Z46.5
- malfunctioning K91.4
- status Z93.3
Colpitis (acute) (*see also* Vaginitis) N76.0
Colpocele N81.1
Colpocystitis (*see also* Vaginitis) N76.0
Column, spinal, vertebral – *see condition*
Coma R40.2
- apoplectic I64
- diabetic (with ketoacidosis)
  (hyperosmolar) – *code to* E10-E14 with
  fourth character .0
- eclamptic (*see also* Eclampsia) O15.9
- epileptic G40.8
- hepatic (*see also* Failure, hepatic) K72.9
- hyperglycemic (diabetic) E14.0
- hyperosmolar (diabetic) E14.0
- hypoglycemic (nondiabetic) E15
- – diabetic – *code to* E10-E14 with fourth
    character .0
- insulin – *code to* E10-E14 with fourth
    character .0
- – drug-induced – *code to* E10-E14 with
    fourth character .0
- – – in nondiabetic E15
- – in nondiabetic (drug-induced) E15
- Kussmaul's – *code to* E10-E14 with fourth
    character .0
- myxedematous E03.5
- newborn P91.5

Coma—*continued*
- prolonged, due to intracranial injury
  S06.7
- uremic N19
Comatose R40.2
Combat fatigue F43.0
Combined – *see condition*
Comedo, comedones (giant) L70.0
Comedocarcinoma (M8501/3) – *see also*
  Neoplasm, breast, malignant
- noninfiltrating (M8501/2)
- – breast D05.7
- – specified site – *see* Neoplasm, in situ
- – unspecified site D05.7
Comedomastitis N60.4
Comminuted fracture – *code as* Fracture,
  closed
Common
- arterial trunk Q20.0
- atrioventricular canal Q21.2
- atrium Q21.1
- truncus (arteriosus) Q20.0
- variable immunodeficiency – *see*
  Immunodeficiency, common variable
- ventricle Q20.4
Commotio, commotion (current)
- brain S06.0
- cerebri S06.0
- retinae S05.8
- spinal cord – *see* Injury, spinal cord, by
  region
- spinalis – *see* Injury, spinal cord, by
  region
Communication
- between
- – base of aorta and pulmonary artery
  Q21.4
- – left ventricle and right atrium Q20.5
- – pericardial sac and pleural sac Q34.8
- – pulmonary artery and pulmonary vein,
  congenital Q25.7
- – uterus and digestive or urinary tract,
  congenital Q51.7
Compensation
- failure – *see* Disease, heart
- neurosis, psychoneurosis F68.0
Complaint – *see also* Disease
- bowel, functional K59.9
- – psychogenic F45.3
- intestine, functional K59.9
- – psychogenic F45.3
- kidney (*see also* Disease, renal) N28.9
Complete – *see condition*

Complex
- Addison-Schilder E71.3
- cardiorenal (*see also* Hypertension, cardiorenal) I13.9
- Costen's K07.6
- Eisenmenger I27.8
- hypersexual F52.7
- jumped process, spine – *see* Dislocation, vertebra
- primary, tuberculous A16.7
- – with bacteriological and histological confirmation A15.7
- Schilder-Addison E71.3
- subluxation (vertebral) M99.1
- Taussig-Bing Q20.1

Complications (from) (of)
- accidental puncture or laceration during procedure T81.2
- amputation stump (late) (surgical) T87.6
- – infection or inflammation T87.4
- – necrosis T87.5
- – neuroma T87.3
- – specified NEC T87.6
- anastomosis (and bypass) NEC T85.9
- – intestinal (internal) NEC K91.8
- – – involving urinary tract N99.8
- – urinary tract (involving intestinal tract) N99.8
- – vascular T82.9
- – – infection or inflammation T82.7
- – – mechanical T82.3
- – – specified NEC T82.8
- anesthesia, anesthetic NEC (*see also* Anesthesia, complication or reaction NEC) T88.5
- – brain, postpartum, puerperal O89.2
- – cardiac
- – – in labor and delivery O74.2
- – – in pregnancy O29.1
- – – postpartum, puerperal O89.1
- – central nervous system
- – – in labor and delivery O74.3
- – – in pregnancy O29.2
- – – postpartum, puerperal O89.2
- – difficult or failed intubation T88.4
- – hyperthermia, malignant T88.3
- – hypothermia NEC T88.5
- – in
- – – abortion – *see* Abortion
- – – labor and delivery O74.9
- – – – specified NEC O74.8
- – – postpartum, puerperal O89.9
- – – – specified NEC O89.8
- – – pregnancy O29.9

Complications—*continued*
- anesthesia, anesthetic NEC—*continued*
- – in—*continued*
- – – pregnancy—*continued*
- – – – specified NEC O29.8
- – malignant hyperthermia T88.3
- – pulmonary NEC
- – – in labor and delivery O74.1
- – – in pregnancy O29.0
- – – postpartum, puerperal O89.0
- – shock T88.2
- – spinal and epidural
- – – in labor and delivery NEC O74.6
- – – – headache O74.5
- – – in pregnancy NEC O29.5
- – – – headache O29.4
- – – postpartum, puerperal NEC O89.5
- – – – headache O89.4
- aortic (bifurcation) graft – *see* Complications, graft, arterial
- aortocoronary (bypass) graft – *see* Complications, coronary artery (bypass) graft
- aortofemoral (bypass) graft – *see* Complications, graft, arterial
- arteriovenous fistula or shunt, surgically created T82.9
- – infection or inflammation T82.7
- – mechanical T82.5
- – specified NEC T82.8
- arthroplasty T84.9
- – specified NEC T84.8
- artificial
- – fertilization or insemination N98.9
- – – attempted introduction (of)
- – – – embryo in embryo transfer N98.3
- – – – ovum following in vitro fertilization N98.2
- – – hyperstimulation of ovaries N98.1
- – – infection N98.0
- – – specified NEC N98.8
- – heart T82.9
- – – infection or inflammation T82.7
- – – mechanical T82.5
- – – specified NEC T82.8
- balloon implant or device
- – gastrointestinal T85.9
- – – infection or inflammation T85.7
- – – mechanical T85.5
- – – specified NEC T85.8
- – vascular (counterpulsation) T82.9
- – – infection or inflammation T82.7
- – – mechanical T82.5
- – – specified NEC T82.8

Complications—*continued*
- bile duct implant (prosthetic) T85.9
- − infection or inflammation T85.7
- − mechanical T85.5
- − specified NEC T85.8
- bladder device (auxiliary) T83.9
- − infection or inflammation T83.5
- − mechanical T83.1
- − specified NEC T83.8
  bone
- − graft T84.9
- − − infection or inflammation T84.7
- − − mechanical T84.3
- − − specified NEC T84.8
- − growth stimulator (electrode) T84.9
- − − infection or inflammation T84.7
- − − mechanical T84.3
- − − specified NEC T84.8
- brain neurostimulator (electrode) T85.9
- − infection or inflammation T85.7
- − mechanical T85.1
- − specified NEC T85.8
- breast implant (prosthetic) T85.9
- − infection or inflammation T85.7
- − mechanical T85.4
- − specified NEC T85.8
- bypass (*see also* Complications, anastomosis) T85.9
- − aortocoronary − *see* Complications, coronary artery (bypass) graft
- − arterial NEC − *see* Complications, graft, arterial
- cardiac (*see also* Disease, heart) I51.9
- − device, implant or graft T82.9
- − − infection or inflammation T82.7
- − − mechanical T82.5
- − − pacemaker (electrode) (pulse generator) T82.9
- − − − infection or inflammation T82.7
- − − − mechanical T82.1
- − − − specified NEC T82.8
- − − specified NEC T82.8
- − − valve graft T82.9
- − − − infection or inflammation T82.7
- − − − mechanical T82.2
- − − − specified NEC T82.8
- − − valve prosthesis T82.9
- − − − infection or inflammation T82.6
- − − − mechanical T82.0
- − − − specified NEC T82.8
- − pacemaker (electrode) (pulse generator) T82.9
- − − infection or inflammation T82.7
- − − mechanical T82.1

Complications—*continued*
- cardiac—*continued*
- − pacemaker—*continued*
- − − − specified NEC T82.8
- − − postoperative I97.9
- − − − specified NEC I97.8
- − − valve
- − − − graft T82.9
- − − − − infection or inflammation T82.7
- − − − − mechanical T82.2
- − − − − specified NEC T82.8
- − − − prosthesis T82.9
- − − − − infection or inflammation T82.6
- − − − − mechanical T82.0
- − − − − specified NEC T82.8
- cardiorenal I13.2
- carotid artery (bypass) graft − *see* Complications, graft, arterial
- catheter (device) NEC T85.9
- − cystostomy − *see* Complications, catheter, urinary
- − infection or inflammation T85.7
- − mechanical T85.6
- − specified NEC T85.8
- − urethral, indwelling − *see* Complications, catheter, urinary
- − urinary (indwelling) T83.9
- − − infection or inflammation T83.5
- − − mechanical T83.0
- − − specified NEC T83.8
- − − urethral stricture N99.1
- cecostomy (stoma) K91.4
- cesarean section wound NEC O90.8
- − disruption O90.0
- − hematoma O90.2
- − infection (following delivery) O86.0
- chin implant (prosthetic) T85.9
- − infection or inflammation T85.7
- − mechanical T85.6
- − specified NEC T85.8
- circulatory I99
- − postoperative I97.9
- − − specified NEC I97.8
- colostomy (stoma) K91.4
- contraceptive device, intrauterine T83.9
- − infection or inflammation T83.6
- − mechanical T83.3
- − specified NEC T83.8
- cord (umbilical) − *see* Complications, umbilical cord NEC
- corneal graft T85.9
- − infection or inflammation T85.7
- − mechanical T85.3
- − specified NEC T85.8

Complications—*continued*
- coronary artery (bypass) graft T82.9
- – infection or inflammation T82.7
- – mechanical T82.2
- – specified NEC T82.8
- counterpulsation device (balloon), intra-aortic T82.9
- – infection or inflammation T82.7
- – mechanical T82.5
- – specified NEC T82.8
- cystostomy (stoma) N99.5
- – catheter – *see* Complications, catheter, urinary
- delivery (*see also* Complications, obstetric) O75.9
- – procedure (instrumental) (manual) (surgical) O75.4
- – specified NEC O75.8
- device NEC T85.8
- dialysis (renal) T80.9
- – catheter (vascular) T82.9
- – – infection or inflammation T82.7
- – – mechanical T82.4
- – – peritoneal, intraperitoneal – *see* Complications, catheter
- – – specified NEC T82.8
- ear H93.9
- – postoperative H95.9
- – – specified NEC H95.8
- electronic stimulator device (electrode(s)) (pulse generator)
- – bladder (urinary) T83.9
- – – infection or inflammation T83.5
- – – mechanical T83.1
- – – specified NEC T83.8
- – bone T84.9
- – – infection or inflammation T84.7
- – – mechanical T84.3
- – – specified NEC T84.8
- – cardiac (defibrillator) (pacemaker) T82.9
- – – infection or inflammation T82.7
- – – mechanical T82.1
- – – specified NEC T82.8
- – muscle T84.9
- – – infection or inflammation T84.7
- – – mechanical T84.4
- – – specified NEC T84.8
- – nervous system (brain) (peripheral nerve) (spinal cord) T85.9
- – – infection or inflammation T85.7
- – – mechanical T85.1
- – – specified NEC T85.8
- electroshock therapy T88.9

Complications—*continued*
- electroshock therapy—*continued*
- – specified NEC T88.8
- endocrine E34.9
- – postoperative E89.9
- – – specified NEC E89.8
- enterostomy (stoma) K91.4
- episiotomy, disruption O90.1
- esophageal anti-reflux device T85.9
- – infection or inflammation T85.7
- – mechanical T85.5
- – specified NEC T85.8
- extracorporeal circulation T80.9
- eye H57.9
- – implant (prosthetic) T85.9
- – – infection or inflammation T85.7
- – – mechanical T85.3
- – – – intraocular lens T85.2
- – – specified NEC T85.8
- – postoperative H59.9
- – – blebitis H59.8
- – – specified NEC H59.8
- female genital N94.9
- – device, implant or graft T83.9
- – – infection or inflammation T83.6
- – – mechanical T83.4
- – – – intrauterine contraceptive device T83.3
- – – specified NEC T83.8
- femoral artery (bypass) graft – *see* Complications, graft, arterial NEC
- fixation device, internal (orthopedic) T84.9
- – infection or inflammation T84.6
- – mechanical T84.2
- – – bones of limb T84.1
- – specified NEC T84.8
- following
- – abortion O08.9
- – – specified NEC O08.8
- – acute myocardial infarction NEC I23.8
- – – aneurysm (false) (of cardiac wall) (of heart wall) (non-ruptured) I23.3
- – – defect
- – – – septal
- – – – – atrial (heart) I23.1
- – – – – ventricular (heart) I23.2
- – – haemopericardium I23.0
- – – rupture
- – – – cardiac wall I23.3
- – – – – with haemopericardium I23.0
- – – – chordae tendineae I23.4
- – – – papillary muscle I23.5

Complications—*continued*
- following—*continued*
- – acute myocardial infarction NEC—*continued*
- – – thrombosis
- – – – atrium I23.6
- – – – – auricular appendage I23.6
- – – – – ventricle (heart) I23.6
- – – ectopic or molar pregnancy O08.9
- – – – specified NEC O08.8
- – gastrointestinal K92.9
- – – postoperative (*see also* Complications, by type and site) K91.9
- – – – specified NEC K91.8
- – gastrostomy (stoma) K91.8
- – genitourinary, postprocedural N99.9
- – – specified NEC N99.8
- – graft (bypass) (patch) T85.9
- – – arterial T82.9
- – – – infection or inflammation T82.7
- – – – mechanical T82.3
- – – – specified NEC T82.8
- – – bone T84.9
- – – – infection or inflammation T84.7
- – – – marrow NEC T86.0
- – – – mechanical T84.3
- – – – specified NEC T84.8
- – – carotid artery – *see* Complications, graft, arterial
- – – cornea T85.9
- – – – infection or inflammation T85.7
- – – – mechanical T85.3
- – – – specified NEC T85.8
- – – coronary (artery) T82.9
- – – – infection or inflammation T82.7
- – – – mechanical T82.2
- – – – specified NEC T82.8
- – – femoral artery (bypass) – *see* Complications, graft, arterial
- – – genital organ or tract T83.9
- – – – infection or inflammation T83.6
- – – – mechanical T83.4
- – – – specified NEC T83.8
- – – muscle T84.9
- – – – infection or inflammation T84.7
- – – – mechanical T84.4
- – – – specified NEC T84.8
- – – nerve T85.9
- – – – infection or inflammation T85.7
- – – – mechanical T85.6
- – – – specified NEC T85.8
- – – organ (immune or nonimmune cause) (partial) (total) – *see* Complications, organ or tissue transplant

Complications—*continued*
- – graft—*continued*
- – – skin (failure) (infection) (rejection) T86.8
- – – specified NEC T85.8
- – – tendon T84.9
- – – – infection or inflammation T84.7
- – – – mechanical T84.4
- – – – specified NEC T84.8
- – – urinary organ T83.9
- – – – infection or inflammation T83.5
- – – – mechanical T83.2
- – – – specified NEC T83.8
- – – vascular – *see* Complications, graft, arterial NEC
- – heart I51.9
- – – postoperative I97.9
- – – – specified NEC I97.8
- – – transplant, failure or rejection (immune or nonimmune cause) T86.2
- – – – and lung(s) T86.3
- – – valve
- – – – graft T82.9
- – – – – infection or inflammation T82.7
- – – – – mechanical T82.2
- – – – – specified NEC T82.8
- – – – prosthesis T82.9
- – – – – infection or inflammation T82.6
- – – – – mechanical T82.0
- – – – – specified NEC T82.8
- – hemodialysis – *see* Complications, dialysis
- – ileostomy (stoma) K91.4
- – immunization (procedure) – *see* Complications, vaccination
- – implant NEC – *see* Complications, by site and type
- – infusion (procedure) NEC T80.9
- – – blood – *see* Complications, transfusion
- – – catheter T82.9
- – – – infection or inflammation T82.7
- – – – mechanical T82.5
- – – – specified NEC T82.8
- – – infection NEC T80.2
- – – pump – *see* Complications, infusion, catheter
- – – sepsis NEC T80.2
- – inhalation therapy NEC T81.8
- – injection (procedure) T80.9
- – – drug reaction (*see also* Reaction, drug) T88.7
- – – infection NEC T80.2
- – – sepsis NEC T80.2

Complications—*continued*
- injection—*continued*
- – serum (prophylactic) (therapeutic) – *see* Complications, vaccination
- – vaccine (any) – *see* Complications, vaccination
- inoculation (any) (*see also* Complications, vaccination) T80.9
- internal device (catheter) (electronic) (fixation) (prosthetic) NEC – *see* Complications, by site and type
- intraocular lens (prosthetic) T85.9
- – infection or inflammation T85.7
- – mechanical T85.2
- – specified NEC T85.8
- intraperitoneal catheter (dialysis) (infusion) T85.9
- – infection or inflammation T85.7
- – mechanical T85.6
- – specified NEC T85.8
- intrauterine
- – contraceptive device T83.9
- – – infection or inflammation T83.6
- – – mechanical T83.3
- – – specified NEC T83.8
- – procedure NEC, affecting fetus or newborn P96.5
- jejunostomy (stoma) K91.4
- joint prosthesis, internal (any site) T84.9
- – infection or inflammation T84.5
- – mechanical T84.0
- – specified NEC T84.8
- kidney transplant, failure or rejection (immune or nonimmune cause) T86.1
- labor O75.9
- – specified NEC O75.8
- liver transplant, failure or rejection (immune or nonimmune cause) T86.4
- lumbar puncture G97.1
- – cerebrospinal fluid leak G97.0
- – headache or reaction G97.1
- lung transplant, failure or rejection (immune or nonimmune cause) T86.8
- – and heart T86.3
- male genital N50.9
- – device, implant or graft T83.9
- – – infection or inflammation T83.6
- – – mechanical T83.4
- – – specified NEC T83.8
- – postprocedural or postoperative N99.9
- – – specified NEC N99.8
- mastoid (process) (postprocedural) H95.9
- – specified NEC H95.8
- mastoidectomy cavity NEC H95.1

Complications—*continued*
- medical procedure T88.9
- – cardiac T81.8
- – – postprocedural (functional) (late) I97.9
- – – – specified NEC I97.8
- – circulatory T81.7
- – – postprocedural (functional) (late) I97.9
- – – – specified NEC I97.8
- – digestive system K91.9
- – – specified NEC K91.8
- – ear H95.9
- – – specified NEC H95.8
- – eye H59.9
- – – specified NEC H59.8
- – gastrointestinal K91.9
- – – specified NEC K91.8
- – mastoidectomy cavity NEC H95.1
- – musculoskeletal M96.9
- – – specified NEC M96.8
- – nervous system (central) (peripheral) G97.9
- – – specified NEC G97.8
- – peripheral vascular T81.7
- – respiratory J95.9
- – – specified NEC J95.8
- – urethral stricture N99.1
- – vascular T81.7
- – – postprocedural (functional) (late) I97.8
- metabolic E88.9
- – postoperative E89.9
- – – specified NEC E89.8
- musculoskeletal M79.9
- – postprocedural M96.9
- – – specified NEC M96.8
- nephrostomy (stoma) N99.5
- nervous system G98
- – central G96.9
- – device, implant or graft T85.9
- – – infection or inflammation T85.7
- – – mechanical T85.6
- – – specified NEC T85.8
- – electronic stimulator (electrode(s)) T85.9
- – – infection or inflammation T85.7
- – – mechanical T85.1
- – – specified NEC T85.8
- – postprocedural G97.9
- – – specified NEC G97.8
- neurostimulator T85.9
- – infection or inflammation T85.7
- – mechanical T85.1

Complications—*continued*
- neurostimulator—*continued*
- – specified NEC T85.8
- nonabsorbable (permanent) sutures NEC T85.9
- – in bone repair NEC – *see* Complications, fixation device, internal
- obstetric O75.9
- – procedure (instrumental) (manual) (surgical) specified NEC O75.4
- – specified NEC O75.8
- – surgical wound NEC O90.8
- – – hematoma O90.2
- – – infection O86.0
- organ or tissue transplant, failure or rejection (immune or nonimmune cause) (partial) (total) T86.9
- – bone T86.8
- – bone marrow T86.0
- – heart T86.2
- – – and lung(s) T86.3
- – intestine T86.8
- – kidney T86.1
- – liver T86.4
- – lung(s) T86.8
- – – and heart T86.3
- – pancreas T86.8
- – skin (allograft) (autograft) T86.8
- – specified NEC T86.8
- orthopedic
- – external device or appliance T88.8
- – interal device, implant or graft T84.9
- – – infection or inflammation T84.5-T84.7
- – – mechanical T84.0-T84.4
- – – specified NEC T84.8
- – fracture (following insertion of implant, joint prosthesis, bone plate) M96.6
- – internal fixation (nail) (plate) (rod) T84.9
- – – infection or inflammation NEC T84.6
- – – mechanical NEC T84.2
- – – – bones of limb T84.1
- – – specified NEC T84.8
- – joint prosthesis T84.9
- – – infection or inflammation T84.5
- – – mechanical T84.0
- – – specified NEC T84.8
- pacemaker (cardiac) (electrode(s)) (pulse generator) T82.9
- – infection or inflammation T82.7
- – mechanical T82.1
- – specified NEC T82.8

Complications—*continued*
- pancreas transplant, failure or rejection (immune or nonimmune cause) T86.8
- penile prosthesis (implant) T83.9
- – infection or inflammation T83.6
- – mechanical T83.4
- – specified NEC T83.8
- perfusion NEC T80.9
- perineal repair (obstetrical) NEC O90.8
- – disruption O90.1
- – hematoma O90.2
- – infection (following delivery) O86.0
- peripheral nerve device, implant or graft T85.9
- – electronic stimulator T85.9
- – – infection or inflammation T85.7
- – – mechanical T85.1
- – – specified NEC T85.8
- – infection or inflammation NEC T85.7
- – mechanical NEC T85.6
- – specified NEC T85.8
- phototherapy T88.9
- – specified NEC T88.8
- postmastoidectomy NEC H95.1
- – recurrent cholesteatoma H95.0
- postoperative (*see also* Complications, surgical procedure) T81.9
- – specified NEC T81.8
- postprocedural
- – ear H95.9
- – – specified NEC H95.8
- – endocrine E89.9
- – – specified NEC E89.8
- – metabolic E89.9
- – – specified NEC E89.8
- pregnancy NEC (*see also* Pregnancy, complicated by) O26.9
- procedure (surgical or medical care) T88.9
- prosthetic device, graft or implant T85.9
- – breast T85.9
- – – infection or inflammation T85.7
- – – mechanical T85.4
- – – specified NEC T85.8
- – cardiac and vascular T82.9
- – eye T85.9
- – – infection or inflammation T85.7
- – – mechanical NEC T85.3
- – – – intraocular lens T85.2
- – – specified NEC T85.8
- – gastrointestinal tract T85.9
- – – infection or inflammation T85.7
- – – mechanical T85.5
- – – specified NEC T85.8

Complications—*continued*
- prosthetic device, graft or implant—
  continued
- - genital organ or tract T83.9
- - - infection or inflammation T83.6
- - - mechanical T83.4
- - - specified NEC T83.8
- - heart valve T82.9
- - - infection or inflammation T82.6
- - - mechanical T82.0
- - - specified NEC T82.8
- - infection or inflammation NEC T85.7
- - joint T84.9
- - - fracture, bone M96.6
- - - infection or inflammation T84.5
- - - mechanical T84.0
- - - specified NEC T84.8
- - mechanical NEC T85.6
- - specified NEC T85.8
- - urinary organ or tract T83.9
- - - infection or inflammation T83.5
- - - mechanical T83.1
- - - specified NEC T83.8
- - vascular T82.9
- - - specified NEC T82.8
- puerperium – *see* Puerperal
- puncture, spinal G97.1
- - cerebrospinal fluid leak G97.0
- - headache or reaction G97.1
- pyelogram N99.8
- radiation T66
- radiotherapy NEC T66
- - kyphosis M96.2
- - scoliosis M96.5
- reattached
- - extremity (infection) (rejection) T87.2
- - - lower T87.1
- - - upper T87.0
- - specified body part NEC T87.2
- reimplant NEC T85.9
- - limb (infection) (rejection) T87.2
- - - lower T87.1
- - - upper T87.0
- - organ, failure or rejection (immune or
  nonimmune cause) (partial) (total) – *see*
  Complications, organ or tissue
  transplant
- - prosthetic device NEC – *see*
  Complications, prosthetic device, graft
  or implant
- renal N28.9
- - allograft T86.1
- - dialysis – *see* Complications, dialysis
- respiratory J98.9

Complications—*continued*
- respiratory—*continued*
- - device, implant or graft T85.9
- - - infection or inflammation T85.7
- - - mechanical T85.6
- - - specified NEC T85.8
- - postoperative J95.9
- - - specified NEC J95.8
- - therapy NEC T81.8
- sedation during labor and delivery O74.9
- - affecting fetus or newborn P04.0
- - cardiac O74.2
- - central nervous system O74.3
- - pulmonary NEC O74.1
- shunt T85.9
- - vascular T82.9
- - - infection or inflammation T82.7
- - - mechanical T82.5
- - - specified NEC T82.8
- - ventricular (communicating) T85.9
- - - infection or inflammation T85.7
- - - mechanical T85.0
- - - specified NEC T85.8
- skin graft (failure) (infection) (rejection)
  T86.8
- spinal
- - anesthesia – *see* Complications,
  anesthesia, spinal and epidural
- - catheter (epidural) (subdural) T85.9
- - - infection or inflammation T85.7
- - - mechanical T85.6
- - - specified NEC T85.8
- - puncture or tap G97.1
- - - cerebrospinal fluid leak G97.0
- - - headache or reaction G97.1
- surgical procedure T81.9
- - accidental puncture or laceration T81.2
- - amputation stump (late) NEC T87.6
- - - infection or inflammation T87.4
- - - necrosis T87.5
- - - neuroma T87.3
- - anoxic brain damage T88.5
- - burst stitches or sutures T81.3
- - cardiac T81.8
- - - long-term effect following cardiac
  surgery I97.1
- - - postprocedural (functional) (late)
  I97.8
- - cholesteatoma, recurrent
  (postmastoidectomy) H95.0
- - circulatory (early) T81.7
- - - functional disturbance NEC I97.8
- - - postprocedural I97.9
- - dehiscence (of wound) T81.3

Complications—*continued*
- surgical procedure—*continued*
- - dehiscence—*continued*
- - - cesarean section O90.0
- - - episiotomy O90.1
- - digestive system K91.9
- - - functional disorder NEC K91.8
- - - specified NEC K91.8
- - disruption of wound T81.3
- - - cesarean section O90.0
- - - episiotomy O90.1
- - dumping syndrome (postgastrectomy) K91.1
- - ear H95.9
- - - specified NEC H95.8
- - elephantiasis or lymphedema I97.8
- - - postmastectomy I97.2
- - emphysema (surgical) T81.8
- - endocrine E89.9
- - - specified NEC E89.8
- - evisceration T81.3
- - eye H59.9
- - - specified NEC H59.8
- - fistula (persistent postoperative) T81.8
- - foreign body inadvertently left in wound (sponge) (suture) (swab) T81.5
- - gastrointestinal K91.9
- - - specified NEC K91.8
- - genitourinary N99.9
- - - specified NEC N99.8
- - hemorrhage or hematoma T81.0
- - hepatic failure K91.8
- - hyperglycemia (postpancreatectomy) E89.1
- - hypoinsulinemia (postpancreatectomy) E89.1
- - hypoparathyroidism (postparathyroidectomy) E89.2
- - hypopituitarism (posthypophysectomy) E89.3
- - hypothyroidism (post-thyroidectomy) E89.0
- - intestinal obstruction K91.3
- - intracranial hypotension following ventricular shunting (ventriculostomy) G97.2
- - malabsorption (postsurgical) NEC K91.2
- - - osteoporosis M81.3
- - mastoidectomy cavity NEC H95.1
- - - recurrent cholesteatoma H95.0
- - metabolic E89.9
- - - specified NEC E89.8
- - musculoskeletal M96.9

Complications—*continued*
- surgical procedure—*continued*
- - musculoskeletal—*continued*
- - - specified NEC M96.8
- - nervous system (central) (peripheral) G97.9
- - - specified NEC G97.8
- - ovarian failure E89.4
- - peripheral vascular T81.7
- - postcardiotomy syndrome I97.0
- - postcholecystectomy syndrome K91.5
- - postcommissurotomy syndrome I97.0
- - postgastrectomy dumping syndrome K91.1
- - postlaminectomy syndrome NEC M96.1
- - - kyphosis M96.3
- - postmastectomy lymphedema syndrome I97.2
- - postvagotomy syndrome K91.1
- - postvalvulotomy syndrome I97.0
- - pulmonary insufficiency (acute) J95.2
- - - chronic J95.3
- - reattached body part (infection) (rejection) NEC T87.2
- - - lower limb T87.1
- - - upper limb T87.0
- - respiratory J95.9
- - - specified NEC J95.8
- - shock (endotoxic) (hypovolemic) (septic) T81.1
- - specified NEC T81.8
- - stitch abscess T81.4
- - subglottic stenosis (postsurgical) J95.5
- - testicular hypofunction E89.5
- - transplant – *see* Complications, organ or tissue transplant
- - urinary N99.9
- - - specified NEC N99.8
- - vaginal vault prolapse (posthysterectomy) N99.3
- - vascular (peripheral) T81.7
- - vitreous (touch) syndrome H59.0
- - wound infection T81.4
- suture, permanent (wire) T85.9
- - infection or inflammation NEC T85.7
- - in repair of bone – *see* Complications, fixation device, internal
- - mechanical T85.6
- - specified NEC T85.8
- tracheostomy J95.0
- transfusion (blood) (lymphocytes) (plasma) T80.9
- - embolism T80.1

Complications—*continued*
- transfusion—*continued*
- – embolism—*continued*
- – – air T80.0
- – hemolysis T80.8
- – incompatibility reaction (ABO) (blood group) T80.3
- – – Rh (factor) T80.4
- – infection T80.2
- – reaction NEC T80.8
- – sepsis T80.2
- – serum (reaction) T80.6
- – – shock, anaphylactic T80.5
- – shock T80.8
- – thromboembolism, thrombus T80.1
- transplant NEC (*see also* Complications, organ or tissue transplant) T86.9
- trauma (early) T79.9
- – specified NEC T79.8
- ultrasound therapy T88.9
- umbilical cord
- – affecting fetus or newborn P02.6
- – complicating delivery O69.9
- – – specified NEC O69.8
- urethral catheter NEC (*see also* Complications, catheter, urinary) T83.9
- vaccination T88.1
- – anaphylaxis NEC T80.5
- – arthropathy M02.2
- – cellulitis T88.0
- – encephalitis or encephalomyelitis G04.0
- – infection (general) (local) NEC T88.0
- – meningitis G03.8
- – myelitis G04.0
- – protein sickness T80.6
- – rash T88.1
- – reaction (allergic) T88.1
- – – Herxheimer's T78.2
- – – serum T80.6
- – sepsis, septicemia T88.0
- – serum intoxication, sickness, rash, or reaction NEC T80.6
- – vaccinia (generalized) (localized) B08.0
- vas deferens device or implant T83.9
- – infection or inflammation T83.6
- – mechanical T83.4
- – specified NEC T83.8
- vascular I99
- – device, implant or graft T82.9
- – – infection or inflammation T82.7
- – – mechanical NEC T82.5
- – – specified NEC T82.8

Complications—*continued*
- vascular—*continued*
- – following
- – – infusion, therapeutic injection or transfusion T80.1
- – – procedure, specified NEC T81.7
- – postoperative I97.8
- vena cava device (filter) (sieve) (umbrella) T82.9
- – infection or inflammation T82.7
- – mechanical T82.5
- – specified NEC T82.8
- venous NEC
- – complicating pregnancy O22.8
- – following
- – – abortion (subsequent episode) O08.7
- – – – current episode – *see* Abortion
- – – ectopic or molar pregnancy O08.7
- ventilation therapy NEC T81.8
- ventricular (communicating) shunt device (catheter) T85.9
- – infection or inflammation T85.7
- – mechanical T85.0
- – specified NEC T85.8
- wire suture, permanent (implanted) – *see* Complications, suture, permanent

Compressed air disease T70.3
Compression
- with injury – *code to* Injury, by type and site
- artery I77.1
- – celiac, syndrome I77.4
- brachial plexus G54.0
- brain (stem) G93.5
- – due to
- – – contusion (diffuse) S06.2
- – – – focal S06.3
- – – injury NEC S06.2
- – – traumatic S06.2
- bronchus J98.0
- cauda equina G83.4
- cerebral – *see* Compression, brain
- cord (umbilical) – *see* Compression, umbilical cord
- diver's squeeze T70.3
- during birth (fetus or newborn) P15.9
- esophagus K22.2
- eustachian tube H68.1
- facies Q67.1
- fracture – *see* Fracture
- heart – *see* Disease, heart
- intestine (*see also* Obstruction, intestine) K56.6
- laryngeal nerve, recurrent G52.2

Compression—*continued*
- laryngeal nerve, recurrent—*continued*
- - with paralysis of vocal cords and larynx J38.0
- lumbosacral plexus G54.1
- lung J98.4
- lymphatic vessel I89.0
- medulla – *see* Compression, brain
- nerve (*see also* Disorder, nerve) G58.9
- - median (in carpal tunnel) G56.0
- - optic H47.0
- - posterior tibial (in tarsal tunnel) G57.5
- - root or plexus NEC (in) G54.9
- - - intervertebral disk disorder NEC M51.1† G55.1*
- - - - with myelopathy M51.0† G99.2*
- - - - cervical M50.1† G55.1*
- - - - - with myelopathy M50.0† G99.2*
- - - neoplastic disease NEC (M8000/1) (*see also* Neoplasm) D48.9† G55.0*
- - - spondylosis M47.2† G55.2*
- - sciatic (acute) G57.0
- - sympathetic G90.8
- - traumatic – *see* Injury, nerve
- - ulnar G56.2
- spinal (cord) G95.2
- - by displacement of intervertebral disk NEC M51.0† G99.2*
- - - cervical M50.0† G99.2*
- - nerve root NEC G54.9
- - - due to displacement of intervertebral disk NEC M51.1† G55.1*
- - - - with myelopathy M51.0† G99.2*
- - - - cervical M50.1† G55.1*
- - - - - with myelopathy M50.0† G99.2*
- - - traumatic – *see* Injury, nerve, spinal
- - spondylogenic (cervical) (lumbar, lumbosacral) (thoracic) M47.1† G99.2*
- - - anterior M47.0† G99.2*
- - traumatic (*see also* Injury, spinal cord, by region) T09.3
- sympathetic nerve NEC G90.8
- syndrome T79.5
- trachea J39.8
- umbilical cord
- - affecting fetus or newborn P02.5
- - - with cord prolapse P02.4
- - complicating delivery O69.2
- - - cord around neck O69.1
- - - prolapse O69.0

Compression—*continued*
- umbilical cord—*continued*
- - complicating delivery—*continued*
- - - specified NEC O69.2
- - vein I87.1
- - vena cava (inferior) (superior) I87.1
Compromised immune (system) NEC D89.9
Compulsion, compulsive
- gambling F63.0
- neurosis F42.1
- personality F60.5
- states F42.1
- - mixed with obsessional thoughts F42.2
- swearing F42.8
- - in Gilles de la Tourette's syndrome F95.2
- tics and spasms F95.9
Concato's disease A19.9
- pleural – *see* Pleurisy, with effusion
Concavity chest wall M95.4
Concealed penis Q55.6
Concrescence (teeth) K00.2
Concretio cordis I31.1
Concretion – *see also* Calculus
- appendicular K38.1
- canaliculus H04.5
- clitoris N90.8
- conjunctiva H11.1
- eyelid H02.8
- lacrimal passages H04.5
- prepuce (male) N47
- seminal vesicle N50.8
- tonsil J35.8
Concussion (current) S06.0
- blast (air) (hydraulic) (immersion) (underwater)
- - abdomen or thorax – *see* Injury, by site
- - brain S06.0
- - ear S09.8
- brain S06.0
- cauda equina S34.3
- cerebral S06.0
- conus medullaris S34.3
- ocular S05.8
- spinal (cord) T09.3
- - cervical S14.0
- - lumbar S34.0
- - thoracic S24.0
- syndrome F07.2
Condition – *see* Disease

Conditions arising in the perinatal period

Note: Conditions arising in the perinatal period, even though death or morbidity occurs later, should, as far as possible, be coded to chapter XVI, which takes precedence over chapters containing codes for diseases by their anatomical site.

These exclude:

Congenital malformations, deformations and chromosomal abnormalities (Q00-Q99)
Endocrine, nutritional and metabolic diseases (E00-E99)
Injury, poisoning and certain other consequences of external causes (S00-T99)
Neoplasms (C00-D48)
Tetanus neonatorum (A33)

- ablatio, ablation
- - placentae, affecting fetus or newborn P02.1
- abnormal, abnormality, abnormalities
- - amnion, amniotic fluid, affecting fetus or newborn P02.9
- - anticoagulation, newborn (transient) P61.6
- - cervix, maternal (acquired) (congenital), in pregnancy or childbirth
- - - affecting fetus or newborn P03.8
- - - causing obstructed labor
- - - - affecting fetus or newborn P03.1
- - chorion, affecting fetus or newborn P02.9
- - coagulation, newborn, transient P61.6
- - fetus, fetal
- - - causing disproportion, affecting fetus or newborn P03.1
- - forces of labor affecting fetus or newborn P03.6
- - labor NEC, affecting fetus or newborn P03.6
- - membranes (fetal)
- - - affecting fetus or newborn P02.9
- - - specified type NEC, affecting fetus or newborn P02.8
- - organs or tissues of maternal pelvis, in pregnancy or childbirth
- - - affecting fetus or newborn P03.8
- - - causing obstructed labor
- - - - affecting fetus or newborn P03.1
- - parturition, affecting fetus or newborn P03.9

Conditions arising in the perinatal period—*continued*

- abnormal, abnormality—*continued*
- - presentation (fetus)
- - - before labor, affecting fetus or newborn P01.7
- - - causing obstructed labour, affecting fetus or newborn (any, except breech) P03.1
- - - - breech P03.0
- - pulmonary
- - - function, newborn P28.8
- - - ventilation, newborn P28.8
- - umbilical cord, affecting fetus or newborn P02.6
- - uterus, maternal, in pregnancy or childbirth
- - - affecting fetus or newborn P03.8
- - - causing obstructed labor
- - - - affecting fetus or newborn P03.1
- - vagina, maternal (acquired) (congenital), in pregnancy or childbirth
- - - causing obstructed labor
- - - - affecting fetus or newborn P03.1
- - vulva and perineum, maternal (acquired) (congenital), in pregnancy or childbirth
- - - causing obstructed labor
- - - - affecting fetus or newborn P03.1
- ABO hemolytic disease (fetus or newborn) P55.1
- aborter, habitual or recurrent NEC
- - current abortion, affecting fetus or newborn P01.8
- abortion (complete) (incomplete)
- - fetus or newborn P96.4
- - habitual or recurrent, with current abortion, fetus P01.8
- - legal (induced), fetus P96.4
- - medical, fetus P96.4
- - spontaneous, fetus P01.8
- - - threatened, affecting fetus or newborn P01.8
- - therapeutic, fetus P96.4
- - threatened (spontaneous), affecting fetus or newborn P01.8
- abruptio placentae, affecting fetus or newborn P02.1
- abscess (embolic) (infective) (metastatic) (multiple) (perforated) (pyogenic) (septic)
- - breast (acute) (chronic) (nonpuerperal), newborn P39.0

**Conditions arising in the perinatal
period**—*continued*
- abscess—*continued*
-   - kidney, maternal, complicating
pregnancy
-   - - affecting fetus or newborn P00.1
-   - navel, newborn P38
-   - umbilicus, newborn P38
- absorption
-   - chemical
-   - - through placenta (fetus or newborn)
P04.8
-   - - - - environmental substance P04.6
-   - - - - nutritional substance P04.5
-   - - - - obstetric anesthetic or analgesic
drug P04.0
-   - drug NEC (fetus or newborn) – *see also*
Conditions originating in the perinatal
period, reaction, drug
-   - - through placenta P04.1
-   - - - addictive P04.4
-   - - - obstetric anesthetic or analgesic
medication P04.0
-   - maternal medication NEC through
placenta (fetus or newborn) P04.1
- accident
-   - birth – *see* Conditions originating in the
perinatal period, birth, injury
-   - during pregnancy, to mother, affecting
fetus or newborn P00.5
- acidosis (lactic) (respiratory)
-   - fetal – *see* Conditions originating in the
perinatal period, distress, fetal
-   - intrauterine – *see* Conditions
originating in the perinatal period,
distress, fetal
-   - metabolic NEC
-   - - late, of newborn P74.0
-   - - newborn – *see* Conditions originating
in the perinatal period, distress, fetal
- acrocyanosis, newborn P28.2
- addiction, maternal
-   - alcohol, alcoholic (ethyl) (methyl)
(wood), complicating pregnancy or
childbirth
-   - - affecting fetus or newborn P04.3
-   - drug NEC, maternal, complicating
pregnancy or childbirth
-   - - affecting fetus or newborn P04.4
-   - - withdrawal symptoms in newborn
P96.1

**Conditions arising in the perinatal
period**—*continued*
- adhesions, adhesive (postinfective)
-   - amnion to fetus, affecting fetus or
newborn P02.8
- adiponecrosis neonatorum P83.8
- aeration lung imperfect, newborn P28.1
- albuminuria, albuminuric (acute) (chronic)
(subacute)
-   - pre-eclamptic, affecting fetus or
newborn P00.0
- alcoholism (acute) (chronic), complicating
pregnancy or childbirth
-   - affecting fetus or newborn P04.3
- amnionitis, affecting fetus or newborn
P02.7
- amputation, any part of fetus, to facilitate
delivery P03.8
- anaerosis of newborn P28.8
- anasarca, fetus or newborn P83.2
- android pelvis, maternal
-   - with disproportion (fetopelvic),
affecting fetus or newborn P03.1
- anemia
-   - congenital P61.4
-   - - due to isoimmunization NEC P55.9
-   - - following fetal blood loss P61.3
-   - due to
-   - - fetal blood loss P61.3
-   - - prematurity P61.2
-   - erythroblastic, fetus or newborn (see
also Conditions originating in the
perinatal period, disease, hemolytic)
P55.9
-   - fetus or newborn P61.4
-   - - due to
-   - - - ABO (antibodies)
(isoimmunization) (maternal/fetal
incompatibility) P55.1
-   - - - Rh (antibodies) (isoimmunization)
(maternal/fetal incompatibility)
P55.0
-   - - following fetal blood loss P61.3
-   - - posthemorrhagic P61.3
-   - hemolytic, acute, fetus or newborn (see
also Conditions originating in the
perinatal period, disease, hemolytic)
P55.9
-   - maternal, of or complicating pregnancy
-   - - affecting fetus or newborn P00.8
-   - of prematurity P61.2
-   - posthemorrhagic (chronic), newborn
P61.3

Conditions arising in the perinatal period—*continued*
- anomaly, anomalous (congenital) (unspecified type)
- – cervix, maternal, in pregnancy or childbirth NEC
- – – affecting fetus or newborn P03.8
- – – causing obstructed labor
- – – – affecting fetus or newborn P03.1
- – uterus, maternal, in pregnancy or childbirth
- – – affecting fetus or newborn P03.8
- – – causing obstructed labor
- – – – affecting fetus or newborn P03.1
- anoxemia – *see* Conditions originating in the perinatal period, anoxia
- anoxia (see also Conditions, originating in the perinatal period, hypoxia)
- – cerebral, newborn (see also Conditions originating in the perinatal period, asphyxia, newborn) P21.9
- – newborn (see also Conditions, originating in the perinatal period, asphyxia, newborn) P21.9
- anteversion
- – uterus, uterine, maternal (cervix) (postinfectional) (postpartal, old), in pregnancy or childbirth
- – – affecting fetus or newborn P03.8
- – – causing obstructed labor
- – – – affecting fetus or newborn P03.1
- anthropoid pelvis, maternal
- – with disproportion (fetopelvic), affecting fetus or newborn P03.1
- antibodies (blood group) (see also Conditions originating in the perinatal period, incompatibility)
- – anti-D, fetus or newborn P55.0
- anuria, newborn P96.0
- apgar (score)
- – low NEC, with asphyxia P21.9
- – 0-3 at 1 minute, with asphyxia P21.0
- – 4-7 at 1 minute, with asphyxia P21.1
- apnea, apneic (spells), newborn NEC P28.4
- – sleep (primary) P28.3
- arrest, arrested
- – active phase of labor, affecting fetus or newborn P03.6
- – cardiac, newborn P29.1
- – coronary, infant P29.1
- – deep transverse, affecting fetus or newborn P03.1
- – development or growth, fetus P05.9

Conditions arising in the perinatal period—*continued*
- arrest, arrested—*continued*
- – respiratory, newborn P28.5
- arrhythmia (cardiac) (ventricular), newborn P29.1
- asphyxia, asphyxiation (by)
- – antenatal (see also Conditions originating in the perinatal period, distress, fetal) P20.9
- – birth (see also Conditions originating in the perinatal period, asphyxia, newborn) P21.9
- – fetal (see also Conditions originating in the perinatal period, distress, fetal) P20.9
- – food or foreign body (in), newborn P24.3
- – intrauterine (see also Conditions originating in the perinatal period, distress, fetal) P20.9
- – mucus (in), newborn P24.1
- – newborn P21.9
- – – with 1-minute Apgar score
- – – – low NEC P21.9
- – – – 0-3 P21.0
- – – – 4-7 P21.1
- – – blue P21.1
- – – livida P21.1
- – – mild or moderate P21.1
- – – pallida P21.0
- – – severe P21.0
- – – white P21.0
- – perinatal – *see* Conditions originating in the perinatal period, asphyxia, newborn
- – postnatal – *see* Conditions originating in the perinatal period, asphyxia, newborn
- – prenatal (see also Conditions originating in the perinatal period, distress, fetal) P20.9
- aspiration
- – amniotic fluid (newborn) P24.1
- – blood, newborn P24.2
- – liquor (amnii) (newborn) P24.1
- – meconium (newborn) P24.0
- – milk (newborn) P24.3
- – mucus, newborn P24.1
- – newborn (massive) (syndrome) P24.9
- – – meconium P24.0
- – vernix caseosa (newborn) P24.8
- asymmetry
- – lumbar spine with disproportion, affecting fetus or newborn P03.1

125

Conditions arising in the perinatal
period—*continued*
- asymmetry—*continued*
- - pelvis with disproportion (fetopelvic),
  affecting fetus or newborn P03.1
- atelcctasis (massive) (partial) (pressure)
  (pulmonary)
- - fetus or newborn (secondary) P28.1
- - - due to resorption P28.1
- - - partial P28 1
- - - primary P28.0
- - - subtotal P28.0
- atonia, atony, atonic
- - congenital P94.2
- - uterus, maternal, during labor
- - - affecting fetus or newborn P03.6
- atresia, atretic
- - cervix, maternal (acquired), in
  pregnancy or childbirth
- - - causing obstructed labor
- - - - affecting fetus or newborn P03.1
- attack
- - cyanotic, newborn P28.2
- - respiration, respiratory, newborn P28.8
- awareness of heart beat
- - fetal P20.9
- - newborn P29.1
- baby, floppy (syndrome) P94.2
- bacteremia
- - due to bacterial organisms NEC –
    see also Conditions originating in the
    perinatal period, infection, by specified
    organism
- - - newborn P36.9
- Bandl's ring (contraction), complicating
  delivery
- - affecting fetus or newborn P03.6
- bicornate or bicornis maternal uterus, in
  pregnancy or childbirth
- - affecting fetus or newborn P03.8
- bigeminal pulse
- - fetal P20.9
- - newborn P29.1
- birth
- - abnormal NEC, affecting fetus or
  newborn P03.9
- - delayed, fetus P03.8
- - difficult NEC, affecting fetus or
  newborn P03.9
- - forced NEC, affecting fetus or newborn
  P03.8
- - forceps, affecting fetus or newborn
  P03.2

Conditions arising in the perinatal
period—*continued*
- birth—*continued*
- - immature (between 28 and 37
  completed weeks) P07.3
- - - extremely (less than 28 completed
  weeks) P07.2
- - induced, affecting fetus or newborn
  P03.8
- - injury P15.9
- - - basal ganglia P11.1
- - - brachial plexus NEC P14.3
- - - brain (compression) (pressure) P11.2
- - - central nervous system NEC P11.9
- - - cerebellum P11.1
- - - cerebral hemorrhage P10.1
- - - external genitalia P15.5
- - - eye P15.3
- - - face P15.4
- - - fracture
- - - - bone P13.9
- - - - - specified NEC P13.8
- - - - clavicle P13.4
- - - - femur P13.2
- - - - humerus P13.3
- - - - long bone, except femur P13.3
- - - - radius and ulna P13.3
- - - - skull P13.0
- - - - spine P11.5
- - - - tibia and fibula P13.3
- - - intracranial P11.2
- - - - laceration or hemorrhage P10.9
- - - - - specified NEC P10.8
- - - intraventricular hemorrhage P10.2
- - - laceration
- - - - brain P10.1
- - - - by scalpel P15.8
- - - - peripheral nerve P14.9
- - - liver P15.0
- - - meninges
- - - - brain P11.1
- - - - spinal cord P11.5
- - - nerve
- - - - brachial plexus P14.3
- - - - cranial NEC (except facial) P11.4
- - - - facial P11.3
- - - - peripheral P14.9
- - - - phrenic (paralysis) P14.2
- - - penis P15.5
- - - scalp P12.9
- - - scalpel wound P15.8
- - - scrotum P15.5
- - - skull NEC P13.1
- - - - fracture P13.0

Conditions arising in the perinatal period—*continued*
- birth—*continued*
- – injury—*continued*
- – – specified site or type NEC P15.8
- – – spinal cord P11.5
- – – spine P11.5
- – – spleen P15.1
- – – sternomastoid (hematoma) P15.2
- – – subarachnoid hemorrhage P10.3
- – – subcutaneous fat necrosis P15.6
- – – subdural hemorrhage P10.0
- – – tentorial tear P10.4
- – – testes P15.5
- – – vulva P15.5
- – instrumental NEC, affecting fetus or newborn P03.8
- – multiple, affecting fetus or newborn P01.5
- – palsy or paralysis, newborn, NEC (birth injury) P14.9
- – post-term (42 weeks or more) P08.2
- – precipitate, affecting fetus or newborn P03.5
- – premature (infant) P07.3
- – prolonged, affecting fetus or newborn P03.8
- – retarded, affecting fetus or newborn P03.8
- – shock, newborn P96.8
- – trauma – *see* Conditions originating in the perinatal period, birth, injury
- – twin, affecting fetus or newborn P01.5
- – vacuum extractor, affecting fetus or newborn P03.3
- – ventouse, affecting fetus or newborn P03.3
- – weight
- – – low (between 1000 and 2499 grams at birth) P07.1
- – – – extremely (999 grams or less at birth) P07.0
- – – 4500 grams or more P08.0
- bleb(s) lung (ruptured), fetus or newborn P25.8
- bleeding (see also Conditions originating in perinatal period, hemorrhage)
- – rectum, rectal, newborn P54.2
- – umbilical stump P51.9
- – vagina, vaginal (abnormal), newborn P54.6
- blood dyscrasia, fetus or newborn P61.9
- born in toilet (see also Birth, precipitate fetus or newborn) P03.5

Conditions arising in the perinatal period—*continued*
- brachycardia
- – fetal P20.9
- – newborn P29.1
- bradycardia (any type) (sinoatrial) (sinus) (vagal)
- – fetal – *see* Conditions originating in the perinatal period, distress, fetal
- – newborn P29.1
- breech
- – delivery NEC, affecting fetus or newborn P03.0
- – extraction, affecting fetus or newborn P03.0
- – presentation
- – – before labor, affecting fetus or newborn P01.7
- – – during labor, affecting fetus or newborn P03.0
- bronze baby syndrome P83.8
- bruise (skin surface intact)
- – fetus or newborn P54.5
- – scalp, due to birth injury, newborn P12.3
- – umbilical cord, affecting fetus or newborn P02.6
- bubbly lung syndrome P27.0
- bulla(e), lung, fetus or newborn P25.8
- candidiasis, candidal
- – congenital P37.5
- – neonatal P37.5
- caput succedaneum P12.8
- catastrophe, catastrophy, cardiorespiratory, newborn P28.8
- caul over face (causing asphyxia) P21.9
- cellulitis (diffuse) (with lymphangitis)
- – navel, newborn P38
- – umbilicus, newborn P38
- cephalematocele, cephal(o)hematocele
- – fetus or newborn P52.8
- – – birth injury P10.8
- cephalematoma, cephalhematoma (calcified)
- – fetus or newborn (birth injury) P12.0
- cervicitis, maternal (acute) (chronic) (nonvenereal) (subacute) (with ulceration)
- – complicating pregnancy, affecting fetus or newborn P00.8
- cesarean operation or section
- – affecting fetus or newborn P03.4
- – post mortem, affecting fetus or newborn P01.6

Conditions arising in the perinatal period—*continued*
- cessation
- - cardiac, newborn P29.0
- - cardiorespiratory, newborn P29.0
- - respiratory, newborn P28.5
- chemotherapy (session) (for)
- - cancer, maternal, affecting fetus or newborn P04.1
- chickenpox, congenital P35.8
- chignon, fetus or newborn (birth injury) (from vacuum extraction) P12.1
- chorioamnionitis, fetus or newborn P02.7
- chorioretinitis, in toxoplasmosis, congenital (active) P37.1† H32.0*
- circulation
- - failure (peripheral)
- - - fetus or newborn P29.8
- - fetal, persistent P29.3
- cirrhosis, cirrhotic (hepatic)
- - liver (chronic) (hepatolienal) (hypertrophic) (nodular) (splenomegalic)
- - - congenital P78.8
- cleidotomy, fetus or newborn P03.8
- clotting, disseminated, intravascular, newborn P60
- coagulation, intravascular (diffuse) (disseminated)
- - antepartum, affecting fetus or newborn P02.1
- - fetus or newborn P60
- coagulopathy (see also Conditions originating in the perinatal period, defect, coagulation)
- - consumption, newborn P60
- cold injury syndrome (newborn) P80.0
- collapse
- - cardiocirculatory, newborn P29.8
- - cardiopulmonary, newborn P29.8
- - cardiovascular, newborn P29.8
- - circulatory (peripheral), fetus or newborn P29.8
- - respiratory, newborn P28.8
- - vascular (peripheral)
- - - during labor and delivery, affecting fetus or newborn P03.8
- - - fetus or newborn P29.8
- coma, newborn P91.5
- complications (from) (of)
- - intrauterine procedure NEC, affecting fetus or newborn P96.5

Conditions arising in the perinatal period—*continued*
- complications—*continued*
- - maternal sedation during labor and delivery, affecting fetus or newborn P04.0
- - umbilical cord, affecting fetus or newborn P02.6
- compression
- - during birth (fetus or newborn) P15.9
- - umbilical cord, affecting fetus or newborn P02.5
- - - with cord prolapse P02.4
- compromise, respiratory, newborn P28.5
- congestion, congestive (chronic) (passive)
- - facial, due to birth injury P15.4
- conjunctivitis (in) (due to)
- - chlamydial, neonatal P39.1
- - neonatal P39.1
- constriction
- - cervix, cervical (canal), in pregnancy or childbirth
- - - causing obstructed labour, affecting fetus or newborn P03.1
- - ring dystocia (uterus), affecting fetus or newborn P03.6
- contraction, contracture, contracted
- - hourglass uterus (complicating delivery), affecting fetus or newborn P03.6
- - pelvis, maternal (acquired) (general)
- - - with disproportion (fetopelvic), affecting fetus or newborn P03.1
- - ring (Bandl's) (complicating delivery), affecting fetus or newborn P03.6
- - uterus, maternal, abnormal NEC, affecting fetus or newborn P03.6
- contusion (skin surface intact)
- - fetus or newborn P54.5
- - scalp, due to birth injury P12.3
- convulsions (idiopathic), newborn P90
- cord – *see also condition*
- - around neck (tightly) (with compression), affecting fetus or newborn P02.5
- coupled rhythm
- - fetal P20.9
- - newborn P29.1
- cranioclasis, fetus P03.8
- craniotabes (cause unknown), neonatal P96.3
- craniotomy, fetus P03.8

Conditions arising in the perinatal period—*continued*

– cretin, cretinism (congenital) (endemic) (nongoitrous) (sporadic)
– – pelvis, maternal, with disproportion (fetopelvic), affecting fetus or newborn P03.1
– cyst (colloid) (mucous) (retention) (simple)
– – periventricular, acquired, newborn P91.1
– cystitis, maternal (exudative) (hemorrhagic) (septic) (suppurative)
– – complicating pregnancy, affecting fetus or newborn P00.1
– cystocele(-rectocele), maternal, in pregnancy or childbirth
– – affecting fetus or newborn P03.8
– – causing obstructed labor
– – – affecting fetus or newborn P03.1
– dacryocystitis (acute) (phlegmonous), neonatal P39.1
– damage
– – brain (nontraumatic)
– – – anoxic, hypoxic
– – – – at birth P21.9
– – – – fetal P20.9
– – – – intrauterine P20.9
– – – – newborn P21.9
– – – due to birth injury P11.2
– – – ischemic, newborn P91.0
– – – newborn P11.2
– – eye, birth injury P15.3
– deadborn fetus P95
– death
– – fetus, fetal (cause not stated) (intrauterine) P95
– – infant, from intrauterine coil P00.7
– – neonatal NEC P96.8
– – obstetric, maternal (cause unknown), affecting fetus or newborn P01.6
– debility (chronic) (general), congenital or neonatal NEC P96.9
– decapitation, fetal (to facilitate delivery) P03.8
– deciduitis (acute), affecting fetus or newborn P00.8
– decompensation, lung (pulmonary), newborn P28.8
– defect, defective coagulation (factor)
– – antepartum with hemorrhage, maternal, affecting fetus or newborn P02.1
– – newborn, transient P61.6

Conditions arising in the perinatal period—*continued*

– defibrination (syndrome)
– – antepartum, maternal, affecting fetus or newborn P02.1
– – fetus or newborn P60
– deficiency, deficient
– – coagulation
– – – antepartum, maternal, affecting fetus or newborn P02.1
– – – newborn, transient P61.6
– – surfactant P28.0
– – vitamin K, of newborn P53
– deformity
– – fetal, causing obstructed labor, affecting fetus or newborn P03.1
– – pelvis, pelvic, maternal (acquired) (bony)
– – – with disproportion (fetopelvic), affecting fetus or newborn P03.1
– – soft parts, maternal organs or tissues (of pelvis), in pregnancy or childbirth NEC
– – – affecting fetus or newborn P03.8
– – – causing obstructed labor
– – – – affecting fetus or newborn P03.1
– dehydration, newborn P74.1
– delay, delayed,
– – birth or delivery NEC, affecting fetus or newborn P03.8
– – closure, ductus arteriosus (Botalli) P29.3
– – delivery, second twin, triplet, etc.
– – – affecting fetus or newborn P03.8
– – primary respiration (see also Conditions originating in the perinatal period, asphyxia, newborn) P21.9
– delivery (single)
– – breech NEC, affecting fetus or newborn P03.0
– – cesarean (for), affecting fetus or newborn P03.4
– – extremely rapid, newborn P03.5
– – forceps, affecting fetus or newborn P03.2
– – precipitate, affecting fetus or newborn P03.5
– – premature or preterm NEC, affecting fetus or newborn P07.3
– – vacuum extractor NEC, affecting fetus or newborn P03.3
– – ventouse NEC, affecting fetus or newborn P03.3
– demise, fetal P95

Conditions arising in the perinatal period—*continued*
- dependence
- – due to drug NEC
- – – maternal, complicating pregnancy or childbirth
- – – – affecting fetus or newborn P04.4
- – – – withdrawal symptoms in newborn P96.1
- depression
- – central nervous system (CNS) NEC, newborn P91.4
- – cerebral, newborn P91.4
- – respiration, respiratory, newborn P28.5
- – vital centers, newborn P91.4
- destruction, live fetus to facilitate delivery (fetus) P03.8
- development
- – arrested, fetus P05.9
- – incomplete P05.9
- device, contraceptive, intrauterine, affecting fetus or newborn P00.8
- diabetes, diabetic (controlled) (familial) (mellitus) (on insulin) (severe) (uncontrolled)
- – arising in pregnancy, maternal, affecting fetus or newborn P70.0
- – complicating pregnancy or childbirth, maternal, affecting fetus or newborn P70.1
- – – arising in pregnancy, affecting fetus or newborn P70.0
- – – gestational, affecting fetus or newborn P70.0
- – neonatal (transient) P70.2
- diarrhea, diarrheal (disease) (endemic) (infantile) (summer) (see also Conditions originating in the perinatal period, enteritis)
- – neonatal (noninfective) P78.3
- difficult, difficulty (in)
- – birth, affecting fetus or newborn P03.9
- – feeding, newborn P92.9
- – – breast P92.5
- – – specified NEC P92.8
- – respiratory, newborn P28.8
- dilatation cervix (uteri), maternal –
  see also Conditions originating in the perinatal period, incompetency, cervix
- – incomplete, poor, slow, affecting fetus or newborn P03.6
- disease, diseased – see also Conditions originating in the perinatal period, syndrome

Conditions arising in the perinatal period—*continued*
- disease, diseased—*continued*
- – breast, inflammatory, fetus or newborn P83.4
- – cardiorespiratory, newborn P96.8
- – cardiovascular, fetus or newborn P29.9
- – – specified NEC P29.8
- – circulatory (system) NEC, fetus or newborn P29.9
- – – maternal, affecting fetus or newborn P00.3
- – facial nerve (seventh), newborn (birth injury) P11.3
- – heart (organic)
- – – congenital
- – – – maternal, affecting fetus or newborn P00.3
- – – rheumatic (chronic) (inactive) (old) (quiescent) (with chorea)
- – – – maternal, affecting fetus or newborn P00.3
- – hemolytic (fetus) (newborn) P55.9
- – – due to
- – – – incompatibility
- – – – – ABO (blood group) P55.1
- – – – – blood (group) (Duffy) (K(ell)) (Kidd) (Lewis) (M) (S) NEC P55.8
- – – – – Rh (blood group) (factor) P55.0
- – – – Rh-negative mother P55.0
- – – specified type NEC P55.8
- – hemorrhagic, fetus or newborn P53
- – hyaline (diffuse) (generalized), membrane (lung) (newborn) P22.0
- – infectious, infective
- – – congenital P37.9
- – – – specified NEC P37.8
- – – maternal, complicating pregnancy or childbirth
- – – – affecting fetus or newborn P00.2
- – maternal, unrelated to pregnancy NEC, affecting fetus or newborn P00.9
- – pelvis, pelvic, maternal
- – – inflammatory (female), complicating pregnancy
- – – – affecting fetus or newborn P00.8
- – placenta, affecting fetus or newborn P02.2
- – renal, maternal (functional) (pelvis)
- – – complicating pregnancy, affecting fetus or newborn P00.1

Conditions arising in the perinatal period—*continued*
− disease, diseased—*continued*
− − respiratory (tract)
− − − chronic NEC, fetus or newborn P27.9
− − − − specified NEC P27.8
− − − newborn P28.9
− − − − specified type NEC P28.8
− − viral, virus NEC
− − − congenital P35.9
− − − − specified NEC P35.8
− disorder (of) − *see also* Conditions originating in the perinatal period, disease
− − amino-acid, neonatal, transitory P74.8
− − coagulation (factor)
− − − antepartum with hemorrhage, maternal, affecting fetus or newborn P02.1
− − − newborn, transient P61.6
− − digestive (system), fetus or newborn P78.9
− − − specified NEC P78.8
− − feeding, newborn P92.9
− − fetus or newborn P96.9
− − − specified NEC P96.8
− − hematological, fetus or newborn P61.9
− − − specified NEC P61.8
− − hemorrhagic NEC, newborn P53
− − integument, fetus or newborn P83.9
− − − specified NEC P83.8
− − membranes or fluid, amniotic, affecting fetus or newborn P02.9
− − muscle tone, newborn P94.9
− − − specified NEC P94.8
− − seizure, newborn P90
− − skin, fetus or newborn P83.9
− − − specified NEC P83.8
− − temperature regulation, fetus or newborn P81.9
− − − specified NEC P81.8
− − thyroid (gland) function NEC, neonatal, transitory P72.2
− disproportion (fetopelvic), affecting fetus or newborn P03.1
− distortion (congenital) lumbar spine, maternal
− − with disproportion, affecting fetus or newborn P03.1
− distress
− − cardiac
− − − congenital P20.9
− − − newborn P29.8
− − cardiopulmonary, newborn P96.8

Conditions arising in the perinatal period—*continued*
− distress—*continued*
− − cardiorespiratory, newborn P96.8
− − circulatory, newborn P96.8
− − fetal (syndrome) P20.-
− − − first noted
− − − − before onset of labor P20.0
− − − − during labor and delivery P20.1
− − intrauterine − *see* Conditions originating in the perinatal period, distress, fetal
− − respiratory, newborn P22.9
− − − specified NEC P22.8
− disturbance − *see also* Conditions originating in the perinatal period, disease
− − cerebral status, newborn P91.9
− − − specified NEC P91.8
− − electrolyte
− − − newborn, transitory P74.4
− − − − potassium balance P74.3
− − − − sodium balance P74.2
− − − − specified type NEC P74.4
− − endocrine (gland), neonatal, transitory P72.9
− − − specified NEC P72.8
− − feeding, newborn P92.9
− − metabolism, neonatal, transitory P74.9
− − − calcium and magnesium P71.9
− − − − specified type NEC P71.8
− − − carbohydrate metabolism P70.9
− − − − specified type NEC P70.8
− − − specified NEC P74.8
− − potassium balance, newborn P74.3
− − sodium balance, newborn P74.2
− − temperature regulation, newborn P81.9
− − − specified NEC P81.8
− double uterus, maternal, in pregnancy or childbirth
− − affecting fetus or newborn P03.8
− Duchenne'sparalysis, birth injury P14.0
− dyscrasia, blood, fetus or newborn P61.9
− − specified type NEC P61.8
− dysfunction uterus, complicating delivery
− − affecting fetus or newborn P03.6
− dysmaturity (see also Conditions originating in the perinatal period, immaturity) P05.0
− − pulmonary (newborn) (Wilson-Mikity) P27.0
− dysplasia − *see also* Conditions originating in the perinatal period, anomaly
− − bronchopulmonary (perinatal) P27.1

131

Conditions arising in the perinatal period—*continued*
- dysplasia—*continued*
- – lung (congenital), associated with short gestation P28.0
- dyspnea (nocturnal) (paroxysmal), newborn P22.8
- dysrhythmia (cardiac), newborn P29.1
- dystocia
- – affecting fetus or newborn P03.1
- – cervical, maternal (hypotonic), affecting fetus or newborn P03.6
- – contraction ring, maternal, affecting fetus or newborn P03.6
- – fetal, fetus, affecting fetus or newborn P03.1
- – maternal, affecting fetus or newborn P03.1
- – positional, affecting fetus or newborn P03.1
- – shoulder (girdle), affecting fetus or newborn P03.1
- – uterine NEC, maternal, affecting fetus or newborn P03.6
- ecchymosis (see also Conditions originating in the perinatal period, hemorrhage)
- – fetus or newborn P54.5
- eclampsia, eclamptic (coma) (convulsions) (delirium) (with pre-existing or pregnancy-related hypertension) NEC
- – pregnancy, affecting fetus or newborn P00.0
- edema, edematous brain
- – due to birth injury P11.0
- – fetus or newborn (anoxia or hypoxia) P52.4
- – – birth injury P11.0
- – fetus or newborn NEC, classifiable to R60.- P83.3
- – newborn, classifiable to R60.- P83.3
- effect, adverse NEC
- – anesthesia in labor and delivery, affecting fetus or newborn P04.0
- effusion, pleura, pleurisy, pleuritic, pleuropericardial
- – fetus or newborn P28.8
- embarrassment, respiratory, newborn – *see* Conditions originating in the perinatal period, distress, respiratory
- embolism (septic), air (any site) (traumatic), newborn NEC P25.8

Conditions arising in the perinatal period—*continued*
- embryotomy (to facilitate delivery), fetus P03.8
- emphysema (atrophic) (chronic) (interlobular) (lung) (obstructive) (pulmonary) (senile)
- – – congenital (interstitial) P25.0
- – – fetus or newborn (interstitial) P25.0
- – – interstitial, congenital P25.0
- – – – perinatal period P25.0
- – – mediastinal, fetus or newborn P25.2
- encephalitis in toxoplasmosis, congenital P37.1† G05.2*
- encephalopathia hyperbilirubinemica, newborn P57.9
- – due to isoimmunization (conditions in P55.-) P57.0
- encephalopathy (acute) (cerebral)
- – hyperbilirubinemic, newborn P57.9
- – – due to isoimmunization (conditions in P55.-) P57.0
- – in birth injury P11.1
- – ischemic
- – – anoxic (hypoxic), newborn P21.9
- – – newborn P91.0
- endometritis (nonspecific) (purulent) (septic) (suppurative)
- – maternal, complicating pregnancy, affecting fetus or newborn P00.8
- engorgement, breast, newborn P83.4
- entanglement umbilical cord(s), affecting fetus or newborn P02.5
- enteritis (acute) (diarrheal) (hemorrhagic) (see also Conditions originating in the perinatal period, diarrhea)
- – necrotizing of fetus or newborn P77
- enterocolitis (see also Conditions originating in the perinatal period, diarrhea)
- – necrotizing (chronic), fetus or newborn P77
- Erb(-Duchenne) paralysis (birth injury) (newborn) P14.0
- Erb's palsy, paralysis (brachial) (birth) (newborn) P14.0
- erythema, erythematous
- – neonatorum P83.8
- – – toxic P83.1
- – rash, newborn P83.8
- – toxic, toxicum NEC, newborn P83.1
- erythroblastosis (fetalis) (newborn) P55.9

Conditions arising in the perinatal period—*continued*
- erythroblastosis—*continued*
- − due to
- − − ABO (antibodies) (incompatibility) (isoimmunization) P55.1
- − − Rh (antibodies) (incompatibility) (isoimmunization) P55.0
- erythroderma neonatorum P83.8
- − toxic P83.1
- evisceration, birth injury P15.8
- excess, excessive, excessively
- − large, fetus or infant P08.0
- − long umbilical cord (entangled), affecting fetus or newborn P02.5
- − short umbilical cord, affecting fetus or newborn P02.6
- exhaustion (physical NEC)
- − fetus or newborn P96.8
- − maternal, complicating delivery, affecting fetus or newborn P03.8
- exsanguination − *see* Conditions originating in the perinatal period, hemorrhage
- extraction
- − with hook (fetus) P03.8
- − breech NEC, affecting fetus or newborn P03.0
- face, facial presentation, affecting fetus or newborn P01.7
- failure, failed
- − cardiac, newborn P29.0
- − cardiopulmonary (acute) (chronic), newborn P29.0
- − cervical dilatation in labor, affecting fetus or newborn P03.6
- − descent of head (at term), affecting fetus or newborn P03.1
- − expansion, terminal respiratory units (newborn) (primary) P28.0
- − fetal head to enter pelvic brim, affecting fetus or newborn P03.1
- − forceps NEC (with subsequent delivery by cesarean section)
- − − affecting fetus or newborn P03.1
- − heart (acute) (sudden), newborn P29.0
- − − congestive P29.0
- − − left (ventricular) P29.0
- − pulmonary, newborn P28.5
- − renal, congenital P96.0
- − respiration, respiratory, newborn P28.5
- − trial of labor (with subsequent cesarean section), affecting fetus or newborn P03.1

Conditions arising in the perinatal period—*continued*
- failure, failed—*continued*
- − vacuum extraction NEC (with subsequent cesarean section), affecting fetus or newborn P03.1
- − ventilatory, newborn P28.5
- − ventouse NEC (with subsequent cesarean section), affecting fetus or newborn P03.1
- − ventricular, left, newborn P29.0
- − vital centers, fetus or newborn P91.8
- fecalith (impaction), congenital P76.8
- feeding problem, newborn P92.9
- − specified NEC P92.8
- fever, newborn P81.9
- − environmental P81.0
- fibroid (tumor), maternal
- − in pregnancy or childbirth, affecting fetus or newborn P03.8
- fibromyoma, maternal
- − uterus (corpus), in pregnancy or childbirth, affecting fetus or newborn P03.8
- fibrosis, fibrotic
- − lung (atrophic) (capillary) (chronic) (confluent) (massive) (perialveolar) (peribronchial), congenital P27.8
- − perineum, maternal, in pregnancy or childbirth
- − − causing obstructed labor, affecting fetus or newborn P03.1
- − pulmonary, congenital P27.8
- fit, newborn P90
- flail chest, newborn (birth injury) P13.8
- flat − *see also* Conditions originating in the perinatal period, anomaly, by site
- − pelvis, maternal
- − − with disproportion (fetopelvic), affecting fetus or newborn P03.1
- floppy baby syndrome (nonspecific) P94.2
- forced birth or delivery NEC, affecting fetus or newborn P03.8
- forceps delivery NEC, affecting fetus or newborn P03.2
- fracture (abduction) (adduction) (avulsion) (comminuted) (compression) (dislocation) (oblique) (separation)
- − bone NEC, birth injury P13.9
- − clavicle (acromial end) (interligamentous) (shaft), birth injury P13.4
- − femur, femoral, birth injury P13.2

133

Conditions arising in the perinatal period—*continued*
- fracture—*continued*
- − − skull, birth injury P13.0
- − − vertebra, vertebral (back) (body) (column) (neural arch) (pedicle) (spinous process) (transverse process), birth injury P11.5
- − funnel pelvis, maternal (acquired)
- − − with disproportion (fetopelvic), affecting fetus or newborn P03.1
- − gallop rhythm
- − − fetal P20.9
- − − newborn P29.1
- − ganglionitis geniculate, newborn (birth injury) P11.3
- − gastro-esophageal reflux in newborn P78.8
- − gestation (period) – *see also* Conditions originating in the perinatal period, pregnancy
- − − less than 28 weeks P07.2
- − − 28 weeks but less than 37 weeks P07.3
- − − 42 or more completed weeks P08.2
- − glaucoma, traumatic, newborn (birth injury) P15.3
- − goiter (plunging) (substernal)
- − − congenital (nontoxic), transitory, with normal functioning P72.0
- − − neonatal NEC P72.0
- − gonococcus, gonococcal (disease) (infection) (see also condition)
- − − maternal, complicating pregnancy or childbirth
- − − − affecting fetus or newborn P00.2
- − gonorrhea (acute) (chronic)
- − − maternal, complicating pregnancy or childbirth
- − − − affecting fetus or newborn P00.2
- − granuloma, umbilicus, newborn P38
- − Gray syndrome (newborn) P93
- − Grey syndrome (newborn) P93
- − heart beat
- − − abnormality
- − − − fetal P20.9
- − − − newborn P29.1
- − − awareness
- − − − fetal P20.9
- − − − newborn P29.1
- − heavy-for-dates NEC (fetus or infant) P08.1
- − − exceptionally (4500 g or more) P08.0
- − hematemesis, newborn, neonatal P54.0
- − − due to swallowed maternal blood P78.2

Conditions arising in the perinatal period—*continued*
- − hematoma (traumatic) (skin surface intact)
- − − birth injury NEC P15.8
- − − brain (traumatic), fetus or newborn NEC P52.4
- − − − birth injury P10.1
- − − face, birth injury P15.4
- − − liver (subcapsular), birth injury P15.0
- − − penis, birth injury P15.5
- − − scrotum, superficial, birth injury P15.5
- − − spinal (cord) (meninges)
- − − − fetus or newborn (birth injury) P11.5
- − − sternocleidomastoid, birth injury P15.2
- − − sternomastoid, birth injury P15.2
- − − subarachnoid, fetus or newborn (nontraumatic) P52.5
- − − − birth injury P10.3
- − − subdural, fetus or newborn (localized) P52.8
- − − − birth injury P10.0
- − − superficial, fetus or newborn P54.5
- − − testis, birth injury P15.5
- − − umbilical cord, complicating delivery, affecting fetus or newborn P02.6
- − − vulva, fetus or newborn (birth injury) P15.5
- − hematomyelia (central), fetus or newborn (birth injury) P11.5
- − hematorachis, hematorrhachis, fetus or newborn (birth injury) P11.5
- − hemiplegia, newborn NEC P91.8
- − − birth injury P11.9
- − hemolysis
- − − autoimmune, newborn P55.9
- − − intravascular NEC, newborn P60
- − − neonatal (excessive) P58.8
- − hemopericardium, newborn P54.8
- − hemoptysis, newborn P26.9
- − hemorrhage, hemorrhagic
- − − accidental antepartum, affecting fetus or newborn P02.1
- − − adrenal (capsule) (gland), newborn P54.4
- − − alveolar, lung, newborn P26.8
- − − antepartum (see also Conditions originating in the perinatal period, hemorrhage, pregnancy)
- − − − affecting fetus or newborn P02.1
- − − bowel, newborn P54.3
- − − brain (miliary) (nontraumatic) (petechial)
- − − − due to birth injury P10.1
- − − − fetus or newborn P52.4

Conditions arising in the perinatal period—*continued*
- hemorrhage, hemorrhagic—*continued*
- – brain—*continued*
- – – fetus or newborn—*continued*
- – – – birth injury P10.1
- – – stem, newborn P52.4
- – cerebellar, cerebellum (nontraumatic), fetus or newborn P52.6
- – cerebral, cerebrum, fetus or newborn (anoxic) P52.4
- – – birth injury P10.1
- – complicating delivery
- – – affecting fetus or newborn P02.1
- – – associated with coagulation defect, maternal, affecting fetus or newborn P03.8
- – – – afibrinogenemia P03.8
- – – due to
- – – – low-lying placenta, affecting fetus or newborn P02.0
- – – – placenta previa, affecting fetus or newborn P02.0
- – – – premature separation of placenta, affecting fetus or newborn P02.1
- – – – trauma, affecting fetus or newborn P03.8
- – – – uterine leiomyoma, affecting fetus or newborn P03.8
- – conjunctiva, newborn P54.8
- – cord, newborn (stump) P51.9
- – cutaneous, fetus or newborn P54.5
- – disease, fetus or newborn P53
- – epicranial subaponeurotic (massive), birth injury P12.2
- – extradural, fetus or newborn (anoxic) (nontraumatic) P52.8
- – – birth injury P10.8
- – fetal, fetus (see also Conditions arising in the perinatal period, hemorrhage, by specified sites) P50.9
- – – from
- – – – cut end of co-twin's cord P50.5
- – – – placenta P50.2
- – – – ruptured cord P50.1
- – – – vasa previa P50.0
- – – into
- – – – co-twin P50.3
- – – – maternal circulation P50.4
- – – specified NEC P50.8
- – fetal-maternal P50.4
- – gastroenteric, newborn P54.3
- – gastrointestinal (tract), newborn P54.3
- – internal (organs) NEC, newborn P54.8

Conditions arising in the perinatal period—*continued*
- hemorrhage, hemorrhagic—*continued*
- – intestine, newborn P54.3
- – intra-alveolar (lung), newborn P26.8
- – intracerebral (nontraumatic), fetus or newborn P52.4
- – – birth injury P10.1
- – intracranial, fetus or newborn (nontraumatic) P52.9
- – – birth injury P10.9
- – – specified NEC P52.8
- – intraventricular, fetus or newborn (nontraumatic) P52.3
- – – birth injury P10.2
- – – grade
- – – – 1 P52.0
- – – – 2 P52.1
- – – – 3 P52.2
- – lung, newborn P26.9
- – – massive P26.1
- – – specified NEC P26.8
- – massive umbilical, newborn P51.0
- – maternal, gestational, affecting fetus or newborn P02.1
- – mucous membrane NEC, newborn P54.8
- – nasal turbinate, newborn P54.8
- – navel, newborn P51.9
- – newborn P54.9
- – – specified NEC P54.8
- – nose, newborn P54.8
- – placenta NEC, affecting fetus or newborn P02.1
- – – from surgical or instrumental damage, affecting fetus or newborn P02.1
- – – previa, affecting fetus or newborn P02.0
- – posterior fossa (nontraumatic), fetus or newborn P52.6
- – pregnancy – see also Conditions originating in the perinatal period, hemorrhage, antepartum
- – – due to
- – – – abruptio placentae, affecting fetus or newborn P02.1
- – – – afibrinogenemia, or other coagulation defect (conditions in category D65-D68), affecting fetus or newborn P02.1
- – – – leiomyoma, uterus, affecting fetus or newborn P02.1

Conditions arising in the perinatal
period—*continued*
- hemorrhage, hemorrhagic—*continued*
- − pregnancy—*continued*
- − − due to—*continued*
- − − − placenta previa , affecting fetus or
  newborn P02.0
- − − − premature separation of placenta
  (normally implanted), affecting
  fetus or newborn P02.1
- − − − threatened abortion, affecting fetus
  or newborn P02.1
- − − − trauma, affecting fetus or newborn
  P02.1
- − − early, affecting fetus or newborn
  P02.1
- − − pulmonary, newborn P26.9
- − − − massive P26.1
- − − − specified NEC P26.8
- − − rectum (sphincter), newborn P54.2
- − − skin, fetus or newborn P54.5
- − − slipped umbilical ligature P51.8
- − − spinal (cord), fetus or newborn (birth
  injury) P11.5
- − − stomach, newborn P54.3
- − − subarachnoid, fetus or newborn
  (nontraumatic) P52.5
- − − − birth injury P10.3
- − − subconjunctival, birth injury P15.3
- − subdural (acute)
- − − − fetus or newborn (nontraumatic)
  (anoxic) (hypoxic) P52.8
- − − − − birth injury P10.0
- − − subependymal, fetus or newborn P52.0
- − − − with intraventricular extension P52.1
- − − − − and intracerebral extension P52.2
- − − suprarenal (capsule) (gland), newborn
  P54.4
- − − tentorium (traumatic) NEC, fetus or
  newborn (birth injury) P10.4
- − − tracheobronchial, newborn P26.0
- − − umbilicus, umbilical
- − − − cord,
- − − − − after birth, newborn P51.9
- − − − − fetus, from ruptured cord P50.1
- − − − newborn P51.9
- − − − − massive P51.0
- − − − − slipped ligature P51.8
- − − − stump P51.9
- − − unavoidable (antepartum) (due to
  placenta previa), affecting fetus or
  newborn P02.0
- − − vagina (abnormal), newborn P54.6

Conditions arising in the perinatal
period—*continued*
- hemorrhage, hemorrhagic—*continued*
- − − vasa previa, affecting fetus or newborn
  P50.0
- − − viscera NEC, newborn P54.8
- − hemothorax (bacterial) (nontuberculous),
  newborn P54.8
- − hepatitis
  fetus or newborn (giant cell)
  (idiopathic) P59.2
- − − in toxoplasmosis, congenital (active)
  P37.1† K77.0∗
- − − neonatal (giant cell) (idiopathic) (toxic)
  P59.2
- − − viral, virus (acute), congenital P35.3
- − herpes simplex, congenital P35.2
- − hyaline membrane (disease) (lung)
  (pulmonary) (newborn) P22.0
- − hydramnios, affecting fetus or newborn
  P01.3
- − hydrocele (spermatic cord) (testis) (tunica
  vaginalis), congenital P83.5
- − − fetus or newborn P83.5
- − hydrocephalus (acquired) (external)
  (internal) (malignant) (recurrent)
- − − causing disproportion, affecting fetus or
  newborn P03.1
- − − due to toxoplasmosis (congenital)
  P37.1
- − hydrops fetal(is) or newborn (idiopathic)
  P83.2
- − − due to
- − − − ABO isoimmunization P56.0
- − − − hemolytic disease NEC P56.9
- − − − isoimmunization (ABO) (Rh) P56.0
- − − − Rh incompatibility P56.0
- − hyperbilirubinemia NEC
- − − neonatal (transient) (see also Conditions
  originating in the perinatal period,
  jaundice, fetus or newborn) P59.9
- − − − of prematurity P59.0
- − hyperemesis (see also Conditions
  originating in the perinatal period,
  vomiting)
- − − gravidarum, maternal (mild), affecting
  fetus or newborn P01.8
- − hypermagnesemia, neonatal P71.8
- − hypermaturity (fetus or newborn) P08.2

Conditions arising in the perinatal period—*continued*

- hypertension, hypertensive (accelerated) (benign) (essential) (idiopathic) (malignant) (primary) (systemic)
- – maternal, complicating pregnancy or childbirth
- – – affecting fetus or newborn P00.0
- – newborn P29.2
- – – pulmonary (persistent) P29.3
- – pulmonary (artery), of newborn (persistent) P29.3
- hyperthermia (of unknown origin), newborn, environmental P81.0
- hyperthyroidism (apathetic) (latent) (pre-adult) (recurrent), neonatal, transitory P72.1
- hypertony, hypertonia, hypertonicity
- – congenital P94.1
- – uterus, uterine (contractions) (complicating delivery), affecting fetus or newborn P03.6
- hypertrophy, hypertrophic breast, fetus or newborn P83.4
- hypocalcemia, neonatal P71.1
- – due to cow's milk P71.0
- – phosphate-loading (newborn) P71.1
- hypoglycemia (spontaneous)
- – in infant of diabetic mother P70.1
- – – gestational diabetes P70.0
- – neonatal (transitory) P70.4
- – – iatrogenic P70.3
- – – maternal diabetes P70.1
- – – – gestational P70.0
- – transitory neonatal P70.4
- hypomagnesemia, neonatal P71.2
- hypoparathyroidism, neonatal, transitory P71.4
- hypoplasia, hypoplastic
- – lung (congenital) (lobe), associated with short gestation P28.0
- – pulmonary, associated with short gestation P28.0
- hypoprothrombinemia (congenital) (hereditary) (idiopathic), newborn, transient P61.6
- hypothermia (accidental) (due to)
- – neonatal P80.9
- – – environmental (mild) NEC P80.8
- – – mild P80.8
- – – severe (chronic) (cold injury syndrome) P80.0
- – – specified NEC P80.8

Conditions arising in the perinatal period—*continued*

- hypothyroidism (acquired), neonatal, transitory P72.2
- hypotonia, hypotonicity, hypotony NEC, congenital (benign) P94.2
- hypoxia – *see also* Conditions originating in the perinatal period, anoxia
- – fetal – *see* Conditions originating in the perinatal period, distress, fetal
- – intrauterine P20.9
- – – first noted
- – – – before onset of labor P20.0
- – – – during labor and delivery P20.1
- – newborn (see also Conditions originating in the perinatal period, asphyxia, newborn) P21.9
- hysterotomy, affecting fetus or newborn P03.8
- icterus neonatorum (see also Conditions originating in the perinatal period, jaundice, fetus or newborn) P59.9
- ileus (bowel) (colon) (inhibitory) (intestine) (neurogenic), newborn, transitory P76.1
- imbalance, electrolyte
- – neonatal, transitory NEC P74.4
- – – potassium P74.3
- – – sodium P74.2
- immature, birth (28 completed weeks or more but less than 37 completed weeks) P07.3
- – extremely (less than 28 completed weeks) P07.2
- immaturity (28 completed weeks or more but less than 37 completed weeks) P07.3
- – extreme (less than 28 completed weeks) P07.2
- – fetal, fetus P07.3
- – fetus or infant light-for-dates – *see* Conditions originating in the perinatal period, light-for-dates
- – gross P07.2
- – infant P07.3
- – newborn P07.3
- – pulmonary, fetus or newborn P28.0
- – respiratory P28.0
- immunization
- – ABO (see also Conditions originating in the perinatal period, isoimmunization, ABO)
- – – affecting management of pregnancy, in fetus or newborn P55.1

Conditions arising in the perinatal period—*continued*
- impaction, impacted shoulder, affecting fetus or newborn P03.1
- imperfect aeration, lung (newborn) NEC P28.1
- improperly tied umbilical cord (causing hemorrhage) P51.8
- inability to breathe properly, newborn P28.8
- inadequate, inadequacy
- – development
- – – fetus P05.9
- – – lungs, associated with short gestation P28.0
- – pulmonary function, newborn P28.5
- – – ventilation, newborn P28.5
- – ventilation, newborn P28.5
- incompatibility
- – ABO, fetus or newborn P55.1
- – blood (group) (Duffy) (K(ell)) (Kidd) (Lewis) (M) (S) NEC
- – – fetus or newborn P55.8
- – Rh (blood group) (factor), fetus or newborn P55.0
- incompatible with life (newborn) (nonviable) P07.2
- incompetency, incompetent cervix, cervical (os), maternal
- – in pregnancy, affecting fetus or newborn P01.0
- incomplete – *see also condition*
- – expansion, lungs (newborn) NEC P28.1
- incoordinate, incoordination
- – uterus (action) (contractions) (complicating delivery)
- – – affecting fetus or newborn P03.6
- induction of labor, affecting fetus or newborn P03.8
- inertia uterus, uterine during labor
- – affecting fetus or newborn P03.6
- infancy, infantile, infantilism – *see also condition*
- – genitalia, genitals, maternal (after puberty)
- – – in pregnancy or childbirth NEC, affecting fetus or newborn P03.8
- – pelvis, maternal
- – – with disproportion (fetopelvic), affecting fetus or newborn P03.1
- infant(s) – *see also* Conditions originating in the perinatal period, infancy
- – of diabetic mother (syndrome of) P70.1

Conditions arising in the perinatal period—*continued*
- infant(s)—*continued*
- – of diabetic mother—*continued*
- – – gestational diabetes P70.0
- infarct, infarction (of), placenta (complicating pregnancy), affecting fetus or newborn P02.2
- infection, infected (opportunistic) (see also Conditions originating in the perinatal period, inflammation)
- – amniotic fluid, sac or cavity, affecting fetus or newborn P02.7
- – Candida (albicans) (tropicalis),
- – – neonatal P37.5
- – – congenital P37.5
- – Citrobacter, newborn P37.8
- – Clostridium, clostridium, congenital P39.8
- – congenital NEC P39.9
- – – Candida (albicans) P37.5
- – – clostridium, other than Clostridium tetani P39.8
- – – cytomegalovirus P35.1
- – – Escherichia coli P39.8
- – – – sepsis P36.4
- – – hepatitis, viral P35.3
- – – herpes simplex P35.2
- – – infectious or parasitic disease P37.9
- – – – specified NEC P37.8
- – – listeriosis (disseminated) P37.2
- – – malaria NEC P37.4
- – – – falciparum P37.3
- – – Plasmodium falciparum P37.3
- – – poliomyelitis P35.8
- – – rubella P35.0
- – – salmonella P39.8
- – – skin P39.4
- – – streptococcal NEC P39.8
- – – – sepsis P36.1
- – – – – group B P36.0
- – – toxoplasmosis (acute) (chronic) (subacute) P37.1
- – – tuberculosis P37.0
- – – urinary (tract) P39.3
- – – vaccinia P35.8
- – – virus P35.9
- – – – specified type NEC P35.8
- – cytomegalovirus, cytomegaloviral, congenital P35.1
- – Enterobacter (cloacae), newborn P37.8
- – Escherichia (E.) coli NEC, congenital P39.8
- – – sepsis P36.4

Conditions arising in the perinatal period—*continued*
- infection, infected—*continued*
- – fetus (see also Conditions originating in the perinatal period, infection, congenital) P39.9
- – – intra-amniotic NEC P39.2
- – genital organ or tract, maternal
- – – complicating pregnancy, affecting fetus or newborn P00.8
- – herpes (simplex), congenital P35.2
- – intra-amniotic, fetus P39.2
- – intrauterine (complicating pregnancy)
- – – fetus or newborn P00.8
- – – specified infection NEC, fetus P39.2
- – kidney, maternal (cortex) (hematogenous)
- – – complicating pregnancy, affecting fetus or newborn P00.1
- – Listeria monocytogenes, congenital P37.2
- – Monilia, neonatal P37.5
- – navel, newborn P38
- – newborn P39.9
- – – skin P39.4
- – – specified type NEC (see also Conditions originating in the perinatal period, infection, congenital) P39.8
- – perinatal period NEC P39.9
- – – specified type NEC P39.8
- – polymicrobial, newborn P37.9
- – respiratory (tract) NEC
- – – fetus P28.8
- – – newborn, neonatal P28.8
- – rubella, congenital P35.0
- – Salmonella (arizonae) (cholerae-suis) (enteritidis) (typhimurium)
- – – congenital P39.8
- – skin (local) (staphylococcal) (streptococcal)
- – – newborn P39.4
- – staphylococcal NEC
- – – hemolytic, newborn P36.3
- – – newborn P37.8
- – streptococcal NEC
- – – congenital P39.8
- – – – sepsis P36.1
- – – – – group B P36.0
- – umbilicus, newborn P38
- – urinary (tract) NEC
- – – maternal, complicating pregnancy, affecting fetus or newborn P00.1
- – – newborn P39.3

Conditions arising in the perinatal period—*continued*
- inflammation, inflamed, inflammatory (with exudation) (see also Conditions originating in the perinatal period, infection)
- – navel, newborn P38
- – umbilicus, newborn P38
- influenza (specific virus not identified)
- – maternal, affecting fetus or newborn P00.2
- inhalation, meconium (newborn) P24.0
- injury, injuries (see also specified injury type)
- – birth (see also Conditions originating in the perinatal period, birth, injury) P15.9
- – brachial plexus, newborn P14.3
- – brain, anoxic
- – – at birth P21.9
- – – newborn P21.9
- – childbirth (fetus or newborn) (see also Conditions originating in the perinatal period, birth, injury) P15.9
- – delivery (fetus or newborn) P15.9
- – maternal, during pregnancy, affecting fetus or newborn P00.5
- – nerve, facial, newborn P11.3
- – scalp, fetus or newborn (birth injury) P12.9
- – – due to monitoring (electrode) (sampling incision) P12.4
- – – specified NEC P12.8
- – skeleton, skeletal, birth injury P13.9
- – – specified part NEC P13.8
- inspissated bile syndrome (newborn) P59.1
- insufficiency, insufficient
- – circulatory NEC, fetus or newborn P29.8
- – heart, newborn P29.0
- – lung, newborn P28.5
- – myocardial, myocardium (acute) (chronic), newborn P29.0
- – placental, affecting fetus or newborn P02.2
- – pulmonary, newborn P28.5
- – respiratory (acute), newborn P28.5
- – ventilation, ventilatory, newborn P28.8
- insufficiently tied umbilical cord P51.8
- interruption (of)
- – oxygen cycle, newborn P28.8
- – respiration, newborn P28.8
- intoxication NEC, drug, newborn P93

Conditions arising in the perinatal period—*continued*
- intrauterine contraceptive device (IUD), affecting fetus or newborn P01.8
- irritable, irritability, cerebral, in newborn P91.3
- ischemia, ischemic
- - cerebral (chronic) (generalized)
- - - newborn P91.0
- - - prenatal P91.0
- - myocardium, myocardial, transient, of newborn P29.4
- isoimmunization NEC (see also Conditions originating in the perinatal period, incompatibility)
- - fetus or newborn P55.9
- - - with
- - - - hydrops fetalis P56.0
- - - - kernicterus P57.0
- - - ABO P55.1
- - - Rh P55.0
- - - specified type NEC P55.8
- jaundice (yellow)
- - breast-milk (inhibitor) P59.3
- - due to or associated with
- - - delivery due to delayed conjugation P59.0
- - - preterm delivery P59.0
- - fetus or newborn (physiological) P59.9
- - - due to or associated with
- - - - ABO
- - - - - antibodies P55.1
- - - - - incompatibility, maternal/fetal P55.1
- - - - - isoimmunization P55.1
- - - - absence or deficiency of enzyme system for bilirubin conjugation (congenital) P59.8
- - - - bleeding P58.1
- - - - breast milk inhibitors to conjugation P59.3
- - - - bruising P58.0
- - - - delayed conjugation P59.8
- - - - - associated with preterm delivery P59.0
- - - - drugs or toxins
- - - - - given to newborn P58.4
- - - - - transmitted from mother P58.4
- - - - excessive hemolysis NEC P58.9
- - - - - specified type NEC P58.8
- - - - hepatocellular damage P59.2
- - - - hereditary hemolytic anemia P58.8

Conditions arising in the perinatal period—*continued*
- jaundice—*continued*
- - fetus or newborn—*continued*
- - - due to or associated with—*continued*
- - - - incompatibility, maternal/fetal NEC P55.9
- - - - infection P58.2
- - - - inspissated bile syndrome P59.1
- - - - isoimmunization NEC P55.9
- - - - polycythemia P58.3
- - - - preterm delivery P59.0
- - - - Rh
- - - - - antibodies P55.0
- - - - - incompatibility, maternal/fetal P55.0
- - - - - isoimmunization P55.0
- - - - swallowed maternal blood P58.5
- - - specified cause NEC P59.8
- - nuclear, newborn – *see* Conditions originating in the perinatal period, kernicterus of newborn
- kernicterus of newborn P57.9
- - due to isoimmunization (conditions in P55.-) P57.0
- - specified type NEC P57.8
- Klumpke(-Déjerine) palsy, paralysis (birth) (newborn) P14.1
- knot (true), umbilical cord, affecting fetus or newborn P02.5
- labor (see also Conditions originating in the perinatal period, delivery)
- - abnormal NEC, affecting fetus or newborn P03.6
- - arrested active phase, affecting fetus or newborn P03.6
- - desultory, affecting fetus or newborn P03.6
- - dyscoordinate, affecting fetus or newborn P03.6
- - forced or induced, affecting fetus or newborn P03.8
- - hypertonic, affecting fetus or newborn P03.6
- - hypotonic, affecting fetus or newborn P03.6
- - incoordinate, affecting fetus or newborn P03.6
- - irregular, affecting fetus or newborn P03.6
- - obstructed
- - - affecting fetus or newborn P03.1

140

Conditions arising in the perinatal period—*continued*
- labor—*continued*
- - obstructed—*continued*
- - - by or due to
- - - - abnormal
- - - - - pelvis (bony), affecting fetus or newborn P03.1
- - - - - presentation or position, affecting fetus or newborn P03.1
- - - - - size, fetus, affecting fetus or newborn P03.1
- - - - cephalopelvic disproportion (normally formed fetus), affecting fetus or newborn P03.1
- - - - disproportion, fetopelvic NEC, affecting fetus or newborn P03.1
- - - - malpresentation, affecting fetus or newborn P03.1
- - precipitate, affecting fetus or newborn P03.5
- - prolonged or protracted, affecting fetus or newborn P03.8
- laceration (see also Conditions originating in the perinatal period, wound)
- - brain (any part) (cortex) (diffuse) (membrane), during birth P10.8
- - - with hemorrhage P10.1
- - cerebral (diffuse), during birth P10.8
- - - with hemorrhage P10.1
- - intracranial NEC, birth injury P10.9
- - spinal cord (meninges), fetus or newborn (birth injury) P11.5
- lack of exchange of gases, newborn P28.5
- large-for-dates NEC (fetus or infant) P08.1
- - exceptionally (4500 g or more) P08.0
- laryngismus (stridulus), congenital P28.8
- lateroversion, uterus, uterine, maternal (cervix) (postinfectional) (postpartal, old)
- - in pregnancy or childbirth, affecting fetus or newborn P03.8
- leak, leakage of air (bronchus) (intrathoracic) (lung) (pleural) (pulmonary) (thorax), newborn P25.1
- lesion, vascular (nontraumatic)
- - umbilical cord, complicating delivery
- - - affecting fetus or newborn P02.6
- leukomalacia, cerebral, newborn P91.2

Conditions arising in the perinatal period—*continued*
- lie, abnormal (maternal care) (see also Conditions originating in the perinatal period, presentation, fetal, abnormal)
- - before labor, affecting fetus or newborn P01.7
- light, fetus or newborn, for gestational age P05.0
- light-for-dates (infant) P05.0
- - and small-for-dates P05.1
- listeriosis, listerellosis, congenital (disseminated) P37.2
- - fetal P37.2
- - neonatal (disseminated) P37.2
- lithopedion P95
- locked twins causing obstructed labor, affecting fetus or newborn P03.1
- long labor, affecting fetus or newborn P03.8
- loss of fluid (acute), fetus or newborn P74.1
- low
- - birthweight (2499 grams or less) (see also Conditions originating in the perinatal period, weight) P07.1
- - - extreme (999 grams or less) P07.0
- - - for gestational age P05.0
- - cardiac, output, newborn P29.8
- lupus erythematosus, systemic (discoid) (local)
- - maternal, affecting fetus or newborn P00.8
- luxation , eyeball, birth injury P15.3
- lymphadenopathy (generalized), due to toxoplasmosis
- - congenital (acute) (chronic) (subacute) P37.1
- maceration of fetus or newborn (cause not stated) P95
- malaria, malarial fever, congenital NEC P37.4
- - falciparum P37.3
- male type pelvis, maternal
- - with disproportion (fetopelvic), affecting fetus or newborn P03.1
- malformation (congenital) – *see also* Conditions originating in the perinatal period, anomaly
- - pelvic organs or tissues NEC, maternal
- - - in pregnancy or childbirth, affecting fetus or newborn P03.8
- - - - causing obstructed labor, affecting fetus or newborn P03.1

Conditions arising in the perinatal period—*continued*
- malformation—*continued*
- − umbilical cord NEC (complicating delivery)
- − − affecting fetus or newborn P02.6
- malnutrition
- − intrauterine or fetal P05.2
- − − light-for-dates P05.0
- − − small-for-dates P05.1
- − maternal, affecting fetus or newborn P00.4
- mastitis (acute) (nonpuerperal) (subacute)
- − infective, newborn or neonatal P39.0
- − noninfective, newborn or neonatal P83.4
- maternal condition, affecting fetus or newborn P00.9
- − acute yellow atrophy of liver P00.8
- − alcohol use P04.3
- − anesthesia or analgesia P04.0
- − blood loss (gestational) P02.1
- − cancer chemotherapy P04.1
- − chorioamnionitis P02.7
- − circulatory disease (conditions in I00-I99, Q20-Q28) P00.3
- − complication of pregnancy NEC P01.9
- − congenital heart disease (conditions in Q20-Q24) P00.3
- − cortical necrosis of kidney P00.1
- − cytotoxic drug P04.1
- − death P01.6
- − diabetes mellitus (conditions in E10-E14) P70.1
- − disease NEC P00.9
- − drug abuse P04.4
- − eclampsia P00.0
- − exposure to environmental chemical substances P04.6
- − genital tract infections NEC P00.8
- − glomerular diseases (conditions in N00-N08) P00.1
- − hemorrhage, gestational P02.1
- − hepatitis, acute, malignant or subacute P00.8
- − hyperemesis (gravidarum) P01.8
- − hypertension (conditions in O10-O11, O13-O16) P00.0
- − infectious and parasitic diseases (conditions in A00-B99, J09-J11) P00.2
- − influenza P00.2
- − − manifest influenza in the infant P35.8

Conditions arising in the perinatal period—*continued*
- maternal condition, affecting fetus or newborn—*continued*
- − injury (conditions in S00-T79) P00.5
- − intrauterine coil P01.8
- − malaria P00.2
- − − manifest malaria NEC in infant or fetus P37.4
- − − − falciparum P37.3
- − malnutrition P00.4
- − necrosis of liver P00.8
- − nephritis, nephrotic syndrome and nephrosis (conditions in N00-N08) P00.1
- − noxious influence transmitted via breast milk or placenta P04.9
- − − specified NEC P04.8
- − nutritional disorder (conditions in E40-E64) P00.4
- − operation unrelated to current pregnancy P00.6
- − pre-eclampsia P00.0
- − previous surgery, uterus or pelvic organs P03.8
- − proteinuria P00.1
- − pyelitis or pyelonephritis P00.1
- − renal disease or failure P00.1
- − respiratory disease (conditions in J00-J99, Q30-Q34) P00.3
- − rheumatic heart disease (chronic) (conditions in I05-I09) P00.3
- − rubella (conditions in B06) P00.2
- − − manifest rubella in the infant or fetus P35.0
- − septate vagina P03.8
- − stenosis or stricture of vagina P03.8
- − surgery unrelated to current pregnancy P00.6
- − − to uterus or pelvic organs P03.8
- − syphilis (conditions in A50-A53) P00.2
- − thrombophlebitis P00.3
- − tobacco use P04.2
- − toxemia (of pregnancy) P00.0
- − toxoplasmosis (conditions in B58.-) P00.2
- − − manifest toxoplasmosis (acute) (chronic) (subacute) in the infant or fetus P37.1
- − transmission of chemical substance through the placenta (see also Conditions originating in the perinatal period, absorption, chemical, through placenta) P04.8

Conditions arising in the perinatal period—*continued*
- maternal condition, affecting fetus or newborn—*continued*
- – uremia P00.1
- – urinary tract conditions (conditions in N00- N39) P00.1
- – vomiting (pernicious) (persistent) (vicious) P01.8
- meconium
- – obstruction, fetus or newborn P76.0
- – peritonitis P78.0
- – plug syndrome (newborn) NEC P76.0
- – stain, fetus or newborn P20.9
- melena, newborn, neonatal P54.1
- – due to swallowed maternal blood P78.2
- membranitis, affecting fetus or newborn P02.7
- meningoencephalitis, in toxoplasmosis, congenital P37.1† G05.2∗
- meningoencephalomyelitis, due to toxoplasma or toxoplasmosis, congenital P37.1† G05.2∗
  microcephalus, microcephalic, microcephaly, due to toxoplasmosis (congenital) P37.1
- Mikity-Wilson disease or syndrome P27.0
- molding, head (during birth) P13.1
- mole (pigmented), hydatid, hydatidiform (benign) (complicating pregnancy) (delivered) (undelivered)
- – newborn P02.2
- moniliasis, neonatal P37.5
- mucus
- – asphyxia or suffocation, newborn P24.1
- – plug
- – – aspiration, newborn P24.1
- – – tracheobronchial, newborn P24.1
- multiple, multiplex – *see also condition*
- – birth, affecting fetus or newborn P01.5
- myasthenia, myasthenic gravis, neonatal, transient P94.0
- necrosis, necrotic (ischemic) (necrotizing)
- – fat (generalized)
- – – subcutaneous, due to birth injury P15.6
- – kidney (bilateral)
- – – tubular, complicating pregnancy , affecting fetus or newborn P00.1
- – liver (cell), maternal
- – – complicating pregnancy or childbirth, affecting fetus or newborn P00.8

Conditions arising in the perinatal period—*continued*
- necrosis, necrotic—*continued*
- – subcutaneous fat, fetus or newborn P83.8
- – umbilical cord, affecting fetus or newborn P02.6
- neonatal esophageal reflux P78.8
- nephritis, nephritic, maternal, complicating pregnancy or childbirth
- – with secondary hypertension, pre-existing, affecting fetus or newborn P00.0
- – affecting fetus or newborn P00.1
- neuritis, cranial nerve
- – seventh or facial, newborn (birth injury) P11.3
- neutropenia, neutropenic (congenital) (cyclic) (drug-induced) (periodic) (primary) (splenic) (toxic)
- – neonatal, transitory (isoimmune) (maternal transfer) P61.5
- nonexpansion, lung (newborn) P28.0
- nonviable P07.2
- nuchal cord, newborn P02.5
- obstetric trauma NEC (complicating delivery), affecting fetus or newborn P03.8
- obstruction, obstructed, obstructive
- – intestine (mechanical) (neurogenic) (paroxysmal) (postinfective) (reflex)
- – – newborn P76.9
- – – – due to
- – – – – fecaliths P76.8
- – – – – inspissated milk P76.2
- – – – – meconium (plug) P76.0
- – – – – specified NEC P76.8
- – labor (see also Conditions originating in the perinatal period, labor, obstructed)
- – – – affecting fetus or newborn P03.1
- – – meconium plug, newborn P76.0
- oligohydramnios, affecting fetus or newborn P01.2
- omphalitis (congenital) (newborn) (with mild hemorrhage) P38
- omphalorrhagia, newborn P51.9
- operation
- – for delivery, affecting fetus or newborn (see also Conditions originating in the perinatal period, delivery, by type, affecting fetus) P03.8
- – maternal, unrelated to current delivery, affecting fetus or newborn P00.6
- ophthalmia neonatorum, newborn P39.1

**Conditions arising in the perinatal
period**—*continued*
– overfeeding, newborn P92.4
– oversize fetus P08.1
– – causing disproportion, affecting fetus or
newborn P03.1
– – exceptionally large (more than 4500 g)
P08.0
– palpitations (heart)
– – fetal P20.9
– – newborn P29.1
– palsy (see also Conditions originating in
the perinatal period, paralysis)
– – brachial plexus NEC
– – – fetus or newborn (birth injury) P14.3
– – Erb's P14.0
– – facial, newborn (birth injury) P11.3
– – Klumpke(-Déjerine) P14.1
– papyraceous fetus P95
– paralysis, paralytic (complete)
(incomplete)
– – birth injury P14.9
– – brachial plexus NEC, birth injury
P14.3
– – – newborn P14.3
– – Duchenne's, birth injury P14.0
– – Erb(-Duchenne) (birth) (newborn)
P14.0
– – facial (nerve), birth injury P11.3
– – – newborn P11.3
– – Klumpke(-Déjerine) (birth injury)
(newborn) P14.1
– – nerve
– – – birth injury P14.9
– – – facial, birth injury (newborn) P11.3
– – – newborn (birth injury) P14.9
– – – phrenic (birth injury) (newborn)
P14.2
– – – radial, birth injury (newborn) P14.3
– – – seventh or facial (birth injury)
(newborn) P11.3
– – newborn P91.8
– – – birth injury P11.9
– – radial nerve, birth injury (newborn)
P14.3
– paraplegia (lower), newborn P91.8
– – birth injury P11.9
– patent cervix, maternal, complicating
pregnancy
– – affecting fetus or newborn P01.0
– pendulous abdomen, maternal, in
pregnancy or childbirth
– – affecting fetus or newborn P03.8

**Conditions arising in the perinatal
period**—*continued*
– perforation, perforated (nontraumatic) (see
also Conditions originating in the
perinatal period, rupture)
– – intestine (bowel) (colon) (ileum)
(jejunum) (rectum) (sigmoid), fetus or
newborn P78.0
– peritonitis (adhesive) (fibrinous) (with
effusion)
– – congenital NEC P78.1
– – meconium (newborn) P78.0
– – neonatal P78.1
– – – meconium P78.0
– persistence, persistent (congenital) fetal
circulation P29.3
– – occipitoposterior or transverse
(position), affecting fetus or newborn
P03.1
– petechia, petechiae, fetus or newborn
P54.5
– pithecoid maternal pelvis, with
disproportion (fetopelvic)
– – affecting fetus or newborn P03.1
– placenta, placental (see also condition)
– – ablatio, affecting fetus or newborn
P02.1
– – abnormal, abnormality NEC
– – – with hemorrhage, affecting fetus or
newborn P02.1
– – – affecting fetus or newborn P02.2
– – abruptio, affecting fetus or newborn
P02.1
– – disease NEC, affecting fetus or
newborn P02.2
– – infarction, affecting fetus or newborn
P02.2
– – insufficiency , affecting fetus or
newborn P02.2
– – marginal (hemorrhage) (rupture),
affecting fetus or newborn P02.0
– – previa (central) (complete) (marginal)
(partial) (total) (with hemorrhage,
affecting fetus or newborn P02.0
– placentitis, affecting fetus or newborn
P02.7
– platypelloid maternal pelvis, with
disproportion (fetopelvic)
– – affecting fetus or newborn P03.1
– plug, meconium (newborn), syndrome
P76.0
– pneumomediastinum, congenital or
perinatal (newborn) P25.2

Conditions arising in the perinatal
period—*continued*
- pneumonia (acute) (community acquired)
  (double) (hemorrhagic) (lobe) (migratory)
  (nosocomial) (primary) (purulent) (septic)
  (unresolved) (see also Conditions
  originating in the perinatal period,
  pneumonitis)
- – aspiration
- – – newborn P24.9
- – – – meconium P24.0
- – chlamydial, congenital P23.1
- – congenital (infective) P23.9
- – – due to
- – – – bacterium NEC P23.6
- – – – Chlamydia P23.1
- – – – Escherichia coli P23.4
- – – – Haemophilus influenzae P23.6
- – – – infective organism NEC P23.8
- – – – Klebsiella pneumoniae P23.6
- – – – Mycoplasma P23.6
- – – – Pseudomonas P23.5
- – – – staphylococcus P23.2
- – – – streptococcus (except group B)
  P23.6
- – – – – group B P23.3
- – – – viral agent P23.0
- – – specified NEC P23.8
- – in (due to), Chlamydia, neonatal P23.1
- – meconium P24.0
- – neonatal P23.9
- – – aspiration P24.9
- – viral, virus (broncho) (interstitial)
  (lobar) , congenital P23.0
- pneumonitis (acute) (primary) (see also
  Conditions originating in the perinatal
  period, pneumonia)
- – due to toxoplasmosis, congenital
  P37.1† J17.3*
- – meconium P24.0
- – neonatal aspiration P24.9
- – rubella, congenital P35.0
- pneumopericardium
- – congenital P25.3
- – fetus or newborn P25.3
- pneumothorax
- – congenital P25.1
- – newborn P25.1
- – perinatal period P25.1
- – spontaneous NEC
- – – fetus or newborn P25.1
- poliomyelitis (acute) (anterior)
  (epidemic), congenital P35.8

Conditions arising in the perinatal
period—*continued*
- polycythemia (primary) (rubra) (vera),
  neonatorum P61.1
- polyhydramnios, affecting fetus or
  newborn P01.3
- polyp, polypus
- – cervix (uteri), maternal, in pregnancy or
  childbirth, affecting fetus or newborn
  P03.8
- – umbilical, newborn P83.6
- – uterus (body) (corpus) (mucous),
  maternal, in pregnancy or childbirth,
  affecting fetus or newborn P03.8
- poor
- – contractions, labor, affecting fetus or
  newborn P03.6
- – fetal growth NEC P05.9
- postmaturity, postmature (fetus or
  newborn) P08.2
- postterm (pregnancy), infant P08.2
- precipitate labor or delivery, affecting
  fetus or newborn P03.5
- pre-eclampsia, affecting fetus or newborn
  P00.0
- pregnancy (single) (uterine)
- – abdominal (ectopic), affecting fetus or
  newborn P01.4
- – cornual, fetus or newborn P01.4
- – ectopic (ruptured), affecting fetus or
  newborn P01.4
- – multiple NEC, affecting fetus or
  newborn P01.5
- – mural, fetus or newborn P01.4
- – ovarian, fetus or newborn P01.4
- – quadruplet, affecting fetus or newborn
  P01.5
- – quintuplet, affecting fetus or newborn
  P01.5
- – sextuplet, affecting fetus or newborn
  P01.5
- – triplet, affecting fetus or newborn
  P01.5
- – tubal (with abortion) (with rupture),
  affecting fetus or newborn P01.4
- – twin, affecting fetus or newborn P01.5
- premature – *see also condition*
- – birth NEC P07.3
- – delivery, newborn NEC P07.3
- – infant NEC P07.3
- – – light-for-dates P05.0
- – labor, newborn NEC P07.3
- – lungs P28.0

Conditions arising in the perinatal period—*continued*
- premature—*continued*
- − − rupture, membranes or amnion, affecting fetus or newborn P01.1
- − prematurity NEC (less than 37 completed weeks) (see also Conditions originating in the perinatal period, immaturity) P07.3
- − − extreme (less than 28 completed weeks) P07.2
- − − gross P07.2
- − − marked P07.2
- − − severe P07.2
- − presentation, fetal
- − − abnormal
- − − − before labor, affecting fetus or newborn P01.7
- − − − causing obstructed labor, affecting fetus or newborn (any, except breech) P03.1
- − − − − breech P03.0
- − − breech
- − − − with external version before labor, affecting fetus or newborn P01.7
- − − − before labor, affecting fetus or newborn P01.7
- − − − causing obstructed labor, fetus or newborn P03.0
- − pressure
- − − birth, fetus or newborn, NEC P15.9
- − − brain injury at birth NEC P11.1
- − − increased, intracranial (benign), injury at birth P11.0
- − preterm infant, newborn NEC P07.3
- − previa
- − − placenta (with hemorrhage), affecting fetus or newborn P02.0
- − − vasa, affecting fetus or newborn P02.6
- − previable P07.2
- − problem (related to) (with) (see also Conditions originating in the perinatal period, disease)
- − − feeding newborn P92.9
- − − − breast P92.5
- − − − overfeeding P92.4
- − − − slow P92.2
- − − − specified NEC P92.8
- − − − underfeeding P92.3
- − procedure (surgical), maternal (unrelated to current delivery), affecting fetus or newborn P00.6
- − − nonsurgical (medical) P00.7
- − prolapse, prolapsed
- − − arm or hand, in fetus or newborn P03.1

Conditions arising in the perinatal period—*continued*
- prolapse, prolapsed—*continued*
- − − fetal limb NEC, in fetus or newborn P03.1
- − − leg, in fetus or newborn P03.1
- − − umbilical cord, affecting fetus or newborn P02.4
- − − uterus (with prolapse of vagina), pregnant, affecting fetus or newborn P03.8
- − prolonged
- − − labor, affecting fetus or newborn P03.8
- − − uterine contractions in labor, affecting fetus or newborn P03.6
- − prominent ischial spine or sacral promontory, with disproportion (fetopelvic)
- − − affecting fetus or newborn P03.1
- − proteinuria, pre-eclamptic, affecting fetus or newborn P00.0
- − pseudomenses (newborn) P54.6
- − pseudomenstruation (newborn) P54.6
- − pseudoparalysis, atonic, congenital P94.2
- − pseudosclerema, newborn P83.8
- − pulse
- − − alternating
- − − − fetal P20.9
- − − − newborn P29.1
- − − bigeminal
- − − − fetal P20.9
- − − − newborn P29.1
- − pulsus alternans or trigeminus
- − − fetal P20.9
- − − newborn P29.1
- − purpura, thrombocytopenic (congenital) (hereditary), neonatal, transitory P61.0
- − pyelitis, maternal (congenital) (uremic), complicating pregnancy, affecting fetus or newborn P00.1
- − pyelonephritis, maternal, complicating pregnancy, affecting fetus or newborn P00.1
- − pyoderma, pyodermia NEC, newborn P39.4
- − pyrexia (of unknown origin), newborn, environmentally-induced P81.0
- − quadriplegia, newborn NEC P11.9
- − quadruplet, affecting fetus or newborn P01.5
- − quintuplet, affecting fetus or newborn P01.5
- − rachitic – *see also condition*

Conditions arising in the perinatal period—*continued*
– rachitic—*continued*
– – pelvis, maternal (late effect), with disproportion (fetopelvic), affecting fetus or newborn P03.1
– radiology, maternal, affecting fetus or newborn P00.7
– rapid
– – heart (beat)
– – – fetal P20.9
– – – newborn P29.1
– – second stage (delivery), affecting fetus or newborn P03.5
– R.D.S. (newborn) P22.0
– reaction – *see also* Conditions originating in the perinatal period, disorder
– – drug NEC
– – – newborn P93
– – – withdrawal
– – – – infant of dependent mother P96.1
– – – – newborn P96.1
– rectocele, maternal, in pregnancy or childbirth
– – causing obstructed labor, affecting fetus or newborn P03.1
– regurgitation, food, newborn P92.1
– respiration, insufficient, or poor, newborn NEC P28.5
– retardation
– – growth, fetus P05.9
– – – intrauterine P05.9
– – physical, fetus P05.9
– retraction, ring, uterus (Bandl's) (pathological), affecting fetus or newborn P03.6
– retroversion, retroverted uterus, uterine, maternal, in pregnancy or childbirth
– – causing obstructed labor, affecting fetus or newborn P03.1
– Rh (factor)
– – hemolytic disease (fetus or newborn) P55.0
– – incompatibility, immunization or sensitization, fetus or newborn P55.0
– – negative mother affecting fetus or newborn P55.0
– rigid, rigidity – *see also condition*
– – cervix, maternal (uteri), in pregnancy or childbirth
– – – affecting fetus or newborn P03.8
– – – causing obstructed labor, affecting fetus or newborn P03.1

Conditions arising in the perinatal period—*continued*
– rigid, rigidity—*continued*
– – pelvic floor, maternal, in pregnancy or childbirth
– – – affecting fetus or newborn P03.8
– – – causing obstructed labor, affecting fetus or newborn P03.1
– – perineum or vulva, maternal, in pregnancy or childbirth
– – – causing obstructed labor, affecting fetus or newborn P03.1
– – vagina, maternal, in pregnancy or childbirth
– – – causing obstructed labor, affecting fetus or newborn P03.8
– ring(s)
– – Bandl's, fetus or newborn P03.6
– – contraction, complicating delivery, affecting fetus or newborn P03.6
– – retraction, uterus, pathological, affecting fetus or newborn P03.6
– rotation, manual, affecting fetus or newborn P03.8
– rubella
– – congenital P35.0
– – maternal, affecting fetus or newborn P00.2
– – – manifest rubella in infant P35.0
– rumination, newborn P92.1
– rupture, ruptured – *see also* Conditions originating in the perinatal period, perforation
– – fontanelle P13.1
– – intestine (bowel) (colon) (ileum) (jejunum) (rectum) (sigmoid), fetus or newborn P78.0
– – kidney, birth injury P15.8
– – liver, birth injury P15.0
– – marginal sinus (placental) (with hemorrhage), affecting fetus or newborn P02.1
– – – with placenta previa, affecting fetus or newborn P02.0
– – membranes
– – – artificial, delayed delivery following
– – – – affecting fetus or newborn P01.1
– – – premature, affecting fetus or newborn P01.1
– – – spontaneous, delayed delivery following
– – – – affecting fetus or newborn P01.1
– – spinal cord, fetus or newborn (birth injury) P11.5

Conditions arising in the perinatal period—*continued*
- rupture, ruptured—*continued*
- - spleen (traumatic)
- - - birth injury P15.1
- - - congenital P15.1
- - umbilical cord, complicating delivery, affecting fetus or newborn P50.1
- - uterus, maternal
  - during or after labor, affecting fetus or newborn P03.8
- salpingo-oophoritis, maternal (purulent) (ruptured) (septic) (suppurative)
- - complicating pregnancy, affecting fetus or newborn P00.8
- scar, scarring,
- - cervix, maternal
- - - in pregnancy or childbirth, affecting fetus or newborn P03.8
- - due to previous cesarean section, complicating pregnancy or childbirth
- - - affecting fetus or newborn P03.8
- - uterus, maternal
- - - in pregnancy or childbirth, affecting fetus or newborn P03.8
- scleredema, newborn P83.0
- sclerema (newborn) P83.0
- - adiposum P83.0
- - edematosum P83.0
- scleroderma, sclerodermia (diffuse) (generalized), newborn P83.8
- scoliotic maternal pelvis with disproportion (fetopelvic)
- - affecting fetus or newborn P03.1
- section, cesarean
- - affecting fetus or newborn P03.4
- - - postmortem P01.6
- - - previous, in pregnancy or childbirth P03.8
- seizure(s), newborn P90
- sepsis (generalized) (see also Conditions originating in the perinatal period, septicemia)
- - bacterial, newborn P36.9
- - - due to
- - - - anaerobes NEC P36.5
- - - - Escherichia coli P36.4
- - - - Staphylococcus NEC P36.3
- - - - - aureus P36.2
- - - - streptococcus NEC P36.1
- - - - - group B P36.0
- - - specified type NEC P36.8
- - newborn NEC P36.9

Conditions arising in the perinatal period—*continued*
- sepsis—*continued*
- - newborn NEC—*continued*
- - - due to
- - - - anaerobes NEC P36.5
- - - - Escherichia coli P36.4
- - - - Staphylococcus NEC P36.3
- - - - - aureus P36.2
- - - - streptococcus NEC P36.1
- - - - - group B P36.0
- - - specified NEC P36.8
- - umbilical (newborn) (organism unspecified) P38
- septic – *see also condition*
- - umbilical cord P38
- septicemia, septicemic (generalized) (suppurative) (see also Conditions originating in the perinatal period, sepsis)
- - Actinobacter, newborn P36.8
- - Bacillus coli, newborn P36.8
- - Citobacter, newborn P36.8
- - Enterobacter (aerogenes) (clocae), newborn P36.8
- - Friedlanders', newborn P36.8
- - newborn NEC (see also Conditions originating in the perinatal period, sepsis, newborn) P36.9
- - Streptococcus, streptococcal, neonatal P36.1
- sextuplet, affecting fetus or newborn P01.5
- shock (acute),
- - birth, fetus or newborn NEC P96.8
- - lung, newborn P22.0
- - septic (see also Conditions originating in the perinatal period, septicemia)
- - - newborn P36.9
- - septicemic, newborn P36.9
- short, shortening, shortness
- - cord (umbilical), complicating delivery, affecting fetus or newborn P02.6
- sinus, marginal, ruptured or bleeding, maternal, affecting fetus or newborn P02.1
- - with placenta previa, affecting fetus or newborn P02.0
- sleep apnea, newborn P28.3
- slipped, slipping ligature, umbilical P51.8
- slow
- - feeding, newborn P92.2
- - fetal growth NEC P05.9
- - heart(beat)
- - - fetal P20.9

Conditions arising in the perinatal period—*continued*
- slow—*continued*
- – heart(beat)—*continued*
- – – newborn P29.1
- small(ness)
- – fetus or newborn for gestational age P05.1
- – pelvis, maternal, with disproportion (fetopelvic), affecting fetus or newborn P03.1
- small-and-light-for-dates (infant) P05.1
- small-for-dates (infant) P05.1
- snuffles (non-syphilitic), newborn P28.8
- spasm(s), spastic, spasticity (*see also condition*)
- – cervix, maternal, complicating delivery, affecting fetus or newborn P03.6
- – uterus, maternal, complicating labor, affecting fetus or newborn P03.6
- spondylolisthesis, maternal (acquired)
- – with disproportion (fetopelvic), affecting fetus or newborn P03.1
- spondylolysis, maternal, lumbosacral region
- – with disproportion (fetopelvic), affecting fetus or newborn P03.1
- spondylosis, maternal
- – with disproportion (fetopelvic), affecting fetus or newborn P03.1
- standstill respiration, respiratory, newborn P28.5
- stenosis (cicatricial)
- – cervix, cervical (canal), maternal, in pregnancy or childbirth
- – – affecting fetus or newborn P03.8
- – – causing obstructed labor, affecting fetus or newborn P03.1
- – vagina, maternal, in pregnancy or childbirth
- – – affecting fetus or newborn P03.8
- – – causing obstructed labor, affecting fetus or newborn P03.1
- stillbirth NEC P95
- strangulation, strangulated, umbilical cord, fetus or newborn P02.5
- – with cord prolapse P02.4
- stricture (see also Conditions originating in the perinatal period, stenosis)
- – cervix, cervical (canal), maternal, in pregnancy or childbirth
- – – affecting fetus or newborn P03.8
- – – causing obstructed labor, affecting fetus or newborn P03.1

Conditions arising in the perinatal period—*continued*
- stridor, congenital (larynx) NEC P28.8
- stroke (apoplectic) (brain) (paralytic), hemorrhagic, newborn P52.4
- surgery, previous, in pregnancy or childbirth
- – cervix, maternal
- – – causing obstructed labor, affecting fetus or newborn P03.1
- – pelvic soft tissues NEC, maternal
- – – affecting fetus or newborn P03.8
- – – causing obstructed labor, affecting fetus or newborn P03.1
- – uterus, maternal
- – – causing obstructed labor, affecting fetus or newborn P03.1
- suspended maternal uterus, in pregnancy or childbirth
- – causing obstructed labor, affecting fetus or newborn P03.1
- syncope, bradycardia
- – fetal P20.9
- – newborn P29.1
- syndrome – *see also* Conditions originating in the perinatal period, disease
- – aspiration, of newborn (massive) P24.9
- – – meconium P24.0
- – bronze baby P83.8
- – bubbly lung P27.0
- – cardiorespiratory distress (idiopathic), newborn P22.0
- – cold injury (newborn) P80.0
- – congenital rubella (manifest) P35.0
- – defibrination, fetus or newborn P60
- – drug withdrawal, infant of dependent mother P96.1
- – fetal transfusion P02.3
- – fetomaternal dysfunctional P02.2
- – floppy, baby P94.2
- – gray (newborn) P93
- – idiopathic cardiorespiratory distress, newborn P22.0
- – infant of diabetic mother P70.1
- – – gestational diabetes P70.0
- – inspissated bile (newborn) P59.1
- – low cardiac output, newborn P29.8
- – lower radicular, newborn (birth injury), P14.8
- – meconium plug (newborn) P76.0
- – perfusion, newborn P28.8
- – placental
- – – dysfunction, affecting fetus or newborn P02.2

Conditions arising in the perinatal period—*continued*
- syndrome—*continued*
- − − placental—*continued*
- − − − insufficiency, affecting fetus or newborn P02.2
- − − − transfusion, in fetus or newborn P02.3
- − − pulmonary dysmaturity (Wilson-Mikity) P27.0
- − radicular NEC, upper limbs, newborn (birth injury) P14.3
- − − respiratory distress (idiopathic) (newborn) P22.0
- − − transfusion, fetomaternal P50.4
- − − twin (to twin) transfusion, in fetus or newborn P02.3
- − − wet lung, newborn P22.1
- − − withdrawal, drug
- − − − infant of dependent mother P96.1
- − − − therapeutic use, newborn P96.2
- − syphilis, syphilitic, maternal (acquired), affecting fetus or newborn P00.2
- − − complicating pregnancy or childbirth P00.2
- − tachycardia
- − − fetal – *see* Conditions originating in the perinatal period, distress, fetal
- − − newborn P29.1
- − tachypnea, transitory, of newborn P22.1
- − tear, torn (traumatic) – *see also* Conditions originating in the perinatal period, wound
- − − tentorial, at birth P10.4
- − − umbilical cord, affecting fetus or newborn P50.1
- − temperature, cold, trauma from, newborn P80.0
- − tetany (due to), neonatal (without calcium or magnesium deficiency) P71.3
- − threatened
- − − abortion, affecting fetus P01.8
- − − labor (see also Complications originating in the perinatal period, labor, false)
- − − − affecting fetus P01.8
- − − miscarriage, affecting fetus P01.8
- − − premature delivery, affecting fetus P01.8
- − thrombocytopenia, thrombocytopenic
- − − due to
- − − − exchange transfusion P61.0
- − − − idiopathic maternal thrombocytopenia P61.0

Conditions arising in the perinatal period—*continued*
- − thrombocytopenia, thrombocytopenic—*continued*
- − − due to—*continued*
- − − − isoimmunization P61.0
- − − neonatal, transitory P61.0
- − thrombophlebitis, maternal
- − − antepartum (superficial), affecting fetus or newborn P00.3
- − − pregnancy (superficial), affecting fetus or newborn P00.3
- − thrombosis, thrombotic (multiple) (progressive) (septic) (vein) (vessel)
- − − umbilical cord (vessels), complicating delivery, affecting fetus or newborn P02.6
- − thyrotoxicosis, neonatal P72.1
- − tobacco (nicotine), maternal use, affecting fetus or newborn P04.2
- − torsion umbilical cord in fetus or newborn P02.5
- − torticollis (intermittent) (spastic), due to birth injury P15.2
- − toxemia, maternal (of pregnancy), affecting fetus or newborn P00.0
- − toxoplasma, toxoplasmosis
- − − congenital (acute) (chronic) (subacute) P37.1
- − − maternal, affecting fetus or newborn P00.2
- − − − manifest toxoplasmosis in infant or fetus (acute) (chronic) (subacute) P37.1
- − transfusion
- − − placental (syndrome) (mother), in fetus or newborn P02.3
- − − twin-to-twin, fetus or newborn P02.3
- − transverse – *see also condition*
- − − arrest (deep), in labor, affecting fetus or newborn P03.1
- − − lie
- − − − before labor, affecting fetus or newborn P01.7
- − − − causing obstructed labor, affecting fetus or newborn P03.1
- − trauma, traumatism (see also Conditions originating in the perinatal period, injury)
- − − birth – *see* Conditions originating in the perinatal period, birth, injury
- − − maternal, during pregnancy, affecting fetus or newborn P00.5
- − trigeminy
- − − fetal P20.9

Conditions arising in the perinatal period—*continued*
- trigeminy—*continued*
- – newborn P29.1
- triplet, affecting fetus or newborn P01.5
- tuberculosis, tubercular, tuberculous (caseous) (degeneration) (gangrene) (necrosis)
- – congenital P37.0
- – maternal, complicating pregnancy or childbirth, affecting fetus or newborn P00.2
- tumor
- – cervix, maternal, in pregnancy or childbirth
- – – affecting fetus or newborn P03.8
- – – causing obstructed labor, affecting fetus or newborn P03.1
- – ovary, maternal, in pregnancy or childbirth
- – – affecting fetus or newborn P03.8
- – pelvic, maternal, in pregnancy or childbirth
- – – affecting fetus or newborn P03.8
- – – causing obstructed labor, affecting fetus or newborn P03.1
- – uterus (body), maternal, in pregnancy or childbirth
- – – affecting fetus or newborn P03.8
- – – causing obstructed labor, affecting fetus or newborn P03.1
- – vagina, maternal, in pregnancy or childbirth
- – – affecting fetus or newborn P03.8
- – – causing obstructed labor, affecting fetus or newborn P03.1
- – vulva or perineum, maternal, in pregnancy or childbirth
- – – affecting fetus or newborn P03.8
- – – causing obstructed labor, affecting fetus or newborn P03.1
- twin (pregnancy) (fetus or newborn) P01.5
- twist, twisted umbilical cord in fetus or newborn P02.5
- tyrosinemia, newborn, transitory P74.5
- ulcer, ulcerated, ulcerating, ulceration, ulcerative
- – intestine, intestinal, perforating, fetus or newborn P78.0
- – peptic (site unspecified), newborn P78.8
- underfeeding, newborn P92.3
- underweight for gestational age P05.0

Conditions arising in the perinatal period—*continued*
- Underwood's disease P83.0
- unstable lie, fetus or newborn, before labor P01.7
- uremia, uremic (coma)
- – congenital P96.0
- – maternal NEC, affecting fetus or newborn P00.1
- – newborn P96.0
- urticaria neonatorum P83.8
- use (of) harmful patent medicines, maternal, affecting fetus or newborn P04.1
- uveitis (anterior), due to toxoplasmosis, congenital P37.1† H22.0*
- vaccinia (generalized) (localized)
- – congenital P35.8
- vaginitis, maternal (acute), complicating pregnancy, affecting fetus or newborn P00.8
- varicella, congenital P35.8
- varicose vein (ruptured), umbilical cord, affecting fetus or newborn P02.6
- varix (ruptured), umbilical cord, affecting fetus or newborn P02.6
- vasa previa
- – affecting fetus or newborn P02.6
- – hemorrhage from, affecting fetus or newborn P50.0
- ventilator lung, newborn P27.8
- ventouse delivery NEC, affecting fetus or newborn P03.3
- version, with extraction, affecting fetus or newborn P01.7
- viremia, newborn P35.9
- vitality, lack of, newborn P96.8
- volvulus (bowel) (colon) (intestine), newborn P76.8
- vomiting (see also Conditions originating in the perinatal period, hyperemesis)
- – newborn P92.0
- weak, weakness, newborn P96.8
- weight
- – 999 grams or less at birth (extremely low) P07.0
- – 1000-2499 grams at birth (low) P07.1
- wet lung, newborn P22.1
- wide cranial sutures, newborn P96.3
- Wilson-Mikity syndrome P27.0
- withdrawal state, symptoms, syndrome, newborn
- – correct therapeutic substance properly administered P96.2

Conditions arising in the perinatal period—*continued*
- withdrawal state, symptoms—*continued*
- – infant of dependent mother P96.1
- – therapeutic substance, neonatal P96.2
- wound (cut) (laceration) (open) (penetrating (puncture wound) (with penetrating foreign body)
- – scalpel, fetus or newborn (birth injury) P15.8

Conduct disorder – *see* Disorder, conduct
Condyloma A63.0
- acuminatum A63.0
- gonorrheal A54.0
- latum A51.3
- syphilitic A51.3
- – congenital A50.0
- venereal, syphilitic A51.3

Conflagration – *see also* Burn
- asphyxia (by inhalation of smoke, gases, fumes or vapors) T59.9
- – specified agent – *see* Table of drugs and chemicals

Conflict (with) – *see also* Discord
- social role NEC Z73.5

Confluent – *see condition*
Confusion, confused R41.0
- epileptic F05.8
- mental state (psychogenic) F44.8
- psychogenic F44.8
- reactive (from emotional stress, psychological trauma) F44.8

Congelation T69.9
Congenital – *see also condition*
- aortic septum Q25.4
- intrinsic factor deficiency D51.0
- malformation – *see* Anomaly

Congestion, congestive (chronic) (passive)
- bladder N32.8
- bowel K63.8
- brain G93.8
- breast N64.5
- bronchial J98.0
- chest (*see also* Edema, lung) J81
- circulatory NEC I99
- duodenum K31.8
- eye H11.4
- facial, due to birth injury P15.4
- general R68.8
- glottis J37.0
- heart (*see also* Failure, heart, congestive) I50.0
- hepatic K76.1

Congestion, congestive—*continued*
- hypostatic, lung (*see also* Edema, lung) J81
- intestine K63.8
- kidney N28.8
- labyrinth H83.8
- larynx J37.0
- liver K76.1
- lung (hypostatic) (*see also* Edema, lung) J81
- – active or acute (*see also* Pneumonia) J18.2
- orbit, orbital H05.2
- – inflammatory (chronic) H05.1
- – – acute H05.0
- ovary N83.8
- pancreas K86.8
- pelvic, female N94.8
- pleural J94.8
- prostate (active) N42.1
- pulmonary – *see* Congestion, lung
- renal N28.8
- retina H35.8
- seminal vesicle N50.1
- spinal cord G95.1
- spleen D73.2
- stomach K31.8
- trachea – *see* Tracheitis
- urethra N36.8
- uterus N85.8
- venous (passive) I87.8
- viscera R68.8

Conical
- cervix (hypertrophic elongation) N88.4
- cornea H18.6
- teeth K00.2

Conjoined twins Q89.4
Conjugal maladjustment Z63.0
Conjunctiva – *see condition*
Conjunctivitis (in) (due to) H10.9
- Acanthamoeba B60.1† H13.1*
- acute H10.3
- – specified NEC H10.2
- adenoviral (acute) (follicular) B30.1† H13.1*
- allergic (acute) H10.1
- Apollo B30.3† H13.1*
- atopic (acute) H10.1
- Béal's B30.2† H13.1*
- blennorrhagic (gonococcal) (neonatorum) A54.3† H13.1*
- chlamydial A74.0† H13.1*
- – neonatal P39.1

Conjunctivitis—*continued*
- chronic (nodosa) (petrificans) (phlyctenular) H10.4
- coxsackievirus 24 B30.3† H13.1∗
- diphtheritic A36.8† H13.1∗
- enterovirus type 70 (hemorrhagic) B30.3† H13.1∗
- epidemic (viral) B30.9† H13.1∗
- − hemorrhagic B30.3† H13.1∗
- gonococcal (neonatorum) A54.3† H13.1∗
- granular (trachomatous) A71.1† H13.1∗
- hemorrhagic (acute) (epidemic) B30.3† H13.1∗
- herpes (simplex) (virus) B00.5† H13.1∗
- − zoster B02.3† H13.1∗
- inclusion A74.0† H13.1∗
- infectious disease NEC B99† H13.1∗
- Koch-Weeks' H10.0
- meningococcal A39.8† H13.1∗
- Morax-Axenfeld H10.2
- mucopurulent H10.0
- neonatal P39.1
- Newcastle B30.8† H13.1∗
- parasitic disease NEC B89† H13.1∗
- Parinaud's H10.8
- rosacea L71.-† H13.2∗
- specified NEC H10.8
- swimming-pool B30.1† H13.1∗
- syphilis (late) A52.7† H13.1∗
- trachomatous A71.1
- tuberculous A18.5† H13.1∗
- tularemic A21.1† H13.1∗
- viral B30.9† H13.1∗
- − specified NEC B30.8† H13.1∗
- zoster (herpes) B02.3† H13.1∗

Connective tissue – *see condition*
Conn's syndrome E26.0
Conradi(-Hunermann) disease Q77.3
Consanguinity Z84.3
- counseling Z71.8
Conscious simulation (of illness) Z76.5
Consecutive – *see condition*
Consolidation lung (base) – *see* Pneumonia, lobar
Constipation (atonic) (simple) (spastic) K59.0
- drug-induced
- − correct substance properly administered K59.0
- − overdose or wrong substance given or taken T50.9
- − − specified drug – *see* Table of drugs and chemicals
- neurogenic K59.0

Constipation—*continued*
- psychogenic F45.3
Constitutional – *see condition*
Constriction – *see also* Stricture
- asphyxiation or suffocation by T71
- bronchial J98.0
- duodenum K31.5
- esophagus K22.2
- external canal, ear H61.3
- gallbladder (*see also* Obstruction, gallbladder) K82.0
- intestine (*see also* Obstruction, intestine) K56.6
- larynx J38.6
- − congenital Q31.8
- − − specified NEC Q31.8
- − − subglottic Q31.1
- organ or site, congenital NEC – *see* Atresia, by site
- prepuce (acquired) N47
- ring dystocia (uterus) O62.4
- − affecting fetus or newborn P03.6
- spastic – *see* Spasm
- ureter N13.5
- − with infection N13.6
- urethra (*see also* Stricture, urethra) N35.9
- visual field (functional) (peripheral) H53.4
Constrictive – *see condition*
Consultation, medical – *see* Counseling medical
- without complaint or sickness Z71.9
Consumption – *see* Tuberculosis
Contact (with)
- acariasis Z20.7
- AIDS virus Z20.6
- cholera Z20.0
- communicable disease Z20.9
- − sexually transmitted Z20.2
- − specified NEC Z20.8
- − viral NEC Z20.8
- German measles Z20.4
- gonorrhea Z20.2
- human immunodeficiency virus (HIV) Z20.6
- infection
- − human immunodeficiency virus (HIV) Z20.6
- − intestinal Z20.0
- − sexually transmitted Z20.2
- − specified NEC Z20.8
- infestation (parasitic) NEC Z20.7
- intestinal infectious disease Z20.0
- parasitic disease Z20.7

Contact—*continued*
- pediculosis Z20.7
- poliomyelitis Z20.8
- rabies Z20.3
- rubella Z20.4
- sexually transmitted disease Z20.2
- smallpox (laboratory) Z20.8
- syphilis Z20.2
- tuberculosis Z20.1
- venereal disease Z20.2
- viral disease NEC Z20.8
- viral hepatitis Z20.5

Contamination, food (*see also* Intoxication, foodborne) A05.9

Contraception, contraceptive
- advice Z30.0
- counseling Z30.0
- device (intrauterine) (in situ) Z97.5
- − causing menorrhagia T83.8
- − checking Z30.5
- − complications, mechanical T83.3
- − in place Z97.5
- − insertion Z30.1
- − reinsertion Z30.5
- − removal Z30.5
- maintenance (drug) Z30.4
- − device (intrauterine) Z30.5
- − examination Z30.4
- management Z30.9
- − specified NEC Z30.8
- prescription Z30.0
- − repeat Z30.4
- surveillance (drug) Z30.4
- − device (intrauterine) Z30.5

Contraction, contracture, contracted
- Achilles tendon M67.0
- − congenital Q66.8
- amputation stump (flexion) (late) (surgical) T87.6
- bile duct (common) (hepatic) K83.8
- bladder N32.8
- − neck or sphincter N32.0
- bowel, cecum, colon or intestine, any part (*see also* Obstruction, intestine) K56.6
- bronchial J98.0
- burn (old) − *see* Cicatrix
- cervix (*see also* Stricture, cervix) N88.2
- cicatricial − *see* Cicatrix
- conjunctiva, trachomatous, active A71.1
- Dupuytren's M72.0
- eyelid H02.5
- finger NEC M20.0
- − congenital Q68.1

Contraction, contracture—*continued*
- finger NEC—*continued*
- − − joint (*see also* Contraction, joint) M24.5
- flaccid − *see* Contraction, paralytic
- gallbladder or cystic duct K82.8
- heart valve − *see* Endocarditis
- hip (*see also* Contraction, joint) M24.5
- hourglass
- − − bladder N32.8
- − − − congenital Q64.7
- − − gallbladder K82.8
- − − − congenital Q44.1
- − − stomach K31.8
- − − − congenital Q40.2
- − − − psychogenic F45.3
- − − uterus (complicating delivery) O62.4
- − − − affecting fetus or newborn P03.6
- hysterical F44.4
- internal os (*see also* Stricture, cervix) N88.2
- joint (abduction) (acquired) (adduction) (flexion) (rotation) M24.5
- − congenital NEC Q68.8
- − − hip Q65.8
- − hysterical F44.4
- kidney (granular) (secondary) (*see also* Sclerosis, renal) N26
- − congenital Q63.8
- − hydronephritic N13.3
- − − with infection N13.6
- − pyelonephritic (*see also* Pyelitis, chronic) N11.9
- − tuberculous A18.1† N29.1*
- ligament M24.2
- − congenital Q79.8
- muscle (postinfective) (postural) NEC M62.4
- − with contracture of joint M24.5
- − congenital Q79.8
- − extraocular H50.8
- − eye (extrinsic) (*see also* Strabismus) H50.8
- − − paralytic H49.9
- − hysterical F44.4
- − ischemic (Volkmann's) T79.6
- − psychogenic F45.8
- − − conversion reaction F44.4
- ocular muscle (*see also* Strabismus) H50.8
- organ or site, congenital NEC − *see* Atresia, by site
- outlet (pelvis) − *see* Contraction, pelvis
- palmar fascia M72.0

Contraction, contracture—*continued*
- paralytic
- – joint (*see also* Contraction, joint)
   M24.5
- – muscle M62.4
- – – ocular (*see also* Strabismus,
      paralytic) H49.9
- pelvis (acquired) (general) M95.5
- – with disproportion (fetopelvic) O33.1
- – – affecting fetus or newborn P03.1
- – – causing obstructed labor O65.1
- – – inlet O33.2
- – – mid-cavity O33.3
- – – outlet O33.3
- plantar fascia M72.2
- premature
- – atrium I49.1
- – auriculoventricular I49.4
- – heart I49.4
- – junctional I49.2
- – ventricular I49.3
- prostate N42.8
- pylorus NEC (*see also* Pylorospasm)
   K31.3
- – psychogenic F45.3
- ring (Bandl's) (complicating delivery)
   O62.4
- – affecting fetus or newborn P03.6
- scar – *see* Cicatrix
- spine M43.9
- sternocleidomastoid (muscle), congenital
   Q68.0
- stomach K31.8
- – hourglass K31.8
- – – congenital Q40.2
- – – psychogenic F45.3
- – psychogenic F45.3
- tendon (sheath) (*see also* Short, tendon)
   M67.1
- – with contracture of joint M24.5
- toe M20.5
- ureterovesical orifice (postinfectional)
   N13.5
- – with infection N13.6
- urethra (*see also* Stricture, urethra) N35.9
- uterus N85.8
- – abnormal NEC O62.9
- – – affecting fetus or newborn P03.6
- – clonic (complicating delivery) O62.4
- – dyscoordinate (complicating delivery)
   O62.4
- – hourglass (complicating delivery)
   O62.4
- – hypertonic O62.4

Contraction, contracture—*continued*
- uterus—*continued*
- – hypotonic NEC O62.2
- – inadequate
- – – primary O62.0
- – – secondary O62.1
- – incoordinate (complicating delivery)
   O62.4
- – poor O62.2
- – tetanic (complicating delivery) O62.4
- – vagina (outlet) N89.5
- – vesical N32.8
- – – neck or urethral orifice N32.0
- – visual field H53.4
- – Volkmann's (ischemic) T79.6
Contusion (skin surface intact) (*see also*
   Injury, superficial) T14.0
- with
- – crush injury – *see* Crush
- – nerve injury – *see* Injury, nerve
- – open wound – *see* Wound, open
- abdomen, abdominal (muscle) (wall)
   S30.1
- adnexa, eye NEC S05.8
- ankle S90.0
- – and foot, multiple S90.7
- arm
- – meaning upper limb T11.0
- – upper (and shoulder) S40.0
- axilla S40.0
- bone NEC T14.0
- brain (diffuse) S06.2
- – focal S06.3
- breast S20.0
- brow S00.1
- buttock S30.0
- canthus, eye S00.1
- cerebellum S06.2
- cerebral (diffuse) S06.2
- – focal S06.3
- chest (wall) S20.2
- clitoris S30.2
- conjunctiva S05.0
- – with foreign body (in conjunctival sac)
   T15.1
- cornea S05.1
- – with foreign body T15.0
- corpus cavernosum S30.2
- cortex (brain) (cerebral) (focal) S06.3
- – diffuse S06.2
- costal region S20.2
- elbow S50.0
- epididymis S30.2
- epigastric region S30.1

Contusion—*continued*
- esophagus (thoracic) S27.8
- − cervical S10.0
- eye NEC S05.8
- eyeball S05.1
- eyebrow S00.1
- eyelid (and periocular area) S00.1
- fetus or newborn P54.5
- finger(s) S60.0
- − with damage to nail (matrix) S60.1
- flank S30.1
- foot (except toe(s) alone) S90.3
- − specified part NEC S90.3
- − toe(s) S90.1
- − − with damage to nail (matrix) S90.2
- forearm S50.1
- − elbow S50.0
- genital organs, external S30.2
- globe (eye) S05.1
- groin S30.1
- hand S60.2
- − finger(s) (alone) S60.0
- − − with damage to nail (matrix) S60.1
- − wrist S60.2
- heel S90.3
- hip S70.0
- iliac region S30.1
- inguinal region S30.1
- interscapular region S20.2
- iris (eye) S05.1
- knee S80.0
- labium (majus) (minus) S30.2
- lacrimal apparatus, gland or sac S05.8
- larynx S10.0
- leg
- − lower S80.1
- − − knee S80.0
- − − multiple S80.7
- − meaning lower limb T13.0
- lens S05.1
- limb
- − lower T13.0
- − upper T11.0
- lower back S30.0
- lumbar region S30.0
- membrane, brain S06.8
- muscle T14.6
- nail
- − finger S60.1
- − toe S90.2
- neck S10.9
- nerve − *see* Injury, nerve
- occipital
- − lobe (brain) S06.3

Contusion—*continued*
- occipital—*continued*
- − region (scalp) S00.0
- orbit (region) (tissues) S05.1
- parietal
- − lobe (brain) S06.3
- − region (scalp) S00.0
- pelvis S30.0
- penis S30.2
- perineum S30.2
- periocular area S00.1
- pharynx S10.0
- popliteal space S80.1
- prepuce S30.2
- pubic region S30.1
- pudendum S30.2
- quadriceps femoris S70.1
- sacral region S30.0
- scalp S00.0
- − due to birth injury P12.3
- scapular region S40.0
- − multiple S40.7
- sclera S05.1
- scrotum S30.2
- shoulder (and arm) S40.0
- − multiple S40.7
- skin NEC T14.0
- spinal cord − *see also* Injury, spinal cord, by region
- − cauda equina S34.3
- − conus medullaris S34.3
- sternal region S20.2
- subconjunctival S05.0
- subcutaneous NEC T14.0
- subperiosteal NEC T14.0
- supraclavicular fossa S10.8
- supraorbital S00.8
- temple (region) S00.8
- temporal
- − lobe (brain) S06.3
- − region S00.8
- testis S30.2
- thigh S70.1
- thorax S20.2
- throat S10.0
- thumb S60.0
- − with damage to nail (matrix) S60.1
- toe(s) S90.1
- − with damage to nail(s) (matrix) S90.2
- trachea (cervical) S10.0
- − thoracic S27.5
- tunica vaginalis S30.2
- vagina S30.2
- vocal cord(s) S10.0

Contusion—*continued*
- vulva S30.2
- wrist S60.2
Conus (congenital) (any type) Q14.8
- acquired H35.3
- – cornea H18.6
- medullaris syndrome G95.8
Convalescence (following) Z54.9
- chemotherapy Z54.2
- psychotherapy Z54.3
- radiotherapy Z54.1
- surgery NEC Z54.0
- treatment (for) Z54.9
- – combined Z54.7
- – fracture Z54.4
- – – surgery Z54.0
- – mental disorder NEC Z54.3
- – specified NEC Z54.8
Conversion hysteria, neurosis or reaction F44.9
Conviction (legal), anxiety concerning Z65.0
- with imprisonment Z65.1
Convulsions (idiopathic) (*see also* Seizure(s)) R56.8
- apoplectiform (cerebral ischemia) I67.8
- dissociative F44.5
- epileptic (*see also* Epilepsy) G40.9
- epileptiform, epileptoid (*see also* Seizure, epileptiform) R56.8
- ether (anesthetic)
- – correct substance properly administered R56.8
- – overdose or wrong substance given T41.0
- febrile R56.0
- generalized R56.8
- hysterical F44.5
- infantile R56.8
- – epilepsy – *see* Epilepsy
- jacksonian G40.1
- myoclonic G40.3
- neonatal, benign (familial) G40.3
- newborn P90
- obstetrical (nephritic) (uremic) – *see* Eclampsia
- paretic A52.1
- psychomotor G40.2
- reflex R25.8
- tetanus, tetanic (*see also* Tetanus) A35
- uremic N19

Convulsive – *see also* Convulsions
- equivalent, abdominal G40.8
Cooley's anemia D56.1
Cooper's
- disease N60.1
- hernia (*see also* Hernia, abdomen, specified site NEC) K45.8
Copra itch B88.0
Coprolith or coprostasis K56.4
Coprophagy F50.8
Coproporphyria, hereditary E80.2
Cor
- biloculare Q20.8
- bovis, bovinum – *see* Hypertrophy, cardiac
- pulmonale (chronic) I27.9
- – acute I26.0
- triatriatum, triatrium Q24.2
- triloculare Q20.8
- – biatrium Q20.4
- – biventriculare Q21.1
Corbus' disease N48.1
Cord – *see also* condition
- around neck (tightly) (with compression)
- – affecting fetus or newborn P02.5
- – complicating delivery O69.1
- bladder G95.8
- – tabetic A52.1
Cordis ectopia Q24.8
Corditis (spermatic) N49.1
Corectopia Q13.2
Cori's disease (glycogen storage) E74.0
Corkhandler's disease or lung J67.3
Corkscrew esophagus K22.4
Corkworker's disease or lung J67.3
Corlett's pyosis L00
Corn (infected) L84
Cornea – *see also* condition
- guttata H18.4
- plana Q13.4
Cornelia de Lange syndrome Q87.1
Cornu cutaneum L85.8
Cornual gestation or pregnancy O00.8
Coronary (artery) – *see* condition
Coronavirus, as cause of disease classified elsewhere B97.2
Corpora – *see also* condition
- amylacea, prostate N42.8
- cavernosa – *see* condition
Corpulence (*see also* Obesity) E66.9
Corpus – *see* condition
Corrected transposition Q20.5

Corrosion (injury) (acid) (caustic) (chemical) (external) (internal) (lime) T30.4

Note: The following fourth-character subdivisions are for use with categories T20-T25, T29 and T30:

.4 Unspecified degree
.5 First degree [Erythema]
.6 Second degree [Blisters, epidermal loss]
.7 Third degree [Deep necrosis of underlying tissue][Full-thickness skin loss]
- abdomen, abdominal (muscle) (wall) T21.-
- alimentary tract NEC T28.7
- ankle (and foot) T25.-
- – with leg T29.-
- anus T21.-
- arm(s) (upper) (meaning upper limb) T22.-
- – with wrist and hand T29.-
- axilla T22.-
- back T21.-
- blisters – *code as* Corrosion, by site, with fourth character .6
- breast(s) T21.-
- buttock(s) T21.-
- cervix T28.8
- chest wall T21.-
- colon T28.7
- conjunctiva (and cornea) T26.6
- cornea (and conjunctiva) T26.6
- deep necrosis of underlying tissue – *code as* Corrosion, by site, with fourth character .7
- ear (auricle) (canal) (drum) (external) T20.-
- entire body – *see* Corrosion, multiple body regions
- epidermal loss – *code as* Corrosion, by site, with fourth character .6
- epiglottis T27.4
- erythema, erythematous – *code as* Corrosion, by site, with fourth character .5
- esophagus T28.6
- extremity – *see* Corrosion, limb
- eye(s) T26.9
- – with resulting rupture and destruction of eyeball T26.7
- – specified part NEC (*see also* Corrosion, by site) T26.8
- eyeball – *see* Corrosion, eye

Corrosion—*continued*
- eyelid(s) T26.5
- face T20.-
- finger(s) (nail) (subungual) T23.-
- first degree – *code as* Corrosion, by site, with fourth character .5
- flank T21.-
- foot (and ankle) (phalanges) T25.-
- – with leg T29.-
- fourth degree – *code as* Corrosion, by site, with fourth character .7
- full-thickness skin loss – *code as* Corrosion, by site, with fourth character .7
- gastrointestinal tract NEC T28.7
- genitourinary organs
- – external T21.-
- – internal T28.8
- groin T21.-
- hand(s) (phalanges) (and wrist) T23.-
- – with arm T29.-
- head (and face) (and neck) T20.-
- – eye(s) only – *see* Corrosion, eye
- hip T24.-
- inhalation (*see also* Corrosion, by site) T27.7
- internal organs NEC (*see also* Corrosion, by site) T28.9
- interscapular region T21.-
- intestine (large) (small) T28.7
- knee T24.-
- labium (majus) (minus) T21.-
- lacrimal apparatus, duct, gland or sac T26.8
- larynx T27.4
- – with lung T27.5
- leg(s) (lower) (meaning lower limb) T24.-
- – with ankle and foot T29.-
- limb(s)
- – lower (except ankle or foot alone) T24.-
- – – with ankle and foot T29.-
- – – upper (except wrist and hand alone) T22.-
- – – with wrist and hand T29.-
- lip(s) T20.-
- lower back T21.-
- lung (with larynx and trachea) T27.5
- mouth T28.5
- multiple body regions (sites classifiable to more than one category in T20-T28) T29.4
- – first degree (only, without second or third degree) T29.5

158

Corrosion—*continued*
- multiple body regions—*continued*
- - second degree (with first degree) T29.6
- - third degree (with first and second degree) T29.7
- neck T20.-
- nose (septum) T20.-
- ocular adnexa T26.9
- palm(s) T23.-
- partial thickness skin damage – *code as* Corrosion, by site, with fourth character .6
- pelvis T21.-
- penis T21.-
- perineum T21.-
- periocular area T26.5
- pharynx T28.5
- rectum T28.7
- respiratory tract T27.7
- - specified part NEC T27.6
- scalp T20.-
- scapular region T22.-
- sclera T26.8
- scrotum T21.-
- second degree – *code as* Corrosion, by site, with fourth character .6
- shoulder(s) T22.-
- skin NEC T30.4
- stomach T28.7
- temple T20.-
- testis T21.-
- thigh(s) T24.-
- third degree – *code as* Corrosion, by site, with fourth character .7
- thorax (external) T21.-
- throat (meaning pharynx) T28.5
- thumb(s) T23.-
- toe(nail) (subungual) T25.-
- tongue T28.5
- tonsil(s) T28.5
- total body – *see* Corrosion, multiple body regions
- trachea T27.4
- - with lung T27.5
- trunk T21.-
- unspecified site with extent of body surface involved specified
- - less than 10 per cent T32.0
- - 10-19 per cent T32.1
- - 20-29 per cent T32.2
- - 30-39 per cent T32.3
- - 40-49 per cent T32.4
- - 50-59 per cent T32.5
- - 60-69 per cent T32.6
- - 70-79 per cent T32.7

Corrosion—*continued*
- unspecified site with extent of body surface involved specified—*continued*
- - 80-89 per cent T32.8
- - 90 per cent or more T32.9
- uterus T28.8
- vagina T28.8
- vulva T21.-
- wrist(s) (and hand) T23.-
- - with arm T29.-
Corrosive burn – *see* Corrosion
Corsican fever (*see also* Malaria) B54
Cortical – *see condition*
Cortico-adrenal – *see condition*
Coryza (acute) J00
- with grippe or influenza (*see also* Influenza, with, respiratory manifestations) J11.1
Costen's syndrome or complex K07.6
Costiveness (*see also* Constipation) K59.0
Costochondritis M94.0
Cotard's syndrome F22.0
Cot death R95
Cough R05
- with hemorrhage (*see also* Hemoptysis) R04.2
- bronchial R05
- - with grippe or influenza (*see also* Influenza, with, respiratory manifestations) J11.1
- chronic R05
- epidemic R05
- functional F45.3
- hysterical F45.3
- laryngeal, spasmodic R05
- nervous R05
- psychogenic F45.3
- smokers' J41.0
- tea taster's B49
Counseling Z71.9
- alcohol abuse Z71.4
- consanguinity Z71.8
- contraceptive Z30.0
- dietary Z71.3
- drug abuse Z71.5
- for non-attending third party Z71.0
- - related to sexual bahavior or orientation Z70.2
- genetic Z31.5
- health (advice) (education) (instruction) (*see also* Counseling, medical) Z71.9
- human immunodeficiency virus (HIV) Z71.7

Counseling—*continued*
- impotence Z70.1
- medical (for) Z71.9
- - boarding school resident Z59.3
- - condition not demonstrated Z71.1
- - consanguinity Z71.8
- - feared complaint and no disease found Z71.1
- - human immunodeficiency virus (HIV) Z71.7
- - institutional resident Z59.3
- - on behalf of another Z71.0
- - - related to sexual behavior or orientation Z70.2
- - person living alone Z60.2
- - specified reason NEC Z71.8
- procreative Z31.6
- promiscuity Z70.1
- sex, sexual (related to) Z70.9
- - attitude(s) Z70.0
- - behavior or orientation Z70.1
- - combined concerns Z70.3
- - non-responsiveness Z70.1
- - on behalf of third party Z70.2
- - specified reason NEC Z70.8
- specified reason NEC Z71.8
- substance abuse Z71.8
- - alcohol Z71.4
- - drug Z71.5
- - tobacco Z71.6
- tobacco use Z71.6
Coupled rhythm R00.8
Couvelaire syndrome or uterus (complicating delivery) (*see also* Abruptio placentae) O45.8
Cowperitis (*see also* Urethritis) N34.2
Cowper's gland – *see condition*
Cowpox B08.0
- eyelid B08.0† H03.1*
Coxa
- plana M91.2
- valga (acquired) M21.0
- - congenital Q65.8
- - late effect of rickets E64.3
- vara (acquired) M21.1
- - congenital Q65.8
- - late effect of rickets E64.3
Coxalgia, coxalgic (nontuberculous) M25.5
- tuberculous A18.0† M01.1*
Coxarthrosis M16.9
- dysplastic (unilateral) M16.3
- - bilateral M16.2
- post-traumatic (unilateral) M16.5

Coxarthrosis—*continued*
- post-traumatic—*continued*
- - bilateral M16.4
- primary (unilateral) M16.1
- - bilateral M16.0
- secondary NEC (unilateral) M16.7
- - bilateral M16.6
Coxitis M13.1
Coxsackievirus NEC (infection) B34.1
- as cause of disease classified elsewhere B97.1
- carditis B33.2† I43.0*
- central nervous system NEC A88.8
- endocarditis B33.2† I39.8*
- enteritis A08.3
- meningitis (aseptic) A87.0† G02.0*
- myocarditis B33.2† I41.1*
- pericarditis B33.2† I32.1*
- pharyngitis B08.5
- pleurodynia B33.0
- specific disease NEC B33.8
- unspecified nature or site B34.1
Crabs, meaning pubic lice B85.3
Cracked nipple N64.0
- puerperal, postpartum, gestational O92.1
Cradle cap L21.0
Craft neurosis F48.8
Cramp(s) R25.2
- abdominal R10.4
- bathing T75.1
- colic R10.4
- - psychogenic F45.3
- fireman T67.2
- heat T67.2
- immersion T75.1
- intestinal R10.4
- - psychogenic F45.3
- limb (lower) (upper) NEC R25.2
- linotypist's F48.8
- - organic G25.8
- muscle (general) (limb) R25.2
- - due to immersion T75.1
- - psychogenic F45.8
- occupational (hand) F48.8
- - organic G25.8
- salt-depletion E87.1
- stoker's T67.2
- swimmer's T75.1
- telegrapher's F48.8
- - organic G25.8
- typist's F48.8
- - organic G25.8
- uterus N94.8

Cramp(s)—*continued*
- uterus—*continued*
- - - menstrual (*see also* Dysmenorrhea) N94.6
- writer's F48.8
- - organic G25.8
Cranial – *see condition*
Cranioclasis, fetus P03.8
Craniocleidodysostosis Q74.0
Craniofenestria (skull) Q75.8
Craniolacunia (skull) Q75.8
Craniopagus Q89.4
Craniopharyngeal – *see condition*
Craniopharyngioma (M9350/1) D44.4
Craniorachischisis (totalis) Q00.1
Cranioschisis Q75.8
Craniostenosis Q75.0
Craniosynostosis Q75.0
Craniotabes (cause unknown) M83.8
- neonatal P96.3
- rachitic E64.3
- syphilitic A50.5
Craniotomy, fetus P03.8
- to facilitate delivery O83.4
Cranium – *see condition*
Craw-craw B73
Creaking joint M24.8
- knee M23.8
Creeping palsy or paralysis G12.2
Crenated tongue K14.8
Crepitus
- caput Q75.8
- joint M24.8
- - knee M23.8
Crescent or conus choroid, congenital Q14.3
CREST syndrome M34.1
Cretin, cretinism (congenital) (endemic) (nongoitrous) (sporadic) E00.9
- pelvis, with disproportion (fetopelvic) O33.0
- - affecting fetus or newborn P03.1
- - causing obstructed labor O65.0
- type
- - hypothyroid E00.1
- - mixed E00.2
- - myxedematous E00.1
- - neurological E00.0
Creutzfeldt-Jakob disease or syndrome A81.0
- with dementia A81.0† F02.1*
Crib death R95
Cribriform hymen Q52.3
Cri-du-chat syndrome Q93.4

Crigler-Najjar disease or syndrome E80.5
Crime, victim of Z65.4
Criminalism F60.2
Crisis
- abdomen R10.4
- acute reaction F43.0
- addisonian E27.2
- adrenal (cortical) E27.2
- emotional F43.2
- - acute reaction to stress F43.0
- - adjustment reaction F43.2
- - specific to childhood and adolescence F93.8
- glaucomatocyclitic H40.4
- nitritoid
- - correct substance properly administered I95.2
- - overdose or wrong substance given or taken T37.8
- oculogyric H51.8
- - psychogenic F45.8
- Pel's (tabetic) A52.1
- renal N28.8
- sickle-cell D57.0
- state (acute reaction) F43.0
- tabetic A52.1
- thyroid E05.5
- thyrotoxic E05.5
Crohn's disease K50.9
- large intestine (colon or rectum) K50.1
- - with small intestine K50.8
- small intestine (duodenum, ileum or jejunum) K50.0
- - with large intestine K50.8
Crooked septum, nasal J34.2
Cross syndrome E70.3
Crossbite (anterior) (posterior) K07.2
Cross-eye H50.0
Croup, croupous (catarrhal) (infectious) (inflammatory) (nondiphtheritic) J05.0
- bronchial J20.9
- diphtheritic A36.2
- false J38.5
- spasmodic J38.5
- - diphtheritic A36.2
- stridulous J38.5
- - diphtheritic A36.2
Crouzon's disease Q75.1
Crowding, tooth, teeth K07.3
CRST syndrome M34.1
Cruchet's disease A85.8
Cruelty in children (*see also* Disorder, conduct) F91.8

Crush, crushed, crushing T14.7
- abdomen S38.1
- ankle S97.0
- - with foot, toe(s) S97.8
- arm
- - meaning upper limb T04.2
- - upper (and shoulder) S47
- axilla S47
- back, lower S38.1
- buttock S38.1
- cheek S07.0
- chest S28.0
- cranium S07.1
- ear S07.0
- elbow S57.0
- face S07.0
- finger(s) (and thumb) S67.0
- - with hand (and wrist) S67.8
- foot S97.8
- - with ankle, toe(s) S97.8
- forearm S57.9
- - specified NEC S57.8
- genitalia, external (female) (male) S38.0
- hand (except fingers alone) S67.8
- head S07.9
- - specified NEC S07.8
- heel S97.8
- hip S77.0
- - with thigh S77.2
- internal organ (abdomen, chest, or pelvis) T14.7
- knee S87.0
- labium (majus) (minus) S38.0
- larynx S17.0
- leg
- - lower S87.8
- - meaning lower limb T04.3
- limb
- - lower T04.3
- - upper T04.2
- lip S07.0
- lower
- - back S38.1
- - limb T04.3
- multiple T04.9
- - body regions NEC T04.8
- - head S07.-
- - - with
- - - - neck T04.0
- - - - other body regions NEC T04.8
- - limb
- - - lower T04.3

Crush, crushed—*continued*
- multiple—*continued*
- - limb—*continued*
- - - lower—*continued*
- - - - with
- - - - - thorax, abdomen, lower back and pelvis T04.7
- - - - - upper limb(s) T04.4
- - - upper T04.2
- - - - with
- - - - - lower limb(s) T04.4
- - - - - thorax, abdomen, lower back and pelvis T04.7
- - neck S17.-
- - - with
- - - - head T04.0
- - - - other body regions T04.8
- - specified sites NEC T04.8
- - thorax S28.0
- - - with
- - - - abdomen, lower back and pelvis T04.1
- - - - - and limb(s) T04.7
- - - - other body regions T04.8
- - trunk T04.1
- - - with
- - - - limb(s) T04.7
- - - - other body regions T04.8
- - upper limb T04.2
- neck S17.9
- - with
- - - head T04.0
- - - other body regions T04.8
- nerve – *see* Injury, nerve
- nose S07.0
- pelvis S38.1
- penis S38.0
- scalp S07.8
- scapular region S47
- scrotum S38.0
- severe, unspecified site T14.7
- shoulder (and upper arm) S47
- skull S07.1
- syndrome (complication of trauma) T79.5
- testis S38.0
- thigh S77.1
- - with hip S77.2
- throat S17.8
- thumb (and finger(s)) S67.0
- - with hand (and wrist) S67.8
- toe(s) S97.1
- - with foot (and ankle) S97.8
- trachea S17.0
- trunk (multiple sites) T04.1

Crush, crushed—*continued*
- trunk—*continued*
- − − with
- − − − limb(s) T04.7
- − − − other body regions T04.8
- − vulva S38.0
- − wrist (and hand) S67.8
Crusta lactea L21.0
Cruveilhier-Baumgarten cirrhosis, disease or syndrome K74.6
Cruveilhier's atrophy or disease G12.8
Cryoglobulinemia, cryoglobulinemic (essential) (idiopathic) (mixed) (primary) (purpura) (secondary) (vasculitis) D89.1
- with lung involvement D89.1† J99.8∗
Cryptitis (anal) (rectal) K62.8
Cryptococcosis, Cryptococcus (infection) (neoformans) B45.9
- bone B45.3† M90.2∗
- cerebral B45.1† G05.2∗
- cutaneous B45.2† L99.8∗
- disseminated B45.7
- generalized B45.7
- meningitis B45.1† G02.1∗
- meningocerebralis B45.1† G02.1∗
- osseous B45.3† M90.2∗
- pulmonary B45.0† J99.8∗
- skin B45.2† L99.8∗
- specified NEC B45.8
Cryptopapillitis (anus) K62.8
Cryptophthalmos Q11.2
- syndrome Q87.0
Cryptorchid, cryptorchism, cryptorchidism Q53.9
- bilateral Q53.2
- unilateral Q53.1
Cryptosporidiosis A07.2
- resulting from HIV disease B20.8
Cryptostromosis J67.6
Crystalluria R82.9
Cubitus
- valgus (acquired) M21.0
- − congenital Q68.8
- − late effect of rickets E64.3
- varus (acquired) M21.1
- − congenital Q68.8
- − late effect of rickets E64.3
Cultural deprivation or shock Z60.3
Curling's ulcer (*see also* Ulcer, peptic, acute) K27.3
Curse, Ondine's G47.3

Curvature
- organ or site, congenital NEC – *see* Distortion
- penis (lateral) Q55.6
- Pott's (spinal) A18.0† M49.0∗
- radius, idiopathic, progressive (congenital) Q74.0
- spine (acquired) (angular) (idiopathic) (incorrect) (postural) M43.9
- − congenital Q67.5
- − due to or associated with
- − − Charcot-Marie-Tooth disease G60.0† M49.4∗
- − − osteitis
- − − − deformans M88.8
- − − − fibrosa cystica E21.0† M49.8∗
- − − tuberculosis (Pott's curvature) A18.0† M49.0∗
- − late effect of rickets E64.3
- − tuberculous A18.0† M49.0∗
Cushingoid due to steroid therapy
- correct substance properly administered E24.2
- overdose or wrong substance given or taken T38.0
Cushing's
- syndrome or disease E24.9
- − drug-induced E24.2
- − iatrogenic E24.2
- − pituitary-dependent E24.0
- − specified NEC E24.8
- ulcer (*see also* Ulcer, peptic, acute) K27.3
Cusp, Carabelli – *see condition*
Cut (external) – *see also* Wound, open
- muscle – *see* Injury, muscle
Cutis – *see also condition*
- hyperelastica Q82.8
- − acquired L57.4
- laxa (hyperelastica) (*see also* Dermatolysis) Q82.8
- − senilis L57.4
- marmorata R23.8
- osteosis L94.2
- pendula – *see* Dermatolysis
- rhomboidalis nuchae L57.2
- verticis gyrata Q82.8
- − acquired L91.8
Cyanosis R23.0
- conjunctiva H11.4
- enterogenous D74.8
- paroxysmal digital I73.0
- retina, retinal H35.8
Cyanotic heart disease I24.9
- congenital Q24.9

163

Cycle
- anovulatory N97.0
- menstrual, irregular N92.6

Cyclencephaly Q04.9

Cyclical vomiting R11
- psychogenic F50.5

Cyclitis (*see also* Iridocyclitis) H20.9
- Fuchs' heterochromic H20.8
- posterior H30.2

Cycloid personality F34.0

Cyclophoria H50.5

Cyclopia, cyclops Q87.0

Cyclopism Q87.0

Cycloplegia H52.5

Cyclospasm H52.5

Cyclothymia F34.0

Cyclothymic personality F34.0

Cyclotropia H50.4

Cylindroma (M8200/3) – *see also*
Neoplasm, malignant
- eccrine dermal (M8200/0) – *see*
Neoplasm, skin, benign
- skin (M8200/0) – *see* Neoplasm, skin,
benign

Cylindruria R82.9

Cyphosis – *see* Kyphosis

Cyst (colloid) (mucous) (retention)
(simple)

Note: In general, cysts are not neoplastic and
are classified either as specific entities or to
the appropriate category for disease of the
specified anatomical site. This generalization
does not apply to certain types of cysts
which are neoplastic in nature, for example
dermoid, or to cysts of certain structures, for
example branchial cleft, which are classified
as developmental anomalies.

The following listing includes some of the
most frequently reported sites of cysts as
well as qualifiers that indicate the type of
cyst. The qualifiers are not usually repeated
under the anatomical sites. Since the code
assignment for a given site may vary
depending on the type of cyst, the coder
should refer to the listings under the
specified type of cyst before considering the
site.

- adenoid (infected) J35.8
- adrenal gland E27.8
- - congenital Q89.1
- air, lung J98.4
- amnion, amniotic O41.8

Cyst—*continued*
- anterior chamber (eye) (exudative)
(implantation) (parasitic) H21.3
- antrum J34.1
- anus K62.8
- apical (tooth) (periodontal) K04.8
- appendix K38.8
- arachnoid, brain (acquired) G93.0
- - congenital Q04.6
- arytenoid J38.7
- Baker's M71.2
- - ruptured M66.0
- - tuberculous A18.0† M01.1*
- Bartholin's gland N75.0
- bile duct (common) (hepatic) K83.5
- bladder (multiple) (trigone) N32.8
- blue dome (breast) N60.0
- bone (local) NEC M85.6
- - aneurysmal M85.5
- - jaw K09.2
- - - developmental (nonodontogenic)
K09.1
- - - - odontogenic K09.0
- - - latent K10.0
- - solitary M85.4
- brain (acquired) G93.0
- - congenital Q04.6
- - hydatid (*see also* Echinococcus)
B67.9† G94.8*
- - third ventricle (colloid), congenital
Q04.6
- branchial (cleft) Q18.0
- branchiogenic Q18.0
- breast (benign) (blue dome)
(pedunculated) N60.0
- - involution N60.8
- - sebaceous N60.8
- broad ligament (benign) N83.8
- bronchogenic (mediastinal)
(sequestration) J98.4
- - congenital Q33.0
- buccal K09.8
- bulbourethral gland N36.8
- bursa, bursal NEC M71.3
- - pharyngeal J39.2
- calcifying odontogenic (M9301/0) D16.5
- - upper jaw (bone) D16.4
- canal of Nuck (female) N94.8
- - congenital Q52.4
- canthus H11.4
- carcinomatous (M8010/3) – *see*
Neoplasm, malignant
- cauda equina G95.8
- cavum septi pellucidi – *see* Cyst, brain

Cyst—*continued*
- celomic (pericardium) Q24.8
- cerebellopontine (angle) – *see* Cyst, brain
- cerebellum – *see* Cyst, brain
- cerebral – *see* Cyst, brain
- cervical lateral Q18.1
- cervix NEC N88.8
- – embryonic Q51.6
- – nabothian N88.8
- chiasmal optic NEC H47.4
- chocolate (ovary) N80.1
- choledochus, congenital Q44.4
- chorion O41.8
- choroid plexus G93.0
- ciliary body (exudative) (implantation) (parasitic) H21.3
- clitoris N90.7
- colon K63.8
- common (bile) duct K83.5
- congenital NEC Q89.8
- – epiglottis Q31.8
- – esophagus Q39.8
- – fallopian tube Q50.4
- – kidney Q61.0
- – – multicystic Q61.4
- – – polycystic Q61.3
- – larynx Q31.8
- – liver Q44.7
- – mediastinum Q34.1
- – ovary Q50.1
- – oviduct Q50.4
- – periurethral (tissue) Q64.7
- – prepuce Q55.6
- – salivary gland (any) Q38.4
- – thymus (gland) Q89.2
- – tongue Q38.3
- – ureterovesical orifice Q62.8
- – vulva Q52.7
- conjunctiva H11.4
- cornea H18.8
- corpora quadrigemina G93.0
- corpus
- – albicans N83.2
- – luteum (hemorrhagic) (ruptured) N83.1
- Cowper's gland (benign) (infected) N36.8
- cranial meninges G93.0
- craniobuccal pouch E23.6
- craniopharyngeal pouch E23.6
- cystic duct K82.8
- cysticercus (*see also* Cysticercosis) B69.9
- Dandy-Walker Q03.1
- dental (root) K04.8
- – eruption K09.0
- – primordial K09.0

Cyst—*continued*
- dentigerous (mandible) (maxilla) K09.0
- dermoid (M9084/0) – *see also* Neoplasm, benign
- – with malignant transformation (M9084/3) C56
- – implantation
- – – external area or site (skin) NEC L72.0
- – – iris H21.3
- – – vagina N89.8
- – – vulva N90.7
- – mouth K09.8
- – oral soft tissue K09.8
- developmental K09.1
- – odontogenic (glandular) K09.0
- – oral region (nonodontogenic) K09.1
- – ovary, ovarian Q50.1
- dura (cerebral) G93.0
- – spinal G96.1
- ear (external) Q18.1
- echinococcal (*see also* Echinococcus) B67.9
- embryonic, fallopian tube Q50.4
- endometrium, endometrial (uterus) N85.8
- – ectopic (*see also* Endometriosis) N80.9
- enterogenous Q43.8
- epidermal, epidermoid (inclusion) (*see also* Cyst, skin) L72.0
- – mouth K09.8
- – oral soft tissue K09.8
- epididymis N50.8
- epiglottis J38.7
- epiphysis cerebri E34.8
- epithelial (inclusion) L72.0
- epoophoron Q50.5
- eruption K09.0
- esophagus K22.8
- ethmoid sinus J34.1
- external female genital organs NEC N90.7
- eye NEC H57.8
- – congenital Q15.8
- eyelid (sebaceous) H02.8
- – infected H00.0
- fallopian tube N83.8
- fimbrial (twisted) Q50.4
- follicle (graafian) (hemorrhagic) N83.0
- – nabothian N88.8
- follicular (atretic) (hemorrhagic) (ovarian) N83.0
- – odontogenic K09.0
- – skin L72.9
- – – specified NEC L72.8

Cyst—*continued*
- frontal sinus J34.1
- gallbladder K82.8
- ganglion M67.4
- Gartner's duct Q50.5
- gingiva K09.0
- gland of Moll H02.8
- globulomaxillary K09.1
- graafian follicle (hemorrhagic) N83.0
- granulosal lutein (hemorrhagic) N83.1
- hemangiomatous (M9120/0) D18.0
- hydatid (*see also* Echinococcus) B67.9
- - liver (*see also* Cyst, liver, hydatid) B67.8† K77.0∗
- - lung NEC B67.9† J99.8∗
- - Morgagni
- - - female Q50.5
- - - male (epididymal) Q55.4
- - - - testicular Q55.2
- - specified site NEC B67.9
- hymen N89.8
- - embryonic Q52.4
- hypopharynx J39.2
- hypophysis, hypophyseal (duct) (recurrent) E23.6
- - cerebri E23.6
- implantation (dermoid)
- - external area or site (skin) NEC L72.0
- - iris H21.3
- - vagina N89.8
- - vulva N90.7
- incisive canal K09.1
- inclusion (epidermal) (epidermoid) (epithelial) (squamous) L72.0
- - not of skin – *see* Cyst, by site
- intestine (large) (small) K63.8
- intracranial – *see* Cyst, brain
- intraligamentous M24.2
- - knee M23.8
- intrasellar E23.6
- iris (exudative) (implantation) (parasitic) H21.3
- jaw (bone) (aneurysmal) (hemorrhagic) (traumatic) K09.2
- - developmental (glandular) (odontogenic) K09.0
- joint NEC M25.8
- kidney (acquired) N28.1
- - congenital Q61.0
- - calyceal (*see also* Hydronephrosis) N13.3
- - multicystic (developmental) Q61.4
- - - acquired N28.1
- - multiple Q61.3

Cyst—*continued*
- kidney—*continued*
- - multiple—*continued*
- - - autosomal dominant (adult type) Q61.2
- - - autosomal recessive (infantile type) Q61.1
- - polycystic Q61.3
- - autosomal dominant (adult type) Q61.2
- - - autosomal recessive (infantile type) Q61.1
- - pyelogenic (*see also* Hydronephrosis) N13.3
- labium (majus) (minus) N90.7
- - sebaceous N90.7
- lacrimal H04.8
- - gland H04.1
- - passages or sac H04.6
- larynx J38.7
- lateral periodontal K09.0
- lens H27.8
- - congenital Q12.8
- lip (gland) K13.0
- liver (idiopathic) K76.8
- - congenital Q44.7
- - hydatid B67.8† K77.0∗
- - - granulosus B67.0† K77.0∗
- - - multilocularis B67.5† K77.0∗
- lung J98.4
- - congenital Q33.0
- - giant bullous J43.9
- lutein N83.1
- lymphangiomatous (M9173/0) D18.1
- lymphoepithelial, oral soft tissue K09.8
- macula H35.3
- malignant (M8000/3) – *see* Neoplasm, malignant
- mammary gland – *see* Cyst, breast
- mandible K09.2
- - dentigerous K09.0
- maxilla K09.2
- - dentigerous K09.0
- - radicular K04.8
- medial, face and neck Q18.8
- median
- - anterior maxillary K09.1
- - palatal K09.1
- mediastinum, congenital Q34.1
- meibomian (gland) H00.1
- - infected H00.0
- membrane, brain G93.0
- meninges (cerebral) G93.0
- - spinal G96.1

Cyst—*continued*
- meniscus, knee M23.0
- mesentery, mesenteric K66.8
- – chyle I89.8
- mesonephric duct
- – female Q50.5
- – male Q55.4
- milk N64.8
- Morgagni (hydatid)
- – female Q50.5
- – male (epididymal) Q55.4
- – – testicular Q55.2
- mouth K09.8
- muellerian duct Q50.4
- multilocular (ovary) (M8000/1) D39.1
- – benign (M8000/0) – *see* Neoplasm, benign
- myometrium N85.8
- nabothian (follicle) (ruptured) N88.8
- nasoalveolar K09.8
- nasolabial K09.8
- nasopalatine (duct) K09.1
- nasopharynx J39.2
- neoplastic (M8000/1) – *see also* Neoplasm, uncertain behavior
- – benign (M8000/0) – *see* Neoplasm, benign
- nervous system NEC G96.8
- neuroenteric (congenital) Q06.8
- nipple N60.0
- nose (turbinates) J34.1
- – sinus J34.1
- odontogenic, developmental (glandular) K09.0
- omentum (lesser) K66.8
- – congenital Q45.8
- ora serrata H33.1
- oral
- – region K09.9
- – – developmental (nonodontogenic) K09.1
- – – specified NEC K09.8
- – soft tissue K09.9
- – – specified NEC K09.8
- orbit H05.8
- ovary, ovarian (twisted) NEC N83.2
- – adherent N83.2
- – chocolate N80.1
- – corpus
- – – albicans N83.2
- – – luteum (hemorrhagic) N83.1
- – dermoid (M9084/0) D27
- – developmental Q50.1
- – due to failure or involution NEC N83.2

Cyst—*continued*
- ovary, ovarian—*continued*
- – follicular (graafian) (hemorrhagic) N83.0
- – hemorrhagic N83.2
- – in pregnancy or childbirth O34.8
- – – with obstructed labor O65.5
- – multilocular (M8000/1) D39.1
- – pseudomucinous (M8470/0) D27
- – retention N83.2
- – serous N83.2
- – theca lutein (hemorrhagic) N83.1
- – tuberculous A18.1† N74.1*
- oviduct N83.8
- palate (fissural) (median) K09.1
- palatine papilla (jaw) K09.1
- pancreas, pancreatic (hemorrhagic) (true) K86.2
- – congenital Q45.2
- – false K86.3
- paramesonephric duct
- – female Q50.4
- – male Q55.2
- paraphysis, cerebri, congenital Q04.6
- parasitic B89
- parathyroid (gland) E21.4
- paratubal N83.8
- paraurethral duct N36.8
- paroophoron Q50.5
- parotid gland K11.6
- parovarian Q50.5
- pelvis, female N94.8
- – in pregnancy or childbirth O34.8
- – – causing obstructed labor O65.5
- penis (sebaceous) N48.8
- periapical K04.8
- pericardial, congenital Q24.8
- periodontal K04.8
- – lateral K09.0
- peritoneum K66.8
- – chylous I89.8
- periventricular, acquired, newborn P91.1
- pharynx (wall) J39.2
- pilar L72.1
- pilonidal (infected) (rectum) L05.9
- – with abscess L05.0
- – malignant (M9084/3) C44.5
- pituitary (duct) (gland) E23.6
- placenta (amniotic) O43.1
- pleura J94.8
- popliteal M71.2
- – ruptured M66.0
- porencephalic Q04.6
- – acquired G93.0

Cyst—*continued*
- postmastoidectomy cavity (mucosal) H95.1
- preauricular Q18.1
- prepuce N48.8
- – congenital Q55.6
- pretragal Q18.1
- primordial (jaw) K09.0
- prostate N42.8
- pseudomucinous (ovary) (M8470/0) D27
- pupillary, miotic H21.2
- radicular (residual) K04.8
- Rathke's pouch E23.6
- rectum (epithelium) (mucous) K62.8
- renal (acquired) N28.1
- – congenital Q61.0
- – – multicystic Q61.4
- – – polycystic Q61.3
- residual (radicular) K04.8
- retina (parasitic) H33.1
- retroperitoneal K66.8
- salivary gland or duct (mucous extravasation or retention) K11.6
- Sampson's N80.1
- sclera H15.8
- scrotum L72.9
- – sebaceous L72.1
- sebaceous (duct) (gland) L72.1
- – breast N60.8
- – eyelid H02.8
    genital organ NEC
- – – female N94.8
- – – male N50.8
- – scrotum L72.1
- semilunar cartilage (knee) (multiple) M23.0
- seminal vesicle N50.8
- sinus (accessory) (nasal) J34.1
- Skene's gland N36.8
- skin L72.9
- – breast N60.8
- – epidermal, epidermoid L72.0
- – epithelial L72.0
- – eyelid H02.8
- – inclusion L72.0
- – genital organ NEC
- – – female N90.7
- – – male N50.8
- – scrotum L72.9
- – sebaceous L72.1
- – sweat gland or duct L74.8
- solitary
- – bone M85.4
- – jaw K09.2

Cyst—*continued*
- spermatic cord N50.8
- sphenoid sinus J34.1
- spinal meninges G96.1
- spleen NEC D73.4
- – hydatid (*see also* Echinococcus) B67.9† D77*
- Stafne's K10.0
- subcutaneous, pheomycotic (chromomycotic) B43.2† I99.8*
- subdural (cerebral) G93.0
- – spinal cord G96.1
- sublingual gland K11.6
- submandibular gland K11.6
- suburethral N36.8
- suprarenal gland E27.8
- suprasellar – *see* Cyst, brain
- sweat gland or duct L74.8
- synovial M71.3
- – ruptured M66.1
- tarsal H00.1
- tendon (sheath) M67.8
- testis N50.8
- Thornwaldt's J39.2
- thymus (gland) E32.8
- thyroglossal duct (infected) (persistent) Q89.2
- thyroid (gland) E04.1
- tongue K14.8
- tonsil J35.8
- tooth – *see* Cyst, dental
- Tornwaldt's J39.2
- trichilemmal L72.1
- trichodermal L72.1
- tubal (fallopian) N83.8
- – inflammatory N70.1
- tunica vaginalis N50.8
- turbinate (nose) J34.1
- Tyson's gland N48.8
- urachus, congenital Q64.4
- ureter N28.8
- ureterovesical orifice N28.8
- urethra, urethral (gland) N36.8
- uterine ligament N83.8
- uterus (body) (corpus) (recurrent) N85.8
- – embryonic Q51.8
- – – cervix Q51.6
- vagina, vaginal (implantation) (inclusion) (squamous cell) (wall) N89.8
- – embryonic Q52.4
- vallecula, vallecular (epiglottis) J38.7
- vesical (orifice) N32.8
- vitreous body H43.8
- vulva (implantation) (inclusion) N90.7

Cyst—*continued*
- vulva—*continued*
- – congenital Q52.7
- – sebaceous gland N90.7
- vulvovaginal gland N90.7
- wolffian
- – female Q50.5
- – male Q55.4

Cystadenocarcinoma (M8440/3) – *see also* Neoplasm, malignant
- bile duct (M8161/3) C22.1
- endometrioid (M8380/3) – *see* Neoplasm, malignant
- – specified site – *see* Neoplasm, malignant
- – unspecified site
- – – female C56
- – – male C61
- mucinous (M8470/3)
- – papillary (M8471/3)
- – – specified site – *see* Neoplasm, malignant
- – – unspecified site C56
- – specified site – *see* Neoplasm, malignant
- – unspecified site C56
- papillary (M8450/3)
- – mucinous (M8471/3)
- – – specified site – *see* Neoplasm, malignant
- – – unspecified site C56
- – pseudomucinous (M8471/3)
- – – specified site – *see* Neoplasm, malignant
- – – unspecified site C56
- – serous (M8460/3)
- – – specified site – *see* Neoplasm, malignant
- – – unspecified site C56
- – specified site – *see* Neoplasm, malignant
- – unspecified site C56
- pseudomucinous (M8470/3)
- – papillary (M8471/3)
- – – specified site – *see* Neoplasm, malignant
- – – unspecified site C56
- – specified site – *see* Neoplasm, malignant
- – unspecified site C56
- serous (M8441/3)
- – papillary (M8460/3)
- – – specified site – *see* Neoplasm, malignant

Cystadenocarcinoma—*continued*
- serous—*continued*
- – papillary—*continued*
- – – unspecified site C56
- – specified site – *see* Neoplasm, malignant
- – unspecified site C56

Cystadenofibroma (M9013/0)
- clear cell (M8313/0) – *see* Neoplasm, benign
- endometrioid (M8381/0) D27
- – borderline malignancy (M8381/1) D39.1
- – malignant (M8381/3) C56
- mucinous (M9015/0)
- – specified site – *see* Neoplasm, benign
- – unspecified site D27
- serous (M9014/0)
- – specified site – *see* Neoplasm, benign
- – unspecified site D27
- specified site – *see* Neoplasm, benign
- unspecified site D27

Cystadenoma (M8440/0) – *see also* Neoplasm, benign
- bile duct (M8161/0) D13.4
- endometrioid (M8380/0) – *see also* Neoplasm, benign
- – borderline malignancy (M8380/1) – *see* Neoplasm, uncertain behavior
- malignant (M8440/3) – *see* Neoplasm, malignant
- mucinous (M8470/0)
- – borderline malignancy (M8472/1)
- – – ovary (M8472/3) C56
- – – specified site NEC – *see* Neoplasm, uncertain behavior
- – – unspecified site C56
- – papillary (M8471/0)
- – – borderline malignancy (M8473/1)
- – – – ovary (M8473/3) C56
- – – – specified site NEC – *see* Neoplasm, uncertain behavior
- – – – unspecified site C56
- – – specified site – *see* Neoplasm, benign
- – – unspecified site D27
- – specified site – *see* Neoplasm, benign
- – unspecified site D27
- papillary (M8450/0)
- – borderline malignancy (M8451/1)
- – – ovary (M8451/3) C56
- – – specified site NEC – *see* Neoplasm, uncertain behavior
- – – unspecified site C56
- – lymphomatosum (M8561/0)

Cystadenoma—*continued*
- papillary—*continued*
- - lymphomatosum—*continued*
- - - specified site – *see* Neoplasm, benign
- - - unspecified site D11.9
- - mucinous (M8471/0)
- - - borderline malignancy (M8473/1)
- - - - ovary (M8473/3) C56
- - - - specified site NEC – *see*
        Neoplasm, uncertain behavior
- - - - unspecified site C56
- - - specified site – *see* Neoplasm, benign
- - - unspecified site D27
- - pseudomucinous (M8471/0)
- - - borderline malignancy (M8473/1)
- - - - ovary (M8473/3) C56
- - - - specified site NEC – *see*
        Neoplasm, uncertain behavior
- - - - unspecified site C56
- - - specified site – *see* Neoplasm, benign
- - - unspecified site D27
- - serous (M8460/0)
- - - borderline malignancy (M8462/1)
- - - - ovary (M8462/3) C56
- - - - specified site NEC – *see*
        Neoplasm, uncertain behavior
- - - - unspecified site C56
- - - specified site – *see* Neoplasm, benign
- - - unspecified site D27
- - specified site – *see* Neoplasm, benign
- - unspecified site D27
- pseudomucinous (M8470/0)
- - borderline malignancy (M8472/1)
- - - ovary (M8472/3) C56
- - - specified site NEC – *see* Neoplasm,
      uncertain behavior
- - - unspecified site C56
- - papillary (M8471/0)
- - - borderline malignancy (M8473/1)
- - - - ovary (M8473/3) C56
- - - - specified site NEC – *see*
        Neoplasm, uncertain behavior
- - - - unspecified site C56
- - - specified site – *see* Neoplasm, benign
- - - unspecified site D27
- - specified site – *see* Neoplasm, benign
- - unspecified site D27
- serous (M8441/0)
- - borderline malignancy (M8442/1)
- - - ovary (M8442/3) C56
- - - specified site NEC – *see* Neoplasm,
      uncertain behavior
- - - unspecified site C56
- - papillary (M8460/0)

Cystadenoma—*continued*
- serous—*continued*
- - papillary—*continued*
- - - borderline malignancy (M8462/1)
- - - - ovary (M8462/3) C56
- - - - specified site NEC – *see*
        Neoplasm, uncertain behavior
- - - - unspecified site C56
- - - specified site – *see* Neoplasm, benign
- - - unspecified site D27
- - specified site – *see* Neoplasm, benign
- - unspecified site D27
Cystathioninemia E72.1
Cystathioninuria E72.1
Cystic – *see also* condition
- breast (chronic) N60.1
- - with epithelial proliferation N60.3
- corpus luteum (hemorrhagic) N83.1
- duct – *see condition*
- eyeball (congenital) Q11.0
- fibrosis (*see also* Fibrosis, cystic) E84.9
- kidney Q61.9
- - medullary Q61.5
- liver, congenital Q44.6
- lung disease J98.4
- - congenital Q33.0
- medullary, kidney Q61.5
- meniscus M23.0
- ovary N83.2
Cysticercosis, cysticerciasis B69.9
- with epileptiform fits B69.0† G94.8∗
- brain B69.0† G94.8∗
- central nervous system B69.0† G99.8∗
- cerebral B69.0† G94.8∗
- ocular B69.1† H45.1∗
- specified NEC B69.8
Cysticercus cellulose infestation – *see*
  Cysticercosis
Cystinosis (malignant) E72.0
Cystinuria E72.0
**Cystitis (exudative) (hemorrhagic) (septic)
  (suppurative)** N30.9
- with prostatitis N41.3
- acute N30.0
- allergic N30.8
- amebic A06.8
- blennorrhagic (gonococcal) A54.0
- bullous N30.8
- calculous N21.0
- chlamydial A56.0
- chronic N30.2
- - interstitial N30.1
- - specified NEC N30.2
- complicating pregnancy O23.1

Cystitis—*continued*
- complicating pregnancy—*continued*
- - affecting fetus or newborn P00.1
- cystic(a) N30.8
- diphtheritic A36.8† N33.8*
- encysted N30.8
- eosinophilic N30.8
- gangrenous N30.8
- gonococcal A54.0
- interstitial (chronic) N30.1
- irradiation N30.4
- puerperal, postpartum O86.2
- specified NEC N30.8
- subacute N30.2
- submucous N30.1
- syphilitic (late) A52.7† N33.8*
- trichomonal A59.0† N33.8*
- tuberculous A18.1† N33.0*
Cystocele(-urethrocele)
- female N81.1
- - with prolapse of uterus – *see* Prolapse, uterus
- in pregnancy or childbirth O34.8
- - affecting fetus or newborn P03.8
- - causing obstructed labor O65.5
- - - affecting fetus or newborn P03.1
- male N32.8
Cystolithiasis N21.0

Cystoma (M8440/0) – *see also* Neoplasm, benign
- mucinous (M8470/0)
- - specified site – *see* Neoplasm, benign
- - unspecified site D27
- serous (M8441/0)
- - specified site – *see* Neoplasm, benign
- - unspecified site D27
Cystoplegia N31.2
Cystoptosis N32.8
Cystopyelitis (*see also* Pyelonephritis) N12
- with calculus (impacted) (recurrent) N20.9
Cystorrhagia N32.8
Cystosarcoma phyllodes (M9020/1) D48.6
- benign (M9020/0) D24
- malignant (M9020/3) – *see* Neoplasm, breast, malignant
Cystostomy
- attention to Z43.5
- status Z93.5
Cystourethritis (*see also* Urethritis) N34.2
Cystourethrocele (*see also* Cystocele)
- female N81.1
- male N32.8
Cytomegalovirus infection B25.9
- maternal, (suspected) damage to fetus affecting management of pregnancy O35.3
Cytomycosis (reticuloendothelial) B39.4

D

Da Costa's syndrome F45.3
Dabney's grip B33.0
Dacryoadenitis, dacryadenitis (acute)
  (chronic) H04.0
Dacryocystitis (acute) (phlegmonous)
  H04.3
– chronic H04.4
– neonatal P39.1
– syphilitic A52.7† H06.0∗
– – congenital (early) A50.0† H06.0∗
– trachomatous, active A71.1
Dacryocystoblenorrhea H04.4
Dacryocystocele H04.6
Dacryolith, dacryolithiasis H04.5
Dacryoma H04.6
Dacryopericystitis (acute) (subacute)
  H04.3
– chronic H04.4
Dacryops H04.1
Dacryostenosis H04.5
– congenital Q10.5
Dactylitis L08.9
– bone (*see also* Osteomyelitis) M86.9
– syphilitic A52.7† M90.1∗
– tuberculous A18.0† M90.0∗
Dactylolysis spontanea (ainhum) L94.6
Dactylosymphysis Q70.9
– fingers Q70.0
– toes Q70.2
Damage
– arteriosclerotic – *see* Arteriosclerosis
– brain (nontraumatic) G93.9
– – anoxic, hypoxic G93.1
– – – resulting from a procedure G97.8
– – child NEC G80.9
– – due to birth injury P11.2
– cardiorenal (vascular) (*see also*
  Hypertension, cardiorenal) I13.9
– cerebral NEC – *see* Damage, brain
– chemical, following abortion (subsequent
  episode) O08.6
– coccyx, complicating delivery O71.6
– coronary (*see also* Ischemia, heart) I25.9
– eye, birth injury P15.3
– liver (nontraumatic) K76.9
– – alcoholic K70.9
– – due to drugs – *see* Disease, liver, toxic
– – toxic – *see* Disease, liver, toxic

Damage—*continued*
– pelvic
– – joint or ligament, during delivery
  O71.6
– – organ NEC
– – – during delivery O71.5
– – – following
– – – – abortion (subsequent episode)
  O08.6
– – – – – current episode – *see* Abortion
– – – – ectopic or molar pregnancy O08.6
– renal (*see also* Disease, renal) N28.9
– subendocardium, subendocardial (*see also*
  Degeneration, myocardial) I51.5
– vascular I99
Dana-Putnam syndrome – *see*
  Degeneration, combined
Dandruff L21.0
Dandy-Walker syndrome Q03.1
Danlos' syndrome Q79.6
Darier(-White) disease (congenital) Q82.8
– meaning erythema annulare centrifugum
  L53.1
Darier-Roussy sarcoid D86.3
Darling's disease or histoplasmosis B39.4
Darwin's tubercle Q17.8
Dawson's (inclusion body) encephalitis
  A81.1
De Beurmann(-Gougerot) disease B42.1
De la Tourette's syndrome F95.2
De Lange's syndrome Q87.1
De Morgan's spots I78.1
De Quervain's
– disease M65.4
– thyroiditis E06.1
De Toni-Fanconi(-Debré) syndrome
  E72.0
Dead
– fetus, retained (mother) O36.4
– – early pregnancy O02.1
– labyrinth H83.2
– ovum, retained O02.0
Deadborn fetus NEC P95
Deaf and dumb NEC H91.3
Deaf mutism (acquired) (congenital) NEC
  H91.3
– hysterical F44.6
– syphilitic, congenital A50.0† H94.8∗

Deafness (acquired) (complete) (hereditary) (partial) H91.9
- with blue sclera and fragility of bone Q78.0
- auditory fatigue H91.8
- aviation T70.0
- boilermaker's H83.3
- central – *see* Deafness, sensorineural
- conductive H90.2
- – and sensorineural, mixed H90.8
- – – bilateral H90.6
- – – unilateral (unrestricted hearing other side) H90.7
- – bilateral H90.0
- – unilateral (unrestricted hearing other side) H90.1
- congenital NEC H90.5
- due to toxic agents H91.0
- emotional (hysterical) F44.6
- functional (hysterical) F44.6
- high frequency H91.9
- hysterical F44.6
- low frequency H91.9
- mental R48.8
- mixed conductive and sensorineural H90.8
- – bilateral H90.6
- – unilateral (unrestricted hearing other side) H90.7
- nerve – *see* Deafness, sensorineural
- neural – *see* Deafness, sensorineural
- noise-induced H83.3
- nonspeaking H91.3
- ototoxic H91.0
- perceptive – *see* Deafness, sensorineural
- psychogenic (hysterical) F44.6
- sensorineural H90.5
- – and conductive, mixed H90.8
- – – bilateral H90.6
- – – unilateral (unrestricted hearing other side) H90.7
- – bilateral H90.3
- – unilateral (unrestricted hearing other side) H90.4
- sensory – *see* Deafness, sensorineural
- specified type NEC H91.8
- sudden (idiopathic) H91.2
- syphilitic A52.1† H94.8*
- transient ischemic H93.0
- word (developmental) F80.2

Death
- after delivery (cause not stated) (sudden) O95

Death—*continued*
- anesthetic
- – due to
- – – correct substance properly administered T88.2
- – – overdose or wrong substance given T41.-
- – – – specified anesthetic – *see* Table of drugs and chemicals
- – during delivery O74.8
- – in pregnancy O29.8
- – postpartum, puerperal O89.8
- cardiac, sudden I46.1
- cause unknown R99
- cot R95
- crib R95
- family member Z63.4
- fetus, fetal (cause not stated) (intrauterine) P95
- – early, with retention O02.1
- – late, affecting management of pregnancy O36.4
- instantaneous unexplained R96.0
- intrauterine (late), complicating pregnancy O36.4
- known not to be violent or instantaneous, cause unknown R96.1
- maternal – *see* Death, obstetric
- neonatal NEC P96.8
- obstetric (cause unknown) O95
- – affecting fetus or newborn P01.6
- – between 42 days and one year after delivery O96.-
- – one year or more after delivery O97.-
- sudden (cause unknown) unexplained R96.0
- – during delivery O95
- – infant R95
- – puerperal, during puerperium O95
- unattended (cause unknown) R98
- under anesthesia NEC
- – due to
- – – correct substance properly administered T88.2
- – – overdose or wrong substance given T41.-
- – – – specified anesthetic – *see* Table of drugs and chemicals
- – during delivery O74.8
- without sign of disease R96.1

Debility (chronic) (general) R53
- congenital or neonatal NEC P96.9
- nervous F48.0
- old age R54

Debility—*continued*
- senile R54
Decalcification
- bone M81.9
- teeth K03.8
Decapitation S18
- fetal (to facilitate delivery) P03.8
Decapsulation, kidney N28.8
Decay
- dental K02.9
  senile R54
- tooth, teeth K02.9
Deciduitis (acute), affecting fetus or newborn P00.8
Decline (general) (*see also* Debility) R53
- cognitive, age-associated R41.8
Decompensation
- cardiac (acute) (chronic) (*see also* Disease, heart) I51.9
- cardiorenal I13.2
- cardiovascular (*see also* Disease, cardiovascular) I51.6
- heart (*see also* Disease, heart) I51.9
- hepatic (*see also* Failure, hepatic) K72.9
- myocardial (acute) (chronic) (*see also* Disease, heart) I51.9
- respiratory J98.8
Decompression sickness T70.3
Decrease(d)
- blood
- - platelets (*see also* Thrombocytopenia) D69.6
- - pressure, due to shock following injury T79.4
- estrogen E28.3
- fragility of erythrocytes D58.8
- function
- - lipase (pancreatic) K90.3
- - ovary in hypopituitarism E23.0
- - parenchyma of pancreas K86.8
- - pituitary (gland) (anterior) (lobe) E23.0
- - - posterior E23.0
- functional activity R68.8
- respiration, due to shock following injury T79.4
- tear secretion NEC H04.1
- tolerance
- - fat K90.4
- - glucose R73.0
- - pancreatic K90.3
Decubitus (ulcer) L89.-
- cervix N86
- stage
- - I L89.0

Decubitus—*continued*
- stage—*continued*
- - II L89.1
- - III L89.2
- - IV L89.3
Defect, defective
- abdominal wall, congenital Q79.5
- antibody immunodeficiency D80.9
- aortopulmonary septum Q21.4
- atrial septal (ostium secundum) (type II) Q21.1
- - following acute myocardial infarction (current complication) I23.1
- - ostium primum (type I) Q21.2
- atrioventricular
- - canal Q21.2
- - septum Q21.2
- auricular septal Q21.1
- bilirubin excretion NEC E80.6
- biosynthesis, androgen (testicular) E29.1
- bulbar septum Q21.0
- catalase E80.3
- cell membrane receptor complex (CR3) D71
- circulation I99
- - congenital Q28.9
- - newborn Q28.9
- coagulation (factor) (*see also* Deficiency, factor) D68.9
- - antepartum with hemorrhage O46.0
- - - affecting fetus or newborn P02.1
- - - premature separation of placenta O45.0
- - intrapartum O67.0
- - newborn, transient P61.6
- - postpartum O72.3
- complement system D84.1
- conduction I45.9
- - bone – *see* Deafness, conductive
- congenital, organ or site not listed – *see* Anomaly, by site
- coronary sinus Q21.1
- cushion, endocardial Q21.2
- degradation, glycoprotein E77.1
- Descemet's membrane, congenital Q13.8
- developmental – *see also* Anomaly
- - cauda equina Q06.3
- diaphragm
- - with elevation, eventration or hernia – *see* Hernia, diaphragm
- - congenital Q79.1
- - - with hernia Q79.0
- - - gross (with hernia) Q79.0
- ectodermal, congenital Q82.9

Defect, defective—*continued*
- Eisenmenger's Q21.8
- enzyme
- – catalase E80.3
- – peroxidase E80.3
- esophagus, congenital Q39.9
- extensor retinaculum M62.8
- filling
- – bladder R93.4
- – kidney R93.4
- – ureter R93.4
- glycoprotein degradation E77.1
- Hageman (factor) D68.2
- hearing (*see also* Deafness) H91.9
- 11-hydroxylase E25.0
- 21-hydroxylase E25.0
- 3beta hydroxysteroid dehydrogenase E25.0
- interatrial septal Q21.1
- interauricular septal Q21.1
- interventricular septal Q21.0
- – with dextroposition of aorta, pulmonary stenosis and hypertrophy of right ventricle Q21.3
- – in tetralogy of Fallot Q21.3
- learning (specific) F81.9
- lymphocyte function antigen-1 (LFA-1) D84.0
- lysosomal enzyme, post-translational modification E77.0
- mental – *see* Retardation, mental
- modification, lysosomal enzymes, post-translational E77.0
- ostium
- – primum Q21.2
- – secundum Q21.1
- peroxidase E80.3
- placental blood supply – *see* Insufficiency, placental
- platelets, qualitative D69.1
- postural NEC, spine M43.9
- renal pelvis Q63.8
- – obstructive Q62.3
- respiratory system, congenital Q34.9
- septal (heart) NEC Q21.9
- – acquired (atrial) (auricular) (ventricular) (old) I51.0
- – atrial
- – – concurrent with acute myocardial infarction – *see* Infarct, myocardium
- – – following acute myocardial infarction (current complication) I23.1

Defect, defective—*continued*
- septal—*continued*
- – ventricular (*see also* Defect, ventricular septal) Q21.0
- sinus venosus Q21.1
- speech NEC R47.8
- – developmental F80.9
- vascular (local) I99
- – congenital Q27.9
- ventricular septal Q21.0
- – concurrent with acute myocardial infarction – *see* Infarct, myocardium
- – following acute myocardial infarction (current complication) I23.2
- – in tetralogy of Fallot Q21.3
- vision NEC H54.9
- visual field H53.4
- voice R49.8
- wedge, tooth, teeth (abrasion) K03.1

Deferentitis N49.1
- gonorrheal (acute) (chronic) A54.2† N51.8*

Defibrination (syndrome) D65
- antepartum O46.0
- – affecting fetus or newborn P02.1
- fetus or newborn P60
- following
- – abortion (subsequent episode) O08.1
- – – current episode – *see* Abortion
- – ectopic or molar pregnancy O08.1
- intrapartum O67.0
- postpartum O72.3

Deficiency, deficient
- abdominal muscle syndrome Q79.4
- AC globulin (congenital) (hereditary) D68.2
- – acquired D68.4
- acid phosphatase E83.3
- adenosine deaminase (ADA) D81.3
- aldolase (hereditary) E74.1
- alpha-1-antitrypsin E88.0
- amino-acids E72.9
- anemia – *see* Anemia
- aneurin E51.9
- antibody with
- – hyperimmunoglobulinemia D80.6
- – near-normal immunoglobins D80.6
- anti-hemophilic globulin NEC D66
- antithrombin D68.5
- ascorbic acid E54
- attention (disorder) (syndrome) F98.8
- – with hyperactivity F90.0
- biotin E53.8
- biotin-dependent carboxylase D81.8

175

Deficiency, deficient—*continued*
- brancher enzyme (amylopectinosis) E74.0
- calciferol E55.9
- – with
- – – – adult osteomalacia M83.8
- – – – rickets (*see also* Rickets) E55.0
- calcium (dietary) E58
- calorie, severe E43
- – with marasmus E41
- – – – and kwashiorkor E42
- cardiac (*see also* Insufficiency, myocardial) I50.0
- carnitine (palmityltransferase), muscle E71.3
- carotene E50.9
- central nervous system G96.8
- ceruloplasmin (Wilson) E83.0
- chromium E61.4
- clotting (blood) (*see also* Deficiency, coagulation factor) D68.9
- clotting factor NEC (hereditary) (*see also* Deficiency, factor) D68.2
- coagulation D68.9
- – acquired (any) D68.4
- – antepartum O46.0
- – – affecting fetus or newborn P02.1
- – clotting factor NEC (*see also* Deficiency, factor) D68.2
- – due to
- – – hyperprothrombinemia D68.4
- – – liver disease D68.4
- – – vitamin K deficiency D68.4
- – newborn, transient P61.6
- – postpartum O72.3
- – specified NEC D68.8
- copper (nutritional) E61.0
- corticoadrenal E27.4
- – primary E27.1
- craniofacial axis Q75.0
- cyanocobalamin E53.8
- C_1 esterase inhibitor (C_1-INH) D84.1
- debrancher enzyme (limit dextrinosis) E74.0
- diet E63.9
- disaccharidase E73.9
- edema (*see also* Malnutrition, severe) E43
- endocrine E34.9
- energy supply (*see also* Malnutrition) E46
- – severe (*see also* Malnutrition, severe) E43
- enzymes, circulating NEC E88.0

Deficiency, deficient—*continued*
- ergosterol E55.9
- – with
- – – adult osteomalacia M83.8
- – – rickets (*see also* Rickets) E55.0
- essential fatty acid (EFA) E63.0
- factor – *see also* Deficiency, coagulation
- – Hageman D68.2
- – multiple (congenital) D68.8
- – – acquired D68.4
- – I (congenital) (hereditary) D68.2
- – II (congenital) (hereditary) D68.2
- – V (congenital) (hereditary) D68.2
- – VII (congenital) (hereditary) D68.2
- – VIII (congenital) (functional) (hereditary) (with functional defect) D66
- – – with vascular defect D68.0
- – IX (congenital) (functional) (hereditary) (with functional defect) D67
- – X (congenital) (hereditary) D68.2
- – XI (congenital) (hereditary) D68.1
- – XII (congenital) (hereditary) D68.2
- – XIII (congenital) (hereditary) D68.2
- femoral, proximal focal (congenital) Q72.4
- fibrin-stabilizing factor (congenital) (hereditary) D68.2
- – acquired D68.4
- fibrinogen (congenital) (hereditary) D68.2
- – acquired D65
- folate E53.8
- folic acid E53.8
- fructokinase E74.1
- fructose 1,6-diphosphatase E74.1
- galactokinase E74.2
- galactose-1-phosphate uridyl transferase E74.2
- gammaglobulin in blood D80.1
- – hereditary D80.0
- glucose-6-phosphatase E74.0
- glucose-6-phosphate dehydrogenase anemia D55.0
- beta-glucoronidase E76.2
- glucuronyl transferase E80.5
- glycogen synthetase E74.0
- gonadotropin (isolated) E23.0
- growth hormone (idiopathic) (isolated) E23.0
- Hageman factor D68.2
- hemoglobin D64.9
- hepatophosphorylase E74.0
- homogentisate 1,2-dioxygenase E70.2

Deficiency, deficient—*continued*
- hormone
- – – anterior pituitary (partial) NEC E23.0
- – – – growth E23.0
- – – growth (isolated) E23.0
- – – pituitary E23.0
- – – testicular E29.1
- – 11-hydroxylase E25.0
- – 21-hydroxylase E25.0
- – 3beta hydroxysteroid dehydrogenase E25.0
- – hypoxanthine(-guanine)-phosphoribosyltransferase (HG-PRT) (total H-PRT) E79.1
- – immunity D84.9
- – – cell-mediated D84.8
- – – combined D81.9
- – – humoral D80.9
- – immuno – *see* Immunodeficiency
- – immunoglobulin, selective
- – – A (IgA) D80.2
- – – G (IgG) (subclasses) D80.3
- – – M (IgM) D80.4
- – intrinsic factor (congenital) D51.0
- – iodine E61.8
- – – congenital syndrome (*see also* Syndrome, iodine-deficiency, congenital) E00.9
- – iron E61.1
- – kalium E87.6
- – kappa light chain D80.8
- – labile factor (congenital) (hereditary) D68.2
- – – acquired D68.4
- – lacrimal fluid (acquired) H04.1
- – – congenital Q10.6
- – lactase
- – – congenital E73.0
- – – secondary E73.1
- – lecithin cholesterol acyltransferase E78.6
- – lipocaic K86.8
- – lipoprotein (familial) (high density) E78.6
- – liver phosphorylase E74.0
- – magnesium E61.2
- – major histocompatibility complex
- – – class I D81.6
- – – class II D81.7
- – manganese E61.3
- – mental (familial) (hereditary) – *see* Retardation, mental
- – mineral NEC E61.8
- – molybdenum (nutritional) E61.5
- – moral F60.2
- – multiple nutrient elements E61.7

Deficiency, deficient—*continued*
- muscle carnitine (palmityltransferase) E71.3
- – myocardial (*see also* Insufficiency, myocardial) I50.0
- – myophosphorylase E74.0
- – NADH diaphorase or reductase (congenital) D74.0
- – NADH-methemoglobin reductase (congenital) D74.0
- – natrium E87.1
- – niacin (amide) (-tryptophan) E52
- – nicotinamide E52
- – nicotinic acid E52
- – number of teeth (*see also* Anodontia) K00.0
- – nutrient element E61.9
- – – multiple E61.7
- – – specified NEC E61.8
- – nutrition, nutritional E63.9
- – – sequelae – *see* Sequelae, nutritional deficiency
- – – specified NEC E63.8
- – ornithine transcarbamylase E72.4
- – oxygen (*see also* Anoxia) R09.0
- – – systemic (by suffocation) (low content in atmosphere) T71
- – pantothenic acid E53.8
- – parathyroid (gland) E20.9
- – phenylalanine hydroxylase E70.1
- – phosphoenolpyruvate carboxykinase E74.4
- – pituitary hormone (isolated) E23.0
- – placenta – *see* Insufficiency, placental
- – plasma thromboplastin
- – – antecedent (PTA) D68.1
- – – component (PTC) D67
- – polyglandular E31.8
- – – autoimmune E31.0
- – potassium (K) E87.6
- – proaccelerin (congenital) (hereditary) D68.2
- – – acquired D68.4
- – proconvertin factor (congenital) (hereditary) D68.2
- – – acquired D68.4
- – protein (*see also* Malnutrition) E46
- – – C D68.5
- – – S D68.5
- – prothrombin (congenital) (hereditary) D68.2
- – – acquired D68.4
- – pseudocholinesterase E88.0

Deficiency, deficient—*continued*
- PTA (plasma thromboplastin antecedent) D68.1
- PTC (plasma thromboplastin component) D67
- purine nucleoside phosphorylase (PNP) D81.5
- pyridoxamine, pyridoxal E53.1
- pyridoxine (derivatives) E53.1
- pyruvate
- – carboxylase E74.4
- – dehydrogenase E74.4
- 5-alpha-reductase (with male pseudohermaphroditism) E29.1
- riboflavin E53.0
- salt E87.1
- secretion
- – ovary E28.3
- – salivary gland (any) K11.7
- – urine R34
- selenium (dietary) E59
- serum antitrypsin, familial E88.0
- sodium (Na) E87.1
- SPCA (factor VII) D68.2
- stable factor (congenital) (hereditary) D68.2
- – acquired D68.4
- Stuart-Prower (factor X) D68.2
- sucrase E74.3
- sulfatase E75.2
- sulfite oxidase E72.1
- thiamine, thiaminic (chloride) E51.9
- – beriberi E51.1
- – specified NEC E51.8
- thyroid (gland) (*see also* Hypothyroidism) E03.9
- tocopherol E56.0
- transcobalamin II (anemia) D51.2
- vanadium E61.6
- vascular I99
- viosterol (*see also* Deficiency, calciferol) E55.9
- vitamin (multiple) E56.9
- – A E50.9
- – – with
- – – – Bitot's spot (corneal) E50.1
- – – – follicular keratosis E50.8† L86*
- – – – keratomalacia E50.4† H19.8*
- – – – manifestations NEC E50.8
- – – – night blindness E50.5† H58.1*
- – – – scar of cornea, xerophthalmic E50.6† H19.8*
- – – – xeroderma E50.8† L86*
- – – – xerophthalmia E50.7† H19.8*

Deficiency, deficient—*continued*
- vitamin—*continued*
- – A—*continued*
- – – with—*continued*
- – – – xerosis
- – – – – conjunctival E50.0† H13.8*
- – – – – and Bitot's spot E50.1† H13.8*
- – – – – cornea E50.2† H19.8*
- – – – – and ulceration E50.3† H19.8*
- – – sequelae E64.1
- – – B (complex) NEC E53.9
- – – with
- – – – beriberi E51.1
- – – – pellagra E52
- – – B₁ E51.9
- – – beriberi E51.1
- – – – with circulatory system manifestations E51.1† I98.8*
- – – B₁₂ E53.8
- – – B₂ (riboflavin) E53.0
- – – B₆ E53.1
- – – C E54
- – – – sequelae E64.2
- – – D E55.9
- – – – with
- – – – – adult osteomalacia M83.8
- – – – – rickets (*see also* Rickets) E55.0
- – – E E56.0
- – – group B E53.9
- – – – specified NEC E53.8
- – – H (biotin) E53.8
- – – K E56.1
- – – – of newborn P53
- – – P E56.8
- – – PP (pellagra-preventing) E52
- – – specified NEC E56.8
- – – thiamine E51.9
- – – – beriberi (*see also* Beriberi) E51.1
- zinc, dietary E60

Deficient perineum (female) N81.8
Deficit – *see also* Deficiency
- attention – *see* Attention, deficit disorder or syndrome
Deflection
- radius M21.8
- septum (acquired) (nasal) (nose) J34.2
- spine – *see* Curvature, spine
- turbinate (nose) J34.2
Defluvium
- capillorum (*see also* Alopecia) L65.9
- ciliorum H02.7
- unguium L60.8

Deformity Q89.9
– abdomen, congenital Q89.9
– abdominal wall
– – acquired M95.8
– – congenital Q79.5
– alimentary tract, congenital Q45.9
– – upper Q40.9
– ankle (joint) (acquired) NEC M21.6
– – congenital Q68.8
– anus (acquired) K62.8
– – congenital Q43.9
– aorta (arch) (congenital) Q25.4
– – acquired I77.8
– aortic cusp or valve (congenital) Q23.8
– – acquired (*see also* Endocarditis, aortic) I35.8
– arm (acquired) M21.9
– – congenital Q68.8
– artery (congenital) (peripheral) NEC Q27.9
– – acquired I77.8
– – coronary (acquired) I25.8
– – – congenital Q24.5
– auditory canal (external) (congenital) (*see also* Deformity, ear) Q17.8
– – acquired H61.8
– auricle
– – ear (congenital) (*see also* Deformity, ear) Q17.3
– – – acquired H61.1
– back (acquired) – *see* Deformity, spine
– bile duct (common) (congenital) (hepatic) Q44.5
– – acquired K83.8
– biliary duct or passage (congenital) Q44.5
– – acquired K83.8
– bladder (neck) (sphincter) (trigone) (acquired) N32.8
– – congenital Q64.7
– bone (acquired) M95.9
– brain (congenital) Q04.9
– – acquired G93.8
– – reduction Q04.3
– breast (acquired) N64.8
– – congenital Q83.9
– bronchus (congenital) Q32.4
– – acquired NEC J98.0
– canaliculi (lacrimalis) (acquired) H04.6
– – congenital Q10.6
– canthus, acquired H02.8
– capillary (acquired) I78.8
– cardiovascular system, congenital Q28.9
– caruncle, lacrimal (acquired) H04.6

Deformity—*continued*
– caruncle, lacrimal—*continued*
– – congenital Q10.6
– cecum (congenital) Q43.9
– – acquired K63.8
– cerebral, acquired G93.8
– cervix (uterus) (acquired) NEC N88.8
– – congenital Q51.9
– cheek (acquired) M95.2
– – congenital Q18.9
– chest (acquired) (wall) M95.4
– – congenital Q67.8
– – late effect of rickets E64.3
– chin (acquired) M95.2
– – congenital Q18.9
– choroid (congenital) Q14.3
– – acquired H31.8
– – plexus Q07.8
– cicatricial – *see* Cicatrix
– cilia, acquired H02.8
– clavicle (acquired) M21.8
– – congenital Q68.8
– clitoris (congenital) Q52.6
– – acquired N90.8
– clubfoot – *see* Clubfoot
– coccyx (acquired) M43.8
– colon (congenital) Q43.9
– – acquired K63.8
– concha (ear), congenital (*see also* Deformity, ear) Q17.3
– – acquired H61.1
– cornea (acquired) H18.7
– – congenital Q13.4
– coronary artery (acquired) I25.8
– – congenital Q24.5
– cranium (acquired) M95.2
– – congenital (*see also* Deformity, skull, congenital) Q75.8
– cricoid cartilage (congenital) Q31.8
– – acquired J38.7
– cystic duct (congenital) Q44.5
– – acquired K82.8
– diaphragm (congenital) Q79.1
– – acquired J98.6
– duodenal bulb K31.8
– duodenum (congenital) Q43.9
– – acquired K31.8
– dura – *see* Deformity, meninges or membrane
– ear (acquired) H61.1
– – congenital Q17.9
– – internal Q16.5
– – middle Q16.4
– ectodermal (congenital) Q82.9

Deformity—*continued*
- ejaculatory duct (congenital) Q55.4
- – acquired N50.8
- elbow (joint) (acquired) M21.9
- – congenital Q68.8
- endocrine gland NEC Q89.2
- epididymis (congenital) Q55.4
- – acquired N50.8
- epiglottis (congenital) Q31.8
- – acquired J38.7
- esophagus (congenital) Q39.9
- – acquired K22.8
- eustachian tube (congenital) NEC Q16.4
- eyelid (acquired) H02.8
- – congenital Q10.3
- face (acquired) M95.2
- – congenital Q18.9
- fallopian tube, acquired N83.8
- femur (acquired) M21.8
- fetal
- – with fetopelvic disproportion O33.7
- – causing obstructed labor O66.3
- – – affecting fetus or newborn P03.1
- finger (acquired) M20.0
- – congenital NEC Q68.1
- flexion (joint) (acquired) M21.2
- – congenital NEC Q68.8
- – hip or thigh (acquired) M21.2
- – – congenital Q65.8
- foot (acquired) NEC M21.6
- – congenital Q66.9
- – valgus M21.0
- – – congenital NEC Q66.6
- – varus M21.1
- – – congenital NEC Q66.3
- forearm (acquired) M21.9
- – congenital Q68.8
- forehead (acquired) M95.2
- – congenital Q75.8
- frontal bone (acquired) M95.2
- – congenital Q75.8
- gallbladder (congenital) Q44.1
- – acquired K82.8
- gastrointestinal tract (congenital) Q45.9
- – acquired K63.8
- genitalia, genital organ(s) or system NEC
- – female (congenital) Q52.9
- – – acquired N94.8
- – – external Q52.7
- – male (congenital) Q55.9
- – – acquired N50.8
- globe (eye) (congenital) Q15.8
- – acquired H44.8
- gum, acquired NEC K06.8

Deformity—*continued*
- hand (acquired) M21.9
- – congenital Q68.1
- head (acquired) M95.2
- – congenital Q75.8
- heart (congenital) Q24.9
- – septum Q21.9
- – valve NEC Q24.8
- – – acquired - *see* Endocarditis
- heel (acquired) M21.6
- – congenital Q66.9
- hepatic duct (congenital) Q44.5
- – acquired K83.8
- hip (joint) (acquired) M21.9
- – congenital Q65.9
- – due to (previous) juvenile
  osteochondrosis M91.2
- hourglass – *see* Contraction, hourglass
- humerus (acquired) M21.8
- – congenital Q74.0
- hypophyseal (congenital) Q89.2
- ileocecal (coil) (valve) (acquired) K63.8
- – congenital Q43.9
- ileum (congenital) Q43.9
- – acquired K63.8
- ilium (acquired) M95.5
- – congenital Q74.2
- integument (congenital) Q84.9
- intervertebral cartilage or disk (acquired)
  M51.8
- intestine (large) (small) (congenital) NEC
  Q43.9
- – acquired K63.8
- intrinsic minus or plus (hand) M21.8
- iris (acquired) H21.5
- – congenital Q13.2
- ischium (acquired) M95.5
- – congenital Q74.2
- jaw (acquired) (congenital) K07.9
- joint (acquired) NEC M21.9
- – congenital Q68.8
- kidney(s) (calyx) (pelvis) (congenital)
  Q63.9
- – acquired N28.8
- – artery Q27.2
- – – acquired I77.8
- Klippel-Feil Q76.1
- knee (acquired) NEC M21.9
- – congenital Q68.2
- labium (majus) (minus) (congenital)
  Q52.7
- – acquired N90.8
- lacrimal passages or duct (congenital)
  NEC Q10.6

Deformity—*continued*
- lacrimal passages or duct—*continued*
- – acquired H04.6
- larynx (muscle) (congenital) Q31.8
- – acquired J38.7
- leg (lower) (upper) (acquired) M21.9
- – congenital Q68.8
- lens (acquired) H27.8
- – congenital Q12.9
- lid (fold) (acquired) H02.8
- – congenital Q10.3
- ligament (acquired) M24.2
- limb (acquired) M21.9
- – congenital, except reduction deformity Q68.8
- – specified NEC M21.8
- lip (acquired) NEC K13.0
- – congenital Q38.0
- liver (congenital) Q44.7
- – acquired K76.8
- lumbosacral (congenital) (joint) (region) Q76.4
- – acquired M43.8
- lung (congenital) Q33.9
- – acquired J98.4
- lymphatic system, congenital Q89.9
- Madelung's (radius) Q74.0
- mandible (acquired) (congenital) K07.9
- maxilla (acquired) (congenital) K07.9
- meninges or membrane (congenital) Q07.9
- – cerebral Q04.8
- – – acquired G96.1
- – spinal cord Q06.9
- – – acquired G96.1
- metacarpus (acquired) M21.9
- – congenital Q74.0
- metatarsus (acquired) M21.6
- – congenital Q66.8
- middle ear (congenital) Q16.4
- mitral (leaflets) (valve) I05.8
- – stenosis, congenital Q23.2
- mouth (acquired) K13.7
- multiple, congenital NEC Q89.7
- muscle (acquired) M62.8
- musculoskeletal system (acquired) M95.9
- – specified NEC M95.8
- nail (acquired) L60.8
- – congenital Q84.6
- nasal – *see* Deformity, nose
- neck (acquired) M95.3
- – congenital Q18.9
- – – sternocleidomastoid Q68.0
- nipple (congenital) Q83.9

Deformity—*continued*
- nipple—*continued*
- – acquired N64.8
- nose (acquired) (cartilage) M95.0
- – bone (turbinate) M95.0
- – congenital Q30.9
- – – bent or squashed Q67.4
- – septum J34.2
- – – congenital Q30.8
- – sinus (wall), congenital Q30.8
- – syphilitic
- – – congenital A50.5
- – – late A52.7† J99.8*
- ocular muscle (congenital) Q10.3
- – acquired H50.6
- oesophagus (congenital) Q39.9
- – acquired K22.8
- opticociliary vessels (congenital) Q13.2
- orbit (eye) (acquired) H05.3
- – congenital Q10.7
- organ of Corti (congenital) Q16.5
- ovary (congenital) Q50.3
- – acquired N83.8
- oviduct, acquired N83.8
- palate (congenital) Q38.5
- – acquired K10.8
- – cleft (*see also* Cleft, palate) Q35.9
- pancreas (congenital) Q45.3
- – acquired K86.8
- parathyroid (gland) Q89.2
- parotid (gland) (congenital) Q38.4
- – acquired K11.8
- patella (acquired) M22.8
- – congenital Q68.2
- pelvis, pelvic (acquired) (bony) M95.5
- – with disproportion (fetopelvic) O33.0
- – – affecting fetus or newborn P03.1
- – – causing obstructed labor O65.0
- – congenital Q74.2
- – rachitic (late effect) E64.3
- penis (glans) (congenital) Q55.6
- – acquired N48.8
- pericardium (congenital) Q24.8
- – acquired – *see* Pericarditis
- pharynx (congenital) Q38.8
- – acquired J39.2
- pinna, acquired H61.1
- pituitary (congenital) Q89.2
- posture – *see* Curvature, spine
- prepuce (congenital) Q55.6
- – acquired N48.8
- prostate (congenital) Q55.4
- – acquired N42.8
- pupil (congenital) Q13.2

Deformity—*continued*
- pupil—*continued*
- – acquired H21.5
- pylorus (congenital) Q40.3
- – acquired K31.8
- rachitic (acquired), old or healed E64.3
- radius (acquired) M21.9
- – congenital Q68.8
- rectum (congenital) Q43.9
- – acquired K62.8
- reduction (extremity) (limb),
  congenital (*see also* condition and site)
  Q73.8
- – brain Q04.3
- – lower Q72.9
- – – specified NEC Q72.8
- – upper Q71.9
- – – specified NEC Q71.8
- renal – *see* Deformity, kidney
- respiratory system (congenital) Q34.9
- rib (acquired) M95.4
- – congenital Q76.6
- – – cervical Q76.5
- rotation (joint) (acquired) M21.8
- – congenital Q74.9
- – hip M21.8
- – – congenital Q65.8
- sacroiliac joint (congenital) Q74.2
- – acquired M43.8
- sacrum (acquired) M43.8
- saddle
- – back M40.5
- – nose M95.0
- – – syphilitic A50.5
- salivary gland or duct (congenital) Q38.4
- – acquired K11.8
- scapula (acquired) M21.8
- – congenital Q68.8
- scrotum (congenital) Q55.2
- – acquired N50.8
- seminal vesicles (congenital) Q55.4
- – acquired N50.8
- shoulder (joint) (acquired) M21.9
- – congenital Q74.0
- sigmoid (flexure) (congenital) Q43.9
- – acquired K63.8
- skin (congenital) Q82.9
- skull (acquired) M95.2
- – congenital Q75.8
- – – with
- – – – anencephaly Q00.0
- – – – encephalocele (*see also*
  Encephalocele) Q01.9
- – – – hydrocephalus Q03.9

Deformity—*continued*
- skull—*continued*
- – congenital—*continued*
- – – with—*continued*
- – – – hydrocephalus—*continued*
- – – – – with spina bifida (*see also* Spina
  bifida, with hydrocephalus)
  Q05.4
- – – – microcephaly Q02
- soft parts, organs or tissues (of pelvis)
- – in pregnancy or childbirth NEC O34.8
- – – affecting fetus or newborn P03.8
- – – causing obstructed labor O65.5
- – – – affecting fetus or newborn P03.1
- spermatic cord (congenital) Q55.4
- – acquired N50.8
- spinal M43.9
- – column (acquired) – *see* Deformity,
  spine
- – congenital Q67.5
- – cord (congenital) Q06.9
- – – acquired G95.8
- – nerve root (congenital) Q07.8
- spine (acquired) M43.9
- – congenital Q67.5
- – rachitic E64.3
- – specified NEC M43.8
- spleen
- – acquired D73.8
- – congenital Q89.0
- Sprengel's (congenital) Q74.0
- sternocleidomastoid (muscle), congenital
  Q68.0
- sternum (acquired) M95.4
- – congenital NEC Q76.7
- stomach (congenital) Q40.3
- – acquired K31.8
- submandibular gland (congenital) Q38.4
- talipes – *see* Talipes
- testis (congenital) Q55.2
- – acquired N50.8
- thigh (acquired) M21.9
- – congenital NEC Q68.8
- thorax (acquired) (wall) M95.4
- – congenital Q67.8
- – sequelae of rickets E64.3
- thumb (acquired) M20.0
- – congenital NEC Q68.1
- thymus (tissue) (congenital) Q89.2
- thyroid (gland) (congenital) Q89.2
- – cartilage Q31.8
- – – acquired J38.7
- tibia (acquired) M21.8
- – congenital NEC Q68.8

Deformity—*continued*
- tibia—*continued*
- – saber (syphilitic) A50.5† M90.2∗
- toe (acquired) M20.6
- – congenital Q66.9
- – specified NEC M20.5
- tongue (congenital) Q38.3
- – acquired K14.8
- tooth, teeth K00.2
- trachea (rings) (congenital) Q32.1
- – acquired J39.8
- transverse aortic arch (congenital) Q25.4
- tricuspid (leaflets) (valve) I07.8
- – Ebstein's Q22.5
- trunk (acquired) M95.8
- – congenital Q89.9
- ulna (acquired) M21.9
- – congenital NEC Q68.8
- urachus, congenital Q64.4
- ureter (opening) (congenital) Q62.8
- – acquired N28.8
- urethra (congenital) Q64.7
- – acquired N36.8
- urinary tract (congenital) Q64.9
- uterus (congenital) Q51.9
- – acquired N85.8
- uvula (congenital) Q38.5
- vagina (acquired) N89.8
- – congenital Q52.4
- valgus NEC M21.0
- valve, valvular (congenital) (heart) Q24.8
- – acquired – *see* Endocarditis
- varus NEC M21.1
- vas deferens (congenital) Q55.4
- – acquired N50.8
- vein (congenital) Q27.9
- – great Q26.9
- vertebra – *see* Deformity, spine
- vesicourethral orifice (acquired) N32.8
- – congenital NEC Q64.7
- vessels of optic papilla (congenital) Q14.2
- visual field (contraction) H53.4
- vitreous body, acquired H43.8
- vulva (congenital) Q52.7
- – acquired N90.8
- wrist (joint) (acquired) M21.9
- – congenital Q68.1

Degeneration, degenerative
- adrenal (capsule) (fatty) (gland) (hyaline) (infectional) E27.8
- amyloid (*see also* Amyloidosis) E85.9
- anterior cornua, spinal cord G12.2
- aorta, aortic I70.0

Degeneration, degenerative—*continued*
- aorta, aortic—*continued*
- – fatty I77.8
- aortic valve (heart) (*see also* Endocarditis, aortic) I35.8
- arteriovascular – *see* Arteriosclerosis
- artery, arterial (atheromatous) (calcareous) (*see also* Arteriosclerosis) I70.9
- – cerebral, amyloid E85.4† I68.0∗
- – medial I70.2
- articular cartilage NEC M24.1
- – knee M23.3
- atheromatous – *see* Arteriosclerosis
- basal nuclei or ganglia G23.9
- – specified NEC G23.8
- bone NEC M89.8
- brain (cortical) (progressive) G31.9
- – alcoholic G31.2
- – arteriosclerotic I67.2
- – childhood G31.9
- – – specified NEC G31.8
- – cystic G31.8
- – – congenital Q04.6
- – in
- – – alcoholism G31.2
- – – beriberi E51.1† G32.8∗
- – – cerebrovascular disease I67.9
- – – congenital hydrocephalus Q03.9
- – – Fabry-Anderson disease E75.2† G32.8∗
- – – Gaucher's disease E75.2† G32.8∗
- – – Hunter's syndrome E76.1† G32.8∗
- – – lipidosis
- – – – cerebral E75.4† G32.8∗
- – – – generalized E75.6† G32.8∗
- – – mucopolysaccharidosis E76.3† G32.8∗
- – – myxedema E03.9† G32.8∗
- – – neoplastic disease NEC (M8000/1) (*see also* Neoplasm) D48.9† G32.8∗
- – – Niemann-Pick disease E75.2† G32.8∗
- – – sphingolipidosis E75.3† G32.8∗
- – – vitamin B_{12} deficiency E53.8† G32.8∗
- – senile NEC G31.1
- breast N64.8
- Bruch's membrane H31.1
- calcareous NEC R89.7
- capillaries (fatty) I78.8
- – amyloid E85.8† I79.8∗

Degeneration, degenerative—*continued*
- cardiac (*see also* Degeneration, myocardial) I51.5
- – valve, valvular – *see* Endocarditis
- cardiorenal (*see also* Hypertension, cardiorenal) I13.9
- cardiovascular (*see also* Disease, cardiovascular) I51.6
- – renal (*see also* Hypertension, cardiorenal) I13.9
- cerebellar G31.9
- alcoholic G31.2
- – primary (hereditary) (sporadic) G11.9
- cerebral – *see* Degeneration, brain
- cerebrovascular I67.9
- cervix N88.8
- – due to radiation (intended effect) N88.8
- – – adverse effect or misadventure N99.8
- changes, spine or vertebra M47.9
- chorioretinal H31.1
- – hereditary H31.2
- choroid (colloid) (drusen) H31.1
- – hereditary H31.2
- ciliary body H21.2
- cochlear H83.8
- combined (spinal cord) (subacute) E53.8† G32.0*
- – with anemia (pernicious) D51.0† G32.0*
- – – due to dietary vitamin B₁₂ deficiency D51.3† G32.0*
- – in (due to)
- – – vitamin B₁₂ deficiency E53.8† G32.0*
- – – – anemia D51.9† G32.0*
- conjunctiva H11.1
- cornea H18.4
- – familial, hereditary H18.5
- – hyaline (of old scars) H18.4
- – senile H18.4
- cortical (cerebellar) (parenchymatous) G31.8
- – alcoholic G31.2
- – diffuse, due to arteriopathy I67.2
- cutis L98.8
- – amyloid E85.4† L99.0*
- dental pulp K04.2
- disk disease – *see* Degeneration, intervertebral disk NEC
- dorsolateral (spinal cord) – *see* Degeneration, combined
- extrapyramidal G25.9

Degeneration, degenerative—*continued*
- eye, macular H35.3
- – congenital or hereditary H35.5
- – posterior pole (eye) H35.3
- facet joints (*see also* Spondylosis) M47.9
- fatty
- – liver NEC K76.0
- – – alcoholic K70.0
- – placenta – *see* Placenta, abnormal
- grey matter (brain) (Alpers') G31.8
- heart (*see also* Degeneration, myocardial) I51.5
- – amyloid E85.4† I43.1*
- – atheromatous I25.1
- hepatolenticular (Wilson's) E83.0
- hepatorenal K76.7
- hyaline (diffuse) (generalized) (localized) – *see* Degeneration, by site
- intervertebral disk NEC M51.3
- – with
- – – myelopathy M51.0† G99.2*
- – – radiculitis or radiculopathy M51.1† G55.1*
- – cervical, cervicothoracic M50.3
- – – with
- – – – myelopathy M50.0† G99.2*
- – – – neuritis, radiculitis or radiculopathy M50.1† G55.1*
- – lumbar, lumbosacral M51.3
- – – with
- – – – myelopathy M51.0† G99.2*
- – – – neuritis, radiculitis, radiculopathy or sciatica M51.1† G55.1*
- – thoracic, thoracolumbar M51.3
- – – with
- – – – myelopathy M51.0† G99.2*
- – – – neuritis, radiculitis, radiculopathy or sciatica M51.1† G55.1*
- intestine, amyloid E85.4† K93.8*
- iris (pigmentary) H21.2
- ischemic – *see* Ischemia
- kidney N28.8
- – amyloid E85.4† N29.8*
- – cystic, congenital Q61.9
- – fatty N28.8
- Kuhnt-Junius H35.3
- lens H27.8
- lenticular (familial) (progressive) (Wilson's) (with cirrhosis of liver) E83.0
- liver (diffuse) NEC K76.8
- – amyloid E85.4† K77.8*
- – cystic K76.8
- – – congenital Q44.6
- – fatty NEC K76.0

Degeneration, degenerative—*continued*
- liver—*continued*
- – fatty NEC—*continued*
- – – alcoholic K70.0
- – hypertrophic K76.8
- – parenchymatous, acute or subacute
 K72.0
- – pigmentary K76.8
- – toxic (acute) K71.9
- lung J98.4
- lymph gland I89.8
- – hyaline I89.8
- macula, macular (acquired) (atrophic)
 (exudative) (senile) H35.3
- – congenital or hereditary H35.5
- membranous labyrinth, congenital
 (causing impairment of hearing) Q16.5
- meniscus (*see also* Derangement,
 meniscus) M23.3
- mitral – *see* Insufficiency, mitral
- Mönckeberg's I70.2
- multi-system G90.3
- mural (*see also* Degeneration, myocardial)
 I51.5
- muscle (fatty) (fibrous) (hyaline)
 (progressive) M62.8
- – heart (*see also* Degeneration,
 myocardial) I51.5
- myelin, central nervous system G37.9
- myocardial, myocardium (fatty) (hyaline)
 (senile) I51.5
- – with rheumatic fever (conditions in I00)
 I09.0
- – – active, acute or subacute I01.2
- – – – with chorea I02.0
- – – inactive or quiescent (with chorea)
 I09.0
- – hypertensive (*see also* Hypertension,
 heart) I11.9
- – rheumatic – *see* Degeneration,
 myocardial, with rheumatic fever
- – syphilitic A52.0† I52.0*
- nerve – *see* Disorder, nerve
- nervous system G31.9
- – alcoholic G31.2
- – amyloid E85.4† G99.8*
- – autonomic G90.9
- – fatty G31.8
- – specified NEC G31.8
- nipple N64.8
- olivopontocerebellar (familial)
 (hereditary) G23.8
- osseous labyrinth H83.8
- ovary N83.8

Degeneration, degenerative—*continued*
- ovary—*continued*
- – cystic N83.2
- – microcystic N83.2
- pallidal pigmentary (progressive) G23.0
- pancreas K86.8
- – tuberculous A18.8† K87.1*
- penis N48.8
- pigmentary (diffuse) (general)
 (localized) – *see* Degeneration, by site
- – pallidal (progressive) G23.0
- pineal gland E34.8
- pituitary (gland) E23.6
- placenta O43.8
- posterolateral (spinal cord) – *see*
 Degeneration, combined
- pulmonary valve (heart) I37.8
- pupillary margin H21.2
- renal N28.8
- retina (lattice) (microcystoid) (palisade)
 (paving stone) (peripheral) (reticular)
 (senile) H35.4
- – hereditary (cerebroretinal) (congenital)
 (juvenile) (macula) (peripheral)
 (pigmentary) H35.5
- – Kuhnt-Junius H35.3
- – macula (cystic) (exudative) (hole)
 (nonexudative) (pseudohole) (senile)
 (toxic) H35.3
- – pigmentary (primary) H35.5
- – posterior pole H35.3
- saccule, congenital (causing impairment
 of hearing) Q16.5
- senile R54
- – brain G31.1
- – cardiac, heart or myocardium (*see also*
 Degeneration, myocardial) I51.5
- – vascular – *see* Arteriosclerosis
- sinus (cystic) (*see also* Sinusitis) J32.9
- – polypoid J33.1
- skin L98.8
- – amyloid E85.4† L99.0*
- – colloid L98.8
- spinal (cord) G31.8
- – amyloid E85.4† G32.8*
- – combined (subacute) – *see*
 Degeneration, combined
- – dorsolateral – *see* Degeneration,
 combined
- – familial NEC G31.8
- – fatty G31.8
- – funicular – *see* Degeneration, combined
- – posterolateral – *see* Degeneration,
 combined

Degeneration, degenerative—*continued*
- spinal—*continued*
- − subacute combined − *see* Degeneration, combined
- − tuberculous A17.8† G07*
- spleen D73.0
- − amyloid F85.4† D77*
- stomach K31.8
- striatonigral G23.2
- suprarenal (capsule) (gland) E27.8
- synovial membrane (pulpy) M67.8
- tapetoretinal H35.5
- thymus (gland) E32.8
- − fatty E32.8
- thyroid (gland) E07.8
- tricuspid (heart) (valve) I07.9
- tuberculous NEC (*see also* Tuberculosis) A16.9
- turbinate J34.8
- uterus (cystic) N85.8
- vascular (senile) − *see* Arteriosclerosis
- − hypertensive − *see* Hypertension
- vitreous (body) H43.8
- Wallerian − *see* Disorder, nerve
- Wilson's hepatolenticular E83.0

Deglutition paralysis R13
- hysterical F44.4

Degos' disease I77.8

Dehiscence
- cesarean wound O90.0
- episiotomy O90.1
- operation wound NEC T81.3
- perineal wound (postpartum) O90.1
- postoperative NEC T81.3

Dehydration E86
- newborn P74.1

Déjerine-Roussy syndrome G93.8

Déjerine-Sottas disease or neuropathy (hypertrophic) G60.0

Déjerine-Thomas atrophy G23.8

Delay, delayed
- birth or delivery NEC O63.9
- − affecting fetus or newborn P03.8
- closure, ductus arteriosus (Botalli) P29.3
- coagulation (*see also* Defect, coagulation) D68.9
- conduction (cardiac) (ventricular) I45.8
- delivery, second twin, triplet, etc. O63.2
- − affecting fetus or newborn P03.8
- development R62.9
- − global F89
- − intellectual (specific) F81.9
- − learning F81.9
- − physiological R62.9

Delay, delayed—*continued*
- development—*continued*
- − physiological—*continued*
- − − specified stage NEC R62.0
- − reading F81.0
- − sexual E30.0
- − speech F80.9
- − spelling F81.1
- menstruation (cause unknown) N91.0
- milestone R62.0
- plane in pelvis, complicating delivery O66.9
- primary respiration (*see also* Asphyxia, newborn) P21.9
- puberty (constitutional) E30.0
- union, fracture M84.2

Deletion
- autosome Q93.9
- − specified NEC Q93.8
- chromosome
- − with complex rearrangements NEC Q93.7
- − part Q93.5
- − seen only at prometaphase Q93.6
- − short arm
- − − specified part NEC Q93.5
- − − − 4 Q93.3
- − − − 5 Q93.4
- − − specified part NEC Q93.5
- long arm chromosome 18 or 21 syndrome Q93.5
- − with complex rearrangements NEC Q93.7
- − specified NEC Q93.8

Delhi boil or button B55.1

Delinquency (juvenile) F91.8
- group F91.2
- neurotic F92.8

Delirium, delirious (acute or subacute) (not alcohol- or drug-induced) F05.9
- alcoholic (acute) (tremens) (withdrawal) F10.4
- − chronic F10.6
- due to (secondary to)
- − alcohol
- − − intoxication F10.0
- − − withdrawal F10.4
- − amfetamine (or related substance) intoxication (acute) F15.0
- − cannabis intoxication (acute) F12.0
- − cocaine intoxication (acute) F14.0
- − general medical condition F05.0
- − hallucinogen intoxication (acute) F16.0
- − inhalant intoxication (acute) F18.0

Delirium, delirious—*continued*
- due to—*continued*
- – multiple etiologies F05.8
- – opioid intoxication (acute) F11.0
- – phencyclidine (or related substance) intoxication (acute) F19.0
- – psychoactive substance NEC
- – – intoxication F19.0
- – – withdrawal F19.4
- – sedative, hypnotic or anxiolytic
- – – intoxication F13.0
- – – withdrawal F13.4
- – unknown etiology F05.9
- – withdrawal state – *code to* F10-F19 with fourth character .4
- exhaustion F43.0
- hysterical F44.8
- mixed origin (dementia and other) F05.8
- not superimposed on dementia F05.0
- postoperative F05.8
- puerperal F05.8
- superimposed on dementia F05.1
- thyroid E05.5
- traumatic (*see also* Injury, intracranial) S06.9
- tremens (alcohol-induced) F10.4
- – drug withdrawal – *code to* F11-F19 with fourth character .4
- uremic N19

Delivery (single) O80.9
- assisted O83.9
- – specified NEC O83.8
- breech NEC O83.1
- – affecting fetus or newborn P03.0
- – assisted NEC O83.1
- – extraction NEC O83.0
- cesarean (for) O82.9
- – with hysterectomy O82.2
- – abnormal
- – – cervix O34.4
- – – pelvis (bony) (deformity) (major) NEC with disproportion (fetopelvic) O33.0
- – – – with obstructed labor O65.0
- – – presentation or position O32.9
- – – – in multiple gestation O32.5
- – – uterus, congenital O34.0
- – – vagina O34.6
- – – vulva O34.7
- – abruptio placentae (*see also* Abruptio placentae) O45.9
- – acromion presentation O32.2
- – affecting fetus or newborn P03.4
- – anteversion, uterus O34.5

Delivery—*continued*
- cesarean—*continued*
- – atony, uterus O62.2
- – breech presentation O32.1
- – brow presentation O32.3
- – cephalopelvic disproportion O33.9
- – cerclage O34.3
- – chin presentation O32.3
- – cicatrix of cervix O34.4
- – contracted pelvis (general)
- – – inlet O33.2
- – – outlet O33.3
- – cord presentation or prolapse O69.0
- – cystocele O34.8
- – deformity (acquired) (congenital)
- – – pelvic organs or tissues NEC O34.8
- – – pelvis (bony) NEC O33.0
- – displacement, uterus NEC O34.5
- – disproportion NEC O33.9
- – distress
- – – fetal O36.3
- – – maternal O75.0
- – eclampsia O15.0
- – elective O82.0
- – emergency O82.1
- – face presentation O32.3
- – failed
- – – forceps O66.5
- – – trial of labour NEC O66.4
- – – vacuum extraction O66.5
- – – ventouse O66.5
- – fetal-maternal hemorrhage O43.0
- – hemorrhage (antepartum) O46.9
- – – intrapartum O67.9
- – high head at term O32.4
- – hydrocephalic fetus O33.6
- – incarceration of uterus O34.5
- – incoordinate uterine action O62.4
- – increased size, fetus O33.5
- – inertia, uterus O62.2
- – – primary O62.0
- – – secondary O62.1
- – lateroversion, uterus O34.5
- – mal lie O32.9
- – malposition
- – – fetus O32.9
- – – – in multiple gestation O32.5
- – – pelvic organs or tissues NEC O34.8
- – – uterus NEC O34.5
- – malpresentation NEC O32.9
- – – in multiple gestation O32.5
- – maternal
- – – diabetes mellitus (*see also* Diabetes, complicating pregnancy) O24.9

Delivery—*continued*
- cesarean—*continued*
- - maternal—*continued*
- - - heart disease NEC O99.4
- - meconium in liquor O36.3
- - oblique presentation O32.2
- - oversized fetus O33.5
- - pelvic tumor NEC O34.8
- - placenta previa (with hemorrhage) O44.1
- - - without hemorrhage O44.0
- placental insufficiency O36.5
- - polyp, cervix O34.4
- - poor dilatation, cervix O62.0
- - pre-eclampsia (*see also* Pre-eclampsia) O14.9
- - preterm NEC O60.1
- - - with spontaneous labor O60.1
- - - without spontaneous labor O60.3
- - previous
- - - cesarean section O34.2
- - - surgery (to)
- - - - cervix O34.4
- - - - gynecological NEC O34.8
- - - - uterus O34.2
- - - - vagina O34.6
- - prolapse
- - - arm or hand O32.2
- - - uterus O34.5
- - prolonged labor NEC O63.9
- - rectocele O34.8
- - repeat NEC O82.0
- - retroversion O34.5
- - - uterus O34.5
- - rigid
- - - cervix O34.4
- - - pelvic floor O34.8
- - - perineum O34.7
- - - vagina O34.6
- - - vulva O34.7
- - sacculation, pregnant uterus O34.5
- - scar(s)
- - - cervix O34.4
- - - cesarean section O34.2
- - - uterus O34.2
- - Shirodkar suture in situ O34.3
- - shoulder presentation O32.2
- - specified NEC O82.8
- - stenosis or stricture, cervix O34.4
- - transverse presentation or lie O32.2
- - tumor, pelvic organs or tissues NEC O34.8
- - - cervix O34.4

Delivery—*continued*
- cesarean—*continued*
- - umbilical cord presentation or prolapse O69.0
- cleidotomy, to facilitate delivery O83.4
- completely normal case (*see also* Note at category O80.-) O80.9
- complicated (by) O75.9
- - abnormal, abnormality of
- - - forces of labor O62.9
- - - - specified type NEC O62.8
- - - uterine contractions NEC O62.9
- - abruptio placentae NEC O45.8
- - adherent placenta (morbidly) O43.2
- - anesthetic death O74.8
- - annular detachment of cervix O71.3
- - apoplexy (cerebral) O99.4
- - atony, uterus O62.2
- - Bandl's ring O62.4
- - bleeding (*see also* Delivery, complicated by, hemorrhage) O67.9
- - cerebral hemorrhage O99.4
- - cervical dystocia (failure of cervical dilatation) O62.0
- - - due to abnormality of cervix O65.5
- - compression of cord (umbilical) NEC O69.2
- - - around neck O69.1
- - contraction, contracted ring O62.4
- - cord (umbilical)
- - - around neck, tightly or with compression O69.1
- - - - without compression O69.8
- - - bruising O69.5
- - - complication O69.9
- - - - specified NEC O69.8
- - - compression NEC O69.82
- - - entanglement O69.2
- - - hematoma O69.5
- - - presentation O69.0
- - - prolapse O69.0
- - - short O69.3
- - - thrombosis (vessels) O69.5
- - - vascular lesion O69.5
- - Couvelaire uterus (*see also* Abruptio placentae) O45.8
- - death (sudden), unknown cause O95
- - delay following rupture of membranes (spontaneous) O75.6
- - diastasis recti (abdominis) O71.8
- - dilatation
- - - bladder O66.8
- - - cervix incomplete, poor or slow O62.0

Delivery—*continued*
- complicated—*continued*
- − diseased placenta O43.9
- − disruptio uteri − *see* Delivery,
  complicated by, rupture, uterus
- − distress
- − − fetal O68.9
- − − − biochemical evidence O68.3
- − − − electrocardiographic evidence
  O68.8
- − − − specified evidence NEC O68.8
- − − − ultrasonic evidence O68.8
- − − maternal O75.0
- − dysfunction, uterus NEC O62.9
- − − hypertonic O62.4
- − − hypotonic O62.2
- − − − primary O62.0
- − − − secondary O62.1
- − − incoordinate O62.4
- − eclampsia O15.1
- − embolism (pulmonary) O88.2
- − − air O88.0
- − − amniotic fluid O88.1
- − − blood-clot O88.2
- − − fat O88.8
- − − pyemic O88.3
- − − septic O88.3
- − fetal
- − − deformity O66.3
- − − distress (*see also* Delivery,
  complicated by, distress, fetal)
  O68.9
- − − heart rate anomaly O68.0
- − − − with meconium in liquor O68.2
- − fever during labor O75.2
- − hematoma O71.7
- − − ischial spine O71.7
- − − pelvic O71.7
- − − subdural O99.4
- − − vagina O71.7
- − − vulva or perineum O71.7
- − hemorrhage (uterine) O67.9
- − − accidental (*see also* Abruptio
  placentae) O45.9
- − − associated with
- − − − afibrinogenemia O67.0
- − − − coagulation defect O67.0
- − − − hyperfibrinolysis O67.0
- − − − hypofibrinogenemia O67.0
- − − cerebral O99.4
- − − due to
- − − − low-lying placenta O44.1
- − − − placenta previa O44.1

Delivery—*continued*
- complicated—*continued*
- − hemorrhage—*continued*
- − − due to—*continued*
- − − − premature separation of placenta
  (normally implanted) (*see also*
  Abruptio placentae) O45.9
- − − − retained placenta O72.0
- − − − trauma (obstetric) O67.8
- − − − uterine leiomyoma O67.8
- − − placenta NEC O67.8
- − − postpartum NEC (atonic)
  (immediate) O72.1
- − − − with retained or trapped placenta
  O72.0
- − − − delayed O72.2
- − − − secondary O72.2
- − − − third stage O72.0
- − hourglass contraction, uterus O62.4
- − hypertension (*see also* Hypertension,
  complicating pregnancy) O16
- − incomplete dilatation (cervix) O62.0
- − incoordinate uterine contractions
  O62.4
- − inertia, uterus O62.2
- − − primary O62.0
- − − secondary O62.1
- − infantile
- − − genitalia NEC O34.8
- − − uterus O34.5
- − injury (to mother) O71.9
- − inversion, uterus O71.2
- − laceration O70.9
- − − anus (sphincter) O70.2
- − − − with mucosa O70.3
- − − bladder (urinary) O71.5
- − − bowel O71.5
- − − cervix (uteri) O71.3
- − − fourchette O70.0
- − − hymen O70.0
- − − labia O70.0
- − − pelvic
- − − − floor O70.1
- − − − organ NEC O71.5
- − − − perineum, perineal O70.9
- − − − − first degree O70.0
- − − − − fourth degree O70.3
- − − − − muscles O70.1
- − − − − second degree O70.1
- − − − − skin O70.0
- − − − − slight O70.0
- − − − − third degree O70.2
- − − peritoneum O71.5

Delivery—*continued*
- complicated—*continued*
- – laceration—*continued*
- – – rectovaginal (septum) (without
  perineal laceration) O71.4
- – – – with perineum O70.2
- – – – – with anal or rectal mucosa
  O70.3
- – – specified NEC O71.8
- – sphincter anl O70.2
- – – – with mucosa O70.3
- – – urethra O71.5
- – – uterus O71.1
- – – – before labour O71.0
- – – vagina, vaginal (deep) (high)
  (without perineal laceration) O71.4
- – – – with perineum O70.0
- – – – – and muscles (perineal) (vaginal)
  O70.1
- – – vulva O70.0
- – malposition
- – – placenta (with hemorrhage) O44.1
- – – – without hemorrhage O44.0
- – – uterus or cervix O65.5
- – meconium in liquor O68.1
- – – with fetal heart rate anomaly O68.2
- – metrorrhexis – *see* Delivery,
  complicated by, rupture, uterus
- – obstetric trauma O71.9
- – – specified NEC O71.8
- – obstruction – *see* Labor, obstructed
- – pathological retraction ring, uterus
  O62.4
- – penetration, pregnant uterus, by
  instrument O71.1
- – perforation – *see* Delivery, complicated
  by, laceration
- – placenta, placental
- – – ablatio (*see also* Abruptio placentae)
  O45.9
- – – abnormality NEC O43.1
- – – abruptio (*see also* Abruptio
  placentae) O45.9
- – – accreta O43.2
- – – adherent (morbidly) O43.2
- – – detachment (premature) (*see also*
  Abruptio placentae) O45.9
- – – disorder O43.9
- – – hemorrhage NEC O67.8
- – – increta O43.2
- – – low (implantation) (with
  hemorrhage) O44.1
- – – – without hemorrhage O44.0
- – – malformation NEC O43.1

Delivery—*continued*
- complicated—*continued*
- – placenta, placental—*continued*
- – – malposition (with hemorrhage)
  O44.1
- – – – without hemorrhage O44.0
- – – percreta O43.2
- – – previa (central) (lateral) (marginal)
  (partial) (with hemorrhage) O44.1
- – – – without hemorrhage O44.0
- – – retained (with hemorrhage) O72.0
- – – – without hemorrhage O73.0
- – – separation (premature) (*see also*
  Abruptio placentae) O45.9
- – – vicious insertion (with hemorrhage)
  O44.1
- – – – without hemorrhage O44.0
- – precipitate labor O62.3
- – premature rupture, membranes (*see also*
  Rupture, membranes, premature)
  O42.9
- – previous
- – – cesarean section O75.7
- – – surgery
- – – – cervix O34.4
- – – – gynecological NEC O34.8
- – – – perineum O34.7
- – – – uterus NEC O34.2
- – – – vagina O34.6
- – – – vulva O34.7
- – primipara, elderly or old – *code as*
  Delivery, complicated by, specific
  condition
- – prolapse
- – – arm or hand O32.2
- – – cord (umbilical) O69.0
- – – foot or leg O32.1
- – – uterus O34.5
- – prolonged labor O63.9
- – – first stage O63.0
- – – second stage O63.1
- – retained membranes or portions of
  placenta O72.2
- – – without hemorrhage O73.1
- – retarded birth O63.9
- – retention of secundines (with
  hemorrhage) O72.0
- – – partial O72.2
- – – – without hemorrhage O73.1
- – – without hemorrhage O73.0
- – rupture
- – – bladder (urinary) O71.5
- – – cervix O71.3
- – – pelvic organ NEC O71.5

Delivery—*continued*
- complicated—*continued*
- - rupture—*continued*
- - - perineum (without mention of other laceration) – *see* Delivery, complicated by, laceration, perineum
- - - urethra O71.5
- - - uterus (during or after labor) O71.1
- - - - before labor O71.0
- - sacculation, pregnant uterus O34.5
- - scar(s)
- - - cervix O34.4
- - - cesarean section O75.7
- - - uterus NEC O34.2
- - separation, pubic bone (symphysis pubis) O71.6
- - shock O75.1
- - shoulder presentation O64.4
- - spasm, cervix O62.4
- - stenosis or stricture, cervix O65.5
- - stress, fetal – *see* Delivery, complicated by, distress, fetal
- - tear – *see* Delivery, complicated by, laceration
- - tetanic uterus O62.4
- - trauma (obstetrical) O71.9
- - tumor, pelvic organs or tissues NEC O65.5
- - uterine inertia O62.2
- - - primary O62.0
- - - secondary O62.1
- - vasa previa O69.4
- - velamentous insertion of cord O69.8
- craniotomy, to facilitate delivery O83.4
- delayed NEC O63.9
- - following rupture of membranes (spontaneous) O75.6
- - - artificial O75.5
- - second twin, triplet, etc. O63.2
- destructive operation O83.4
- difficult NEC
- - previous, affecting management of pregnancy Z35.2
- early onset NEC O60.1
- - with spontaneous labor O60.1
- - without spontaneous labor (cesarean section) (induction) O60.3
- embryotomy, to facilitate delivery O83.4
- forceps NEC O81.3
- - with ventouse (vacuum extractor) O81.5
- - affecting fetus or newborn P03.2
- - low O81.0

Delivery—*continued*
- forceps NEC—*continued*
- - low—*continued*
- - - following failed vacuum extraction O66.5
- - mid-cavity O81.1
- - - with rotation O81.2
- manipulation-assisted NEC O83.2
- missed (at or near term) O36.4
- multiple O84.9
- - all (by)
- - - cesarean section O84.2
- - - forceps O84.1
- - - spontaneous O84.0
- - - vacuum extractor O84.1
- - combination of methods O84.8
- - specified NEC O84.8   O80.-
- normal (*see also* Note at category O80.9) O80.9
- postoperative F05.8
- precipitate O62.3
- - affecting fetus or newborn P03.5
- premature or preterm NEC O60.1
- - with spontaneous labor O60.1
- - without spontaneous labor (cesarean section) (induction) O60.3
- - previous, affecting management of pregnancy Z35.2
- spontaneous O80.9
- - breech O80.1
- - specified NEC O80.8
- - vertex O80.0
- threatened premature (before 37 weeks of gestation) O47.0
- uncomplicated (*see also* Note at category O80.9) O80.9
- vacuum extractor NEC O81.4
- - with forceps O81.5
- - affecting fetus or newborn P03.3
- vaginal, following previous cesarean section O75.7
- ventouse NEC O81.4
- - affecting fetus or newborn P03.3
- version with extraction O83.2
- viable fetus in abdominal pregnancy O83.3

Delusions (paranoid) – *see* Disorder, delusional
Dementia (persisting) F03
- alcoholic F10.7
- Alzheimer's type G30.9† F00.9∗
- arteriosclerotic (*see also* Dementia, vascular) F01.9
- atypical, Alzheimer's type G30.8† F00.2∗

Dementia—*continued*
- degenerative (primary) F03
- frontal lobe G31.0† F02.0*
- frontotemporal G31.0† F02.0*
- in (due to)
- - alcohol F10.7
- - Alzheimer's disease G30.9† F00.9*
- - - with onset
- - - - early G30.0† F00.0*
- - - - late G30.1† F00.1*
- - - atypical G30.8† F00.2*
- - - mixed type G30.8† F00.2*
- - arteriosclerotic brain disease F01.9
- - cerebral lipidoses E75.-† F02.8*
- - Creutzfeldt-Jakob disease A81.0†
  F02.1*
- - drugs (residual) – *code to* F10-F19 with
  fourth character .7
- - epilepsy G40.-† F02.8*
- - general paralysis of the insane A52.1†
  F02.8*
- - hepatolenticular degeneration E83.0†
  F02.8*
- - human immunodeficiency virus (HIV)
  disease B22.0† F02.4*
- - Huntington's disease or chorea G10†
  F02.2*
- - hypercalcemia E83.5† F02.8*
- - hypothyroidism, acquired E03.-†
  F02.8*
- - - due to iodine-deficiency E01.-†
  F02.8*
- - inhalants F18.7
- - intoxication (*see also* Table of drugs
  and chemicals) T65.9† F02.8*
- - multiple
- - - etiologies F03
- - - sclerosis G35† F02.8*
- - neurosyphilis A52.1† F02.8*
- - niacin deficiency E52† F02.8*
- - paralysis agitans G20† F02.3*
- - Parkinson's disease (parkinsonism)
  G20† F02.3*
- - pellagra E52† F02.8*
- - Pick's disease G31.0† F02.0*
- - polyarteritis nodosa M30.0† F02.8*
- - sedatives, hypnotics or anxiolytics
  F13.7
- - systemic lupus erythematosus M32.-†
  F02.8*
- - trypanosomiasis, African B56.-†
  F02.8*
- - unknown etiology F03
- - vitamin B12 deficiency E53.8† F02.8*

Dementia—*continued*
- in—*continued*
- - volatile solvents F18.7
- infantile, infantilis F84.3
- Lewy body G31.8
- multi-infarct F01.1
- old age F03
- paralytica, paralytic (syphilitic) A52.1†
  F02.8*
- - juvenilis A50.4
- paretic A52.1† F02.8*
- praecox (*see also* Schizophrenia) F20.9
- presenile F03
- - Alzheimer's type G30.0† F00.0*
- primary degenerative F03
- progressive, syphilitic A52.1† F02.8*
- resulting from HIV disease B22.0†
  F02.4*
- senile F03
- - with acute confusional state F05.1
- - Alzheimer's type G30.1† F00.1*
- - depressed or paranoid type F03
- uremic N18.5† F02.8*
- vascular (of) F01.9
- - acute onset F01.0
- - mixed cortical and subcortical F01.3
- - multi-infarct F01.1
- - predominantly cortical F01.1
- - specified NEC F01.8
- - subcortical F01.2
Demineralization, bone (*see also*
  Osteoporosis) M81.9
Demodex folliculorum (infestation) B88.0
Demoralization R45.3
Demyelination, demyelinization
- central nervous system G37.9
- - specified NEC G37.8
- corpus callosum (central) G37.1
- disseminated, acute G36.9
- - specified NEC G36.8
- in optic neuritis G36.0
Dengue (classical) (fever) A90
- hemorrhagic A91
Dennie-Marfan syphilitic syndrome
  A50.4
Dens evaginatus, in dente or invaginatus
  K00.2
Density
- increased, bone (disseminated)
  (generalized) (spotted) M85.8
- lung (nodular) J98.4
Dental – *see also* condition
- examination Z01.2
Dentia praecox K00.6

Denticles (pulp) K04.2
Dentigerous cyst K09.0
Dentin
– irregular (in pulp) K04.3
– secondary (in pulp) K04.3
– sensitive K03.8
Dentinogenesis imperfecta K00.5
Dentinoma (M9271/0) D16.5
– upper jaw (bone) D16.4
Dentition (syndrome) K00.7
– delayed K00.6
– difficult K00.7
– precocious K00.6
– premature K00.6
– retarded K00.6
Dependence
– due to
– – alcohol (ethyl) (methyl) F10.2
– – – counseling and surveillance Z71.4
– – – detoxification therapy Z50.2
– – – rehabilitation measures Z50.2
– – amfetamine(s) (type) F15.2
– – amobarbital F13.2
– – amytal (sodium) F13.2
– – anxiolytic NEC F13.2
– – barbital(s) F13.2
– – barbiturate(s) (compounds) (drugs
classifiable to T42.3) F13.2
– – bhang F12.2
– – bromide(s) NEC F13.2
– – caffeine F15.2
– – Cannabis (indica) (sativa) (derivatives)
(resin) (type) F12.2
– – chlordiazepoxide F13.2
– – cloral (betaine) (hydrate) F13.2
– – coca (leaf) (derivatives) F14.2
– – cocaine F14.2
– – codeine F11.2
– – combinations of drugs F19.2
– – dagga F12.2
– – dexamfetamine(s) (type) F15.2
– – dextromethorphan F11.2
– – dextromoramide F11.2
– – dextrorphan F11.2
– – diazepam F13.2
– – drug NEC F19.2
– – – combinations NEC F19.2
– – – complicating pregnancy, childbirth or
puerperium O99.3
– – – – affecting fetus or newborn P04.4
– – – – withdrawal symptoms in newborn
P96.1
– – – counseling and surveillance Z71.5
– – – soporific NEC F13.2

Dependence—*continued*
– due to—*continued*
– – drug NEC—*continued*
– – – suspected damage to fetus, affecting
management of pregnancy O35.5
– – – synthetic, with morphine-like effect
F11.2
– – ethyl
– – – alcohol F10.2
– – – bromide F13.2
– – – carbamate F19.2
– – – chloride F19.2
– – – morphine F11.2
– – ganja F12.2
– – glue (airplane) (sniffing) F18.2
– – glutethimide F13.2
– – hallucinogenics F16.2
– – hashish F12.2
– – hemp F12.2
– – heroin (salt) (any) F11.2
– – hypnotic NEC F13.2
– – Indian hemp F12.2
– – inhalants F18.2
– – khat F15.2
– – laudanum F11.2
– – LSD(-25) (derivatives) F16.2
– – luminal F13.2
– – lysergide, lysergic acid, D-lysergic acid
diethylamide F16.2
– – maconha F12.2
– – marihuana, marijuana F12.2
– – meprobamate F13.2
– – mescaline F16.2
– – metamfetamine(s) F15.2
– – methadone F11.2
– – methaqualone F13.2
– – methyl
– – – alcohol F10.2
– – – bromide F13.2
– – – morphine F11.2
– – – phenidate F15.2
– – morphine (sulfate) (sulfite) (type)
F11.2
– – narcotic (drug) NEC F19.2
– – nicotine F17.2
– – nitrous oxide F19.2
– – nonbarbiturate sedatives and
tranquilizers with similar effect F13.2
– – opiate F11.2
– – opioids F11.2
– – opium (alkaloids) (derivatives)
(tincture) F11.2
– – paraldehyde F13.2
– – paregoric F11.2

Dependence—*continued*
− due to—*continued*
− − PCP (phencyclidine) F19.2
− − pentobarbital, pentobarbitone (sodium) F13.2
− − peyote F16.2
− − phencyclidine (PCP) (and related substances) F19.2
− − phenmetrazine F15.2
− − phenobarbital F13.2
− − polysubstance F19.2
− − psilocin, psilocybine F16.2
− − psychostimulant NEC F15.2
− − secobarbital (sodium) F13.2
− − sedative NEC F13.2
− − specified drug NEC F19.2
− − stimulant NEC F15.2
− − substance NEC F19.2
− − tobacco F17.2
− − − counseling and surveillance Z71.6
− − tranquilizer NEC F13.2
− − volatile solvents F18.2
− on
− − aspirator Z99.0
− − care provider (because of) Z74.9
− − − impaired mobility Z74.0
− − − need for
− − − − assistance with personal care Z74.1
− − − − continuous supervision Z74.3
− − − no other household member able to render care Z74.2
− − − specified reason NEC Z74.8
− − machine Z99.9
− − − enabling NEC Z99.8
− − − specified type NEC Z99.8
− − renal dialysis Z99.2
− − respirator Z99.1
− − wheelchair Z99.3
− syndrome – *code to* F10-F19 with fourth character .2
Dependency
− care-provider Z74.9
− passive F60.7
− reactions (persistent) F60.7
Depersonalization (in neurotic state) (neurotic) (syndrome) F48.1
Depletion
− potassium E87.6
− salt or sodium E87.1
− − causing heat exhaustion or prostration T67.4
− volume
− − extracellular fluid E86

Depletion—*continued*
− volume—*continued*
− − plasma E86
Depolarization, premature I49.4
− atrial I49.1
− junctional I49.2
− specified NEC I49.4
− ventricular I49.3
Deposit
− bone in Boeck's sarcoid D86.8
− calcareous, calcium – *see* Calcification
− cholesterol
− − retina H35.8
− − vitreous (body) (humor) H43.2
− conjunctiva H11.1
− cornea H18.0
− crystallin, vitreous (body) (humor) H43.2
− hemosiderin in old scars of cornea H18.0
− metallic in lens H26.8
− skin R23.8
− tooth, teeth (betel) (black) (green) (materia alba) (orange) (tobacco) K03.6
− urate, kidney (*see also* Calculus, kidney) N20.0
Depraved appetite F50.8
− in childhood F98.3
Depression F32.9
− acute F32.9
− agitated (single episode) F32.2
− anxiety F41.2
− − persistent F34.1
− arches M21.4
− − congenital Q66.5
− atypical (single episode) F32.8
− basal metabolic rate R94.8
− bone marrow D61.9
− cerebral R29.8
− − newborn P91.4
− cerebrovascular I67.9
− chest wall M95.4
− climacteric (single episode) F32.8
− endogenous (without psychotic symptoms) F33.2
− − with psychotic symptoms F33.3
− functional activity R68.8
− hysterical F44.8
− involutional (single episode) F32.8
− major (without psychotic symptoms) F32.2
− − with psychotic symptoms F32.3
− − recurrent – *see* Disorder, depressive, recurrent
− manic-depressive – *see* Disorder, depressive, recurrent

Depression—*continued*
- masked (single episode) F32.8
- medullary G93.8
- menopausal (single episode) F32.8
- mental F32.9
- metatarsus – *see* Depression, arches
- monopolar F33.9
- nervous F34.1
- neurotic F34.1
- nose M95.0
- postnatal F53.0
- postpartum F53.0
- post-psychotic of schizophrenia F20.4
- post-schizophrenic F20.4
- psychogenic (reactive) (single episode) F32.9
- psychoneurotic F34.1
- psychotic (single episode) F32.3
- – recurrent F33.3
- reactive (psychogenic) (single episode) F32.9
- – psychotic F32.3
- recurrent (*see also* Disorder, depressive, recurrent) F33.9
- respiration, respiratory, newborn P28.5
- respiratory center G93.8
- seasonal (*see also* Disorder, depressive, recurrent) F33.9
- senile F03
- severe, single episode F32.2
- skull Q67.4
- specified NEC (single episode) F32.8
- sternum M95.4
- visual field H53.4
- vital (recurrent) (without psychotic symptoms) F33.2
- – with psychotic symptoms F33.3
- – single episode F32.2

Deprivation (effects) T73.9
- cultural Z60.3
- emotional NEC Z65.8
- – affecting infant or child T74.3
- food T73.0
- protein (*see also* Malnutrition) E46
- – severe (*see also* Malnutrition, severe) E43
- social Z60.4
- – affecting infant or child T74.3
- specified NEC T73.8
- symptoms, syndrome, drug (narcotic) – *code to* F10-F19 with fourth character .3
- vitamins (*see also* Deficiency, vitamin) E56.9
- water T73.1

Derangement
- cartilage (articular) NEC M24.1
- – knee, meniscus (*see also* Derangement, meniscus) M23.3
- – – recurrent M24.4
- – recurrent M24.4
- elbow (internal) M24.9
- – recurrent M24.4
- joint (internal) M24.9
- – current injury (*see also* Dislocation) T14.3
- – – knee, cartilage or meniscus S83.2
- – elbow M24.9
- – knee M23.9
- – – current injury S83.2
- – – specified NEC M23.8
- – – recurrent M24.4
- – shoulder M24.9
- – specified NEC M24.8
- – temporomandibular K07.6
- knee M23.9
- – current injury S83.2
- – recurrent M24.4
- – specified NEC M23.8
- low back NEC M53.8
- meniscus (anterior horn) (posterior horn) (lateral) (medial) M23.3
- – due to old tear or injury M23.2
- – recurrent M24.4
- mental (*see also* Psychosis) F29
- patella, specified NEC M22.3
- semilunar cartilage (knee) M23.3
- – recurrent M24.4
- shoulder (internal) M24.9
- – current injury (*see also* Dislocation, shoulder) S43.0

Dercum's disease E88.2
Derealization (neurotic) F48.1
Dermal – *see condition*
Dermaphytid – *see* Dermatophytosis
Dermatitis L30.9
- ab igne L59.0
- acarine B88.0
- actinic (due to sun) L57.8
- – other than from sun L59.8
- allergic (contact) (*see also* Dermatitis, due to) L23.9
- ambustionis, due to burn or scald – *see* Burn
- amebic A06.7
- arsenical (ingested) L27.8
- artefacta L98.1
- atopic L20.9
- – specified NEC L20.8

Dermatitis—*continued*
- berlock, berloque L56.2
- blastomycetic B40.3† L99.8*
- blister beetle L24.8
- bullous, bullosa L13.9
- – mucosynechial, atrophic L12.1
- – seasonal L30.8
- – specified NEC L13.8
- calorica L59.0
- – due to burn or scald – *see* Burn
- caterpillar L24.8
- cercarial B65.3
- combustionis L59.0
- – due to burn or scald – *see* Burn
- congelationis T69.1
- contact (occupational) (*see also* Dermatitis, due to) L25.9
- – allergic L23.9
- – irritant L24.9
- diabetic (*see also* E10-E14 with fourth character .6) E14.6† L99.8*
- diaper L22
- diphtheritica A36.3
- dry skin L85.3
- due to
- – acetone (contact) (irritant) L24.2
- – acids (contact) (irritant) L24.5
- – adhesives (allergic) (contact) (plaster) L23.1
- – – irritant L24.5
- – alcohols (irritant) (skin contact) (substances in T51.-) L24.2
- – – taken internally L27.8
- – alkalis (contact) (irritant) L24.5
- – arsenic (ingested) L27.8
- – carbon disulfide (contact) (irritant) L24.2
- – caustics (contact) (irritant) L24.5
- – cement (contact) L25.3
- – – allergic L23.5
- – – irritant L24.5
- – chemicals NEC L25.3
- – – in contact with skin L25.3
- – – – allergic L23.5
- – – – irritant NEC L24.5
- – – taken internally L27.8
- – chromium (allergic) (contact) L23.0
- – – irritant L24.8
- – cold weather L30.8
- – cosmetics (contact) L25.0
- – – allergic L23.2
- – – irritant L24.3
- – Demodex species B88.0
- – Dermanyssus gallinae B88.0

Dermatitis—*continued*
- due to—*continued*
- – detergents (contact) (irritant) L24.0
- – dichromate (allergic) L23.0
- – – irritant L24.5
- – drugs and medicaments (correct substance properly administered) (generalized) (internal use) L27.0
- – – external (*see also* Dermatitis, due to, drugs, in contact with skin) L25.1
- – – – wrong substance given or taken T49.9
- – – – – specified substance – *see* Table of drugs and chemicals
- – – in contact with skin L25.1
- – – – allergic L23.3
- – – – irritant L24.4
- – – localized skin eruption L27.1
- – – wrong substance given or taken T50.9
- – – – specified substance – *see* Table of drugs and chemicals
- – dyes (contact) L25.2
- – – allergic L23.4
- – – irritant L24.8
- – epidermophytosis – *see* Dermatophytosis
- – external irritant NEC L24.9
- – food (ingested) L27.2
- – – in contact with skin L25.4
- – – – allergic L23.6
- – – – irritant L24.6
- – furs (allergic) (contact) L23.8
- – – irritant L24.8
- – glues – *see* Dermatitis, due to, adhesives
- – greases NEC (contact) (irritant) L24.1
- – hot
- – – objects and materials – *see* Burn
- – – weather or places L59.0
- – infrared rays L59.8
- – ingestion, ingested substance L27.9
- – – chemicals NEC L27.8
- – – drugs and medicaments (correct substance properly administered) (generalized) (*see also* Dermatitis, due to, drugs) L27.0
- – – – localized skin eruption L27.1
- – – – wrong substance given or taken T50.9
- – – – – specified substance – *see* Table of drugs and chemicals
- – – food L27.2
- – – specified NEC L27.8

Dermatitis—*continued*
- due to—*continued*
- - insecticide, in contact with skin L25.3
- - - allergic L23.5
- - - irritant L24.5
- - internal agent L27.9
- - - drugs and medicaments (generalized) (*see also* Dermatitis, due to, drugs) L27.0
- - - food L27.2
- - irradiation – *see* Dermatitis, due to, radioactive substances
- - lacquer tree (allergic) (contact) L23.7
- - light (sun) NEC L57.8
- - - acute L56.8
- - - other L59.8
- - Liponyssoides sanguineus B88.0
- - low temperature L30.8
- - metals, metal salts (allergic) (contact) L23.0
- - - irritant L24.8
- - nickel (allergic) (contact) L23.0
- - - irritant L24.8
- - nylon (allergic) (contact) L23.5
- - - irritant L24.5
- - oils NEC (contact) (irritant) L24.1
- - paint solvents (contact) (irritant) L24.2
- - petroleum products (contact) (irritant) (substances in T52.-) L24.2
- - plants NEC (contact) L25.5
- - - allergic L23.7
- - - irritant L24.7
- - plasters (adhesive) (any) (allergic) (contact) L23.1
- - - irritant L24.5
- - plastic (allergic) (contact) L23.5
- - - irritant L24.5
- - preservatives (contact) – *see* Dermatitis, due to, chemicals, in contact with skin
- - primrose (allergic) (contact) L23.7
- - primula (allergic) (contact) L23.7
- - radiation L59.8
- - - nonionizing (chronic exposure) L57.8
- - - sun NEC L57.8
- - - - acute L56.8
- - radioactive substances L58.9
- - - acute L58.0
- - - chronic L58.1
- - radium L58.9
- - - acute L58.0
- - - chronic L58.1
- - ragweed (allergic) (contact) L23.7

Dermatitis—*continued*
- due to—*continued*
- - Rhus (diversiloba) (radicans) (toxicodendron) (venenata) (verniciflua) (allergic) (contact) L23.7
- - rubber (allergic) (contact) L23.5
- - Senecio jacobaea (allergic) (contact) L23.7
- - solvents (contact) (irritant) (substances in T52-T53) L24.2
- - specified agent NEC (contact) L25.8
- - - allergic L23.8
- - - irritant L24.8
- - sunshine NEC L57.8
- - - acute L56.8
- - tetrachlorethylene (contact) (irritant) L24.2
- - toluene (contact) (irritant) L24.2
- - turpentine (contact) L25.3
- - - allergic L23.5
- - - irritant L24.2
- - ultraviolet rays (sun NEC) (chronic exposure) L57.8
- - - acute L56.8
- - vaccine or vaccination (correct substance properly administered) L27.0
- - - wrong substance given or taken T50.9
- - varicose veins I83.1
- - X-rays L58.9
- - - acute L58.0
- - - chronic L58.1
- dysmenorrheica N94.6
- eczematous NEC L30.9
- escharotica – *see* Burn
- exfoliative, exfoliativa (generalized) L26
- eyelid (allergic) (contact) (eczematous) H01.1
- - due to
- - - Demodex species B88.0† H03.0*
- - - herpes (zoster) B02.3† H03.1*
- - - - simplex B00.5† H03.1*
- facta, factitia, factitial L98.1
- flexural NEC L20.8
- friction L30.4
- fungus B36.9
- - specified type NEC B36.8
- gangrenosa, gangrenous infantum L08.0
- harvest mite B88.0† L99.8*
- heat L59.0
- herpesviral, vesicular (ear) (lip) B00.1
- herpetiformis (bullous) (erythematous) (pustular) (vesicular) L13.0

Dermatitis—*continued*
- herpetiformis—*continued*
- – juvenile L12.2
- – senile L12.0
- hiemalis L30.8
- hypostatic, hypostatica I83.1
- – with ulcer I83.2
- infectious eczematoid L30.3
- infective L30.3
- irritant (contact) (*see also* Dermatitis, due to) L24.9
- Jacquet's L22
- Leptus B88.0† L99,8∗
- lichenified NEC L28.0
- medicamentosa (correct substance properly administered) (generalized) (internal use) (*see also* Dermatitis, due to, drugs) L27.0
- – due to contact with skin L25.1
- – – allergic L23.3
- – – irritant L24.4
- – localized skin eruption L27.1
- mite B88.0† L99.8∗
- napkin L22
- nummular L30.0
- papillaris capillitii L73.0
- pellagrous E52
- perioral L71.0
- photocontact L56.2
- pruritic NEC L30.8
- purulent L08.0
- pustular
- – contagious B08.0
- – subcorneal L13.1
- pyococcal L08.0
- pyogenica L08.0
- repens L40.2
- Schamberg's L81.7
- schistosome B65.3
- seasonal bullous L30.8
- seborrheic L21.9
- – infantile L21.1
- – specified NEC L21.8
- sensitization NEC L23.9
- septic L08.0
- solare L57.8
- specified NEC L30.8
- stasis I83.1
- – with ulcer I83.2
- suppurative L08.0
- traumatic NEC L30.4
- ultraviolet (sun) (chronic exposure) L57.8
- – acute L56.8
- varicose I83.1

Dermatitis—*continued*
- varicose—*continued*
- – with ulcer I83.2
- vegetans L10.1
- verrucosa B43.0† L99.8∗
- vesicular, herpesviral B00.1
Dermatoarthritis, lipoid E78.8† M14.3∗
Dermatofibroma (lenticulare) (M8832/0) – *see* Neoplasm, skin, benign
Dermatofibrosarcoma (M8832/3) – *see also* Neoplasm, skin, malignant
- protuberans (M8832/3) C44.9
- – pigmented (M8833/3) C80.-
Dermatographia L50.3
Dermatolysis (exfoliativa) (congenital) Q82.8
- acquired L57.4
- eyelids H02.3
- palpebrarum H02.3
- senile L57.4
Dermatomegaly NEC Q82.8
Dermatomucosomyositis M33.1
Dermatomycosis B36.9
- furfuracea B36.0
- specified type NEC B36.8
Dermatomyositis (acute) (chronic) M33.1
- with lung involvement M33.-† J99.1∗
- in (due to) neoplastic disease NEC (M8000/1) (*see also* Neoplasm) D48.9† M36.0∗
- juvenile M33.0
Dermatoneuritis of children T56.1
Dermatophilosis A48.8
Dermatophytid L30.2
Dermatophytide – *see* Dermatophytosis
Dermatophytosis (epidermophyton) (infection) (Microsporum) (tinea) (Trichophyton) B35.9
- beard B35.0
- body B35.4
- capitis B35.0
- corporis B35.4
- deep-seated B35.8
- disseminated B35.8
- foot B35.3
- granulomatous B35.8
- groin B35.6
- hand B35.2
- nail B35.1
- perianal (area) B35.6
- scalp B35.0
- specified NEC B35.8

Dermatopolymyositis M33.9
- in neoplastic disease NEC
  (M8000/1) (*see also* Neoplasm) D48.9†
  M36.0∗
Dermatopolyneuritis T56.1
Dermatorrhexis Q82.8
- acquired L57.4
Dermatosclerosis (*see also* Scleroderma)
  M34.9
- localized L94.0
Dermatosis L98.9
- Bowen's (M8081/2) – *see* Neoplasm, skin,
  in situ
- bullous L13.9
- – specified NEC L13.8
- exfoliativa L26
- eyelid (noninfectious) H01.1
- factitial L98.1
- febrile neutrophilic L98.2
- gonococcal A54.8† L99.8∗
- herpetiformis L13.0
- menstrual NEC L98.8
- neutrophilic, febrile L98.2
- occupational (*see also* Dermatitis, due to)
  L25.9
- papulosa nigra L82
- pigmentary L81.9
- – progressive L81.7
- – Schamberg's L81.7
- psychogenic F54
- purpuric, pigmented L81.7
- pustular, subcorneal L13.1
- transient acantholytic L11.1
Dermographia, dermographism L50.3
Dermoid (cyst) (M9084/0) – *see also*
  Neoplasm, benign
- with malignant transformation (M9084/3)
  C56
- due to radiation (nonionizing) L57.8
Dermophytosis – *see* Dermatophytosis
Descemetocele H18.7
Descemet's membrane – *see* condition
Descending – *see* condition
Descensus uteri – *see* Prolapse, uterus
Desensitization to allergens Z51.6
Desert
- rheumatism B38.0† J99.8∗
- sore (*see also* Ulcer, skin) L98.4
Desertion (newborn) T74.0
Desmoid (extra-abdominal) (tumor)
  (M8821/1) – *see also* Neoplasm,
  connective tissue, uncertain behavior
- abdominal (M8822/1) D48.1
Desquamation, skin R23.4

Destruction, destructive – *see also* Damage
- articular facet M24.8
- – knee M23.8
- – vertebra (*see also* Spondylosis) M47.9
- bone M89.8
- – syphilitic A52.7† M90.2∗
- joint M24.8
- – sacroiliac M53.3
- live fetus to facilitate delivery (mother)
  O83.4
- – fetus P03.8
- operation to facilitate delivery O83.4
- rectal sphincter K62.8
- septum (nasal) J34.8
- tympanum, tympanic membrane
  (nontraumatic) H73.8
- vertebral disk – *see* Degeneration,
  intervertebral disk
Destructiveness (*see also* Disorder,
  conduct) F91.8
- adjustment reaction F43.2
Detachment
- cartilage (*see also* Sprain) T14.3
- cervix, annular O71.3
- – complicating delivery O71.3
- choroid (old) (postinfectional) (simple)
  (spontaneous) H31.4
- ligament – *see* Sprain
- meniscus (knee) (due to) M23.3
- – current injury S83.2
- – old tear or injury M23.2
- placenta (premature) (*see also* Abruptio
  placentae) O45.9
- retina (without retinal break) H33.2
- – with retinal break H33.0
- – pigment epithelium H35.7
- – rhegmatogenous H33.0
- – serous H33.2
- – specified NEC H33.5
- – traction H33.4
- vitreous (body) H43.8
Deterioration
- epileptic F06.8
- general physical R53
- heart, cardiac (*see also* Degeneration,
  myocardial) I51.5
- mental (*see also* Psychosis) F29
- myocardial, myocardium (*see also*
  Degeneration, myocardial) I51.5
- senile (simple) R54
De Toni-Fanconi syndrome E72.0
Detoxification therapy (for)
- alcohol Z50.2
- drug Z50.3

Deuteranomaly (anomalous trichromat)
H53.5
Deuteranopia (complete) (incomplete)
H53.5
Development
- arrested R62.8
- - bone M89.2
- - child R62.8
- - due to malnutrition E45
- - fetus P05.9
- - - affecting management of pregnancy O36.5
- defective, congenital – *see also* Anomaly, by site
- - cauda equina Q06.3
- - left ventricle Q24.8
- - - in hypoplastic left heart syndrome Q23.4
- - valve Q24.8
- - - pulmonary Q22.2
- delayed (*see also* Delay, development) R62.8
- - arithmetical skills F81.2
- - language (skills) (expressive) F80.1
- - learning skills F81.9
- - mixed skills F83
- - motor coordination F82
- - reading F81.0
- - specified learning skill NEC F81.8
- - speech F80.9
- - spelling F81.1
- imperfect, congenital – *see also* Anomaly, by site
- - heart Q24.9
- - lungs Q33.6
- incomplete P05.9
- - bronchial tree Q32.4
- - organ or site not listed – *see* Hypoplasia, by site
- - respiratory system Q34.8
- tardy, mental (*see also* Retardation, mental) F79.-
Developmental – *see condition*
Devergie's disease L44.0
Deviation
- conjugate (eye) (spastic) H51.8
- esophagus (acquired) K22.8
- eye, skew H51.8
- midline (dental arch) (jaw) (teeth) K07.2
- - specified site NEC – *see* Malposition
- nasal septum J34.2
- - congenital Q67.4
- organ or site, congenital NEC – *see* Malposition, congenital

Deviation—*continued*
- septum (nasal) (acquired) J34.2
- - congenital Q67.4
- sexual F65.9
- - bestiality F65.8
- - erotomania F52.7
- - exhibitionism F65.2
- - fetishism, fetishistic F65.0
- - - transvestism F65.1
- - frotteurism F65.8
- - masochism F65.5
- - multiple F65.6
- - necrophilia F65.8
- - nymphomania F52.7
- - pederosis F65.4
- - pedophilia F65.4
- - sadism, sadomasochism F65.5
- - satyriasis F52.7
- - specified type NEC F65.8
- - transvestism F64.1
- - voyeurism F65.3
- teeth, midline K07.2
- trachea J39.8
- ureter, congenital Q62.6
Device
- cerebral ventricle (communicating), in situ Z98.2
- contraceptive – *see* Contraception, device
- drainage, cerebrospinal fluid, in situ Z98.2
Devic's disease G36.0
Devil's grip B33.0
Devitalized tooth K04.9
Devonshire colic T56.0
Dextraposition, aorta Q20.3
- in tetralogy of Fallot Q21.3
Dextrinosis, limit (debrancher enzyme deficiency) E74.0
Dextrocardia (true) Q24.0
- with
- - complete transposition of viscera Q89.3
- - situs inversus Q89.3
Dextrotransposition, aorta Q20.3
Dhat syndrome F48.8
Dhobi itch B35.6
Di George's syndrome D82.1
Di Guglielmo's disease C94.0
Diabetes, diabetic (mellitus) (controlled) (familial) (severe) E14.-
- acetonemia – *code to* E10-E14 with fourth character .1 E14.1
- acidosis – *code to* E10-E14 with fourth character .1 E14.1

Diabetes, diabetic—*continued*
- adult-onset (nonobese) (obese) E11.-
- arising in pregnancy O24.4
- − affecting fetus or newborn P70.0
- bone change – *code to* E10-E14 with fourth character .6E14.6M90.8
- brittle E10.-
- bronze, bronzed E83.1
- cataract – *code to* E10-E14 with fourth character .3E14.3H28.0
- chemical R73.0
- coma (hyperglycemic) (hyperosmolar) – *code to* E10-E14 with fourth character .0E14.0
- complicating pregnancy, childbirth or puerperium (maternal) O24.-
- − affecting fetus or newborn P70.1
- − arising in pregnancy O24.4
- − − affecting fetus or newborn P70.0
- − gestational O24.4
- − − affecting fetus or newborn P70.0
- − pre-existing O24.3
- − − insulin-dependent O24.0
- − − malnutrition-related O24.2
- − − non-insulin-dependent O24.1
- congenital E10.-
- dietary counseling and surveillance Z71.3
- gangrene – *code to* E10 E14 with fourth character .5E14.5
- gestational O24.4
- hemochromatosis E83.1
- insipidus E23.2
- − nephrogenic N25.1
- − pituitary E23.2
- − vasopressin resistant N25.1
- insulin-dependent E10.-
- intracapillary glomerulosclerosis – *code to* E10-E14 with fourth character .2E14.2N08.3
- iritis – *code to* E10-E14 with fourth character .3E14.3H22.1
- juvenile-onset E10.-
- ketosis, ketoacidosis – *code to* E10-E14 with fourth character .1E14.1
- ketosis-prone E10.-
- Lancereaux's E14.6
- latent R73.0
- malnutrition-related (insulin-or non-insulin-dependent) E12.-
- maturity-onset (nonobese) (obese) E11.-
- neonatal (transient) P70.2
- nephropathy – *code to* E10-E14 with fourth character .2E14.2N08.3

Diabetes, diabetic—*continued*
- nephrosis – *code to* E10-E14 with fourth character .2E14.2N08.3
- neuralgia – *code to* E10-E14 with fourth character .4E14.4G63.2
- neuritis – *code to* E10-E14 with fourth character .4E14.4G63.2
- neuropathy E14.4† G63.2*
- − peripheral autonomic – *code to* E10-E14 with fourth character .4E14.4G99.0
- − polyneuropathy E14.4† G63.2*
- non-insulin-dependent (of the young) E11.-
- nonketotic E11.-
- phosphate E83.3
- renal E74.8
- retinal hemorrhage – *code to* E10-E14 with fourth character .3E14.3H36.0
- retinitis – *code to* E10-E14 with fourth character .3E14.3H36.0
- retinopathy – *code to* E10-E14 with fourth character .3E14.3H36.0
- specified NEC E13.-
- stable E11.-
- steroid-induced
- − correct substance properly administered E13.-
- − overdose or wrong substance given or taken T38.0
- type I E10.-
- type II (nonobese) (obese) E11.-
- unstable E10.-

Diagnosis deferred R69
Dialysis (intermittent) (treatment)
- extracorporeal Z49.1
- − preparatory care only (without treatment) Z49.0
- peritoneal Z49.2
- − preparatory care only (without treatment) Z49.0
- renal Z49.1
- − preparatory care only (without treatment) Z49.0
- retina, retinal H33.0
- specified type NEC Z49.2
- − preparatory care only (without treatment) Z49.0

Diaphragm – *see condition*
Diaphragmatitis, diaphragmitis J98.6
Diaphysial aclasis Q78.6
Diaphysitis M86.8
Diarrhea, diarrheal (disease) (infantile) A09.- A099
- achlorhydric K31.8

Diarrhea, diarrheal—*continued*
- acute A09.9
- – bloody A09.9 0
- – hemorrhagic A09.9 0
- – watery A09.9 0
- allergic K52.2
- amebic (*see also* Amebiasis) A06.0
- – with abscess – *see* Abscess, amebic
- – acute A06.0
- – chronic A06.1
- – nondysenteric A06.2
- and vomiting, epidemic A08.1
- bacillary – *see* Dysentery, bacillary
- balantidial A07.0
- cachectic NEC K52.8
- Chilomastix A07.8
- chronic (noninfectious) K52.9
- coccidial A07.3
- Cochin-China B78.0
- Dientamoeba A07.8
- dietetic K52.2
- due to
- – bacteria A04.9
- – – specified NEC A04.8
- – Campylobacter A04.5
- – Clostridium difficile A04.7
- – Clostridium perfringens (C) (F) A04.8
- – Cryptosporidium A07.2
- – Escherichia coli A04.4
- – – enteroaggregative A04.4
- – – enterohemorrhagic A04.3
- – – enteroinvasive A04.2
- – – enteropathogenic A04.0
- – – enterotoxigenic A04.1
- – – specified NEC A04.4
- – food hypersensitivity K52.2
- – specified organism NEC A08.5
- – – bacterial A04.8
- – – viral A08.3
- – – Staphylococcus A04.8
- – virus (*see also* Enteritis, viral) A08.4
- – Yersinia enterocolitica A04.6
- dysenteric A09.0
- endemic A09.0
- epidemic A09.0
- flagellate A07.9
- functional K59.1
- – following gastrointestinal surgery K91.8
- – psychogenic F45.3
- Giardia lamblia A07.1
- giardial A07.1
- infectious A09.0
- inflammatory A09.9

Diarrhea, diarrheal—*continued*
- inflammatory—*continued*
- – infectious A09.0
- – noninfectious K52.9
- mycotic NEC B49† K93.8*
- neonatal (noninfectious) P78.3
- nervous F45.3
- noninfectious K52.9
- protozoal A07.9
- – specified NEC A07.8
- psychogenic F45.3
- specified
- – bacterium NEC A04.8
- – virus NEC A08.3
- strongyloidiasis B78.0
- toxic K52.1 *—due to drugs*
- trichomonal A07.8
- tropical K90.1
- tuberculous A18.3† K93.0*
- viral (*see also* Enteritis, viral) A08.4
Diastasis
- cranial bones M84.8
- – congenital NEC Q75.8
- joint (traumatic) – *see* Dislocation
- muscle M62.0
- – congenital Q79.8
- recti (abdomen)
- – complicating delivery O71.8
- – congenital Q79.5
Diastema, tooth, teeth K07.3
Diastematomyelia Q06.2
Diataxia, cerebral, infantile G80.4
Diathesis
- gouty M10.9
- hemorrhagic (familial) D69.9
Diaz's disease or osteochondrosis (juvenile) (talus) M92.6
Dibothriocephalus, dibothriocephaliasis (latus) (infection) (infestation) B70.0
- larval B70.1
Dicephalus, dicephaly Q89.4
Dichotomy, teeth K00.2
Dichromat, dichromatopsia (congenital) H53.5
Dichuchwa A65
Dicroceliasis B66.2
Didelphia, didelphys (*see also* Double uterus) Q51.2
Didymytis (*see also* Orchitis) N45.9
Died – *see also* Death
- without
- – medical attention (cause unknown) R98
- – sign of disease R96.1

DiGeorge Syndrome D82.1

Dietary
- counseling and surveillance Z71.3
- inadequacy or deficiency E63.9

Dieulafoy's disease or ulcer K25.0

Difficult, difficulty (in)
- acculturation Z60.3
- birth, affecting fetus or newborn P03.9
- feeding R63.3
- – newborn P92.9
- – – breast P92.5
- – – specified NEC P92.8
- – nonorganic, infant or child F98.2
- intubation, in anesthesia T88.4
- mechanical, gastroduodenal stoma K91.8
- reading (developmental) F81.0
- – secondary to emotional disorders F93.-
- spelling (specific) F81.1
- – with reading disorder F81.3
- – due to inadequate teaching Z55.8
- swallowing (*see also* Dysphagia) R13
- walking R26.2
- work
- – conditions NEC Z56.5
- – schedule Z56.3

Diffuse – *see condition*

Digestive – *see condition*

Diktyoma (M9501/3) – *see* Neoplasm, malignant

Dilaceration, tooth K00.4

Dilatation
- anus K59.8
- – venule – *see* Hemorrhoids
- aorta (focal) (general) (*see also* Aneurysm, aorta) I71.9
- – congenital Q25.4
- – ruptured I71.8
- – syphilitic A52.0† I79.0*
- artery (*see also* Aneurysm) I72.9
- bladder (sphincter) N32.8
- – congenital Q64.7
- blood vessel I99
- bronchial J47
- calyx (due to obstruction) N13.3
- capillaries I78.8
- cardiac (acute) (chronic) (*see also* Hypertrophy, cardiac) I51.7
- – congenital (valve) Q24.8
- – valve – *see* Endocarditis
- cavum septi pellucidi Q06.8
- cecum K59.3
- cervix (uteri) – *see also* Incompetency, cervix
- – incomplete, poor, slow
- – – affecting fetus or newborn P03.6

Dilatation—*continued*
- cervix—*continued*
- – incomplete, poor—*continued*
- – – complicating delivery O62.0
- colon K59.3
- – congenital Q43.2
- common duct (acquired) K83.8
- – congenital Q44.5
- cystic duct (acquired) K82.8
- – congenital Q44.5
- duodenum K59.8
- esophagus K22.8
- – congenital Q39.5
- eustachian tube, congenital Q16.4
- gallbladder K82.8
- gastric – *see* Dilatation, stomach
- heart (acute) (chronic) (*see also* Hypertrophy, cardiac) I51.7
- – congenital Q24.8
- – valve – *see* Endocarditis
- ileum K59.8
- jejunum K59.8
- kidney (calyx) (collecting structures) (cystic) (parenchyma) (pelvis) (idiopathic) N28.8
- lacrimal passages or duct H04.6
- lymphatic vessel I89.0
- mammary duct N60.4
- Meckel's diverticulum (congenital) Q43.0
- myocardium (acute) (chronic) (*see also* Hypertrophy, cardiac) I51.7
- organ or site, congenital NEC – *see* Distortion
- pancreatic duct K86.8
- pericardium – *see* Pericarditis
- pharynx J39.2
- prostate N42.8
- pulmonary artery (idiopathic) I28.8
- pupil H57.0
- rectum K59.3
- saccule, congenital Q16.5
- sphincter ani K62.8
- stomach K31.8
- – acute K31.0
- – psychogenic F45.3
- trachea, congenital Q32.1
- ureter (idiopathic) N28.8
- – congenital Q62.2
- urethra (acquired) N36.8
- vasomotor I73.9
- vein I86.8
- ventricular, ventricle (acute) (chronic) (*see also* Hypertrophy, cardiac) I51.7

Dilatation—*continued*
- ventricular, ventricle—*continued*
- – cerebral, congenital Q04.8
- venule NEC I86.8
- vesical orifice N32.8
Dilated, dilation – *see* Dilatation
Diminished, diminution
- hearing (acuity) (*see also* Deafness) H91.9
- sense or sensation (cold) (heat) (tactile) (vibratory) R20.8
Dimitri-Sturge-Weber disease Q85.8
Dimple
- parasacral, pilonidal or postanal L05.9
- – with abscess L05.0
Dioctophyme renalis (infection) (infestation) B83.8
Dipetalonemiasis B74.4
Diphallus Q55.6
Diphtheria, diphtheritic (gangrenous) (hemorrhagic) A36.9
- cutaneous A36.3
- faucial A36.0
- infection of wound A36.3
- laryngeal A36.2
- myocarditis A36.8† I41.0*
- nasal, anterior A36.8
- nasopharyngeal A36.1
- neurological complication
- – neuritis A36.8† G59.8*
- – paralysis A36.8† G63.0*
- pharyngeal A36.0
- specified site NEC A36.8
- tonsillar A36.0
Diphyllobothriasis (intestine) B70.0
- larval B70.1
Diplacusis H93.2
Diplegia (upper limbs) G83.0
- congenital (cerebral) G80.8
- – spastic G80.1
- lower limbs G82.2
Diplococcus, diplococcal – *see* condition
Diplopia H53.2
Dipsomania F10.2
- with psychosis (*see also* Psychosis, alcoholic) F10.5
Dipylidiasis B71.1
Dirofilariasis B74.8
Dirt-eating child F98.3
Disability
- heart – *see* Disease, heart
- knowledge acquisition F81.9
- learning F81.9
- limiting activities Z73.6

Disability—*continued*
- spelling, specific F81.1
Disappearance of family member Z63.4
Disarticulation – *see* Amputation
- meaning traumatic amputation – *see* Amputation, traumatic
Discharge (from)
- abnormal finding in – *see* Abnormal, specimen
- breast (female) (male) N64.5
- diencephalic autonomic idiopathic G90.5
- ear H92.1
- excessive urine R35
- nipple N64.5
- penile R36
- postnasal – *see* Sinusitis
- prison, anxiety concerning Z65.2
- urethral R36
- vaginal N89.8
Discitis, diskitis M46.4
- pyogenic M46.3
Discoid
- meniscus (congenital) M23.1
- semilunar cartilage (congenital) M23.1
Discoloration, nails L60.8
Discontinuity, ossicles, ear H74.2
Discord (with)
- boss Z56.4
- classmates Z55.4
- counselor Z64.4
- employer Z56.4
- family Z63.8
- fellow employees Z56.4
- landlord Z59.2
- lodgers Z59.2
- neighbors Z59.2
- parents and in-laws Z63.1
- probation officer Z64.4
- social worker Z64.4
- spouse or partner Z63.0
- teachers Z55.4
- workmates Z56.4
Discordant connection
- atrioventricular (congenital) Q20.5
- ventriculoarterial Q20.3
Discrepancy, leg length (acquired) M21.7
- congenital Q72.9
Discrimination
- ethnic Z60.5
- political Z60.5
- racial Z60.5
- religious Z60.5
- sex Z60.5

Disease, diseased – *see also* Syndrome
- adenoids (and tonsils) J35.9
- adrenal (capsule) (cortex) (gland) (medullary) E27.9
- – specified NEC E27.8
- ainhum L94.6
- airway, obstructive, chronic J44.9
- – with
- – – exacerbation (acute) NEC J44.1
- – – lower respiratory infection (except influenza) J44.0
- – due to
- – – cotton dust J66.0
- – – specific organic dusts NEC J66.8
- alimentary canal K63.9
- alligator-skin Q80.9
- – acquired L85.0
- alpha heavy chain C88.3
- alveolar ridge
- – edentulous K06.9
- – – specified NEC K06.8
- alveoli, teeth K08.9
- amyloid (*see also* Amyloidosis) E85.9
- Andes T70.2
- angiospastic I73.9
- – cerebral G45.9
- – vein I87.8
- anterior
- – chamber H21.9
- – horn cell G12.2
- antiglomerular basement membrane (anti-GBM) antibody M31.0† N08.5*
- – tubulo-interstitial nephritis N12
- anus K62.9
- – specified NEC K62.8
- aorta (nonsyphilitic) I77.9
- – syphilitic NEC A52.0† I79.1*
- aortic (heart) (valve) I35.9
- Apollo B30.3† H13.1*
- aponeuroses M77.9
- appendix K38.9
- – specified NEC K38.8
- aqueous (chamber) H21.9
- arterial (*see also* Disease, artery)
- – occlusive I77.1
- – – mesenteric (chronic) K55.1
- – – – acute K55.0
- arteriocardiorenal (*see also* Hypertension, cardiorenal) I13.9
- arteriolar (generalized) (obliterative) I77.9
- arteriorenal – *see* Hypertension, kidney
- arteriosclerotic (*see also* Arteriosclerosis) I70.9

Disease, diseased—*continued*
- arteriosclerotic—*continued*
- – cardiovascular I25.0
- – coronary (artery) I25.1
- – heart I25.1
- artery I77.9
- – cerebral I67.9
- – coronary I25.1
- arthropod-borne NEC (viral) A94
- – specified type NEC A93.8
- atticoantral, chronic H66.2
- auditory canal H61.9
- auricle, ear NEC H61.1
- Australian X A83.4
- autoimmune (systemic) NEC M35.9
- – hemolytic (cold type) (warm type) D59.1
- – – drug-induced D59.0
- aviator's (*see also* Effect, adverse, high altitude) T70.2
- bacterial A49.9
- – specified NEC A48.8
- – zoonotic A28.9
- – – specified type NEC A28.8
- balloon (*see also* Effect, adverse, high altitude) T70.2
- Bartholin's gland N75.9
- basal ganglia G25.9
- – degenerative G23.9
- – – specified NEC G23.8
- – specified NEC G25.8
- behavioral, organic F07.9
- bile duct (common) (hepatic) K83.9
- – with calculus, stones K80.5
- – specified NEC K83.8
- biliary (tract) K83.9
- – specified NEC K83.8
- bird fancier's J67.2
- bladder N32.9
- – in (due to)
- – – schistosomiasis (bilharziasis) B65.0† N33.8*
- – specified NEC N32.8
- blood D75.9
- – forming organs D75.9
- – vessel I99
- bone M89.9
- – aluminium M83.4
- bone-marrow D75.9
- Bornholm B33.0
- bowel K63.9
- – functional (*see also* Disorder, colon, functional) K59.9
- brain G93.9

Disease, diseased—*continued*
- brain—*continued*
- − arterial, artery I67.9
- − arteriosclerotic I67.2
- − congenital Q04.9
- − degenerative − *see* Degeneration, brain
- − inflammatory − *see* Encephalitis
- − organic G93.9
- − − arteriosclerotic I67.2
- − parasitic NEC B71.9† G94.8*
- − Pick's G31.0
- − − dementia in G31.0† F02.0*
- − senile NEC G31.1
- − specified NEC G93.8
- brazier's T56.8
- breast N64.9
- − cystic (chronic) N60.1
- − − with epithelial proliferation N60.3
- − fibrocystic N60.1
- − − with epithelial proliferation N60.3
- − Paget's (M8540/3) C50.0
- − puerperal, postpartum NEC O92.2
- − specified NEC N64.8
- broad ligament (noninflammatory) N83.9
- − inflammatory − *see* Disease, pelvis, inflammatory
- − specified NEC N83.8
- bronchopulmonary J98.4
- bronchus NEC J98.0 ··
- bronze Addison's E27.1
- − tuberculous A18.7† E35.1*
- budgerigar fancier's J67.2
- bullous L13.9
- − chronic, of childhood L12.2
- − specified NEC L13.8
- bursa M71.9
- − specified NEC M71.8
- caisson T70.3
- California (*see also* Coccidioidomycosis) B38.9
- capillaries I78.9
- − specified NEC I78.8
- Carapata A68.0
- cardiac − *see* Disease, heart
- cardiopulmonary, chronic I27.9
- cardiorenal (hepatic) (hypertensive) (vascular) (*see also* Hypertension, cardiorenal) I13.9
- cardiovascular I51.6
- − congenital Q28.9
- − fetus or newborn P29.9
- − − specified NEC P29.8
- − hypertensive − *see* Hypertension, heart

Disease, diseased—*continued*
- cardiovascular—*continued*
- − renal (hypertensive) (*see also* Hypertension, cardiorenal) I13.9
- − syphilitic (asymptomatic) A52.0† I98.0*
- cartilage M94.9
- − specified NEC M94.8
- cat-scratch A28.1
- cecum K63.9
- celiac (adult) (infantile) K90.0
- cellular tissue L98.9
- central core G71.2
- cerebellar, cerebellum − *see* Disease, brain
- cerebral (*see also* Disease, brain) G93.9
- − degenerative − *see* Degeneration, brain
- cerebrospinal G96.9
- cerebrovascular I67.9
- − acute I67.8
- − − embolic I63.4
- − − thrombotic I63.3
- − arteriosclerotic I67.2
- − complicating pregnancy, childbirth or puerperium O99.4
- − embolic I66.9
- − occlusive I66.9
- − specified NEC I67.8
- − thrombotic I66.9
- cervix (uteri) (noninflammatory) N88.9
- − inflammatory (*see also* Cervicitis) N72
- − specified NEC N88.8
- chest J98.9
- Chicago B40.9
- Chignon B36.8
- chigo, chigoe B88.1
- chlamydial A74.9
- − specified NEC A74.8
- cholecystic (*see also* Disease, gallbladder) K82.9
- choroid H31.9
- − specified NEC H31.8
- Christmas D67
- chronic bullous of childhood L12.2
- ciliary body H21.9
- − specified NEC H21.8
- circulatory (system) NEC I99
- − fetus or newborn P29.9
- − maternal, affecting fetus or newborn P00.3
- − syphilitic A52.0† I98.0*
- − − congenital A50.5† I98.0*
- climacteric (female) N95.1
- − male N50.8

Disease, diseased—*continued*
- coagulation factor deficiency
  (congenital) (*see also* Defect, coagulation)
  D68.9
- coccidioidal – *see* Coccidioidomycosis
- cold
- – agglutinin or hemoglobinuria D59.1
- – – paroxysmal D59.6
- – hemagglutinin (chronic) D59.1
- collagen (nonvascular) (vascular) M35.9
- – specified NEC M35.8
- colon K63.9
- – functional (*see also* Disorder, colon,
  functional) K59.9
- combined system – *see* Degeneration,
  combined
- compressed air T70.3
- conjunctiva H11.9
- – chlamydial A74.0† H13.1*
- – specified NEC H11.8
- – viral B30.9† II13.1*
- – – specified NEC B30.8† H13.1*
- connective tissue, systemic M35.9
- – in (due to)
- – – hypogammaglobulinemia D80.1†
  M36.8*
- – – ochronosis E70.2† M36.8*
- – specified NEC M35.8
- corkhandler's or corkworker's J67.3
- cornea H18.9
- – specified NEC H18.8
- coronary (artery) I25.1
- – congenital Q24.5
- – ostial, syphilitic A52.0† I52.0*
- – – aortic A52.0† I39.1*
- – – mitral A52.0† I39.0*
- – – pulmonary A52.0† I39.3*
- corpus cavernosum N48.9
- – specified NEC N48.8
- coxsackie (virus) NEC B34.1
- – as cause of disease classified elsewhere
  B97.1
- – unspecified nature or site B34.1
- cystic
- – breast (chronic) N60.1
- – – with epithelial proliferation N60.3
- – kidney, congenital Q61.9
- – liver, congenital Q44.6
- – lung J98.4
- – – congenital Q33.0
- cystine storage (with renal sclerosis)
  E72.0
- cytomegalic inclusion (generalized)
  B25.9

Disease, diseased—*continued*
- cytomegalic inclusion—*continued*
- – with pneumonia B25.0† J17.1*
- cytomegaloviral B25.9
- – resulting from HIV disease B20.2
- – specified NEC B25.8
- demyelinating, demyelinizating (nervous
  system) G37.9
- – specified NEC G37.8
- dense deposit – *code to* N00-N07 with
  fourth character .6̶N̶0̶5̶.̶6̶
- deposition, hydroxyapatite M11.0
- diaphorase deficiency D74.0
- diaphragm J98.6
- diarrheal, infectious NEC A09.0
- digestive system K92.9
- – specified NEC K92.8
- discogenic M51.2
- – with myelopathy M51.0† G99.2*
- disk, degenerative – *see* Degeneration,
  intervertebral disk
- diverticular – *see* Diverticula
- ductless glands E34.9
- duodenum K31.9
- – specified NEC K31.8
- ear H93.9
- – degenerative H93.0
- – external H61.9
- – inner H83.9
- – – specified NEC H83.8
- – specified NEC H93.8
- – vascular H93.0
- Ebola (virus) A98.4
- Echinococcus (*see also* Echinococcus)
  B67.9
- echovirus NEC B34.1
- – as cause of disease classified elsewhere
  B97.1
- – unspecified nature or site B34.1
- edentulous (alveolar) ridge K06.9
- – specified NEC K06.8
- end-stage kidney N18.5
- endocrine glands or system NEC E34.9
- endomyocardial (eosinophilic) I42.3
- enteroviral, enterovirus NEC B34.1
- – as cause of disease classified elsewhere
  B97.1
- – central nervous system NEC A88.8
- – unspecified nature or site B34.1
- epidemic NEC B99
- epididymis N50.9
- esophagus K22.9
- – psychogenic F45.3
- – specified NEC K22.8

Disease, diseased—*continued*
- eustachian tube H69.9
- external
- - auditory canal H61.9
- - ear H61.9
- extrapyramidal G25.9
- - specified NEC G25.8
- eye H57.9
- - anterior chamber H21.9
- - inflammatory NEC H57.8
- - muscle (external) H50.9
- - specified NEC H57.8
- syphilitic – *see* Oculopathy, syphilitic
- eyeball H44.9
- - specified NEC H44.8
- eyelid H02.9
- - specified NEC H02.8
- eyeworm of Africa B74.3
- facial nerve (seventh) G51.9
- - newborn (birth injury) P11.3
- fallopian tube (noninflammatory) N83.9
- - inflammatory – *see* Salpingo-oophoritis
- - specified NEC N83.8
- fascia M62.9
- - inflammatory M60.9
- - specified NEC M62.8
- female pelvic inflammatory (*see also*
  Disease, pelvis, inflammatory) N73.9
- - tuberculous A18.1† N74.1*
- fetal NEC, known or suspected, affecting
  management of pregnancy O35.8
- fibrocaseous of lung (*see also*
  Tuberculosis, pulmonary) A16.2
- fibrocystic – *see* Fibrocystic disease
- fifth B08.3
- file-cutter's T56.0
- fish-skin Q80.9
- - acquired L85.0
- flax-dresser's J66.1
- fluke – *see* Infestation, fluke
- foot and mouth B08.8
- fourth B08.8
- fungus NEC B49
- gallbladder K82.9
- - specified NEC K82.8
- gamma heavy chain C88.2
- ganister J62.8
- gastric (*see also* Disease, stomach) K31.9
- gastrointestinal (tract) K92.9
- - amyloid E85.4† K93.8*
- - functional (*see also* Disorder,
  gastrointestinal) K59.9
- - specified NEC K92.8

Disease, diseased—*continued*
- genital organs
- - female N94.9
- - male N50.9
- gingiva K06.9
- - specified NEC K06.8
- gland (lymph) I89.9
- glass-blower's (cataract) H26.8
- globe H44.9
- - specified NEC H44.8
- glomerular (*see also* Glomerulonephritis)
  N05.-
- - with edema – *see* Nephrosis
- - chronic N03.-
- - microscopic polyangiitis M31.7†
  N08.5*
- - rapidly progressive N01.-
- glycogen storage (Andersen's) (Cori's)
  (Forbes') (Hers') (McArdle-Schmid-
  Pearson) (Pompe's) (Tauri's) (von
  Gierke's) E74.0
- - generalized E74.0
- - glucose-6-phosphatase deficiency
  E74.0
- - heart E74.0† I43.1*
- - hepatorenal E74.0
- - liver and kidney E74.0
- - myocardium E74.0† I43.1*
- gonococcal NEC A54.9
- graft-versus-host (GVH) (bone marrow)
  T86.0
- grainhandler's J67.8
- granulomatous (childhood) (chronic) D71
- gum K06.9
- gynecological N94.9
- H (Hartnup's) E72.0
- hair (color) (shaft) L67.9
- - follicles L73.9
- - - specified NEC L73.8
- hand, foot and mouth B08.4
- Hand-Schüller-Christian C96.5
- Hb (*see also* Disease, hemoglobin) D58.2
- heart (organic) I51.9
- - with
- - - pulmonary edema (acute) (*see also*
  Failure, ventricular, left) I50.1
- - - rheumatic fever (conditions in I00)
- - - - active I01.9
- - - - - specified NEC I01.8
- - - - inactive or quiescent (with chorea)
  I09.9
- - - - - specified NEC I09.8
- - amyloid E85.4† I43.1*
- - aortic (valve) I35.9

Disease, diseased—*continued*
− heart—*continued*
− − arteriosclerotic or sclerotic (senile) I25.1
− − artery, arterial I25.1
− − beriberi (wet) E51.1† I43.2*
− − black I27.0
− − congenital Q24.9
− − − cyanotic Q24.9
− − − maternal, affecting fetus or newborn P00.3
− − − specified NEC Q24.8
− − congestive (*see also* Failure, heart, congestive) I50.0
− − coronary (*see also* Ischemia, heart) I25.9
− − fibroid (*see also* Myocarditis) I51.4
− − glycogen storage E74.0† I43.1*
− − gonococcal A54.8† I52.0*
− − hypertensive (*see also* Hypertension, heart) I11.9
− − hyperthyroid (*see also* Hyperthyroidism) E05.9† I43.8*
− − ischemic (chronic or with a stated duration of over 4 weeks) I25.9
− − − acute or with a stated duration of 4 weeks or less I24.9
− − − − specified NEC I24.8
− − − asymptomatic I25.6
− − − diagnosed on ECG or other special investigation, but currently presenting no symptoms I25.6
− − − − specified form NEC I25.8
− − kyphoscoliotic I27.1
− − meningococcal A39.5† I52.0*
− − mitral I05.9
− − − specified NEC I05.8
− − muscular (*see also* Degeneration, myocardial) I51.5
− − psychogenic (functional) F45.3
− − pulmonary (chronic) I27.9
− − − acute I26.0
− − − in (due to) schistosomiasis B65.-† I52.1*
− − − specified NEC I27.8
− − rheumatic (chronic) (inactive) (old) (quiescent) (with chorea) I09.9
− − − active or acute I01.9
− − − − with chorea (acute) (rheumatic) (Sydenham's) I02.0
− − − maternal, affecting fetus or newborn P00.3
− − − specified NEC I09.8
− − senile (*see also* Myocarditis) I51.4

Disease, diseased—*continued*
− heart—*continued*
− − syphilitic A52.0† I52.0*
− − − aortic A52.0† I39.1*
− − − − aneurysm A52.0† I79.0*
− − − congenital A50.5† I52.0*
− − thyrotoxic (*see also* Thyrotoxicosis) E05.9† I43.8*
− − valve, valvular (obstructive) (regurgitant) (*see also* Endocarditis) I38
− − − congenital NEC Q24.8
− − − − pulmonary Q22.3
− − vascular – *see* Disease, cardiovascular
− heavy chain
− − alpha C88.3
− − gamma C88.2
− − Mu C88.2
− − NEC C88.2
− hematopoietic organs D75.9
− hemoglobin or Hb
− − abnormal (mixed) NEC D58.2
− − − with thalassemia D56.9
− − C (Hb-C) D58.2
− − − with other abnormal hemoglobin NEC D58.2
− − − elliptocytosis D58.1
− − − Hb-S D57.2
− − − sickle-cell D57.2
− − − thalassemia D56.9
− − D (Hb-D) D58.2
− − − with other abnormal hemoglobin NEC D58.2
− − − Hb-S D57.2
− − − sickle-cell D57.2
− − − thalassemia D56.9
− − E (Hb-E) D58.2
− − − with other abnormal hemoglobin NEC D58.2
− − − Hb-S D57.2
− − − sickle-cell D57.2
− − − thalassemia D56.9
− − elliptocytosis D58.1
− − H (Hb-H) (thalassemia) D56.0
− − − with other abnormal hemoglobin NEC D56.9
− − I thalassemia D56.9
− − M D74.0
− − S or SS – *see* Disease, sickle-cell
− − SC D57.2
− − SD D57.2
− − SE D57.2
− − spherocytosis D58.0
− − unstable, hemolytic D58.2

Disease, diseased—*continued*
- hemolytic (fetus) (newborn) P55.9
- – autoimmune (cold type) (warm type) D59.1
- – drug-induced D59.0
- – due to
- – – incompatibility
- – – – ABO (blood group) P55.1
- – – – blood (group) (Duffy) (K(ell)) (Kidd) (Lewis) (M) (S) NEC P55.8
- – – – Rh (blood group) (factor) P55.0
- – – – Rh-negative mother P55.0
- – specified type NEC P55.8
- hemorrhagic D69.9
- – fetus or newborn P53
- hepatic – *see* Disease, liver
- herpesviral, disseminated B00.7
- high fetal gene or hemoglobin thalassemia D56.9
- hip (joint) M25.9
- – congenital Q65.8
- – suppurative M00.9
- – tuberculous A18.0† M01.1*
- hookworm B76.9
- – specified NEC B76.8
- human immunodeficiency virus (HIV) – *see* Human, immunodeficiency virus (HIV) disease
- hyaline (diffuse) (generalized)
- – membrane (lung) (newborn) P22.0
- – – adult J80
- hydatid (*see also* Echinococcus) B67.9
- hydroxyapatite deposition M11.0
- hyperkinetic (*see also* Hyperkinesia) F90.9
- hypertensive (*see also* Hypertension) I10
- hypophysis E23.7
- Iceland G93.3
- I-cell E77.0
- ill-defined R68.8
- immune D89.9
- immunoproliferative (malignant) C88.9
- – small intestinal C88.3
- – specified NEC C88.7
- inclusion B25.9
- – salivary gland B25.9
- infectious, infective B99
- – complicating pregnancy, childbirth or puerperium O98.9
- – – affecting fetus or newborn P00.2
- – congenital P37.9
- – – specified NEC P37.8

Disease, diseased—*continued*
- infectious, infective—*continued*
- – resulting from HIV disease B20.9
- – – specified NEC B20.8
- intervertebral disk M51.9
- – with myelopathy M51.0† G99.2*
- – cervical, cervicothoracic (with) M50.9
- – – myelopathy M50.0† G99.2*
- – – neuritis, radiculitis or radiculopathy M50.1† G55.1*
- – – specified NEC M50.8
- – lumbar, lumbosacral (with) M51.9
- – – myelopathy M51.0† G99.2*
- – – neuritis, radiculitis, radiculopathy or sciatica M51.1† G55.1*
- – – specified NEC M51.8
- – specified NEC M51.8
- – thoracic, thoracolumbar (with) M51.9
- – – myelopathy M51.0† G99.2*
- – – neuritis, radiculitis or radiculopathy M51.1† G55.1*
- – – specified NEC M51.8
- intestine K63.9
- – functional (*see also* Disorder, intestine, functional) K59.9
- – – specified NEC K59.8
- – organic K63.9
- – protozoal A07.9
- – specified NEC K63.8
- iris H21.9
- – specified NEC H21.8
- iron metabolism or storage E83.1
- itai-itai T56.3
- jaw K10.9
- – specified NEC K10.8
- jigger B88.1
- joint M25.9
- – Charcot's (tabetic) A52.1† M14.6*
- – – diabetic (*see also* E10-E14 with fourth character .6) E14.6† M14.6*
- – – nonsyphilitic NEC G98† M14.6*
- – – syringomyelic G95.0† M49.4*
- – degenerative M19.9
- – – multiple M15.9
- – – spine M47.9
- – sacroiliac M53.3
- – specified NEC M25.8
- – spine NEC M53.9
- – suppurative M00.9
- Katayama B65.2
- Keshan E59

Disease, diseased—*continued*
– kidney (functional) (pelvis) N28.9

Note: Where a term is indexed only at the three-character level, e.g. N01.-, reference should be made to the list of fourth-character subdivisions in Volume 1 at N00-N08.

– – *//* with
– – – edema – *see* Nephrosis
– – – glomerular lesion – *see* Glomerulonephritis
– – – – with edema – *see* Nephrosis
– – – interstitial nephritis N12
– – acute – *see* Nephritis, acute
– – chronic N18.9
– – – end-stage N18.5
– – – stage 1 N18.1
– – – stage 2 N18.2
– – – stage 3 N18.3
– – – stage 4 N18.4
– – – stage 5 N18.5
– – complicating pregnancy O26.8
– – – with hypertension (pre existing) O10.2
– – – – secondary O10.4
– – cystic (congenital) Q61.9
– – – multicystic Q61.4
– – – polycystic Q61.3
– – end-stage (failure) N18.5
– – fibrocystic (congenital) Q61.8
– – hypertensive (*see also* Hypertension, kidney) I12.9
– – – end-stage (failure) I12.0
– – in (due to) schistosomiasis (bilharziasis) B65.-† N29.1*
– – rapidly progressive N01.-
– – tubular (*see also* Nephritis, tubulo-interstitial) N12
– kissing B27.9
– kuru A81.8
– Kyasanur Forest A98.2
– labyrinth, ear H83.9
– – specified NEC H83.8
– lacrimal system H04.9
– – specified NEC H04.8
– larynx J38.7
– legionnaire's A48.1
– – nonpneumonic A48.2
– lens H27.9
– – specified NEC H27.8
– Lewy body (dementia) G31.8
– lip K13.0
– lipid-storage E75.6

Disease, diseased—*continued*
– lipid-storage—*continued*
– – specified NEC E75.5
– liver (chronic) (organic) K76.9
– – alcoholic (chronic) K70.9
– – cystic, congenital Q44.6
– – drug-induced (idiosyncratic) (toxic) (predictable) (unpredictable) – *see* Disease, liver, toxic
– – fatty, nonalcoholic K76.0
– – fibrocystic (congenital) Q44.6
– – fluke
– – – Chinese B66.1
– – – oriental B66.1
– – – sheep B66.3
– – glycogen storage E74.0† K77.8*
– – in (due to) schistosomiasis (bilharziasis) B65.-† K77.0*
– – inflammatory K75.9
– – – alcoholic K70.1
– – – specified NEC K75.8
– – nonalcoholic, fatty K76.0
– – polycystic (congenital) Q44.6
– – toxic K71.9
– – – with
– – – – cholestasis K71.0
– – – – cirrhosis (liver) K71.7
– – – – fibrosis (liver) K71.7
– – – – focal nodular hyperplasia K71.8
– – – – hepatic granuloma K71.8
– – – – hepatic necrosis K71.1
– – – – hepatitis NEC K71.6
– – – – – acute K71.2
– – – – – chronic
– – – – – – active K71.5
– – – – – – lobular K71.4
– – – – – – persistent K71.3
– – – – – lupoid K71.5
– – – – peliosis hepatis K71.8
– – – – veno-occlusive disease (VOD) of liver K71.8
– – veno-occlusive K76.5
– luetic – *see* Syphilis
– lumbosacral region M53.8
– lung J98.4
– – cystic J98.4
– – – congenital Q33.0
– – fibroid (chronic) (*see also* Fibrosis, lung) J84.1
– – fluke B66.4
– – – oriental B66.4
– – in
– – – amyloidosis E85.4† J99.8*
– – – sarcoidosis D86.0

Disease, diseased—*continued*
- lung—*continued*
- – in—*continued*
- – – Sjögren's syndrome M35.0† J99.1*
- = – systemic
- – – – lupus erythematosus M32.1†
  J99.1*
- – – – sclerosis M34.8† J99.1*
- – interstitial J84.9
- – – specified NEC J84.8
- – obstructive (chronic) J44.9
- – – with
- – – – exacerbation J44.1
- – – – lower respiratory infection (except
  influenza) J44.0
- – – – alveolitis, allergic J67.-
- – – – asthma J44.-
- – – – bronchitis J44.8
- – – – – emphysematous J44.8
- – – – – – with acute exacerbation
  J44.1
- – – – – – with acute lower respiratory
  infection J44.0
- – – – emphysema J44.-
- – – – exacerbation (acute) J44.1
- – – – hypersensitivity pneumonitis J67.-
- – – polycystic J98.4
- – – congenital Q33.0
- – – rheumatoid (diffuse) (interstitial)
  M05.1† J99.0*
- – Lyme A69.2
- – lymphatic (channel) (gland) (system)
  (vessel) I89.9
- – lymphoproliferative D47.9
- – – T-gamma D47.9
- – – X-linked D82.3
- – malarial (*see also* Malaria) B54
- – malignant (M8000/3) – *see also*
  Neoplasm, malignant
- – – previous, affecting management of
  pregnancy Z35.8
- – maple-syrup-urine E71.0
- – Marburg (virus) A98.3
- – mastoid (process) H74.9
- – – specified NEC H74.8
- – maternal, unrelated to pregnancy NEC,
  affecting fetus or newborn P00.9
- – mediastinum J98.5
- – Mediterranean D56.9
- – meningeal – *see* Meningitis
- – meningococcal NEC A39.9
- – mental F99
- – – organic F06.9

Disease, diseased—*continued*
- – metabolic, metabolism E88.9
- – – bilirubin E80.7
- – metal-polisher's J62.8
- – metastatic (M8000/6) – *see* Metastasis
- – middle ear H74.9
- – – adhesive H74.1
- – – specified NEC H74.8
- – minicore G71.2
- – mitral (valve) (rheumatic) I05.9
- – – nonrheumatic I34.9
- – mixed connective tissue M35.1
- – moldy hay J67.0
- – motor neuron (bulbar) (familial) (mixed
  type) (spinal) G12.2
- – moyamoya I67.5
- – multicore G71.2
- – muscle M62.9
- – – inflammatory M60.9
- – – ocular (external) H50.9
- – musculoskeletal system, soft tissue
  M79.9
- – – specified NEC M79.8
- – mycotic B49
- – myelodysplastic and myeloproliferative,
  not classifiable C94.6
- – myeloproliferative (chronic) D47.1
- – myocardium, myocardial (*see also*
  Degeneration, myocardial) I51.5
- – – primary (idiopathic) I42.9
- – myoneural G70.9
- – nails L60.9
- – – specified NEC L60.8
- – Nairobi (sheep virus) A93.8
- – nasal J34.8
- – nemaline body G71.2
- – neoplastic (malignant), generalized
  (M8000/6) C79.9
- – – ~~primary site not indicated C80.9~~
- – – ~~primary site unknown, so stated C80.0~~
- – nerve – *see* Disorder, nerve
- – nervous system G98
- – – affecting management of pregnancy,
  childbirth or puerperium O99.3
- – – autonomic G90.9
- – – central G96.9
- – – – specified NEC G96.8
- – – parasympathetic G90.9
- – – specified NEC G98
- – – sympathetic G90.9
- – – vegetative G90.9
- – neuromuscular system G70.9
- – Newcastle B30.8† H13.1*

Disease, diseased—*continued*
- nipple N64.9
- – Paget's (M8540/3) C50.0
- nonarthropod-borne NEC (viral) B34.9
- – as cause of disease classified elsewhere B97.1
- – enterovirus NEC B34.1
- – unspecified nature or site B34.1
- nonautoimmune hemolytic D59.4
- – drug-induced D59.2
- nose J34.8
- nucleus pulposus – *see* Disease, intervertebral disk
- nutritional E63.9
- oast-house-urine E72.1
- ocular
- – herpesviral B00.5
- – zoster B02.3
- optic nerve NEC H47.0
- orbit H05.9
- – specified NEC H05.8
- Oropouche virus A93.0
- osteofibrocystic E21.0
- outer ear H61.9
- ovary (noninflammatory) N83.9
- – cystic N83.2
- – inflammatory – *see* Salpingo-oophoritis
- – polycystic E28.2
- – specified NEC N83.8
- ovum (complicating pregnancy) O02.0
- pancreas K86.9
- – cystic K86.2
- – fibrocystic E84.9
- – specified NEC K86.8
- panvalvular (unspecified origin) I08.9
- – specified NEC (unspecified origin) I08.8
- parametrium (noninflammatory) N83.9
- parasitic B89
- – cerebral NEC B71.9† G94.8*
- – complicating pregnancy, childbirth or puerperium O98.9
- – intestinal NEC B82.9
- – mouth B37.0
- – skin NEC B88.9
- – specified type – *see* Infestation
- – tongue B37.0
- parathyroid (gland) E21.5
- – specified NEC E21.4
- parodontal K05.6
- pearl-worker's M86.8
- pelvis, pelvic
- – female NEC N94.9
- – – specified NEC N94.8

Disease, diseased—*continued*
- pelvis, pelvic—*continued*
- – gonococcal (acute) (chronic) A54.2
- – inflammatory (female) N73.9
- – – acute N73.0
- – – chronic N73.1
- – – complicating pregnancy O23.5
- – – – affecting fetus or newborn P00.8
- – – following
- – – – abortion (subsequent episode) O08.0
- – – – – current episode – *see* Abortion
- – – – ectopic or molar pregnancy O08.0
- – – specified NEC N73.8
- – – tuberculous A18.1† N74.1*
- – organ, female N94.9
- – peritoneum, female NEC N94.8
- penis N48.9
- – inflammatory N48.2
- – specified NEC N48.8
- periapical tissues NEC K04.9
- periodontal K05.6
- – specified NEC K05.5
- periosteum M89.8
- peripheral
- – arterial I73.9
- – autonomic nervous system G90.9
- – nerves – *see* Polyneuropathy
- – vascular NEC I73.9
- peritoneum K66.9
- – pelvic, female NEC N94.8
- – specified NEC K66.8
- pharynx J39.2
- – specified NEC J39.2
- pigeon fancier's J67.2
- pineal gland E34.8
- pink T56.1
- pinna (noninfective) H61.1
- pinworm B80
- Piry virus A93.8
- pituitary (gland) E23.7
- pituitary-snuff-taker's J67.8
- placenta
- – affecting fetus or newborn P02.2
- – complicating pregnancy or childbirth O43.9
- pleura (cavity) J94.9
- – specified NEC J94.8
- pneumatic drill (hammer) T75.2
- polycystic
- – liver or hepatic Q44.6
- – lung or pulmonary J98.4
- – – congenital Q33.0
- – ovary, ovaries E28.2

Disease, diseased—*continued*
- pregnancy NEC (*see also* Pregnancy) O26.9
- prion, central nervous system A81.9
- – specified NEC A81.8
- prostate N42.9
- – specified NEC N42.8
- protozoal B64
- – complicating pregnancy, childbirth or puerperium O98.6
- – intestine, intestinal A07.9
- – specified NEC B60.8
- pseudo-Hurler's E77.0
- psychiatric F99
- psychotic (*see also* Psychosis) F29
- puerperal NEC (*see also* Puerperal) O90.9
- pulmonary – *see also* Disease, lung
- – artery I28.9
- – heart I27.9
- – – specified NEC I27.8
- – valve I37.9
- pulp (dental) NEC K04.9
- pulseless M31.4
- ragpicker's or ragsorter's A22.1
- rectum K62.9
- – specified NEC K62.8
- renal – *see* Disease, kidney
- renovascular (arteriosclerotic) (*see also* Hypertension, kidney) I12.9
- respiratory (tract) J98.9
- – acute or subacute NEC
- – – due to
- – – – chemicals, gases, fumes or vapors (inhalation) J68.3
- – – – external agent J70.9
- – – – – specified NEC J70.8
- – – – radiation J70.0
- – chronic NEC J98.9
- – – due to
- – – – chemicals, gases, fumes or vapors J68.4
- – – – external agent J70.9
- – – – – specified NEC J70.8
- – – – radiation J70.1
- – – fetus or newborn P27.9
- – – – specified NEC P27.8
- – – due to
- – – – chemicals, gases, fumes or vapors J68.9
- – – – acute or subacute NEC J68.3
- – – – chronic J68.4
- – – external agent J70.9
- – – – specified NEC J70.8

Disease, diseased—*continued*
- respiratory—*continued*
- – – newborn P28.9
- – – – specified type NEC P28.8
- – – upper J39.9
- – – – acute or subacute J06.9
- – – – – multiple sites NEC J06.8
- – – – noninfectious NEC J39.8
- – – – specified NEC J39.8
- – – – streptococcal J06.9
- – retina, retinal H35.9
- – – Batten's or Batten-Mayou E75.4† H36.8*
- – – specified NEC H35.8
- – – vascular lesion H35.0
- – rheumatoid – *see* Arthritis, rheumatoid
- – rickettsial NEC A79.9
- – – specified type NEC A79.8
- – Ross River B33.1
- – salivary gland or duct K11.9
- – – inclusion B25.9
- – – specified NEC K11.8
- – – virus B25.9
- – sandworm B76.9
- – sclera H15.9
- – – specified NEC H15.8
- – scrofulous (tuberculous) A18.2
- – scrotum N50.9
- – sebaceous glands L73.9
- – semilunar cartilage, cystic M23.0
- – seminal vesicle N50.9
- – serum NEC T80.6
- – shipyard B30.0† H19.2*
- – sickle-cell D57.1
- – – with
- – – – crisis D57.0
- – – – other abnormal hemoglobin NEC D57.2
- – – elliptocytosis D57.8
- – – spherocytosis D57.8
- – – thalassemia D57.2
- – silo-filler's J68.8
- – simian B B00.4† G05.1*
- – sinus (*see also* Sinusitis) J32.9
- – sixth B08.2
- – skin L98.9
- – – due to metabolic disorder NEC E88.9† L99.8*
- – – specified NEC L98.8
- – slim (HIV) B22.2
- – spinal (cord) G95.9
- – – congenital Q06.9
- – – specified NEC G95.8

Disease, diseased—*continued*
- spine M48.9
- – joint M53.9
- – tuberculous A18.0† M49.0∗
- spinocerebellar (hereditary) G11.9
- – specified NEC G11.8
- spleen D73.9
- – amyloid E85.4† D77∗
- – organic D73.9
- – postinfectional D73.8
- sponge-diver's T63.6
- stomach K31.9
- – functional, psychogenic F45.3
- – specified NEC K31.8
- stonemason's J62.8
- storage
- – glycogen (*see also* Disease, glycogen storage) E74.0
- – mucopolysaccharide E76.3
- striatopallidal system NEC G25.8
- subcutaneous tissue (*see also* Disease, skin) L98.9
- supporting structures of teeth K08.9
- – specified NEC K08.8
- suprarenal (capsule) (gland) E27.9
- – specified NEC E27.8
- sweat glands L74.9
- – specified NEC L74.8
- swimming-pool granuloma A31.1
- sympathetic nervous system G90.9
- synovium M67.9
- – specified NEC M67.8
- syphilitic – *see* Syphilis
- systemic tissue mast cell D47.0
- Tangier E78.6
- tear duct H04.9
- tendon, tendinous M67.9
- – inflammatory NEC M65.9
- – nodular M65.3
- – specified NEC M67.8
- testis N50.9
- throat J39.2
- – septic J02.0
- thromboembolic (*see also* Embolism) I74.9
- thymus (gland) E32.9
- – specified NEC E32.8
- thyroid (gland) E07.9
- – heart (*see also* Hyperthyroidism) E05.9† I43.8∗
- – specified NEC E07.8
- tongue K14.9
- – specified NEC K14.8
- tonsils, tonsillar (and adenoids) J35.9

Disease, diseased—*continued*
- tooth, teeth K08.9
- – hard tissues K03.9
- – – specified NEC K03.8
- – pulp NEC K04.9
- – specified NEC K08.8
- trachea NEC J39.8
- tricuspid (valve) (rheumatic) I07.9
- – nonrheumatic I36.9
- triglyceride-storage E75.5
- trophoblastic (M9100/0) (*see also* Mole, hydatidiform) O01.9
- tsutsugamushi A75.3
- tube (fallopian) (noninflammatory) N83.9
- – inflammatory (*see also* Salpingo-oophoritis) N70.9
- – specified NEC N83.8
- tuberculous NEC (*see also* Tuberculosis) A16.9
- tubo-ovarian (noninflammatory) N83.9
- – inflammatory (*see also* Salpingo-oophoritis) N70.9
- – specified NEC N83.8
- tubotympanic, chronic H66.1
- tubulo-interstitial N15.9
- – specified NEC N15.8
- tympanum H73.9
- – specified NEC H73.8
- ureter N28.9
- – due to (in) schistosomiasis (bilharziasis) B65.0† N29.1∗
- urethra N36.9
- – specified NEC N36.8
- urinary (tract) N39.9
- – bladder N32.9
- – – specified NEC N32.8
- – specified NEC N39.8
- uterus (noninflammatory) N85.9
- – infective (*see also* Endometritis) N71.9
- – inflammatory (*see also* Endometritis) N71.9
- – specified NEC N85.8
- uveal tract (anterior) H21.9
- – posterior H31.9
- vagina, vaginal (noninflammatory) N89.9
- – inflammatory NEC N76.8
- – specified NEC N89.8
- valve, valvular I38
- – multiple (unspecified origin) I08.9
- – – specified NEC (unspecified origin) I08.8
- vas deferens N50.9
- vascular I99
- – arteriosclerotic – *see* Arteriosclerosis

Disease, diseased—*continued*
- vascular—*continued*
- – ciliary body NEC H21.1
- – hypertensive – *see* Hypertension
- – iris NEC H21.1
- – obliterative I77.1
- – – peripheral I73.9
- – occlusive I99
- – peripheral (occlusive) I73.9
- – vasomotor I73.9
- – vasospastic I73.9
- – vein I87.9
- – venereal A64
- – specified nature or type NEC A63.8
- – vertebra, vertebral M48.9
- – disk – *see* Disease, intervertebral disk
- – vibration NEC T75.2
- – viral, virus (*see also* Disease, by type of virus) B34.9
- – arbovirus NEC A94
- – arthropod-borne NEC A94
- – congenital P35.9
- – – specified NEC P35.8
- – Hanta (with renal manifestations) (Dobrava) (Puumala) (Seoul) A98.5† N08.0*
- – – with pulmonary manifestations (Andes) (Bayou) (Bermejo) (Black Creek Canal) (Choclo) (Juquitiba) (Laguna negra) (Lechiguanas) (New York) (Oran) (Sin Nombre) B33.4† J17.1*
- – Hantaan (Korean hemorrhagic fever) A98.5† N08.0*
- – human immunodeficiency (HIV) – *see* Human, immunodeficiency virus (HIV) disease
- – Kunjin A83.4
- – nonarthropod-borne NEC B34.9
- – Powassan A84.8
- – Rocio (encephalitis) A83.6
- – Sin Nombre (Hantavirus (cardio-)pulmonary syndrome) B33.4† J17.1*
- – suspected damage to fetus affecting management of pregnancy O35.3
- – Tahyna B33.8
- – vesicular stomatitis A93.8
- – vitreous H43.9
- – – specified NEC H43.8
- – vocal cord J38.3
- – vulva (noninflammatory) N90.9
- – – inflammatory NEC N76.8
- – – specified NEC N90.8
- – wasting NEC R64

Disease, diseased—*continued*
- whipworm B79
- white blood cells D72.9
- – specified NEC D72.8
- white-spot, meaning lichen sclerosus et atrophicus L90.0
- – penis N48.0
- – vulva N90.4
- white matter NEC R90.8
- winter vomiting (epidemic) A08.1
- woolsorter's A22.1† J17.0*
- zoonotic, bacterial A28.9
- – specified type NEC A28.8

Disfigurement (due to scar) L90.5
Disgerminoma – *see* Dysgerminoma
DISH (diffuse idiopathic skeletal hyperostosis) M48.1
Disinsertion, retina H33.0
Disintegration, complete, of the body R68.8
Dislocatable hip, congenital Q65.6
Dislocation (articular) T14.3
- with fracture – *see* Fracture
- acromioclavicular (joint) S43.1
- ankle S93.0
- – navicular bone S93.3
- arm, meaning upper limb – *see* Dislocation, limb, upper
- astragalus S93.0
- atlantoaxial S13.1
- atlas S13.1
- axis S13.1
- back T09.2
- breast bone S23.2
- capsule, joint – *code as* Dislocation, by site
- carpal (bone) S63.0
- carpometacarpal (joint) S63.0
- cartilage (joint) – *code as* Dislocation, by site
- cervical spine (vertebra) S13.1
- cervicothoracic (spine) (vertebra) T03.8
- chronic – *see* Dislocation, recurrent
- clavicle S43.1
- coccyx S33.2
- congenital NEC Q68.8
- coracoid S43.0
- costal cartilage S23.2
- costochondral S23.2
- cricoarytenoid articulation S13.2
- cricothyroid articulation S13.2
- dorsal vertebra S23.1
- elbow S53.1
- – congenital Q68.8

Dislocation—*continued*
- elbow—*continued*
- − − recurrent M24.4
- eye, eyeball, nontraumatic H44.8
- femur
- − − distal end S83.1
- − − proximal end S73.0
- fibula
- − − distal end S93.0
- − − proximal end S83.1
- finger S63.1
- − − multiple S63.2
- foot S93.3
- forearm T11.2
- fracture − *see* Fracture
- glenohumeral (joint) S43.0
- glenoid S43.0
- habitual − *see* Dislocation, recurrent
- head, part NEC S03.3
- hip S73.0
- − − congenital Q65.2
- − − − bilateral Q65.1
- − − − unilateral Q65.0
- − − recurrent M24.4
- humerus, proximal end S43.0
- infracoracoid S43.0
- innominate (pubic junction) (sacral junction) S33.3
- − − acetabulum S73.0
- interphalangeal (joint(s))
- − − finger or hand S63.1
- − − foot or toe S93.1
- jaw (cartilage) (meniscus) S03.0
- knee S83.1
- − − cap S83.0
- − − congenital Q68.2
- − − old M23.8
- − − pathological M24.3
- − − recurrent M24.4
- lacrimal gland H04.1
- leg, meaning lower limb − *see* Dislocation, limb, lower
- lens (complete) (crystalline) (partial) H27.1
- − − congenital Q12.1
- − − traumatic S05.8
- ligament − *code as* Dislocation, by site
- limb
- − − lower T13.2
- − − − with upper limb(s) T03.4
- − − − multiple sites T03.3
- − − upper T11.2
- − − − with lower limb(s) T03.4
- − − − multiple sites T03.2

Dislocation—*continued*
- lumbar (vertebra) S33.1
- lumbosacral (vertebra) S33.1
- − − congenital Q76.4
- mandible S03.0
- meniscus (knee) − *see* Tear, meniscus
- − − sites specified, other than knee − *code as* Dislocation, by site
- metacarpal (bone) S63.7
- − − distal end S63.1
- − − proximal end S63.0
- metacarpophalangeal (joint) S63.1
- metatarsal (bone) S93.3
- metatarsophalangeal (joint(s)) S93.1
- midcarpal (joint) S63.0
- midtarsal (joint) S93.3
- multiple T03.9
- − − body regions NEC T03.8
- − − fingers S63.2
- − − head S03.5
- − − − with
- − − − − neck T03.0
- − − − − other body regions T03.8
- − − limb
- − − − lower T03.3
- − − − − with
- − − − − − thorax, lower back and pelvis T03.8
- − − − − − upper limb(s) T03.4
- − − − upper T03.2
- − − − − with
- − − − − − lower limb(s) T03.4
- − − − − − thorax, lower back and pelvis T03.8
- − − neck S13.3
- − − − with
- − − − − head T03.0
- − − − − other body regions T03.8
- − − specified NEC T03.8
- − − thorax S23.2
- − − − with lower back and pelvis T03.1
- − − − − with limbs T03.8
- − − trunk T03.1
- neck S13.1
- − − multiple S13.3
- nose (septal cartilage) S03.1
- occiput from atlas S13.1
- old M24.8
- − − knee M23.8
- ossicles, ear H74.2
- patella S83.0
- − − congenital Q74.1
- − − recurrent M22.0

Dislocation—*continued*
- pathological NEC M24.3
- – lumbosacral joint M53.2
- – sacroiliac M53.2
- – spine M53.2
- phalanx
- – finger or hand S63.1
- – foot or toe S93.1
- prosthesis, internal – *see* Complications, prosthetic device, by site, mechanical
- radiocarpal (joint) S63.0
- radiohumeral (joint) S53.0
- radioulnar (joint)
- – distal S63.0
- – proximal S53.1
- radius
- – distal end S63.0
- – proximal end S53.0
- recurrent M24.4
- – elbow M24.4
- – hip M24.4
- – joint NEC M24.4
- – knee M24.4
- – patella M22.0
- – sacroiliac M53.2
- – shoulder M24.4
- rib (cartilage) S23.2
- sacrococcygeal S33.2
- sacroiliac (joint) (ligament) S33.2
- – congenital Q74.2
- – recurrent M53.2
- sacrum S33.2
- scaphoid (bone) (hand) (wrist) S63.0
- – foot S93.3
- scapula S43.3
- semilunar cartilage, knee – *see* Tear, meniscus
- septal cartilage (nose) S03.1
- septum (nasal) (old) J34.2
- sesamoid bone – *code as* Dislocation, by site
- shoulder (blade) (joint) (ligament) S43.0
- – chronic M24.4
- – congenital Q68.8
- – girdle S43.3
- – recurrent M24.4
- spine T09.2
- – cervical S13.1
- – congenital Q76.4
- – lumbar S33.1
- – thoracic S23.1
- spontaneous M24.3
- sternoclavicular (joint) S43.2
- sternum S23.2

Dislocation—*continued*
- subglenoid S43.0
- symphysis pubis S33.3
- – obstetric (traumatic) O71.6
- talus S93.0
- tarsal (bone(s)) (joint(s)) S93.3
- tarsometatarsal (joint(s)) S93.3
- temporomandibular (joint) S03.0
- thigh, proximal end S73.0
- thoracic (vertebra) S23.1
- thumb S63.1
- thyroid cartilage S13.2
- tibia
- – distal end S93.0
- – proximal end S83.1
- tibiofibular (joint)
- – distal S93.0
- – proximal S83.1
- toe(s) S93.1
- tooth S03.2
- trachea S23.2
- ulna
- – distal end S63.0
- – proximal end S53.1
- ulnohumeral (joint) S53.1
- vertebra (articular process) (body) T09.2
- – cervical S13.1
- – cervicothoracic T03.8
- – congenital Q76.4
- – lumbar S33.1
- – thoracic S23.1
- wrist (carpal bone) (scaphoid) (semilunar) S63.0
- xiphoid cartilage S23.2

Disorder (of) – *see also* Disease
- acantholytic L11.9
- – specified NEC L11.8
- accommodation H52.5
- acute
- – psychotic (*see also* Psychosis, acute) F23.9
- – – with schizophrenia-like features F23.2
- – – – specified NEC F23.8
- – – stress F43.0
- adjustment F43.2
- adrenal (capsule) (gland) (medullary) E27.9
- – specified NEC E27.8
- adrenogenital E25.9
- – drug-induced E25.8
- – iatrogenic E25.8
- – idiopathic E25.8
- adult personality (and behavior) F69

Disorder—*continued*
- adult personality—*continued*
- – specified NEC F68.8
- affective (mood) (*see also* Disorder, mood) F39
- – bipolar (*see also* Disorder, bipolar, affective) F31.9
- – organic (mixed) F06.3
- – persistent F34.9
- – – specified NEC F34.8
- – recurrent NEC F38.1
- – right hemisphere, organic F07.8
- – specified NEC F38.8
- aggressive, unsocialized F91.1
- alcohol use F10.9
- allergic – *see* Allergy
- alveolar NEC J84.0
- amino-acid
- – metabolism NEC (*see also* Disturbance, metabolism, amino-acid) E72.9
- – – specified NEC E72.8
- – neonatal, transitory P74.8
- – renal transport NEC E72.0
- – transport NEC E72.0
- amnesic, amnestic
- – alcohol-induced F10.6
- – drug-induced – *code to* F11-F19 with fourth character .6F1X.6
- – due to (secondary to) general medical condition F04
- – sedative, hypnotic or anxiolytic-induced F13.6
- amfetamine (or related substance) use F15.9
- anaerobic glycolysis with anemia D55.2
- anxiety F41.9
- – due to (secondary to)
- – – alcohol F10.8
- – – amfetamine (or related substance) F15.8
- – – caffeine F15.8
- – – cannabis F12.8
- – – cocaine F14.8
- – – general medical condition F06.4
- – – hallucinogen F16.8
- – – inhalant F18.8
- – – phencyclidine (or related substance) F19.8
- – – psychoactive substance NEC F19.8
- – – sedative, hypnotic or anxiolytic F13.8
- – – volatile solvents F18.8
- – generalized F41.1

Disorder—*continued*
- anxiety—*continued*
- – mixed
- – – with depression (mild) F41.2
- – – specified NEC F41.3
- – organic F06.4
- – phobic F40.9
- – – of childhood F93.1
- – – specified NEC F41.8
- anxiolytic use F13.9
- aromatic amino-acid metabolism E70.9
- – specified NEC E70.8
- articulation – *see* Disorder, joint
- attachment (childhood)
- – disinhibited F94.2
- – reactive F94.1
- attention deficit, with hyperactivity F90.0
- autistic F84.0
- autonomic nervous system G90.9
- – specified NEC G90.8
- avoidant, child or adolescent F93.2
- balance
- – acid-base (mixed) E87.4
- – electrolyte E87.8
- – fluid NEC E87.8
- beta-amino-acid metabolism E72.8
- bilirubin excretion E80.6
- binocular
- – movement H51.9
- – – specified NEC H51.8
- – vision NEC H53.3
- bipolar F31.9
- – affective F31.9
- – – current episode
- – – – hypomanic F31.0
- – – – manic (without psychotic symptoms) F31.1
- – – – – with psychotic symptoms F31.2
- – – – mild or moderate depression F31.3
- – – – mixed F31.6
- – – – severe depression (without psychotic symptoms) F31.4
- – – – – with psychotic symptoms F31.5
- – – in remission (currently) F31.7
- – – specified NEC F31.8
- – I F31.9
- – – most recent episode
- – – – depressed
- – – – – mild or moderate severity F31.3
- – – – – severe (without psychotic symptoms) F31.4
- – – – – – with psychotic symptoms F31.5

Disorder—*continued*
- bipolar—*continued*
- – I—*continued*
- – – most recent episode—*continued*
- – – – hypomanic F31.0
- – – – manic (without psychotic symptoms) F31.1
- – – – – with psychotic symptoms F31.2
- – – – mixed F31.6
- – – II F31.8
- – organic F06.3
- – single manic episode F30.9
- – – mild F30.0
- – – moderate F30.1
- – – severe (without psychotic symptoms) F30.1
- – – – with psychotic symptoms F30.2
- bladder N32.9
- – functional NEC N31.9
- – in schistosomiasis B65.0† N33.8*
- – specified NEC N32.8
- body dysmorphic F45.2
- bone M89.9
- – continuity M84.9
- – – specified NEC M84.8
- – density and structure M85.9
- – – specified NEC M85.8
- – development and growth NEC M89.2
- – specified NEC M89.8
- brachial plexus G54.0
- branched-chain amino-acid metabolism E71.2
- – specified NEC E71.1
- breast N64.9
- – puerperal, postpartum O92.2
- – specified NEC N64.8
- Briquet's F45.0
- caffeine use F15.9
- cannabis use F12.9
- carbohydrate
- – absorption, intestinal NEC E74.3
- – metabolism (congenital) E74.9
- – – specified NEC E74.8
- cardiac, functional I51.8
- cardiovascular system I51.6
- – psychogenic F45.3
- cartilage M94.9
- – articular NEC M24.1
- catatonic
- – due to (secondary to) general medical condition F06.1
- – organic F06.1
- – schizophrenia F20.2

Disorder—*continued*
- cervical
- – region NEC M53.8
- – root (nerve) NEC G54.2
- character NEC F68.8
- childhood disintegrative NEC F84.3
- coagulation (factor) (*see also* Defect, coagulation) D68.9
- – newborn, transient P61.6
- cocaine use F14.9
- coccyx NEC M53.3
- cognitive
- due to (secondary to) general medical condition F06.9
- – – mixed F06.8
- – – mild F06.7
- colon K63.9
- – functional K59.9
- – – congenital Q43.2
- – – psychogenic F45.3
- conduct (childhood) F91.9
- – with emotional disorder F92.9
- – – specified NEC F92.8
- – adjustment reaction F43.2
- – compulsive F63.9
- – confined to the family context F91.0
- – depressive F92.0
- – group type F91.2
- – hyperkinetic F90.1
- – oppositional defiance F91.3
- – socialized F91.2
- – solitary aggressive type F91.1
- – specified NEC F91.8
- – unsocialized F91.1
- connective tissue, localized L94.9
- – specified NEC L94.8
- conversion (*see also* Disorder, dissociative) F44.9
- convulsive (secondary) (*see also* Convulsions) R56.8
- corpus cavernosum N48.9
- cranial nerve (*see also* Disorder, nerve, cranial) G52.9
- cyclothymic F34.0
- defiant oppositional F91.3
- delusional F22.0
- – induced F24
- – persistent F22.9
- – – specified NEC F22.8
- – systematized F22.0
- depersonalization F48.1
- depressive (*see also* Depression) F32.9
- – major
- – – recurrent F33.9

Disorder—*continued*
– depressive—*continued*
– – major—*continued*
– – – single episode
– – – – mild F32.0
– – – – moderate F32.1
– – – – severe (without psychotic
      symptoms) F32.2
– – – – – with psychotic symptoms F32.3
– – organic F06.3
– – recurrent F33.9
– – – current episode
– – – – mild F33.0
– – – – moderate F33.1
– – – – severe (without psychotic
      symptoms) F33.2
– – – – – with psychotic symptoms F33.3
– – – in remission F33.4
– – – specified NEC F33.8
– – single episode – *see* Episode,
   depressive
– developmental (global delay) F89
– – arithmetical skills F81.2
– – coordination (motor) F82
– – expressive writing F81.8
– – language (receptive type) F80.2
– – – expressive F80.1
– – learning F81.9
– – – arithmetical F81.2
– – – reading F81.0
– – mixed F83
– – motor coordination or function F82
– – pervasive F84.9
– – – specified NEC F84.8
– – phonological F80.0
– – reading F81.0
– – scholastic skills F81.9
– – – mixed F81.3
– – – specified NEC F81.8
– – specified NEC F88
– – speech F80.9
– – – and language disorder F80.9
– – – articulation F80.0
– – written expression F81.8
– digestive (system) K92.9
– – fetus or newborn P78.9
– – – specified NEC P78.8
– – postprocedural K91.9
– – – specified NEC K91.8
– – psychogenic F45.3
– disinhibited attachment (childhood) F94.2
– disintegrative, childhood NEC F84.3
– disk (intervertebral) M51.9
– disruptive behavior F98.9

Disorder—*continued*
– dissocial personality F60.2
– dissociative F44.9
– – affecting
– – – motor function F44.4
– – – – and sensation F44.7
– – – sensation F44.6
– – brief reactive F43.0
– – due to (secondary to) general medical
   condition F06.5
– – mixed F44.7
– – organic F06.5
– double heterozygous sickling D57.2
– dream anxiety F51.5
– drug-related, residual F19.7
– dysphoric, premenstrual F38.8
– dysthymic F34.1
– ear, postprocedural H95.9
– – specified NEC H95.8
– eating (psychogenic) F50.9
– – specified NEC F50.8
– electrolyte (balance) NEC E87.8
– elimination, transepidermal L87.9
– – specified NEC L87.8
– emotional (persistent) F34.9
– – with conduct disorder F92.9
– – of childhood F93.9
– – – specified NEC F93.8
– endocrine E34.9
– – postprocedural E89.9
– – – specified NEC E89.8
– erythematous – *see* Erythema
– esophagus K22.9
– – psychogenic F45.3
– eustachian tube H69.9
– – specified NEC H69.8
– extrapyramidal G25.9
– – specified type NEC G25.8
– eye, postprocedural H59.9
– – specified NEC H59.8
– factitious F68.1
– factor, coagulation (*see also* Defect,
   coagulation) D68.9
– fatty acid metabolism E71.3
– feeding (infant or child) F98.2
– feigned (with obvious motivation) Z76.5
– – without obvious motivation F68.1
– female
– – hypoactive sexual desire F52.0
– – orgasmic F52.3
– – sexual arousal F52.2
– fetus or newborn P96.9
– – specified NEC P96.8

Disorder—*continued*
- fibroblastic M72.9
- – specified NEC M72.8
- fluid balance E87.8
- follicular (skin) L73.9
- – specified NEC L73.8
- fructose metabolism E74.1
- functional, polymorphonuclear
  neutrophils D71
- gamma-glutamyl cycle E72.8
- gastric (functional) K31.9
- – psychogenic F45.3
  gastrointestinal (functional) NEC K92.9
- – psychogenic F45.3
- gender-identity or -role F64.9
- – childhood F64.2
- – effect on relationship F66.2
- – egodystonic F66.1
- – of adolescence or adulthood
    (nontranssexual) F64.1
- – specified NEC F64.8
- – uncertainty F66.0
- genitourinary system
- – female N94.9
- – male N50.9
- – psychogenic F45.3
- glomerular (in) N05.9
- – amyloidosis E85.4† N08.4*
- – cryoglobulinemia D89.1† N08.2*
- – disseminated intravascular coagulation
    D65† N08.2*
- – Fabry's disease E75.2† N08.4*
- – familial lecithin cholesterol
    acyltransferase deficiency E78.6†
    N08.4*
- – Goodpasture's syndrome M31.0†
    N08.5*
- – hemolytic-uremic syndrome D59.3†
    N08.2*
- – Henoch(-Schönlein) purpura D69.0†
    N08.2*
- – malariae malaria B52.0† N08.0*
- – microscopic polyangiits M31.7†
    N08.5*
- – multiple myeloma C90.0† N08.1*
- – mumps B26.8† N08.0*
- – schistosomiasis B65.-† N08.0*
- – septicemia NEC A41.-† N08.0*
- – – streptococcal A40.-† N08.0*
- – sickle-cell disorders D57.-† N08.2*
- – strongyloidiasis B78.9† N08.0*
- – subacute bacterial endocarditis I33.0†
    N08.8*
- – syphilis A52.7† N08.0*

Disorder—*continued*
- glomerular—*continued*
- – systemic lupus erythematosus M32.1†
    N08.5*
- – thrombotic thrombocytopenic purpura
    M31.1† N08.5*
- – Waldenström macroglobulinemia
    C88.0† N08.1*
- – Wegener's granulomatosis M31.3†
    N08.5*
- gluconeogenesis E74.4
- glucosaminoglycan E76.9
- – specified NEC E76.8
- glycine metabolism E72.5
- glycoprotein metabolism E77.9
- – specified NEC E77.8
- habit (and impulse) F63.9
- – involving sexual behavior NEC F65.9
- – specified NEC F63.8
- hallucinogen use F16.9
- heart action I49.9
- hematological D75.9
- – fetus or newborn P61.9
- – – specified NEC P61.8
- hematopoietic organs D75.9
- hemorrhagic NEC D69.9
- – due to circulating
    anticoagulants (*see also* Circulating
    anticoagulants) D68.3
- hemostasis (*see also* Defect, coagulation)
    D68.9
- histidine metabolism E70.8
- hyperkinetic F90.9
- – specified NEC F90.8
- hyperleucine-isoleucinemia E71.1
- hypervalinemia E71.1
- hypnotic use F13.9
- hypoactive sexual desire F52.0
- hypochondriacal F45.2
- identity
- – dissociative F44.8
- – of childhood F93.8
- immune mechanism (immunity) D89.9
- – specified type NEC D89.8
- impaired renal tubular function N25.9
- – specified NEC N25.8
- impulse (control) F63.9
- inhalant use F18.9
- integument, fetus or newborn P83.9
- – specified NEC P83.8
- intermittent explosive F63.8
- internal secretion, pancreas – *see* Increase,
    secretion, pancreas, endocrine

Disorder—*continued*
- intestine, intestinal
- – carbohydrate absorption NEC E74.3
- – – postoperative K91.2
- – functional K59.9
- – – psychogenic F45.3
- – vascular K55.9
- – – chronic K55.1
- – – specified NEC K55.8
- isovaleric acidemia E71.1
- jaw, developmental K10.0
- – temporomandibular K07.6
- joint M25.9
- – psychogenic F45.8
- kidney N28.9
- – functional (tubular) N25.9
- – in schistosomiasis B65.-† N29.1∗
- – tubular function N25.9
- – – specified NEC N25.8
- lactation O92.7
- language (developmental) F80.9
- – expressive F80.1
- – mixed receptive and expressive F80.2
- – receptive F80.2
- late luteal phase dysphoric N94.8
- learning F81.9
- ligament M24.2
- ligamentous attachments (*see also* Enthesopathy) M77.9
- – spine M46.0
- lipid
- – metabolism, congenital E78.9
- – storage E75.6
- – – specified NEC E75.5
- lipoprotein
- – deficiency (familial) E78.6
- – metabolism E78.9
- – – specified NEC E78.8
- liver K76.9
- – malarial B54† K77.0∗
- low back M53.8
- – psychogenic F45.4
- lumbosacral
- – plexus G54.1
- – root (nerve) NEC G54.4
- lung, interstitial, drug-induced J70.4
- – acute J70.2
- – chronic J70.3
- lysine and hydroxylysine metabolism E72.3
- male
- – erectile F52.2
- – – organic origin NEC N48.4
- – – – psychogenic F52.2

Disorder—*continued*
- male—*continued*
- – hypoactive sexual desire F52.0
- – organic origin NEC N48.4
- – orgasmic F52.3
- – psychogenic F52.2
- manic F30.9
- – organic F06.3
- mastoid process, postprocedural H95.9
- – specified NEC H95.8
- membranes or fluid, amniotic O41.9
- – affecting fetus or newborn P02.9
- meniscus NEC M23.9
- menopausal N95.9
- – specified NEC N95.8
- menstrual N92.6
- – psychogenic F45.8
- – specified NEC N92.5
- mental (or behavioral) (nonpsychotic) F99
- – affecting management of pregnancy, childbirth or puerperium O99.3
- – due to (secondary to)
- – – amfetamine (or related substance) withdrawal F15.9
- – – brain disease, damage or dysfunction F06.9
- – – caffeine use F15.9
- – – cannabis use F12.9
- – – general medical condition F06.9
- – – sedative or hypnotic use F13.9
- – – tobacco (nicotine) use F17.9
- – following organic brain damage F07.9
- – – frontal lobe syndrome F07.0
- – – personality change F07.0
- – – postconcussional syndrome F07.2
- – – specified NEC F07.8
- – infancy, childhood or adolescence F98.9
- – neurotic (*see also* Neurosis) F48.9
- – organic or symptomatic F06.9
- – presenile, psychotic F03
- – previous, affecting management of pregnancy Z35.8
- – psychoneurotic (*see also* Neurosis) F48.9
- – psychotic – *see* Psychosis
- – puerperal F53.9
- – – mild F53.0
- – – psychotic F53.1
- – – severe F53.1
- – – specified NEC F53.8
- – senile, psychotic NEC F03
- metabolism NEC E88.9

Disorder—*continued*
- metabolism—*continued*
- – amino-acid straight-chain E72.8
- – bilirubin E80.7
- – – specified NEC E80.6
- – calcium E83.5
- – carbohydrate E74.9
- – – specified NEC E74.8
- – cholesterol E78.9
- – congenital E88.9
- – copper E83.0
- – following abortion O08.5
- – fructose E74.1
- – galactose E74.2
- – glutamine E72.8
- – glycine E72.5
- – glycoprotein E77.9
- – – specified NEC E77.8
- – glycosaminoglycan E76.9
- – – specified NEC E76.8
- – in labor and delivery O75.8
- – iron E83.1
- – isoleucine E71.1
- – leucine E71.1
- – lipoid E78.9
- – lipoprotein E78.9
- – – specified NEC E78.8
- – magnesium E83.4
- – mineral E83.9
- – – specified NEC E83.8
- – ornithine E72.4
- – phosphatases E83.3
- – phosphorus E83.3
- – plasma protein NEC E88.0
- – porphyrin E80.2
- – postprocedural E89.9
- – – specified NEC E89.8
- – purine E79.9
- – – specified NEC E79.8
- – pyrimidine E79.9
- – – specified NEC E79.8
- – pyruvate E74.4
- – serine E72.8
- – specified NEC E88.8
- – threonine E72.8
- – valine E71.1
- – zinc E83.2
- methylmalonic acidemia E71.1
- micturition NEC R39.1
- – psychogenic F45.3
- mild cognitive F06.7
- mixed
- – anxiety and depressive F41.2

Disorder—*continued*
- mixed—*continued*
- – of scholastic skills (developmental) F81.3
- – receptive expressive language F80.2
- mood (*see also* Disorder, affective) F39
- – due to (secondary to)
- – – alcohol F10.8
- – – amfetamine (or related substance) F15.8
- – – cannabis F12.8
- – – cocaine F14.8
- – – general medical condition F06.3
- – – hallucinogen F16.8
- – – inhalant F18.8
- – – opioid F11.8
- – – phencyclidine (or related substance) F19.8
- – – psychoactive substance NEC F19.8
- – – sedative, hypnotic or anxiolytic F13.8
- – – volatile solvents F18.8
- – organic F06.3
- movement G25.9
- – hysterical F44.4
- – specified NEC G25.8
- – stereotyped F98.4
- – treatment-induced G25.9
- multiple personality F44.8
- muscle M62.9
- – psychogenic F45.8
- – specified NEC M62.8
- – tone, newborn P94.9
- – – specified NEC P94.8
- muscular attachments (*see also* Enthesopathy) M77.9
- – spine M46.0
- musculoskeletal system, soft tissue M79.9
- – postprocedural M96.9
- – psychogenic F45.8
- myoneural G70.9
- – due to lead G70.1
- – specified NEC G70.8
- – toxic G70.1
- myotonic G71.1
- neck region NEC M53.8
- nerve G58.9
- – abducent NEC H49.2
- – accessory G52.8
- – acoustic H93.3
- – auditory H93.3
- – cerebral – *see* Disorder, nerve, cranial

Disorder—*continued*
- nerve—*continued*
- − cranial G52.9
- − − eighth H93.3
- − − eleventh G52.8
- − − fifth G50.9
- − − first G52.0
- − − fourth NEC H49.1
- − − multiple G52.7
- − − ninth G52.1
- − − second NEC H47.0
- − − seventh NEC G51.9
- − − sixth NEC H49.2
- − − specified NEC G52.8
- − − tenth G52.2
- − − third NEC H49.0
- − − twelfth G52.3
- − facial G51.9
- − − specified NEC G51.8
- − femoral G57.2
- − glossopharyngeal NEC G52.1
- − hypoglossal G52.3
- − intercostal G58.0
- − lateral
- − − cutaneous of thigh G57.1
- − − popliteal G57.3
- − lower limb G57.9
- − − specified NEC G57.8
- − medial popliteal G57.4
- − median NEC G56.1
- − multiple G58.7
- − oculomotor NEC H49.0
- − olfactory G52.0
- − optic NEC H47.0
- − peroneal G57.3
- − phrenic G58.8
- − plantar G57.6
- − pneumogastric G52.2
- − radial G56.3
- − recurrent laryngeal G52.2
- − root G54.9
- − − specified NEC G54.8
- − sciatic NEC G57.0
- − specified NEC G58.8
- − − lower limb G57.8
- − − upper limb G56.8
- − sympathetic G90.9
- − tibial G57.4
- − trigeminal G50.9
- − − specified NEC G50.8
- − trochlear NEC H49.1
- − ulnar G56.2
- − upper limb G56.9
- − vagus G52.2

Disorder—*continued*
- nervous system G98
- − autonomic (peripheral) G90.9
- − − specified NEC G90.8
- − central G96.9
- − − specified NEC G96.8
- − parasympathetic G90.9
- − specified NEC G98
- − sympathetic G90.9
- − vegetative G90.9
- neurohypophysis NEC E23.3
- neurological NEC R29.8
- neuromuscular G70.9
- − hereditary NEC G71.9
- − specified NEC G70.8
- − toxic G70.1
- neurotic F48.9
- − specified NEC F48.8
- nicotine use F17.9
- nightmare F51.5
- nose NEC J34.8
- obsessive-compulsive F42.9
- − mixed obsessions and compulsions F42.2
- − predominantly with
- − − compulsions F42.1
- − − obsessions F42.0
- − specified NEC F42.8
- odontogenesis NEC K00.9
- oesophagus – *see* Disorder, esophagus
- opioid use F11.9
- oppositional defiant F91.3
- optic
- − chiasm H47.4
- − disk H47.3
- − radiations H47.5
- − tracts H47.5
- organic
- − anxiety F06.4
- − catatonic F06.1
- − delusional F06.2
- − dissociative F06.5
- − emotionally labile (asthenic) F06.6
- − mood (affective) F06.3
- − schizophrenia-like F06.2
- orgasmic (female) (male) F52.3
- ornithine metabolism E72.4
- overactive, associated with mental retardation and stereotyped movements F84.4
- overanxious, of childhood F93.8
- pain
- − associated with psychological factors F45.4

Disorder—*continued*
- pain—*continued*
- – due to general medical condition
  (secondary) R52.9
- pancreatic internal secretion E16.9
- – specified NEC E16.8
- panic F41.0
- – with agoraphobia F40.0
- papulosquamous L44.9
- – specified NEC L44.8
- paranoid F22.0
- – induced F24
- parathyroid (gland) E21.5
- – specified NEC E21.4
- parietoalveolar NEC J84.0
- paroxysmal, mixed R56.8
- patella M22.9
- – specified NEC M22.8
- patellofemoral M22.2
- pentose phosphate pathway with anemia
  D55.1
- perception, due to hallucinogens F16.7
- peripheral nervous system NEC G64
- persistent
- – affective (mood) F34.9
- – pain (somatoform) F45.4
- persisting
- – amnestic
- – – alcoholic F10.6
- – – sedative-induced F13.6
- – cognitive impairment R41.8
- – – due to
- – – – alcohol F10.7
- – – – cannabis F12.7
- – – – hallucinogens F16.7
- – – – sedatives, hypnotics or anxiolytics
  F13.7
- – – – specified substance NEC F19.7
- personality (*see also* Personality) F60.9
- – affective F34.0
- – aggressive F60.3
- – amoral F60.2
- – anankastic F60.5
- – antisocial F60.2
- – anxious F60.6
- – asocial F60.2
- – asthenic F60.7
- – avoidant F60.6
- – borderline F60.3
- – change (secondary) due to general
  medical condition F07.0
- – compulsive F60.5
- – cyclothymic F34.0
- – dependent F60.7

Disorder—*continued*
- personality—*continued*
- – depressive F34.1
- – dissocial F60.2
- – emotional instability F60.3
- – expansive paranoid F60.0
- – explosive F60.3
- – following organic brain damage F07.0
- – histrionic F60.4
- – hyperthymic F34.0
- – hypothymic F34.1
- – hysterical F60.4
- – immature F60.8
- – inadequate F60.7
- – labile F60.3
- – mixed (nonspecific) F61
- – moral deficiency F60.2
- – narcissistic F60.8
- – negativistic F60.8
- – obsessional F60.5
- – obsessive(-compulsive) F60.5
- – organic F07.9
- – paranoid F60.0
- – passive(-dependent) F60.7
- – passive-aggressive F60.8
- – pathological NEC F60.9
- – psychopathic F60.2
- – schizoid F60.1
- – schizotypal F21
- – self-defeating F60.7
- – sociopathic F60.2
- – specified NEC F60.8
- – unstable (emotional) F60.3
- pervasive, developmental F84.9
- phencyclidine use F19.9
- phobic anxiety, childhood F93.1
- phosphate-losing tubular N25.0
- pigmentation L81.9
- – choroid, congenital Q14.3
- – diminished melanin formation L81.6
- – iron L81.8
- – specified NEC L81.8
- pituitary gland E23.7
- – iatrogenic (postprocedural) E89.3
- – specified NEC E23.6
- plexus G54.9
- – specified NEC G54.8
- porphyrin metabolism E80.2
- postconcussional F07.2
- posthallucinogen perception F16.7
- postmenopausal N95.9
- – specified NEC N95.8
- post-traumatic stress F43.1
- propionic acidemia E71.1

Disorder—*continued*
- prostate N42.9
- - - specified NEC N42.8
- psychoactive substance use F19.9
- psychogenic NEC (*see also condition*) F45.9
- - anxiety F41.8
- - appetite F50.8
- - asthenic F48.0
- - cardiovascular (system) F45.3
- - compulsive F42.1
- - cutaneous F54
- - depressive F32.9
- - digestive (system) F45.3
- - dysmenorrheic F45.8
- - dyspneic F45.3
- - endocrine (system) F54
- - eye NEC F45.8
- - feeding F50.8
- - functional NEC F45.8
- - gastric F45.3
- - gastrointestinal (system) F45.3
- - genitourinary (system) F45.3
- - heart (function) (rhythm) F45.3
- - hyperventilatory F45.3
- - hypochondriacal F45.2
- - intestinal F45.3
- - joint F45.8
- - learning F81.9
- - limb F45.8
- - lymphatic (system) F45.8
- - menstrual F45.8
- - micturition F45.3
- - monoplegic NEC F44.4
- - motor F44.4
- - muscle F45.8
- - musculoskeletal F45.8
- - neurocirculatory F45.3
- - obsessive F42.0
- - occupational F48.8
- - organ or part of body NEC F45.8
- - paralytic NEC F44.4
- - phobic F40.9
- - physical NEC F45.8
- - rectal F45.3
- - respiratory (system) F45.3
- - rheumatic F45.8
- - sexual (function) F52.9
- - skin (allergic) (eczematous) F54
- - sleep F51.9
- - specified part of body NEC F45.8
- - stomach F45.3

Disorder—*continued*
- psychological F99
- - associated with
- - - disease classified elsewhere F54
- - - egodystonic orientation F66.1
- - - sexual
- - - - development F66.9
- - - - relationship F66.2
- - - uncertainty about gender identity F66.0
- psychomotor NEC F44.4
- - hysterical F44.4
- psychoneurotic (*see also* Neurosis) F48.9
- - mixed NEC F48.8
- psychophysiologic (*see also* Disorder, somatoform) F45.9
- psychosexual F65.9
- - development F66.9
- - - specified NEC F66.8
- - identity, of childhood F64.2
- psychosomatic NEC (*see also* Disorder, somatoform) F45.9
- - multiple F45.0
- - undifferentiated F45.1
- psychotic (duc to) (*see also* Psychosis) F29
- - acute F23.9
- - - specified NEC F23.8
- - alcohol(-induced), alcoholic (immediate) F10.5
- - - intoxication (acute) F10.5
- - - residual and late onset F10.7
- - amfetamine (or related substance) (intoxication) F15.5
- - brief
- - - with schizophrenia-like features F23.2
- - - without schizophrenia-like features F23.3
- - cannabis F12.5
- - cocaine (intoxication) F14.5
- - delusional F22.0
- - - acute F23.3
- - drug induced (immediate) (*see also* F11-F19 with fourth character .5) F19.5
- - - residual and late onset (*see also* F11-F19 with fourth character .7) F19.7
- - general medical condition (secondary) with
- - - delusions F06.2
- - - hallucinations F06.0

Disorder—*continued*
- psychotic—*continued*
- − hallucinogens F16.5
- − − intoxication (acute) F16.0
- − − withdrawal F16.4
- − induced F24
- − inhalant (intoxication) F18.5
- − opioid intoxication (acute) F11.5
- − phencyclidine (PCP) (or related substance) F19.5
- − − acute intoxication F19.0
- − polymorphic, acute (without symptoms of schizophrenia) F23.0
- − − with symptoms of schizophrenia F23.1
- − psychoactive substance NEC
- − − intoxication F19.5
- − − withdrawal F19.3
- − residual and late-onset
- − − alcohol-induced F10.7
- − − drug-induced (*see also* F11-F19 with fourth character .7) F19.7
- − sedative, hypnotic or anxiolytic (intoxication) F13.5
- − transient (acute) F23.9
- − − specified NEC F23.8
- puberty E30.9
- − specified NEC E30.8
- purine metabolism E79.9
- pyrimidine metabolism E79.9
- pyruvate metabolism E74.4
- reactive attachment (childhood) F94.1
- reading R48.0
- − developmental (specific) F81.0
- receptive language F80.2
- receptor, hormonal, peripheral E34.5
- recurrent brief depressive F38.1
- reflex R29.2
- refraction H52.7
- − specified NEC H52.6
- relationship F68.8
- − due to sexual orientation F66.2
- renal function, impaired (tubular) N25.9
- respiratory function, impaired J96.9
- − postprocedural J95.8
- − psychogenic F45.3
- right hemisphere organic affective F07.8
- rumination (infant or child) F98.2
- sacroiliac NEC M53.3
- sacrum, sacrococcygeal NEC M53.3
- schizoaffective F25.9
- − bipolar type F25.2
- − depressive type F25.1
- − manic type F25.0

Disorder—*continued*
- schizoaffective—*continued*
- − mixed type F25.2
- − specified NEC F25.8
- schizoid, of childhood F84.5
- schizophreniform F20.8
- − brief F23.2
- schizotypal (personality) F21
- sedative use F13.9
- seizure R56.8
- sense of smell R43.1
- − psychogenic F45.8
- separation anxiety, of childhood F93.0
- sexual
- − arousal, female F52.2
- − aversion F52.1
- − function, psychogenic F52.9
- − maturation F66.0
- − nonorganic F52.9
- − orientation (preference)
- − − effect on relationship F66.2
- − − egodystonic F66.1
- − − uncertainty F66.0
- − preference (*see also* Deviation, sexual) F65.9
- − − fetishistic transvestism F65.1
- − relationship F66.2
- sibling rivalry F93.3
- sickle-cell (sickling) (homozygous) D57.1
- − with crisis D57.0
- − double heterozygous D57.2
- − heterozygous D57.3
- − specified type NEC D57.8
- − trait D57.3
- sinus (nasal) NEC J34.8
- skin L98.9
- − atrophic L90.9
- − − specified NEC L90.8
- − fetus or newborn P83.9
- − − specified NEC P83.8
- − granulomatous L92.9
- − − specified NEC L92.8
- − hypertrophic L91.9
- − − specified NEC L91.8
- − infiltrative NEC L98.6
- − psychogenic (allergic) (eczematous) F54
- sleep G47.9
- − breathing-related G47.3
- − circadian rhythm G47.2
- − − psychogenic F51.2
- − due to
- − − alcohol F10.8

Disorder—*continued*
- sleep—*continued*
- – due to—*continued*
- – – amfetamine (or related substance) F15.8
- – – caffeine F15.8
- – – cannabis F12.8
- – – cocaine F14.8
- – – opioid F11.8
- – – psychoactive substance NEC F19.8
- – – sedative, hypnotic or anxiolytic F13.8
- – emotional F51.9
- – excessive somnolence G47.1
- – hypersomnia type G47.1
- – initiating or maintaining G47.0
- – insomnia type G47.0
- – mixed type G47.8
- – nonorganic F51.9
- – – specified NEC F51.8
- – parasomnia type G47.8
- – specified NEC G47.8
- – terrors F51.4
- – walking F51.3
- sleep-wake pattern or schedule G47.2
- – psychogenic F51.2
- social
- – anxiety, of childhood F93.2
- – functioning, in childhood F94.9
- – – specified NEC F94.8
- soft tissue M79.9
- – specified NEC M79.8
- somatization F45.0
- somatoform F45.9
- – pain (persistent) F45.4
- – somatization (long-lasting) (multiple) F45.0
- – specified NEC F45.8
- – undifferentiated F45.1
- somnolence, excessive G47.1
- specific
- – arithmetical F81.2
- – developmental, of motor F82
- – reading F81.0
- – speech and language F80.9
- – spelling F81.1
- – written expression F81.8
- speech NEC R47.8
- – articulation (functional) (specific) F80.0
- – developmental F80.9
- spelling (specific) F81.1

Disorder—*continued*
- spine M53.9
- – ligamentous or muscular attachments, peripheral M46.0
- – specified NEC M53.8
- stereotyped, habit or movement F98.4
- stomach (functional) (*see also* Disorder, gastric) K31.9
- stress F43.9
- – post-traumatic F43.1
- sulfur-bearing amino-acid metabolism E72.1
- sweat gland (eccrine) L74.9
- – apocrine L75.9
- – – specified NEC L75.8
- – specified NEC L74.8
- temperature regulation, fetus or newborn P81.9
- – specified NEC P81.8
- temporomandibular joint K07.6
- tendon M67.9
- – shoulder region M75.8
- thoracic root (nerve) NEC G54.3
- thyrocalcitonin hypersecretion E07.0
- thyroid (gland) E07.9
- – function NEC, neonatal, transitory P72.2
- – iodine-deficiency-related E01.8
- – specified NEC E07.8
- tic – *see* Tic
- tobacco use F17.9
- tooth
- – development K00.9
- – – specified NEC K00.8
- – eruption K00.6
- – – with abnormal position K07.3
- Tourette's F95.2
- trance and possession F44.3
- tryptophan metabolism E70.8
- tubular, phosphate-losing N25.0
- tubulo-interstitial (in)
- – brucellosis A23.-† N16.0∗
- – cystinosis E72.0† N16.3∗
- – diphtheria A36.8† N16.0∗
- – glycogen storage disease E74.0† N16.3∗
- – leukemia NEC C95.9† N16.1∗
- – lymphoma NEC C85.9† N16.1∗
- – mixed cryoglobulinemia D89.1† N16.2∗
- – multiple myeloma C90.0† N16.1∗
- – Salmonella infection A02.2† N16.0∗
- – sarcoidosis D86.8† N16.2∗

Disorder—*continued*
- tubulo-interstitial—*continued*
- - septicemia A41.-† N16.0*
- - - streptococcal A40.-† N16.0*
- - systemic lupus erythematosus M32.1†
  N16.4*
- - toxoplasmosis B58.8† N16.0*
- - transplant rejection T86.-† N16.5*
- - Wilson's disease E83.0† N16.3*
- tubulo-renal function, impaired N25.9
- - specified NEC N25.8
- tympanic membrane H73.9
  unsocialized aggressive F91.1
- urea cycle metabolism E72.2
- ureter (in) N28.9
- - schistosomiasis B65.0† N29.1*
- - tuberculosis A18.1† N29.1*
- urethra N36.9
- - specified NEC N36.8
- urinary system N39.9
- - specified NEC N39.8
- vestibular function H81.9
- - specified NEC H81.8
- visual
- - cortex H47.6
- - pathways H47.7
- - - specified NEC H47.5
- voice R49.8
- volatile solvent use F18.9
- withdrawing, child or adolescent F93.2

Disorientation R41.0
- psychogenic F44.8

Displacement, displaced
- acquired traumatic of bone, cartilage,
  joint, tendon NEC (without fracture) – *see*
  Dislocation
- adrenal gland (congenital) Q89.1
- appendix, retrocecal (congenital) Q43.8
- auricle (congenital) Q17.4
- bladder (acquired) N32.8
- - congenital Q64.1
- brachial plexus (congenital) Q07.8
- brain stem, caudal (congenital) Q04.8
- canuliculus (lacrimalis), congenital Q10.6
- cardia through esophageal hiatus
  (congenital) Q40.1
- cerebellum, caudal (congenital) Q04.8
- cervix (*see also* Malposition, uterus)
  N85.4
- colon (congenital) Q43.3
- device, implant or graft (*see also*
  Complications, by site and type,
  mechanical) T85.6

Displacement, displaced—*continued*
- device, implant or graft—*continued*
- - arterial graft NEC T82.3
- - - coronary (bypass) T82.2
- - breast (implant) T85.4
- - catheter NEC T85.6
- - - dialysis (renal) T82.4
- - - - intraperitoneal T85.6
- - - infusion NEC T82.5
- - - - spinal (epidural) (subdural) T85.6
- - - urinary (indwelling) T83.0
- - electronic (electrode) (pulse generator)
  (stimulator)
- - - bone T84.3
- - - cardiac T82.1
- - - nervous system (brain) (peripheral
  nerve) (spinal) T85.1
- - - urinary T83.1
- - fixation, internal (orthopedic) NEC
  T84.2
- - - bones of limb T84.1
- - gastrointestinal (bile duct) (esophagus)
  T85.5
- - genital NEC T83.4
- - - intrauterine contraceptive device
  T83.3
- - heart NEC T82.5
- - - valve (prosthesis) T82.0
- - - - graft T82.2
- - joint prosthesis T84.0
- - ocular (corneal graft) (orbital implant)
  NEC T85.3
- - - intraocular lens T85.2
- - orthopedic NEC T84.4
- - - bone graft T84.3
- - specified NEC T85.6
- - urinary NEC T83.1
- - - graft T83.2
- - vascular NEC T82.5
- - ventricular intracranial shunt T85.0
- epithelium
- - columnar, of cervix N87.9
- - cuboidal, beyond limits of external os
  Q51.8
- esophageal mucosa into cardia of
  stomach, congenital Q39.8
- esophagus (acquired) K22.8
- - congenital Q39.8
- eyeball (acquired) (lateral) (old) H05.2
- - congenital Q15.8
- fallopian tube (acquired) N83.4
- - congenital Q50.6
- - opening (congenital) Q50.6
- gallbladder (congenital) Q44.1

Displacement, displaced—*continued*
- gastric mucosa (congenital) Q40.2
- globe (acquired) (lateral) (old) H05.2
- heart (congenital) Q24.8
- – acquired I51.8
- hymen (upward) (congenital) Q52.4
- intervertebral disk NEC M51.2
- – with myelopathy M51.0† G99.2*
- – cervical, cervicothoracic (with) M50.2
- – – with myelopathy M50.0† G99.2*
- – – neuritis, radiculitis or radiculopathy M50.1† G55.1*
- – due to major trauma – *see* Dislocation, vertebra
- – lumbar, lumbosacral (with) M51.2
- – – myelopathy M51.0† G99.2*
- – – neuritis, radiculitis, radiculopathy or sciatica M51.1† G55.1*
- – – specified NEC M51.2
- – thoracic, thoracolumbar (with) M51.2
- – – due to major trauma S23.1
- – – myelopathy M51.0† G99.2*
- – – neuritis, radiculitis, radiculopathy M51.1† G55.1*
- – – specified NEC M51.2
- kidney (acquired) N28.8
- – congenital Q63.2
- lacrymal, lacrimal apparatus or duct (congenital) Q10.6
- lens, congenital Q12.1
- macula (congenital) Q14.1
- nail (congenital) Q84.6
- – acquired L60.8
- oesophagus (acquired) – *see* Displacement, esophagus
- opening of Wharton's duct in mouth Q38.4
- organ or site, congenital NEC – *see* Malposition, congenital
- ovary (acquired) N83.4
- – congenital Q50.3
- – free in peritoneal cavity (congenital) Q50.3
- – into hernial sac N83.4
- oviduct (acquired) N83.4
- – congenital Q50.6
- punctum lacrimale (congenital) Q10.6
- sacroiliac (joint) (congenital) Q74.2
- – current injury S33.2
- – old M53.2
- salivary gland (any) (congenital) Q38.4
- spleen (congenital) Q89.0
- stomach, congenital Q40.2
- tongue (downward) (congenital) Q38.3

Displacement, displaced—*continued*
- tooth, teeth K07.3
- trachea (congenital) Q32.1
- ureter or ureteric opening or orifice (congenital) Q62.6
- uterine opening of oviducts or fallopian tubes Q50.6
- uterus, uterine (*see also* Malposition, uterus) N85.4
- ventricular septum Q21.0
- – with rudimentary ventricle Q20.4

Disproportion (fetopelvic) O33.9
- affecting fetus or newborn P03.1
- caused by
- – conjoined twins O33.7
- – contraction pelvis (general) O33.1
- – – causing obstruction O65.1
- – – inlet O33.2
- – – outlet O33.3
- – fetal
- – – ascites O33.7
- – – deformity NEC O33.7
- – – hydrocephalus O33.6
- – – hydrops O33.7
- – – meningomyelocele O33.7
- – – sacral teratoma O33.7
- – – tumor O33.7
- – hydrocephalic fetus O33.6
- – pelvis, pelvic, abnormality (bony) NEC O33.0
- – – causing obstructed labor O65.0
- – unusually large fetus O33.5
- causing obstructed labor O65.4
- cephalopelvic O33.9
- – causing obstructed labor O65.4
- fetal (with normally formed fetus) O33.5
- fiber-type G71.2
- mixed maternal and fetal origin O33.4
- specified NEC O33.8

Disruptio uteri – *see* Rupture, uterus
Disruption
- ciliary body NEC H21.5
- family Z63.8
- – involving divorce or separation Z63.5
- iris NEC H21.5
- ligament(s) – *see also* Sprain
- – knee
- – – current injury – *see* Dislocation, knee
- – – old (chronic) M23.5
- – – spontaneous NEC M23.6
- marital Z63.0
- – involving divorce Z63.5
- wound
- – episiotomy O90.1

Disruption—*continued*
– wound—*continued*
– – operation T81.3
– – – cesarean O90.0
– – perineal (obstetric) O90.1
Dissatisfaction with
– employment Z56.7
– school environment Z55.4
Dissecting – *see condition*
Dissection
– aorta (any part) (ruptured) I71.0
– artery NEC I72.9
– – carotid I72.0
– – cerebral (nonruptured) I67.0
– – – ruptured (*see also* Hemorrhage, subarachnoid) I60.7
– – iliac (ruptured) I72.3
– – limb (ruptured)
– – – lower I72.4
– – – upper I72.1
– – precerebral NEC I72.5
– – – acquired (ruptured) I72.5
– – – – carotid I72.0
– – – – vertebral I72.5
– – – congenital (nonruptured) Q28.1
– – renal (ruptured) I72.2
– – specified (ruptured) NEC I72.8
– traumatic (complication)(early), specified site – *see* Injury, blood vessel, vascular
– vascular NEC I72.9
– wound – *see* Wound, open
Disseminated – *see condition*
Dissocial behavior, without manifest psychiatric disorder Z03.2
Dissociation
– auriculoventricular or atrioventricular (AV) (any degree) I45.8
– interference I45.8
Dissociative reaction, state F44.9
Dissolution, vertebra M81.9
Distal intestinal obstruction (syndrome) E84.1
Distension
– abdomen R14
– bladder N32.8
– cecum K63.8
– colon K63.8
– gallbladder K82.8
– intestine K63.8
– kidney N28.8
– liver K76.8
– seminal vesicle N50.8
– stomach K31.8
– – acute K31.0

Distension—*continued*
– stomach—*continued*
– – psychogenic F45.3
– ureter N28.8
– uterus N85.8
Distoma hepaticum infestation B66.3
Distomiasis B66.9
– hemic B65.9
– hepatic B66.3† K77.0*
– – due to Clonorchis sinensis B66.1† K77.0*
– intestinal B66.5
– liver B66.3† K77.0*
– – due to Clonorchis sinensis B66.1† K77.0*
– lung B66.4† J99.8*
– pulmonary B66.4† J99.8*
Distomolar (fourth molar) K00.1
– causing crowding K07.3
Disto-occlusion K07.2
Distortion (congenital)
– arm NEC Q68.8
– bile duct or passage Q44.5
– bladder Q64.7
– brain Q04.9
– cervix (uteri) Q51.9
– chest (wall) Q67.8
– – bones Q76.8
– clavicle Q74.0
– clitoris Q52.6
– coccyx Q76.4
– common duct Q44.5
– cystic duct Q44.5
– ear (auricle) (external) Q17.3
– – inner Q16.5
– – ossicles Q16.3
– eustachian tube Q16.4
– eye (adnexa) Q15.8
– face bone(s) NEC Q75.8
– fallopian tube Q50.6
– femur NEC Q68.8
– fibula NEC Q68.8
– finger(s) Q68.1
– foot Q66.9
– gyri Q04.8
– hand bone(s) Q68.1
– heart (auricle) (ventricle) Q24.8
– – valve (cusp) Q24.8
– hepatic duct Q44.5
– humerus NEC Q68.8
– hymen Q52.4
– intrafamilial communications Z63.8
– knee (joint) Q68.2
– labium (majus) (minus) Q52.7

Distortion—*continued*
- leg NEC Q68.8
- lens Q12.8
- liver Q44.7
- lumbar spine Q76.4
- – with disproportion O33.8
- – – affecting fetus or newborn P03.1
- – – causing obstructed labor O65.0
- lumbosacral (joint) (region) Q76.4
- nerve Q07.8
- nose Q30.8
- organ
- – of Corti Q16.5
- – – or site not listed – *see* Anomaly, by site
- oviduct Q50.6
- pancreas Q45.3
- patella Q68.2
- radius NEC Q68.8
- sacroiliac joint Q74.2
- sacrum Q76.4
- scapula Q74.0
- shoulder girdle Q74.0
- skull bone(s) NEC Q75.8
- – with
- – – encephalocele (*see also*
     Encephalocele) Q01.9
- – – hydrocephalus Q03.9
- – – – with spina bifida (*see also* Spina
       bifida, with hydrocephalus) Q05.4
- – – microcephaly Q02
- spinal cord Q06.8
- spine Q76.4
- spleen Q89.0
- sternum NEC Q76.7
- thorax (wall) Q67.8
- – bony Q76.8
- tibia NEC Q68.8
- toe(s) Q66.9
- tongue Q38.3
- trachea (cartilage) Q32.1
- ulna NEC Q68.8
- ureter Q62.8
- urethra Q64.7
- – causing obstruction Q64.3
- uterus Q51.9
- vagina Q52.4
- vertebra Q76.4
- vulva Q52.7
- wrist (bones) (joint) Q68.8
Distress
- abdominal R10.4
- epigastric R10.1
- fetal (syndrome) P20.-

Distress—*continued*
- fetal—*continued*
- – affecting
- – – labor and delivery O68.-
- – – management of pregnancy (unrelated
     to labor or delivery) O36.3
- – complicating labor and delivery O68.-
- – first noted
- – – before onset of labor P20.0
- – – during labor and delivery P20.1
- gastrointestinal (functional) K30
- – psychogenic F45.3
- intestinal (functional) NEC K59.9
- – psychogenic F45.3
- intrauterine – *see* Distress, fetal
- maternal, during labor and delivery O75.0
- respiratory R06.0
- – adult J80
- – newborn P22.9
- – – specified NEC P22.8
- – psychogenic F45.3
- – syndrome (idiopathic) (newborn) P22.0
- – – adult J80
Distribution vessel, atypical Q27.9
- precerebral Q28.1
Districhiasis L68.8
Disturbance – *see also* Disease
- absorption K90.9
- – calcium E58
- – carbohydrate K90.4
- – fat K90.4
- – – pancreatic K90.3
- – protein K90.4
- – starch K90.4
- – vitamin (*see also* Deficiency, vitamin)
     E56.9
- acid-base equilibrium (mixed) E87.4
- activity and attention (with hyperkinesis)
     F90.0
- assimilation, food K90.9
- auditory nerve, except deafness H93.3
- behavior – *see* Disorder, conduct
- blood clotting (mechanism) (*see also*
     Defect, coagulation) D68.9
- cerebral
- – nerve – *see* Disorder, nerve, cranial
- – status, newborn P91.9
- – – specified NEC P91.8
- circulatory I99
- conduct (*see also* Disorder, conduct)
     F91.9
- – with emotional disorder F92.9
- – adjustment reaction F43.2
- – compulsive F63.9

Disturbance—*continued*
- conduct—*continued*
- – disruptive F91.9
- – hyperkinetic F90.1
- – socialized F91.2
- – specified NEC F91.8
- – unsocialized F91.1
- coordination R27.8
- cranial nerve – *see* Disorder, nerve, cranial
- deep sensibility – *see* Disturbance, sensation
- digestive K30
- – psychogenic F45.3
- electrolyte (*see also* Imbalance, electrolyte) E87.8
- – newborn, transitory P74.4
- – – potassium balance P74.3
- – – sodium balance P74.2
- – – specified type NEC P74.4
- emotions specific to childhood and adolescence F93.9
- – with
- – – anxiety and fearfulness NEC F93.8
- – – sensitivity (withdrawal) F93.2
- – – shyness F93.2
- – – social withdrawal F93.2
- – involving relationship problems F93.8
- – mixed F93.8
- – specified NEC F93.8
- endocrine (gland) E34.9
- – neonatal, transitory P72.9
- – – specified NEC P72.8
- equilibrium R42
- feeding R63.3
- – newborn P92.9
- – nonorganic origin (infant or child) F98.2
- – psychogenic NEC F50.8
- fructose metabolism E74.1
- gait R26.8
- – hysterical F44.4
- – psychogenic F44.4
- gastrointestinal (functional) K30
- – psychogenic F45.3
- habit, child F98.9
- hearing, except deafness and tinnitus H93.2
- heart, functional (conditions in I44-I50)
- – due to presence of (cardiac) prosthesis I97.1
- – postoperative I97.8
- – – cardiac surgery I97.1
- hormones E34.9

Disturbance—*continued*
- innervation uterus (parasympathetic) (sympathetic) N85.8
- keratinization NEC
- – lip K13.0
- – oral (mucosa) (soft tissue) K13.2
- – tongue K13.2
- learning (specific) F81.9
- memory (*see also* Amnesia) R41.3
- – mild, following organic brain damage F06.7
- mental F99
- – associated with diseases classified elsewhere F54
- metabolism E88.9
- – amino-acid E72.9
- – – aromatic E70.9
- – – branched-chain E71.2
- – – straight-chain E72.8
- – – sulfur-bearing E72.1
- – ammonia E72.2
- – arginine E72.2
- – arginosuccinic acid E72.2
- – carbohydrate E74.9
- – cholesterol E78.9
- – citrulline E72.2
- – cystathionine E72.1
- – general E88.9
- – glutamine E72.8
- – histidine E70.8
- – homocystine E72.1
- – hydroxylysine E72.3
- – in labor or delivery O75.8
- – iron E83.1
- – lipoid E78.9
- – lysine E72.3
- – methionine E72.1
- – neonatal, transitory P74.9
- – – calcium and magnesium P71.9
- – – – specified type NEC P71.8
- – – carbohydrate metabolism P70.9
- – – – specified type NEC P70.8
- – – specified NEC P74.8
- – ornithine E72.4
- – phosphate E83.3
- – sodium NEC E87.8
- – threonine E72.8
- – tryptophan E70.8
- – tyrosine E70.2
- – urea cycle E72.2
- motor R29.2
- nervous, functional R45.0
- neuromuscular mechanism, eye, due to syphilis A52.1† H58.8*

Disturbance—*continued*
- nutritional E63.9
- − − nail L60.3
- ocular motion H51.9
- − − psychogenic F45.8
- oculogyric H51.8
- − − psychogenic F45.8
- oculomotor H51.9
- − − psychogenic F45.8
- olfactory nerve R43.1
- optic nerve NEC H47.0
- oral epithelium, including tongue K13.2
- perceptual due to
- − − alcohol withdrawal F10.3
- − − amfetamine (or related substance) intoxication (acute) F15.0
- − − cannabis intoxication (acute) F12.0
- − − cocaine intoxication (acute) F14.0
- − − hallucinogen intoxication (acute) F16.0
- − − opioid intoxication (acute) F11.0
- − − phencyclidine (or related substance) intoxication (acute) F19.0
- − − sedative, hypnotic or anxiolytic intoxication F13.0
- personality (pattern) (trait) (*see also* Disorder, personality) F60.9
- − − following organic brain damage F07.0
- polyglandular E31.9
- − − specified NEC E31.8
- potassium balance, newborn P74.3
- psychogenic F45.9
- psychomotor F44.4
- pupillary H57.0
- reflex R29.2
- rhythm, heart I49.9
- salivary secretion K11.7
- sensation (cold) (heat) (localization) (tactile discrimination) (texture) (vibratory) NEC R20.8
- − − hysterical F44.6
- − − skin R20.8
- − − smell R43.1
- − − − and taste (mixed) R43.8
- − − taste R43.2
- sensory − *see* Disturbance, sensation
- situational (transient) (*see also* Reaction, adjustment) F43.2
- − − acute F43.0
- sleep G47.9
- − − nonorganic origin F51.9
- smell R43.1
- − − and taste (mixed) R43.8
- sociopathic F60.2
- sodium balance, newborn P74.2

Disturbance—*continued*
- speech NEC R47.8
- − − developmental F80.9
- stomach (functional) K31.9
- sympathetic (nerve) G90.9
- taste R43.8
- temperature
- − − regulation, newborn P81.9
- − − − specified NEC P81.8
- − − sense R20.8
- − − − hysterical F44.6
- tooth
- − − eruption K00.6
- − − formation K00.4
- − − structure, hereditary NEC K00.5
- touch − *see* Disturbance, sensation
- vascular I99
- − − arteriosclerotic − *see* Arteriosclerosis
- vasomotor I73.9
- vasospastic I73.9
- vision, visual H53.9
- − − specified NEC H53.8
- voice R49.8
- − − psychogenic F44.4

Diuresis R35

Diver's palsy, paralysis or squeeze T70.3

Diverticula, diverticulitis, diverticulosis, diverticulum (acute) (multiple) K57.9
- appendix (noninflammatory) K38.2
- bladder (sphincter) N32.3
- − − congenital Q64.6
- bronchus (congenital) Q32.4
- − − acquired J98.0
- calyx, calyceal (kidney) N28.8
- cardia (stomach) K22.5
- cecum (*see also* Diverticula, intestine, large) K57.3
- − − congenital Q43.8
- colon (*see also* Diverticula, intestine, large) K57.3
- − − congenital Q43.8
- duodenum (*see also* Diverticula, intestine, small) K57.1
- − − congenital Q43.8
- esophagus (congenital) Q39.6
- − − acquired (epiphrenic) (pulsion) (traction) K22.5
- eustachian tube H69.8
- fallopian tube N83.8
- gastric K31.4
- heart (congenital) Q24.8
- ileum (*see also* Diverticula, intestine, small) K57.1

235

Diverticula—*continued*
- intestine K57.9
- – with abscess, perforation or peritonitis K57.8
- – both large and small K57.5
- – – with abscess, perforation or peritonitis K57.4
- – congenital Q43.8
- – large K57.3
- – – with abscess, perforation or peritonitis K57.2
- – small K57.1
- – – with abscess, perforation or peritonitis K57.0
- jejunum (*see also* Diverticula, intestine, small) K57.1
- Meckel's (displaced) (hypertrophic) Q43.0
- pericardium (congenital) (cyst) Q24.8
- pharyngoesophageal (congenital) Q39.6
- – acquired K22.5
- pharynx (congenital) Q38.7
- rectosigmoid (*see also* Diverticula, intestine, large) K57.3
- – congenital Q43.8
- rectum (*see also* Diverticula, intestine, large) K57.3
- seminal vesicle N50.8
- sigmoid (*see also* Diverticula, intestine, large) K57.3
- – congenital Q43.8
- stomach (acquired) K31.4
- – congenital Q40.2
- trachea (acquired) J39.8
- ureter (acquired) N28.8
- – congenital Q62.8
- ureterovesical orifice N28.8
- urethra (acquired) N36.1
- – congenital Q64.7
- ventricle, left (congenital) Q24.8
- vesical N32.3
- – congenital Q64.6
- Zenker's (esophagus) K22.5
Division
- cervix uteri (acquired) N88.8
- external os into two openings by frenum Q51.8
- glans penis Q55.6
- labia minora (congenital) Q52.7
- ligament (current) (partial or complete) (*see also* Sprain) T14.3
- – with open wound – *see* Wound, open
- muscle (current) (partial or complete) (*see also* Injury, muscle) T14.6

Division—*continued*
- muscle—*continued*
- – with open wound – *see* Wound, open
- nerve (traumatic) – *see* Injury, nerve
- spinal cord – *see* Injury, spinal cord, by region
- vein I87.8
Divorce, causing family disruption Z63.5
Dizziness R42
- hysterical F44.8
- psychogenic F45.8
Doehle-Heller aortitis A52.0† I79.1*
Dog bite – *see* Wound, open
Dolichocephaly Q67.2
Dolichocolon Q43.8
Dolichostenomelia Q74.0
Donohue's syndrome E34.8
Donor (organ or tissue) Z52.9
- blood (components) Z52.0
- bone Z52.2
- – marrow Z52.3
- cornea Z52.5
- heart Z52.7
- kidney Z52.4
- liver Z52.6
- lymphocytes Z52.0
- platelets Z52.0
- potential, examination of Z00.5
- skin Z52.1
- specified organ or tissue NEC Z52.8
- stem cells Z52.0
Donovanosis A58
Dorsalgia M54.9
- psychogenic F45.4
- specified NEC M54.8
Dorsopathy M53.9
- deforming M43.9
- – specified NEC M43.8
- specified NEC M53.8
Double
- albumin E88.0
- aortic arch Q25.4
- auditory canal Q17.8
- auricle (heart) Q20.8
- bladder Q64.7
- cervix Q51.8
- – with doubling of uterus (and vagina) Q51.1
- external os Q51.8
- inlet ventricle Q20.4
- kidney with double pelvis (renal) Q63.0
- meatus urinarius Q64.7
- monster Q89.4

Double—*continued*
– outlet
– – left ventricle Q20.2
– – right ventricle Q20.1
– pelvis (renal) with double ureter Q62.5
– tongue Q38.3
– ureter (one or both sides) Q62.5
– – with double pelvis (renal) Q62.5
– urethra Q64.7
– urinary meatus Q64.7
– uterus Q51.2
– – with
– – – double cervix (and vagina) Q51.1
– – – double vagina (and cervix) Q51.1
– – in pregnancy or childbirth O34.0
– – – affecting fetus or newborn P03.8
– – – causing obstructed labor O65.5
– vagina Q52.1
– – with double uterus (and cervix) Q51.1
– vision H53.2
– vulva Q52.7
Douglas' pouch or cul-de-sac – *see condition*
Down's disease or syndrome (*see also* Trisomy, 21) Q90.9
Dracontiasis B72
Dracunculiasis, dracunculosis B72
Dream state, hysterical F44.8
Drechslera (hawaiiensis) (infection) B43.8
Drepanocytic anemia (*see also* Disease, sickle-cell) D57.1
Dressler's syndrome I24.1
Drift, ulnar M21.8
Drinking (alcohol)
– excessive, to excess NEC F10.0
– – habitual (continual) F10.2
Drop
– finger M20.0
– foot M21.3
– toe M20.5
– wrist M21.3
Dropped
– dead, unexplained R96.0
– heart beats I45.9
Dropsy, dropsical (*see also* Hydrops) R60.9
– abdomen R18
– brain – *see* Hydrocephalus
– cardiac, heart (*see also* Failure, heart, congestive) I50.0
– cardiorenal I13.2
– gangrenous (*see also* Gangrene) R02
– lung (*see also* Edema, lung) J81
– pericardium (*see also* Pericarditis) I31.9

Drowned, drowning T75.1
Drowsiness R40.0
Drug
– abuse counseling and surveillance Z71.5
– addiction (*see also* Dependence) – *code to* F10-F19 with fourth character .2
– adverse effect NEC, correct substance properly administered T88.7
– dependence – *code to* F10-F19 with fourth character .2
– detoxification therapy Z50.3
– fever R50.2
– habit – *code to* F10-F19 with fourth character .2
– harmful use – *code to* F10-F19 with fourth character .1F1X.1
– overdose – *see* Table of drugs and chemicals
– poisoning – *see* Table of drugs and chemicals
– rehabilitation measures Z50.3
– resistant bacterial agent in bacterial infection – *see* Resistance, antibiotic, by bacterial agent
– use NEC Z72.2
– wrong substance given or taken in error – *see* Table of drugs and chemicals
Drunkenness F10.0
– acute in alcoholism F10.0
– chronic F10.2
– pathological F10.0
Drusen
– macula (degenerative) (retina) H35.3
– optic disk H47.3
Dry, dryness – *see also condition*
– socket (teeth) K10.3
Duane's syndrome H50.8
Dubin-Johnson disease or syndrome E80.6
Dubois' disease (thymus gland) A50.5† E35.8*
Dubowitz' syndrome Q87.1
Duchenne-Aran muscular atrophy G12.2
Duchenne-Griesinger disease G71.0
Duchenne's
– disease or syndrome
– – motor neuron disease G12.2
– – due to or associated with
– – – motor neuron disease G12.2
– – – muscular dystrophy G71.0
– locomotor ataxia (syphilitic) A52.1
– paralysis
– – birth injury P14.0

237

Duchenne's—*continued*
– paralysis—*continued*
– – due to or associated with
– – – motor neuron disease G12.2
– – – muscular dystrophy G71.0
Ducrey's chancre A57
Duct, ductus – *see condition*
Duhring's disease L13.0
Dullness, cardiac (decreased) (increased)
R01.2
Dumbness (*see also* Aphasia) R47.0
Dumdum fever B55.0
Dumping syndrome (postgastrectomy)
K91.1
Duodenitis (nonspecific) (peptic) K29.8
Duodenocholangitis (*see also* Cholangitis)
K83.0
Duodenum, duodenal – *see condition*
Duplay's bursitis or periarthritis M75.0
Duplex, duplication – *see also* Accessory
– alimentary tract NEC Q45.8
– anus Q43.4
– appendix (and cecum) Q43.4
– biliary duct (any) Q44.5
– bladder Q64.7
– cecum (and appendix) Q43.4
– chromosome NEC
– – with complex rearrangements NEC
Q92.5
– – seen only at prometaphase Q92.4
– cystic duct Q44.5
– digestive organs NEC Q45.8
– esophagus Q39.8
– frontonasal process Q75.8
– intestine (large) (small) Q43.4
– kidney Q63.0
– liver Q44.7
– oesophagus Q39.8
– pancreas Q45.3
– penis Q55.6
– placenta O43.1
– respiratory organs NEC Q34.8
– salivary duct Q38.4
– spinal cord (incomplete) Q06.8
– stomach Q40.2
Dupuytren's contraction or disease M72.0
Durand-Nicolas-Favre disease A55
Duroziez' disease Q23.2
Dust exposure (inorganic) Z58.1
– occupational Z57.2
– reticulation (*see also* Pneumoconiosis)
J64
– – organic dusts J66.8

Dutton's relapsing fever (West African)
A68.1
Dwarfism E34.3
– achondroplastic Q77.4
– congenital E34.3
– constitutional E34.3
– hypochondroplastic Q77.4
– hypophyseal E23.0
– infantile E34.3
– Laron-type E34.3
– Lorain(-Levi) type E23.0
– metatropic Q77.8
– nephrotic-glycosuric (with
hypophosphatemic rickets) E72.0†
N16.3*
– nutritional E45
– pancreatic K86.8
– pituitary E23.0
– psychosocial E34.3
– renal N25.0
– thanatophoric Q77.1
Dyke-Young anemia (secondary)
(symptomatic) D59.1
Dysacusis H93.2
Dysadrenocortism E27.9
Dysarthria R47.1
Dysautonomia (familial) G90.1
Dysbarism T70.3
Dysbasia R26.2
– angiosclerotica intermittens I73.9
– hysterical F44.4
– lordotica (progressiva) G24.1
– nonorganic origin F44.4
– psychogenic F44.4
Dyscalculia R48.8
– developmental F81.2
Dyschezia R19.8
Dyschondroplasia (with hemangiomata)
Q78.4
Dyschromia (skin) L81.9
Dyscranio-pygo-phalangy Q87.0
Dyscrasia
– blood (with) D75.9
– – antepartum hemorrhage O46.0
– – fetus or newborn P61.9
– – – specified type NEC P61.8
– – intrapartum hemorrhage O67.0
– – puerperal, postpartum O72.3
– polyglandular, pluriglandular E31.9
Dysendocrinism E34.9
Dysentery, dysenteric (catarrhal)
(diarrhea) (epidemic) (hemorrhagic)
(infectious) (sporadic) (tropical) A09.0

Dysentery—*continued*
- amebic (*see also* Amebiasis) A06.0
- - with abscess – *see* Abscess, amebic
- - acute A06.0
- - chronic A06.1
- arthritis A09.9† M03.-*
- - bacillary A03.9† M03.-*
- - infectious A09.0† M03.-*
- bacillary A03.9
- - arthritis A03.9† M01.3*
- - Boyd A03.2
- - Flexner A03.1
- - Schmitz(-Stutzer) A03.0
- - Shiga(-Kruse) A03.0
- - Shigella A03.9
- - - boydii A03.2
- - - dysenteriae A03.0
- - - flexneri A03.1
- - - group A A03.0
- - - group B A03.1
- - - group C A03.2
- - - group D A03.3
- - - sonnei A03.3
- - - specified type NEC A03.8
- - Sonne A03.3
- - specified type NEC A03.8
- balantidial A07.0
- Balantidium coli A07.0
- Boyd's A03.2
- candidal B37.8
- Chilomastix A07.8
- coccidial A07.3
- Dientamoeba (fragilis) A07.8
- Embadomonas A07.8
- Entamoeba, entamebic – *see* Dysentery, amebic
- Flexner's A03.1
- Giardia lamblia A07.1
- Hiss-Russell A03.1
- Lamblia A07.1
- leishmanial B55.0
- metazoal B82.0
- monilial B37.8
- protozoal A07.9
- Salmonella A02.0
- schistosomal B65.1
- Schmitz(-Stutzer) A03.0
- Shiga(-Kruse) A03.0
- Shigella NEC (*see also* Dysentery, bacillary) A03.9
- Sonne A03.3
- strongyloidiasis B78.0
- trichomonal A07.8
- viral (*see also* Enteritis, viral) A08.4

Dysesthesia R20.8
- hysterical F44.6
Dysfibrinogenemia (congenital) D68.2
Dysfunction
- adrenal E27.9
- ambulatory (transient) following surgery Z48.8
- autonomic
- - due to alcohol G31.2
- - somatoform F45.3
- bladder N31.9
- - neurogenic NEC (*see also* Dysfunction, bladder, neuromuscular) N31.9
- - neuromuscular NEC N31.9
- - - atonic (motor) (sensory) N31.2
- - - autonomous N31.2
- - - flaccid N31.2
- - - nonreflex N31.2
- - - reflex N31.1
- - - specified NEC N31.8
- - - uninhibited N31.0
- bleeding, uterus N93.8
- cerebral G93.8
- colon K59.9
- - psychogenic F45.3
- colostomy or enterostomy K91.4
- cystic duct K82.8
- cystostomy (stoma) N99.5
- endocrine NEC E34.9
- endometrium N85.8
- enteric stoma K91.4
- erectile (psychogenic) F52.2
- - organic origin NEC N48.4
- gallbladder K82.8
- gastrostomy (stoma) K91.8
- gland, glandular NEC E34.9
- heart I51.8
- hemoglobin D58.2
- hepatic K76.8
- hypophysis E23.3
- hypothalamic NEC E23.3
- ileostomy (stoma) K91.4
- jejunostomy (stoma) K91.4
- kidney (*see also* Disease, renal) N28.9
- labyrinthine H83.2
- liver K76.8
- orgasmic F52.3
- ovary E28.9
- - specified NEC E28.8
- papillary muscle I51.8
- physiological NEC R68.8
- - psychogenic F59
- pineal gland E34.8
- pituitary (gland) E23.3

Dysfunction—*continued*
- placental O43.8
- polyglandular E31.9
- - specified NEC E31.8
- psychophysiological F59
- rectum K59.9
- - psychogenic F45.3
- segmental M99.0
- senile R54
- sexual (due to)
- - alcohol F10.8
- - amfetamine (or related substance) F15.8
- - anxiolytic, hypnotic or sedative F13.8
- - cannabis F12.8
- - cocaine F14.8
- - excessive sexual drive F52.7
- - failure of genital response F52.2
- - inhibited orgasm (female) (male) F52.3
- - lack
- - - of sexual enjoyment F52.1
- - - or loss of sexual desire F52.0
- - nonorganic F52.9
- - - specified NEC F52.8
- - opioid F11.8
- - orgasmic dysfunction (female) (male) F52.3
- - premature ejaculation F52.4
- - psychoactive substances NEC F19.8
- - psychogenic F52.9
- - sexual aversion F52.1
- - vaginismus (nonorganic) (psychogenic) F52.5
- somatic M99.0
- somatoform autonomic F45.3
- stomach K31.8
- - psychogenic F45.3
- suprarenal E27.9
- symbolic NEC R48.8
- temporomandibular (joint) (joint-pain syndrome) K07.6
- testicular (endocrine) E29.9
- - specified NEC E29.8
- thyroid E07.9
- ureterostomy (stoma) N99.5
- urethrostomy (stoma) N99.5
- uterus, complicating delivery O62.9
- - affecting fetus or newborn P03.6
- - hypertonic O62.4
- - hypotonic O62.2
- - - primary O62.0
- - - secondary O62.1

Dysgenesis—*continued*
- gonadal (due to chromosomal anomaly) Q96.9
- - pure Q99.1
- renal Q60.5
- - bilateral Q60.4
- - unilateral Q60.3
- reticular D72.0
Dysgerminoma (M9060/3)
- specified site – *see* Neoplasm, malignant
- unspecified site
- - female C56
- - male C62.9
Dysgeusia R43.2
Dysgraphia R27.8
Dyshidrosis, dysidrosis L30.1
Dyskaryotic cervical smear R87.6
Dyskeratosis L85.8
- cervix (*see also* Dysplasia, cervix) N87.9
- congenital Q82.8
- uterus NEC N85.8
Dyskinesia G24.9
- biliary (cystic duct or gallbladder) K82.8
- esophagus K22.4
- hysterical F44.4
- intestinal K59.8
- neuroleptic-induced (tardive) G24.0
- nonorganic origin F44.4
- orofacial (idiopathic) G24.4
- psychogenic F44.4
- trachea J39.8
- tracheobronchial J98.0
Dyslalia (developmental) F80.0
Dyslexia R48.0
- developmental F81.0
Dyslipidemia E78.-
- depressed HDL cholesterol E78.6
- elevated fasting triglycerides E78.1
Dysmaturity (*see also* Immaturity) P05.0
- pulmonary (newborn) (Wilson-Mikity) P27.0
Dysmenorrhea (essential) (exfoliative) N94.6
- congestive (syndrome) N94.6
- primary N94.4
- psychogenic F45.8
- secondary N94.5
Dysmetria R27.8
Dysmorphism (due to)
- alcohol Q86.0
- exogenous cause NEC Q86.8
- hydantoin Q86.1
- warfarin Q86.2

240

Dysmorphophobia (nondelusional) F45.2
– delusional F22.8
Dysnomia R47.0
Dysorexia R63.0
– psychogenic F50.8
Dysostosis
– cleidocranial, cleidocranialis Q74.0
– craniofacial Q75.1
– mandibulofacial (incomplete) Q75.4
– multiplex E76.0
– oculomandibular Q75.5
Dyspareunia (female) N94.1
– male N48.8
– nonorganic F52.6
– psychogenic F52.6
– secondary N94.1
Dyspepsia (allergic) (congenital)
(functional) (gastrointestinal)
(occupational) (reflex) K30
– atonic K30
– nervous F45.3
– neurotic F45.3
– psychogenic F45.3
Dysphagia R13
– functional (hysterical) F45.8
– hysterical F45.8
– nervous (hysterical) F45.8
– psychogenic F45.8
– sideropenic D50.1
Dysphagocytosis, congenital D71
Dysphasia R47.0
– developmental
– – expressive type F80.1
– – receptive type F80.2
Dysphonia R49.0
– functional F44.4
– hysterical F44.4
– psychogenic F44.4
– spastica J38.3
Dyspituitarism E23.3
Dysplasia – *see also* Anomaly
– acetabular, congenital Q65.8
– arterial, fibromuscular I77.3
– arrhythmogenic right ventricular I42.8
– asphyxiating thoracic (congenital) Q77.2
– bronchopulmonary, perinatal P27.1
– cervix (uteri) N87.9
– – mild N87.0
– – moderate N87.1
– – severe NEC N87.2
– chondroectodermal Q77.6
– dentinal K00.5
– diaphyseal, progressive Q78.3
– dystrophic Q77.5

Dysplasia—*continued*
– ectodermal (anhidrotic) (congenital)
    (hereditary) Q82.4
– – hydrotic Q82.8
– epiphysis, epiphysealis
– – multiple, multiplex Q77.3
– – punctata Q77.3
– epithelial, uterine cervix (*see also*
    Dysplasia, cervix) N87.9
– eye (congenital) Q11.2
– fibrous
– – bone NEC M85.0
– – diaphyseal, progressive Q78.3
– – jaw K10.8
– – monostotic M85.0
– – polyostotic Q78.1
– florid osseous (M9275/0) D16.5
– – upper jaw (bone) D16.4
– hip, congenital Q65.8
– joint, congenital Q74.8
– kidney (multicystic) Q61.4
– leg Q74.2
– lung, congenital (not associated with short
    gestation) Q33.6
– mammary (gland) (benign) N60.9
– – cystic N60.1
– – specified NEC N60.8
– metaphyseal (Jansen's) (McKusick's)
    (Schmid's) Q78.5
– muscle Q79.8
– oculodentodigital Q87.0
– periapical (cemental) (cemento-osseous)
    (M9272/0) D16.5
– – upper jaw (bone) D16.4
– periosteum M89.8
– polyostotic fibrous Q78.1
– prostate (low grade) N42.3
– – high grade D07.5
– renal (multicystic) Q61.4
– retinal, congenital Q14.1
– right ventricular, arrhythmogenic I42.8
– septo-optic Q04.4
– spinal cord Q06.1
– spondyloepiphyseal Q77.7
– thymic, with immunodeficiency D82.1
– vagina N89.3
– – mild N89.0
– – moderate N89.1
– – severe NEC N89.2
– vulva N90.3
– – mild N90.0
– – moderate N90.1
– – severe NEC N90.2

Dyspnea (nocturnal) (paroxysmal) R06.0
- asthmatic (bronchial) J45.9
- - with bronchitis J45.9
- - - chronic J44.8
- - cardiac (*see also* Failure, ventricular, left) I50.1
- cardiac (*see also* Failure, ventricular, left) I50.1
- functional F45.3
- hyperventilation R06.0
- hysterical F45.3
- newborn P22.8
- psychogenic F45.3
- uremic N19
Dyspraxia R27.8
- developmental (syndrome) F82
Dysproteinemia E88.0
Dysreflexia
- autonomic G90.4
Dysrhythmia
- cardiac I49.9
- - newborn P29.1
- - postoperative I97.8
- - - long-term effect of cardiac surgery I97.1
- cerebral or cortical (*see also* Epilepsy) G40.9
Dyssomnia (*see also* Disorder, sleep) G47.9
Dyssynergia
- biliary K83.8
- cerebellaris myoclonica (Hunt's ataxia) G11.1
Dysthymia F34.1
Dysthyroidism E07.9
Dystocia O66.9
- affecting fetus or newborn P03.1
- cervical (failure of cervical dilatation) O62.0
- - affecting fetus or newborn P03.6
- - due to abnormality of cervix O65.5
- contraction ring O62.4
- - affecting fetus or newborn P03.6
- fetal, fetus O66.9
- - abnormality NEC O66.3
- - affecting fetus or newborn P03.1
- - oversized O66.2
- maternal O66.9
- - affecting fetus or newborn P03.1
- positional O64.9
- - affecting fetus or newborn P03.1
- shoulder (girdle) O66.0
- - affecting fetus or newborn P03.1
- - causing obstructed labor O66.0

Dystocia—*continued*
- uterine NEC O62.4
- - affecting fetus or newborn P03.6
Dystonia G24.9
- deformans progressive G24.1
- drug-induced G24.0
- idiopathic G24.1
- - familial G24.1
- - nonfamilial G24.2
- - orofacial G24.4
- lenticularis G24.8
- musculorum deformans G24.1
- orofacial (idiopathic) G24.4
- specified NEC G24.8
- torsion (idiopathic) G24.1
- - symptomatic (nonfamilial) G24.2
Dystonic movements R25.8
Dystrophy, dystrophia
- adiposogenital E23.6
- Becker's type G71.0
- choroid (central areolar) (generalized) (gyrate) (hereditary) (peripapillary) H31.2
- cornea (endothelial) (epithelial) (granular) (hereditary) (lattice) (macular) H18.5
- Duchenne's type G71.0
- due to malnutrition E45
- Erb's G71.0
- Fuchs' H18.5
- Gower's muscular G71.0
- hair L67.8
- Landouzy-Déjerine G71.0
- Leyden-Moebius G71.0
- muscular G71.0
- - benign (Becker type) G71.0
- - congenital (hereditary) (progressive) G71.2
- - - myotonic G71.1
- - distal G71.0
- - Duchenne type G71.0
- - Emery-Dreifuss G71.0
- - Erb type G71.0
- - facioscapulohumeral G71.0
- - Gower's G71.0
- - hereditary (progressive) G71.0
- - Landouzy-Déjerine type G71.0
- - limb-girdle G71.0
- - myotonic G71.1
- - progressive (hereditary) G71.0
- - - Charcot-Marie(-Tooth) type G60.0
- - pseudohypertrophic (infantile) G71.0
- - severe (Duchenne type) G71.0
- myocardium, myocardial (*see also* Degeneration, myocardial) I51.5

Dystrophy—*continued*
- myotonic, myotonica G71.1
- nail L60.3
- – congenital Q84.6
- nutritional E45
- ocular G71.0
- oculocerebrorenal E72.0
- oculopharyngeal G71.0
- ovarian N83.8
- polyglandular E31.8
- reflex (sympathetic) M89.0
- retinal (albipunctate) (pigmentary)
  (vitelliform) (hereditary) H35.5
- – in
- – – lipid storage disorders E75.-†
  H36.8∗

Dystrophy—*continued*
- retinal—*continued*
- – in—*continued*
- – – systemic lipidoses E75.6† H36.8∗
- Salzmann's nodular H18.4
- scapuloperoneal G71.0
- skin NEC L98.8
- sympathetic (reflex) M89.0
- tapetoretinal H35.5
- thoracic, asphyxiating Q77.2
- unguium L60.3
- – congenital Q84.6
- vitreoretinal H35.5
- vulva N90.4
- yellow (liver) – *see* Failure, hepatic
Dysuria R30.0
- psychogenic F45.3

E

Eales' disease H35.0
Ear – *see also condition*
– piercing Z41.3
– wax (impacted) H61.2
Earache H92.0
Eaton-Lambert syndrome (*see also*
Neoplasm) C80.-† G73.1*
– unassociated with neoplasm G70.8
Eberth's disease (typhoid fever) A01.0
Ebola virus disease A98.4
Ebstein's
– anomaly or syndrome (heart) Q22.5
– disease (renal tubular degeneration in
diabetes) E14.2† N16.3*
Eccentro-osteochondrodysplasia E76.2
Ecchondroma (M9210/0) – *see* Neoplasm,
bone, benign
Ecchondrosis (M9210/1) D48.0
Ecchymosis R58
– conjunctiva H11.3
– eye (traumatic) S05.1
– eyelid (traumatic) S00.1
– fetus or newborn P54.5
– spontaneous R23.3
– traumatic – *see* Contusion
Echinococciasis – *see* Echinococcus
Echinococcosis – *see* Echinococcus
Echinococcus (infection) B67.9
– granulosus B67.4
– – bone B67.2† M90.2*
– – liver B67.0† K77.0*
– – lung B67.1† J99.8*
– – multiple sites B67.3
– – specified site NEC B67.3
– – thyroid B67.3† E35.0*
– liver NEC B67.8† K77.0*
– – granulosus B67.0† K77.0*
– – multilocularis B67.5† K77.0*
– multilocularis B67.7
– – liver B67.5† K77.0*
– – multiple sites B67.6
– – specified site NEC B67.6
– orbit B67.-† H06.1*
– specified site NEC B67.9
– – granulosus B67.3
– – multilocularis B67.6
Echinorhynchiasis B83.8
Echinostomiasis B66.8
Echolalia R48.8

**Echovirus, as cause of disease classified
elsewhere** B97.1
**Eclampsia, eclamptic (coma) (convulsions)
(delirium) (with pre-existing or
pregnancy-related hypertension) NEC**
O15.9
– during labor and delivery O15.1
– not associated with pregnancy or
childbirth R56.8
– postpartum O15.2
– pregnancy O15.0
– – affecting fetus or newborn P00.0
– puerperal O15.2
Economic circumstances affecting care
Z59.9
Economo's disease A85.8
Ectasia, ectasis
– aorta (*see also* Aneurysm, aorta) I71.9
– – ruptured I71.8
– breast N60.4
– capillary I78.8
– cornea H18.7
– mammary duct N60.4
– sclera H15.8
Ecthyma L08.0
– contagiosum B08.0
– gangrenosum L08.0
– infectiosum B08.0
Ectocardia Q24.8
Ectodermal dysplasia (anhidrotic) Q82.4
Ectodermosis erosiva pluriorificialis
L51.1
Ectopic, ectopia (congenital)
– abdominal viscera Q45.8
– – due to defect in anterior abdominal wall
Q79.5
– ACTH syndrome E24.3
– anus Q43.5
– atrial beats I49.1
– beats I49.4
– – atrial I49.1
– – ventricular I49.3
– bladder Q64.1
– bone and cartilage in lung Q33.5
– brain Q04.8
– breast tissue Q83.8
– cardiac Q24.8
– cerebral Q04.8
– cordis Q24.8

Ectopic, ectopia—*continued*
- endometrium (*see also* Endometriosis) N80.9
- gastric mucosa Q40.2
- gestation (*see also* Pregnancy, by site) O00.9
- heart Q24.8
- hormone secretion NEC E34.2
- kidney (crossed) (pelvis) Q63.2
- lens, lentis Q12.1
- mole (*see also* Pregnancy, by site) O00.9
- organ or site NEC – *see* Malposition, congenital
- pancreas Q45.3
- pregnancy (*see also* Pregnancy, by site) O00.9
- pupil H21.5
- renal Q63.2
- testis (bilateral) (unilateral) Q53.0
- tissue in lung Q33.5
- ureter Q62.6
- ventricular beats I49.3
- vesicae Q64.1

Ectromelia Q73.8
- lower limb Q72.9
- upper limb Q71.9

Ectropion H02.1
- cervix N86
- – with cervicitis N72
- – congenital Q51.8
- congenital Q10.1
- eyelid (cicatricial) (paralytic) (senile) (spastic) H02.1
- – congenital Q10.1
- iris H21.8
- lip (acquired) K13.0
- – congenital Q38.0
- urethra N36.3
- uvea H21.8

Eczema (acute) (chronic) (erythematous) (fissum) (rubrum) (squamous) (*see also* Dermatitis) L30.9
- dyshydrotic L30.1
- external ear H60.5
- herpeticum B00.0
- hypertrophicum L28.0
- hypostatic I83.1
- impetiginous L01.1
- infantile (due to any substance) L20.8
- – intertriginous L21.1
- – seborrheic L21.1
- intertriginous NEC L30.4
- – infantile L21.1
- intrinsic (allergic) L20.8

Eczema—*continued*
- lichenified NEC L28.0
- marginatum (hebrae) B35.6
- pustular L30.3
- stasis I83.1
- vaccination, vaccinatum T88.1
- varicose I83.1

Eczematid L30.2

Eddowes(-Spurway) syndrome Q78.0

Edema, edematous R60.9
- with nephritis (*see also* Nephrosis) N04.-
- amputation stump (surgical) T87.6
- angioneurotic (allergic) (any site) (with urticaria) T78.3
- – hereditary D84.1
- angiospastic I73.9
- Berlin's (traumatic) S05.8
- brain G93.6
- – due to birth injury P11.0
- – fetus or newborn (anoxia or hypoxia) P52.4
- – – birth injury P11.0
- – traumatic S06.1
- cardiac (*see also* Failure, heart, congestive) I50.0
- cardiovascular (*see also* Failure, heart, congestive) I50.0
- cerebral – *see* Edema, brain
- cerebrospinal – *see* Edema, brain
- cervix (uteri) (acute) N88.8
- – puerperal, postpartum O90.8
- circumscribed, acute T78.3
- – hereditary D84.1
- complicating pregnancy O12.0
- conjunctiva H11.4
- cornea NEC H18.2
- due to lymphatic obstruction I89.0
- epiglottis – *see* Edema, glottis
- essential, acute T78.3
- – hereditary D84.1
- extremities, lower – *see* Edema, legs
- eyelid NEC H02.8
- famine (*see also* Malnutrition, severe) E43
- fetus or newborn NEC P83.3
- generalized R60.1
- gestational O12.0
- – with proteinuria O12.2
- glottis, glottic, glottidis (obstructive) (passive) J38.4
- – allergic T78.3
- – – hereditary D84.1
- heart (*see also* Failure, heart, congestive) I50.0

Edema, edematous—*continued*
- heat T67.7
- inanition (*see also* Malnutrition, severe) E43
- infectious R60.9
- iris H21.8
- joint M25.4
- larynx (*see also* Edema, glottis) J38.4
- legs R60.0
-   - due to venous obstruction I87.1
- localized R60.0
-   - due to venous obstruction I87.1
- lower limbs - *see* Edema, legs
- lung (acute) J81
-   - with heart condition or failure (*see also* Failure, ventricular, left) I50.1
-   - due to
-     - chemicals, fumes or vapors (inhalation) J68.1
-     - external agent J70.9
-      - specified NEC J70.8
-     - radiation J70.0
-   - meaning failure, left ventricle I50.1
-   - chemical (acute) J68.1
-     - chronic J68.4
-   - chronic J81
-     - due to
-      - chemicals, gases, fumes or vapors (inhalation) J68.4
-      - external agent J70.9
-       - specified NEC J70.8
-   - due to
-     - external agent J70.9
-      - specified NEC J70.8
-     - high altitude T70.2
-     - near drowning T75.1
-   - terminal J81
- lymphatic I89.0
-   - due to mastectomy I97.2
- macula H35.8
- Milroy's Q82.0
- nasopharynx J39.2
- newborn P83.3
- nutritional (*see also* Malnutrition, severe) E43
-   - with dyspigmentation, skin and hair E40
- optic disk or nerve H47.1
- orbit H05.2
- papilla, optic H47.1
- penis N48.8
- periodic T78.3
-   - hereditary D84.1
- pharynx J39.2

Edema, edematous—*continued*
- pitting R60.9
- pulmonary - *see* Edema, lung
- Quincke's T78.3
-   - hereditary D84.1
- retina H35.8
- salt E87.0
- scrotum N50.8
- seminal vesicle N50.8
- spermatic cord N50.8
- spinal (cord) (nontraumatic) (vascular) G95.1
-   - traumatic T09.3
- starvation (*see also* Malnutrition, severe) E43
- subglottic (*see also* Edema, glottis) J38.4
- supraglottic (*see also* Edema, glottis) J38.4
- testis N50.8
- toxic NEC R60.9
- tunica vaginalis N50.8
- vas deferens N50.8
- vulva (acute) N90.8

Educational handicap Z55.9
- specified NEC Z55.8

Edward's syndrome (*see also* Trisomy, 18) Q91.3

Effect, adverse NEC T78.9
- abnormal gravitational (G) forces or states T75.8
- abuse of
-   - adult T74.9
-   - child T74.9
- air pressure T70.9
-   - specified NEC T70.8
- altitude (high) - *see* Effect, adverse, high altitude
- anesthesia (*see also* Anesthesia) T88.5
-   - in
-     - labor and delivery O74.9
-      - affecting fetus or newborn P04.0
-     - pregnancy O29.9
-   - local, toxic
-     - in
-      - labor and delivery O74.4
-      - pregnancy O29.3
-     - postpartum, puerperal O89.3
-   - postpartum, puerperal O89.9
-   - specified NEC T88.5
-     - in
-      - labor and delivery O74.8
-      - pregnancy O29.8
-     - postpartum, puerperal O89.8
-   - spinal and epidural T88.5

Effect, adverse NEC—*continued*
- anesthesia—*continued*
- – – spinal and epidural—*continued*
- – – – headache T88.5
- – – – – in
- – – – – – labor and delivery O74.5
- – – – – – pregnancy O29.4
- – – – – postpartum, puerperal O89.4
- – – – in
- – – – – labor and delivery O74.6
- – – – – pregnancy O29.5
- – – – postpartum, puerperal O89.5
- antitoxin – *see* Complications, vaccination
- atmospheric pressure T70.9
- – – due to explosion T70.8
- – – high T70.3
- – – low – *see* Effect, adverse, high altitude
- – – specified effect NEC T70.8
- biological, correct substance properly administered (*see also* Effect, adverse, drug) T88.7
- blood (derivatives) (serum) (transfusion) – *see* Complications, transfusion
- chemical substance NEC T65.9
- – – specified – *see* Table of drugs and chemicals
- cobalt, radioactive T66
- cold (temperature) (weather) T69.9
- – – chilblains T69.1
- – – frostbite – *see* Frostbite
- – – specified effect NEC T69.8
- drugs and medicaments NEC T88.7
- – – correct substance properly administered T88.7
- – – overdose or wrong substance given or taken T50.9
- – – – specified drug – *see* Table of drugs and chemicals
- electric current, electricity (shock) T75.4
- – – burn – *see* Burn
- exertion (excessive) T73.3
- exposure – *see* Exposure
- external cause NEC T75.8
- fallout (radioactive) NEC T66
- fluoroscopy NEC T66
- foodstuffs
- – – allergic reaction (*see also* Allergy, food) T78.1
- – – noxious T62.9
- – – – specified type NEC (*see also* Poisoning, by name of noxious foodstuff) T62.8
- gases, fumes or vapors T59.9

Effect, adverse NEC—*continued*
- gases, fumes or vapors—*continued*
- – – specified NEC – *see* Table of drugs and chemicals
- glue (airplane) sniffing F18.1
- heat (*see also* Heat) T67.9
- high altitude NEC T70.2
- – anoxia T70.2
- – on
- – – ears T70.0
- – – sinuses T70.1
- – – polycythemia D75.1
- high-pressure fluids T70.4
- hot weather (*see also* Heat) T67.9
- hunger T73.0
- immunization – *see* Complications, vaccination
- immunological agents – *see* Complications, vaccination
- implantation (removable) of isotope or radium NEC T66
- infrared (radiation) (rays) NEC T66
- – – dermatitis or eczema L59.8
- infusion – *see* Complications, infusion
- ingestion or injection of isotope (therapeutic) NEC T66
- irradiation NEC T66
- isotope (radioactive) NEC T66
- lack of care of infants T74.0
- lightning T75.0
- – – burn – *see* Burn
- medical care T88.9
- – – specified NEC T88.8
- medicinal substance, correct, properly administered (*see also* Effect, adverse, drug) T88.7
- mesothorium NEC T66
- motion T75.3
- noise, on inner ear H83.3
- overheated places (*see also* Heat) T67.9
- polonium NEC T66
- psychosocial, of work environment Z56.5
- radiation (diagnostic) (fallout) (infrared) (natural source) (therapeutic) (tracer) (ultraviolet) (X-ray) NEC T66
- – – dermatitis or eczema – *see* Dermatitis, due to, radiation
- – – fibrosis of lung J70.1
- – – pneumonitis J70.0
- – – pulmonary manifestations
- – – – acute J70.0
- – – – chronic J70.1
- – – skin L59.9

Effect, adverse NEC—*continued*
- radiation—*continued*
- - suspected damage to fetus, affecting management of pregnancy O35.6
- radioactive substance NEC T66
- - dermatitis or eczema (*see also* Radiodermatitis) L58.9
- radioactivity NEC T66
- radiotherapy NEC T66
- - dermatitis or eczema (*see also* Radiodermatitis) L58.9
- radium NEC T66
- reduced temperature T69.9
- - specified effect NEC T69.8
- roentgen rays, roentgenography, roentgenoscopy NEC T66
- serum (prophylactic) (therapeutic) NEC T80.6
- specified NEC T78.8
- - external cause NEC T75.8
- teletherapy NEC T66
- thirst T73.1
- toxic – *see* Poisoning
- transfusion – *see* Complications, transfusion
- ultraviolet (radiation) (rays) NEC T66
- - burn – *see* Burn
- - dermatitis or eczema – *see* Dermatitis, due to, ultraviolet rays
- - - acute L56.8
- uranium NEC T66
- vaccine (any) – *see* Complications, vaccination
- vibration T75.2
- water pressure NEC T70.9
- - specified NEC T70.8
- weightlessness T75.8
- whole blood – *see* Complications, transfusion
- work environment Z56.5
- X-rays NEC T66
- - dermatitis or eczema (*see also* Radiodermatitis) L58.9
Effect(s) (of) (from) – *see* Effect, adverse
Effects, late – *see* Sequelae
Effluvium
- anagen L65.1
- telogen L65.0
Effort syndrome (psychogenic) F45.3
Effusion
- amniotic fluid – *see* Rupture, membranes, premature
- brain (serous) G93.6
- cerebral G93.6

Effusion—*continued*
- cerebrospinal (*see also* Meningitis) G03.9
- chest – *see* Effusion, pleura
- chylous, chyliform (pleura) J94.0
- intracranial G93.6
- joint M25.4
- meninges (*see also* Meningitis) G03.9
- pericardium, pericardial (noninflammatory) I31.3
- - acute (*see also* Pericarditis, acute) I30.9
- peritoneal (chronic) R18
- pleura, pleurisy, pleuritic, pleuropericardial J90
- - chylous, chyliform J94.0
- - fetus or newborn P28.8
- - influenzal (*see also* Influenza, with, respiratory manifestations) J11.1
- - malignant NEC C78.2
- - tuberculous NEC A16.5
- - - primary (progressive) A16.7
- - - - with bacteriological and histological confirmation A15.7
- spinal (*see also* Meningitis) G03.9
- thorax, thoracic – *see* Effusion, pleura
Egg shell nails L60.3
- congenital Q84.6
Egyptian splenomegaly B65.1
Ehlers-Danlos syndrome Q79.6
Eichstedt's disease B36.0
Eisenmenger's
- complex or syndrome I27.8
- defect Q21.8
Ejaculation
- premature F52.4
- semen, painful N48.8
- - psychogenic F52.6
Ekbom's syndrome (restless legs) G25.8
Elastic skin Q82.8
- acquired L57.4
Elastofibroma (M8820/0) – *see* Neoplasm, connective tissue, benign
Elastoma (juvenile) Q82.8
- Miescher's L87.2
Elastomyofibrosis I42.4
Elastosis
- actinic, solar L57.8
- atrophicans (senile) L57.4
- perforans serpiginosa L87.2
- senilis L57.4
Elbow – *see condition*

Electric current, electricity, effects (concussion) (fatal) (nonfatal) (shock) T75.4
– burn – *see* Burn
Electrocution T75.4
Electrolyte imbalance E87.8
Elephantiasis (nonfilarial) I89.0
– bancroftian B74.0
– congenital (any site) (hereditary) Q82.0
– due to
– – Brugia (malayi) B74.1
– – – timori B74.2
– – mastectomy I97.2
– – Wuchereria (bancrofti) B74.0
– eyelid H02.8
– filarial, filariensis (*see also* Filaria, filarial, filariasis) B74.9
– glandular I89.0
– graecorum A30.5
– lymphangiectatic I89.0
– lymphatic vessel I89.0
– – due to mastectomy I97.2
– scrotum (nonfilarial) I89.0
– surgical I97.8
– – postmastectomy I97.2
– telangiectodes I89.0
– vulva (nonfilarial) N90.8
Elevated, elevation
– antibody titer R76.0
– basal metabolic rate R94.8
– blood pressure (*see also* Hypertension) I10
– – reading (incidental) (isolated) (nonspecific), no diagnosis of hypertension R03.0
– body temperature (of unknown origin) R50.9
– diaphragm, congenital Q79.1
– erythrocyte sedimentation rate R70.0
– immunoglobulin level R76.8
– lactic acid dehydrogenase (LDH) level R74.0
– leukocyte count R72
– scapula, congenital Q74.0
– sedimentation rate R70.0
– transaminase level R74.0
– urine level of
– – catecholamines R82.5
– – indoleacetic acid R82.5
– – 17-ketosteroids R82.5
– – steroids R82.5
– venous pressure I87.8
– white blood cells NEC R72

Elliptocytosis (congenital) (hereditary) D58.1
– Hb C (disease) D58.1
– hemoglobin disease D58.1
– sickle-cell (disease) D57.8
Ellison-Zollinger syndrome E16.4
Ellis-van Creveld syndrome Q77.6
Elongated, elongation (congenital) –
see also Distortion
– cervix (uteri) Q51.8
– – hypertrophic N88.4
– colon Q43.8
– common bile duct Q44.5
– cystic duct Q44.5
– frenulum, penis Q55.6
– labia minora (acquired) N90.6
– ligamentum patellae Q74.1
– petiolus (epiglottidis) Q31.8
– tooth, teeth K00.2
Eltor cholera A00.1
Emaciation (due to malnutrition) E41
Embadomoniasis A07.8
Embedded tooth, teeth K01.0
– with abnormal position (same or adjacent tooth) K07.3
Embolic – *see condition*
Embolism (septic) I74.9
– air (any site) (traumatic) T79.0
– – following
– – – abortion – *see* Embolism, following, abortion
– – – infusion, therapeutic injection or transfusion T80.0
– – – procedure NEC T81.7
– – in pregnancy, childbirth or puerperium O88.0
– amniotic fluid (pulmonary) O88.1
– – following abortion – *see* Embolism, following, abortion
– aorta, aortic I74.1
– – abdominal I74.0
– – bifurcation I74.0
– – saddle I74.0
– – thoracic I74.1
– artery I74.9
– – auditory, internal I65.8
– – basilar (*see also* Occlusion, artery, basilar) I65.1
– – carotid (common) (internal) (*see also* Occlusion, artery, carotid) I65.2
– – cerebellar (anterior inferior) (posterior inferior) (superior) (*see also* Occlusion, artery, cerebellar) I66.3

Embolism—*continued*
- artery—*continued*
- - cerebral (*see also* Occlusion, artery, cerebral) I66.9
- - choroidal (anterior) I66.8
- - communicating posterior I66.8
- - coronary (*see also* Infarct, myocardium) I21.9
- - - not resulting in infarction I24.0
- - hypophyseal I66.8
- - iliac I74.5
- - limb I74.4
- - - lower I74.3
- - - upper I74.2
- - mesenteric (with gangrene) K55.0
- - ophthalmic H34.2
- - peripheral I74.4
- - pontine I66.8
- - precerebral (*see also* Occlusion, artery, precerebral) I65.9
- - pulmonary – *see* Embolism, pulmonary
- - renal N28.0
- - retinal H34.2
- - specified NEC I74.8
- - vertebral (*see also* Occlusion, artery, vertebral) I65.0
- birth, mother – *see* Embolism, obstetric
- blood clot
- - following
- - - abortion O08.2
- - in pregnancy, childbirth or puerperium O88.2
- brain (*see also* Occlusion, artery, cerebral) I66.9
- - in pregnancy, childbirth or puerperium O88.2
- capillary I78.8
- cardiac (*see also* Infarct, myocardium) I21.9
- - not resulting in infarction I24.0
- carotid (artery) (common) (internal) (*see also* Occlusion, artery, carotid) I65.2
- cavernous sinus (venous) – *see* Embolism, intracranial venous sinus
- cerebral (*see also* Occlusion, artery, cerebral) I66.9
- coronary (artery or vein) (systemic) (*see also* Infarct, myocardium) I21.9
- - not resulting in infarction I24.0
- due to device, implant or graft (*see also* Complications, by site and type, specified NEC) T85.8

Embolism—*continued*
- due to device, implant or graft—*continued*
- - arterial graft NEC T82.8
- - breast (implant) T85.8
- - catheter NEC T85.8
- - - dialysis (renal) T82.8
- - - - intraperitoneal T85.8
- - - infusion NEC T82.8
- - - - spinal (epidural) (subdural) T85.8
- - - urinary (indwelling) T83.8
- - electronic (electrode) (pulse generator) (stimulator)
- - - bone T84.8
- - - cardiac T82.8
- - - nervous system (brain) (peripheral nerve) (spinal) T85.8
- - - urinary T83.8
- - fixation, internal (orthopedic) NEC T84.8
- - gastrointestinal (bile duct) (esophagus) T85.8
- - genital NEC T83.8
- - heart (graft) (valve) T82.8
- - joint prosthesis T84.8
- - ocular (corneal graft) (orbital implant) T85.8
- - orthopedic (bone graft) NEC T84.8
- - specified NEC T85.8
- - urinary (graft) NEC T83.8
- - vascular NEC T82.8
- - ventricular intracranial shunt T85.8
- eye H34.2
- fat (cerebral) (pulmonary) (systemic) T79.1
- - complicating delivery O88.8
- femoral I74.3
- - vein (superficial) I80.1
- following
- - abortion (subsequent episode) O08.2
- - - current episode – *see* Abortion
- - ectopic or molar pregnancy O08.2
- - infusion, therapeutic injection or transfusion
- - - air T80.0
- - - thrombus T80.1
- heart (fatty) (*see also* Infarct, myocardium) I21.9
- - not resulting in infarction I24.0
- hepatic (vein) I82.0
- in pregnancy, childbirth or puerperium (*see also* Embolism, obstetric) O88.2
- intestine (artery) (vein) (with gangrene) K55.0

Embolism—*continued*
- intracranial (*see also* Occlusion, artery, cerebral) I66.9
- – venous sinus (any) G08
- – – nonpyogenic I67.6
- intraspinal venous sinuses or veins G08
- – nonpyogenic G95.1
- kidney (artery) N28.0
- lateral sinus (venous) – *see* Embolism, intracranial, venous sinus
- leg I80.3
- longitudinal sinus (venous) – *see* Embolism, intracranial, venous sinus
- lower extremity I80.3
- – arterial I74.3
- lung (massive) – *see* Embolism, pulmonary
- meninges I66.8
- mesenteric (artery) (vein) (with gangrene) K55.0
- multiple NEC I74.9
- obstetric (pulmonary) O88.2
- – air O88.0
- – amniotic fluid O88.1
- – blood clot O88.2
- – fat O88.8
- – pyemic O88.3
- – septic O88.3
- – specified NEC O88.8
- ophthalmic H34.2
- paradoxical NEC I74.9
- penis N48.8
- peripheral artery NEC I74.4
- pituitary E23.6
- portal (vein) I81
- postoperative T81.7
- precerebral artery (*see also* Occlusion, artery, precerebral) I65.9
- puerperal – *see* Embolism, obstetric
- pulmonary (artery) (vein) I26.9
- – with acute cor pulmonale I26.0
- – in pregnancy, childbirth or puerperium – *see* Embolism, obstetric
- pyemic (multiple) (*see also* Sepsis) A41.9
- – following
- – – abortion (subsequent episode) O08.2
- – – – current episode – *see* Abortion
- – – ectopic or molar pregnancy O08.2
- – pneumococcal A40.3
- – – with pneumonia J13
- – puerperal, postpartal or in childbirth (any organism) O88.3
- – specified organism NEC A41.8
- – staphylococcal A41.2

Embolism—*continued*
- pyemic—*continued*
- – streptococcal A40.9
- renal (artery) N28.0
- – vein I82.3
- retina, retinal H34.2
- septicemic – *see* Sepsis
- sinus – *see* Embolism, intracranial, venous sinus
- soap, following abortion O08.2
- spinal cord G95.1
- – pyogenic origin G06.1
- spleen, splenic (artery) I74.8
- thrombus (thromboembolism), following infusion, therapeutic injection or transfusion T80.1
- vein I82.9
- – cerebral I67.6
- – coronary (*see also* Infarct, myocardium) I21.9
- – – not resulting in infarction I24.0
- – hepatic I82.0
- – mesenteric (with gangrene) K55.0
- – portal I81
- – pulmonary – *see* Embolism, pulmonary
- – renal I82.3
- – specified NEC I82.8
- – vena cava I82.2
- vessels of brain (*see also* Occlusion, artery, cerebral) I66.9
Embolus – *see* Embolism
Embryoma (M9080/1) – *see also* Neoplasm, uncertain behavior
- benign (M9080/0) – *see* Neoplasm, benign
- kidney (M8960/3) C64
- liver (M8970/3) C22.0
- malignant (M9080/3) – *see also* Neoplasm, malignant
- – kidney (M8960/3) C64
- – liver (M8970/3) C22.0
- – testis (M9070/3) C62.9
- – – descended (scrotal) C62.1
- – – undescended C62.0
- testis (M9070/3) C62.9
- – descended (scrotal) C62.1
- – undescended C62.0
Embryonic
- circulation Q28.9
- heart Q28.9
- vas deferens Q55.4
Embryotomy (mother) (to facilitate delivery) O83.4
- fetus P03.8
Embryotoxon Q13.4

Emesis (*see also* Vomiting) R11
- gravidarum – *see* Hyperemesis, gravidarum
Emotionality, pathological F60.3
Emphysema (atrophic) (chronic) (interlobular) (lung) (obstructive) (pulmonary) (senile) J43.9
- bullous J43.9
- cellular tissue (traumatic) T79.7
- – surgical T81.8
- centrilobular J43.2
- compensatory J98.3
- congenital (interstitial) P25.0
- conjunctiva H11.8
- connective tissue (traumatic) T79.7
- – surgical T81.8
- due to chemicals, gases, fumes or vapors J68.4
- eyelid(s) H02.8
- – surgical T81.8
- – traumatic T79.7
- fetus or newborn (interstitial) P25.0
- interstitial J98.2
- – congenital P25.0
- – perinatal period P25.0
- laminated tissue T79.7
- – surgical T81.8
- mediastinal J98.2
- – fetus or newborn P25.2
- orbit, orbital H05.8
- panacinar J43.1
- panlobular J43.1
- specified NEC J43.8
- subcutaneous (traumatic) T79.7
- – postprocedural T81.8
- – surgical T81.8
- surgical T81.8
- traumatic (subcutaneous) T79.7
- unilateral J43.0
- vesicular J43.9
Empty nest syndrome Z60.0
Empyema (chest) (double) (pleura) (supradiaphragmatic) (thorax) J86.9
- with fistula J86.0
- accessory sinus (chronic) (*see also* Sinusitis) J32.9
- antrum (chronic) (*see also* Sinusitis, maxillary) J32.0
- brain (any part) (*see also* Abscess, brain) G06.0
- ethmoidal (sinus) (chronic) (*see also* Sinusitis, ethmoidal) J32.2
- extradural (*see also* Abscess, extradural) G06.2

Empyema—*continued*
- frontal (sinus) (chronic) (*see also* Sinusitis, frontal) J32.1
- gallbladder K81.0
- mastoid (process) (acute) H70.0
- maxillary sinus (chronic) (*see also* Sinusitis, maxillary) J32.0
- nasal sinus (chronic) (*see also* Sinusitis) J32.9
- sinus (accessory) (nasal) (chronic) (*see also* Sinusitis) J32.9
- sphenoidal (sinus) (chronic) (*see also* Sinusitis, sphenoidal) J32.3
- subarachnoid (*see also* Abscess, extradural) G06.2
- subdural (*see also* Abscess, subdural) G06.2
- tuberculous A16.5
- – with bacteriological and histological confirmation A15.6
- ureter (*see also* Ureteritis) N28.8
- ventricular (*see also* Abscess, brain) G06.0
En coup de sabre lesion L94.1
Enamel pearls K00.2
Enameloma K00.2
Enanthema, viral B09
Encephalitis (chronic) (hemorrhagic) (idiopathic) (nonepidemic) (spurious) (subacute) G04.9
- acute (*see also* Encephalitis, viral) A86
- – disseminated (postimmunization) (postinfectious) (postvaccination) G04.0
- arboviral, arbovirus NEC A85.2
- arthropod-borne NEC (viral) A85.2
- Australian A83.4
- California (virus) A83.5
- Central European (tick-borne) A84.1
- Czechoslovakian A84.1
- Dawson's (inclusion body) A81.1
- disseminated, acute G04.0
- endemic (viral) A86
- epidemic NEC (viral) A86
- equine (acute) (infectious) (viral) A83.9
- – Eastern A83.2
- – Venezuelan A92.2† G05.1*
- – Western A83.1
- Far Eastern (tick-borne) A84.0
- following vaccination or other immunization procedure G04.0
- herpes zoster B02.0† G05.1*
- herpesviral B00.4† G05.1*
- Ilheus (virus) A83.8

Encephalitis—*continued*
- in (due to)
- – actinomycosis A42.8† G05.0*
- – adenovirus A85.1† G05.1*
- – African trypanosomiasis B56.-†
  G05.2*
- – Chagas' disease (chronic) B57.4†
  G05.2*
- – cytomegalovirus B25.8† G05.1*
- – enterovirus A85.0† G05.1*
- – herpes (simplex) virus B00.4† G05.1*
- – human metapneumovirus A85.8†
  G05.1*
- – infectious disease NEC B99† G05.2*
- – influenza (specific virus not identified)
  J11.8† G05.1*
- – – avian influenza virus identified J09†
  G05.1*
- – – other influenza virus identified
  J10.8† G05.1*
- – listeriosis A32.1† G05.0*
- – measles B05.0† G05.1*
- – mumps B26.2† G05.1*
- – naegleriasis B60.2† G05.2*
- – parasitic disease NEC B89† G05.2*
- – poliovirus A80.9† G05.1*
- – rubella B06.0† G05.1*
- – syphilis
- – – congenital A50.4† G05.0*
- – – late A52.1† G05.0*
- – systemic lupus erythematosus M32.1†
  G05.8*
- – toxoplasmosis (acquired) B58.2†
  G05.2*
- – – congenital P37.1† G05.2*
- – tuberculosis A17.8† G05.0*
- – zoster B02.0† G05.1*
- infectious (acute), viral NEC A86
- Japanese (B type) A83.0
- La Crosse A83.5
- lead T56.0
- lethargica (acute) (infectious) A85.8
- louping ill A84.8
- lupus erythematosus, systemic M32.1†
  G05.8*
- lymphatica A87.2† G05.1*
- Mengo A85.8
- meningococcal A39.8† G05.0*
- Murray Valley A83.4
- otitic NEC H66.4† G05.8*
- periaxialis (concentrica) (diffuse) G37.5
- postchickenpox B01.1† G05.1*
- postimmunization G04.0
- postinfectious NEC G04.8

Encephalitis—*continued*
- postmeasles B05.0† G05.1*
- postvaccinal G04.0
- postvaricella B01.1† G05.1*
- postviral NEC A86
- Powassan A84.8
- Rio Bravo A85.8
- Russian
- – autumnal A83.0
- – spring-summer (taiga) A84.0
- saturnine T56.0
- specified NEC G04.8
- St Louis A83.3
- suppurative G04.8
- Torula, torular (cryptococcal) B45.1†
  G05.2*
- toxic NEC G92
- trichinosis B75† G05.2*
- type
- – B A83.0
- – C A83.3
- Venezuelan equine A92.2† G05.1*
- Vienna A85.8
- viral, virus A86
- – arthropod-borne NEC A85.2
- – mosquito-borne A83.9
- – – specified NEC A83.8
- – specified type NEC A85.8
- – tick-borne A84.9
- – – specified NEC A84.8

Encephalocele Q01.9
- frontal Q01.0
- nasofrontal Q01.1
- occipital Q01.2
- specified NEC Q01.8

Encephalomalacia (brain) (cerebellar) (cerebral) (*see also* Softening, brain) G93.8

Encephalomeningitis – *see* Meningoencephalitis

Encephalomeningocele (*see also* Encephalocele) Q01.9

Encephalomeningomyelitis – *see* Meningoencephalitis

Encephalomyelitis (*see also* Encephalitis) G04.9
- acute disseminated (postimmunization) G04.0
- – postinfectious G04.0
- benign myalgic G93.3
- due to or resulting from vaccination (any) G04.0
- equine Venezuelan A92.2† G05.1*
- myalgic, benign G93.3

Encephalomyelitis—*continued*
- postchickenpox B01.1† G05.1*
- postinfectious NEC G04.8
- postmeasles B05.0† G05.1*
- postvaccinal G04.0
- postvaricella B01.1† G05.1*
- rubella B06.0† G05.1*
- specified NEC G04.8
- Venezuelan equine A92.2† G05.1*
Encephalomyelocele (*see also*
Encephalocele) Q01.9
Encephalomyelomeningitis – *see*
Meningoencephalitis
Encephalomyelopathy G96.9
**Encephalomyeloradiculoneuritis (acute)
(Guillain-Barré)** G61.0
Encephalomyeloradiculopathy G96.9
**Encephalopathia hyperbilirubinemica,
newborn** P57.9
- due to isoimmunization (conditions in
P55.-) P57.0
Encephalopathy (acute) G93.4
- alcoholic G31.2
- anoxic – *see* Damage, brain, anoxic
- arteriosclerotic I67.2
- centrolobar progressive (Schilder) G37.0
- demyelinating callosal G37.1
- hepatic (*see also* Failure, hepatic) K72.9
- hyperbilirubinemic, newborn P57.9
- – due to isoimmunization (conditions in
P55.-) P57.0
- hypertensive I67.4
- hypoxic – *see* Damage, brain, anoxic
- – ischemic of newborn P91.6
- in (due to)
- – birth injury P11.1
- – hyperinsulinism E16.1† G94.8*
- – influenza (specific virus not identified)
J11.8† G94.8*
- – – avian influenza virus identified J09†
G94.8*
- – – other influenza virus identified
J10.8† G94.8*
- – lack of vitamin (*see also* Deficiency,
vitamin) E56.9† G32.8*
- – neoplastic disease NEC
(M8000/1) (*see also* Neoplasm)
D48.9† G13.1*
- – serum (nontherapeutic) (therapeutic)
T80.6
- – syphilis A52.1† G94.8*
- – trauma (postconcussional) F07.2
- – – current injury – *see* Contusion, brain
- – vaccination T80.6

Encephalopathy—*continued*
- lead T56.0
- myoclonic, early, symptomatic G40.4
- necrotizing, subacute (Leigh) G31.8
- pellagrous E52† G32.8*
- portosystemic (*see also* Failure, hepatic)
K72.9
- postcontusional F07.2
- – current injury – *see* Contusion, brain
- posthypoglycemic (coma) E16.1† G94.8*
- postradiation G93.8
- resulting from HIV disease B22.0
- saturnine T56.0
- spongiform, subacute (viral) A81.0
- toxic G92
- traumatic (postconcussional) F07.2
- – current injury S06.0
- vitamin B deficiency NEC E53.9†
G32.8*
- Wernicke's E51.2† G32.8*
Encephalorrhagia (*see also* Hemorrhage,
intracerebral) I61.9
Enchondroma (M9220/0) – *see* Neoplasm,
bone, benign
**Enchondromatosis (cartilaginous)
(multiple)** Q78.4
Encopresis R15
- functional F98.1
- nonorganic origin F98.1
- psychogenic F98.1
Encounter with health service (for) Z76.9
- administrative purpose only Z02.9
- – specified reason NEC Z02.8
- specified NEC Z76.8
Encystment – *see* Cyst
**Endarteritis (bacterial) (infective) (septic)
(subacute)** I77.6
- brain I67.7
- cerebral or cerebrospinal I67.7
- deformans – *see* Arteriosclerosis
- embolic (*see also* Embolism) I74.9
- obliterans (*see also* Arteriosclerosis)
I70.9
- – pulmonary I28.8
- retina H35.0
- senile – *see* Arteriosclerosis
- syphilitic A52.0† I79.8*
- – brain or cerebral A52.0† I68.1*
- – congenital A50.5† I79.8*
- tuberculous A18.8† I79.8*
Endemic – *see condition*

Endocarditis (chronic) (nonbacterial) (thrombotic) (valvular) I38
– with rheumatic fever (conditions in I00)
– – active – *see* Endocarditis, acute, rheumatic
– – inactive or quiescent – *see* condition, by valve, rheumatic
– acute or subacute I33.9
– – infective I33.0
– – rheumatic (aortic) (mitral) (pulmonary) (tricuspid) I01.1
– – – with chorea (acute) (rheumatic) (Sydenham's) I02.0
– aortic (heart) (nonrheumatic) (valve) I35.8
– – with
– – – mitral disease (unspecified origin) I08.0
– – – – with tricuspid (valve) disease (unspecified origin) I08.3
– – – – active or acute I01.1
– – – – – with chorea (acute) (rheumatic) (Sydenham's) I02.0
– – – rheumatic fever (conditions in I00)
– – – – active – *see* Endocarditis, acute, rheumatic
– – – – inactive or quiescent (with chorea) I06.9
– – – tricuspid (valve) disease (unspecified origin) I08.2
– – – – with mitral (valve) disease (unspecified origin) I08.3
– – acute or subacute I33.9
– – arteriosclerotic I35.8
– – rheumatic I06.9
– – – with mitral disease I08.0
– – – – with tricuspid (valve) disease I08.3
– – – – active or acute I01.1
– – – – – with chorea (acute) (rheumatic) (Sydenham's) I02.0
– – – active or acute I01.1
– – – – with chorea (acute) (rheumatic) (Sydenham's) I02.0
– – – specified NEC I06.8
– – specified cause NEC I35.8
– – syphilitic A52.0† I39.1*
– arteriosclerotic I38
– atypical verrucous (Libman-Sacks) M32.1† I39.8*
– bacterial (acute) (any valve) (subacute) I33.0
– candidal B37.6† I39.8*
– congenital I42.4

Endocarditis—*continued*
– Coxiella burnetii A78† I39.8*
– coxsackie virus B33.2† I39.8*
– due to prosthetic cardiac valve T82.6
– fetal I42.4
– gonococcal A54.8† I39.8*
– infectious or infective (acute) (any valve) (subacute) I33.0
– lenta (acute) (any valve) (subacute) I33.0
– Libman-Sacks M32.1† I39.8*
– listerial A32.8† I39.8*
– Löffler's I42.3
– malignant (acute) (any valve) (subacute) I33.0
– meningococcal A39.5† I39.8*
– mitral (chronic) (double) (fibroid) (heart) (inactive) (valve) (with chorea) I05.9
– – with
– – – aortic (valve) disease (unspecified origin) I08.0
– – – – with tricuspid (valve) disease (unspecified origin) I08.3
– – – – active or acute I01.1
– – – – – with chorea (acute) (rheumatic) (Sydenham's) I02.0
– – – rheumatic fever (conditions in I00)
– – – – active – *see* Endocarditis, acute, rheumatic
– – – – inactive or quiescent (with chorea) I05.9
– – – tricuspid (valve) disease (unspecified origin) I08.1
– – – – with aortic (valve) disease (unspecified origin) I08.3
– – active or acute I01.1
– – – with chorea (acute) (rheumatic) (Sydenham's) I02.0
– – arteriosclerotic I34.8
– – nonrheumatic I34.8
– – – acute or subacute I33.9
– – specified NEC I05.8
– monilial B37.6† I39.8*
– multiple valves (unspecified origin) I08.9
– – specified disorders (unspecified origin) I08.8
– mycotic (acute) (any valve) (subacute) I33.0
– pneumococcal (acute) (any valve) (subacute) I33.0
– pulmonary (chronic) (heart) (valve) I37.8
– – with rheumatic fever (conditions in I00)
– – – active – *see* Endocarditis, acute, rheumatic

Endometrioma = Endometriosis of ovary N80.1

Endocarditis—*continued*
- pulmonary—*continued*
- - with rheumatic fever—*continued*
- - - inactive or quiescent (with chorea)
    I09.8
- - - - with aortic, mitral or tricuspid
      disease (unspecified origin) I08.8
- - acute or subacute I33.9
- - - rheumatic I01.1
- - - with chorea (acute) (rheumatic)
      (Sydenham's) I02.0
- - arteriosclerotic I37.8
- - rheumatic (chronic) (inactive) (with
    chorea) I09.8
- - - active or acute I01.1
- - - - with chorea (acute) (rheumatic)
      (Sydenham's) I02.0
- - syphilitic A52.0† I39.3*
- purulent (acute) (any valve) (subacute)
  I33.0
- Q fever A78† I39.8*
- rheumatic (chronic) (inactive) – *see also*
  condition, by valve, rheumatic
- - active or acute (aortic) (mitral)
    (pulmonary) (tricuspid) I01.1
- - - with chorea (acute) (rheumatic)
      (Sydenham's) I02.0
- septic (acute) (any valve) (subacute)
  I33.0
- streptococcal (acute) (any valve)
  (subacute) I33.0
- subacute – *see* Endocarditis, acute
- suppurative (acute) (any valve) (subacute)
  I33.0
- syphilitic NEC A52.0† I39.8*
- toxic I33.9
- tricuspid (chronic) (heart) (inactive)
  (rheumatic) (valve) (with chorea) I07.8
- - with
- - - aortic (valve) disease (unspecified
      origin) I08.2
- - - - mitral (valve) disease (unspecified
      origin) I08.3
- - - mitral (valve) disease (unspecified
      origin) I08.1
- - - - aortic (valve) disease (unspecified
      origin) I08.3
- - - rheumatic fever (conditions in I00)
- - - - active – *see* Endocarditis, acute,
      rheumatic
- - - - inactive or quiescent (with chorea)
      I07.8
- - active or acute I01.1

Endocarditis—*continued*
- tricuspid—*continued*
- - active or acute—*continued*
- - - with chorea (acute) (rheumatic)
      (Sydenham's) I02.0
- - arteriosclerotic I36.8
- - nonrheumatic I36.8
- - - acute or subacute I33.9
- - specified cause, except rheumatic I36.8
- tuberculous (*see also* Tuberculosis,
  endocarditis) A18.8† I39.8*
- typhoid A01.0† I39.8*
- ulcerative (acute) (any valve) (subacute)
  I33.0
- vegetative (acute) (any valve) (subacute)
  I33.0
- verrucous (atypical) (nonbacterial)
  (nonrheumatic) M32.1† I39.8*
Endocardium, endocardial – *see also*
  condition
- cushion defect Q21.2
Endocervicitis (*see also* Cervicitis) N72
- due to intrauterine (contraceptive) device
  T83.6
- hyperplastic N72
Endocrine – *see condition*
Endomastoiditis – *see* Mastoiditis
Endometriosis N80.9
- fallopian tube N80.2
- intestine N80.5
- ovary N80.1
- pelvic peritoneum N80.3
- rectovaginal septum N80.4
- skin (scar) N80.6
- specified site NEC N80.8
- stromal (M8931/1) D39.0
- uterus N80.0
- vagina N80.4
Endometritis (nonspecific) (purulent)
  (septic) (suppurative) N71.9
- acute N71.0
- blenorrhagic (acute) (chronic) A54.2†
  N74.3*
- cervix, cervical (with erosion or
  ectropion) (*see also* Cervicitis) N72
- - hyperplastic N72
- chlamydial A56.1† N74.4*
- chronic N71.1
- complicating pregnancy O23.5
- - affecting fetus or newborn P00.8
- following
- - abortion (subsequent episode) O08.0
- - - current episode – *see* Abortion
- - ectopic or molar pregnancy O08.0

Endometritis—*continued*
- gonococcal, gonorrheal (acute) (chronic) A54.2† N74.3*
- hyperplastic N85.0
- – cervix N72
- puerperal, postpartum O85
- senile (atrophic) N71.9
- subacute N71.0
- tuberculous A18.1† N74.1*

Endometrium – *see condition*
Endomyocarditis – *see* Endocarditis
Endomyofibrosis I42.3
Endomyometritis (*see also* Endometritis) N71.9
Endoperineuritis – *see* Disorder, nerve
Endophlebitis (*see also* Phlebitis) I80.9
Endophthalmia H44.0
Endophthalmitis (acute) (infective) (metastatic) (subacute) H44.0
- with associated postprocedural bleb H59.8
- gonorrheal A54.3† H45.1*
- in (due to)
- – cysticercosis B69.1† H45.1*
- – onchocerciasis B73† H45.1*
- – toxocariasis B83.0† H45.1*
- parasitic NEC H44.1
- purulent H44.0
- specified NEC H44.1
- sympathetic H44.1

Endosalpingioma (M8932/0) D28.2
Endosteitis – *see* Osteomyelitis
Endothelioma, bone (M9260/3) – *see* Neoplasm, bone, malignant
Endotheliosis (hemorrhagic infectious) D69.8
Endotrachelitis (*see also* Cervicitis) N72
Engelmann(-Camurati) syndrome Q78.3
Engman's disease L30.3
Engorgement
- breast N64.5
- – newborn P83.4
- – puerperal, postpartum O92.2
- lung (passive) (*see also* Edema, lung) J81
- pulmonary (passive) (*see also* Edema, lung) J81
- stomach K31.8
- venous, retina H34.8

Enlargement, enlarged – *see also* Hypertrophy
- adenoids J35.2
- – with tonsils J35.3
- alveolar ridge K08.8

Enlargement, enlarged—*continued*
- apertures of diaphragm (congenital) Q79.1
- blind spot, visual field H53.4
- gingival K06.1
- heart, cardiac (*see also* Hypertrophy, cardiac) I51.7
- lacrimal gland, chronic H04.0
- liver (*see also* Hypertrophy, liver) R16.0
- lymph gland or node R59.9
- – generalized R59.1
- – localized R59.0
- organ or site, congenital NEC – *see* Anomaly, by site
- parathyroid (gland) E21.0
- prostate N40
- spleen – *see* Splenomegaly
- thymus (gland) (congenital) E32.0
- thyroid (gland) (*see also* Goiter) E04.9
- tongue K14.8
- tonsils J35.1
- – with adenoids J35.3
- uterus N85.2

Enophthalmos H05.4
Entamebic, entamebiasis – *see* Amebiasis
Entanglement
- umbilical cord(s) O69.2
- – with compression O69.2
- – affecting fetus or newborn P02.5
- – around neck (with compression) O69.1
- – – without compression O69.8
- – of twins in monoamniotic sac O69.2

Enteralgia R10.4
Enteric – *see condition*
Enteritis (diarrheal) (hemorrhagic) A09.9
- with septicemia NEC A09.0
- acute A09.9
- – bloody A09.0
- – hemorrhagic A09.0
- allergic K52.2
- amebic (*see also* Amebiasis) A06.0
- – acute A06.0
- – – with abscess – *see* Abscess, amebic
- – – nondysenteric A06.2
- – chronic A06.1
- – – with abscess – *see* Abscess, amebic
- – – nondysenteric A06.2
- – nondysenteric A06.2
- bacillary NEC A03.9
- bacterial A04.9
- – specified NEC A04.8
- candidal B37.8
- Chilomastix A07.8
- chronic (noninfectious) K52.9

Enteritis—*continued*
- chronic—*continued*
- - ulcerative K51.9
- coccidial A07.3
- dietetic K52.2
- due to
- - food hypersensitivity K52.2
- - infectious organism (bacterial) (viral) –
  see Enteritis, infectious
- - Yersinia enterocolitica A04.6
- eltor A00.1
- epidemic A09.0
- gangrenous (*see also* Enteritis, infectious)
  A09.0
- giardial A07.1
- infectious NEC A09.0
- - due to
- - - adenovirus A08.2
- - - Aerobacter aerogenes A04.8
- - - Arizona (bacillus) A02.0
- - - bacteria NEC A04.9
- - - - specified NEC A04.8
- - - Campylobacter A04.5
- - - Clostridium perfringens A04.8
- - - Enterobacter aerogenes A04.8
- - - enterovirus A08.3
- - - Escherichia coli A04.4
- - - - enteroaggregative A04.4
- - - - enterohemorrhagic A04.3
- - - - enteroinvasive A04.2
- - - - enteropathogenic A04.0
- - - - enterotoxigenic A04.1
- - - - specified NEC A04.4
- - - specified
- - - - bacteria NEC A04.8
- - - - virus NEC A08.3
- - - Staphylococcus A04.8
- - - virus NEC A08.4
- - - - specified type NEC A08.3
- - - Yersinia enterocolitica A04.6
- - specified organism NEC A08.5
- influenzal (specific virus not identified)
  J11.8
- - avian influenza virus identified J09
- - other influenza virus identified J10.8
- ischemic K55.9
- - acute K55.0
- - chronic K55.1
- microsporidial A07.8
- mucomembranous, myxomembranous –
  see Syndrome, irritable bowel
- mucous – *see* Syndrome, irritable bowel
- necroticans A05.2
- necrotizing of fetus or newborn P77

Enteritis—*continued*
- neurogenic – *see* Syndrome, irritable
  bowel
- noninfectious K52.9
- parasitic NEC B82.9
- paratyphoid (fever) (*see also* Fever,
  paratyphoid) A01.4
- protozoal A07.9
- - specified NEC A07.8
- regional (of) K50.9
- - intestine K50.9
- - - large (colon or rectum) K50.1
- - - - with small intestine K50.8
- - - small (duodenum, ileum or jejunum)
  K50.0
- - - - with large intestine K50.8
- rotaviral A08.0
- Salmonella, salmonellosis (arizonae)
  (cholerae-suis) (enteritidis) (typhimurium)
  A02.0
- segmental K50.9
- septic A09.0
- Shigella (*see also* Infection, Shigella)
  A03.9
- spasmodic, spastic – *see* Syndrome,
  irritable bowel
- staphylococcal A04.8
- toxic K52.1
- trichomonal A07.8
- tuberculous (*see also* Tuberculosis)
  A18.3† K93.0*
- typhosa A01.0
- ulcerative (chronic) K51.9
- - specified NEC K51.8
- viral A08.4
- - adenovirus A08.2
- - enterovirus A08.3
- - Rotavirus A08.0
- - small round structured A08.1
- - virus specified NEC A08.3
Enterobiasis B80
Enterobius vermicularis (infection)
  (infestation) B80
Enterocele (*see also* Hernia, abdomen)
  K46.9
- vagina, vaginal (acquired) (congenital)
  NEC N81.5
Enterocolitis (*see also* Enteritis) A09.9
- due to Clostridium difficile A04.7
- fulminant ischemic K55.0
- hemorrhagic (acute) K55.0
- infectious NEC A09.0
- ischemic K55.9

Enterocolitis—*continued*
- necrotizing
- - due to Clostridium difficile A04.7
- - fetus or newborn P77
- noninfectious NEC K52.9
- ulcerative (chronic) K51.0
Enterogastritis – *see* Enteritis
Enterolith, enterolithiasis (impaction)
  K56.4
Enteropathy K63.9
- gluten-sensitive K90.0
- protein-losing K90.4
Enteroptosis K63.4
Enterorrhagia K92.2
Enterostenosis (*see also* Obstruction,
  intestine) K56.6
Enterostomy, malfunctioning K91.4
**Enterovirus, as cause of disease classified
  elsewhere** B97.1
Enthesopathy M77.9
- ankle and tarsus M77.5
- elbow region M77.8
- foot NEC M77.5
- hip M76.8
- knee M76.8
- lower limb M76.9
- - specified NEC M76.8
- peripheral NEC M77.9
- shoulder region M75.9
- - adhesive M75.0
- - specified NEC M75.8
- specified NEC M77.8
- spinal M46.0
- wrist and carpus NEC M77.8
Entomophthoromycosis B46.8
Entrance, air into vein – *see* Embolism, air
Entrapment, nerve – *see* Neuropathy,
  entrapment
**Entropion (cicatricial) (eyelid) (paralytic)
  (senile) (spastic)** H02.0
- congenital Q10.2
- - eyelid Q10.2
Enucleated eye (traumatic, current) S05.7
Enuresis R32
- functional F98.0
- nocturnal R32
- - psychogenic F98.0
- nonorganic origin F98.0
- psychogenic F98.0
Eosinopenia D72.8
Eosinophilia (allergic) (hereditary) D72.1
- pulmonary NEC J82
- tropical (pulmonary) J82
Eosinophilia-myalgia syndrome M35.8

**Ependymitis (acute) (cerebral) (chronic)
  (granular)** (*see also* Encephalomyelitis)
  G04.9
Ependymoblastoma (M9392/3)
- specified site – *see* Neoplasm, malignant
- unspecified site C71.9
Ependymoma (epithelial) (malignant)
  (M9391/3)
- anaplastic (M9392/3)
- - specified site – *see* Neoplasm,
  malignant
- - unspecified site C71.9
- myxopapillary (M9394/1) D43.2
- - specified site – *see* Neoplasm, uncertain
  behavior
- - unspecified site D43.2
- papillary (M9393/1) D43.2
- - specified site – *see* Neoplasm, uncertain
  behavior
- - unspecified site D43.2
- specified site – *see* Neoplasm, malignant
- unspecified site C71.9
Ependymopathy G93.8
Ephelis, ephelides L81.2
Epiblepharon (congenital) Q10.3
**Epicanthus, epicanthic fold (eyelid)
  (congenital)** Q10.3
Epicondylitis (elbow)
- lateral M77.1
- medial M77.0
Epicystitis (*see also* Cystitis) N30.9
Epidemic – *see condition*
Epidermidalization, cervix (*see also*
  Dysplasia, cervix) N87.9
Epidermis, epidermal – *see condition*
Epidermodysplasia verruciformis B07
Epidermolysis
- bullosa (congenital) Q81.9
- - acquired L12.3
- - dystrophica Q81.2
- - letalis Q81.1
- - simplex Q81.0
- - specified NEC Q81.8
- necroticans combustiformis L51.2
- - due to drug
- - - correct substance properly
  administered L51.2
- - - overdose or wrong substance given
  or taken T50.9
- - - - specified drug – *see* Table of drugs
  and chemicals
Epidermophytid – *see* Dermatophytosis
Epidermophytosis (infected) – *see*
  Dermatophytosis

Epididymis – *see condition*
Epididymitis (acute) (nonvenereal) (recurrent) (residual) N45.9
– with abscess N45.0
– blennorrhagic (gonococcal) A54.2† N51.1*
– caseous (tuberculous) A18.1† N51.1*
– chlamydial A56.1† N51.1*
– gonococcal A54.2† N51.1*
– syphilitic A52.7† N51.1*
– tuberculous A18.1† N51.1*
Epididymo-orchitis (*see also* Epididymitis) N45.9
– with abscess N45.0
Epidural – *see condition*
Epigastrium, epigastric – *see condition*
Epigastrocele – *see* Hernia, ventral
Epiglottis – *see condition*
Epiglottitis, epiglottiditis (acute) J05.1
– chronic J37.0
Epignathus Q89.4
Epilepsy, epileptic, epilepsia G40.9
– with
– – complex partial seizures G40.2
– – grand mal seizures on awakening G40.3
– – myoclonic absences G40.4
– – myoclonic-astatic seizures G40.4
– – simple partial seizures G40.1
– abdominal G40.8
– absence (juvenile) (childhood) G40.3
– akinetic G40.3
– attack G40.9
– – with alteration of consciousness G40.2
– – without alteration of consciousness G40.1
– automatism G40.2
– Bravais-jacksonian G40.1
– cerebral G40.9
– childhood (benign) (with)
– – centrotemporal EEG spikes G40.0
– – occipital EEG paroxysms G40.0
– climacteric G40.8
– clonic G40.3
– clouded state G40.8
– coma G40.8
– convulsions G40.9
– cortical (focal) (motor) G40.1
– cysticercosis B69.0† G94.8*
– deterioration (mental) F06.8
– due to syphilis A52.1† G94.8*
– equivalent G40.8
– fits G40.9
– focal (motor) G40.1

Epilepsy, epileptic—*continued*
– generalized G40.3
– – convulsive G40.3
– – flexion G40.3
– – idiopathic G40.3
– – nonconvulsive G40.3
– – specified NEC G40.4
– grand mal (seizures) G40.6
– – on awakening G40.3
– idiopathic G40.9
– – generalized G40.3
– – localization-related G40.0
– jacksonian (motor) (sensory) G40.1
– Kozhevnikof's G40.5
– limbic system G40.2
– localization-related (focal) (partial) G40.8
– – idiopathic G40.0
– – symptomatic G40.1
– – – with
– – – – alteration of consciousness G40.2
– – – – complex partial seizures G40.2
– – – – simple partial seizures G40.1
– – – without alteration of consciousness G40.1
– major G40.3
– minor G40.3
– mixed (type) G40.3
– motor partial G40.1
– musicogenic G40.8
– myoclonus, myoclonic G40.3
– – benign, of infancy G40.3
– – juvenile G40.3
– – progressive (familial) G40.3
– parasitic NEC B71.9† G94.8*
– partial (localized) G40.1
– – with
– – – alteration of consciousness G40.2
– – – memory and ideational disturbances G40.2
– – secondarily generalized G40.1
– partialis continua G40.5
– peripheral G40.8
– petit mal (juvenile) (childhood) G40.3
– procursiva G40.2
– progressive (familial) myoclonic G40.3
– psychomotor G40.2
– psychosensory G40.2
– reflex G40.8
– related to
– – alcohol G40.5
– – drugs G40.5
– – external cause NEC G40.5
– – hormonal changes G40.5
– – sleep deprivation G40.5

Epilepsy, epileptic—*continued*
– related to—*continued*
– – stress G40.5
– seizure (*see also* Seizure, epileptic) G40.9
– senile G40.8
– somatomotor G40.1
– somatosensory G40.1
– specified type NEC G40.8
– status G41.9
– – absence G41.1
– – complex partial G41.2
– – focal motor G41.8
– – grand mal G41.0
– – petit mal G41.1
– – psychomotor G41.2
– – specified NEC G41.8
– – temporal lobe G41.2
– – tonic-clonic G41.0
– symptomatic NEC G40.8
– – with
– – – complex partial seizures G40.2
– – – simple partial seizures G40.1
– syndrome
– – with
– – – complex partial seizures G40.2
– – – seizures of localized onset G40.0
– – – simple partial seizures G40.1
– – generalized G40.4
– – – idiopathic G40.3
– – special NEC G40.5
– temporal lobe G40.2
– tonic(-clonic) G40.3
– traumatic (injury unspecified) T90.5
– – injury specified – *code to* Sequelae of specified injury
– twilight F05.8
– uncinate (gyrus) G40.2
– Unverricht(-Lundborg) (familial myoclonic) G40.3
– visceral G40.8
– visual G40.8
Epiloia Q85.1
Epimenorrhea N92.0
Epipharyngitis (*see also* Nasopharyngitis) J00
Epiphora H04.2
Epiphyseolysis, epiphysiolysis (*see also* Osteochondrosis) M93.9
Epiphysitis (*see also* Osteochondrosis) M93.9
– juvenile M92.9
– syphilitic (congenital) A50.0† M90.2*
Epiplocele (*see also* Hernia, abdomen) K46.9

Epiploitis (*see also* Peritonitis) K65.9
Epiplosarcomphalocele Q79.2
Episcleritis H15.1
– in (due to)
– – syphilis A52.7† H19.0*
– – tuberculosis A18.5† H19.0*
– periodica fugax H15.1
– suppurative H15.1
– syphilitic (late) A52.7† H19.0*
– tuberculous A18.5† H19.0*
Episode
– affective, mixed F38.0
– brain (apoplectic) I64
– cerebral (apoplectic) I64
– depressive F32.9
– – major (*see also* Disorder, depressive, major) F32.9
– – mild F32.0
– – moderate F32.1
– – recurrent – *see also* Disorder, depressive, recurrent
– – – brief F38.1
– – severe (without psychotic symptoms) F32.2
– – – with psychotic symptoms F32.3
– – specified NEC F32.8
– hypomanic F30.0
– manic F30.9
– – recurrent F31.8
– psychotic (*see also* Psychosis) F23.9
– – organic F06.8
– schizophrenic (acute) NEC, brief F23.2
Epispadias (female) (male) Q64.0
Episplenitis D73.8
Epistaxis (multiple) R04.0
– vicarious menstruation N94.8
Epithelioma (malignant) (M8011/3) –
   see also Neoplasm, malignant
– adenoides cysticum (M8100/0) – *see*
   Neoplasm, skin, benign
– basal cell (M8090/3) – *see* Neoplasm,
   skin, malignant
– benign (M8011/0) – *see* Neoplasm, benign
– Bowen's (M8081/2) – *see* Neoplasm, skin,
   in situ
– calcifying, of Malherbe (M8110/0) – *see*
   Neoplasm, skin, benign
– external site – *see* Neoplasm, skin,
   malignant
– intraepidermal, Jadassohn (M8096/0) –
   see Neoplasm, skin, benign
– squamous cell (M8070/3) – *see* Neoplasm,
   malignant
Epitheliomatosis, pigmented Q82.1

Epithelium, epithelial – *see condition*
Epituberculosis (with atelectasis) (allergic) A16.7
– with bacteriological and histological confirmation A15.7
Eponychia Q84.6
Epstein's
– nephrosis or syndrome (*see also* Nephrosis) N04.-
– pearl K09.8
Epulis (fibrous) (giant cell) (gingiva) K06.8
Equinia A24.0
Equinovarus (congenital) (talipes) Q66.0
– acquired M21.5
Equivalent
– convulsive (abdominal) G40.8
– epileptic (psychic) G40.2
Erb(-Duchenne) paralysis (birth injury) (newborn) P14.0
Erb-Goldflam disease or syndrome G70.0
Erb's
– disease G71.0
– palsy, paralysis (brachial) (birth) (newborn) P14.0
– – spinal (spastic), syphilitic A52.1
– pseudohypertrophic muscular dystrophy G71.0
Erection, painful (persistent) N48.3
Ergosterol deficiency (vitamin D) E55.9
– with
– – adult ostcomalacia M83.8
– – rickets (*see also* Rickets) E55.0
Ergotism T62.2
– from ergot used as drug (migraine therapy)
– – correct substance properly administered G92
– – overdose or wrong substance given or taken T48.0
Erosio interdigitalis blastomycetica B37.2
Erosion
– artery I77.8
– bone M85.8
– bronchus J98.0
– cartilage (joint) M94.8
– cervix (uteri) (acquired) (chronic) (congenital) N86
– – with cervicitis N72
– cornea (nontraumatic) H16.0
– – recurrent H18.8
– – traumatic S05.0
– dental (due to diet, drugs or vomiting) (idiopathic) (occupational) K03.2

Erosion—*continued*
– duodenum, postpyloric – *see* Ulcer, duodenum
– esophagus K22.1
– gastric – *see* Ulcer, stomach
– gastrojejunal – *see* Ulcer, gastrojejunal
– intestine K63.3
– lymphatic vessel I89.8
– pylorus, pyloric (ulcer) – *see* Ulcer, stomach
– spine, aneurysmal A52.0† I68.8*
– stomach – *see* Ulcer, stomach
– teeth (due to diet, drugs or vomiting) (idiopathic) (occupational) K03.2
– urethra N36.8
– uterus N85.8
Erotomania F52.7
Error
– metabolism, inborn – *see* Disorder, metabolism
– refractive H52.7
Eructation R14
– nervous or psychogenic F45.3
Eruption
– creeping B76.9
– drug (generalized) (taken internally) L27.0
– – in contact with skin – *see* Dermatitis, due to, drugs, in contact with skin
– – localized L27.1
– Hutchinson, summer L56.4
– Kaposi's varicelliform B00.0
– napkin L22
– polymorphous light (sun) L56.4
– ringed R23.8
– skin (nonspecific) R21
– – creeping (meaning hookworm) B76.9
– – due to prophylactic inoculation or vaccination (generalized) (*see also* Dermatitis, due to, vaccine) L27.0
– – – localized L27.1
– – erysipeloid A26.0
– – feigned L98.1
– – Kaposi's varicelliform B00.0
– – lichenoid L28.0
– – meaning dermatitis – *see* Dermatitis
– – toxic NEC L53.0
– tooth, teeth, abnormal (incomplete) (late) (premature) (sequence) K00.6
– vesicular R23.8
Erysipelas (gangrenous) (infantile) (newborn) (phlegmonous) (suppurative) A46
– external ear A46† H62.0*

Erysipelas—*continued*
- puerperal, postpartum O86.8
Erysipeloid A26.9
- cutaneous (Rosenbach's) A26.0
- disseminated A26.8
- septicemia A26.7
- specified NEC A26.8
Erythema, erythematous L53.9
- ab igne L59.0
- annulare (centrifugum) (rheumaticum) L53.1
- chronic figurate NEC L53.3
- chronicum migrans (Borrelia burgdorferi) A69.2
- diaper L22
- due to
- - chemical NEC L53.0
- - - in contact with skin L25.3
- - drug (internal use) – *see* Dermatitis, due to, drugs
- elevatum diutinum L95.1
- endemic E52
- epidemic, arthritic A25.1
- figuratum perstans L53.3
- gluteal L22
- heat – *code as* Burn, by site, with fourth character .1
- ichthyosiforme congenitum bullous Q80.3
- induratum (nontuberculous) L52
- - tuberculous A18.4
- infectiosum B08.3
- inflammation NEC L53.9
- intertrigo L30.4
- iris L51.1† H22.8*
- marginatum L53.2
- - in (due to) acute rheumatic fever I00† L54.0*
- medicamentosum – *see* Dermatitis, due to, drugs
- migrans A26.0
- - tongue K14.1
- multiforme L51.9
- - bullous, bullosum L51.1
- - conjunctiva L51.1† H13.8*
- - nonbullous L51.0
- - pemphigoides L12.0
- - specified NEC L51.8
- napkin L22
- neonatorum P83.8
- - toxic P83.1
- nodosum L52
- - tuberculous A18.4
- palmar L53.8

Erythema, erythematous—*continued*
- pernio T69.1
- rash, newborn P83.8
- scarlatiniform (exfoliative) (recurrent) L53.8
- solare L55.0
- specified NEC L53.8
- toxic, toxicum NEC L53.0
- - newborn P83.1
- tuberculous (primary) A18.4
Erythematous, erythematosus – *see condition*
Erythermalgia (primary) I73.8
Erythralgia I73.8
Erythrasma L08.1
Erythredema (polyneuropathy) T56.1
Erythremia (acute) C94.0
- chronic D45
- secondary D75.1
Erythroblastopenia (*see also* Aplasia, red cell) D60.9
Erythroblastosis (fetalis) (newborn) P55.9
- due to
- - ABO (antibodies) (incompatibility) (isoimmunization) P55.1
- - Rh (antibodies) (incompatibility) (isoimmunization) P55.0
Erythrocyanosis (crurum) I73.8
Erythrocythemia – *see* Erythremia
Erythrocytosis (megalosplenic) (secondary) D75.1
- familial D75.0
- oval, hereditary (*see also* Elliptocytosis) D58.1
Erythroderma (*see also* Erythema) L53.9
- bullous ichthyosiform, congenital Q80.3
- desquamativum L21.1
- ichthyosiform, congenital (bullous) Q80.3
- neonatorum P83.8
- psoriaticum L40.8
- secondary L53.9
Erythrogenesis imperfecta D61.0
Erythroleukemia C94.0
Erythromelalgia I73.8
Erythrophagocytosis D75.8
Erythrophobia F40.2
Erythroplakia, oral epithelium and tongue K13.2
Erythroplasia (Queyrat) (M8080/2)
- specified site – *see* Neoplasm, skin, in situ
- unspecified site D07.4
Escherichia (E.) coli, as cause of disease classified elsewhere B96.2
Esophagismus K22.4

Esophagitis (acute) (alkaline) (chemical) (chronic) (infectional) (necrotic) (peptic) (postoperative) K20
- due to gastrointestinal reflux disease K21.0
- reflux K21.0
- tuberculous A18.8† K23.0*
- ulcerative K22.1

Esophagomalacia K22.8
Esophagostomiasis B81.8
Esophagotracheal – *see condition*
Esophagus – *see condition*
Esophoria H50.5
- convergence, excess H51.1
- divergence, insufficiency H51.8

Esotropia (alternating) (monocular) H50.0
- intermittent H50.3

Espundia B55.2
Essential – *see condition*
Esthesioneuroblastoma (M9522/3) C30.0
Esthesioneurocytoma (M9521/3) C30.0
Esthesioneuroepithelioma (M9523/3) C30.0
Esthiomene A55
Estivo-autumnal malaria (fever) B50.9
Estrangement Z63.5
Estriasis (*see also* Myiasis) B87.9
Ethanolism (*see also* Alcoholism) F10.2
Etherism F18.2
Ethmoid, ethmoidal – *see condition*
Ethmoiditis (chronic) (nonpurulent) (purulent) (*see also* Sinusitis, ethmoidal) J32.2
- influenzal (*see also* Influenza, with, respiratory manifestations) J11.1
- Woakes' J33.1

Ethylism (*see also* Alcoholism) F10.2
Eulenburg's disease G71.1
Eumycetoma B47.0
Eunuchoidism E29.1
- hypogonadotropic E23.0

European blastomycosis (*see also* Cryptococcosis) B45.9
Eustachian – *see condition*
Evaluation (for) (of)
- development state
- - adolescent Z00.3
- - infant or child Z00.1
- - period of rapid growth in childhood Z00.2
- - puberty Z00.3
- growth and developmental state (period of rapid growth) Z00.2

Evaluation—*continued*
- growth and developmental state— *continued*
- - child Z00.1
- mental health (status) Z00.4
- - requested by authority Z04.6
- period of rapid growth in childhood Z00.2
- suspected condition (*see also* Observation) Z03.9

Evans' syndrome D69.3
Eventration K43.9
- colon into chest – *see* Hernia, diaphragm
- diaphragm (congenital) Q79.1

Eversion
- bladder N32.8
- cervix (uteri) N86
- - with cervicitis N72
- foot NEC M21.0
- - congenital Q66.6
- punctum lacrimale (postinfectional) (senile) H04.5
- ureter (meatus) N28.8
- urethra (meatus) N36.3
- uterus N81.4

Evisceration
- birth injury P15.8
- operative wound T81.3
- traumatic NEC T06.5
- - eye S05.7

Evulsion – *see* Avulsion
Ewing's sarcoma or tumor (M9260/3) – *see* Neoplasm, bone, malignant

Examination (general) (routine) (of) (for) Z00.0
- adolescent (development state) Z00.3
- allergy Z01.5
- annual (periodic) (physical) Z00.0
- - gynecological Z01.4
- blood pressure Z01.3
- cancer staging – *see* Neoplasm, malignant
- cervical Papanicolaou smear Z12.4
- - as part of routine gynecological examination Z01.4
- chest X-ray Z01.6
- - for suspected tuberculosis Z03.0
- clinical research control or normal comparison Z00.6
- contraceptive (drug) maintenance (routine) Z30.4
- - device (intrauterine) Z30.5
- dental Z01.2
- donor (potential) Z00.5
- ear Z01.1

Examination—*continued*
- eye Z01.0
- following
- - accident NEC Z04.3
- - - transport Z04.1
- - - work Z04.2
- - motor vehicle accident Z04.1
- - treatment (for) Z09.9
- - - combined NEC Z09.7
- - - - fracture Z09.4
- - - - malignant neoplasm Z08.7
- - - malignant neoplasm Z08.9
- - - - chemotherapy Z08.2
- - - - combined treatment Z08.7
- - - - radiotherapy Z08.1
- - - - specified treatment NEC Z08.8
- - - - surgery Z08.0
- - - specified condition NEC Z09.8
- follow-up (routine) (following) Z09.9
- - chemotherapy NEC Z09.2
- - - malignant neoplasm Z08.2
- - fracture Z09.4
- - malignant neoplasm Z08.9
- - - chemotherapy Z08.2
- - - combined treatment Z08.7
- - - radiotherapy Z08.1
- - - specified treatment NEC Z08.8
- - - surgery Z08.0
- - postpartum Z39.2
- - psychotherapy Z09.3
- - radiotherapy NEC Z09.1
- - - malignant neoplasm Z08.1
- - surgery NEC Z09.0
- - - malignant neoplasm Z08.0
- gynecological Z01.4
- - for contraceptive (drug) maintenance Z30.4
- - - device (intrauterine) Z30.5
- health – *see* Examination, medical
- hearing Z01.1
- infant or child Z00.1
- inflicted injury (victim or culprit) NEC Z04.5
- laboratory Z01.7
- lactating mother Z39.1
- medical (for) (of) Z00.0
- - administrative purpose only Z02.9
- - - specified NEC Z02.8
- - admission to
- - - armed forces Z02.3
- - - old age home Z02.2
- - - prison Z02.8
- - - residential institution Z02.2
- - - school Z02.0

Examination—*continued*
- medical—*continued*
- - admission to—*continued*
- - - summer camp Z02.8
- - adoption Z02.8
- - armed forces personnel Z10.2
- - athletes Z10.3
- - camp (summer) Z02.8
- - control subject in clinical research Z00.6
- - defined sub-population NEC Z10.8
- - donor (potential) Z00.5
- - driving licence Z02.4
- - general Z00.0
- - immigration Z02.8
- - infant or child Z00.1
- - inhabitants of institutions Z10.1
- - insurance purposes Z02.6
- - marriage Z02.8
- - medicolegal reasons NEC Z04.8
- - naturalization Z02.8
- - occupational Z10.0
- - participation in sport Z02.5
- - population survey Z00.8
- - pre-employment Z02.1
- - preschool children Z10.8
- - - for admission to school Z02.0
- - prisoners Z10.8
- - - for entrance into prison Z02.8
- - prostitutes Z10.8
- - recruitment for armed forces Z02.3
- - refugees Z10.8
- - schoolchildren Z10.8
- - specified NEC Z00.8
- - sport competition Z02.5
- - sports teams Z10.3
- - students Z10.8
- medicolegal reason NEC Z04.8
- pelvic (annual) (periodic) Z01.4
- period of rapid growth in childhood Z00.2
- postpartum
- - immediately after delivery Z39.0
- - routine follow-up Z39.2
- pregnancy (possible) (unconfirmed) Z32.0
- - confirmed Z32.1
- psychiatric NEC Z00.4
- - requested by authority Z04.6
- radiological NEC Z01.6
- rape or seduction, alleged (victim or culprit) Z04.4
- sensitization Z01.5
- skin (hypersensitivity) Z01.5

Examination—*continued*
- special (*see also* Examination, by type) Z01.9
- – specified type NEC Z01.8
- specified type or reason NEC Z04.8
- teeth Z01.2
- vision Z01.0
- well baby Z00.1

Exanthem, exanthema (*see also* Rash) R21
- with enteroviral vesicular stomatitis B08.4
- Boston A88.0
- epidemic with meningitis A88.0† G02.0*
- subitum B08.2
- viral, virus B09
- – specified type NEC B08.8

Excess, excessive, excessively
- alcohol level in blood R78.0
- androgen (ovarian) E28.1
- attrition, tooth, teeth K03.0
- carotene, carotin (dietary) E67.1
- cold, effects of T69.9
- – specified effect NEC T69.8
- convergence H51.1
- development, breast N62
- divergence H51.8
- drinking (alcohol) NEC F10.0
- – habitual (continual) F10.2
- eating R63.2
- estrogen E28.0
- fat E66.9
- – in heart (*see also* Degeneration, myocardial) I51.5
- – localized E65
- foreskin N47
- heat (*see also* Heat) T67.9
- kalium E87.5
- large
- – colon K59.3
- – – congenital Q43.8
- – fetus or infant P08.0
- – – with obstructed labor O66.2
- – – affecting management of pregnancy O36.6
- – – causing disproportion O33.5
- – organ or site, congenital NEC – *see* Anomaly, by site
- long
- – organ or site, congenital NEC – *see* Anomaly, by site
- – umbilical cord (entangled)
- – – affecting fetus or newborn P02.5
- – – complicating labor or delivery O69.2
- menstruation (with regular cycle) N92.0

Excess, excessive—*continued*
- menstruation—*continued*
- – – with irregular cycle N92.1
- natrium E87.0
- number of teeth K00.1
- – causing crowding K07.3
- nutrient (dietary) NEC E67.8
- potassium (K) E87.5
- salivation K11.7
- secretion (*see also* Hypersecretion)
- – milk O92.6
- – sputum R09.3
- – sweat R61.9
- sexual drive F52.7
- short
- – organ or site, congenital NEC – *see* Anomaly, by site
- – umbilical cord
- – – affecting fetus or newborn P02.6
- – – complicating labor or delivery O69.3
- skin, eyelid (acquired) H02.3
- – congenital Q10.3
- sodium (Na) E87.0
- sputum R09.3
- sweating R61.9
- thirst R63.1
- – due to deprivation of water T73.1
- vitamin
- – A (dietary) E67.0
- – – administered as drug (chronic) (prolonged excessive intake) E67.0
- – – reaction to sudden overdose T45.2
- – D (dietary) E67.3
- – – administered as drug (chronic) (prolonged excessive intake) E67.3
- – – – reaction to sudden overdose T45.2

Excitability, abnormal, under minor stress (personality disorder) F60.3
Excitation
- psychogenic F30.8
- reactive (from emotional stress, psychological trauma) F30.8
Excitement
- hypomanic F30.0
- manic F30.9
- mental, reactive (from emotional stress, psychological trauma) F30.8
- state, reactive (from emotional stress, psychological trauma) F30.8
Excoriation (traumatic) (*see also* Injury, superficial) T14.0
- neurotic L98.1
Excyclophoria H50.5
Excyclotropia H50.4

Exercise
- breathing Z50.1
- remedial NEC Z50.1
- therapeutic NEC Z50.1

Exfoliation, teeth, due to systemic causes K08.0

Exfoliative – *see condition*

Exhaustion (physical NEC) R53
- battle F43.0
- cardiac (*see also* Failure, heart) I50.9
- complicating pregnancy O26.8
- delirium F43.0
- due to
- – cold T69.8
- – excessive exertion T73.3
- – exposure T73.2
- – neurasthenia F48.0
- – pregnancy O26.8
- fetus or newborn P96.8
- heart (*see also* Failure, heart) I50.9
- heat (*see also* Heat, exhaustion) T67.5
- maternal, complicating delivery O75.8
- – affecting fetus or newborn P03.8
- mental F48.0
- myocardium, myocardial (*see also* Failure, heart) I50.9
- nervous F48.0
- old age R54
- psychogenic F48.0
- psychosis F43.0
- senile R54
- vital NEC Z73.0

Exhibitionism F65.2

Exocervicitis (*see also* Cervicitis) N72

Exomphalos Q79.2
- meaning hernia – *see* Hernia, umbilicus

Exophoria H50.5
- convergence, insufficiency H51.1
- divergence, excess H51.8

Exophthalmos H05.2
- congenital Q15.8
- due to thyrotoxicosis (hyperthyroidism) E05.0† H06.2∗
- dysthyroid E05.0† H06.2∗
- goiter E05.0† H06.2∗
- intermittent NEC H05.2
- pulsating H05.2
- thyrotoxic, thyrotropic E05.0† H06.2∗

Exostosis M89.9
- cartilaginous (M9210/0) – *see* Neoplasm, bone, benign
- congenital (multiple) Q78.6
- external ear canal H61.8
- gonococcal A54.4† M90.2∗

Exostosis—*continued*
- jaw (bone) K10.8
- multiple, congenital Q78.6
- orbit H05.3
- osteocartilaginous (M9210/0) – *see* Neoplasm, bone, benign
- syphilitic A52.7† M90.2∗

Exotropia (alternating) (monocular) H50.1
- intermittent H50.3

Explanation of
- investigation finding Z71.2
- medication Z71.8

Exposure (to) (*see also* Contact, with) T75.8
- acariasis Z20.7
- agricultural toxic agents (gases) (liquids) (solids) (vapors) Z57.4
- – nonoccupational Z58.5
- AIDS virus Z20.6
- air
- – contaminants NEC Z58.1
- – – occupational NEC Z57.3
- – – – dust Z57.2
- – – tobacco smoke Z58.7
- – pollution NEC Z58.1
- – – occupational NEC Z57.3
- – – – dust Z57.2
- – – tobacco smoke Z58.7
- cholera Z20.0
- cold, effects of T69.9
- – specified effect NEC T69.8
- communicable disease Z20.9
- – specified NEC Z20.8
- disaster Z65.5
- discrimination Z60.5
- dust NEC Z58.1
- – occupational Z57.2
- exhaustion, due to T73.2
- extreme temperature (occupational) Z57.6
- – nonoccupational Z58.5
- German measles Z20.4
- gonorrhea Z20.2
- human immunodeficiency virus (HIV) Z20.6
- human T-lymphotropic virus type 1 (HTLV-1) Z20.8
- industrial toxic agents (gases) (liquids) (solids) (vapors) Z57.5
- – nonoccupational Z58.5
- infestation (parasitic) NEC Z20.7
- intestinal infectious disease Z20.0
- noise Z58.0

Exposure—*continued*
– noise—*continued*
– – occupational Z57.0
– occupational risk factor Z57.9
– – specified NEC Z57.8
– parasitic disease NEC Z20.7
– pediculosis Z20.7
– persecution Z60.5
– poliomyelitis Z20.8
– pollution NEC Z58.5
– – air contaminants NEC Z58.1
– – – occupational Z57.3
– – – tobacco smoke Z58.7
– – dust NEC Z58.1
– – – occupational Z57.2
– – noise NEC Z58.0
– – – occupational Z57.0
– – occupational Z57.8
– – soil Z58.3
– – – occupational Z57.8
– – specified NEC Z58.5
– – – occupational Z57.8
– – water Z58.2
– rabies Z20.3
– radiation NEC Z58.4
– – occupational Z57.1
– rubella Z20.4
– sexually transmitted disease Z20.2
– smallpox (laboratory) Z20.8
– soil pollution Z58.3
– – occupational Z57.8
– syphilis Z20.2
– terrorism Z65.4
– torture Z65.4
– toxic agents (gases) (liquids) (solids) (vapors)
– – agricultural Z57.4
– – – nonoccupational Z58.5
– – industrial NEC Z57.5
– – – nonoccupational Z58.5
– tuberculosis Z20.1
– vibration Z58.8
– – occupational Z57.7
– viral disease NEC Z20.8
– – hepatitis Z20.5
– war Z65.5

Exposure—*continued*
– water pollution Z58.2
Exsanguination – *see* Hemorrhage
Exstrophy (congenital)
– abdominal contents Q45.8
– bladder Q64.1
Extensive *see condition*
Extra (*see also* Accessory)
– marker chromosomes Q92.6
– rib Q76.6
– – cervical Q76.5
Extraction
– with hook (fetus) P03.8
– after version O83.2
– breech NEC O83.0
– – affecting fetus or newborn P03.0
– manual NEC O83.2
– menstrual Z30.3
– vacuum (delivery) O81.4
Extrasystoles(supraventricular) I49.4
– atrial I49.1
– auricular I49.1
– junctional I49.2
– ventricular I49.3
Extrauterine gestation or
  pregnancy (*see also* Pregnancy, by site)
  O00.9
Extravasation
– blood R58
– chyle into mesentery I89.8
– urine R39.0
Extremity – *see* condition, by site
Extrophy – *see* Exstrophy
Extroversion
– bladder Q64.1
– uterus (sequela, obstetric) N81.4
– – complicating delivery O71.2
Extrusion
– eye implant (ball) (globe) T85.3
– intervertebral disk – *see* Displacement, intervertebral disk
Exudate, pleural – *see* Effusion, pleura
Exudative – *see condition*
Eye, eyeball, eyelid – *see condition*
Eyestrain H53.1
Eyeworm disease of Africa B74.3

F

Faber's syndrome D50.9
Fabry(-Anderson) disease E75.2
Face, facial – *see also condition*
- presentation, affecting fetus or newborn P01.7
Faciocephalalgia, autonomic (*see also* Neuropathy, peripheral, autonomic) G90.0
Factor(s)
- psychic, associated with diseases classified elsewhere F54
- psychological
- – affecting physical conditions F54
- – or behavioral
- – – affecting general medical condition F54
Fahr-Volhard disease (of kidney) I12.9
- with renal insufficiency I12.0
Fahr's disease (of brain) G23.8
Failure, failed
- aortic (valve) I35.8
- – rheumatic I06.8
- attempted abortion – *see* Abortion, attempted
- biventricular I50.0
- cardiac (*see also* Failure, heart) I50.9
- – newborn P29.0
- cardiorenal (chronic) I50.9
- – hypertensive I13.2
- cardiorespiratory (*see also* Failure, heart) R09.2
- – specified, during or due to a procedure T81.8
- – – long-term effect of cardiac surgery I97.1
- cerebrovascular I67.9
- cervical dilatation in labor O62.0
- – affecting fetus or newborn P03.6
- circulation, circulatory (peripheral) R57.9
- compensation – *see* Disease, heart
- compliance with medical treatment or regimen Z91.1
- congestive (*see also* Failure, heart, congestive) I50.0
- coronary (*see also* Insufficiency, coronary) I24.8
- descent of head (at term) (mother) O32.4
- – affecting fetus or newborn P03.1

Failure, failed—*continued*
- engagement of head NEC (at term) (mother) O32.4
- erection (penile) F52.2
- examination(s), anxiety concerning Z55.2
- expansion, terminal respiratory units (newborn) (primary) P28.0
- fetal head to enter pelvic brim (mother) O32.4
- – affecting fetus or newborn P03.1
- forceps NEC (with subsequent delivery by cesarean section) O66.5
- – affecting fetus or newborn P03.1
- genital response F52.2
- heart (acute) (sudden) (senile) I50.9
- – with
- – – acute pulmonary edema – *see* Failure, ventricular, left
- – – decompensation (*see also* Failure, heart, congestive) I50.9
- – – dilatation – *see* Disease, heart
- – – other organ failure (*see also* Failure organ multiple NEC) – *code* each site
- – complicating
- – – anesthesia (general) (local) or other sedation
- – – – during labor and delivery O74.2
- – – – in pregnancy O29.1
- – – – postpartum, puerperal O89.1
- – – delivery (cesarean) (instrumental) O75.4
- – – surgery T81.8
- – congestive I50.0
- – – hypertensive (*see also* Hypertension, heart) I11.0
- – – – with renal disease I13.0
- – – – – with renal failure I13.2
- – – – newborn P29.0
- – degenerative (*see also* Degeneration, myocardial) I51.5
- – due to presence of cardiac prosthesis I97.1
- – high output – *see* Disease, heart
- – hypertensive (*see also* Hypertension, heart) I11.0
- – – with renal disease I13.0
- – – – with renal failure I13.2
- – ischemic I25.5

Failure, failed—*continued*
- heart—*continued*
-   – left (ventricular) (*see also* Failure, ventricular, left) I50.1
-   – newborn P29.0
-   – organic – *see* Disease, heart
-   – postoperative I97.8
-   – – cardiac surgery I97.1
-   – rheumatic (chronic) (inactive) – *see* condition, by valve, rheumatic
-   – right (ventricular) (secondary to left heart failure, conditions in I50.1) (*see also* Failure, heart, congestive) I50.0
-   – specified, during or due to a procedure T81.8
-   – – long-term effect of cardiac surgery I97.1
-   – thyrotoxic (*see also* Thyrotoxicosis) E05.9† I43.8*
-   – valvular – *see* Endocarditis
- hepatic K72.9
-   – with other organ failure (*see also* Failure organ multiple NEC) – code *each* site
-   – acute or subacute K72.0
-   – alcoholic (acute) (chronic) (subacute) (with or without hepatic coma) K70.4
-   – chronic K72.1
-   – due to drugs (acute) (chronic) (subacute) K71.1
-   – postoperative K91.8
- hepatorenal K76.7
- induction (of labor) O61.9
-   – abortion – *see* Abortion, attempted
-   – by
-   – – oxytocic drugs O61.0
-   – – prostaglandins O61.0
-   – instrumental O61.1
-   – mechanical O61.1
-   – medical O61.0
-   – specified NEC O61.8
-   – surgical O61.1
- intubation during anesthesia T88.4
-   – during pregnancy O29.6
-   – in labor and delivery O74.7
-   – postpartum, puerperal O89.6
- involution, thymus (gland) E32.0
- kidney N19
-   – with
-   – – hypertension (*see also* Hypertension, kidney) I12.0

Failure, failed—*continued*
- kidney—*continued*
-   – with—*continued*
-   – – hypertensive
-   – – – heart disease (conditions in I11) I13.1
-   – – – with heart failure (congestive) I13.2
-   – – – kidney disease (*see also* Hypertension, kidney) I12.0
-   – – tubular necrosis (acute) N17.0
-   – acute N17.9
-   – with
-   – – cortical necrosis N17.1
-   – – medullary necrosis N17.2
-   – – tubular necrosis N17.0
-   – with
-   – – following labour and delivery O90.4
-   – – specified NEC N17.8
-   – chronic N18.9
-   – end-stage N18.5
-   – hypertensive (*see also* Hypertension, kidney) I12.0
-   – stage 1 N18.1
-   – stage 2 N18.2
-   – stage 3 N18.3
-   – stage 4 N18.4
-   – stage 5 N18.5
- congenital P96.0
- end-stage (chronic) N18.5
- following
-   – abortion (subsequent episode) O08.4
-   – – current episode – *see* Abortion
-   – crushing T79.5
-   – ectopic or molar pregnancy O08.4
-   – labour and delivery (acute) O90.4
-   – hypertensive (*see also* Hypertension, kidney) I12.0
-   – postprocedural N99.0
- lactation (complete) O92.3
-   – partial O92.4
- liver – *see* Failure, hepatic
- menstruation at puberty (*see also* Amenorrhea, primary) N91.0
- mitral I05.8
- myocardial, myocardium (*see also* Failure, heart) I50.9
- organ – *see* Failure, by site
-   – multiple NEC R68.8
- orgasm (female) (male) (psychogenic) F52.3
- ovarian (primary) E28.3
-   – iatrogenic E89.4

Failure, failed—*continued*
- ovarian—*continued*
- – postprocedural (postablative)
  (postirradiation) (postsurgical) E89.4
- ovulation causing infertility N97.0
- polyglandular, autoimmune E31.0
- renal – *see* Failure, kidney
- respiration, respiratory J96.9
- – with other organ failure (*see also* ~~each~~
  Failure organ multiple NEC) – *code* ~~to~~
  site
- – acute J96.0
- – center G93.8
- – chronic J96.1
- – newborn P28.5
- – postprocedural J95.8
- rotation
- – cecum Q43.3
- – colon Q43.3
- – intestine Q43.3
- – kidney Q63.2
- segmentation – *see also* Fusion
- – fingers Q70.0
- – toes Q70.2
- – vertebra Q76.4
- – – with scoliosis Q76.3
- senile (general) R54
- sexual arousal (female) (male) F52.2
- testicular endocrine function E29.1
- to
- – gain weight R62.8
- – thrive R62.8
- – – resulting from HIV disease B22.2
- transplant T86.9
- – bone T86.8
- – – marrow T86.0
- – heart T86.2
- – – with lung(s) T86.3
- – intestine T86.8
- – kidney T86.1
- – liver T86.4
- – lung(s) T86.8
- – – with heart T86.3
- – pancreas T86.8
- – skin (allograft) (autograft) T86.8
- – specified organ or tissue NEC T86.8
- trial of labor (with subsequent cesarean
  section) O66.4
- – affecting fetus or newborn P03.1
- urinary – *see* Failure, kidney
- vacuum extraction NEC (with subsequent
  cesarean section) O66.5
- – affecting fetus or newborn P03.1

Failure, failed—*continued*
- ventouse NEC (with subsequent cesarean
  section) O66.5
- – affecting fetus or newborn P03.1
- ventricular (*see also* Failure, heart) I50.9
- – left I50.1
- – – with rheumatic fever (conditions in
  I00)
- – – – active I01.8
- – – – – with chorea I02.0
- – – – inactive or quiescent (with chorea)
  I09.8
- – – hypertensive (*see also* Hypertension,
  heart) I11.0
- – – rheumatic (chronic) (inactive) (with
  chorea) I09.8
- – – – active or acute I01.8
- – – – – with chorea I02.0
- – right (*see also* Failure, heart,
  congestive) I50.0
- vital centers, fetus or newborn P91.8
Fainting (fit) R55
Fallen arches M21.4
Falling, any organ or part – *see* Prolapse
Fallopian
- insufflation Z31.4
- tube – *see condition*
Fallot's
- pentalogy Q21.8
- tetrad or tetralogy Q21.3
Fallout, radioactive (adverse effect) NEC
T66
Falls
- repeated R29.6
False – *see also condition*
- joint M84.1
- labor (pains) O47.9
- – after 37 completed weeks of gestation
  O47.1
- – before 37 completed weeks of gestation
  O47.0
- passage, urethra (prostatic) N36.0
- positive serological test for syphilis
  (Wassermann reaction) R76.2
- pregnancy F45.8
Family, familial – *see also condition*
- disruption Z63.8
- – involving divorce or separation Z63.5
- planning advice Z30.0
- problem Z63.9
- – specified NEC Z63.8
Famine (effects of) T73.0
- edema (*see also* Malnutrition, severe)
  E43

Fanconi (-de Toni) (-Debré) syndrome
E72.0
Fanconi's anemia D61.0
Farber's disease or syndrome E75.2
Farcy A24.0
Farmer's
– lung J67.0
– skin L57.8
Farsightedness H52.0
Fascia – *see condition*
Fasciculation R25.3
Fasciculitis optica H46
Fasciitis M72.9
– diffuse (eosinophilic) M35.4
– necrotizing M72.6
– nodular M72.4
– perirenal (with ureteral obstruction)
  N13.5
– – with infection N13.6
– plantar M72.2
– specified NEC M72.8
– traumatic (old) M72.8
– – current – *code as* Sprain, by site
Fascioliasis B66.3
**Fasciolopsiasis (intestinal), fasciolopsis
(buski)** B66.5
Fat
– excessive E66.9
– – in heart (*see also* Degeneration,
  myocardial) I51.5
– in stool R19.5
– localized (pad) E65
– – heart (*see also* Degeneration,
  myocardial) I51.5
– – knee M79.4
– – retropatellar M79.4
– pad E65
– – knee M79.4
Fatal syncope, unexplained R96.0
Fatigue R53
– combat F43.0
– complicating pregnancy O26.8
– heat (transient) T67.6
– muscle M62.6
– myocardium (*see also* Failure, heart)
  I50.9
– nervous, neurosis F48.0
– operational F48.8
– psychogenic (general) F48.0
– senile R54
– syndrome F48.0
– voice R49.8
Fatness E66.9

Fatty – *see also* condition
– apron E65
– degeneration – *see* Degeneration, fatty
– heart (enlarged) (*see also* Degeneration,
  myocardial) I51.5
– liver (nonalcoholic) NEC K76.0
– – alcoholic K70.0
– necrosis – *see* Degeneration, fatty
Fauces – *see condition*
Faucitis J02.9
Favism (anemia) D55.0
Favus – *see* Dermatophytosis
Fazio-Londe disease or syndrome G12.1
Fear complex or reaction F40.9
Feared complaint unfounded Z71.1
Febricula (continued) (simple) R50.9
Febris, febrile (*see also* Fever) R50.9
– flava (*see also* Fever, yellow) A95.9
– melitensis A23.0
– puerperalis O85
– recurrens (*see also* Fever, relapsing)
  A68.9
– rubra A38
Fecal – *see condition*
Fecalith (impaction) K56.4
– appendix K38.1
– congenital P76.8
**Feeble rapid pulse due to shock following
injury** T79.4
Feeble-minded F70.-
Feeding
– difficulties and mismanagement R63.3
– faulty R63.3
– formula check (infant) Z00.1
– improper R63.3
– problem R63.3
– – newborn P92.9
– – – specified NEC P92.8
– – nonorganic F50.8
Feer's disease T56.1
Feet – *see condition*
Feigned illness Z76.5
Feil-Klippel syndrome Q76.1
Felon (with lymphangitis) L03.0
Felty's syndrome M05.0
Femur, femoral – *see condition*
Fenestration, fenestrated – *see also*
  Imperfect, closure
– aortopulmonary Q21.4
– cusps, heart valve NEC Q24.8
– – pulmonary Q22.2
– pulmonic cusps Q22.2
Fertile eunuch syndrome E23.0

Fertilization (assisted) NEC Z31.3
– in vitro Z31.2
Fetal – *see* Fetus
Fetalis uterus Q51.8
Fetid
– breath R19.6
– sweat L75.0
Fetishism F65.0
– transvestic F65.1
Fetus, fetal – *see also condition*
– alcohol syndrome (dysmorphic) Q86.0
– compressus (mother) O31.0
– hydantoin syndrome Q86.1
– papyraceous (mother) O31.0
Fever R50.9
– with
– – chills R50.8
– – – in malarial regions B54
– – rigors R50.8
– – – in malarial regions B54
– abortus A23.1
– Aden (dengue) A90
– African tick-borne A68.1
– American
– – mountain (tick) A93.2
– – spotted A77.0
– aphthous B08.8
– arbovirus, arboviral A94
– – hemorrhagic A94
– – specified NEC A93.8
– Argentinian hemorrhagic A96.0
– Assam B55.0
– Australian Q A78
– Bangkok hemorrhagic A91
– Barmah forest A92.8
– Bartonella A44.0
– bilious, hemoglobinuric B50.8
– blackwater B50.8
– blister B00.1
– Bolivian hemorrhagic A96.1
– Bonvale dam T73.3
– boutonneuse A77.1
– brain (*see also* Encephalitis) G04.9
– Brazilian purpuric A48.4
– breakbone A90
– Bullis A77.0
– Bunyamwera A92.8
– Burdwan B55.0
– Bwamba A92.8
– Cameroon (*see also* Malaria) B54
– cat-scratch A28.1
– Central Asian hemorrhagic A98.0
– cerebral (*see also* Encephalitis) G04.9

Fever—*continued*
– cerebrospinal meningococcal A39.0†
G01*
– Chagres B50.9
– Chandipura A92.8
– Changuinola A93.8
– Charcot's (biliary) (hepatic) (intermittent)
K80.5
– Chikungunya (virus) (hemorrhagic)
A92.0
– Chitral A93.1
– Colorado tick (virus) A93.2
– congestive (remittent) (*see also* Malaria)
B54
– Congo virus A98.0
– continued malarial B50.9
– Corsican (*see also* Malaria) B54
– Crimean-Congo hemorrhagic A98.0
– Cyprus A23.0
– dandy A90
– deer fly (*see also* Tularemia) A21.9
– dengue (virus) A90
– – hemorrhagic A91
– – sandfly A93.1
– desert B38.0† J99.8*
– due to heat T67.0
– dumdum B55.0
– enteroviral exanthematous (Boston
exanthem) A88.0
– ephemeral (of unknown origin) R50.9
– epidemic hemorrhagic A98.5† N08.0*
– erysipelatous (*see also* Erysipelas) A46
– estivo-autumnal (malarial) B50.9
– famine A75.0
– following delivery O86.4
– Fort Bragg A27.8
– gastromalarial (*see also* Malaria) B54
– Gibraltar A23.0
– glandular B27.9
– Guama (viral) A92.8
– Haverhill A25.1
– hay (allergic) J30.1
– – with asthma (bronchial) J45.0
– – due to
– – – allergen other than pollen J30.3
– – – pollen, any plant or tree J30.1
– heat (effects) T67.0
– hematuric, bilious B50.8
– hemoglobinuric (bilious) (malarial) B50.8
– hemorrhagic (arthropod-borne) NEC A94
– – with renal syndrome A98.5† N08.0*
– – arenaviral A96.9
– – – specified NEC A96.8
– – Argentinian A96.0

273

Fever—*continued*
- hemorrhagic—*continued*
- - Bangkok A91
- - Bolivian A96.1
- - Central Asian A98.0
- - Chikungunya A92.0
- - Crimean-Congo A98.0
- - dengue (virus) A91
- - epidemic A98.5† N08.0*
- - Junin (virus) A96.0
- - Korean A98.5† N08.0*
- - Machupo (virus) A96.1
- - mite-borne A93.8
- - mosquito-borne A92.8
- - Omsk A98.1
- - Philippine A91
- - Russian A98.5† N08.0*
- - Singapore A91
- - Southeast Asia A91
- - Thailand A91
- - tick-borne NEC A93.8
- - viral A99
- - - specified NEC A98.8
- herpetic B00.1
- inanition R50.9
- Indiana A93.8
- infective NEC B99
- intermittent (bilious) (*see also* Malaria) B54
- - of unknown origin R50.9
- - pernicious B50.9
- iodide
- - correct substance properly administered R50.2
- - overdose or wrong substance given or taken T48.4
- Japanese river A75.3
- jungle (*see also* Malaria) B54
- Junin (virus) hemorrhagic A96.0
- Katayama B65.2
- kedani A75.3
- Kenya (tick) A77.1
- Kew Garden A79.1
- Korean hemorrhagic A98.5† N08.0*
- Lassa A96.2
- Lone Star A77.0
- Machupo (virus) hemorrhagic A96.1
- Malta A23.9
- Marseilles A77.1
- marsh (*see also* Malaria) B54
- Mayaro (viral) A92.8
- Mediterranean A23.0
- - familial E85.0
- - tick A77.1

Fever—*continued*
- meningeal – *see* Meningitis
- metal fume T56.8
- Meuse A79.0
- Mexican A75.2
- mianeh A68.1
- miasmatic (*see also* Malaria) B54
- mosquito-borne (viral) A92.9
- - hemorrhagic A92.8
- mountain A23.0
- - meaning Rocky Mountain spotted fever A77.0
- - tick (American) (viral) A93.2
- Mucambo (viral) A92.8
- mud A27.9
- Neapolitan A23.0
- newborn P81.9
- - environmental P81.0
- Nine Mile A78
- non-exanthematous tick A93.2
- North Asian tick-borne A77.2
- Omsk hemorrhagic A98.1
- O'nyong-nyong (viral) A92.1
- Oropouche (viral) A93.0
- Oroya A44.0
- paludal (*see also* Malaria) B54
- Panama (malarial) B50.9
- Pappataci A93.1
- paratyphoid A01.4
- - A A01.1
- - B A01.2
- - C A01.3
- parrot A70
- periodic (Mediterranean) E85.0
- persistent (of unknown origin) R50.8
- pharyngoconjunctival B30.2† H13.1*
- Philippine hemorrhagic A91
- phlebotomus A93.1
- Piry (virus) A93.8
- Pixuna (viral) A92.8
- Plasmodium ovale B53.0
- polioviral (nonparalytic) A80.4
- polymer fume T59.8
- Pontiac A48.2
- postoperative (due to infection) T81.4
- pretibial A27.8
- puerperal O85
- putrid – *see* Sepsis
- pyemic – *see* Sepsis
- Q A78
- quadrilateral A78
- quartan (malaria) B52.9
- Queensland (coastal) (tick) A77.3
- quintan A79.0

Fever—*continued*
- rabbit (*see also* Tularemia) A21.9
- rat-bite A25.9
- – due to
- – – Spirillum A25.0
- – – Streptobacillus moniliformis A25.1
- recurrent – *see* Fever, relapsing
- relapsing (Borrelia) A68.9
- – Carter's (Asiatic) A68.1
- – Dutton's (West African) A68.1
- – louse-borne A68.0
- – Novy's
- – – louse-borne A68.0
- – – tick-borne A68.1
- – Obermeyer's (European) A68.0
- – tick-borne A68.1
- remittent (congestive) (*see also* Malaria) B54
- rheumatic (active) (acute) (chronic) (subacute) I00
- – with central nervous system involvement I02.9
- – active with heart involvement I01.-
- – inactive or quiescent with
- – – cardiac hypertrophy I09.8
- – – carditis I09.9
- – – endocarditis I09.1
- – – – aortic (valve) I06.9
- – – – – with mitral (valve) disease I08.0
- – – – mitral (valve) I05.9
- – – – – with aortic (valve) disease I08.0
- – – – pulmonary (valve) I09.8
- – – – tricuspid (valve) I07.8
- – – heart disease NEC I09.8
- – – heart failure (congestive) (conditions in I50.0, I50.9) I09.8
- – – left ventricular failure (conditions in I50.1) I09.8
- – – myocarditis, myocardial degeneration (conditions in I51.4) I09.0
- – – pancarditis I09.9
- – – pericarditis I09.2
- Rift Valley (viral) A92.4
- Rocky Mountain spotted A77.0
- Ross River B33.1
- Russian hemorrhagic A98.5† N08.0*
- San Joaquin (Valley) B38.0† J99.8*
- sandfly A93.1
- Sao Paulo A77.0
- scarlet A38
- septic – *see* Sepsis

Fever—*continued*
- seven-day (autumnal) (Japanese) (leptospirosis) A27.8
- – dengue A90
- shin bone A79.0
- Singapore hemorrhagic A91
- solar A90
- Songo A98.5† N08.0*
- sore B00.1
- South African tick-bite A68.1
- Southeast Asia hemorrhagic A91
- spinal – *see* Meningitis
- spirillary A25.0
- spotted A77.9
- – American A77.0
- – cerebrospinal meningitis A39.0† G01*
- – Colombian A77.0
- – due to Rickettsia
- – – australis A77.3
- – – conorii A77.1
- – – rickettsii A77.0
- – – sibirica A77.2
- – – specified type NEC A77.8
- – Rocky Mountain A77.0
- steroid
- – correct substance properly administered R50.2
- – overdose or wrong substance given or taken T38.0
- streptobacillary A25.1
- subtertian B50.9
- Sumatran mite A75.3
- sun A90
- swamp A27.9
- Tahyna B33.8
- tertian – *see* Malaria, tertian
- Thailand hemorrhagic A91
- thermic T67.0
- three-day A93.1
- tick-bite NEC A93.8
- tick-borne A93.8
- – American mountain A93.2
- – Colorado A93.2
- – Kemerovo A93.8
- – Quaranfil A93.8
- – specified NEC A93.8
- trench A79.0
- tsutsugamushi A75.3
- typhogastric A01.0
- typhoid (abortive) (hemorrhagic) (intermittent) (malignant) A01.0
- – with
- – – gastro-intestinal perforation A01.0† K93.8*

Fever—*continued*
- typhoid—*continued*
- – with—*continued*
- – – gastro-intestinal perforation—
  continued
- – – – with peritonitis A01.0† K67.8*
- – – – pneumopathy A01.0† J17.0*
- typhus – *see* Typhus (fever)
- undulant (*see also* Brucella) A23.9
- unknown origin R50.9
- uremic N19
- uveoparotid D86.8
- valley B38.0† J99.8*
- Venezuelan equine A92.2
- vesicular stomatitis A93.8
- viral hemorrhagic – *see* Fever,
  hemorrhagic, by type of virus
- Wesselsbron (viral) A92.8
- West
- – African B50.8
- – Nile (viral) A92.3
- Whitmore's (*see also* Melioidosis) A24.4
- Wolhynian A79.0
- yellow A95.9
- – jungle A95.0
- – sylvatic A95.0
- – urban A95.1
- Zika (viral) A92.8
Fibrillation
- atrial or auricular (established) I48
- cardiac I49.8
- heart I49.8
- muscular M62.8
- ventricular I49.0
Fibrin
- ball or bodies, pleural (sac) J94.1
- chamber, anterior (eye) (gelatinous
  exudate) H20.0
Fibrinogenolysis – *see* Fibrinolysis
Fibrinogenopenia D68.8
- acquired D65
- congenital D68.2
Fibrinolysis (acquired) (hemorrhagic)
  D65
- antepartum O46.0
- following
- – abortion (subsequent episode) O08.1
- – – current episode – *see* Abortion
- – ectopic or molar pregnancy O08.1
- intrapartum O67.0
- postpartum O72.3
Fibrinopenia (hereditary) (*see also*
  Afibrinogenemia) D68.2
- acquired D68.4

Fibrinopurulent – *see* condition
Fibrinous – *see* condition
Fibroadenoma (M9010/0)
- cellular intracanalicular (M9020/0) D24
- giant (M9016/0) D24
- intracanalicular (M9011/0)
- – cellular (M9020/0) D24
- – giant (M9020/0) D24
- – specified site – *see* Neoplasm, benign
- – unspecified site D24
- juvenile (M9030/0) D24
- pericanalicular (M9012/0)
- – specified site – *see* Neoplasm, benign
- – unspecified site D24
- phyllodes (M9020/0) D24
- prostate D29.1
- specified site NEC – *see* Neoplasm,
  benign
- unspecified site D24
Fibroadenosis, breast (chronic) (cystic)
  (diffuse) (periodic) (segmental) N60.2
Fibroangioma (M9160/0) – *see also*
  Neoplasm, benign
- juvenile (M9160/0)
- – specified site – *see* Neoplasm, benign
- – unspecified site D10.6
Fibrochondrosarcoma (M9220/3) – *see*
  Neoplasm, cartilage, malignant
Fibrocystic
- disease (*see also* Fibrosis, cystic) E84.9
- – breast N60.1
- – – with epithelial proliferation N60.3
- – liver Q44.6
- – lung (congenital) E84.0
- – pancreas E84.9
- kidney (congenital) Q61.8
Fibrodysplasia ossificans progressiva
  M61.1
Fibroelastosis (cordis) (endocardial)
  (endomyocardial) I42.4
Fibroid (tumor) (M8890/0) – *see also*
  Neoplasm, connective tissue, benign
- disease, lung (chronic) (*see also* Fibrosis,
  lung) J84.1
- heart (disease) (*see also* Myocarditis)
  I51.4
- in pregnancy or childbirth O34.1
- – affecting fetus or newborn P03.8
- – causing obstructed labor O65.5
- induration, lung (chronic) (*see also*
  Fibrosis, lung) J84.1
- lung (*see also* Fibrosis, lung) J84.1
- pneumonia (chronic) (*see also* Fibrosis,
  lung) J84.1

Fibroid—*continued*
- uterus D25.9
Fibrolipoma (M8851/0) – *see* Lipoma
Fibroliposarcoma (M8850/3) – *see*
  Neoplasm, connective tissue, malignant
Fibroma (M8810/0) – *see also* Neoplasm,
  connective tissue, benign
- ameloblastic (M9330/0) D16.5
- – upper jaw (bone) D16.4
- bone (nonossifying) M89.8
- – ossifying (M9262/0) – *see* Neoplasm,
  bone, benign
- cementifying (M9274/0) – *see* Neoplasm,
  bone, benign
- chondromyxoid (M9241/0) – *see*
  Neoplasm, bone, benign
- desmoplastic (M8823/1) – *see* Neoplasm,
  connective tissue, uncertain behavior
- durum (M8810/0) – *see* Neoplasm,
  connective tissue, benign
- fascial (M8813/0) – *see* Neoplasm,
  connective tissue, benign
- invasive (M8821/1) – *see* Neoplasm,
  connective tissue, uncertain behavior
- molle (M8851/0) – *see* Lipoma
- myxoid (M8811/0) – *see* Neoplasm,
  connective tissue, benign
- nasopharynx, nasopharyngeal (juvenile)
  (M9160/0) D10.6
- nonosteogenic (nonossifying) – *see*
  Dysplasia, fibrous
- odontogenic (central) (M9321/0) D16.5
- – peripheral (M9322/0) D16.5
- – – upper jaw (bone) D16.4
- – upper jaw (bone) D16.4
- ossifying (M9262/0) – *see* Neoplasm,
  bone, benign
- periosteal (M8812/0) – *see* Neoplasm,
  bone, benign
- prostate D29.1
- soft (M8851/0) – *see* Lipoma
Fibromatosis M72.9
- abdominal (M8822/1) – *see* Neoplasm,
  connective tissue, uncertain behavior
- aggressive (M8821/1) – *see* Neoplasm,
  connective tissue, uncertain behavior
- congenital, generalized (M8824/1) – *see*
  Neoplasm, connective tissue, uncertain
  behavior
- gingival K06.1
- palmar (fascial) M72.0
- plantar (fascial) M72.2
- pseudosarcomatous (proliferative)
  (subcutaneous) M72.4

Fibromatosis—*continued*
- retroperitoneal D48.3
- specified NEC M72.8
Fibromyalgia M79.7
Fibromyoma (M8890/0) – *see also*
  Neoplasm, connective tissue, benign
- uterus (corpus) (*see also* Leiomyoma)
  D25.9
- – in pregnancy or childbirth O34.1
- – – affecting fetus or newborn P03.8
- – – causing obstructed labor O65.5
Fibromyositis M79.7
Fibromyxolipoma (M8852/0) D17.9
Fibromyxoma (M8811/0) – *see* Neoplasm,
  connective tissue, benign
Fibromyxosarcoma (M8811/3) – *see*
  Neoplasm, connective tissue, malignant
Fibro-odontoma, ameloblastic (M9290/0)
  D16.5
- upper jaw (bone) D16.4
Fibro-osteoma (M9262/0) – *see* Neoplasm,
  bone, benign
Fibroplasia, retrolental H35.1
Fibropurulent – *see condition*
Fibrosarcoma (M8810/3) – *see also*
  Neoplasm, connective tissue, malignant
- ameloblastic (M9330/3) C41.1
- – upper jaw (bone) C41.0
- congenital (M8814/3) C49.9
- fascial (M8813/3) C49.9
- infantile (M8814/3) C49.9
- odontogenic (M9330/3) C41.1
- – upper jaw (bone) C41.0
- periosteal (M8812/3) – *see* Neoplasm,
  bone, malignant
Fibrosclerosis
- breast N60.3
- multifocal M35.5
- penis (corpora cavernosa) N48.6
Fibrosis, fibrotic
- adrenal (gland) E27.8
- alcoholic K70.2
- amnion O41.8
- anal papillae K62.8
- arteriocapillary – *see* Arteriosclerosis
- bladder N32.8
- breast N60.3
- capillary, lung (chronic) (*see also*
  Fibrosis, lung) J84.1
- cardiac (*see also* Myocarditis) I51.4
- cervix N88.8
- chorion O41.8
- corpus cavernosum (sclerosing) N48.6
- cystic (of pancreas) E84.9

Fibrosis, fibrotic—*continued*
- cystic—*continued*
- – with
- – – combined manifestations E84.8
- – – distal intestinal obstruction
  (syndrome) E84.1
- – – intestinal manifestations E84.1
- – – pulmonary manifestations E84.0
- – specified NEC E84.8
- due to device, implant or graft (*see also*
  Complications, by site and type, specified
  NEC) T85.8
- – arterial graft NEC T82.8
- – breast (implant) T85.8
- – catheter NEC T85.8
- – – dialysis (renal) T82.8
- – – – intraperitoneal T85.8
- – – infusion NEC T82.8
- – – – spinal (epidural) (subdural) T85.8
- – – urinary (indwelling) T83.8
- – electronic (electrode) (pulse generator)
  (stimulator)
- – – bone T84.8
- – – cardiac T82.8
- – – nervous system (brain) (peripheral
  nerve) (spinal) T85.8
- – – urinary T83.8
- – fixation, internal (orthopedic) NEC
  T84.8
- – gastrointestinal (bile duct) (esophagus)
  T85.8
- – genital NEC T83.8
- – heart NEC T82.8
- – joint prosthesis T84.8
- – ocular (corneal graft) (orbital implant)
  NEC T85.8
- – orthopedic NEC T84.8
- – specified NEC T85.8
- – urinary NEC T83.8
- – vascular NEC T82.8
- – ventricular intracranial shunt T85.8
- ejaculatory duct N50.8
- endocardium (*see also* Endocarditis) I38
- endomyocardial (tropical) I42.3
- epididymis N50.8
- eye muscle H50.6
- heart (*see also* Myocarditis) I51.4
- hepatic – *see* Fibrosis, liver
- hepatolienal (portal hypertension) K76.6
- hepatosplenic (portal hypertension)
  K76.6
- intrascrotal N50.8
- kidney (*see also* Sclerosis, renal) N26
- liver K74.0

Fibrosis, fibrotic—*continued*
- liver—*continued*
- – with sclerosis K74.2
- – – alcoholic K70.2
- – alcoholic K70.2
- lung (atrophic) (capillary) (chronic)
  (confluent) (massive) (perialveolar)
  (peribronchial) J84.1
- – with
- – – aluminosis J63.0
- – – amianthosis J61
- – – anthracosilicosis J60
- – – anthracosis J60
- – – asbestosis J61
- – – bagassosis J67.1
- – – berylliosis J63.2
- – – byssinosis J66.0
- – – calcicosis J62.8
- – – chalicosis J62.8
- – – dust reticulation J64
- – – farmer's lung J67.0
- – – gannister disease J62.8
- – – pneumoconiosis NEC J64
- – – siderosis J63.4
- – – silicosis J62.8
- – – stannosis J63.5
- – congenital P27.8
- – diffuse (idiopathic) (interstitial) J84.1
- – due to
- – – bauxite J63.1
- – – chemicals, gases, fumes or vapors
  (inhalation) J68.4
- – – graphite J63.3
- – – talc J62.0
- – following radiation J70.1
- – idiopathic J84.1
- – postinflammatory J84.1
- – silicotic J62.8
- – tuberculous – *see* Tuberculosis,
  pulmonary
- lymphatic gland I89.8
- median bar N40
- mediastinum (idiopathic) J98.5
- meninges G96.1
- myocardium, myocardial (*see also*
  Myocarditis) I51.4
- oviduct N83.8
- pancreas K86.8
- penis NEC N48.6
- perineum, in pregnancy or childbirth
  O34.7
- – causing obstructed labor O65.5
- – – affecting fetus or newborn P03.1
- placenta O43.8

Fibrosis, fibrotic—*continued*
– pleura J94.1
– prostate (chronic) N40
– pulmonary (*see also* Fibrosis, lung) J84.1
– – congenital P27.8
– rectal sphincter K62.8
– retroperitoneal, idiopathic (with ureteral obstruction) N13.5
– – with infection N13.6
– scrotum N50.8
– seminal vesicle N50.8
– senile R54
– skin NEC L90.5
– spermatic cord N50.8
– spleen D73.8
– – in schistosomiasis (bilharziasis) B65.-† D77*
– subepidermal nodular (M8832/0) – *see* Neoplasm, skin, benign
– submucous (oral) (tongue) K13.5
– testis N50.8
– – chronic, due to syphilis A52.7† N51.1*
– thymus (gland) E32.8
– tongue, submucous K13.5
– tunica vaginalis N50.8
– uterus (non-neoplastic) N85.8
– vagina N89.8
– valve, heart (*see also* Endocarditis) I38
– vas deferens N50.8
– vein I87.8
Fibrositis (periarticular) (rheumatoid) M79.7
Fibrothorax J94.1
Fibrotic – *see* Fibrosis
Fibrous – *see condition*
Fibroxanthoma (M8830/0) – *see also* Neoplasm, connective tissue, benign
– atypical (M8830/1) – *see* Neoplasm, connective tissue, uncertain behavior
– malignant (M8830/3) – *see* Neoplasm, connective tissue, malignant
Fibroxanthosarcoma (M8830/3) – *see* Neoplasm, connective tissue, malignant
Fiedler's
– disease (icterohemorrhagic leptospirosis) A27.0
– myocarditis (acute) I40.1
Fifth disease B08.3
Filaria, filarial, filariasis B74.9
– bancroftian B74.0
– due to
– – Brugia (malayi) B74.1
– – – timori B74.2
– – Mansonella ozzardi B74.4

Filaria, filarial—*continued*
– due to—*continued*
– – Wuchereria (bancrofti) B74.0
– Malayan B74.1
– specified type NEC B74.8
Filatov's disease B27.0
File-cutter's disease T56.0
Fimbrial cyst Q50.4
Financial problem affecting care NEC Z59.9
– bankruptcy Z59.8
– foreclosure on loan Z59.8
Finding in blood (of substance not normally found in blood) R78.9
– addictive drug NEC R78.4
– alcohol (excessive level) R78.0
– cocaine R78.2
– hallucinogen R78.3
– heavy metals (abnormal level) R78.7
– lithium (abnormal level) R78.8
– opiate drug R78.1
– psychotropic drug R78.5
– specified substance NEC R78.8
– steroid agent R78.6
Finger – *see condition*
Fire, Saint Anthony's (*see also* Erysipelas) A46
Fire-setting
– pathological (compulsive) F63.1
– without manifest psychiatric disorder Z03.2
Fish-hook stomach K31.8
Fishmeal-worker's lung J67.8
Fissure, fissured
– anus, anal K60.2
– – acute K60.0
– – chronic K60.1
– – congenital Q43.8
– ear, lobule, congenital Q17.8
– epiglottis (congenital) Q31.8
– larynx J38.7
– – congenital Q31.8
– lip K13.0
– nipple N64.0
– – puerperal, postpartum or gestational O92.1
– nose Q30.2
– palate (congenital) (*see also* Cleft, palate) Q35.9
– skin R23.4
– spine (congenital) (*see also* Spina bifida) Q05.9
– – with hydrocephalus (*see also* Spina bifida, with hydrocephalus) Q05.4

Remember Malformaha v cangenital

Fissure, fissured—*continued*
- tongue (acquired) K14.5
- - congenital Q38.3
Fistula L98.8
- abdomen (wall) K63.2
- - bladder N32.2
   intestine NEC K63.2
- - ureter N28.8
- - uterus N82.5
- abdominothoracic J86.0
- abdominouterine N82.5
- - congenital Q51.7
- accessory sinuses (*see also* Sinusitis)
  J32.9
- actinomycotic – *see* Actinomycosis
- alveolar antrum (*see also* Sinusitis,
  maxillary) J32.0
- anorectal K60.5
- antrobuccal (*see also* Sinusitis, maxillary)
  J32.0
- antrum (*see also* Sinusitis, maxillary)
  J32.0
- anus, anal (infectional) (recurrent) K60.3
- - congenital Q43.6
- - - with absence, atresia and stenosis
    Q42.2
- - tuberculous A18.3† K93.0*
- aorta-duodenal I77.2
- appendix, appendicular K38.3
- arteriovenous (acquired) (nonruptured)
  I77.0
- - brain I67.1
- - - congenital Q28.2
- - - - ruptured I60.8
- - - ruptured I60.8
- - congenital (peripheral) Q27.3
- - - brain Q28.2
- - - - ruptured I60.8
- - - pulmonary Q25.7
- - coronary I25.4
- - - congenital Q24.5
- - pulmonary I28.0
- - - congenital Q25.7
- - surgically created (for dialysis) Z99.2
- - - complication NEC T82.9
- - - - infection or inflammation T82.7
- - - - mechanical T82.5
- - - - specified NEC T82.8
- - traumatic – *see* Injury, blood vessel
- artery I77.2
- aural (mastoid) H70.1
- auricle H61.1
- - congenital Q18.1
- Bartholin's gland N82.9

Fistula—*continued*
- bile duct (common) (hepatic) K83.3
- - with calculus, stones K80.5
- biliary (tract) (*see also* Fistula, bile duct)
  K83.3
- bladder (sphincter) NEC (*see also* Fistula,
  vesico-) N32.2
- - into seminal vesicle N32.2
- bone M89.8
- - with osteomyelitis, chronic M86.4
- brain G96.0
- - arteriovenous (acquired) I67.1
- - - congenital Q28.2
- branchial (cleft) Q18.0
- branchiogenous Q18.0
- breast N61
- - puerperal, postpartum or gestational,
  due to mastitis (purulent) O91.1
- bronchial J86.0
- bronchocutaneous, bronchomediastinal,
  bronchopleural, bronchopleuromediastinal
  (infective) J86.0
- - tuberculous NEC A16.4
- - - with bacteriological and histological
    confirmation A15.5
- bronchoesophageal J86.0
- - congenital Q39.2
- - - with atresia of esophagus Q39.1
- bronchovisceral J86.0
- buccal cavity (infective) K12.2
- cecosigmoidal K63.2
- cecum K63.2
- cerebrospinal (fluid) G96.0
- cervical, lateral Q18.1
- cervicoaural Q18.1
- cervicosigmoidal N82.4
- cervicovesical N82.1
- cervix N82.9
- chest (wall) J86.0
- cholecystenteric (*see also* Fistula,
  gallbladder) K82.3
- cholecystocolic (*see also* Fistula,
  gallbladder) K82.3
- cholecystocolonic (*see also* Fistula,
  gallbladder) K82.3
- cholecystoduodenal (*see also* Fistula,
  gallbladder) K82.3
- cholecystogastric (*see also* Fistula,
  gallbladder) K82.3
- cholecystointestinal (*see also* Fistula,
  gallbladder) K82.3
- choledochoduodenal (*see also* Fistula, bile
  duct) K83.3
- coccyx L05.9

Fistula—*continued*
- coccyx—*continued*
- – with abscess L05.0
- colon K63.2
- colostomy K91.4
- common duct (*see also* Fistula, bile duct) K83.3
- congenital, site not listed – *see* Anomaly, by site
- coronary, arteriovenous I25.4
- – congenital Q24.5
- costal region J86.0
- cul-de-sac, Douglas' N82.9
- cutaneous L98.8
- cystic duct (*see also* Fistula, gallbladder) K82.3
- – congenital Q44.5
- duodenum K31.6
- ear (external) (canal) H61.8
- enterocolic K63.2
- enterocutaneous K63.2
- enterouterine N82.4
- – congenital Q51.7
- enterovaginal N82.4
- – congenital Q52.2
- – large intestine N82.3
- – small intestine N82.2
- epididymis N50.8
- – tuberculous A18.1† N51.1*
- esophagobronchial J86.0
- – congenital Q39.2
- – – with atresia of esophagus Q39.1
- esophagocutaneous K22.8
- esophagopleural-cutaneous J86.0
- esophagotracheal J86.0
- – congenital Q39.2
- – – with atresia of esophagus Q39.1
- esophagus K22.8
- – congenital Q39.2
- – – with atresia of esophagus Q39.1
- ethmoid (*see also* Sinusitis, ethmoidal) J32.2
- eyeball (cornea) (sclera) H44.4
- eyelid H01.8
- fallopian tube, external N82.5
- fecal K63.2
- – congenital Q43.6
- from periapical abscess K04.6
- frontal sinus (*see also* Sinusitis, frontal) J32.1
- gallbladder K82.3
- – with calculus, cholelithiasis, stones (*see also* Cholelithiasis) K80.2
- gastric K31.6

Fistula—*continued*
- gastrocolic K31.6
- – congenital Q40.2
- – tuberculous A18.3† K93.0*
- gastroenterocolic K31.6
- gastrojejunal K31.6
- gastrojejunocolic K31.6
- genital tract (female) N82.9
- – specified NEC N82.8
- – to
- – – intestine NEC N82.4
- – – skin N82.5
- hepatic artery-portal vein, congenital Q26.6
- hepatopleural J86.0
- hepatopulmonary J86.0
- ileorectal or ileosigmoidal K63.2
- ileovaginal N82.2
- ileovesical N32.1
- ileum K63.2
- in ano K60.3
- – tuberculous A18.3† K93.0*
- inner ear (labyrinth) H83.1
- intestine NEC K63.2
- intestinocolonic (abdominal) K63.2
- intestinoureteral N28.8
- intestinouterine N82.4
- intestinovaginal N82.4
- – large intestine N82.3
- – small intestine N82.2
- intestinovesical N32.1
- ischiorectal (fossa) K61.3
- jejunum K63.2
- joint M25.1
- – tuberculous – *see* Tuberculosis, joint
- kidney N28.8
- labium (majus) (minus) N82.9
- labyrinth H83.1
- lacrimal (gland) (sac) H04.6
- lacrimonasal duct H04.6
- laryngotracheal, congenital Q34.8
- larynx J38.7
- lip K13.0
- – congenital Q38.0
- lumbar, tuberculous A18.0† M49.0*
- lung J86.0
- lymphatic I89.8
- mammary (gland) N61
- mastoid (process) (region) H70.1
- maxillary J32.0
- medial, face and neck Q18.8
- mediastinal J86.0
- mediastinobronchial J86.0
- mediastinocutaneous J86.0

Fistula—*continued*
- middle ear H74.8
- mouth K12.2
- nasal J34.8
- – sinus (*see also* Sinusitis) J32.9
- nasopharynx J39.2
- nipple N64.0
- nose J34.8
- oesophago- – *see* Fistula, esophago-
- oesophagus – *see* Fistula, esophagus
- oral (cutaneous) K12.2
- – maxillary J32.0
- – nasal (with cleft palate) (*see also* Cleft, palate) Q35.9
- orbit, orbital H05.8
- oroantral J32.0
- oviduct, external N82.5
- pancreatic K86.8
- pancreaticoduodenal K86.8
- parotid (gland) K11.4
- penis N48.8
- perianal K60.3
- pericardium (pleura) (sac) – *see* Pericarditis
- perineorectal K60.4
- perineum, perineal (with urethral involvement) NEC N36.0
- – tuberculous A18.1† N37.8*
- – ureter N28.8
- perirectal K60.4
- – tuberculous A18.3† K93.0*
- peritoneum K65.9
- pharyngoesophageal J39.2
- pharynx J39.2
- – branchial cleft (congenital) Q18.0
- pilonidal (infected) (rectum) L05.9
- – with abscess L05.0
- pleura, pleural, pleurocutaneous or pleuroperitoneal J86.0
- – tuberculous NEC A16.5
- – – with bacteriological and histological confirmation A15.6
- portal vein-hepatic artery, congenital Q26.6
- postauricular H70.1
- postoperative, persistent T81.8
- – specified site – *see* Fistula, by site
- preauricular (congenital) Q18.1
- prostate N42.8
- pulmonary J86.0
- – arteriovenous I28.0
- – – congenital Q25.7
- – tuberculous (*see also* Tuberculosis, pulmonary) A16.2

Fistula—*continued*
- pulmonoperitoneal J86.0
- rectolabial N82.4
- rectosigmoid (intercommunicating) K63.2
- rectoureteral N28.8
- rectourethral N36.0
- – congenital Q64.7
- rectouterine N82.4
- – congenital Q51.7
- rectovaginal N82.3
- – congenital Q52.2
- – tuberculous A18.1† N74.1*
- rectovesical N32.1
- – congenital Q64.7
- rectovesicovaginal N82.3
- rectovulval N82.4
- – congenital Q52.7
- rectum (to skin) K60.4
- – congenital Q43.6
- – – with absence, atresia and stenosis Q42.0
- – tuberculous A18.3† K93.0*
- renal N28.8
- retroauricular H70.1
- salivary duct or gland (any) K11.4
- – congenital Q38.4
- scrotum (urinary) N50.8
- – tuberculous A18.1† N51.8*
- semicircular canals H83.1
- sigmoid K63.2
- – to bladder N32.1
- sinus (*see also* Sinusitis) J32.9
- skin L98.8
- – to genital tract (female) N82.5
- splenocolic D73.8
- stercoral K63.2
- stomach K31.6
- sublingual gland K11.4
- submandibular gland K11.4
- thoracic J86.0
- – duct I89.8
- thoracoabdominal J86.0
- thoracogastric J86.0
- thoracointestinal J86.0
- thorax J86.0
- thyroglossal duct Q89.2
- thyroid E07.8
- trachea, congenital (external) (internal) Q32.1
- tracheoesophageal J86.0
- – congenital Q39.2
- – – with atresia of esophagus Q39.1
- – following tracheostomy J95.0

Fistula—*continued*
- traumatic arteriovenous (*see also* Injury, blood vessel) T14.5
- tuberculous – *code as* Tuberculosis, by site
- umbilicourinary Q64.8
- urachus, congenital Q64.4
- ureter (persistent) N28.8
- ureteroabdominal N28.8
- ureterorectal N28.8
- ureterosigmoido-abdominal N28.8
- ureterovaginal N82.1
- ureterovesical N32.2
- urethra N36.0
- – congenital Q64.7
- – tuberculous A18.1† N37.8*
- urethroperineal N36.0
- urethroperineovesical N32.2
- urethrorectal N36.0
- – congenital Q64.7
- urethroscrotal N50.8
- urethrovaginal N82.1
- urethrovesical N32.2
- urinary (tract) (persistent) (recurrent) N36.0
- uteroabdominal N82.5
- – congenital Q51.7
- uteroenteric, uterointestinal N82.4
- – congenital Q51.7
- uterorectal N82.4
- – congenital Q51.7
- uteroureteric N82.1
- uterourethral Q51.7
- uterovaginal N82.8
- uterovesical N82.1
- – congenital Q51.7
- uterus N82.9
- vagina (wall) N82.9
- vaginocutaneous (postpartal) N82.5
- vaginointestinal NEC N82.4
- – large intestine N82.3
- – small intestine N82.2
- vaginoperineal N82.5
- vesical NEC N32.2
- vesicoabdominal N32.2
- vesicocervicovaginal N82.1
- vesicocolic N32.1
- vesicoenteric N32.1
- vesicointestinal N32.1
- vesicometrorectal N82.4
- vesicoperineal N32.2
- vesicorectal N32.1
- – congenital Q64.7
- vesicosigmoidal N32.1

Fistula—*continued*
- vesicosigmoidovaginal N82.3
- vesicoureteral N32.2
- vesicoureterovaginal N82.1
- vesicourethral N32.2
- vesicourethrorectal N32.1
- vesicouterine N82.1
- – congenital Q51.7
- vesicovaginal N82.0
- vulvorectal N82.4
- – congenital Q52.7

Fit R56.8
- epileptic (*see also* Epilepsy) G40.9
- fainting R55
- hysterical F44.5
- newborn P90

Fitting (of)
- artificial
- – arm (complete) (partial) Z44.0
- – breast Z44.3
- – eye Z44.2
- – leg (complete) (partial) Z44.1
- colostomy belt Z46.5
- contact lenses Z46.0
- dentures Z46.3
- device NEC (related to) Z46.9
- – abdominal Z46.5
- – nervous system Z46.2
- – orthodontic Z46.4
- – orthotic Z46.7
- – prosthetic (external) Z44.9
- – – breast Z44.3
- – – dental Z46.3
- – – specified NEC Z44.8
- – special senses Z46.2
- – specified NEC Z46.8
- – substitution
- – – auditory Z46.2
- – – visual Z46.2
- – urinary Z46.6
- glasses (reading) Z46.0
- hearing aid Z46.1
- ileostomy device Z46.5
- intestinal appliance NEC Z46.5
- orthopedic device (brace) (cast) (corset) (shoes) Z46.7
- pacemaker (cardiac) Z45.0
- prosthesis (external) Z44.9
- – breast Z44.3
- – specified NEC Z44.8
- spectacles Z46.0
- wheelchair Z46.8

Fitz Hugh and Curtis syndrome A54.8†
  K67.1∗
– chlamydial A74.8† K67.0∗
– gonococcal A54.8† K67.1∗
Fixation
– joint – *see* Ankylosis
– larynx J38.7
– stapes H74.3
– – deafness (*see also* Deafness,
  conductive) H90.2
– uterus (acquired) – *see* Malposition, uterus
– vocal cord J38.3
Flabby ridge K06.8
Flaccid – *see also condition*
– palate, congenital Q38.5
Flail
– chest S22.5
– – newborn (birth injury) P13.8
– joint (paralytic) M25.2
Flajani's disease E05.0
**Flashbacks (residual to alcohol or drug
  use)** – *code to* F10-F19 with fourth
  character .7
Flat – *see also* Anomaly, by site
– chamber (eye) H44.4
– chest, congenital Q67.8
– foot (acquired) (fixed type) (painful)
  (postural) M21.4
– – congenital Q66.5
– – rachitic (late effect) E64.3
– – rigid Q66.5
– – spastic (everted) Q66.5
– pelvis M95.5
– – with disproportion (fetopelvic) O33.0
– – – affecting fetus or newborn P03.1
– – – causing obstructed labor O65.0
– – congenital Q74.2
Flatau-Schilder disease G37.0
Flatback syndrome M40.3
Flattening
– head, femur M89.8
– hip M91.2
– nose (congenital) Q67.4
Flatulence R14
– psychogenic F45.3
Flatus R14
– vaginalis N89.8
Flax-dresser's disease J66.1
Flea bite – *see* Injury, superficial
Flecks, glaucomatous (subcapsular)
  H26.2
Fleischer-Kayser ring (cornea) H18.0
Fleshy mole O02.0
Flexibilitas cerea – *see* Catalepsy

Flexion
– cervix (*see also* Malposition, uterus)
  N85.4
– contracture, joint (*see also* Contraction,
  joint) M24.5
– deformity, joint M21.2
– – hip, congenital Q65.8
– uterus (*see also* Malposition, uterus)
  N85.4
– – lateral – *see* Lateroversion, uterus
Flexner's dysentery A03.1
Flexure – *see* Flexion
Flint murmur (aortic insufficiency) I35.1
Floater, vitreous H43.3
Floating
– cartilage (joint) M24.0
– – knee M23.4
– gallbladder, congenital Q44.1
– kidney N28.8
– – congenital Q63.8
– spleen D73.8
Floor – *see condition*
Floppy baby syndrome (nonspecific)
  P94.2
Flu – *see* Influenza
Fluctuating blood pressure I99
Fluid
– abdomen R18
– chest J94.8
– heart (*see also* Failure, heart, congestive)
  I50.0
– joint M25.4
– loss (acute) E86
– peritoneal cavity R18
– pleural cavity J94.8
Flukes NEC (*see also* Infestation, fluke)
  B66.9
– blood NEC (*see also* Schistosomiasis)
  B65.9
– liver B66.3
Fluor (vaginalis) N89.8
– trichomonal or due to Trichomonas
  (vaginalis) A59.0
Fluorosis
– dental K00.3
– skeletal M85.1
Flushing R23.2
Flutter
– atrial or auricular I48
– heart I49.8
– – atrial I48
– – ventricular I49.0
– ventricular I49.0
Fochier's abscess – *code as* Abscess, by site

Focus, Assmann's (*see also* Tuberculosis, pulmonary) A16.2
Fogo selvagem L10.3
Fold, folds (anomalous) – *see also* Anomaly, by site
– Descemet's membrane H18.3
– epicanthic Q10.3
– heart Q24.8
Folie à deux F24
Follicle
– cervix (nabothian) (ruptured) N88.8
– nabothian N88.8
Follicular – *see condition*
Folliculitis L73.9
– abscedens et suffodiens L66.3
– decalvans L66.2
– gonococcal (acute) (chronic) A54.0
– keloid, keloidalis L73.0
– pustular L01.0
– ulerythematosa reticulata L66.4
Folliculome lipidique (M8641/0)
– specified site – *see* Neoplasm, benign
– unspecified site
– – female D27
– – male D29.2
Fölling's disease E70.0
Food
– asphyxia (from aspiration or inhalation) (*see also* Asphyxia, food) T17.9
– choked on (*see also* Asphyxia, food) T17.9
– deprivation T73.0
– – specified kind of food NEC E63.8
– lack of T73.0
– strangulation or suffocation (*see also* Asphyxia, food) T17.9
Foot – *see condition*
Foramen ovale (nonclosure) (patent) (persistent) Q21.1
Forbes' glycogen storage disease E74.0
Forced birth or delivery NEC O83.9
– affecting fetus or newborn P03.8
Forceps delivery NEC O81.3
– affecting fetus or newborn P03.2
Fordyce-Fox disease L75.2
Fordyce's disease (mouth) Q38.6
Forearm – *see condition*
Foreign body
– accidently left during a procedure T81.5
– anterior chamber (eye) S05.5
– ciliary body (eye) S05.5
– entering through orifice
– – accessory sinus T17.0

Foreign body—*continued*
– entering through orifice—*continued*
– – alimentary canal T18.9
– – – multiple parts T18.8
– – – specified part NEC T18.8
– – alveolar process T18.0
– – antrum (Highmore's) T17.0
– – anus T18.5
– – appendix T18.4
– – asphyxia due to (*see also* Asphyxia, food) T17.9
– – auditory canal T16
– – auricle T16
– – bladder T19.1
– – bronchioles T17.8
– – bronchus (main) T17.5
– – buccal cavity T18.0
– – canthus (inner) T15.1
– – cecum T18.4
– – cervix (canal) (uteri) T19.3
– – colon T18.4
– – conjunctiva, conjunctival sac T15.1
– – cornea T15.0
– – digestive organ or tract NEC T18.9
– – – multiple parts T18.8
– – – specified part NEC T18.8
– – duodenum T18.3
– – ear (external) T16
– – esophagus T18.1
– – eye (external) NEC T15.9
– – – multiple parts T15.8
– – – specified part NEC T15.8
– – eyeball T15.8
– – eyelid T15.1
– – gastrointestinal tract T18.9
– – – multiple parts T18.8
– – – specified part NEC T18.8
– – genitourinary tract T19.9
– – – multiple parts T19.8
– – – specified part NEC T19.8
– – globe T15.8
– – gum T18.0
– – Highmore's antrum T17.0
– – hypopharynx T17.2
– – ileum T18.3
– – intestine (small) T18.3
– – – large T18.4
– – lacrimal apparatus, duct, gland or sac T15.8
– – large intestine T18.4
– – larynx T17.3
– – lung T17.8
– – maxillary sinus T17.0
– – mouth T18.0

Foreign body—*continued*
- entering through orifice—*continued*
- – nasal sinus T17.0
- – nasopharynx T17.2
- – nose (passage) T17.1
- – nostril T17.1
- – oral cavity T18.0
- – palate T18.0
- – penis T19.8
- – pharynx T17.2
- – piriform sinus T17.2
- – rectosigmoid (junction) T18.5
- – rectum T18.5
- – respiratory tract T17.9
- – – multiple parts T17.8
- – – specified part NEC T17.8
- – sinus (accessory) (frontal) (maxillary) (nasal) T17.0
- – – piriform T17.2
- – small intestine T18.3
- – stomach T18.2
- – suffocation by (*see also* Asphyxia, food) T17.9
- – tear ducts or glands T15.8
- – throat T17.2
- – tongue T18.0
- – tonsil, tonsillar (fossa) T17.2
- – trachea T17.4
- – ureter T19.8
- – urethra T19.0
- – uterus (any part) T19.3
- – vagina T19.2
- – vulva T19.2
- granuloma (old) (soft tissue) M60.2
- – skin L92.3
- in
- – puncture wound – *see* Wound, open, by site
- – soft tissue (residual) M79.5
- inadvertently left in operation wound (causing adhesions, obstruction or perforation) T81.5
- ingestion, ingested NEC T18.9
- inhalation or inspiration (*see also* Asphyxia, food) T17.9
- internal organ, not entering through a natural orifice – *code as* Injury, by site
- intraocular S05.5
- – old, retained (nonmagnetic) H44.7
- – – magnetic H44.6
- iris S05.5
- lens S05.5
- lid (eye) T15.1
- ocular muscle S05.4

Foreign body—*continued*
- ocular muscle—*continued*
- – old, retained H05.5
- old or residual, soft tissue M79.5
- operation wound, left accidentally T81.5
  orbit S05.4
- – old, retained H05.5
- respiratory tract T17.9
- – multiple parts T17.8
- – specified part NEC T17.8
- retained (nonmagnetic) (old) (in)
- – anterior chamber (eye) H44.7
- – – magnetic H44.6
- – ciliary body H44.7
- – – magnetic H44.6
- – eyelid H02.8
- – globe H44.7
- – – magnetic H44.6
- – intraocular H44.7
- – – magnetic H44.6
- – iris H44.7
- – – magnetic H44.6
- – lens H44.7
- – – magnetic H44.6
- – muscle M79.5
- – orbit H05.5
- – posterior wall of globe H44.7
- – – magnetic H44.6
- – retrobulbar H05.5
- – soft tissue M79.5
- – vitreous H44.7
- – – magnetic H44.6
- retina S05.5
- superficial, without major open wound (*see also* Injury, superficial) T14.0
- swallowed T18.9
- vitreous (humor) S05.5

Forestier's disease (rhizomelic pseudopolyarthritis) M35.3
- ankylosing hyperostosis M48.1

Formation
- hyalin in cornea H18.4
- sequestrum in bone (due to infection) M86.6
- valve
- – colon, congenital Q43.8
- – ureter (congenital) Q62.3

Formication R20.2

Fort Bragg fever A27.8

Fossa – *see condition*
- pyriform – *see condition*

Fothergill's
- disease (scarlatina anginosa) A38

Fothergill's—*continued*
- syndrome (trigeminal neuralgia) (*see also* Neuralgia, trigeminal) G50.0

Foul breath R19.6

Found dead (cause unknown) R98

Foundling Z76.1

Fournier's disease or gangrene N49.8
- female N76.8

Fourth
- cranial nerve – *see condition*
- molar K00.1

Foville's (peduncular) disease or syndrome I67.8† G46.3∗

Fox(-Fordyce) disease L75.2

Fracture (abduction) (adduction) (avulsion) (comminuted) (compression) (dislocation) (oblique) (separation) T14.2
- acetabulum S32.4
- acromion (process) S42.1
- alveolus S02.8
- ankle (bimalleolar) (trimalleolar) S82.8
- – talus S92.1
- arm
- – meaning upper limb – *see* Fracture, limb, upper
- – upper S42.3
- – – specified NEC S42.8
- astragalus S92.1
- axis S12.1
- back – *see* Fracture, vertebra
- Barton's S52.5
- base of skull S02.1
- Bennett's S62.2
- bimalleolar S82.8
- blow-out S02.3
- bone T14.2
- – birth injury P13.9
- – following insertion of orthopedic implant, joint prosthesis or bone plate M96.6
- – in (due to) neoplastic disease NEC (M8000/1) (*see also* Neoplasm) D48.0† M90.7∗
- – pathological (cause unknown) (*see also* Fracture, pathological) M84.4
- bucket handle (semilunar cartilage) – *see* Tear, meniscus
- calcaneus S92.0
- carpal bone(s) NEC S62.1
- cervical (*see also* Fracture, vertebra, cervical) S12.9
- clavicle (acromial end) (interligamentous) (shaft) S42.0

Fracture—*continued*
- clavicle—*continued*
- – with other bone(s) or shoulder and upper arm S42.7
- – birth injury P13.4
- coccyx S32.2
- collar bone (*see also* Fracture, clavicle) S42.0
- Colles' (reversed) S52.5
- costochondral, costosternal junction S22.3
- – multiple S22.4
- – – with flail chest S22.5
- cranium – *see* Fracture, skull
- cricoid cartilage S12.8
- cuboid (ankle) S92.2
- cuneiform
- – foot S92.2
- – wrist S62.1
- delayed union M84.2
- due to birth injury – *see* Birth injury, fracture
- Dupuytren's S82.6
- elbow S52.0
- ethmoid (bone) (sinus) S02.1
- face bone S02.9
- – with skull bone(s) (multiple) S02.7
- – specified NEC S02.8
- fatigue M84.3
- – vertebra M48.4
- femur, femoral S72.9
- – birth injury P13.2
- – condyles, epicondyles S72.4
- – distal end S72.4
- – epiphysis
- – – head S72.0
- – – lower S72.4
- – – upper S72.0
- – head S72.0
- – intertrochanteric S72.1
- – intratrochanteric S72.1
- – lower (end or extremity) S72.4
- – multiple S72.7
- – neck S72.0
- – pertrochanteric S72.1
- – shaft (lower third) (middle third) (upper third) S72.3
- – specified NEC S72.8
- – subtrochanteric (region) (section) S72.2
- – transcervical S72.0
- – transtrochanteric S72.1
- fibula (alone) (styloid) S82.4
- – with tibia – *see* Fracture, tibia

Fracture—*continued*
- fibula—*continued*
- – involving ankle or malleolus S82.6
- finger (except thumb) S62.6
- – multiple (of one hand) S62.7
- foot S92.9
- – multiple S92.7
- forearm S52.9
- – multiple S52.7
- – specified NEC S52.8
- fossa (anterior) (middle) (posterior) S02.1
- frontal (bone) (skull) S02.0
- – sinus S02.0
- glenoid (cavity) (scapula) S42.1
- greenstick – *see* Fracture, by site
- hallux S92.4
- hand NEC S62.8
- – carpal (capitate) (hamate) (lunate) S62.1
- – – navicular (scaphoid) S62.0
- – – specified NEC S62.1
- – metacarpal S62.3
- – – first S62.2
- – – multiple S62.4
- – – specified NEC S62.3
- – phalanx S62.6
- – scaphoid (navicular, hand) S62.0
- healed or old with complications – *see* Nature of the complication
- heel bone S92.0
- hip (*see also* Fracture, femur, neck) S72.0
- humerus S42.3
- – anatomical neck S42.2
- – and clavicle, scapula (multiple) S42.7
- – articular process S42.4
- – distal end S42.4
- – epiphysis
- – – lower S42.4
- – – upper S42.2
- – external condyle S42.4
- – great tuberosity S42.2
- – intercondylar S42.4
- – internal epicondyle S42.4
- – lesser tuberosity S42.2
- – lower end (articular process) or extremity S42.4
- – proximal end S42.2
- – shaft S42.3
- – supracondylar S42.4
- – surgical neck S42.2
- – tuberosity S42.2
- – upper end or extremity S42.2
- hyoid bone S12.8
- ilium S32.3

Fracture—*continued*
- impaction, impacted – *code as* Fracture, by site
- innominate bone S32.3
- ischium S32.8
- jaw (bone) (condyle) (coronoid (process)) (ramus) (symphysis) (lower) S02.6
- – upper S02.4
- knee cap S82.0
- larynx S12.8
- late effects – *see* Sequelae, fracture
- leg
- – lower S82.9
- – – multiple S82.7
- – meaning lower limb – *see* Fracture, limb, lower
- limb
- – lower T12
- – – both T02.5
- – – multiple (same limb) NEC T02.3
- – upper T10
- – – both T02.4
- – – multiple (same limb) NEC T02.2
- lumbar spine S32.0
- – with pelvis (multiple) S32.7
- lumbosacral spine S32.8
- malar bone S02.4
- Malgaigne's S32.7
- malleolus S82.8
- – lateral S82.6
- – medial S82.5
- malunion M84.0
- mandible (condylar) (lower jaw) S02.6
- manubrium (sterni) S22.2
- march S92.3
- maxilla, maxillary (bone) (sinus) (superior) (upper jaw) S02.4
- – inferior S02.6
- metacarpal S62.3
- – first S62.2
- – multiple S62.4
- – specified NEC S62.3
- metastatic (M8000/6) C79.5† M90.7*
- – vertebra C79.5† M49.5*
- metatarsal bone S92.3
- Monteggia's S52.0
- multiple T02.9
- – arm
- – – meaning upper limb – *see* Fracture, multiple, limb, upper
- – – upper S42.7
- – body regions NEC T02.8
- – bones of trunk NEC T02.1
- – clavicle, scapula and humerus S42.7

Fracture—*continued*
– multiple—*continued*
– – face bone(s) (with skull) S02.7
– – femur S72.7
– – fingers S62.7
– – foot S92.7
– – forearm NEC S52.7
– – hand (and wrist) NEC S62.8
– – – fingers alone S62.7
– – – metacarpal bones S62.4
– – head S02.7
– – – with
– – – – neck T02.0
– – – – other body regions T02.8
– – leg
– – – lower S82.7
– – – meaning lower limb – *see* Fracture,
     multiple, limb, lower
– – limb
– – – lower (one) T02.3
– – – – with
– – – – – other lower limb T02.5
– – – – – thorax, lower back and pelvis
         T02.7
– – – – – upper limb(s) T02.6
– – – upper (one) T02.2
– – – – with
– – – – – lower limb(s) T02.6
– – – – – other upper limb T02.4
– – – – – thorax, lower back and pelvis
         T02.7
– – metacarpal bones S62.4
– – neck S12.7
– – – with
– – – – head T02.0
– – – – other body regions T02.8
– – pelvis (and lumbar spine) S32.7
– – ribs S22.4
– – – with flail chest S22.5
– – skull S02.7
– – – with facial bones S02.7
– – specified NEC T02.8
– – spine (*see also* Fracture, multiple,
     vertebrae) T02.1
– – thorax S22.8
– – – with
– – – – limb(s) T02.7
– – – – lower back and pelvis T02.1
– – – – other body regions NEC T02.8
– – trunk T02.1
– – – with
– – – – limb(s) T02.7
– – – – other body regions NEC T02.8
– – unspecified sites T02.9

Fracture—*continued*
– multiple—*continued*
– – vertebrae T02.1
– – – cervical S12.7
– – – lumbar (and pelvis) S32.7
– – – thoracic S22.1
– – wrist (and hand) NEC S62.8
– nasal (bone(s)) S02.2
– navicular (scaphoid, foot) S92.2
– – hand S62.0
– neck S12.9
– neoplastic NEC (M8000/1) (*see also*
     Neoplasm) D48.9† M90.7*
– neural arch – *see* Fracture, vertebra
– nonunion M84.1
– nose, nasal (bone) (septum) S02.2
– occiput S02.1
– odontoid process S12.1
– olecranon (process) (ulna) S52.0
– orbit, orbital (bone) (region) S02.8
– – floor (blow-out) S02.3
– – roof S02.1
– os
– – calcis S92.0
– – magnum S62.1
– – pubis S32.5
– palate S02.8
– parietal bone (skull) S02.0
– patella S82.0
– pathological (cause unknown) M84.4
– – with osteoporosis M80.9
– – – disuse M80.2
– – – drug-induced M80.4
– – – idiopathic M80.5
– – – postmenopausal M80.0
– – – postoophorectomy M80.1
– – – postsurgical malabsorption M80.3
– – – specified NEC M80.8
– – due to neoplastic disease NEC
     (M8000/1) (*see also* Neoplasm)
     D48.9† M90.7*
– pedicle (of vertebral arch) – *see* Fracture,
     vertebra
– pelvis, pelvic (bone) S32.8
– – multiple S32.7
– phalanx
– – foot S92.5
– – toe (except great) (*see also* Fracture,
     toe) S92.5
– pisiform S62.1
– pond S02.9
– prosthetic device, internal – *see*
     Complications, prosthetic device, by site,
     mechanical

Fracture—*continued*
- pubis S32.5
- radius S52.8
- – and ulna S52.7
- – – lower or distal ends S52.6
- – – shafts S52.4
- – head S52.1
- – lower or distal end S52.5
- – multiple NEC S52.7
- – neck S52.1
- – shaft S52.3
- – upper or proximal end S52.1
- ramus
- – inferior or superior, pubis S32.5
- – mandible S02.6
- rib S22.3
- – with flail chest S22.5
- – multiple S22.4
- – – with flail chest S22.5
- root, tooth S02.5
- sacrum S32.1
- scaphoid (hand) S62.0
- – foot S92.2
- scapula (acromial process) (body) (glenoid (cavity)) (neck) S42.1
- – with other bone(s) of shoulder and upper arm S42.7
- semilunar bone, wrist S62.1
- sequelae – *see* Sequelae, fracture
- sesamoid bone
- – foot S92.4
- – hand S62.1
- – other – *code as* Fracture, by site
- shoulder (girdle) S42.9
- – blade S42.1
- – specified NEC S42.8
- skull S02.9
- – with face bone(s) (multiple) S02.7
- – base S02.1
- – birth injury P13.0
- – frontal bone S02.0
- – parietal bone S02.0
- – vault S02.0
- Smith's S52.5
- sphenoid (bone) (sinus) S02.1
- spine – *see* Fracture, vertebra
- spinous process – *see* Fracture, vertebra
- spontaneous (cause unknown) (*see also* Fracture, pathological) M84.4
- stave (of thumb) S62.2
- sternum S22.2
- – with flail chest S22.5
- stress M84.3
- – vertebra M48.4

Fracture—*continued*
- supracondylar, elbow S42.4
- symphysis pubis S32.5
- talus (ankle bone) S92.1
- tarsus, tarsal bone(s) S92.2
- temporal bone (styloid) S02.1
- thorax (bony) S22.9
- – specified NEC S22.8
- thumb (of one hand) S62.5
- thyroid cartilage S12.8
- tibia (shaft) (with fibula) S82.2
- – condyles S82.1
- – distal end S82.3
- – epiphysis
- – – lower S82.3
- – – upper S82.1
- – head (involving knee joint) S82.1
- – intercondyloid eminence S82.1
- – involving ankle or malleolus S82.5
- – lower end (with fibula) S82.3
- – proximal end S82.1
- – tuberosity S82.1
- – upper end or extremity S82.1
- toe (except great) S92.5
- – great S92.4
- tooth (root) S02.5
- trachea (cartilage) S12.8
- transverse process – *see* Fracture, vertebra
- trapezium or trapezoid bone S62.1
- trimalleolar S82.8
- triquetrum (cuneiform of carpus) S62.1
- trochanter (greater) (lesser) S72.1
- trunk (multiple) T02.1
- – with limb(s) (multiple) T02.7
- tuberosity (external) – *code as* Fracture, by site
- ulna (shaft) S52.2
- – and radius
- – – lower or distal ends S52.6
- – – shafts S52.4
- – coronoid process S52.0
- – head S52.8
- – lower (distal) end S52.8
- – multiple NEC S52.7
- – upper or proximal end S52.0
- unciform S62.1
- vault of skull S02.0
- vertebra, vertebral (back) (body) (column) (neural arch) (pedicle) (spinous process) (transverse process) T08
- – atlas S12.0
- – axis S12.1
- – birth injury P11.5
- – cervical (teardrop) S12.9

Fracture—*continued*
- vertebra, vertebral—*continued*
- – cervical—*continued*
- – – axis S12.1
- – – first (atlas) S12.0
- – – multiple S12.7
- – – second (axis) S12.1
- – – specified NEC S12.2
- – coccyx S32.2
- – dorsal S22.0
- – – multiple S22.1
- – fetus or newborn (birth injury) P11.5
- – lumbar S32.0
- – – multiple S32.7
- – metastatic (M8000/6) C79.5† M49.5*
- – sacrum S32.1
- – thoracic S22.0
- – – multiple S22.1
- vertex S02.0
- vomer (bone) S02.2
- wrist NEC S62.8
- xiphisternum, xiphoid (process) S22.2
- zygoma S02.4

Fragile, fragility
- autosomal site Q95.5
- bone, congenital (with blue sclera) Q78.0
- capillary (hereditary) D69.8
- hair L67.8
- nails L60.3
- non-sex chromosome site Q95.5
- X chromosome Q99.2

Fragilitas
- crinium L67.8
- ossium (with blue sclerae) (hereditary) Q78.0
- unguium L60.3
- – congenital Q84.6

Frambesia, frambesial (tropica) (*see also* Yaws) A66.9
- initial lesion or ulcer A66.0
- primary A66.0

Frambeside
- gummatous A66.4
- of early yaws A66.2

Frambesioma A66.1

Franceschetti-Klein(-Wildervanck) disease or syndrome Q75.4

Francis' disease (*see also* Tularemia) A21.9

Franklin disease C88.2

Frank's essential thrombocytopenia D69.3

Fraser's syndrome Q87.0

Freckle(s) L81.2
- malignant melanoma in (M8742/3) – *see* Melanoma
- melanotic (Hutchinson's) (M8742/2) – *see* Melanoma, in situ

Frederickson's hyperlipoproteinemia, type
- I and V E78.3
- IIA E78.0
- IIb and III E78.2
- IV E78.1

Freeman-Sheldon syndrome Q87.0

Freezing (*see also* Effect, adverse, cold) T69.9

Freiberg's disease (infraction of metatarsal head or osteochondrosis) M92.7

Frei's disease A55

Fremitus, friction, cardiac R01.2

Frenum, frenulum
- external os Q51.8
- tongue (shortening) (congenital) Q38.1

Frequency of micturition (nocturnal) R35
- psychogenic F45.3

Frey's syndrome G50.8

Friction
- burn – *see* Burn, by site
- fremitus, cardiac R01.2
- precordial R01.2
- sounds, chest R09.8

Friderichsen-Waterhouse syndrome or disease A39.1† E35.1*

Friedländer's B (bacillus) NEC (*see also condition*) A49.8

Friedreich's
- ataxia G11.1
- combined systemic disease G11.1
- facial hemihypertrophy Q67.4
- sclerosis (cerebellum) (spinal cord) G11.1

Frigidity F52.0

Fröhlich's syndrome E23.6

Frontal – *see also condition*
- lobe syndrome F07.0

Frostbite T35.7
- with
- – partial thickness skin loss – *see* Frostbite, by site, superficial
- – tissue necrosis – *see* Frostbite, by site, with tissue necrosis
- abdominal wall T35.3
- – with tissue necrosis T34.3
- – superficial T33.3
- ankle (and foot) (alone) T35.5

Frostbite—*continued*
- ankle—*continued*
- – with
- – – leg – *see* Frostbite, limb, lower
- – – tissue necrosis T34.8
- – superficial T33.8
- arm (meaning upper limb) (upper) – *see* Frostbite, limb, upper
- face T35.2
- – with tissue necrosis T34.0
- – superficial T33.0
- fingers T35.4
- – with tissue necrosis T34.5
- – superficial T33.5
- foot (and toes) (alone) T35.5
- – with
- – – leg – *see* Frostbite, limb, lower
- – – tissue necrosis T34.8
- – superficial T33.8
- hand (and fingers) (alone) T35.4
- – with
- – – arm – *see* Frostbite, limb, upper
- – – tissue necrosis T34.5
- – superficial T33.5
- head T35.2
- – with tissue necrosis T34.0
- – superficial T33.0
- hip (and thigh) T35.5
- – with tissue necrosis T34.6
- – superficial T33.6
- knee T35.5
- – with tissue necrosis T34.7
- – superficial T33.7
- leg
- – lower
- – – with tissue necrosis T34.7
- – – superficial T33.7
- – meaning lower limb – *see* Frostbite, limb, lower
- limb
- – lower T35.5
- – – with tissue necrosis T34.9
- – – superficial T33.9
- – upper T35.4
- – – with tissue necrosis T34.4
- – – superficial T33.4
- multiple body regions T35.6
- – with tissue necrosis T35.1
- – superficial T35.0
- neck T35.2
- – with tissue necrosis T34.1
- – superficial T33.1
- pelvis T35.3
- – with tissue necrosis T34.3

Frostbite—*continued*
- pelvis—*continued*
- – superficial T33.3
- superficial T33.9
- – multiple body regions T35.0
- – specified site NEC T33.9
- thigh T35.5
- – with tissue necrosis T34.6
- – superficial T33.6
- thorax T35.3
- – with tissue necrosis T34.2
- – superficial T33.2
- toes T35.5
- – with tissue necrosis T34.8
- – superficial T33.8
- trunk T35.3
- – with tissue necrosis T34.9
- – superficial T33.9
- wrist (and hand) (alone) T35.4
- – with
- – – arm – *see* Frostbite, limb, upper
- – – tissue necrosis T34.5
- – superficial T33.5

Frotteurism F65.8
Frozen (*see also* Effect, adverse, cold) T69.9
- pelvis (female) N94.8
- – male K66.8
- shoulder M75.0
Fructose-1,6-diphosphatase deficiency E74.1
Fructosemia (benign) (essential) E74.1
Fructosuria (essential) E74.1
Fuchs'
- dystrophy (corneal endothelium) H18.5
- heterochromic cyclitis H20.8
Fucosidosis E77.1
Fugue R68.8
- dissociative F44.1
- hysterical F44.1
- postictal in epilepsy G40.9
- reaction to exceptional stress (transient) F43.0
Fulminant, fulminating – *see condition*
Functional – *see also condition*
- bleeding (uterus) N93.8
Functioning, intellectual, borderline R41.8
Fundus – *see condition*
Fungemia NEC B49
Fungus, fungous
- cerebral G93.5
- disease NEC B49
- infection – *see* Infection, fungus

Funiculitis (acute) (chronic) (endemic) N49.1
– gonococcal (acute) (chronic) A54.2† N51.8*
– tuberculous A18.1† N51.8*
Funnel
– breast (acquired) M95.4
– – congenital Q67.6
– – late effect of rickets E64.3
– chest (acquired) M95.4
– – congenital Q67.6
– – late effect of rickets E64.3
– pelvis (acquired) M95.5
– – with disproportion (fetopelvic) O33.3
– – – affecting fetus or newborn P03.1
– – – causing obstructed labor O65.3
– – congenital Q74.2
FUO (fever of unknown origin) R50.9
Furfur L21.0
Furrier's lung J67.8
Furrowed K14.5
– nail(s) (transverse) L60.4
– – congenital Q84.6
– tongue K14.5
– – congenital Q38.3
Furuncle (*see also* Abscess, by site) L02.9
– auricle (ear) H60.0
– ear, external H60.0
– external auditory canal H60.0
– eyelid H00.0
– labium (majus) (minus) N76.4
– lacrimal
– – gland H04.0
– – passages (duct) (sac) H04.3
– nose J34.0
– orbit, orbital H05.0
– vulva N76.4
Furunculosis (*see also* Abscess, cutaneous) L02.9
Fusion, fused (congenital)
– astragaloscaphoid Q74.2
– auditory canal Q16.1
– binocular with defective stereopsis H53.3
– cervical spine – *see* Fusion, spine
– choanal Q30.0

Fusion, fused—*continued*
– cusps, heart valve NEC Q24.8
– – mitral Q23.2
– – pulmonary Q22.1
– – tricuspid Q22.4
– ear ossicles Q16.3
– fingers Q70.0
– hymen Q52.3
– joint (acquired) – *see also* Ankylosis
– – congenital Q74.8
– kidneys (incomplete) Q63.1
– labium (majus) (minus) Q52.5
– larynx and trachea Q34.8
– limb, congenital Q74.8
– – lower Q74.2
– – upper Q74.0
– lobes, lung Q33.8
– lumbosacral (acquired) M43.2
– – arthrodesis status Z98.1
– – congenital Q76.4
– – postprocedural status Z98.1
– nares, nose, nasal, nostril(s) Q30.0
– organ or site not listed – *see* Anomaly, by site
– ossicles Q79.9
– – auditory Q16.3
– ribs Q76.6
– sacroiliac (joint) (acquired) M43.2
– – arthrodesis status Z98.1
– – congenital Q74.2
– – postprocedural status Z98.1
– spine (acquired) NEC M43.2
– – arthrodesis status Z98.1
– – congenital Q76.4
– – postoperative status Z98.1
– sublingual duct with submaxillary duct Q38.4
– testis Q55.1
– toes Q70.2
– tooth, teeth K00.2
– trachea and esophagus Q39.8
– twins Q89.4
– vagina Q52.4
– vertebra (arch) – *see* Fusion, spine
– vulva Q52.5
Fusospirillosis A69.1

G

Gain in weight (abnormal)
(excessive) (*see also* Weight, gain) R63.5
– pregnancy O26.0
Gaisböck's disease D75.1
Gait
– abnormality R26.8
– ataxic R26.0
– disturbance R26.8
– paralytic R26.1
– spastic R26.1
– staggering R26.0
Galactocele (breast) N64.8
– puerperal, postpartum O92.7
Galactophoritis N61
– gestational, puerperal, postpartum O91.2
Galactorrhea O92.6
– not associated with childbirth N64.3
Galactosemia E74.2
Galactosuria E74.2
Galacturia R82.0
– schistosomiasis (bilharziasis) B65.0
Galen's vein – *see condition*
Gall duct – *see condition*
Gallbladder – *see condition*
Gallop rhythm R00.8
Gallstone (colic) (cystic duct)
(gallbladder) (impacted) (multiple)
K80.2
– with cholecystitis (chronic) K80.1
– – acute K80.0
– bile duct (common) (hepatic) K80.5
– causing intestinal obstruction K56.3
– specified NEC K80.8
Gambling Z72.6
– pathological (compulsive) F63.0
Gammopathy
– associated with lymphoplasmacytic
  dyscrasia D47.2
– monoclonal (of undetermined
  significance) D47.2
– polyclonal D89.0
Gamna's disease D73.1
Gandy-Nanta disease D73.1
Gang
– activity, without manifest psychiatric
  disorder Z03.2
– membership with dissocial behavior
  F91.2
Gangliocytoma (M9490/0) D36.1

Ganglioglioma (M9505/1) – *see* Neoplasm,
  uncertain behavior
Ganglion (compound) (diffuse) (joint)
(tendon (sheath)) M67.4
– of yaws (early) (late) A66.6
– tuberculous A18.0† M68.0*
Ganglioneuroblastoma (M9490/3) – *see*
  Neoplasm, nerve, malignant
Ganglioneuroma (M9490/0) D36.1
– malignant (M9490/3) – *see* Neoplasm,
  nerve, malignant
Ganglioneuromatosis (M9491/0) D36.1
Ganglionitis
– fifth nerve (*see also* Neuralgia, trigeminal)
  G50.0
– gasserian (postherpetic) (postzoster)
  B02.3† H58.8*
– geniculate G51.1
– – newborn (birth injury) P11.3
– – postherpetic, postzoster B02.2† G53.0*
– herpes zoster B02.2† G53.0*
– postherpetic geniculate B02.2† G53.0*
Gangliosidosis E75.1
– GM₁ E75.1
– GM₂ (adult) (infantile) (juvenile) E75.0
– GM₃ E75.1
Gangosa A66.5† J99.8*
Gangrene, gangrenous (dry) (moist) (skin)
(ulcer) (*see also* Necrosis) R02
– with diabetes (mellitus) – *code to* E10-
  E14 with fourth character .5
– abdomen (wall) R02
– alveolar K10.3
– appendix K35.8
– – with
– – – peritoneal abscess K35.3
– – – peritonitis, generalized K35.2
– – – – with mention of perforation or
        rupture K35.2
– – – peritonitis, localized K35.3
– – – – with mention of perforation or
        rupture K35.3
– arteriosclerotic (general) (senile) I70.2
– auricle R02
– Bacillus welchii A48.0
– bladder (infectious) N30.8
– bowel, cecum or colon – *see* Gangrene,
  intestine
– Clostridium perfringens or welchii A48.0

Gangrene, gangrenous—*continued*
- connective tissue R02
- cornea H18.8
- corpora cavernosa N48.2
- – noninfective N48.8
- cutaneous, spreading R02
- decubital – *see* Ulcer, decubitus
- diabetic (any site) – *code to* E10-E14 with fourth character .5
- dropsical R02
- epidemic T62.2
- epididymis (infectional) (*see also* Epididymitis) N45.9
- Fournier's N49.8
- – female N76.8
- fusospirochetal A69.0
- gallbladder (*see also* Cholecystitis, acute) K81.0
- gas (bacillus) A48.0
- hernia – *see* Hernia, by site, with gangrene
- intestine, intestinal (hemorrhagic) (massive) K55.0
- – with
- – – mesenteric embolism K55.0
- – – obstruction (*see also* Obstruction, intestine) K56.6
- limb (lower) (upper) R02
- lung J85.0
- Meleney's (synergistic) L98.4
- mesentery K55.0
- – with intestinal obstruction (*see also* Obstruction, intestine) K56.6
- mouth A69.0
- ovary (*see also* Salpingo-oophoritis) N70.9
- pancreas K85.-
- penis N48.2
- – noninfective N48.8
- perineum R02
- pharynx (*see also* Pharyngitis) J02.9
- – Vincent's A69.1
- presenile I73.1
- pulmonary J85.0
- pulpal (dental) K04.1
- Raynaud's I73.0
- retropharyngeal J39.2
- scrotum N49.2
- – noninfective N50.8
- senile (atherosclerotic) I70.2
- spermatic cord N49.1
- – noninfective N50.8
- spine R02
- spreading cutaneous R02
- stomatitis A69.0

Gangrene, gangrenous—*continued*
- symmetrical I73.0
- testis (infectional) (*see also* Orchitis) N45.9
- – noninfective N50.8
- throat (*see also* Pharyngitis) J02.9
- – Vincent's A69.1
- thyroid (gland) E07.8
- tuberculous NEC (*see also* Tuberculosis) A16.9
- tunica vaginalis N49.1
- – noninfective N50.8
- umbilicus R02
- uterus (*see also* Endometritis) N71.9
- vas deferens N49.1
- – noninfective N50.8
- vulva N76.8

Gannister disease J62.8
Ganser's syndrome (hysterical) F44.8
Gardner-Diamond syndrome D69.2
Gargoylism E76.0
Garré's disease, osteitis (sclerosing), osteomyelitis M86.8
Garrod's pad, knuckle M72.1
Gartner's duct
- cyst Q50.5
- persistent Q50.6
Gas
- asphyxia, asphyxiation, inhalation, poisoning, suffocation NEC T59.9
- – specified gas – *see* Table of drugs and chemicals
- gangrene A48.0
- on stomach R14
- pain R14
Gastralgia R10.1
- psychogenic F45.4
Gastrectasis K31.8
- psychogenic F45.3
Gastric – *see condition*
Gastrinoma (M8153/1)
- malignant (M8153/3)
- – pancreas C25.4
- – specified site NEC – *see* Neoplasm, malignant
- – unspecified site C25.4
- specified site – *see* Neoplasm, uncertain behavior
- unspecified site D37.7
Gastritis (simple) K29.7
- acute (erosive) K29.1
- – hemorrhagic K29.0
- alcoholic K29.2
- allergic K29.6

Gastropathy, Portal K 31.8 (Inish)

Gastritis—*continued*
- atrophic (chronic) K29.4
- chronic (antral) (fundal) K29.5
- – atrophic K29.4
- – superficial K29.3
- dietary counseling and surveillance Z71.3
- due to nutritional deficiency E63.9†
  K93.8*
- eosinophilic K52.8
- giant hypertrophic K29.6
  granulomatous K29.6
- hypertrophic (mucosa) K29.6
- nervous F54
- specified NEC K29.6
- superficial chronic K29.3
- tuberculous A18.8† K93.8*
- viral NEC A08.4

Gastrocarcinoma (M8010/3) – *see*
  Neoplasm, malignant, stomach

Gastrocolic – *see condition*

Gastrodisciasis, gastrodiscoidiasis B66.8

Gastroduodenitis K29.9
- virus, viral A08.4
- – specified type NEC A08.3

Gastrodynia R10.1

Gastroenteritis (acute) (*see also* Enteritis)
  A09.9
- with septicemia NEC A09.0
- allergic K52.2
- chronic (noninfectious) K52.9
- dietetic K52.2
- due to
- – Cryptosporidium A07.2
- – food poisoning (*see also* Intoxication,
  foodborne) A05.9
- – radiation K52.0
- eosinophilic K52.8
- epidemic A09.0
- food hypersensitivity K52.2
- infectious (*see also* Enteritis, infectious)
  A09.0
- nonbacterial, of infancy A08.5
- noninfectious K52.9
- – specified NEC K52.8
- rotaviral A08.0
- salmonella A02.0
- septic A09.0
- toxic K52.1
- viral A08.4
- – acute infectious A08.3
- – epidemic A08.1
- – – type Norwalk A08.1
- – infantile (acute) A08.3
- – Norwalk agent A08.1

Gastroenteritis—*continued*
- viral—*continued*
- – rotaviral A08.0
- – severe, of infants A08.3
- – specified type NEC A08.3

Gastroenteropathy (*see also*
  Gastroenteritis) A09.9
- acute, due to Norwalk agent A08.1
- infectious A09.0
- noninfectious K52.9

Gastroenteroptosis K63.4

Gastrointestinal – *see condition*

Gastrojejunal – *see condition*

Gastrojejunitis, noninfectious (*see also*
  Enteritis) K52.9

Gastrojejunocolic – *see condition*

Gastroliths K31.8

Gastromalacia K31.8

Gastroptosis K31.8

Gastrorrhagia K92.2
- psychogenic F45.3

Gastroschisis (congenital) Q79.3

Gastrospasm (neurogenic) (reflex) K31.8
- neurotic F45.3
- psychogenic F45.3

Gastrostaxis K92.2

Gastrostenosis K31.8

Gastrostomy
- attention to Z43.1
- status Z93.1

Gastrosuccorrhea (continuous)
  (intermittent) K31.8
- neurotic F45.3
- psychogenic F45.3

Gaucher's disease or splenomegaly (adult)
  (infantile) E75.2

Gee (-Herter) (-Thaysen) disease K90.0

Gélineau's syndrome G47.4

Gemination, tooth, teeth K00.2

Gemistocytoma (M9411/3)
- specified site – *see* Neoplasm, malignant
- unspecified site C71.9

General, generalized – *see condition*

Genital – *see condition*

Genito-anorectal syndrome A55

Genitourinary system – *see condition*

Genu
- extrorsum (acquired) M21.1
- – congenital Q68.2
- – late effect of rickets E64.3
- rachitic (old) E64.3
- recurvatum (acquired) M21.8
- – congenital Q68.2
- – late effect of rickets E64.3

Genu—*continued*
- valgum (acquired) M21.0
- – congenital Q74.1
- – late effect of rickets E64.3
- varum (acquired) M21.1
- – congenital Q74.1
- – late effect of rickets E64.3
Geographic tongue K14.1
Geotrichosis B48.3
Gephyrophobia F40.2
Gerhardt's syndrome J38.0
German measles (*see also* Rubella) B06.9
Germinoblastoma (diffuse) C85.9
- follicular C82.9
Germinoma (M9064/3) – *see* Neoplasm, malignant
Gerontoxon H18.4
Gerstmann's syndrome (developmental) F81.2
Gestation (period) – *see also* Pregnancy
- ectopic – *see* Pregnancy, by site
- multiple O30.9
- – specified NEC O30.8
Ghon tubercle, primary infection A16.7
- with bacteriological and histological confirmation A15.7
Ghost vessels (cornea) H16.4
Ghoul hand A66.3
Giannotti-Crosti disease L44.4
Giant
- cell
- – epulis K06.8
- – peripheral granuloma K06.8
- esophagus, congenital Q39.5
- kidney, congenital Q63.3
- urticaria T78.3
- – hereditary D84.1
Giardiasis A07.1
Gibert's disease or pityriasis L42
Giddiness R42
- hysterical F44.8
- psychogenic F45.8
Gierke's disease E74.0
Gigantism (pituitary) E22.0
- constitutional E34.4
Gilbert's disease or syndrome E80.4
Gilchrist's disease B40.9
Gilford-Hutchinson disease E34.8
Gilles de la Tourette's disease or syndrome F95.2
Gingivitis K05.1
- acute K05.0
- – necrotizing A69.1

Gingivitis—*continued*
- chronic (desquamative) (hyperplastic) (simple marginal) (ulcerative) K05.1
- necrotizing ulcerative (acute) A69.1
- pellagrous E52† K93.8*
- – acute necrotizing A69.1
- Vincent's A69.1
Gingivoglossitis K14.0
Gingivosis K05.1
Gingivostomatitis K05.1
- herpesviral B00.2
- necrotizing ulcerative (acute) A69.1
Gland, glandular – *see condition*
Glanders A24.0
Glanzmann's disease or thrombasthenia D69.1
Glass-blower's disease (cataract) H26.8
Glaucoma H40.9
- with pseudoexfoliation of lens H40.1
- absolute H44.5
- acute H40.2
- – narrow angle H40.2
- – secondary NEC H40.5
- angle-closure (acute) (chronic) (intermittent) (primary) (residual state) H40.2
- borderline H40.0
- capsular (with pseudoexfoliation of lens) H40.1
- chronic H40.1
- – angle-closure H40.2
- – noncongestive H40.1
- – open-angle H40.1
- – simple H40.1
- closed angle H40.2
- congenital Q15.0
- corticosteroid-induced H40.6
- hypersecretion H40.8
- in (due to)
- – amyloidosis E85.-† H42.0*
- – aniridia Q13.1† H42.8*
- – concussion of globe H40.3
- – dislocation of lens H40.5
- – disorder of lens NEC H40.5
- – drugs H40.6
- – endocrine disease NEC E34.9† H42.0*
- – eye
- – – inflammation H40.4
- – – trauma H40.3
- – hypermature cataract H40.5
- – iridocyclitis H40.4
- – Lowe's syndrome E72.0† H42.0*
- – metabolic disease NEC E88.9† H42.0*
- – ocular disorders NEC H40.5

Glaucoma—*continued*
- in—*continued*
- – – onchocerciasis B73† H42.8*
- – – retinal vein occlusion H40.5
- – – Rieger's anomaly Q13.8† H42.8*
- – – rubeosis of iris H40.5
- – tumor of globe H40.5
- – infantile Q15.0
- – low-tension H40.1
- – malignant H40.2
- – narrow angle H40.2
- – newborn Q15.0
- – noncongestive (chronic) H40.1
- – nonobstructive H40.1
- – obstructive H40.2
- – – due to lens changes H40.5
- – open-angle (primary) (residual stage) H40.1
- – phacolytic H40.5
- – pigmentary H40.1
- – postinfectious H40.4
- – secondary NEC (*see also* Glaucoma, in) H40.5
- – simple (chronic) H40.1
- – simplex H40.1
- – specified NEC H40.8
- – suspect H40.0
- – syphilitic A52.7† H42.8*
- – traumatic H40.3
- – – newborn (birth injury) P15.3
- – tuberculous A18.5† H42.8*

Glaucomatous flecks (subcapsular) H26.2
Gleet (gonococcal) A54.0
Glénard's disease K63.4
Glioblastoma (multiforme) (M9440/3)
- with sarcomatous component (M9442/3)
- – specified site – *see* Neoplasm, malignant
- – unspecified site C71.9
- – giant cell (M9441/3)
- – specified site – *see* Neoplasm, malignant
- – unspecified site C71.9
- specified site – *see* Neoplasm, malignant
- unspecified site C71.9

Glioma (malignant) (M9380/3)
- astrocytic (M9400/3)
- – specified site – *see* Neoplasm, malignant
- – unspecified site C71.9
- mixed (M9382/3)
- – specified site – *see* Neoplasm, malignant
- – unspecified site C71.9

Glioma—*continued*
- nose Q30.8
- specified site NEC – *see* Neoplasm, malignant
- subependymal (M9383/1) D43.2
- – specified site – *see* Neoplasm, uncertain behavior
- – unspecified site D43.2
- unspecified site C71.9

Gliomatosis cerebri (M9381/3) C71.0
Glioneuroma (M9505/1) – *see* Neoplasm, uncertain behavior
Gliosarcoma (M9442/3)
- specified site – *see* Neoplasm, malignant
- unspecified site C71.9

Gliosis (cerebral) G93.8
- spinal G95.8

Globinuria R82.3
Globus (hystericus) F45.8
Glomangioma (M8712/0) D18.0
Glomangiomyoma (M8713/0) D18.0
Glomangiosarcoma (M8710/3) – *see* Neoplasm, connective tissue, malignant
Glomerular
- disease in syphilis A52.7† N08.0*
- nephritis (*see also* Glomerulonephritis) N05.-

Glomerulitis (*see also* Glomerulonephritis) N05.-
Glomerulonephritis (*see also* Nephritis) N05.-

Note: Where a term is indexed only at the three-character level, e.g. N01.-, reference should be made to the list of fourth-character subdivisions in Volume 1 at N00-N08.

- with edema (*see also* Nephrosis) N04.-
- acute N00.-
- chronic N03.-
- crescentic (diffuse) NEC – *code to* N00-N07 with fourth character .7
- dense deposit – *code to* N00-N07 with fourth character .6
- diffuse
- – crescentic – *code to* N00-N07 with fourth character .7
- – endocapillary proliferative – *code to* N00-N07 with fourth character .4
- – membranous – *code to* N00-N07 with fourth character .2
- – mesangial proliferative – *code to* N00-N07 with fourth character .3
- – mesangiocapillary – *code to* N00-N07 with fourth character .5

Glomerulonephritis—*continued*
- diffuse—*continued*
- - sclerosing (*see also* Failure, renal, chronic) N18.9
- endocapillary proliferative (diffuse) NEC – *code to* N00-N07 with fourth character .4
- extracapillary NEC – *code to* N00-N07 with fourth character .7
- focal (and segmental) – *code to* N00-N07 with fourth character .1
- hypocomplementemic – *see* Glomerulonephritis, membranoproliferative
- IgA – *see* Nephropathy, IgA
- immune complex (circulating) NEC N05.8
- in (due to)
- - amyloidosis E85.-† N08.4*
- - bilharziasis B65.-† N08.0*
- - cryoglobulinemia D89.1† N08.2*
- - defibrination syndrome D65† N08.2*
- - diabetes mellitus (*see also* E10-E14 with fourth character .2) E14.2† N08.3*
- - disseminated intravascular coagulation D65† N08.2*
- - Fabry(-Anderson) disease E75.2† N08.4*
- - Goodpasture's syndrome M31.0† N08.5*
- - hemolytic-uremic syndrome D59.3† N08.2*
- - Henoch(-Schönlein) purpura D69.0† N08.2*
- - lecithin cholesterol acyltransferase deficiency E78.6† N08.4*
- - microscopic polyangiitis M31.7† N08.5*
- - multiple myeloma C90.0† N08.1*
- - Plasmodium malariae B52.0† N08.0*
- - schistosomiasis B65.-† N08.0*
- - sepsis A41.-† N08.0*
- - - streptococcal A40.-† N08.0*
- - sickle-cell disorders D57.-† N08.2*
- - strongyloidiasis B78.9† N08.0*
- - subacute bacterial endocarditis I33.0† N08.8*
- - systemic lupus erythematosus M32.1† N08.5*
- - thrombotic thrombocytopenic purpura M31.1† N08.5*
- - Waldenström macroglobulinemia C88.0† N08.1*

Glomerulonephritis—*continued*
- in—*continued*
- - Wegener's granulomatosis M31.3† N08.5*
- lobular, lobulonodular – *see* Glomerulonephritis, membranoproliferative
- membranoproliferative (diffuse) (type 1) (type 3) – *code to* N00-N07 with fourth character .5N0.5
- - dense deposit (type 2) NEC – *code to* N00-N07 with fourth character .6
- membranous (diffuse) NEC – *code to* N00-N07 with fourth character .2
- mesangial
- - IgA/IgG – *see* Nephropathy, IgA
- - proliferative (diffuse) NEC – *code to* N00-N07 with fourth character .3
- mesangiocapillary (diffuse) NEC – *code to* N00-N07 with fourth character .5
- necrotic, necrotizing NEC – *code to* N00-N07 with fourth character .8
- nodular – *see* Glomerulonephritis, membranoproliferative
- poststreptococcal NEC N05.9
- - acute N00.-
- - chronic N03.-
- - rapidly progressive N01.-
- proliferative NEC – *code to* N00-N07 with fourth character .8
- - diffuse (lupus) M32.1† N08.5*
- rapidly progressive N01.-
- sclerosing, diffuse (*see also* Failure, kidney, chronic) N18.9
- specified pathology NEC – *code to* N00-N07 with fourth character .8
- subacute – *see* Nephritis, rapidly progressive
Glomerulopathy (*see also* Glomerulonephritis) N05.-
Glomerulosclerosis (*see also* Sclerosis, renal) N26
- intracapillary E14.2† N08.3*
Glossalgia K14.6
Glossitis K14.0
- areata exfoliativa K14.1
- atrophic K14.4
- benign migratory K14.1
- chronic superficial K14.0
- cortical superficial, sclerotic K14.0
- Hunter's D51.0
- interstitial, sclerous K14.0
- median rhomboid K14.2
- Moeller's K14.0

Glossitis—*continued*
- pellagrous E52† K93.8∗
- superficial, chronic K14.0
Glossodynia K14.6
- exfoliativa K14.0
Glossopathy K14.9
Glossophytia K14.3
Glossoplegia K14.8
Glossopyrosis K14.6
Glossy skin L90.8
Glottis – *see condition*
Glottitis (*see also* Laryngitis) J04.0
Glucagonoma
- malignant (M8152/3)
- – pancreas C25.4
- – specified site NEC – *see* Neoplasm, malignant
- – unspecified site C25.4
- pancreas
- – benign (M8152/0) D13.7
- – uncertain or unknown behavior (M8152/1) D37.7
- – malignant (M8152/3) C25.4
- specified site NEC
- – benign (M8152/0) – *see* Neoplasm, benign
- – uncertain or unknown behavior (M8152/1) – *see* Neoplasm, uncertain or unknown behavior
- – malignant (M8152/3) – *see* Neoplasm, malignant
- unspecified site
- – benign (M8152/0) D13.7
- – uncertain or unknown behavior (M8152/1) D37.7
- – malignant (M8152/3) C25.4
Glucoglycinuria E72.5
Glucose-galactose malabsorption E74.3
Glue
- ear H65.3
- sniffing (airplane) F18.1
- – dependence F18.2
Glycinemia E72.5
Glycinuria (renal) E72.0
Glycogen
- infiltration (*see also* Disease, glycogen storage) E74.0
- storage disease (*see also* Disease, glycogen storage) E74.0
Glycogenosis (diffuse) (generalized) (with hepatic cirrhosis) (*see also* Disease, glycogen storage) E74.0
- cardiac E74.0† I43.1∗
Glycopenia E16.2

Glycosuria R81
- renal E74.8
Gnathostoma spinigerum (infection) (infestation), gnathostomiasis (wandering swelling) B83.1
Goiter (plunging) (substernal) E04.9
- with
- – hyperthyroidism (recurrent) (*see also* Goiter, toxic) E05.0
- – – adenomatous E05.2
- – – nodular E05.2
- – thyrotoxicosis (*see also* Goiter, toxic) E05.0
- – – adenomatous E05.2
- – – nodular E05.2
- adenomatous (*see also* Goiter, nodular) E04.9
- congenital (nontoxic) E03.0
- – diffuse E03.0
- – parenchymatous E03.0
- – transitory, with normal functioning P72.0
- cystic E04.2
- – due to iodine-deficiency E01.1
- due to
- – enzyme defect in synthesis of thyroid hormone E07.1
- – iodine-deficiency (endemic) E01.2
- dyshormogenetic (familial) E07.1
- endemic (iodine-deficiency) E01.2
- – diffuse E01.0
- – multinodular E01.1
- exophthalmic E05.0
- iodine-deficiency (endemic) E01.2
- – diffuse E01.0
- – multinodular E01.1
- – nodular E01.1
- lymphadenoid E06.3
- multinodular (cystic) (nontoxic) E04.2
- – toxic or with hyperthyroidism E05.2
- neonatal NEC P72.0
- nodular (nontoxic) (due to) E04.9
- – with
- – – hyperthyroidism E05.2
- – – thyrotoxicosis E05.2
- – endemic E01.1
- – iodine-deficiency E01.1
- – sporadic E04.9
- – toxic E05.2
- nontoxic E04.9
- – diffuse (colloid) E04.0
- – multinodular E04.2
- – simple E04.0
- – specified NEC E04.8

Goiter—*continued*
- nontoxic—*continued*
- - uninodular E04.1
- simple E04.0
- toxic E05.0
- - adenomatous E05.2
- - multinodular E05.2
- - nodular E05.2
- - uninodular E05.1
- - tumor, malignant (M8000/3) C73
- uninodular (nontoxic) E04.1
- - toxic or with hyperthyroidism E05.1
Goiter-deafness syndrome E07.1
Goldberg-Maxwell syndrome E34.5
Goldblatt's hypertension or kidney I70.1
Goldenhar(-Gorlin) syndrome Q87.0
Goldflam-Erb disease or syndrome G70.0
Goldscheider's disease Q81.8
Goldstein's disease I78.0
Golfer's elbow M77.0
Gonadoblastoma (M9073/1)
- specified site – *see* Neoplasm, uncertain behavior
- unspecified site
- - female D39.1
- - male D40.1
Gonarthrosis M17.9
- post-traumatic (unilateral) M17.3
- - bilateral M17.2
- primary (unilateral) M17.1
- - bilateral M17.0
- secondary NEC (unilateral) M17.5
- - bilateral M17.4
Gonecystitis (*see also* Vesiculitis) N49.0
Gongylonemiasis B83.8
Goniosynechiae H21.5
Gonococcemia A54.8
Gonococcus, gonococcal (disease) (infection) (*see also condition*) A54.9
- anus A54.6
- bursa, bursitis A54.4† M73.0∗
- complicating pregnancy, childbirth or puerperium O98.2
- - affecting fetus or newborn P00.2
- conjunctiva, conjunctivitis (neonatorum) A54.3† H13.1∗
- endocardium A54.8† I39.8∗
- eye, newborn A54.3† H13.1∗
- fallopian tubes (acute) (chronic) A54.2† N74.3∗
- genitourinary (organ) (system) (tract) (acute)
- - lower A54.0

Gonococcus, gonococcal—*continued*
- genitourinary—*continued*
- - lower—*continued*
- - - with abscess (accessory gland) (periurethral) A54.1
- - upper (*see also condition*) A54.2
- heart A54.8† I52.0∗
- iridocyclitis A54.3† H22.0∗
- joint A54.4† M01.3∗
- lymphatic (gland) (node) A54.8
- meninges, meningitis A54.8† G01∗
- pelviperitonitis A54.2† N74.3∗
- pelvis (acute) (chronic) A54.2
- pharynx A54.5
- pyosalpinx (acute) (chronic) A54.2† N74.3∗
- rectum A54.6
- skin A54.8† L99.8∗
- specified site NEC A54.8
- tendon sheath A54.4† M68.0∗
- urethra (acute) (chronic) A54.0
- - with abscess (accessory gland) (periurethral) A54.1
- vulva (acute) (chronic) A54.0
Gonocytoma (M9073/1)
- specified site – *see* Neoplasm, uncertain behavior
- unspecified site
- - female D39.1
- - male D40.1
Gonorrhea (acute) (chronic) A54.9
- Bartholin's gland (acute) (chronic) (purulent) A54.0
- - with abscess (accessory gland) (periurethral) A54.1
- bladder A54.0
- cervix A54.0
- complicating pregnancy, childbirth or puerperium O98.2
- - affecting fetus or newborn P00.2
- conjunctiva, conjunctivitis (neonatorum) A54.3† H13.1∗
- Cowper's gland (with abscess) A54.1
- fallopian tube (acute) (chronic) A54.2† N74.3∗
- kidney (acute) (chronic) A54.2† N29.1∗
- lower genitourinary tract A54.0
- - with abscess (accessory gland) (periurethral) A54.1
- ovary (acute) (chronic) A54.2† N74.3∗
- pelvis (acute) (chronic) A54.2
- - female pelvic inflammatory disease A54.2† N74.3∗
- penis A54.0

Gonorrhea—*continued*
- prostate (acute) (chronic) A54.2† N51.0∗
- seminal vesicle (acute) (chronic) A54.2†
  N51.8∗
- specified site not listed (*see also*
  Gonococcus) A54.8
- spermatic cord (acute) (chronic) A54.2†
  N51.8∗
- urethra A54.0
- – with abscess (accessory gland)
  (periurethral) A54.1
- vagina A54.0
- vas deferens (acute) (chronic) A54.2†
  N51.8∗
- vulva A54.0
Goodall's disease A08.1
Goodpasture's syndrome M31.0
Gopalan's syndrome E53.9
Gorlin-Chaudry-Moss syndrome Q87.0
Gottron's papules L94.4
Gougerot-Carteaud disease or syndrome
  L83
Goundou A66.6
Gout, gouty M10.9
- drug-induced M10.2
- idiopathic M10.0
- in (due to) renal impairment M10.3
- lead-induced M10.1
- primary M10.0
- saturnine M10.1
- secondary NEC M10.4
- syphilitic A52.7† M14.8∗
- tophi NEC M10.0
- – ear M10.0† H62.8∗
- – heart M10.0† I43.8∗
Gower's muscular dystrophy G71.0
Gradenigo's syndrome H66.0
Graefe's disease H49.4
Graft-versus-host (GVH) disease (bone
  marrow) T86.0
Grainhandler's disease or lung J67.8
Grand mal
- epilepsy (idiopathic) G40.6
- – on awakening G40.3
- seizure (with or without petit mal) G40.6
- – on awakening G40.3
- status (epilepticus) G41.0
Granite worker's lung J62.8
Granular – *see condition*
Granulation tissue (abnormal) (excessive)
  L92.9
- postmastoidectomy cavity H95.1
Granulocytopenia (malignant) (primary)
  D70

Granuloma L92.9
- abdomen K66.8
- actinic L57.5
- annulare (perforating) L92.0
- apical K04.5
- aural H60.4
- beryllium (skin) L92.3
- bone M86.8
- – eosinophilic C96.6
- – from residual foreign body M86.8
- brain (any site) G06.0
- – in schistosomiasis B65.-† G07∗
- canaliculus lacrimalis H04.6
- candidal (cutaneous) B37.2
- cerebral (any site) G06.0
- coccidioidal (primary) (progressive)
  B38.7
- – lung B38.1† J99.8∗
- – meninges B38.4† G02.1∗
- colon K63.8
- conjunctiva H10.4
- dental K04.5
- ear, middle H71
- eosinophilic C96.6
- – bone C96.6
- – lung C96.6
- – oral mucosa K13.4
- – skin L92.2
- eyelid H01.8
- facial(e) L92.2
- foreign body (in soft tissue) NEC M60.2
- – in operation wound T81.5
- – skin L92.3
- gangraenescens M31.2
- genito-inguinale A58
- giant cell (central) (jaw) (reparative)
  K10.1
- – gingiva (peripheral) K06.8
- gland (lymph) I88.8
- hepatic NEC K75.3
- – in (due to)
- – – berylliosis J63.2† K77.8∗
- – – sarcoidosis D86.8† K77.8∗
- Hodgkin C81.9
- ileum K63.8
- infectious NEC B99
- inguinale (Donovan) (venereal) A58
- intestine NEC K63.8
- intracranial (any site) G06.0
- intraspinal (any part) G06.1
- iridocyclitis H20.1
- jaw (bone) (central) K10.1
- – reparative giant cell K10.1
- kidney (*see also* Infection, kidney) N15.8

Granuloma—*continued*
- lacrimal sac (nonspecific) H04.6
- larynx J38.7
- lethal midline (facial) M31.2
- liver NEC (*see also* Granuloma, hepatic) K75.3
- lung (infectious) (*see also* Fibrosis, lung) J84.1
- − − coccidioidal B38.1† J99.8*
- − − eosinophilic C96.6
- − Majocchi's B35.8
- − malignant (facial(e)) M31.2
- − mandible (central) K10.1
- − midline (lethal) M31.2
- − monilial (cutaneous) B37.2
- − operation wound T81.8
- − − foreign body T81.5
- − − stitch T81.8
- − − talc T81.6
- − oral mucosa K13.4
- − orbit, orbital H05.1
- − paracoccidioidal B41.8
- − periapical K04.5
- − peritoneum K66.8
- − − due to ova of helminths NEC (*see also* Helminthiasis) B83.9† K67.8*
- − postmastoidectomy cavity H95.0
- − prostate N42.8
- − pudendi (ulcerating) A58
- − pulp, internal (tooth) K03.3
- − pyogenic, pyogenicum (of) (skin) L98.0
- − − gingiva K06.8
- − − maxillary alveolar ridge K04.5
- − − oral mucosa K13.4
- − rectum K62.8
- − reticulohistiocytic D76.3
- − rubrum nasi L74.8
- − septic (skin) L98.0
- − silica (skin) L92.3
- − sinus (accessory) (infective) (nasal) (*see also* Sinusitis) J32.9
- − spine
- − − syphilitic (epidural) A52.1† G07*
- − − tuberculous A18.0† M49.0*
- − stitch (postoperative) T81.8
- − suppurative (skin) L98.0
- − swimming pool A31.1
- − talc M60.2
- − − in operation wound T81.6
- − telangiectaticum (skin) L98.0
- − trichophyticum B35.8
- − umbilicus L92.8
- − − newborn P38
- − urethra N36.8

Granuloma—*continued*
- venereum A58
- vocal cord J38.3

Granulomatosis L92.9
- lymphoid C83.8
- lymphomatoid C83.8
- miliary (listerial) A32.8
- necrotizing, respiratory M31.3
- progressive septic D71
- specified NEC L92.8
- Wegener's M31.3

Granulomatous tissue (abnormal) (excessive) L92.9
Granulosis rubra nasi L74.8
Graphite fibrosis (of lung) J63.3
Graphospasm F48.8
- organic G25.8
Grating scapula M89.8
Gravel (urinary) (*see also* Calculus) N20.9
Graves' disease E05.0
Gravis – *see condition*
Grawitz tumor (M8312/3) C64
Gray syndrome (newborn) P93
Grayness, hair (premature) L67.1
- congenital Q84.2
Green sickness D50.8
Greenfield's disease
- meaning
- − concentric sclerosis (encephalitis periaxialis concentrica) G37.5
- − metachromatic leukodystrophy E75.2
Greenstick fracture – *code as* Fracture, by site
Grey syndrome (newborn) P93
Griesinger's disease B76.9
Grinder's lung or pneumoconiosis J62.8
Grinding, teeth F45.8
Grip
- Dabney's B33.0
- devil's B33.0
Grippe, grippal – *see also* Influenza
- Balkan A78
- summer, of Italy A93.1
Groin – *see condition*
Grover's disease or syndrome L11.1
Growing pains, children R29.8
Growth (fungoid) (neoplastic) (new) (M8000/1) – *see also* Neoplasm, uncertain behavior
- adenoid (vegetative) J35.8
- benign (M8000/0) – *see* Neoplasm, benign
- malignant (M8000/3) – *see* Neoplasm, malignant
- rapid, childhood Z00.2

Growth—*continued*
- secondary (M8000/6) – *see* Neoplasm, secondary
Gruby's disease B35.0
Gubler-Millard paralysis or syndrome I67.9† G46.3*
Guerin-Stern syndrome Q74.3
Guillain-Barré disease or syndrome G61.0
Guinea worm (infection) (infestation) B72
Gull's disease E03.4
Gum – *see condition*
Gumboil K04.7
- with sinus K04.6
Gumma (syphilitic) A52.7
- artery A52.0† I79.8*
- – cerebral A52.0† I68.8*
- bone A52.7† M90.2*
- – of yaws (late) A66.6† M90.2*
- brain A52.1† G07*
- cauda equina A52.1† G07*
- central nervous system A52.3
- ciliary body A52.7† H22.8*
- congenital A50.5
- eyelid A52.7† H03.1*
- heart A52.0† I52.0*
- intracranial A52.1† G07*
- iris A52.7† H22.8*
- kidney A52.7† N29.0*
- larynx A52.7† J99.8*
- leptomeninges A52.1† G07*
- liver A52.7† K77.0*
- meninges A52.1† G07*
- myocardium A52.0† I41.0*
- nasopharynx A52.7† J99.8*
- neurosyphilitic A52.3

Gumma—*continued*
- nose A52.7† J99.8*
- orbit A52.7† H06.3*
- palate (soft) A52.7† K93.8*
- penis A52.7† N51.8*
- pericardium A52.0† I32.0*
- pharynx A52.7† J99.8*
- pituitary A52.7† E35.8*
- scrofulous (tuberculous) A18.4
- skin A52.7† L99.8*
- specified site NEC A52.7
- spinal cord A52.1† G07*
- tongue A52.7† K93.8*
- tonsil A52.7† J99.8*
- trachea A52.7† J99.8*
- tuberculous A18.4
- ulcerative due to yaws A66.4
- ureter A52.7† N29.1*
- yaws A66.4
- – bone A66.6† M90.2*
Gunn's syndrome Q07.8
Gunshot wound – *see also* Wound, open
- fracture – *code as* Fracture, by site
- internal organs – *see* Injury, by site
Gynandrism Q56.0
Gynandroblastoma (M8632/1)
- specified site – *see* Neoplasm, uncertain behavior
- unspecified site
- – female D39.1
- – male D40.1
Gynecological examination (periodic) (routine) Z01.4
Gynecomastia N62
Gynephobia F40.1
Gyrate scalp Q82.8

H

H (Hartnup's) disease E72.0
Haas' disease or osteochondrosis (juvenile) (head of humerus) M92.0
Habit, habituation
– chorea F95.8
– disturbance, child F98.9
– drug – *see* Dependence, drug
– laxative F55
Haemophilus (H.) influenzae, as cause of disease classified elsewhere B96.3
Haff disease T61.2
Hageman's factor defect, deficiency or disease D68.2
Haglund's disease or osteochondrosis (juvenile) (os tibiale externum) M92.6
Hailey-Hailey disease Q82.8
Hair – *see also* condition
– plucking F63.3
– – in stereotyped movement disorder F98.4
Hairball in stomach T18.2
Hair-pulling, pathological (compulsive) F63.3
Hairy black tongue K14.3
Half vertebra Q76.4
Halitosis R19.6
Hallerman-Streiff syndrome Q87.0
Hallervorden-Spatz disease G23.0
Hallopeau's acrodermatitis or disease L40.2
Hallucination R44.3
– auditory R44.0
– gustatory R44.2
– olfactory R44.2
– specified NEC R44.2
– tactile R44.2
– visual R44.1
Hallucinosis (chronic) F28
– alcoholic (acute) F10.5
– induced by drug – *code to* F11-F19 with fourth character .5
– organic F06.0
Hallux
– deformity (acquired) NEC M20.3
– malleus (acquired) NEC M20.3
– rigidus (acquired) M20.2
– – congenital Q74.2
– – late effect of rickets E64.3
– valgus (acquired) M20.1

Hallux—*continued*
– valgus—*continued*
– – congenital Q66.6
– varus (acquired) M20.3
– – congenital Q66.3
Halo, visual H53.1
Hamartoma, hamartoblastoma Q85.9
– epithelial (gingival), odontogenic, central or peripheral (M9321/0) D16.5
– – upper jaw (bone) D16.4
Hamartosis Q85.9
Hamman-Rich syndrome J84.1
Hammer toe (acquired) NEC M20.4
– congenital Q66.8
– late effect of rickets E64.3
Hand – *see* condition
Handicap, handicapped
– educational Z55.9
– – specified NEC Z55.8
Hand-Schüller-Christian disease or syndrome C96.5
Hanging (asphyxia) (strangulation) (suffocation) T71
Hangnail (with lymphangitis) L03.0
Hangover (alcohol) F10.0
Hanhart's syndrome Q87.0
Hanot-Chauffard(-Troisier) syndrome E83.1
Hanot's cirrhosis or disease K74.3
Hansen's disease (*see also* Leprosy) A30.9
Hantaan virus disease (Korean hemorrhagic fever) A98.5† N08.0*
Hantavirus disease (with renal manifestations) (Dobrava) (Puumala) (Seoul) A98.5† N08.0*
– with pulmonary manifestations (Andes) (Bayou) (Bermejo) (Black Creek Canal) (Choclo) (Juquitiba) (Laguna negra) (Lechiguanas) (New York) (Oran) (Sin Nombre) B33.4† J17.1*
Happy puppet syndrome Q93.5
Harada's disease or syndrome H30.8
Hardening
– artery – *see* Arteriosclerosis
– brain G93.8
Harelip (complete) (incomplete) (*see also* Cleft, lip) Q36.9
Harlequin (fetus) Q80.4
Harley's disease D59.6

Harmful use (of)
- alcohol F10.1
- anxiolytics F13.1
- cannabinoids F12.1
- cocaine F14.1
- drug – *code to* F11-F19 with fourth character .1
- hallucinogens F16.1
- hypnotics F13.1
- opioids F11.1
- phencyclidine (PCP) F19.1
- sedatives F13.1
- stimulants NEC F15.1

Harris' lines M89.1
Hartnup's disease E72.0
Harvester's lung J67.0
Harvesting ovum for in vitro fertilization Z31.2
Hashimoto's disease or thyroiditis E06.3
Hashitoxicosis (transient) E06.3
Hassal-Henle bodies or warts (cornea) H18.4
Haut mal G40.6
Haverhill fever A25.1
Hay fever J30.1
Hayem-Widal syndrome D59.8
Haygarth's nodes M15.8
Haymaker's lung J67.0
Hb (abnormal)
- disease – *see* Disease, hemoglobin
- trait – *see* Trait

Head – *see condition*
Headache R51
- allergic NEC G44.8
- cluster (chronic) (episodic) G44.0
- drug-induced NEC G44.4
- emotional F45.4
- histamine G44.0
- lumbar puncture G97.1
- migraine (type) G43.9
- nonorganic origin F45.4
- postspinal puncture G97.1
- post-traumatic, chronic G44.3
- psychogenic F45.4
- specified syndrome NEC G44.8
- spinal and epidural anesthesia-induced (in) T88.5
- – labor and delivery O74.5
- – postpartum, puerperal O89.4
- – pregnancy O29.4
- spinal fluid loss (from puncture) G97.1
- tension (chronic) (episodic) G44.2
- vascular G44.1

Health
- advice Z71.9
- check-up (routine) Z00.0
- – infant or child Z00.1
- – occupational Z10.0
- education Z71.9
- instruction Z71.9
- services provided because (of)
- – bedfast status Z74.0
- – boarding school residence Z59.3
- – holiday relief for person providing home care Z75.5
- – inadequate
- – – economic resources NEC Z59.9
- – – housing Z59.1
- – lack of housing Z59.0
- – need for
- – – assistance with personal care Z74.1
- – – continuous supervision Z74.3
- – no care available in home Z74.2
- – person living alone Z60.2
- – poverty NEC Z59.6
- – – extreme Z59.5
- – reduced mobility Z74.0
- – residence in institution Z59.3
- – specified cause NEC Z59.8

Healthy
- infant
- – accompanying sick mother Z76.3
- – receiving care Z76.2
- person accompanying sick person Z76.3

Hearing examination Z01.1
Heart – *see condition*
Heart beat
- abnormality R00.8
- awareness R00.2
- rapid R00.0
- slow R00.1

Heartburn R12
- psychogenic F45.3

Heat (effects) T67.9
- apoplexy T67.0
- burn – *see* Burn
- collapse T67.1
- cramps T67.2
- dermatitis or eczema L59.0
- edema T67.7
- erythema – *code as* Burn, by site, with fourth character .1
- excessive T67.9
- – specified effect NEC T67.8
- exhaustion T67.5
- – anhydrotic T67.3

Heat—*continued*
- exhaustion—*continued*
- – due to
- – – salt (and water) depletion T67.4
- – – water depletion T67.3
- – – – with salt depletion T67.4
- fatigue (transient) T67.6
- fever T67.0
- hyperpyrexia T67.0
- prickly L74.0
- prostration – *see* Heat, exhaustion
- pyrexia T67.0
- rash L74.0
- specified effect NEC T67.8
- stroke T67.0
- sunburn (*see also* Sunburn) L55.9
- syncope T67.1

Heavy-for-dates NEC (fetus or infant)
  P08.1
- exceptionally (4500 g or more) P08.0

Hebephrenia, hebephrenic
  (schizophrenia) F20.1

Heberden's disease or nodes (with
  arthropathy) M15.1

Hebra's
- pityriasis L26
- prurigo L28.2

Heel – *see condition*

Heerfordt's disease D86.8

Hegglin's anomaly or syndrome D72.0

Heilmeyer-Schoner disease D45

Heine-Medin disease A80.9

Heinz body anemia, congenital D58.2

✗ **Helicobacter pylori, as cause of disease**
  classified elsewhere B98.0

Heller's disease or syndrome F84.3

HELLP syndrome (hemolysis, elevated
  liver enzymes and low platelet count)
  O14.2

Helminthiasis (*see also* Infestation) B83.9
- Ancylostoma B76.0
- intestinal B82.0
- – mixed types (types classifiable to more
  than one of the titles B65.0-B81.3 and
  B81.8) B81.4
- – specified type NEC B81.8
- mixed types (intestinal) (types classifiable
  to more than one of the titles B65.0-B81.3
  and B81.8) B81.4
- Necator (americanus) B76.1
- specified type NEC B83.8

Heloma L84

Hemangioblastoma (M9161/1) – *see*
  Neoplasm, connective tissue, uncertain
  behavior

Hemangioendothelioma (M9130/1) –
  see also Neoplasm, uncertain behavior
- benign (M9130/0) D18.0
- bone (diffuse) (M9130/3) – *see* Neoplasm,
  bone, malignant
- epithelioid (M9133/1) – *see also*
  Neoplasm, uncertain behavior
- – malignant (M9133/3) – *see* Neoplasm,
  malignant
- malignant (M9130/3) – *see* Neoplasm,
  connective tissue, malignant
- nervous system (M9130/0) D18.0

Hemangiofibroma (M9160/0) – *see*
  Neoplasm, benign

Hemangiolipoma (M8861/0) – *see* Lipoma

Hemangioma (M9120/0) D18.0
- arteriovenous (M9123/0) D18.0
- capillary (M9131/0) D18.0
- cavernous (M9121/0) D18.0
- epithelioid (M9125/0) D18.0
- histiocytoid (M9126/0) D18.0
- infantile (M9131/0) D18.0
- intramuscular (M9132/0) D18.0
- juvenile (M9131/0) D18.0
- malignant (M9120/3) – *see* Neoplasm,
  connective tissue, malignant
- plexiform (M9131/0) D18.0
- racemose (M9123/0) D18.0
- sclerosing (M8832/0) – *see* Neoplasm,
  skin, benign
- simplex (M9131/0) D18.0
- venous (M9122/0) D18.0
- verrucous keratotic (M9142/0) D18.0

Hemangiomatosis (systemic) Q82.8
- involving single site (M9120/0) – *see*
  Hemangioma

Hemangiopericytoma (M9150/1) – *see also*
  Neoplasm, connective tissue, uncertain
  behavior
- benign (M9150/0) – *see* Neoplasm,
  connective tissue, benign
- malignant (M9150/3) – *see* Neoplasm,
  connective tissue, malignant

Hemangiosarcoma (M9120/3) – *see*
  Neoplasm, connective tissue, malignant

Hemarthrosis (nontraumatic) M25.0
- traumatic – *see* Sprain, by site

Hematemesis K92.0
- with ulcer – *code as* Ulcer, by site, with
  hemorrhage
- newborn, neonatal P54.0

Pylori (when not the cause of disease
  classified to another chapter)
  A04.8

Hematemesis—*continued*
- newborn, neonatal—*continued*
- – due to swallowed maternal blood P78.2

Hematidrosis L74.8

Hematinuria (*see also* Hemoglobinuria) R82.3
- malarial B50.8

Hematobilia K83.8

Hematocele
- female NEC N94.8
- – with ectopic pregnancy O00.9
- – ovary N83.8
- male N50.1

Hematochyluria, in schistosomiasis (bilharziasis) B65.0

Hematocolpos (with hematometra or hematosalpinx) N89.7

Hematocornea H18.0

Hematogenous – *see condition*

Hematoma (traumatic) (skin surface intact) (*see also* Injury, superficial) T14.0
- with
- – injury of internal organs – *see* Injury, by site
- – open wound – *see* Wound, open
- amputation stump (surgical) T87.6
- aorta, dissecting I71.0
- arterial (complicating trauma) (*see also* Injury, blood vessel) T14.5
- auricle S00.4
- – nontraumatic H61.1
- birth injury NEC P15.8
- brain (traumatic) S06.8
- – with cerebral laceration or contusion (diffuse) S06.2
- – – focal S06.3
- – fetus or newborn NEC P52.4
- – – birth injury P10.1
- – nontraumatic (*see also* Hemorrhage, intracerebral) I61.9
- – – epidural or extradural I62.1
- – – subarachnoid (*see also* Hemorrhage, subarachnoid) I60.9
- – – subdural (*see also* Hemorrhage, subdural) I62.0
- – subarachnoid, arachnoid, traumatic S06.6
- – subdural, traumatic S06.5
- breast (nontraumatic) N64.8
- broad ligament (nontraumatic) N83.7
- – traumatic S37.8
- cerebral – *see* Hematoma, brain
- cesarean section wound O90.2

Hematoma—*continued*
- complicating delivery (pelvic) (perineal) (vagina) (vulva) O71.7
- corpus cavernosum (nontraumatic) N48.8
- epididymis (nontraumatic) N50.1
- epidural (traumatic) S06.4
- – spinal – *see* Injury, spinal cord, by region
- episiotomy O90.2
- face, birth injury P15.4
- genital organ NEC (nontraumatic)
- – female (nonobstetric) N94.8
- – male N50.1
- – traumatic (external site), superficial S30.2
- – – internal – *see* Injury, by site
- internal organs – *see* Injury, by site
- labia (nonobstetric) (nontraumatic) N90.8
- liver (subcapsular) (nontraumatic) K76.8
- – birth injury P15.0
- mediastinum S27.8
- mesosalpinx (nontraumatic) N83.7
- – traumatic S37.8
- muscle – *code as* Contusion, by site
- obstetrical surgical wound O90.2
- orbit, orbital (nontraumatic) H05.2
- – traumatic S05.1
- pelvis (female) (nonobstetric) (nontraumatic) N94.8
- – obstetric O71.7
- – traumatic (*see also* Injury, by site) S37.9
- – – specified organ NEC (*see also* Injury, by site) S37.8
- penis (nontraumatic) N48.8
- – birth injury P15.5
- perianal (nontraumatic) I84.3
- perineal S30.2
- – complicating delivery O71.7
- perirenal S37.0
- pinna S00.4
- – nontraumatic H61.1
- placenta O43.8
- postoperative T81.0
- retroperitoneal (nontraumatic) K66.1
- – traumatic S36.8
- scrotum, superficial S30.2
- – birth injury P15.5
- seminal vesicle (nontraumatic) N50.1
- – traumatic S37.8
- spermatic cord (traumatic) S37.8
- – nontraumatic N50.1
- spinal (cord) (meninges) (*see also* Injury, spinal cord, by region) T09.3

Hematoma—*continued*
- spinal—*continued*
- − − fetus or newborn (birth injury) P11.5
- − sternocleidomastoid, birth injury P15.2
- − sternomastoid, birth injury P15.2
- − subarachnoid (traumatic) S06.6
- − − fetus or newborn (nontraumatic) P52.5
- − − − birth injury P10.3
- − − nontraumatic (*see also* Hemorrhage, subarachnoid) I60.9
- − subdural (traumatic) S06.5
- − − fetus or newborn (localized) P52.8
- − − − birth injury P10.0
- − − nontraumatic (*see also* Hemorrhage, subdural) I62.0
- − superficial, fetus or newborn P54.5
- − testis (nontraumatic) N50.1
- − − birth injury P15.5
- − tunica vaginalis (nontraumatic) N50.1
- − umbilical cord, complicating delivery O69.5
- − − affecting fetus or newborn P02.6
- − uterine ligament (broad) (nontraumatic) N83.7
- − − traumatic S37.8
- − vagina (nontraumatic) N89.8
- − − complicating delivery O71.7
- − vas deferens (nontraumatic) N50.1
- − − traumatic S37.8
- − vitreous H43.1
- − vulva (nonobstetric) (nontraumatic) N90.8
- − − complicating delivery O71.7
- − − fetus or newborn (birth injury) P15.5
Hematometra N85.7
- with hematocolpos N89.7
Hematomyelia (central) G95.1
- fetus or newborn (birth injury) P11.5
- traumatic T14.4
Hematomyelitis G04.9
Hematoperitoneum – *see* Hemoperitoneum
Hematopneumothorax – *see* Hemothorax
Hematoporphyria – *see* Porphyria
Hematorachis, hematorrhachis G95.1
- fetus or newborn (birth injury) P11.5
Hematosalpinx N83.6
- with
- − hematocolpos N89.7
- − hematometra N85.7
- − − with hematocolpos N89.7
- infectional (*see also* Salpingo-oophoritis) N70.9
Hematospermia N50.1
Hematothorax – *see* Hemothorax

Hematuria (essential) R31
- benign (familial) (of childhood) (*see also* Hematuria, idiopathic) N02.-
- endemic (*see also* Schistosomiasis) B65.0
- idiopathic N02.-
- − with glomerular lesion
- − − focal and segmental hyalinosis or sclerosis N02.1
- − − membranoproliferative (diffuse) N02.5
- − − membranous (diffuse) N02.2
- − − mesangial proliferative (diffuse) N02.3
- − − mesangiocapillary (diffuse) N02.5
- − − proliferative NEC N02.8
- − − specified pathology NEC N02.8
- intermittent (*see also* Hematuria, idiopathic) N02.-
- malarial B50.8
- paroxysmal (*see also* Hematuria, idiopathic) N02.-
- − nocturnal D59.5
- persistent (*see also* Hematuria, idiopathic) N02.-
- recurrent (*see also* Hematuria, idiopathic) N02.-
- sulfonamide(s)
- − correct substance properly administered R31
- − overdose or wrong substance given or taken T37.0
- tropical (*see also* Schistosomiasis) B65.0
- tuberculous A18.1
Hemeralopia (day blindness) H53.1
- vitamin A deficiency E50.5† H58.1∗
Hemianalgesia R20.0
Hemianencephaly Q00.0
Hemianesthesia R20.0
Hemianopia, hemianopsia (binasal) (bitemporal) (heteronymous) (homonymous) (nasal) (peripheral) H53.4
- syphilitic A52.7† H58.1∗
Hemiathetosis R25.8
Hemiatrophy R68.8
- cerebellar G31.9
- face, facial, progressive (Romberg) G51.8
- tongue K14.8
Hemiballism(us) G25.5
Hemicardia Q24.8
Hemicephalus, hemicephaly Q00.0
Hemichorea G25.5
Hemicolitis, left K51.5

Hemicrania
- congenital malformation Q00.0
- meaning migraine G43.9
- paroxysmal, chronic G44.0
Hemidystrophy – *see* Hemiatrophy
Hemiectromelia Q73.8
Hemihypalgesia R20.8
Hemihypesthesia R20.1
Hemimelia Q73.8
- lower limb Q72.8
- upper limb Q71.8
Hemiparalysis (*see also* Hemiplegia)
  G81.9
Hemiparesis (*see also* Hemiplegia) G81.9
Hemiparesthesia R20.2
Hemiparkinsonism G20
Hemiplegia G81.9
- alternans facialis G83.8
- ascending NEC G81.9
- – spinal G95.8
- congenital (cerebral) G80.8
- – spastic G80.2
- embolic (current episode) I63.4
- flaccid G81.0
- hysterical F44.4
- newborn NEC P91.8
- – birth injury P11.9
- spastic G81.1
- – congenital G80.2
- spinal G81.1
- thrombotic (current episode) I63.3
Hemisection, spinal cord – *see* Injury,
  spinal cord, by region
Hemispasm (facial) R25.2
Hemisporosis B48.8
Hemitremor R25.1
Hemivertebra Q76.4
- failure of segmentation with scoliosis
  Q76.3
- fusion with scoliosis Q76.3
Hemochromatosis (diabetic) (hereditary)
  (liver) (myocardium) (primary
  idiopathic) (secondary) E83.1
- with refractory anemia (related to
  alkylating agent) (related to
  Epipodophyllotoxin) (related to therapy)
  NEC D46.1
Hemodialysis Z49.1
- preparatory care only (without treatment)
  Z49.0
Hemoglobin – *see also* condition
- abnormal (disease) – *see* Disease,
  hemoglobin
- AS genotype D57.3

Hemoglobin—*continued*
- fetal, hereditary persistence (HPFH)
  D56.4
- low NEC D64.9
- S (Hb S), heterozygous D57.3
Hemoglobinemia D59.9
  due to blood transfusion T80.8
- paroxysmal D59.6
- – nocturnal D59.5
Hemoglobinopathy (mixed) NEC D58.2
- with thalassemia D56.9
- sickle-cell D57.1
- – with thalassemia D57.2
Hemoglobinuria R82.3
- with anemia, hemolytic, acquired
  (chronic) NEC D59.6
- cold agglutinin (disease) D59.1
- – paroxysmal (with Raynaud's syndrome)
  D59.6
- due to exertion or hemolysis NEC D59.6
- intermittent D59.6
- malarial B50.8
- march D59.6
- nocturnal (paroxysmal) D59.5
- paroxysmal (cold) D59.6
- – nocturnal D59.5
Hemolymphangioma (M9175/0) D18.1
Hemolysis
- intravascular
- – with
- – – abortion (subsequent episode) O08.1
- – – – current episode – *see* Abortion
- – – ectopic or molar pregnancy O08.1
- – – hemorrhage
- – – – antepartum – *see* Hemorrhage,
  antepartum
- – – – intrapartum (*see also* Hemorrhage,
  complicating, delivery) O67.0
- – postpartum O72.3
- neonatal (excessive) P58.8
Hemolytic – *see* condition
Hemopericardium I31.2
- following acute myocardial infarction
  (current complication) I23.0
- newborn P54.8
- traumatic S26.0
Hemoperitoneum K66.1
- infectional K65.9
- traumatic S36.8
Hemophilia (familial) (hereditary) D66
- A D66
- B D67
- C D68.1

Hemophilia—*continued*
- calcipriva (*see also* Defect, coagulation) D68.4
- classical D66
- nonfamilial (*see also* Defect, coagulation) D68.4
- vascular D68.0

Hemophthalmos H44.8

Hemopneumothorax – *see also* Hemothorax
- traumatic S27.2

Hemoptysis R04.2
- newborn P26.9
- tuberculous – *see* Tuberculosis, pulmonary

Hemorrhage, hemorrhagic R58
- abdomen R58
- accidental antepartum O46.9
- – affecting fetus or newborn P02.1
- adenoid J35.8
- adrenal (capsule) (gland) E27.4
- – medulla E27.8
- – newborn P54.4
- after delivery – *see* Hemorrhage, postpartum
- alveolar
- – lung, newborn P26.8
- – process K08.8
- alveolus K08.8
- amputation stump (surgical) T81.0
- – secondary, delayed T87.6
- anemia (chronic) D50.0
- – acute D62
- antepartum (*see also* Hemorrhage, pregnancy) O46.9
- – with
- – – afibrinogenemia O46.0
- – – coagulation defect O46.0
- – – disseminated intravascular coagulation O46.0
- – affecting fetus or newborn P02.1
- anus (sphincter) K62.5
- apoplexy (stroke) (*see also* Hemorrhage, intracerebral) I61.9
- arachnoid – *see* Hemorrhage, subarachnoid
- artery R58
- – brain (*see also* Hemorrhage, intracerebral) I61.9
- basilar (ganglion) I61.0
- bladder N32.8
- bowel K92.2
- – newborn P54.3
- brain (miliary) (nontraumatic) I61.9

Hemorrhage, hemorrhagic—*continued*
- brain—*continued*
- – due to
- – – birth injury P10.1
- – – rupture of aneurysm (congenital) (*see also* Hemorrhage, subarachnoid) I60.9
- – – syphilis A52.0† I68.8*
- – epidural or extradural (traumatic) S06.4
- – fetus or newborn P52.4
- – – birth injury P10.1
- – puerperal, postpartum or in childbirth or pregnancy O99.4
- – subarachnoid – *see* Hemorrhage, subarachnoid
- – subdural – *see* Hemorrhage, subdural
- – traumatic S06.8
- breast N64.5
- bronchial tube – *see* Hemorrhage, lung
- bronchopulmonary – *see* Hemorrhage, lung
- bronchus – *see* Hemorrhage, lung
- bulbar I61.5
- capillary I78.8
- – primary D69.8
- cecum K92.2
- cerebellar, cerebellum (nontraumatic) I61.4
- – fetus or newborn P52.6
- – traumatic S06.8
- cerebral, cerebrum (*see also* Hemorrhage, intracerebral) I61.9
- – fetus or newborn (anoxic) P52.4
- – – birth injury P10.1
- – lobe I61.1
- cerebromeningeal I61.8
- cerebrospinal (*see also* Hemorrhage, intracerebral) I61.9
- cervix (uteri) (stump) NEC N88.8
- chamber, anterior (eye) H21.0
- childbirth – *see* Hemorrhage, complicating, delivery
- choroid (expulsive) H31.3
- ciliary body H21.0
- cochlea H83.8
- colon K92.2
- complicating
- – delivery O67.9
- – – affecting fetus or newborn P02.1
- – – associated with coagulation defect (afibrinogenemia) (hyperfibrinolysis) (hypofibrinogenemia) O67.0
- – – – affecting fetus or newborn P03.8

Hemorrhage, hemorrhagic—*continued*
- complicating—*continued*
- – delivery—*continued*
- – – due to
- – – – low-lying placenta O44.1
- – – – – affecting fetus or newborn P02.0
- – – – placenta previa O44.1
- – – – – affecting fetus or newborn P02.0
- – – – premature separation of placenta (*see also* Abruptio placentae) O45.9
- – – – – affecting fetus or newborn P02.1
- – – – retained
- – – – – placenta O72.0
- – – – – products of conception O72.2
- – – – – secundines O72.2
- – – – – – partial O72.2
- – – – trauma O67.8
- – – – – affecting fetus or newborn P03.8
- – – – uterine leiomyoma O67.8
- – – – – affecting fetus or newborn P03.8
- – ectopic or molar pregnancy (subsequent episode) O08.1
- – surgical procedure T81.0
- concealed NEC R58
- – conjunctiva H11.3
- – newborn P54.8
- cord, newborn (stump) P51.9
- corpus luteum (ruptured) cyst N83.1
- cortical (brain) I61.1
- cranial (*see also* Hemorrhage, intracranial) I62.9
- cutaneous R23.3
- – due to autosensitivity, erythrocyte D69.2
- – fetus or newborn P54.5
- delayed
- – following
- – – abortion (subsequent episode) O08.1
- – – ectopic or molar pregnancy O08.1
- – postpartum O72.2
- diathesis (familial) D69.9
- disease D69.9
- – fetus or newborn P53
- – specified type NEC D69.8

Hemorrhage, hemorrhagic—*continued*
- due to or associated with
- – afibrinogenemia or other coagulation defect (conditions in category D65-D69)
- – – antepartum O46.0
- – – intrapartum O67.0
- – device, implant or graft (*see also* Complications, by site and type) T85.8
- – – arterial graft NEC T82.8
- – – breast T85.8
- – – catheter NEC T85.8
- – – – dialysis (renal) T82.8
- – – – – intraperitoneal T85.8
- – – – infusion NEC T82.8
- – – – – spinal (epidural) (subdural) T85.8
- – – – urinary (indwelling) T83.8
- – – electronic (electrode) (pulse generator) (stimulator)
- – – – bone T84.8
- – – – cardiac T82.8
- – – – nervous system (brain) (peripheral nerve) (spinal) T85.8
- – – – urinary T83.8
- – – fixation, internal (orthopedic) NEC T84.8
- – – gastrointestinal (bile duct) (esophagus) T85.8
- – – genital NEC T83.8
- – – heart NEC T82.8
- – – joint prosthesis T84.8
- – – ocular (corneal graft) (orbital implant) NEC T85.8
- – – orthopedic NEC T84.8
- – – specified NEC T85.8
- – – urinary NEC T83.8
- – – vascular NEC T82.8
- – – ventricular intracranial shunt T85.8
- duodenum, duodenal K92.2
- – ulcer – *see* Ulcer, duodenum, with hemorrhage
- dura mater – *see* Hemorrhage, subdural
- endotracheal – *see* Hemorrhage, lung
- epicranial subaponeurotic (massive), birth injury P12.2
- epidural (traumatic) S06.4
- esophagus K22.8
- – varix I85.0
- excessive, following abortion or ectopic pregnancy (subsequent episode) O08.1
- extradural (traumatic) S06.4
- – birth injury P10.8

Hemorrhage, hemorrhagic—*continued*
- extradural—*continued*
- – fetus or newborn (anoxic)
  (nontraumatic) P52.8
- – nontraumatic I62.1
- eye NEC H57.8
- – fundus H35.6
- fallopian tube N83.6
- fetal, fetus P50.9
- – from
- – – cut end of co-twin's cord P50.5
- – – placenta P50.2
- – – ruptured cord P50.1
- – – vasa previa P50.0
- – into
- – – co-twin P50.3
- – – maternal circulation P50.4
- – – – affecting management of
       pregnancy or puerperium O43.0
- – specified NEC P50.8
- fetal-maternal P50.4
- – affecting management of pregnancy or
  puerperium O43.0
- fibrinogenolysis (*see also* Fibrinolysis)
  D65
- fibrinolytic (acquired) (*see also*
  Fibrinolysis) D65
- following abortion (subsequent episode)
  O08.1
- – current episode – *see* Abortion
- from
- – ear (nontraumatic) H92.2
- – tracheostomy stoma J95.0
- fundus, eye H35.6
- funis – *see* Hemorrhage, umbilicus, cord
- gastric – *see* Hemorrhage, stomach
- gastroenteric K92.2
- – newborn P54.3
- gastrointestinal (tract) K92.2
- – newborn P54.3
- genitourinary (tract) NEC R31
- gingiva K06.8
- globe (eye) H44.8
- graafian follicle cyst (ruptured) N83.0
- gum K06.8
- heart (*see also* Carditis) I51.8
- hypopharyngeal (throat) R58
- intermenstrual (regular) N92.3
- – irregular N92.1
- internal (organs) NEC R58
- – capsule I61.0
- – ear H83.8
- – newborn P54.8
- intestine K92.2

Hemorrhage, hemorrhagic—*continued*
- intestine—*continued*
- – newborn P54.3
- intra-abdominal R58
- intra-alveolar (lung), newborn P26.8
- intracerebral (nontraumatic) I61.9
- – complicating pregnancy, childbirth or
  puerperium O99.4
- – deep I61.0
- – fetus or newborn P52.4
- – – birth injury P10.1
- – in
- – – brain stem I61.3
- – – cerebellum I61.4
- – – hemisphere I61.2
- – – – cortical I61.1
- – – – subcortical I61.0
- – – intraventricular I61.5
- – – multiple localized I61.6
- – – specified NEC I61.8
- – – superficial I61.1
- – traumatic (diffuse) S06.2
- – – focal S06.3
- intracranial (nontraumatic) I62.9
- – birth injury P10.9
- – fetus or newborn P52.9
- – – specified NEC P52.8
- – traumatic S06.8
- intramedullary NEC G95.1
- intraocular H44.8
- intrapartum (*see also* Hemorrhage,
  complicating, delivery) O67.9
- intrapelvic
- – female N94.8
- – male K66.1
- intraperitoneal K66.1
- intrapontine I61.3
- intrauterine N85.7
- – complicating delivery (*see also*
  Hemorrhage, complicating, delivery)
  O67.9
- – postpartum – *see* Hemorrhage,
  postpartum
- intraventricular I61.5
- – fetus or newborn (nontraumatic) P52.3
- – – birth injury P10.2
- – – grade
- – – – 1 P52.0
- – – – 2 P52.1
- – – – 3 P52.2
- intravesical N32.8
- iris (postinfectional) (postinflammatory)
  (toxic) H21.0
- joint (nontraumatic) M25.0

313

Hemorrhage, hemorrhagic—*continued*
- kidney N28.8
- knee (joint) (nontraumatic) M25.0
- labyrinth H83.8
- lenticular striate artery I61.0
- ligature, vessel T81.0
- liver K76.8
- lung R04.8
- – newborn P26.9
- – – massive P26.1
- – – specified NEC P26.8
- – tuberculous – *see* Tuberculosis, pulmonary
- massive umbilical, newborn P51.0
- maternal gestational, affecting fetus or newborn P02.1
- mediastinum – *see* Hemorrhage, lung
- medulla I61.3
- membrane (brain) I60.8
- – spinal cord – *see* Hemorrhage, spinal cord
- meninges, meningeal (brain) (middle) I60.8
- – spinal cord – *see* Hemorrhage, spinal cord
- mesentery K66.1
- metritis (*see also* Endometritis) N71.9
- mouth K13.7
- mucous membrane NEC R58
- – newborn P54.8
- muscle M62.8
- nail (subungual) L60.8
- nasal turbinate R04.0
- – newborn P54.8
- navel, newborn P51.9
- newborn P54.9
- – specified NEC P54.8
- nipple N64.5
- nose R04.0
- – newborn P54.8
- omentum K66.1
- optic nerve (sheath) H47.0
- orbit, orbital H05.2
- ovary NEC N83.8
- oviduct N83.6
- pancreas K86.8
- parathyroid (gland) (spontaneous) E21.4
- parturition – *see* Hemorrhage, complicating, delivery
- penis N48.8
- pericardium, pericarditis I31.2
- peritoneum, peritoneal K66.1
- peritonsillar tissue J35.8
- – due to infection J36

Hemorrhage, hemorrhagic—*continued*
- petechial R23.3
- – due to autosensitivity, erythrocyte D69.2
- pituitary (gland) E23.6
- placenta NEC O46.8
- – affecting fetus or newborn P02.1
- – antepartum O46.8
- – from surgical or instrumental damage O46.8
- – – affecting fetus or newborn P02.1
- – – antepartum O46.8
- – – intrapartum O67.8
- – intrapartum O67.8
- – previa O44.1
- – – affecting fetus or newborn P02.0
- pleura – *see* Hemorrhage, lung
- polioencephalitis, superior E51.2† G32.8*
- polymyositis – *see* Polymyositis
- pons, pontine I61.3
- posterior fossa (nontraumatic) I61.8
- – fetus or newborn P52.6
- postmenopausal N95.0
- postnasal R04.0
- postoperative T81.0
- postpartum NEC (following delivery of placenta) O72.1
- – delayed or secondary O72.2
- – retained placenta O72.0
- – third stage O72.0
- pregnancy – *see also* Hemorrhage, antepartum
- – due to
- – – abruptio placentae O45.9
- – – – affecting fetus or newborn P02.1
- – – afibrinogenemia, or other coagulation defect (conditions in category D65-D68) O46.0
- – – – affecting fetus or newborn P02.1
- – – leiomyoma, uterus O46.8
- – – – affecting fetus or newborn P02.1
- – – placenta previa O44.1
- – – – affecting fetus or newborn P02.0
- – – premature separation of placenta (normally implanted) – *see also* Abruptio placentae
- – – – affecting fetus or newborn P02.1
- – – threatened abortion O20.0
- – – – affecting fetus or newborn P02.1
- – – trauma, affecting fetus or newborn P02.1
- – early O20.9
- – – affecting fetus or newborn P02.1

Hemorrhage, hemorrhagic—*continued*
- pregnancy—*continued*
- – – previous, affecting management of pregnancy, childbirth Z35.2
- – – unavoidable – *see* Hemorrhage, pregnancy, due to, placenta previa
- preretinal H35.6
- prostate N42.1
- puerperal (*see also* Hemorrhage, postpartum) O72.1
- – – delayed or secondary O72.2
- pulmonary R04.8
- – newborn P26.9
- – – massive P26.1
- – – specified NEC P26.8
- – – tuberculous – *see* Tuberculosis, pulmonary
- purpura (primary) D69.3
- rectum (sphincter) K62.5
- – newborn P54.2
- recurrent traumatic, following initial hemorrhage at time of injury T79.2
- renal N28.8
- respiratory passage or tract R04.9
- – specified NEC R04.8
- retina, retinal (vessels) H35.6
- – diabetic (*see also* E10-E14 with fourth character .3) E14.3† H36.0*
- retroperitoneal R58
- scalp R58
- scrotum N50.1
- secondary (nontraumatic) R58
- – following initial hemorrhage at time of injury T79.2
- seminal vesicle N50.1
- skin R23.3
- – fetus or newborn P54.5
- slipped umbilical ligature P51.8
- spermatic cord N50.1
- spinal (cord) G95.1
- – fetus or newborn (birth injury) P11.5
- spleen D73.5
- stomach K92.2
- – newborn P54.3
- – ulcer – *see* Ulcer, stomach, with hemorrhage
- subarachnoid (nontraumatic) I60.9
- – fetus or newborn P52.5
- – – birth injury P10.3
- – from
- – – anterior communicating artery I60.2
- – – basilar artery I60.4
- – – carotid siphon and bifurcation I60.0
- – – cavernous sinus I60.8

Hemorrhage, hemorrhagic—*continued*
- subarachnoid—*continued*
- – from—*continued*
- – – intracranial artery I60.7
- – – – specified NEC I60.6
- – – middle
- – – – cerebral artery I60.1
- – – – meningeal artery I60.8
- – – multiple intracranial arteries I60.6
- – – posterior communicating artery I60.3
- – – vertebral artery I60.5
- – puerperal, postpartum or in childbirth or pregnancy O99.4
- – specified NEC I60.8
- – traumatic S06.6
- subconjunctival H11.3
- – birth injury P15.3
- subcortical (brain) I61.0
- subcutaneous R23.3
- subdiaphragmatic R58
- subdural (acute) (nontraumatic) I62.0
- – birth injury P10.0
- – fetus or newborn (anoxic) (hypoxic) P52.8
- – – birth injury P10.0
- – spinal G95.1
- – traumatic S06.5
- subependymal
- – fetus or newborn P52.0
- – – with intraventricular extension P52.1
- – – – and intracerebral extension P52.2
- subhyaloid H35.6
- subperiosteal M89.8
- subretinal H35.6
- subtentorial (*see also* Hemorrhage, subdural) I62.0
- subungual L60.8
- suprarenal (capsule) (gland) E27.4
- – newborn P54.4
- tentorium (traumatic) NEC S06.8
- – fetus or newborn (birth injury) P10.4
- – nontraumatic – *see* Hemorrhage, subdural
- testis N50.1
- third stage (postpartum) O72.0
- thorax – *see* Hemorrhage, lung
- throat R04.1
- thymus (gland) E32.8
- thyroid (cyst) (gland) E07.8
- tongue K14.8
- tonsil J35.8   T81.0
- trachea – *see* Hemorrhage, lung
- tracheobronchial R04.8

315

Hemorrhage, hemorrhagic—*continued*
- tracheobronchial—*continued*
- – newborn P26.0
- traumatic – *code as* Injury, by type and site
- – cerebellar S06.8
- – intracranial S06.8
- – recurrent or secondary (following initial hemorrhage at time of injury) T79.2
- tuberculous NEC – *see* Tuberculosis, pulmonary
- tunica vaginalis N50.1
- ulcer – *code as* Ulcer, by site, with hemorrhage
- umbilicus, umbilical
- – cord
- – – after birth, newborn P51.9
- – – complicating delivery O69.5
- – – fetus, from ruptured cord P50.1
- – newborn P51.9
- – – massive P51.0
- – – slipped ligature P51.8
- – stump P51.9
- unavoidable (antepartum) (due to placenta previa) O44.1
- – affecting fetus or newborn P02.0
- urethra (idiopathic) N36.8
- uterus, uterine (abnormal) N93.9
- – climacteric N92.4
- – complicating delivery – *see* Hemorrhage, complicating, delivery
- – dysfunctional or functional N93.8
- – intermenstrual (regular) N92.3
- – – irregular N92.1
- – postmenopausal N95.0
- – postpartum – *see* Hemorrhage, postpartum
- – preclimacteric or premenopausal N92.4
- – prepubertal N93.8
- – pubertal N92.2
- vagina (abnormal) N93.9
- – newborn P54.6
- vas deferens N50.1
- vasa previa O69.4
- – affecting fetus or newborn P50.0
- ventricular I61.5
- vesical N32.8
- viscera NEC R58
- – newborn P54.8
- vitreous (humor) (intraocular) H43.1
- vulva N90.8

Hemorrhoids I84.9
- bleeding, prolapsed, strangulated or ulcerated NEC I84.8

Hemorrhoids—*continued*
- complicating
- – pregnancy O22.4
- – puerperium O87.2
- external I84.5
- – bleeding, prolapsed, strangulated or ulcerated I84.4
- – thrombosed I84.3
- internal I84.2
- – bleeding, prolapsed, strangulated or ulcerated I84.1
- – thrombosed I84.0
- thrombosed NEC I84.7

Hemosalpinx N83.6
- with
- – hematocolpos N89.7
- – hematometra N85.7
- – – with hematocolpos N89.7

Hemosiderosis E83.1
- dietary E83.1
- pulmonary, idiopathic E83.1† J99.8*
- transfusion T80.8

Hemothorax (bacterial) (nontuberculous) J94.2
- newborn P54.8
- traumatic S27.1
- – with pneumothorax S27.2
- tuberculous NEC A16.5
- – with bacteriological and histological confirmation A15.6

Henoch(-Schönlein) disease or syndrome (purpura) D69.0

Henpue, henpuye A66.6

Hepar lobatum (syphilitic) A52.7† K77.0*

Hepatalgia K76.8

Hepatitis K75.9
- acute NEC B17.9
- – with hepatic failure (*see also* Failure, hepatic) K72.9
- – alcoholic K70.1
- – infectious B15.9
- – – with hepatic coma B15.0
- – viral (unspecified) B17.9
- alcoholic (acute) (chronic) K70.1
- amebic (*see also* Abscess, liver, amebic) A06.4
- anicteric, acute (viral) – *see* Hepatitis, viral
- antigen-associated (HAA) (*see also* Hepatitis, viral, type B) B16.9
- Australia-antigen (positive) (*see also* Hepatitis, viral, type B) B16.9
- autoimmune K75.4
- bacterial NEC K75.8

Hepatitis—*continued*
- catarrhal (acute) B15.9
- − with hepatic coma B15.0
- cholangiolitic K75.8
- cholestatic K75.8
- chronic K73.9
- − active NEC K73.2
- − lobular NEC K73.1
- − persistent NEC K73.0
- − specified NEC K73.8
- cytomegaloviral B25.1† K77.0*
- due to ethanol (acute) (chronic) K70.1
- epidemic B15.9
- − with hepatic coma B15.0
- fetus or newborn (giant cell) (idiopathic) P59.2
- from injection, inoculation or transfusion (blood) (plasma) (serum) (other substance) (*see also* Hepatitis, viral, type B) B16.9
- fulminant NEC (viral) – *see* Hepatitis, viral
- granulomatous NEC K75.3
- herpesviral B00.8† K77.0*
- homologous serum (*see also* Hepatitis, viral, type B) B16.9
- in (due to)
- − mumps B26.8† K77.0*
- − toxoplasmosis (acquired) B58.1† K77.0*
- − − congenital (active) P37.1† K77.0*
- infectious, infective
- − acute (subacute) B15.9
- − chronic B18.9
- − − with hepatic coma B15.0
- inoculation (*see also* Hepatitis, viral, type B) B16.9
- interstitial (chronic) K74.6
- lupoid NEC K73.2
- malignant NEC (with hepatic failure) K72.9
- neonatal (giant cell) (idiopathic) (toxic) P59.2
- postimmunization (*see also* Hepatitis, viral, type B) B16.9
- post-transfusion (*see also* Hepatitis, viral, by type) B19.-
- reactive, nonspecific K75.2
- serum (*see also* Hepatitis, viral, type B) B16.9
- syphilitic (late) A52.7† K77.0*
- − congenital (early) A50.0† K77.0*
- − − late A50.5† K77.0*
- − secondary A51.4† K77.0*

Hepatitis—*continued*
- toxic (*see also* Disease, liver, toxic) K71.6
- tuberculous A18.8† K77.0*
- viral, virus (acute) B19.9
- − with hepatic coma B19.0
- − acute (unspecified) B17.9
- − chronic B18.9
- − − specified NEC B18.8
- − − type
- − − − B B18.1
- − − − − with delta-agent B18.0
- − − − C B18.2
- − − complicating pregnancy, childbirth or puerperium O98.4
- − − congenital P35.3
- − − coxsackie B33.8† K77.0*
- − − cytomegalic inclusion B25.1† K77.0*
- − − non-A, non-B B17.8
- − − specified type NEC (with or without coma) B17.8
- − − type
- − − − A B15.9
- − − − − with hepatic coma B15.0
- − − − B B16.9
- − − − − with
- − − − − − delta-agent (coinfection) (without hepatic coma) B16.1
- − − − − − − with hepatic coma B16.0
- − − − − − hepatic coma (without delta-agent coinfection) B16.2
- − − − C B18.2
- − − − − acute or a stated duration of less than six months B17.1
- − − − − chronic (stated duration of six months or more) B18.2
- − − − E B17.2
- − − − non-A, non-B B17.8
- − − − unspecified
- − − − − with hepatic coma B19.0
- − − − − without hepatic coma B19.9
- − − unspecified
- − − − with hepatic coma B19.0
- − − − without hepatic coma B19.9
- − − − acute B17.9

Hepatization, lung (acute) (*see also* Pneumonia, lobar) J18.1
Hepatoblastoma (M8970/3) C22.2
Hepatocarcinoma (M8170/3) C22.0
Hepatocholangiocarcinoma (M8180/3) C22.0
Hepatocholangitis K75.8
Hepatolenticular degeneration E83.0

Hepatoma (malignant) (M8170/3) C22.0
- benign (M8170/0) D13.4
- embryonal (M8970/3) C22.0
Hepatomegalia glycogenica diffusa
E74.0† K77.8*
Hepatomegaly (*see also* Hypertrophy, liver)
R16.0
- congenital Q44.7
- with splenomegaly R16.2
- in infectious mononucleosis
(gammaherpesviral) B27.0† K77.0*
Hepatoptosis K76.8
**Hepatorenal syndrome, following labor
and delivery** O90.4
Hepatosis K76.8
Hepatosplenomegaly R16.2
- hyperlipemic (Bürger-Grütz type) E78.3†
K77.8*
Hereditary – *see condition*
Heredodegeneration, macular H35.5
Heredopathia atactica polyneuritiformis
G60.1
Heredosyphilis (*see also* Syphilis,
congenital) A50.9
Herlitz' syndrome Q81.1
Hermansky-Pudlak syndrome E70.3
Hermaphrodite, hermaphroditism (true)
Q56.0
- chimera 46,XX/46,XY Q99.0
- 46,XX with streak gonads Q99.1
- 46,XX/46,XY Q99.0
- 46,XY with streak gonads Q99.1
Hernia, hernial (acquired) (recurrent)
K46.9
- with
- - gangrene (*see also* Hernia, by site, with,
gangrene) K46.1
- - obstruction (*see also* Hernia, by site,
with, obstruction) K46.0
- abdomen, abdominal K46.9
- - specified site NEC K45.8
- - - with
- - - - gangrene (and obstruction) K45.1
- - - - obstruction K45.0
- - wall – *see* Hernia, ventral
- appendix – *see* Hernia, abdomen
- bladder (mucosa) (sphincter)
- - congenital (female) (male) Q64.7
- - female N81.1
- - male N32.8
- brain, congenital (*see also* Encephalocele)
Q01.9
- cartilage, vertebra – *see* Displacement,
intervertebral disk

Hernia, hernial—*continued*
- cerebral, congenital (*see also*
Encephalocele) Q01.9
- - endaural Q01.8
- ciliary body (traumatic) S05.2
- colon – *see* Hernia, abdomen
Cooper's *see* Hernia, abdomen, specifid
site NEC
- crural – *see* Hernia, femoral
- diaphragm, diaphragmatic K44.9
- - with
- - - gangrene (and obstruction) K44.1
- - - obstruction K44.0
- - congenital Q79.0
- direct (inguinal) – *see* Hernia, inguinal
- diverticulum, intestine – *see* Hernia,
abdomen
- double (inguinal) – *see* Hernia, inguinal,
bilateral
- epigastric – *see* Hernia, ventral
- esophageal hiatus – *see also* Hernia, hiatal
- - congenital Q40.1
- external (inguinal) – *see* Hernia, inguinal
- fallopian tube N83.4
- fascia M62.8
- femoral K41.9
- - with
- - - gangrene (and obstruction) K41.4
- - - obstruction K41.3
- - bilateral K41.2
- - - with
- - - - gangrene (and obstruction) K41.1
- - - - obstruction K41.0
- - unilateral K41.9
- - - with
- - - - gangrene (and obstruction) K41.4
- - - - obstruction K41.3
- foramen magnum G93.5
- - congenital Q01.8
- funicular (umbilical) – *see also* Hernia,
umbilicus
- - spermatic (cord) – *see* Hernia, inguinal
- gastrointestinal tract – *see* Hernia,
abdomen
- Hesselbach's – *see* Hernia, femoral, by
type
- hiatal (esophageal) (sliding) K44.9
- - with
- - - gangrene (and obstruction) K44.1
- - - obstruction K44.0
- - congenital Q40.1
- incarcerated – *see also* Hernia, by site,
with obstruction

Hernia, hernial—*continued*
− incarcerated—*continued*
− − with gangrene − *see* Hernia, by site,
  with gangrene
− incisional − *see* Hernia, ventral
− indirect (inguinal) − *see* Hernia, inguinal
− inguinal (direct) (external) (funicular)
  (indirect) (internal) (oblique) (scrotal)
  (sliding) K40.9
− − with
− − − gangrene (and obstruction) K40.4
− − − obstruction K40.3
− − bilateral K40.2
− − − with
− − − − gangrene (and obstruction) K40.1
− − − − obstruction K40.0
− − unilateral K40.9
− − − with
− − − − gangrene (and obstruction) K40.4
− − − − obstruction K40.3
− interstitial − *see* Hernia, abdomen
− intervertebral cartilage or disk − *see*
  Displacement, intervertebral disk
− intestine, intestinal − *see* Hernia, by site
− intra-abdominal − *see* Hernia, abdomen
− iris (traumatic) S05.2
− irreducible (*see also* Hernia, by site, with
  obstruction) K46.0
− − with gangrene (*see also* Hernia, by site,
  with gangrene) K46.1
− ischiatic − *see* Hernia, abdomen, specified
  site NEC
− ischiorectal − *see* Hernia, abdomen,
  specified site NEC
− lens (traumatic) S05.2
− linea (alba) (semilunaris) − *see* Hernia,
  ventral
− Littre's − *see* Hernia, abdomen
− lumbar − *see* Hernia, abdomen, specified
  site NEC
− lung (subcutaneous) J98.4
− mediastinum J98.5
− mesenteric (internal) − *see* Hernia,
  abdomen
− muscle (sheath) M62.8
− nucleus pulposus − *see* Displacement,
  intervertebral disk
− oblique (inguinal) − *see* Hernia, inguinal
− obstructive (*see also* Hernia, by site, with
  obstruction) K46.0
− − with gangrene (*see also* Hernia, by site,
  with gangrene) K46.1
− obturator − *see* Hernia, abdomen,
  specified site NEC

Hernia, hernial—*continued*
− omental − *see* Hernia, abdomen
− ovary N83.4
− oviduct N83.4
− paraesophageal − *see also* Hernia,
  diaphragm
− − congenital Q40.1
− paraumbilical − *see* Hernia, umbilicus
− perineal − *see* Hernia, abdomen, specified
  site NEC
− Petit's − *see* Hernia, abdomen, specified
  site NEC
− postoperative − *see* Hernia, ventral
− pregnant uterus O34.5
− prevesical N32.8
− pudendal − *see* Hernia, abdomen,
  specified site NEC
− rectovaginal N81.6
− retroperitoneal − *see* Hernia, abdomen,
  specified site NEC
− Richter's − *see* Hernia, abdomen, with
  obstruction
− Rieux's, Riex's − *see* Hernia, abdomen,
  specified site NEC
− sciatic − *see* Hernia, abdomen, specified
  site NEC
− scrotum, scrotal − *see* Hernia, inguinal
− sliding (inguinal) − *see also* Hernia,
  inguinal
− − hiatus − *see* Hernia, hiatal
− spigelian − *see* Hernia, ventral
− spinal (*see also* Spina bifida) Q05.9
− − with hydrocephalus (*see also* Spina
  bifida, with hydrocephalus) Q05.4
− strangulated (*see also* Hernia, by site, with
  obstruction) K46.0
− − with gangrene (*see also* Hernia, by site,
  with gangrene) K46.1
− supra-umbilicus − *see* Hernia, ventral
− tendon M67.8
− Treitz's (fossa) − *see* Hernia, abdomen,
  specified site NEC
− tunica vaginalis Q55.2
− umbilicus, umbilical K42.9
− − with
− − − gangrene (and obstruction) K42.1
− − − obstruction K42.0
− ureter N28.8
− urethra, congenital Q64.7
− urinary meatus, congenital Q64.7
− uterus N81.4
− − pregnant O34.5
− vaginal (anterior) (wall) N81.1
− Velpeau's − *see* Hernia, femoral

Hernia, hernial—*continued*
- ventral K43.9
- – with
- – – gangrene (and obstruction) K43.1
- – – obstruction K43.0
- vesical
- – – congenital (female) (male) Q64.7
- – – female N81.1
- – – male N32.8
- vitreous (into wound) S05.2
- – – into anterior chamber H43.0

Herniation – *see also* Hernia
- brain (stem) G93.5
- cerebral G93.5
- mediastinum J98.5
- nucleus pulposus – *see* Displacement, intervertebral disk

Herpangina B08.5

Herpes, herpetic B00.9
- anogenital A60.9
- blepharitis (zoster) B02.3† H03.1*
- – simplex B00.5† H03.1*
- circinatus B35.4
- – bullosus L12.0
- conjunctivitis (simplex) B00.5† H13.1*
- – zoster B02.3† H13.1*
- cornea – *see* Herpes, keratitis
- encephalitis B00.4† G05.1*
- eye (zoster) B02.3† H58.8*
- – simplex B00.5† H58.8*
- eyelid (zoster) B02.3† H03.1*
- – simplex B00.5† H03.1*
- facialis B00.1
- febrilis B00.1
- geniculate ganglionitis B02.2† G53.0*
- genital, genitalis A60.0
- – female A60.0† N77.-*
- – male A60.0† N51.-*
- gestational, gestationis O26.4
- gingivostomatitis B00.2
- iridocyclitis (simplex) B00.5† H22.0*
- – zoster B02.3† H22.0*
- iris (vesicular erythema multiforme) L51.1
- iritis (simplex) B00.5† H22.0*
- keratitis (simplex) (dendritic) (disciform) (interstitial) B00.5† H19.1*
- – zoster (interstitial) B02.3† H19.2*
- keratoconjunctivitis (simplex) B00.5† H19.1*
- – zoster B02.3† H19.2*
- labialis B00.1
- lip B00.1
- meningitis (simplex) B00.3† G02.0*

Herpes, herpetic—*continued*
- meningitis—*continued*
- – zoster B02.1† G02.0*
- ophthalmicus (zoster) NEC B02.3† H58.8*
- – simplex B00.5† H58.8*
- penis A60.0† N51.8*
- perianal skin A60.1
- pharyngitis, pharyngotonsillitis B00.2
- rectum A60.1† K93.8*
- resulting from HIV disease B20.3
- scrotum A60.0† N51.8*
- sepsis B00.7
- simplex B00.9
- – complicated NEC B00.8
- – congenital P35.2
- – conjunctivitis B00.5† H13.1*
- – external ear B00.1† H62.1*
- – eyelid B00.5† H03.1*
- – hepatitis B00.8† K77.0*
- – keratitis (interstitial) B00.5† H19.1*
- – specified complication NEC B00.8
- – visceral B00.8
- stomatitis B00.2
- tonsurans B35.0
- visceral B00.8
- vulva A60.0† N77.1*
- whitlow B00.8
- zoster (*see also condition*) B02.9
- – auricularis B02.2† H94.0*
- – complicated NEC B02.8
- – conjunctivitis B02.3† H13.1*
- – disseminated B02.7
- – encephalitis B02.0† G05.1*
- – eye(lid) B02.3† H03.1*
- – geniculate ganglionitis B02.2† G53.0*
- – keratitis (interstitial) B02.3† H19.2*
- – meningitis B02.1† G02.0*
- – neuritis, neuralgia B02.2† G53.0*
- – ophthalmicus NEC B02.3† H58.8*
- – oticus B02.2† H94.0*
- – polyneuropathy B02.2† G63.0*
- – specified complication NEC B02.8
- – trigeminal neuralgia B02.2† G53.0*

Herrick's anemia (*see also* Disease, sickle-cell) D57.1

Hers' disease E74.0

Herter-Gee syndrome K90.0

Herxheimer's reaction T78.2

Hesitancy of micturition R39.1

Hesselbach's hernia – *see* Hernia, femoral, specified site NEC

Heterochromia (congenital) Q13.2
- cataract H26.2

Heterochromia—*continued*
- cyclitis (Fuchs) H20.8
- hair L67.1
- iritis H20.8
- retained metallic foreign body (nonmagnetic) H44.7
- – magnetic H44.6
- uveitis H20.8
Heterophoria H50.5
Heterophyes, heterophyiasis (small intestine) B66.8
Heterotopia, heterotopic – *see also* Malposition, congenital
- cerebralis Q04.8
Heterotropia H50.4
- intermittent H50.3
- vertical H50.2
Heubner-Herter disease K90.0
Hexadactylism Q69.9
Hibernoma (M8880/0) – *see* Lipoma
Hiccup, hiccough R06.6
- epidemic B33.0
- psychogenic F45.3
Hidradenitis (axillaris) (suppurative) L73.2
Hidradenoma (nodular) (M8400/0) – *see also* Neoplasm, skin, benign
- clear cell (M8402/0) D23.9
- papillary (M8405/0) D23.9
Hidrocystoma (M8404/0) – *see* Neoplasm, skin, benign
High
- altitude effects T70.2
- – anoxia T70.2
- – on
- – – ears T70.0
- – – sinuses T70.1
- – polycythemia D75.1
- arch
- – foot Q66.7
- – palate, congenital Q38.5
- arterial tension (*see also* Hypertension) I10
- basal metabolic rate R94.8
- blood pressure (*see also* Hypertension) I10
- – reading (incidental) (isolated) (nonspecific), without diagnosis of hypertension R03.0
- diaphragm (congenital) Q79.1
- expressed emotional level within family Z63.8
- head at term O32.4
- palate, congenital Q38.5

High—*continued*
- risk
- – environment (physical) NEC Z58.9
- – – occupational NEC Z57.9
- – – – specified NEC Z57.8
- – – specified NEC Z58.8
- – infant NEC Z76.2
- – sexual behavior Z72.5
- temperature (of unknown origin) R50.9
- thoracic rib Q76.6
Hildenbrand's disease A75.0
Hilum – *see condition*
Hip – *see condition*
Hippel's disease Q85.8
Hippus H57.0
Hirschsprung's disease or megacolon Q43.1
Hirsutism, hirsuties L68.0
Hirudiniasis
- external B88.3
- internal B83.4
Hiss-Russell dysentery A03.1
Histidinemia, histidinuria E70.8
Histiocytoma (M8832/0) – *see also* Neoplasm, skin, benign
- fibrous (M8830/0) – *see also* Neoplasm, skin, benign
- – atypical (M8830/1) – *see* Neoplasm, connective tissue, uncertain behavior
- – malignant (M8830/3) – *see* Neoplasm, connective tissue, malignant
Histiocytosis D76.3
- acute differentiated progressive C96.0
- Langerhans' cell NEC C96.6
- – multifocal (X)
- – – multisystemic (disseminated) C96.0
- – – unisystemic C96.5
- – unifocal (X) C96.6
- malignant C96.8
- mononuclear phagocytes NEC D76.1
- – Langerhans' cells C96.6
- sinus, with massive lymphadenopathy D76.3
- syndrome NEC C96.6 D76.3
- X NEC C96.6
- – acute (progressive) C96.0
- – chronic D76.3
- – multifocal C96.5
- – unifocal C96.6
- – multisystemic C96.0
Histoplasmosis B39.9
- with pneumonia NEC B39.2† J17.2*
- African B39.5
- American – *see* Histoplasmosis, capsulati

Histoplasmosis—*continued*
- capsulati B39.4
- − disseminated B39.3
- − generalized B39.3
- − pulmonary B39.2† J99.8∗
- − − acute B39.0† J99.8∗
- − − chronic B39.1† J99.8∗
- Darling's B39.4
- duboisii B39.5
- lung NEC B39.2† J99.8∗

History (personal) (of)
- abuse Z91.8
- alcohol abuse Z86.4
- allergy to
- − analgesic agent NEC Z88.6
- − anesthetic NEC Z88.4
- − antibiotic agent NEC Z88.1
- − anti-infective agent NEC Z88.3
- − drugs, medicaments and biological substances Z88.9
- − − specified NEC Z88.8
- − medicinal agents Z88.9
- − − specified NEC Z88.8
- − narcotic agent NEC Z88.5
- − nonmedicinal agents Z91.0
- − penicillin Z88.0
- − serum Z88.7
- − sulfonamides Z88.2
- − vaccine Z88.7
- anticoagulant use (current) (long-term) Z92.1
- arthritis Z87.3
- aspirin use (current) (long-term) Z92.2
- benign neoplasm Z86.0
- chemotherapy for neoplastic disease Z92.6
- chromosomal abnormality Z87.7
- congenital malformation Z87.7
- contraception Z92.0
- disease or disorder (of) Z87.8
- − blood and blood-forming organs Z86.2
- − circulatory system Z86.7
- − digestive system Z87.1
- − ear Z86.6
- − endocrine Z86.3
- − eye Z86.6
- − genital system Z87.4
- − hematological Z86.2
- − immune mechanism Z86.2
- − infectious Z86.1
- − mental NEC Z86.5
- − metabolic Z86.3
- − musculoskeletal Z87.3
- − nervous system Z86.6

History—*continued*
- disease or disorder—*continued*
- − nutritional Z86.3
- − obstetric Z87.5
- − parasitic Z86.1
- − respiratory system Z87.0
- − sense organs Z86.6
- − skin Z87.2
- − specified site or type NEC Z87.8
- − subcutaneous tissue Z87.2
- − trophoblastic Z87.5
- − urinary system Z87.4
- drug abuse Z86.4
- family, of
- − alcohol abuse Z81.1
- − allergy NEC Z84.8
- − anemia Z83.2
- − arthritis Z82.6
- − asthma Z82.5
- − blindness Z82.1
- − chromosomal anomaly Z82.7
- − chronic
- − − disabling disease NEC Z82.8
- − − lower respiratory disease Z82.5
- − congenital malformations and deformations Z82.7
- − consanguinity Z84.3
- − deafness Z82.2
- − diabetes mellitus Z83.3
- − disability NEC Z82.8
- − disease or disorder (of)
- − − allergic NEC Z84.8
- − − behavioral NEC Z81.8
- − − blood and blood-forming organs Z83.2
- − − cardiovascular NEC Z82.4
- − − chronic disabling NEC Z82.8
- − − digestive Z83.7
- − − ear NEC Z83.5
- − − endocrine Z83.4
- − − eye NEC Z83.5
- − − genitourinary NEC Z84.2
- − − hematological Z83.2
- − − immune mechanism Z83.2
- − − infectious NEC Z83.1
- − − ischemic heart Z82.4
- − − kidney Z84.1
- − − mental NEC Z81.8
- − − metabolic Z83.4
- − − musculoskeletal Z82.6
- − − neurological NEC Z82.0
- − − nutritional NEC Z83.4
- − − parasitic NEC Z83.1
- − − psychiatric NEC Z81.8

History—*continued*
- family, of—*continued*
- – disease or disorder—*continued*
- – – respiratory NEC Z83.6
- – – skin and subcutaneous tissue NEC
  Z84.0
- – – specified NEC Z84.8
- – drug abuse NEC Z81.3
- – epilepsy Z82.0
- – hearing loss Z82.2
- – human immunodeficiency virus (HIV)
  infection Z83.0
- – Huntington's chorea Z82.0
- – leukemia Z80.6
- – malignant neoplasm (of) NEC Z80.9
- – – breast Z80.3
- – – bronchus Z80.1
- – – digestive organ Z80.0
- – – gastrointestinal tract Z80.0
- – – genital organ Z80.4
- – – hematopoietic NEC Z80.7
- – – intrathoracic organ NEC Z80.2
- – – lung Z80.1
- – – lymphatic NEC Z80.7
- – – respiratory organ NEC Z80.2
- – – specified site NEC Z80.8
- – – trachea Z80.1
- – – urinary organ or tract Z80.5
- – mental
- – – disorder NEC Z81.8
- – – retardation Z81.0
- – psychiatric disorder Z81.8
- – psychoactive substance abuse NEC
  Z81.3
- – respiratory condition, chronic NEC
  Z82.5
- – self-harmful behavior Z81.8
- – skin condition Z84.0
- – specified condition NEC Z84.8
- – stroke (cerebrovascular) Z82.3
- – substance abuse NEC Z81.4
- – – alcohol Z81.1
- – – drug NEC Z81.3
- – – psychoactive NEC Z81.3
- – – tobacco Z81.2
- – tobacco abuse Z81.2
- – violence, violent behavior Z81.8
- – visual loss Z82.1
- hyperthermia, malignant Z88.4
- in situ neoplasm Z86.0
- injury NEC Z91.6
- irradiation Z92.3
- leukemia Z85.6
- malignant neoplasm (of) Z85.9

History—*continued*
- malignant neoplasm—*continued*
- – breast Z85.3
- – bronchus Z85.1
- – digestive organ Z85.0
- – gastrointestinal tract Z85.0
- – genital organ Z85.4
- – hematopoietic NEC Z85.7
- – intrathoracic organ NEC Z85.2
- – lung Z85.1
- – lymphatic NEC Z85.7
- – respiratory organ NEC Z85.2
- – skin Z85.8
- – specified site NEC Z85.8
- – trachea Z85.1
- – urinary organ or tract Z85.5
- maltreatment Z91.8
- medical treatment Z92.9
- – specified type NEC Z92.8
- noncompliance with medical treatment or
  regimen Z91.1
- nutritional deficiency Z86.3
- parasuicide (attempt) Z91.5
- perinatal problems Z87.6
- physical trauma NEC Z91.6
- – self-harm or suicide attempt Z91.5
- poisoning NEC Z91.8
- – self-harm or suicide attempt Z91.5
- poor personal hygiene Z91.2
- psychiatric disorder NEC Z86.5
- psychological trauma NEC Z91.4
- – in childhood Z61.7
- radiation therapy Z92.3
- rehabilitation (measures) Z92.5
- respiratory condition Z87.0
- risk factors NEC Z91.8
- self-harm Z91.5
- self-poisoning attempt Z91.5
- sleep-wake cycle problem Z91.3
- substance abuse NEC Z86.4
- suicide attempt Z91.5
- surgery (major) NEC Z92.4
- – transplant – *see* Transplant
- tobacco abuse Z86.4
- trauma NEC Z91.6
- – psychological NEC Z91.4
- – self-harm Z91.5
- unhealthy sleep-wake cycle Z91.3
- use of medicaments (current) (long-term)
  NEC Z92.2
- – anticoagulants Z92.1
- – aspirin Z92.2

His-Werner disease A79.0

HIV – *see also* Human, immunodeficiency virus (HIV) disease
– laboratory evidence (nonconclusive) R75
– nonconclusive test in infants R75
- positive, seropositive Z21
Hives (bold) (*see also* Urticaria) L50.9
Hoarseness R49.0
Hobo Z59.0
Hodgkin
– disease C81.9
– – lymphocytic depletion C81.3
– – lymphocyte rich C81.4
– – mixed cellularity C81.2
– – nodular
– – – sclerosis C81.1
– – – lymphocyte predominant C81.0
– – – mixed cellularity C81.2
– granuloma C81.9
– lymphocyte predominant, nodular C81.0
– lymphoma, malignant (classical) C81.9
– – lymphocytic depletion C81.3
– – lymphocyte-rich C81.4
– – mixed cellularity C81.2
– – nodular
– – – sclerosis C81.1
– – – lymphocyte predominant C81.0
– – – mixed cellularity C81.2
– – type not specified C81.7
– paragranuloma (nodular) C81.0
– sarcoma C81.3
Hodgson's disease I71.2
– ruptured I71.1
Hoffa-Kastert disease E88.8
Hoffa's disease E88.8
Hoffmann-Bouveret syndrome I47.9
Hoffmann's syndrome E03.9† G73.5*
Hole (round)
– macula H35.3
– retina (without detachment) H33.3
– – with detachment H33.0
Holiday relief care Z75.5
Hollenhorst's plaque H34.2
Hollow foot (congenital) Q66.7
– acquired M21.6
Holoprosencephaly Q04.2
Holt-Oram syndrome Q87.2
Homelessness Z59.0
Homesickness F43.2
Homocystinemia, homocystinuria E72.1
Homogentisate l,2-dioxygenase deficiency E70.2
Homologous serum hepatitis (prophylactic) (therapeutic) (*see also* Hepatitis, viral, type B) B16.9

Honeycomb lung J98.4
– congenital Q33.0
Hooded
– clitoris Q52.6
– penis Q55.6
Hookworm (anemia) (disease) (infection) (infestation) B76.9
– specified NEC B76.8
Hordeolum (eyelid) (external) (internal) (recurrent) H00.0
Horn
– cutaneous L85.8
– nail L60.2
– – congenital Q84.6
Horner(-Claude Bernard) syndrome G90.2
– traumatic S14.5
Horseshoe kidney (congenital) Q63.1
Horton's headache or neuralgia G44.0
Hospital hopper syndrome F68.1
Hospitalism in children F43.2
Hostility R45.5
– towards child Z62.3
Hourglass (contracture) – *see also* Contraction, hourglass
– stomach K31.8
– – congenital Q40.2
– – stricture K31.2
Household, housing circumstance affecting care Z59.9
– specified NEC Z59.8
Housemaid's knee M70.4
Hudson(-Stähli) line (cornea) H18.0
Human
– bite (open wound) – *see also* Wound, open
– – intact skin surface – *see* Contusion
– immunodeficiency virus (HIV) disease (infection) B24
– – asymptomatic status Z21
– – complicating pregnancy, childbirth or the puerperium O98.7
– – contact Z20.6
– – counseling Z71.7
– – dementia B22.0† F02.4*
– – exposure to Z20.6
– – laboratory evidence R75
– – resulting in
– – – acute HIV infection syndrome B23.0
– – – bacterial infection NEC B20.1
– – – Burkitt lymphoma B21.1
– – – candidiasis B20.4
– – – chronic lymphadenopathy, generalized (persistent) B23.1

Human—*continued*
– immunodeficiency virus—*continued*
– – resulting in—*continued*
– – – cryptosporidiosis B20.8
– – – cytomegaloviral disease B20.2
– – – dementia B22.0† F02.4*
– – – encephalopathy B22.0
– – – failure to thrive B22.2
– – – generalized lymphadenopathy
    (persistent) B23.1
– – – hematological abnormality NEC
    B23.2
– – – herpesviral infections B20.3
– – – immunological abnormality NEC
    B23.2
– – – infection B20.9
– – – – bacterial NEC B20.1
– – – – candidal B20.4
– – – – Cryptosporidium B20.8
– – – – cytomegaloviral B20.2
– – – – fungus NEC B20.5
– – – – herpesvirus B20.3
– – – – multiple B20.7
– – – – mycobacterial B20.0
– – – – mycotic NEC B20.5
– – – – papovavirus B20.3
– – – – parasitic NEC B20.8
– – – – Pneumocystis carinii (pneumonia)
    B20.6
– – – – Pneumocystis jirovecii
    (pneumonia) B20.6
– – – – specified NEC B20.8
– – – – tuberculous B20.0
– – – – viral NEC B20.3
– – – infectious disease NEC B20.9
– – – – specified NEC B20.8
– – – Kaposi's sarcoma B21.0
– – – lymphadenopathy
– – – – generalized (persistent) B23.1
– – – lymphoid interstitial pneumonitis
    B22.1
– – – lymphoma (malignant) B21.2
– – – – Burkitt B21.1
– – – – non-Hodgkin NEC B21.2
– – – multiple
– – – – diseases classified elsewhere
    B22.7
– – – – infections B20.7
– – – – malignant neoplasms B21.7
– – – mycobacterial infection B20.0
– – – mycosis NEC B20.5
– – – neoplasm, malignant B21.9
– – – – hematopoietic tissue NEC B21.3
– – – – lymphoid tissue NEC B21.3

Human—*continued*
– immunodeficiency virus—*continued*
– – resulting in—*continued*
– – – neoplasm, malignant—*continued*
– – – – multiple B21.7
– – – – specified NEC B21.8
– – – non-Hodgkin lymphoma NEC B21.2
– – – papovavirus infection B20.3
– – – parasitic disease NEC B20.9
– – – – specified NEC B20.8
– – – Pneumocystis carinii pneumonia
    B20.6
– – – Pneumocystis jirovecii pneumonia
    B20.6
– – – pneumonitis, interstitial, lymphoid
    B22.1
– – – sarcoma NEC B21.9
– – – – Kaposi's B21.0
– – – specified condition NEC B23.8
– – – toxoplasmosis B20.8
– – – tuberculosis B20.0
– – – viral infection NEC B20.3
– – – wasting syndrome B22.2
– metapneumovirus B97.8
– – resulting in
– – – bronchiolitis J21.1
– – – bronchitis J20.8
– – – encephalitis A85.8† G05.1*
– – – pneumonia J12.3
– T-cell lymphotropic virus type-1 (HTLV-
    1) infection B33.3
– – as cause of disease classified elsewhere
    B97.3
– – carrier Z22.6
Humidifier lung or pneumonitis J67.7
Humiliation (experience) in childhood
    Z61.3
Humpback (acquired) M40.2
– congenital Q76.4
Hunchback (acquired) M40.2
– congenital Q76.4
Hunger T73.0
– air, psychogenic F45.3
Hunner's ulcer N30.1
Hunter's
– glossitis D51.0
– syndrome E76.1
Huntington's disease or chorea G10
– with dementia G10† F02.2*
Hunt's
– disease or syndrome (herpetic geniculate
    ganglionitis) B02.2† G53.0*
– – dyssynergia cerebellaris myoclonica
    G11.1

Hunt's—*continued*
- neuralgia B02.2† G53.0∗
Hurler(-Scheie) disease or syndrome
E76.0
Hurst's disease G36.1
Hurthle cell
- adenocarcinoma (M8290/3) C73
- adenoma (M8290/0) D34
- carcinoma (M8290/3) C73
- tumor (M8290/0) D34
Hutchinson-Boeck disease or
syndrome (*see also* Sarcoidosis) D86.9
Hutchinson-Gilford disease or syndrome
E34.8
Hutchinson's
- disease meaning
- - angioma serpiginosum L81.7
- - pompholyx L30.1
- - prurigo estivalis L56.4
- - summer eruption or summer prurigo
L56.4
- melanotic freckle (M8742/2) – *see*
Melanoma, in situ
- - malignant melanoma in (M8742/3) –
see Melanoma
- teeth or incisors (congenital syphilis)
A50.5
- triad (congenital syphilis) A50.5
Hyalin plaque, sclera, senile H15.8
Hyaline membrane (disease) (lung)
(pulmonary) (newborn) P22.0
Hyalinosis
- cutis (et mucosae) E78.8
- focal and segmental (glomerular) – *code*
to N00-N07 with fourth character .1
Hyalitis, hyalosis, asteroid H43.2
- syphilitic (late) A52.7† H45.8∗
Hydatid
- cyst or tumor – *see* Echinococcus
- mole – *see* Hydatidiform mole
- Morgagni's
- - female Q50.5
- - male (epididymal) Q55.4
- - - testicular Q55.2
Hydatidiform mole (benign) (complicating
pregnancy) (delivered) (undelivered)
(M9100/0) (*see also* Mole, hydatidiform)
O01.9
- classical (M9100/0) O01.0
- complete (M9100/0) O01.0
- invasive (M9100/1) D39.2
- malignant (M9100/1) D39.2
- partial (M9103/0) O01.1

Hydatidiform mole—*continued*
- previous, affecting management of
pregnancy Z35.1
Hydatidosis – *see* Echinococcus
Hydradenitis (axillaris) (suppurative)
L73.2
Hydradenoma (M8400/0) – *see*
Hidradenoma
Hydramnios O40
- affecting fetus or newborn P01.3
Hydrancephaly, hydranencephaly Q04.3
- with spina bifida (*see also* Spina bifida,
with hydrocephalus) Q05.4
Hydrargyrism NEC T56.1
Hydrarthrosis M25.4
- gonococcal A54.4† M14.8∗
- intermittent M12.4
- of yaws (early) (late) A66.6† M14.8∗
- syphilitic (late) A52.7† M14.8∗
- - congenital A50.5† M03.1∗
Hydremia D64.8
Hydrencephalocele (congenital) (*see also*
Encephalocele) Q01.9
Hydrencephalomeningocele
(congenital) (*see also* Encephalocele)
Q01.9
Hydroa R23.8
- estivale L56.4
vacciniforme L56.4
Hydroadenitis (axillaris) (suppurative)
L73.2
Hydrocalycosis (*see also* Hydronephrosis)
N13.3
Hydrocele (spermatic cord) (testis) (tunica
vaginalis) N43.3
- canal of Nuck N94.8
- congenital P83.5
- encysted N43.0
- female NEC N94.8
- fetus or newborn P83.5
- infected N43.1
- round ligament N94.8
- specified NEC N43.2
- spinalis (*see also* Spina bifida) Q05.9
- - with hydrocephalus (*see also* Spina
bifida, with hydrocephalus) Q05.4
- vulva N90.8
Hydrocephalus (acquired) (external)
(internal) (malignant) (recurrent)
G91.9
- aqueduct Sylvius stricture (*see also*
Hydrocephalus, congenital) Q03.0
- causing disproportion O33.6
- - with obstructed labor O66.3

Hydrocephalus—*continued*
– causing disproportion—*continued*
– – affecting fetus or newborn P03.1
– communicating G91.0
– congenital (external) (internal) Q03.9
– – with spina bifida – *see also* Spina
    bifida, with hydrocephalus
– – – cervical Q05.0
– – – dorsal Q05.1
– – – lumbar Q05.2
– – – lumbosacral Q05.2
– – – sacral Q05.3
– – – thoracic Q05.1
– – – thoracolumbar Q05.1
– – specified NEC Q03.8
– due to toxoplasmosis (congenital) P37.1
– fetus (suspected), affecting management
    of pregnancy O35.0
– foramen Magendie block (acquired)
    G91.1
– – congenital (*see also* Hydrocephalus,
    congenital) Q03.1
– in (due to)
– – infectious disease NEC B99† G94.0∗
– – neoplastic disease NEC
    (M8000/1) (*see also* Neoplasm)
    D48.9† G94.1∗
– – parasitic disease B89† G94.0∗
– newborn Q03.9
– – with spina bifida (*see also* Spina bifida,
    with hydrocephalus) Q05.4
– noncommunicating G91.1
– normal-pressure G91.2
– obstructive G91.1
– post-traumatic NEC G91.3
– specified NEC G91.8
– syphilitic, congenital A50.4† G94.0∗
Hydrocolpos (congenital) N89.8
Hydrocystoma (M8404/0) – *see* Neoplasm,
skin, benign
Hydroencephalocele (congenital) (*see also*
Encephalocele) Q01.9
Hydroencephalomeningocele
(congenital) (*see also* Encephalocele)
Q01.9
Hydrohematopneumothorax – *see*
Hemothorax
Hydromeningitis – *see* Meningitis
Hydromeningocele (spinal) (*see also* Spina
bifida) Q05.9
– cranial (*see also* Encephalocele) Q01.9
Hydrometra N85.8
Hydrometrocolpos N89.8
Hydromicrocephaly Q02

Hydromphalos (since birth) Q45.8
Hydromyelia Q06.4
Hydromyelocele (*see also* Spina bifida)
Q05.9
– with hydrocephalus (*see also* Spina bifida,
    with hydrocephalus) Q05.4
Hydronephrosis (atrophic) (early)
(functionless) (intermittent) (primary)
(secondary) NEC N13.3
– with
– – infection N13.6
– – obstruction (by) (of)
– – – renal calculus N13.2
– – – – with infection N13.6
– – – ureteral NEC N13.1
– – – – with infection N13.6
– – – – calculus N13.2
– – – – – with infection N13.6
– – – – ureteropelvic junction N13.0
– – – – with infection N13.6
– – ureteral stricture NEC N13.1
– – – with infection N13.6
– congenital Q62.0
– tuberculous A18.1† N29.1∗
Hydropericarditis (*see also* Pericarditis)
I31.9
Hydropericardium (*see also* Pericarditis)
I31.9
Hydroperitoneum R18
Hydrophobia – *see* Rabies
Hydrophthalmos Q15.0
Hydropneumohemothorax – *see*
Hemothorax
Hydropneumopericarditis (*see also*
Pericarditis) I31.9
Hydropneumopericardium (*see also*
Pericarditis) I31.9
Hydropneumothorax J94.8
– traumatic S27.3
– tuberculous NEC A16.5
Hydrops R60.9
– abdominis R18
– amnii (complicating pregnancy) (*see also*
    Hydramnios) O40
– articulorum intermittens M12.4
– cardiac (*see also* Failure, heart,
    congestive) I50.0
– causing obstructed labor (mother) O66.3
– endolymphatic H81.0
– fetal(is) or newborn (idiopathic) P83.2
– – affecting management of pregnancy
    O36.2
– – due to
– – – ABO isoimmunization P56.0

Hydrops—*continued*
– fetal(is) or newborn—*continued*
– – due to—*continued*
– – – ABO isoimmunization—*continued*
– – – – affecting management of
    pregnancy O36.1
– – – hemolytic disease NEC P56.9
– – – isoimmunization (ABO) (Rh) P56.0
– – – Rh incompatibility P56.0
– – – – affecting management of
    pregnancy O36.0
– gallbladder K82.1
– joint (*see also* Hydrarthrosis) M25.4
– labyrinth H81.0
– nutritional (*see also* Malnutrition, severe)
    E43
– pericardium – *see* Pericarditis
– pleura (*see also* Hydrothorax) J94.8
– spermatic cord (*see also* Hydrocele)
    N43.3
Hydropyonephrosis N13.6
Hydrorachis Q06.4
Hydrorrhea (nasal) J34.8
– pregnancy – *see* Rupture, membranes,
    premature
Hydrosadenitis (axillaris) (suppurative)
    L73.2
Hydrosalpinx (fallopian tube)
    (follicularis) N70.1
Hydrothorax (double) (pleura) J94.8
– chylous (nonfilarial) I89.8
– – filarial (*see also* Filaria, filarial,
    filariasis) B74.9† J91∗
– traumatic S27.8
– tuberculous – *see* Tuberculosis
Hydroureter (*see also* Hydronephrosis)
    N13.4
– with infection N13.6
– congenital Q62.3
Hydroureteronephrosis (*see also*
    Hydronephrosis) N13.3
– with infection N13.6
Hydrourethra N36.8
Hydroxykynureninuria E70.8
Hydroxylysinemia E72.3
Hydroxyprolinemia E72.5
Hygroma (congenital) (cystic) (M9173/0)
    D18.1
– praepatellare, prepatellar M70.4
Hymen – *see* condition
Hymenolepis, hymenolepiasis (diminuta)
    (infection) (infestation) (nana) B71.0
Hypalgesia R20.8

Hyperacidity (gastric) K31.8
– psychogenic F45.3
Hyperactive, hyperactivity
– basal cell, uterine cervix (*see also*
    Dysplasia, cervix) N87.9
– bowel sounds R19.1
– cervix epithelial (basal) (*see also*
    Dysplasia, cervix) N87.9
– child F90.9
– – attention deficit F90.0
– detrusor muscle N32.8
– gastrointestinal K31.8
– – psychogenic F45.3
– nasal mucous membrane J34.3
– stomach K31.8
– thyroid (gland) (*see also*
    Hyperthyroidism) E05.9
Hyperacusis H93.2
Hyperadrenalism E27.5
Hyperadrenocorticism E24.9
– congenital E25.0
– iatrogenic
– – correct substance properly administered
    E24.2
– – overdose or wrong substance given or
    taken T38.0
– not associated with Cushing's syndrome
    E27.0
– pituitary-dependent E24.0
Hyperaldosteronism E26.9
– primary (due to (bilateral) adrenal
    hyperplasia) E26.0
– secondary E26.1
– specified NEC E26.8
Hyperalgesia R20.8
Hyperalimentation R63.2
– carotene, carotin E67.1
– specified NEC E67.8
– vitamin
– – A E67.0
– – D E67.3
Hyperaminoaciduria
– arginine E72.2
– cystine E72.0
– lysine E72.3
– ornithine E72.4
Hyperammonemia (congenital) E72.2
Hyperazotemia – *see* Uremia
Hyperbetalipoproteinemia (familial)
    E78.0
– with prebetalipoproteinemia E78.2
Hyperbilirubinemia
– constitutional E80.6
– familial conjugated E80.6

Hyperbilirubinemia—*continued*
- neonatal (transient) (*see also* Jaundice, fetus or newborn) P59.9
- – of prematurity P59.0

Hypercalcemia, hypocalciuric, familial E83.5

Hypercalciuria, idiopathic E83.5

Hypercapnia R06.8

Hypercarotenemia, hypercarotinemia (dietary) E67.1

Hypercementosis K03.4

Hyperchloremia E87.8

Hyperchlorhydria K31.8
- neurotic F45.3
- psychogenic F45.3

Hypercholesterinemia – *see* Hypercholesterolemia

Hypercholesterolemia (essential) (familial) (hereditary) (primary) (pure) E78.0
- with hyperglyceridemia, endogenous E78.2
- dietary counseling and surveillance Z71.3

Hyperchylia gastrica, psychogenic F45.3

Hyperchylomicronemia (familial) (primary) E78.3
- with hyperbetalipoproteinemia E78.3

Hypercorticalism, pituitary-dependent E24.0

Hypercorticosteronism
- correct substance properly administered E24.2
- overdose or wrong substance given or taken T38.0

Hypercortisonism
- correct substance properly administered E24.2
- overdose or wrong substance given or taken T38.0

Hyperelectrolytemia E87.8

Hyperemesis (*see also* Vomiting) R11
- gravidarum (mild) O21.0
- – with
- – – carbohydrate depletion O21.1
- – – dehydration O21.1
- – – electrolyte imbalance O21.1
- – – metabolic disturbance O21.1
- – affecting fetus or newborn P01.8
- – severe (with metabolic disturbance) O21.1
- psychogenic F45.3

Hyperemia (acute) (passive) R68.8
- anal mucosa K62.8
- bladder N32.8
- cerebral I67.8

Hyperemia—*continued*
- conjunctiva H11.4
- ear, internal, acute H83.0
- enteric K59.8
- eye H11.4
- eyelid (active) (passive) H02.8
- intestine K59.8
- iris H21.1
- kidney N28.8
- labyrinth H83.0
- liver (active) K76.8
- lung (passive) (*see also* Edema, lung) J81
- pulmonary (passive) (*see also* Edema, lung) J81
- renal N28.8
- retina H35.8
- stomach K31.8

Hyperesthesia (body surface) R20.3
- larynx (reflex) J38.7
- – hysterical F44.8
- pharynx (reflex) J39.2
- – hysterical F44.8

Hyperestrogenism (drug-induced) (iatrogenic) E28.0

Hyperfibrinolysis – *see* Fibrinolysis

Hyperfructosemia E74.1

Hyperfunction
- adrenal cortex, not associated with Cushing's syndrome E27.0
- – medulla E27.5
- – – adrenomedullary E27.5
- – virilism E25.9
- – – congenital E25.0
- ovarian E28.8
- pancreas K86.8
- parathyroid (gland) E21.3
- pituitary (gland) (anterior) E22.9
- – specified NEC E22.8
- polyglandular E31.1
- testicular E29.0

Hypergammaglobulinemia D89.2
- polyclonal D89.0
- Waldenström's D89.0

Hypergastrinemia E16.4

Hyperglobulinemia R77.1

Hyperglycemia, hyperglycemic R73.9
- coma – *code to* E10-E14 with fourth character .0
- postpancreatectomy E89.1

Hyperglyceridemia (endogenous) (essential) (familial) (hereditary) (pure) E78.1
- mixed E78.3

Hyperglycinemia (non-ketotic) E72.5

Hypergonadism
- ovarian E28.8
- testicular (infantile) (primary) E29.0

Hyperheparinemia (*see also* Circulating anticoagulants) D68.3

Hyperhidrosis, hyperidrosis R61.9
- generalized R61.1
- localized R61.0
- psychogenic F45.8

Hyperhistidinemia E70.8

Hyperhomocysteinemia E72.1

Hyperhydroxyprolinemia E72.5

Hyperinsulinism (functional) E16.1
- with coma (hypoglycemic) E15
- ectopic E16.1
- therapeutic misadventure (from administration of insulin) T38.3

Hyperkalemia E87.5

Hyperkeratosis (*see also* Keratosis) L85.9
- cervix (*see also* Dysplasia, cervix) N87.9
- due to yaws (early) (late) (palmar or plantar) A66.3
- follicularis Q82.8
- − penetrans (in cutem) L87.0
- palmoplantaris climacterica L85.1
- pinta A67.1
- senile (with pruritus) L57.0
- universalis congenita Q80.8
- vocal cord J38.3
- vulva N90.4

Hyperkinesia, hyperkinetic (disease) (reaction) (syndrome) (adolescence) (childhood) F90.9
- with
- − conduct disorder F90.1
- − disturbance of activity and attention F90.0
- − mental retardation and stereotyped movements F84.4
- − specified manifestation NEC F90.8
- heart I51.8

Hyperleucine-isoleucinemia E71.1

Hyperlipemia, hyperlipidemia E78.5
- combined familial E78.4
- group
- − A E78.0
- − B E78.1
- − C E78.2
- − D E78.3
- mixed E78.2
- specified NEC E78.4

Hyperlipidosis E75.6
- hereditary NEC E75.5

Hyperlipoproteinemia E78.5
- Fredrickson's type
- − I E78.3
- − IIa E78.0
- − IIb E78.2
- − III E78.2
- − IV E78.1
- − V E78.3
- low-density-lipoprotein-type (LDL) E78.0
- very-low-density-lipoprotein-type (VLDL) E78.1

Hyperlysinemia E72.3

Hypermagnesemia E83.4
- neonatal P71.8

Hypermaturity (fetus or newborn) P08.2

Hypermenorrhea N92.0

Hypermethioninemia E72.1

Hypermetropia (congenital) H52.0

Hypermobility, hypermotility
- coccyx M53.2
- meniscus (knee) M23.3
- scapula M25.3
- stomach K31.8
- − psychogenic F45.3
- syndrome M35.7

Hypernasality R49.2

Hypernatremia E87.0

Hypernephroma (M8312/3) C64

Hyperopia H52.0

Hyperorexia nervosa F50.2

Hyperornithinemia E72.4

Hyperosmia R43.1

Hyperosmolality E87.0

Hyperostosis M85.8
- ankylosing (spine) M48.1
- cortical (skull) M85.2
- − infantile M89.8
- frontal, internal of skull M85.2
- interna frontalis M85.2
- monomelic M85.8
- skeletal, diffuse idiopathic M48.1
- skull M85.2
- − congenital Q75.8
- vertebral, ankylosing M48.1

Hyperovarism E28.8

Hyperoxaluria (primary) E74.8

Hyperoxia T59.8

Hyperparathyroidism E21.3
- primary E21.0
- secondary NEC E21.1
- − renal N25.8
- specified NEC E21.2
- tertiary E21.2

Hyperpathia R20.8
Hyperperistalsis R19.2
– psychogenic F45.3
Hyperpermeability, capillary I78.8
Hyperphagia R63.2
Hyperphenylalaninemia NEC E70.1
Hyperphoria (alternating) H50.5
Hyperphosphatemia E83.3
Hyperpiesis, hyperpiesia – *see*
  Hypertension
Hyperpigmentation NEC (*see also*
  Pigmentation) L81.8
– melanin NEC L81.4
– postinflammatory L81.0
Hyperpinealism E34.8
Hyperpituitarism E22.9
Hyperplasia, hyperplastic
– adenoids J35.2
– adrenal (capsule) (cortex) (gland) E27.8
– – with
– – – sexual precocity (male) E25.9
– – – – congenital E25.0
– – – virilism, adrenal E25.9
– – – – congenital E25.0
– – – virilization (female) E25.9
– – – – congenital E25.0
– – congenital E25.0
– – – salt-losing E25.0
– adrenomedullary E27.5
– appendix (lymphoid) K38.0
– artery, fibromuscular I77.3
– bone M89.3
– – marrow D75.8
– breast (*see also* Hypertrophy, breast) N62
– C-cell, thyroid E07.0
– cementation (tooth) (teeth) K03.4
– cervical gland R59.0
– cervix (uteri) (basal cell) (endometrium)
  (polypoid) (*see also* Dysplasia, cervix)
  N87.9
– – congenital Q51.8
– clitoris, congenital Q52.6
– denture K06.2
– endocervicitis N72
– endometrium, endometrial (cystic)
  (glandular) (glandular-cystic) (polypoid)
  N85.0
– – cervix – *see* Dysplasia, cervix
– epithelial L85.9
– – focal, oral, including tongue K13.2
– – nipple N62
– – skin L85.9
– – tongue K13.2
– – vaginal wall N89.3

Hyperplasia, hyperplastic—*continued*
– erythroid D75.8
– genital
– – female NEC N94.8
– – male N50.8
– gingiva K06.1
– glandularis cystica uteri (interstitialis)
  N85.0
– gum K06.1
– hymen, congenital Q52.4
– irritative, edentulous (alveolar) K06.2
– kidney (congenital) Q63.3
– labia N90.6
– – epithelial N90.3
– liver (congenital) Q44.7
– – nodular, focal K76.8
– lymph gland or node R59.9
– mandible, mandibular K07.0
– – unilateral condylar K10.8
– maxilla, maxillary K07.0
– myometrium, myometrial N85.2
– nose
– – lymphoid J34.8
– – polypoid J33.9
– oral mucosa (irritative) K13.6
– organ or site, congenital NEC – *see*
  Anomaly, by site
– ovary N83.8
– palate, papillary (irritative) K13.6
– pancreatic islet cells E16.9
– – alpha E16.8
– – – with excess
– – – – gastrin E16.4
– – – – glucagon E16.3
– – beta E16.1
– parathyroid (gland) E21.0
– pharynx (lymphoid) J39.2
– prostate (adenofibromatous) (nodular)
  N40
– renal artery I77.8
– reticulo-endothelial (cell) D75.8
– salivary gland (any) K11.1
– Schimmelbusch's N60.1
– suprarenal capsule (gland) E27.8
– thymus (gland) (persistent) E32.0
– thyroid (gland) (*see also* Goiter) E04.9
– tonsils (faucial) (infective) (lingual)
  (lymphoid) J35.1
– – with adenoids J35.3
– unilateral condylar K10.8
– uterus, uterine N85.2
– – endometrium (glandular) N85.0
– – – adenomatous N85.1
– – – atypical (adenomatous) N85.1

Hyperplasia, hyperplastic—*continued*
- vulva N90.6
- – epithelial N90.3
Hyperpnea (*see also* Hyperventilation) R06.4
Hyperpotassemia E87.5
Hyperprebetalipoproteinemia (familial) E78.1
Hyperprolactinemia E22.1
Hyperprolinemia (type I) (type II) E72.5
Hyperproteinemia E88.0
Hyperprothrombinemia, causing coagulation factor deficiency D68.4
Hyperpyrexia R50.9
- heat (effects) T67.0
- malignant, due to anesthetic T88.3
- rheumatic – *see* Fever, rheumatic
- unknown origin R50.9
Hyper-reflexia R29.2
Hypersalivation K11.7
Hypersecretion
- ACTH (not associated with Cushing's syndrome) E27.0
- – pituitary E24.0
- adrenaline E27.5
- adrenomedullary E27.5
- androgen (testicular) E29.0
- – ovarian (drug-induced) (iatrogenic) E28.1
- calcitonin E07.0
- catecholamine E27.5
- corticoadrenal E24.9
- cortisol E24.9
- epinephrine E27.5
- estrogen E28.0
- gastric K31.8
- – psychogenic F45.3
- gastrin E16.4
- glucagon E16.3
- hormone(s)
- – ACTH (not associated with Cushing's syndrome) E27.0
- – – pituitary E24.0
- – antidiuretic E22.2
- – growth E22.0
- – intestinal NEC E34.1
- – ovarian androgen E28.1
- – pituitary E22.9
- – testicular E29.0
- – thyroid stimulating E05.8
- insulin – *see* Hyperinsulinism
- lacrimal glands H04.2
- medulloadrenal E27.5
- milk O92.6

Hypersecretion—*continued*
- ovarian androgens E28.1
- salivary gland (any) K11.7
- thyrocalcitonin E07.0
- upper respiratory J39.8
Hypersegmentation, leukocytic, hereditary D72.0
Hypersensitive, hypersensitiveness, hypersensitivity – *see also* Allergy
- carotid sinus G90.0
- drug (*see also* Allergy, drug) T88.7
- gastrointestinal K52.2
- – psychogenic F45.3
- labyrinth H83.2
- pain R20.8
- pneumonitis (*see also* Pneumonitis, allergic) J67.9
- reaction T78.4
- – upper respiratory tract NEC J39.3
Hypersomnia (organic) G47.1
- nonorganic origin F51.1
- primary F51.1
Hypersplenia, hypersplenism D73.1
Hyperstimulation, ovaries (associated with induced ovulation) N98.1
Hypersusceptibility – *see* Allergy
Hypertelorism (ocular) (orbital) Q75.2
Hypertension, hypertensive (accelerated) (benign) (essential) (idiopathic) (malignant) (primary) (systemic) I10
- with
- – heart involvement (conditions in I51.4-I51.9 due to hypertension) (*see also* Hypertension, heart) I11.9
- – kidney involvement (*see also* Hypertension, kidney) I12.9
- – renal sclerosis (conditions in N26.-) (*see also* Hypertension, kidney) I12.9
- – – with
- – – – failure (conditions in N18.-, N19.-) I12.0
- – – – heart involvement (conditions in I51.4-I51.9) – *see* Hypertension, cardiorenal
- benign, intracranial G93.2
- cardiorenal (disease) I13.9
- – with
- – – renal failure I13.1
- – – – and heart failure (congestive) I13.2
- cardiovascular
- – disease (arteriosclerotic) (sclerotic) (*see also* Hypertension, heart) I11.9

Hypertension, hypertensive—*continued*
- cardiovascular—*continued*
- - disease—*continued*
- - - with heart failure
    (congestive) (*see also* Hypertension,
    heart) I11.0
- - - - with renal failure I13.2
- - renal (disease) (sclerosis) (*see also*
    Hypertension, cardiorenal) I13.9
- - - with renal failure I13.1
- - - - with heart failure I13.2
- complicating pregnancy, childbirth or
    puerperium O16
- - with
- - - albuminuria (and edema) (*see also*
    Pre-eclampsia) O14.9
- - - - severe O14.1
- - - edema (*see also* Pre-eclampsia)
    O14.9
- - - - severe O14.1
- - - heart disease O10.1
- - - - and renal disease, pre-existing
    O10.3
- - - renal disease, pre-existing O10.2
- - affecting fetus or newborn P00.0
- - essential (benign), pre-existing O10.0
- - - with superimposed proteinuria O11
- - - malignant, pre-existing O10.0
- - malignant, pre-existing O10.0
- - - with superimposed proteinuria O11
- - pre-existing O10.9
- - - with superimposed proteinuria O11
- - - malignant O10.0
- - pregnancy-induced (*see also*
    Hypertension, gestational) O13
- - secondary to renal disease, pre-existing
    O10.4
- - transient – *see* Hypertension,
    gestational
- due to
- - endocrine disorders I15.2
- - pheochromocytoma I15.2
- - renal disorders NEC I15.1
- - - arterial I15.0
- - renovascular disorders I15.0
- - specified disease NEC I15.8
- encephalopathy I67.4
- gestational (pregnancy-induced) (without
    significant proteinuria) O13
- - with significant proteinuria or
    albuminuria (and edema) (*see also* Pre-
    eclampsia) O14.9
- Goldblatt's I70.1

Hypertension, hypertensive—*continued*
- heart (disease) (conditions in I51.4-I51.9
    due to hypertension) I11.9
- - with
- - - heart failure (congestive) (~~see also~~
    ~~Hypertension, heart~~) I11.0
- - - hypertensive kidney disease
    (conditions in I12) (*see also*
    Hypertension, cardiorenal) I13.9
- - - renal sclerosis (*see also*
    Hypertension, cardiorenal) I13.9
- intracranial (benign) G93.2
- kidney I12.9
- - with
- - - heart involvement (conditions in
    I51.4-I51.9 due to
    Hypertension) (*see also*
    Hypertension, cardiorenal) I13.9
- - - - with heart failure (congestive)
    I13.0
- - - - - with renal failure I13.2
- - - hypertensive heart disease
    (conditions in I11.-) (*see also*
    Hypertension, cardiorenal) I13.9
- - - - with heart failure (congestive)
    I13.0
- - - - - with renal failure I13.2
- - - renal failure I12.0
- lesser circulation I27.0
- maternal (of pregnancy) NEC (*see also*
    Hypertension, complicating pregnancy)
    O16
- newborn P29.2
- - pulmonary (persistent) P29.3
- ocular H40.0
- portal (due to chronic liver disease)
    (idiopathic) K76.6
- - in (due to) schistosomiasis (bilharziasis)
    B65.-† K77.0*
- psychogenic F45.3
- pulmonary (artery) (secondary) NEC
    I27.2
- - of newborn (persistent) P29.3
- - primary (idiopathic) I27.0
- renal (*see also* Hypertension, kidney)
    I12.9
- renovascular I15.0
- secondary NEC I15.9
- - due to
- - - endocrine disorders I15.2
- - - pheochromocytoma I15.2
- - - renal disorders NEC I15.1
- - - - arterial I15.0
- - - renovascular disorders I15.0

Hypertension, hypertensive—*continued*
− secondary NEC—*continued*
− − specified NEC I15.8
Hyperthecosis ovary E28.8
Hyperthermia (of unknown
origin) (*see also* Hyperpyrexia) R50.9
− malignant, due to anesthesia T88.3
  newborn, environmental P81.0
Hyperthyroid (recurrent) – *see*
Hyperthyroidism
Hyperthyroidism (latent) (pre-adult)
(recurrent) E05.9
− with
− − goiter (diffuse) E05.0
− − − adenomatous E05.2
− − − multinodular E05.2
− − − nodular E05.2
− − − uninodular E05.1
− − thyroid nodule (single) E05.1
− neonatal, transitory P72.1
Hypertony, hypertonia, hypertonicity
− bladder N31.8
− congenital P94.1
− stomach K31.8
− − psychogenic F45.3
− uterus, uterine (contractions)
  (complicating delivery) O62.4
− − affecting fetus or newborn P03.6
Hypertrichosis L68.9
− congenital Q84.2
− eyelid H02.8
− lanuginosa Q84.2
− − acquired L68.1
− localized L68.2
− specified NEC L68.8
Hypertriglyceridemia, essential E78.1
Hypertrophy, hypertrophic
− adenofibromatous, prostate N40
− adenoids (infective) J35.2
− − with tonsils J35.3
− adrenal cortex E27.8
− alveolar process or ridge K08.8
− anal papillae K62.8
− artery I77.8
− − congenital NEC Q27.8
− arthritis (*see also* Arthrosis) M19.9
− auricular – *see* Hypertrophy, cardiac
− Bartholin's gland N75.8
− bile duct (common) (hepatic) K83.8
− bladder (sphincter) (trigone) N32.8
− bone M89.3
− brain G93.8
− breast N62
− − cystic N60.1

Hypertrophy, hypertrophic—*continued*
− breast—*continued*
− − cystic—*continued*
− − − with epithelial proliferation N60.3
− − fetus or newborn P83.4
− − pubertal, massive N62
− − puerperal, postpartum O92.2
− − senile (parenchymatous) N62
− cardiac (chronic) (idiopathic) I51.7
− − with rheumatic fever (conditions in I00)
− − − active I01.8
− − − inactive or quiescent (with chorea)
      I09.8
− − congenital NEC Q24.8
− − fatty (*see also* Degeneration,
    myocardial) I51.5
− − hypertensive (*see also* Hypertension,
    heart) I11.9
− − rheumatic (with chorea) I09.8
− − − active or acute I01.8
− − − − with chorea I02.0
− − valve (*see also* Endocarditis) I38
− cartilage M94.8
− cecum (*see also* Megacolon) K59.3
− cervix (uteri) N88.8
− − congenital Q51.8
− − elongation N88.4
− clitoris (cirrhotic) N90.8
− − congenital Q52.6
− colon (*see also* Megacolon) K59.3
− − congenital Q43.2
− conjunctiva, lymphoid H11.8
− corpora cavernosa N48.8
− cystic duct K82.8
− duodenum K31.8
− endometrium (glandular) N85.0
− − atypical (adenomatous) N85.1
− − cervix N88.8
− epididymis N50.8
− esophageal hiatus (congenital) Q79.1
− − with hernia – *see* Hernia, hiatal
− eyelid H02.8
− fat pad E65
− − knee (infrapatellar) (popliteal)
    (prepatellar) (retropatellar) M79.4
− foot (congenital) Q74.2
− frenulum, frenum (tongue) K14.8
− − lip K13.0
− gallbladder K82.8
− gastric mucosa K29.6
− gland, glandular R59.9
− − generalized R59.1
− − localized R59.0
− gum (mucous membrane) K06.1

Hypertrophy, hypertrophic—*continued*
- heart (idiopathic) – *see also* Hypertrophy, cardiac
- – valve – *see* Endocarditis
- hemifacial Q67.4
- hepatic – *see* Hypertrophy, liver
- hiatus (esophageal) Q79.1
- hilus gland R59.0
- hymen, congenital Q52.4
- ileum K63.8
- intestine NEC K63.8
- jejunum K63.8
- kidney (compensatory) N28.8
- – congenital Q63.3
- labium (majus) (minus) N90.6
- ligament M24.2
- lingual tonsil (infective) J35.1
- – with adenoids J35.3
- lip K13.0
- – congenital Q18.6
- liver R16.0
- – acute K76.8
- – cirrhotic – *see* Cirrhosis, liver
- – fatty – *see* Fatty, liver
- lymph, lymphatic gland R59.9
- – generalized R59.1
- – localized R59.0
- – tuberculous – *see* Tuberculosis, lymph gland
- mammary gland – *see* Hypertrophy, breast
- Meckel's diverticulum (congenital) Q43.0
- median bar N40
- meibomian gland H00.1
- meniscus, knee, congenital Q74.1
- metatarsal head M89.3
- metatarsus M89.3
- mucous membrane
- – alveolar ridge K06.2
- – gum K06.1
- – nose (turbinate) J34.3
- muscle M62.8
- muscular coat, artery I77.8
- myocardium (*see also* Hypertrophy, cardiac) I51.7
- – idiopathic I42.2
- myometrium N85.2
- nail L60.2
- – congenital Q84.5
- nasal J34.8
- – alae J34.8
- – bone J34.8
- – cartilage J34.8
- – mucous membrane (septum) J34.8
- – sinus J34.8

Hypertrophy, hypertrophic—*continued*
- nasal—*continued*
- – turbinate J34.3
- nasopharynx, lymphoid (infectional) (tissue) (wall) J35.2
- nipple N62
- organ or site, congenital NEC – *see* Anomaly, by site
- ovary N83.8
- palate (hard) K10.8
- – soft K13.7
- pancreas, congenital Q45.3
- parathyroid (gland) E21.0
- parotid gland K11.1
- penis N48.8
- pharyngeal tonsil J35.2
- pharynx J39.2
- – lymphoid (infectional) (tissue) (wall) J35.2
- pituitary (anterior) (fossa) (gland) E23.6
- prepuce (congenital) N47
- – female N90.8
- prostate (adenofibromatous) (asymptomatic) (benign) (early) (recurrent) N40
- – congenital Q55.4
- pseudomuscular G71.0
- pylorus (adult) (muscle) (sphincter) K31.1
- – congenital or infantile Q40.0
- rectal, rectum (sphincter) K62.8
- rhinitis (turbinate) J31.0
- salivary gland (any) K11.1
- – congenital Q38.4
- scaphoid (tarsal) M89.3
- scar L91.0
- scrotum N50.8
- seminal vesicle N50.8
- sigmoid (*see also* Megacolon) K59.3
- spermatic cord N50.8
- spleen – *see* Splenomegaly
- spondylitis M47.9
- stomach K31.8
- sublingual gland K11.1
- submandibular gland K11.1
- suprarenal cortex (gland) E27.8
- synovial NEC M67.2
- tendon M67.8
- testis N50.8
- – congenital Q55.2
- thymic, thymus (gland) (congenital) E32.0
- thyroid (gland) (*see also* Goiter) E04.9
- toe (congenital) Q74.2

Hypertrophy, hypertrophic—*continued*
- toe—*continued*
- – acquired M20.5
- tongue K14.8
- – congenital Q38.2
- – papillae (foliate) K14.3
- tonsils (faucial) (infective) (lingual) (lymphoid) J35.1
- – with adenoids J35.3
- tunica vaginalis N50.8
- ureter N28.8
- urethra N36.8
- uterus N85.2
- – neck (with elongation) N88.4
- – puerperal O90.8
- uvula K13.7
- vagina N89.8
- vas deferens N50.8
- vein I87.8
- ventricle, ventricular (heart) – *see also* Hypertrophy, cardiac
- – congenital Q24.8
- – in tetralogy of Fallot Q21.3
- verumontanum N36.8
- vocal cord J38.3
- vulva N90.6
- – stasis (nonfilarial) N90.6
Hypertropia H50.2
Hypertyrosinemia E70.2
Hyperuricemia (asymptomatic) E79.0
Hypervalinemia E71.1
Hyperventilation (tetany) R06.4
- hysterical F45.3
- psychogenic F45.3
- syndrome F45.3
Hypervitaminosis (dietary) NEC E67.8
- A E67.0
- – reaction to sudden overdose T45.2
- B$_6$ E67.2
- D E67.3
- – reaction to sudden overdose T45.2
- from excessive administration or use of vitamin preparations (chronic) E67.8
- – reaction to sudden overdose T45.2
- K E67.8
- – overdose or wrong substance given or taken T45.7
Hypervolemia E87.7
Hypesthesia R20.1
- cornea H18.8
Hyphema H21.0
- traumatic S05.1
Hypnotherapy NEC Z50.4

Hypoacidity, gastric K31.8
- psychogenic F45.3
Hypoadrenalism, hypoadrenia E27.4
- primary E27.1
- tuberculous A18.7† E35.1*
Hypoadrenocorticism E27.4
- pituitary E23.0
- primary E27.1
Hypoalbuminemia E88.0
Hypoaldosteronism E27.4
Hypoalphalipoproteinemia E78.6
Hypobarism T70.2
Hypobaropathy T70.2
Hypobetalipoproteinemia (familial) E78.6
Hypocalcemia E83.5
- dietary E58
- neonatal P71.1
- – due to cow's milk P71.0
- phosphate-loading (newborn) P71.1
Hypochloremia E87.8
Hypochlorhydria K31.8
- neurotic F45.3
- psychogenic F45.3
Hypochondria, hypochondriac, hypochondriasis (reaction) F45.2
Hypochondrogenesis Q77.0
Hypochondroplasia Q77.4
Hypochromasia, blood cells D50.8
Hypodontia (*see also* Anodontia) K00.0
Hypoeosinophilia D72.8
Hypoesthesia R20.1
Hypofibrinogenemia D68.8
- acquired D65
- congenital (hereditary) D68.2
Hypofunction
- adrenocortical E27.4
- – drug-induced E27.3
- – postprocedural E89.6
- – primary E27.1
- adrenomedullary, postprocedural E89.6
- cerebral R29.8
- corticoadrenal NEC E27.4
- intestinal K59.8
- labyrinth H83.2
- ovary E28.3
- pituitary (gland) (anterior) E23.0
- testicular E29.1
- – postprocedural (iatrogenic) (postirradiation) (postsurgical) E89.5
Hypogalactia O92.4
Hypogammaglobulinemia (*see also* Agammaglobulinemia) D80.1
- hereditary D80.0
- nonfamilial D80.1

Hypogammaglobulinemia—*continued*
– transient, of infancy D80.7
Hypogenitalism (congenital) – *see*
  Hypogonadism
Hypoglossia Q38.3
Hypoglycemia (spontaneous) E16.2
– coma E15
– – diabetic – *code to* E10-E14 with fourth
    character .0
– dietary counseling and surveillance Z71.3
– drug-induced E16.0
– – with coma (nondiabetic) E15
– due to insulin E16.0
– – with coma (nondiabetic) E15
– – therapeutic misadventure T38.3
– functional, nonhyperinsulinemic E16.1
– iatrogenic E16.0
– – with coma (nondiabetic) E15
– in infant of diabetic mother P70.1
– – gestational diabetes P70.0
– infantile E16.1
– leucine-induced E71.1
– neonatal (transitory) P70.4
– – iatrogenic P70.3
– – maternal diabetes P70.1
– – – gestational P70.0
– reactive (not drug-induced) E16.1
– transitory neonatal P70.4
Hypogonadism
– female E28.3
– hypogonadotropic E23.0
– male E29.1
– ovarian (primary) E28.3
– pituitary E23.0
– testicular (primary) E29.1
Hypohidrosis, hypoidrosis L74.4
Hypoinsulinemia, postprocedural E89.1
Hypokalemia E87.6
Hypoleukocytosis D70
Hypolipoproteinemia (alpha) (beta) E78.6
Hypomagnesemia E83.4
– neonatal P71.2
Hypomania, hypomanic reaction F30.0
Hypomenorrhea (*see also* Oligomenorrhea)
  N91.5
Hypometabolism R63.8
Hypomotility
– gastrointestinal (tract) K31.8
– – psychogenic F45.3
– intestine K59.8
– – psychogenic F45.3
– stomach K31.8
– – psychogenic F45.3
Hyponasality R49.2

Hyponatremia E87.1
Hypo-osmolality E87.1
Hypo-ovarianism, hypo-ovarism E28.3
Hypoparathyroidism E20.9
– familial E20.8
– idiopathic E20.0
– neonatal, transitory P71.4
– postprocedural E89.2
– specified NEC E20.8
Hypopharyngitis (*see also*
  Laryngopharyngitis) J06.0
Hypophoria H50.5
**Hypophosphatemia, hypophosphatasia
  (acquired) (congenital) (familial) (renal)**
  E83.3
Hypophyseal, hypophysis – *see also*
  condition
– dwarfism E23.0
– gigantism E22.0
Hypopiesis – *see* Hypotension
Hypopinealism E34.8
Hypopituitarism (juvenile) E23.0
– drug-induced E23.1
– due to
– – hypophysectomy E89.3
– – radiotherapy E89.3
– iatrogenic NEC E23.1
– postirradiation E89.3
– postpartum E23.0
– postprocedural E89.3
Hypoplasia, hypoplastic
– adrenal (gland), congenital Q89.1
– alimentary tract, congenital Q45.8
– – upper Q40.8
– anus, anal (canal) Q42.3
– – with fistula Q42.2
– aorta, aortic Q25.4
– – ascending, in hypoplastic left heart
    syndrome Q23.4
– – valve Q23.1
– – – in hypoplastic left heart syndrome
      Q23.4
– areola, congenital Q83.8
– arm, meaning upper limb (congenital)
  Q71.9
– artery (peripheral) Q27.8
– – brain (congenital) Q28.3
– – coronary Q24.5
– – pulmonary Q25.7
– – retinal (congenital) Q14.1
– – umbilical Q27.0
– auditory canal Q17.8
– – causing impairment of hearing Q16.9
– biliary duct or passage Q44.5

Hypoplasia, hypoplastic—*continued*
- bone NEC Q79.9
- – face Q75.8
- – marrow D61.9
- – – megakaryocytic D69.4
- – skull (*see also* Hypoplasia, skull)
  Q75.8
- brain Q02
- – gyri Q04.3
- – part of Q04.3
- breast (areola), congenital Q83.8
- bronchus Q32.4
- cardiac Q24.8
- carpus Q71.8
- cartilage-hair – *see* Dysplasia,
  metaphyseal
- cecum Q42.8
- cementum K00.4
- cephalic Q02
- cerebellum Q04.3
- cervix (uteri), congenital Q51.8
- clavicle (congenital) Q74.0
- coccyx Q76.4
- colon Q42.9
- – specified NEC Q42.8
- corpus callosum Q04.0
- cricoid cartilage Q31.2
- digestive organ(s) or tract NEC Q45.8
- – upper (congenital) Q40.8
- ear (auricle) (lobe) Q17.2
- – middle Q16.4
- enamel of teeth (neonatal) (postnatal)
  (prenatal) K00.4
- endocrine (gland) NEC Q89.2
- endometrium N85.8
- epididymis (congenital) Q55.4
- epiglottis Q31.2
- erythroid, congenital D61.0
- esophagus (congenital) Q39.8
- eustachian tube Q16.4
- eye Q11.2
- eyelid (congenital) Q10.3
- face Q18.8
- – bone(s) Q75.8
- femur (congenital) Q72.8
- fibula (congenital) Q72.8
- finger (congenital) Q71.8
- focal dermal Q82.8
- foot Q72.8
- gallbladder Q44.0
- genitalia, genital organ(s)
- – female, congenital Q52.8
- – – external Q52.7
- – – internal NEC Q52.8

Hypoplasia, hypoplastic—*continued*
- genitalia, genital organ(s)—*continued*
- – in adiposogenital dystrophy E23.6
- glottis Q31.2
- hair Q84.2
- hand (congenital) Q71.8
- heart Q24.8
- humerus (congenital) Q71.8
- intestine (small) Q41.9
- – large Q42.9
- – – specified NEC Q42.8
- jaw K07.0
- kidney(s) Q60.5
- – bilateral Q60.4
- – unilateral Q60.3
- labium (majus) (minus), congenital Q52.7
- larynx Q31.2
- left heart syndrome Q23.4
- leg, meaning lower limb (congenital)
  Q72.9
- limb Q73.8
- – lower (congenital) Q72.9
- – upper (congenital) Q71.9
- liver Q44.7
- lung (lobe) (not associated with short
  gestation) Q33.6
- – with immaturity, prematurity or low
  birth weight P28.0
- – associated with short gestation P28.0
- mammary (areola), congenital Q83.8
- mandible, mandibular K07.0
- – unilateral condylar K10.8
- maxillary K07.0
- medullary D61.9
- megakaryocytic D69.4
- metacarpus Q71.8
- metatarsus Q72.8
- muscle Q79.8
- nail(s) Q84.6
- nose, nasal Q30.1
- osseous meatus (ear) Q17.8
- ovary, congenital Q50.3
- pancreas Q45.0
- parathyroid (gland) Q89.2
- parotid gland Q38.4
- patella Q74.1
- pelvis, pelvic girdle Q74.2
- penis (congenital) Q55.6
- peripheral vascular system Q27.8
- pituitary (gland) (congenital) Q89.2
- pulmonary (not associated with short
  gestation) Q33.6
- – associated with short gestation P28.0
- radioulnar Q71.8

Hypoplasia, hypoplastic—*continued*
- radius Q71.8
- rectum Q42.1
- – with fistula Q42.0
- respiratory system NEC Q34.8
- rib Q76.6
- right heart syndrome Q22.6
- sacrum Q76.4
- scapula Q74.0
- scrotum Q55.1
- shoulder girdle Q74.0
- skin Q82.8
- skull (bone) Q75.8
- – with
- – – anencephaly Q00.0
- – – encephalocele (*see also*
    Encephalocele) Q01.9
- – – hydrocephalus Q03.9
- – – – with spina bifida (*see also* Spina
    bifida, with hydrocephalus) Q05.4
- – – microcephaly Q02
- spinal (cord) (ventral horn cell) Q06.1
- spine Q76.4
- sternum Q76.7
- tarsus Q72.8
- testis Q55.1
- thymic, with immunodeficiency D82.1
- thymus (gland) Q89.2
- – with immunodeficiency D82.1
- thyroid (gland) E03.1
- – cartilage Q31.2
- tibiofibular (congenital) Q72.8
- toe Q72.8
- tongue Q38.3
- Turner's K00.4
- ulna (congenital) Q71.8
- umbilical artery Q27.0
- unilateral condylar K10.8
- ureter Q62.8
- uterus, congenital Q51.8
- vagina Q52.4
- vascular, peripheral NEC Q27.8
- – brain Q28.3
- vein(s) (peripheral) Q27.8
- – brain Q28.3
- – great Q26.8
- vena cava (inferior) (superior) Q26.8
- vertebra Q76.4
- vulva, congenital Q52.7
- zonule (ciliary) Q12.8
Hypopotassemia E87.6
**Hypoproconvertinemia, congenital
    (hereditary)** D68.2
Hypoproteinemia E77.8

**Hypoprothrombinemia (congenital)
    (hereditary) (idiopathic)** D68.2
- acquired D68.4
- newborn, transient P61.6
Hypoptyalism K11.7
Hypopyon (eye) (anterior chamber)
    H20.0
Hypopyrexia R68.0
Hyporeflexia R29.2
Hyposecretion
- ACTH E23.0
- antidiuretic hormone E23.2
- ovary E28.3
- salivary gland (any) K11.7
- vasopressin E23.2
Hyposegmentation, leukocytic, hereditary
    D72.0
Hyposiderinemia D50.9
Hyposomnia G47.0
- nonorganic origin F51.0
Hypospadias Q54.9
- balanic Q54.0
- coronal Q54.0
- glandular Q54.0
- penile Q54.1
- penoscrotal Q54.2
- perineal Q54.3
- specified NEC Q54.8
Hypospermatogenesis N46
Hyposplenism D73.0
Hypostasis, pulmonary, passive (*see also*
    Edema, lung) J81
Hypostatic – *see condition*
Hyposthenuria N28.8
Hypotension (arterial) (constitutional)
    I95.9
- chronic I95.8
- drug-induced I95.2
- idiopathic (permanent) I95.0
- intracranial, following ventricular
    shunting (ventriculostomy) G97.2
- maternal, syndrome (following labor and
    delivery) O26.5
- neurogenic, orthostatic G90.3
- orthostatic (chronic) I95.1
- – neurogenic G90.3
- postural I95.1
- specified NEC I95.8
Hypothermia (accidental) (due to) T68
- anesthesia T88.5
- low environmental temperature T68
- neonatal P80.9
- – environmental (mild) NEC P80.8
- – mild P80.8

Hypothermia—*continued*
– neonatal—*continued*
– – severe (chronic) (cold injury syndrome)
   P80.0
– – specified NEC P80.8
– not associated with low environmental
   temperature R68.0
Hypothyroidism (acquired) E03.9
– congenital (without goiter) E03.1
– – with goiter (diffuse) E03.0
– due to
– – exogenous substance NEC E03.2
– – iodine-deficiency (acquired) NEC
   E01.8
– – – subclinical E02
– – irradiation therapy E89.0
– – medicament NEC E03.2
– – P-aminosalicylic acid (PAS) E03.2
– – phenylbutazone E03.2
– – resorcinol E03.2
– – sulfonamide E03.2
– – surgery E89.0
– – thiourea group drugs E03.2
– iatrogenic NEC E03.2
– iodine-deficiency (acquired) NEC E01.8
– – congenital (*see also* Syndrome, iodine-
   deficiency, congenital) E00.9
– – subclinical E02
– neonatal, transitory P72.2
– postinfectious E03.3
– postirradiation E89.0
– postprocedural E89.0
– postsurgical E89.0
– specified NEC E03.8
– subclinical, iodine-deficiency-related E02
Hypotonia, hypotonicity, hypotony
– bladder N31.2
– congenital (benign) P94.2

Hypotonia, hypotonicity—*continued*
– eye H44.4
Hypotrichosis (*see also* Alopecia) L65.9
– congenital Q84.0
– due to cytotoxic drugs NEC L65.8
– postinfective NEC L65.8
Hypotropia H50.2
Hypoventilation R06.8
Hypovitaminosis (*see also* Deficiency,
   vitamin) E56.9
– A E50.9
Hypovolemia E86
– surgical shock T81.1
– traumatic (shock) T79.4
Hypoxia – *see also* Anoxia
– cerebral, during or resulting from a
   procedure NEC G97.8
– fetal – *see* Distress, fetal
– – affecting management of pregnancy
   (unrelated to labor or delivery) O36.3
– intrauterine P20.9
– – first noted
– – – before onset of labor P20.0
– – – during labor and delivery P20.1
– myocardial (*see also* Insufficiency,
   coronary) I24.8
– newborn (*see also* Asphyxia, newborn)
   P21.9
Hypsarhythmia G40.4
Hysteralgia, pregnant uterus O26.8
Hysterectomy, cesarean O82.2
Hysteria, hysterical (conversion)
   (dissociative state) F44.9
– anxiety F41.8
– convulsions F44.5
– psychosis, acute F44.9
Hysteroepilepsy F44.5
Hysterotomy, affecting fetus or newborn
   P03.8

I

Ichthyoparasitism due to Vandellia cirrhosa B88.8
Ichthyosis (congenital) Q80.9
– acquired L85.0
– fetalis Q80.4
– hystrix Q80.8
– lamellar Q80.2
– palmaris and plantaris Q82.8
– simplex Q80.0
– vera Q80.8
– vulgaris Q80.0
– X-linked Q80.1
Ichthyotoxism T61.2
– bacterial (*see also* Intoxication, foodborne) A05.9
– due to
– – ciguatera T61.0
– – scombroid T61.1
– – seafood NEC T61.8
– – shellfish NEC T61.2
Icteroanemia, hemolytic (acquired) D59.9
– congenital (*see also* Spherocytosis) D58.0
Icterus (*see also* Jaundice) R17
– hematogenous (acquired) D59.9
– hemolytic (acquired) D59.9
– – congenital (*see also* Spherocytosis) D58.0
– hemorrhagic (acute) (leptospiral) (spirochetal) A27.0
– neonatorum (*see also* Jaundice, fetus or newborn) P59.9
Ictus solaris, solis T67.0
Ideation, suicidal R45.8
– constituting part of a mental disorder – *see condition*
Id reaction (due to bacteria) L30.2
Idioglossia F80.0
Idiopathic – *see condition*
Idiosyncrasy (*see also* Allergy) T78.4
– drug, medicament and biological – *see* Allergy, drug
Idiot, idiocy (congenital) F73.-
– amaurotic (Bielschowsky(-Jansky)) (familial) (infantile (late)) (juvenile (late)) (Vogt-Spielmeyer) E75.4
Ileitis (*see also* Enteritis) A09.9
– backwash K51.0
– infectious A09.0
– noninfectious K52.9

Ileitis—*continued*
– regional or terminal (ulcerative) K50.0
Ileocolitis (*see also* Enteritis) A09.9
– infectious A09.0
– noninfectious K52.9
– ulcerative (chronic) K51.0
Ileostomy
– attention to Z43.2
– malfunctioning K91.4
– status Z93.2
Ileotyphus A01.0
Ileum – *see condition*
Ileus (bowel) (colon) (inhibitory) (intestine) (neurogenic) K56.7
– adynamic K56.0
– due to gallstone (in intestine) K56.3
– duodenal (chronic) K31.5
– mechanical NEC K56.6
– meconium (with cystic fibrosis) E84.1† P75*
– – meaning meconium plug P76.0
– – without cystic fibrosis P76.0
– neurogenic K65.0
– – Hirschsprung's disease or megacolon Q43.1
– newborn
– – due to meconium (with cystic fibrosis) E84.1† P75*
– – – meaning meconium plug P76.0
– – – without cystic fibrosis P76.0
– – transitory P76.1
– obstructive NEC K56.6
– paralytic K56.0
Iliac – *see condition*
Illegitimacy (unwanted pregnancy) Z64.0
– supervision of high-risk pregnancy Z35.7
Illiteracy Z55.0
Illness (*see also* Disease) R69
Imbalance R26.8
– autonomic G90.8
– constituents of food intake E63.1
– electrolyte E87.8
– – due to hyperemesis gravidarum O21.1
– – following abortion O08.5
– – neonatal, transitory NEC P74.4
– – – potassium P74.3
– – – sodium P74.2
– endocrine E34.9
– eye muscle NEC H50.9

Imbalance—*continued*
- hormone E34.9
- hysterical F44.4
- labyrinth H83.2
- posture R29.3
- protein-energy (*see also* Malnutrition) E46
- sympathetic G90.8

Imbecile, imbecility (I.Q. 35-49) F71.-
Imbrication, teeth K07.3
Imerslund(-Gräsbeck) syndrome D51.1
Immature – *see also* Immaturity
- birth (28 completed weeks or more but less than 37 completed weeks) P07.3
- – extremely (less than 28 completed weeks) P07.2
- personality F60.8

Immaturity (28 completed weeks or more but less than 37 completed weeks) P07.3
- extreme (less than 28 completed weeks) P07.2
- fetus or infant light-for-dates – *see* Light-for-dates
- organ or site NEC – *see* Hypoplasia
- pulmonary, fetus or newborn P28.0
- reaction F61
- sexual (female) (male), after puberty E30.0

Immersion T75.1
- foot or hand T69.0

Immobility
- due to prolonged bedrest R26.3
- syndrome (paraplegic) M62.3

Immune compromised NEC D89.9
Immune reconstitution syndrome D89.3
Immunization (*see also* Vaccination) Z26.9
- ABO (*see also* Isoimmunization, ABO)
- – affecting management of pregnancy O36.1
- – – in fetus or newborn P55.1
- complication – *see* Complications, vaccination
- Rh factor – *see also* Isoimmunization, Rh
- – affecting management of pregnancy O36.0
- – from transfusion T80.4

Immunocytoma C83.0
Immunodeficiency D84.9
- with
- – antibody defects D80.9
- – – specified type NEC D80.8
- – increased immunoglobulin in M (IgM) D80.5

Immunodeficiency—*continued*
- with—*continued*
- – major defect D82.9
- – – specified type NEC D82.8
- – partial albinism D82.8
- – short-limbed stature D82.2
- – thrombocytopenia and eczema D82.0
- antibody with
- – hyperimmunoglobulinemia D80.6
- – near-normal immunoglobulins D80.6
- combined D81.9
- – severe (SCID) D81.9
- – – with
- – – – low or normal B-cell numbers D81.2
- – – – low T- and B-cell numbers D81.1
- – – – reticular dysgenesis D81.0
- – specified type NEC D81.8
- common variable D83.9
- – with
- – – abnormalities of B-cell numbers and function D83.0
- – – autoantibodies to B- or T-cells D83.2
- – – immunoregulatory T-cell disorders D83.1
- – specified type NEC D83.8
- following hereditary defective response to Epstein-Barr virus (EBV) D82.3
- selective, immunoglobulin
- – A (IgA) D80.2
- – G (IgG) (subclasses) D80.3
- – M (IgM) D80.4
- specified type NEC D84.8

Immunotherapy, prophylactic Z29.1
Impaction, impacted
- bowel, colon or rectum (fecal) K56.4
- calculus – *see* Calculus
- cerumen (ear) (external) H61.2
- dental K01.1
- fecal, feces K56.4
- fracture – *see* Fracture, by site
- gallbladder (*see also* Cholelithiasis) K80.2
- gallstone(s) (*see also* Cholelithiasis) K80.2
- – bile duct (common) (hepatic) K80.5
- – cystic duct K80.2
- – in intestine, with obstruction (any part) K56.3
- intestine (calculous) (fecal) NEC K56.4
- – gallstone, with ileus K56.3
- molar – *see* Impaction, tooth
- shoulder O66.0

Impaction, impacted—*continued*
– shoulder—*continued*
– – affecting fetus or newborn P03.1
– – causing obstructed labor O66.0
– tooth, teeth K01.1
– – with abnormal position (same or
    adjacent tooth) K07.3
– turbinate J34.8
Impaired, impairment (function)
– auditory discrimination H93.2
– cognitive   *see also*
– – mild F06.7   *decline*
– – persisting (due to)
– – – alcohol F10.7
– – – hallucinogen use F16.7
– – – sedatives F13.7
– glucose tolerance R73.0
– hearing – *see* Deafness
– heart – *see* Disease, heart
– kidney (*see also* Failure, kidney) N19
– – acute N17.-
– – chronic N18.9
– – – end-stage N18.5
– – – stage 1 N18.1
– – – stage 2 N18.2
– – – stage 3 N18.3
– – – stage 4 N18.4
– – – stage 5 N18.5
– – end-stage N18.5
– – tubular function disorder N25.9
– – neonatal, transient P74.8
– liver K72.9
– mastication K08.8
– mobility
– – ear ossicles H74.3
– – requiring care provider Z74.0
– myocardium, myocardial (*see also*
    Insufficiency, myocardial) I50.9
– rectal sphincter R19.8
– renal – *see* Impaired, kidney
– – acute N17.-
– – disorder resulting from N25.9
– tolerance, glucose R73.0
– vision NEC H54.9
– visual
– – binocular H54.9
– – – mild H54.3
– – – moderate H54.2
– – – severe H54.1
– – monocular
– – – moderate H54.6
– – – severe H54.5
Impediment, speech NEC R47.8
– psychogenic (childhood) F98.8

Imperception auditory
  (acquired) (*see also* Deafness) H91.9
– congenital F80.2
Imperfect
– aeration, lung (newborn) NEC P28.1
– closure (congenital)
– – atrioventricular ostium Q21.2
– – branchial cleft or sinus Q18.0
– – choroid Q14.3
– – cricoid cartilage Q31.8
– – cusps, heart valve NEC Q24.8
– – ductus
– – – arteriosus Q25.0
– – – Botalli Q25.0
– – ear drum (causing impairment of
    hearing) Q16.4
– – esophagus with communication to
    bronchus or trachea Q39.1
– – eyelid Q10.3
– – foramen
–   botalli Q21.1
– – – ovale Q21.1
– – genitalia, genital organ(s) or system
– – – female Q52.8
– – – – external Q52.7
– – – – internal NEC Q52.8
– – – male Q55.8
– – glottis Q31.8
– – larynx Q31.8
– – lip (*see also* Cleft, lip) Q36.9
– – nasal septum Q30.3
– – nose Q30.2
– – omphalomesenteric duct Q43.0
– – optic nerve entry Q14.2
– – organ or site not listed – *see* Anomaly,
    by site
– – ostium
– – – interatrial Q21.1
– – – interauricular Q21.1
– – palate (*see also* Cleft, palate) Q35.9
– – preauricular sinus Q18.1
– – retina Q14.1
– – roof of orbit Q75.8
– – septum
– – – aortopulmonary Q21.4
– – – atrial Q21.1
– – – between aorta and pulmonary artery
        Q21.4
– – – heart Q21.9
– – – interatrial Q21.1
– – – interauricular Q21.1
– – – interventricular Q21.0
– – – – in tetralogy of Fallot Q21.3
– – – nasal Q30.3

Imperfect—*continued*
- closure—*continued*
- − septum—*continued*
- − − ventricular Q21.0
- − − − in tetralogy of Fallot Q21.3
- − − skull Q75.0
- − − with
- − − − anencephaly Q00.0
- − − − encephalocele (*see also*
      Encephalocele) Q01.9
- − − − hydrocephalus Q03.9
- − − − − with spina bifida (*see also* Spina
        bifida, with hydrocephalus)
        Q05.4
- − − − microcephaly Q02
- − − spine (with meningocele) (*see also*
      Spina bifida) Q05.9
- − − trachea Q32.1
- − − tympanic membrane (causing
      impairment of hearing) Q16.4
- − − uterus Q51.8
- − − vitelline duct Q43.0
- − erection N48.4
- − fusion – *see* Imperfect, closure
- − posture R29.3
- − rotation, intestine Q43.3
- − septum, ventricular Q21.0

Imperfectly descended testis Q53.9
- bilateral Q53.2
- unilateral Q53.1

Imperforate (congenital) – *see also* Atresia
- anus Q42.3
- − with fistula Q42.2
- cervix (uteri) Q51.8
- esophagus Q39.0
- − with tracheoesophageal fistula Q39.1
- hymen Q52.3
- jejunum Q41.1
- pharynx Q38.8
- rectum Q42.1
- − with fistula Q42.0
- urethra Q64.3
- vagina Q52.4

Impervious (congenital) – *see also* Atresia
- anus Q42.3
- − with fistula Q42.2
- bile duct Q44.2
- esophagus Q39.0
- − with tracheoesophageal fistula Q39.1
- intestine (small) Q41.9
- − large Q42.9
- − − specified NEC Q42.8
- rectum Q42.1
- − with fistula Q42.0

Impervious—*continued*
- ureter Q62.1
- urethra Q64.3

Impetiginization of dermatoses NEC
  L01.1

Impetigo (any organism) (any site)
  (circinate) (contagiosa) (simplex) L01.0
- Bockhart's L01.0
- bullous, bullosa L01.0
- external ear L01.0† H62.4∗
- eyelid L01.0† H03.8∗
- follicularis L01.0
- herpetiformis L40.1
- neonatorum L01.0
- ulcerative L01.0
- vulgaris L01.0

Implantation
- anomalous – *see* Anomaly, by site
- − ureter Q62.6
- cyst
- − external area or site (skin) NEC L72.0
- − iris H21.3
- − vagina N89.8
- − vulva N90.7
- dermoid (cyst) – *see* Implantation, cyst
- ovum (in vitro fertilization) Z31.2
- placenta, low or marginal (*see also*
  Placenta, previa) O44.1

Impotence (sexual) (psychogenic) F52.2
- counseling Z70.1
- organic origin NEC N48.4

Impression, basilar Q75.8
Imprisonment, anxiety concerning Z65.1
Improper care (child) (newborn) T74.0
Improperly tied umbilical cord (causing
  hemorrhage) P51.8
Inaccessible, inaccessibility
- health care NEC Z75.3
- − due to
- − − waiting period Z75.2
- − − − for admission to facility elsewhere
      Z75.1
- other helping agencies Z75.4

Inactive – *see* condition
Inadequate, inadequacy
- biologic, constitutional, functional or
  social F60.7
- development
- − child R62.8
- − fetus P05.9
- − − affecting management of pregnancy
      O36.5
- − genitalia
- − − after puberty NEC E30.0

Inadequate, inadequacy—*continued*
- development—*continued*
- – genitalia—*continued*
- – – congenital
- – – – female Q52.8
- – – – – external Q52.7
- – – – – internal Q52.8
- – – – male Q55.8
- – lungs Q33.6
- – – associated with short gestation P28.0
- – organ or site not listed – *see* Anomaly, by site
- diet (causing nutritional deficiency) E63.9
- drinking-water supply Z58.6
- eating habits Z72.4
- family support Z63.2
- food (supply) NEC Z59.4
- – hunger effects T73.0
- household care, due to
- – family member
- – – handicapped or ill Z74.2
- – – on vacation Z75.5
- – – temporarily away from home Z74.2
- – technical defects in home Z59.1
- – temporary absence from home of person rendering care Z74.2
- housing (heating) (space) Z59.1
- income (financial) Z59.6
- intrafamilial communication Z63.8
- material resources Z59.6
- mental (*see also* Retardation, mental) F79.-
- parental supervision or control of child Z62.0
- personality F60.7
- prenatal care, affecting management of pregnancy Z35.3
- pulmonary
- – function R06.8
- – – newborn P28.5
- – ventilation, newborn P28.5
- social
- – insurance Z59.7
- – skills NEC Z73.4
- supervision of child by parent Z62.0
- teaching affecting education Z55.8
- welfare support Z59.7

Inanition R64
- with edema (*see also* Malnutrition, severe) E43
- due to
- – deprivation of food T73.0

Inanition—*continued*
- due to—*continued*
- – malnutrition (*see also* Malnutrition) E46
- fever R50.9

Inappropriate diet or eating habits Z72.4

Inattention at or after birth T74.0

Incarceration, incarcerated
- hernia (*see also* Hernia, by site, with obstruction) K46.0
- – with gangrene (*see also* Hernia, by site, with gangrene) K46.1
- iris, in wound S05.2
- lens, in wound S05.2
- prison, anxiety concerning Z65.1
- uterus N85.8
- – gravid O34.5
- – – causing obstructed labor O65.5

Incineration (entire body) (from fire, conflagration, electricity or lightning) T29.-

Incised wound
- external – *see* Wound, open
- internal organs – *see* Injury, by site

Incision, incisional
- hernia – *see* Hernia, ventral
- surgical, complication – *see* Complications, surgical procedure
- traumatic
- – external – *see* Wound, open
- – internal organs – *see* Injury, by site

Inclusion, gallbladder in liver (congenital) Q44.1

Incompatibility
- ABO
- – affecting management of pregnancy O36.1
- – fetus or newborn P55.1
- – infusion or transfusion reaction T80.3
- blood (group) (Duffy) (K(ell)) (Kidd) (Lewis) (M) (S) NEC
- – affecting management of pregnancy O36.1
- – fetus or newborn P55.8
- – infusion or transfusion reaction T80.3
- Rh (blood group) (factor)
- – affecting management of pregnancy O36.0
- – fetus or newborn P55.0
- – infusion or transfusion reaction T80.4
- rhesus – *see* Incompatibility, Rh

Incompetency, incompetent
- annular
- − − aortic (valve) (*see also* Insufficiency, aortic) I35.1
- − − mitral (valve) I34.0
- − − pulmonary valve (heart) I37.1
- aortic (valve) (*see also* Insufficiency, aortic) I35.1
- − − syphilitic A52.0† I39.1*
- cardiac valve − *see* Endocarditis
- cervix, cervical (os) N88.3
- − − in pregnancy O34.3
- − − − affecting fetus or newborn P01.0
- mitral (valve) − *see* Insufficiency, mitral
- pelvic fundus N81.8
- pulmonary valve (heart) I37.1
- tricuspid (annular) (valve) (*see also* Insufficiency, tricuspid) I07.1
- − − nonrheumatic (*see also* Insufficiency, tricuspid, nonrheumatic) I36.1
- valvular − *see* Endocarditis

Incomplete − *see also condition*
- expansion, lungs (newborn) NEC P28.1
- rotation, intestine Q43.3

Incontinence R32
- anal sphincter R15
- feces, fecal R15
- − − nonorganic origin F98.1
- overflow N39.4
- psychogenic F45.8
- reflex N39.4
- stress (female) (male) N39.3
- urethral sphincter R32
- urge N39.4
- urine, urinary R32
- − − nonorganic origin F98.0
- − − specified NEC N39.4
- − − stress (female) (male) N39.3

Incontinentia pigmenti Q82.3

Incoordinate, incoordination
- muscular R27.8
- uterus (action) (contractions) (complicating delivery) O62.4
- − − affecting fetus or newborn P03.6

Increase, increased
- anticoagulants (antithrombin) (anti-VIIIa) (anti-IXa) (anti-Xa) (anti-XIa) (*see also* Circulating anticoagulants) D68.3
- cold sense R20.8
- estrogen E28.0
- function
- − adrenal
- − − cortex − *see* Cushing's syndrome
- − − medulla E27.5

Increase, increased—*continued*
- function—*continued*
- − − pituitary (gland) (anterior) (lobe) E22.9
- heat sense R20.8
- intracranial pressure (benign) G93.2
- permeability, capillaries I78.8
- secretion
- − − gastrin E16.4
- − − glucagon E16.3
- − − pancreas, endocrine E16.9
- − − − growth hormone-releasing hormone E16.8
- − − − pancreatic polypeptide E16.8
- − − − somatostatin E16.8
- − − − vasoactive-intestinal polypeptide E16.8
- sphericity, lens Q12.4
- splenic activity D73.1
- venous pressure I87.8

Incrustation, cornea, foreign body T15.0

Incyclophoria H50.5

Incyclotropia H50.4

Indeterminate sex Q56.4

India rubber skin Q82.8

Indigestion (acid) (bilious) (functional) K30
- nervous F45.3
- psychogenic F45.3

Indirect − *see condition*

Induction of labor, affecting fetus or newborn P03.8

Induratio penis plastica N48.6

Induration, indurated
- brain G93.8
- breast (fibrous) N64.5
- − − puerperal, postpartum O92.2
- broad ligament N83.8
- corpora cavernosa (penis) (plastic) N48.6
- liver (chronic) K76.8
- lung (chronic) (fibroid) (*see also* Fibrosis, lung) J84.1
- penile (plastic) N48.6
- phlebitic − *see* Phlebitis
- skin R23.4

Inebriety F10.0

Inefficiency, kidney (*see also* Failure, renal) N19

Inequality, leg (length) (acquired) M21.7
- congenital Q72.9

Inertia
- bladder (neurogenic) N31.2
- stomach K31.8
- − − psychogenic F45.3
- uterus, uterine during labor O62.2

Inertia—*continued*
- uterus, uterine during labor—*continued*
- − − affecting fetus or newborn P03.6
- − − primary O62.0
- − − secondary O62.1
- − vesical (neurogenic) N31.2

Infancy, infantile, infantilism – *see also* condition
- celiac K90.0
- genitalia, genitals (after puberty) E30.0
- − − in pregnancy or childbirth NEC O34.8
- − − − affecting fetus or newborn P03.8
- − − − causing obstructed labor O65.5
- Lorain(-Levi) E23.0
- pancreatic K86.8
- pelvis M95.5
- − − with disproportion (fetopelvic) O33.1
- − − − affecting fetus or newborn P03.1
- − − − causing obstructed labor O65.1
- pituitary E23.0
- renal N25.0
- uterus (*see also* Infancy, genitalia) E30.0

Infant(s) – *see also* Infancy
- excessive crying R68.1
- irritable child R68.1
- lack of care T74.0
- liveborn (singleton) Z38.2
- − born
- − − − in hospital Z38.0
- − − − outside hospital Z38.1
- − multiple NEC Z38.8
- − − − born
- − − − − in hospital Z38.6
- − − − − outside hospital Z38.7
- − − twin Z38.5
- − − − born
- − − − − in hospital Z38.3
- − − − − outside hospital Z38.4
- of diabetic mother (syndrome of) P70.1
- − − gestational diabetes P70.0

Infarct, infarction (of)
- adrenal (capsule) (gland) E27.4
- bowel K55.0
- brain (*see also* Infarct, cerebral) I63.9
- − − embolic I63.4
- − − puerperal, postpartum or in chilbirth or pregnancy O99.4
- breast N64.8
- cardiac (*see also* Infarct, myocardium) I21.9
- cerebellar (*see also* Infarct, cerebral) I63.9
- − − embolic I63.4
- cerebral (hemorrhagic) I63.9

Infarct, infarction—*continued*
- cerebral—*continued*
- − − due to
- − − − cerebral venous thrombosis, nonpyogenic I63.6
- − − − embolism (hemorrhagic)
- − − − − cerebral arteries I63.4
- − − − − precerebral arteries I63.1
- − − − occlusion NEC
- − − − − cerebral arteries I63.5
- − − − − precerebral arteries I63.2
- − − − stenosis NEC
- − − − − cerebral arteries I63.5
- − − − − precerebral arteries I63.2
- − − − thrombosis (hemorrhagic)
- − − − − cerebral arteries I63.3
- − − − − precerebral arteries I63.0
- − − specified NEC I63.8
- colon K55.0
- coronary artery (*see also* Infarct, myocardium) I21.9
- embolic (*see also* Embolism) I74.9
- fallopian tube N83.8
- heart (*see also* Infarct, myocardium) I21.9
- hepatic K76.3
- hypophysis (anterior lobe) E23.6
- intestine (acute) (agnogenic) (hemorrhagic) (nonocclusive) (transmural) K55.0
- kidney N28.0
- liver K76.3
- lung (embolic) (thrombotic) (*see also* Embolism, pulmonary) I26.9
- lymph node I89.8
- mesentery, mesenteric (embolic) (thrombotic) K55.0
- muscle (ischemic) M62.2
- myocardium, myocardial (acute or with a stated duration of 4 weeks or less) I21.9
- − − chronic or with a stated duration of over 4 weeks I25.8
- − − healed or old I25.2
- − − nontransmural I21.4
- − − past (diagnosed on ECG or other special investigation, but currently presenting no symptoms) I25.2
- − − subsequent (extension) (recurrent) (reinfarction) I22.9
- − − − anterior (wall) I22.0
- − − − diaphragmatic (wall) I22.1
- − − − inferior (wall) I22.1
- − − − specified NEC I22.8
- − − syphilitic A52.0† I52.0*

Infarct, infarction—*continued*
- myocardium, myocardial—*continued*
- - transmural I21.3
- - - anterior (wall) (anteroapical)
(anterolateral) (anteroseptal) I21.0
- - - inferior (wall) (diaphragmatic)
(inferolateral) (inferoposterior) I21.1
- - - lateral (wall) I21.2
- - - posterior (true) I21.2
- - - septal I21.2
- - - specified NEC I21.2
- nontransmural I21.4
- omentum K55.0
- ovary N83.8
- papillary muscle – *see* Infarct,
myocardium
- pituitary (gland) E23.6
- placenta (complicating pregnancy) O43.8
- - affecting fetus or newborn P02.2
- prostate N42.8
- pulmonary (artery) (vein)
(hemorrhagic) (*see also* Embolism,
pulmonary) I26.9
- - complicating pregnancy, childbirth or
puerperium – *see* Embolism, obstetric
- renal (embolic) (thrombotic) N28.0
- retina, retinal (artery) H34.2
- spinal (cord) (acute) (embolic)
(nonembolic) G95.1
- spleen D73.5
- - embolic or thrombotic I74.8
- subchorionic – *see* Infarct, placenta
- subendocardial (acute) (nontransmural)
I21.4
- suprarenal (capsule) (gland) E27.4
- thrombotic (*see also* Thrombosis) I82.9
- - artery, arterial – *see* Embolism
- thyroid (gland) E07.8
- ventricle (heart) (*see also* Infarct,
myocardium) I21.9

Infecting – *see* condition
Infection, infected (opportunistic) B99

Note: Parasitic diseases may be described as
either "infections" or "infestations"; both
lead terms should therefore be consulted.

- with
- - antibiotic-resistant bacterial agent
(resistant to) U89.9
- - - methicillin U80.1
- - - multiple antibiotics U88
- - - penicillin U80.0
- - - penicillin-related antibiotic U80.8

Infection, infected—*continued*
- with—*continued*
- - antibiotic-resistant bacterial agent—
continued
- - - specified antibiotic (single) NEC
U89.8
- - - - multiple antibiotics U88
- - - vancomycin U81.0
- - - vancomycin-related antibiotics
U81.8
- - lymphangitis – *see* Lymphangitis
- abortion (subsequent episode) O08.0
- - current episode – *see* Abortion
- abscess (skin) – *see* Abscess, by site
- Absidia (*see also* Mucormycosis) B46.5
- Acanthocheilonema (perstans)
(streptocerca) B74.4
- accessory sinus (chronic) (*see also*
Sinusitis) J32.9
- achorion – *see* Dermatophytosis
- Acremonium falciforme B47.0
- acromioclavicular M00.9
- Actinobacillus (actinomycetem-comitans)
A28.8
- Actinomadura B47.1
- Actinomyces (israelii) (*see also*
Actinomycosis) A42.9
- - actinomycetoma B47.1
- Actinomycetales – *see* Actinomycosis
- actinomycotic NEC (*see also*
Actinomycosis) A42.9
- adenoid (and tonsil) J03.9
- - chronic J35.0
- adenovirus NEC
- - as cause of disease classified elsewhere
B97.0
- - unspecified nature or site B34.0
- alimentary canal NEC (*see also* Enteritis,
infectious) A09.0
- Allescheria boydii B48.2
- Alternaria B48.7
- alveolus, alveolar (process) K04.7
- amebic – *see* Amebiasis
- amniotic fluid, sac or cavity O41.1
- - affecting fetus or newborn P02.7
- Amoeba (histolytica), amoebiasis – *see*
Amebiasis
- amputation stump (surgical) T87.4
- Ancylostoma (duodenale) B76.0
- Angiostrongylus
- - cantonensis B83.2
- - costaricensis B81.3
- anisakiasis, Anisakis larvae B81.0
- anthrax (*see also* Anthrax) A22.9

Infection, infected—*continued*
- antrum (chronic) (*see also* Sinusitis, maxillary) J32.0
- anus, anal (papillae) (sphincter) K62.8
- arbovirus (arborvirus) A94
- – specified type NEC A93.8
- artificial insemination N98.0
- Ascaris lumbricoides (*see also* Ascariasis) B77.9
- Ascomycetes B47.0
- Aspergillus (flavus) (fumigatus) (terreus) (*see also* Aspergillosis) B44.9
- atypical mycobacteria – *see* Mycobacterium, atypical
- auditory meatus (diffuse) (external) H60.3
- auricle (ear) H60.3
- axillary gland (lymph) L04.2
- Bacillus, bacillus NEC A49.9
- – anthracis (*see also* Anthrax) A22.9
- – Ducrey's (any location) A57
- – Flexner's A03.1
- – fragilis, as cause of disease classified elsewhere B96.6
- – Friedländer's NEC A49.8
- – gas (gangrene) A48.0
- – Shiga(-Kruse) A03.0
- – welchii (*see also* Gangrene, gas) A48.0
- bacterial NEC A49.9
- – agent NEC
- – – as cause of disease classified elsewhere B96.8
- – – resistant to antibiotic – *see* Resistance (to), antibiotic(s), by antibiotic agent
- – resulting from HIV disease B20.1
- – specified NEC A48.8
- Bacteroides NEC A49.8
- Balantidium coli A07.0
- Bartholin's gland N75.8
- Basidiobolus B46.8
- bile duct (common) (hepatic) (*see also* Cholangitis) K83.0
- bladder (*see also* Cystitis) N30.9
- Blastomyces, blastomycotic (*see also* Blastomycosis) B40.9
- – brasiliensis (*see also* Paracoccidioidomycosis) B41.9
- – dermatitidis (*see also* Blastomycosis) B40.9
- – European (*see also* Cryptococcosis) B45.9
- – North American B40.9

Infection, infected—*continued*
- Blastomyces, blastomycotic—*continued*
- – – South American (*see also* Paracoccidioidomycosis) B41.9
- bleb
- – postprocedural H59.8
- bloodstream – *see* Sepsis
- bone NEC M86.9
- Bordetella – *see also* Whooping cough
- – pertussis A37.0
- brain (*see also* Encephalitis) G04.9
- – membranes (*see also* Meningitis) G03.9
- – septic G06.0
- – – meninges (*see also* Meningitis) G00.9
- branchial cyst Q18.0
- breast – *see* Mastitis
- bronchus (*see also* Bronchitis) J40
- Brucella A23.9
- – abortus A23.1
- – canis A23.3
- – melitensis A23.0
- – mixed A23.8
- – specified NEC A23.8
- – suis A23.2
- Brugia (malayi) B74.1
- – timori B74.2
- Burkholderia NEC A49.8
- – mallei A24.0
- – – as the cause of disease classified elsewhere B96.8
- – pseudomallei (*see also* Melioidosis) A24.4
- – – as the cause of disease classified elsewhere B96.8
- bursa – *see* Bursitis, infective
- buttocks (skin) L08.9
- Campylobacter, intestinal A04.5
- Candida (albicans) (tropicalis) (*see also* Candidiasis) B37.9
- – neonatal P37.5
- – resulting from HIV disease B20.4
- candiru B88.8
- Capillaria (intestinal) B81.1
- – hepatica B83.8
- – philippinensis B81.1
- cartilage M94.8
- cat liver fluke B66.0
- cellulitis – *see* Cellulitis, by site
- Cephalosporium falciforme B47.0
- cervical gland (lymph) L04.0
- cervix (*see also* Cervicitis) N72

Infection, infected—*continued*
- cesarean section wound (puerperal)
  O86.0
- cestodes – *see* Infestation, cestodes
- chest J22
- Chilomastix (intestinal) A07.8
- Chlamydia, chlamydial A74.9
- – anus A56.3
- – genitourinary tract A56.2† N29.1*
- – – lower A56.0
- – – specified NEC A56.1† N29.1*
- – lymphogranuloma A55
- – pharynx A56.4
- – psittaci A70
- – rectum A56.3
- – sexually transmitted NEC A56.8
- Cladosporium
- – bantianum (brain abscess) B43.1†
  G07*
- – carrionii B43.0† L99.8*
- – castellanii B36.1
- – trichoides (brain abscess) B43.1† G07*
- – werneckii B36.1
- Clonorchis (sinensis) (liver) B66.1
- Clostridium, clostridium
- – bifermentans A48.0
- – botulinum A05.1
- – congenital P39.8
- – difficile
- – – as cause of disease classified
  elsewhere B96.8
- – – foodborne (disease) A04.7
- – – gas gangrene A48.0
- – – necrotizing enterocolitis A04.7
- – – sepsis A41.4
- – gas-forming NEC A48.0
- – histolyticum A48.0
- – novyi, causing gas gangrene A48.0
- – perfringens
- – – as cause of disease classified
  elsewhere B96.7
- – – foodborne (disease) A05.2
- – – gas gangrene A48.0
- – – sepsis A41.4
- – septicum, causing gas gangrene A48.0
- – sordellii, causing gas gangrene A48.0
- – welchii – *see* Infection, Clostridium
  perfringens
- Coccidioides (immitis) (*see also*
  Coccidioidomycosis) B38.9
- colon (*see also* Enteritis, infectious)
  A09.0
- common duct (*see also* Cholangitis)
  K83.0

Infection, infected—*continued*
- congenital NEC P39.9
- – Candida (albicans) P37.5
- – clostridium, other than Clostridium
  tetani P39.8
- – cytomegalovirus P35.1
- – Escherichia coli P39.8
- – – sepsis P36.4
- – hepatitis, viral P35.3
- – herpes simplex P35.2
- – infectious or parasitic disease P37.9
- – – specified NEC P37.8
- – listeriosis (disseminated) P37.2
- – malaria NEC P37.4
- – – falciparum P37.3
- – Plasmodium falciparum P37.3
- – poliomyelitis P35.8
- – rubella P35.0
- – salmonella P39.8
- – skin P39.4
- – streptococcal NEC P39.8
- – – sepsis P36.1
- – – – group B P36.0
- – toxoplasmosis (acute) (chronic)
  (subacute) P37.1
- – tuberculosis P37.0
- – urinary (tract) P39.3
- – vaccinia P35.8
- – virus P35.9
- – – specified type NEC P35.8
- Conidiobolus B46.8
- coronavirus NEC B34.2
- – as cause of disease classified elsewhere
  B97.2
- – severy acute respiratory syndrome
  (SARS) U04.9
- – unspecified nature or site B34.2
- corpus luteum (*see also* Salpingo-
  oophoritis) N70.9
- Corynebacterium diphtheriae – *see*
  Diphtheria
- Coxiella burnetii A78
- Coxsackie(virus) (*see also*
  Coxsackievirus) B34.1
- – as cause of disease classified elsewhere
  B97.1
- – meningitis A87.0† G02.0*
- – myocardium B33.2† I41.1*
- – pericardium B33.2† I32.1*
- – pharynx B08.5
- – specified disease NEC B33.8
- – unspecified nature or site B34.1
- Cryptococcus neoformans (*see also*
  Cryptococcosis) B45.9

Infection, infected—*continued*
- Cryptosporidium A07.2
- - - resulting from HIV disease B20.8
- Cunninghamella (*see also* Mucormycosis) B46.5
- cyst – *see* Cyst
- cystic duct (*see also* Cholecystitis) K81.9
- Cysticercus cellulosae (*see also* Cysticercosis) B69.9
- cytomegalovirus, cytomegaloviral B25.9
- - congenital P35.1
- - maternal, maternal care for (suspected) damage to fetus O35.3
- - mononucleosis B27.1
- - resulting from HIV disease B20.2
- delta-agent (acute), in hepatitis B carrier B17.0
- dental K04.7
- Deuteromycetes B47.0
- Dicrocoelium dendriticum B66.2
- Dipetalonema (perstans) (streptocerca) B74.4
- diphtherial – *see* Diphtheria
- Diphyllobothrium (adult) (latum) (pacificum) B70.0
- - larval B70.1
- Diplogonoporus (grandis) B71.8
- Dipylidium caninum B71.1
- Dirofilaria B74.8
- Dracunculus medinensis B72
- Drechslera (hawaiiensis) B43.8
- Ducrey's (bacillus) (any location) A57
- due to or resulting from
- - artificial insemination N98.0
- - device, implant or graft (*see also* Complications, by site and type) T85.7
- - - arterial graft NEC T82.7
- - - breast (implant) T85.7
- - - catheter NEC T85.7
- - - - dialysis (renal) T82.7
- - - - - intraperitoneal T85.7
- - - - infusion NEC T82.7
- - - - - spinal (epidural) (subdural) T85.7
- - - - urinary (indwelling) T83.5
- - - electronic (electrode) (pulse generator) (stimulator)
- - - - bone T84.7
- - - - cardiac T82.7
- - - - nervous system (brain) (peripheral nerve) (spinal) T85.7
- - - - urinary T83.5
- - - fixation, internal (orthopedic) NEC T84.6

Infection, infected—*continued*
- due to or resulting from—*continued*
- - device, implant or graft—*continued*
- - - gastrointestinal (bile duct) (esophagus) T85.7
- - - genital NEC T83.6
- - - heart NEC T82.7
- - - - valve prosthesis T82.6
- - - joint prosthesis T84.5
- - - ocular (corneal graft) (orbital implant) NEC T85.7
- - - orthopedic NEC T84.7
- - - specified NEC T85.7
- - - urinary NEC T83.5
- - - vascular NEC T82.7
- - - ventricular intracranial shunt T85.7
- - immunization or vaccination T88.0
- - infusion, injection or transfusion NEC T80.2
- - injury NEC – *see* Injury, by site and type
- during labor NEC O75.3
- ear (middle) (*see also* Otitis media) H66.9
- - external H60.3
- - inner H83.0
- Echinococcus (*see also* Echinococcus) B67.9
- echo(virus)
- - as cause of disease classified elsewhere B97.1
- - unspecified nature or site B34.1
- endocardium – *see* Endocarditis, bacterial
- endocervix (*see also* Cervicitis) N72
- Entamoeba – *see* Amebiasis
- enteric (*see also* Enteritis, infectious) A09.0
- Enterobius vermicularis B80
- enterovirus NEC B34.1
- - as cause of disease classified elsewhere B97.1
- - unspecified nature or site B34.1
- Entomophthora B46.8
- Epidermophyton – *see* Dermatophytosis
- epididymis – *see condition*
- episiotomy (puerperal) O86.0
- Erysipelothrix (insidiosa) (rhusiopathiae) (*see also* Erysipeloid) A26.9
- Escherichia (E.) coli NEC A49.8
- - as cause of disease classified elsewhere B96.2
- - congenital P39.8
- - - sepsis P36.4

Infection, infected—*continued*
- Escherichia—*continued*
- – generalized A41.5
- – intestinal (*see also* Enteritis, infectious) A04.4
- ethmoidal (chronic) (sinus) (*see also* Sinusitis, ethmoidal) J32.2
- eustachian tube (ear) H68.0
- external auditory canal (meatus) NEC H60.3
- eye (purulent) H44.0
- eyelid H01.9
- fallopian tube (*see also* Salpingo-oophoritis) N70.9
- Fasciola (gigantica) (hepatica) (indica) B66.3
- Fasciolopsis (buski) B66.5
- fetus P39.9
- – intra-amniotic NEC P39.2
- filarial – *see* Filaria, filarial, filariasis
- finger (skin) L08.9
- fish tapeworm B70.0
- – larval B70.1
- flagellate, intestinal A07.9
- fluke – *see* Infestation, fluke
- focal, teeth K04.7
- Fonsecaea (compacta) (pedrosoi) B43.0† L99.8*
- food (*see also* Intoxication, foodborne) A05.9
- foot (skin) L08.9
- – dermatophytic fungus B35.3
- Francisella tularensis (*see also* Tularemia) A21.9
- fungus NEC B49
- – beard B35.0
- – dermatophytic – *see* Dermatophytosis
- – foot B35.3
- – groin B35.6
- – hand B35.2
- – nail B35.1
- – pathogenic to compromised host only B48.7
- – perianal (area) B35.6
- – resulting from HIV disease B20.5
- – scalp B35.0
- – skin B36.9
- Fusarium B48.7
- gallbladder (*see also* Cholecystitis) K81.9
- gastrointestinal (*see also* Enteritis, infectious) A09.0
- generalized NEC (*see also* Sepsis) A41.9
- genital organ or tract
- – complicating pregnancy O23.5

Infection, infected—*continued*
- genital organ or tract—*continued*
- – complicating pregnancy—*continued*
- – – affecting fetus or newborn P00.8
- – female (*see also* Disease, pelvis, inflammatory) N73.9
- – following
- – – abortion (subsequent episode) O08.0
- – – – current episode – *see* Abortion
- – – ectopic or molar pregnancy O08.0
- – male N49.9
- – – multiple sites N49.8
- – – specified NEC N49.8
- – puerperal, postpartum, childbirth NEC O86.1
- – – major or generalized O85
- – – minor or localized O86.1
- genitourinary tract NEC
- – in pregnancy O23.9
- – puerperal O86.3
- Ghon tubercle, primary A16.7
- – with bacteriological and histological confirmation A15.7
- Giardia lamblia A07.1
- gingiva K05.1
- Gnathostoma (spinigerum) B83.1
- Gongylonema B83.8
- gonococcal NEC (*see also* Gonococcus) A54.9
- Gram-negative bacilli NEC A49.9
- guinea worm B72
- gum K05.1
- Haemophilus
- – aegyptius, systemic A48.4
- – ducreyi (any location) A57
- – influenzae NEC A49.2
- – – as cause of disease classified elsewhere B96.3
- – – unspecified nature or site A49.2
- heart (*see also* Carditis) I51.8
- Heliobacter pylori, as cause of disease classified elsewhere B98.0
- helminths B83.9
- – intestinal B82.0
- – – mixed (types classifiable to more than one of the rubrics B65.0-B81.3 and B81.8) B81.4
- – – specified type NEC B81.8
- – specified type NEC B83.8
- herpes (simplex) (*see also* Herpes) B00.9
- – congenital P35.2
- – disseminated B00.7
- herpesvirus, herpesviral (*see also* Herpes) B00.9

Infection, infected—*continued*
- herpesvirus, herpesviral—*continued*
- - - resulting from HIV disease B20.3
- Heterophyes (heterophyes) B66.8
- Histoplasma (*see also* Histoplasmosis) B39.9
- hookworm B76.9
- human T-cell lymphotropic virus type-1 (HTLV-1) B33.3
- Hymenolepis (nana) B71.0
- hypopharynx (*see also* Pharyngitis) J02.9
- inguinal (lymph) glands L04.1
- - due to soft chancre A57
- intervertebral disk, pyogenic M46.3
- intestine, intestinal (*see also* Enteritis, infectious) A09.0
- intra-amniotic, fetus P39.2
- intrauterine (complicating pregnancy) O23.5
- - puerperal (postpartum) (with sepsis) O85
- - specified infection NEC, fetus P39.2
- Isospora belli or hominis A07.3
- jaw (bone) (lower) (upper) K10.2
- joint – *see* Arthritis, infectious
- kidney (cortex) (hematogenous) N15.9
- - with calculus N20.0
- - - with hydronephrosis N13.6
- - complicating pregnancy O23.0
- - - affecting fetus or newborn P00.1
- - following
- - - abortion (subsequent episode) O08.8
- - - - current episode – *see* Abortion
- - - ectopic gestation O08.8
- - pelvis and ureter (cystic) N28.8
- - puerperal (postpartum) O86.2
- - specified NEC N15.8
- Klebsiella (K.) pneumoniae NEC A49.8
- - as cause of disease classified elsewhere B96.1
- knee (skin) NEC L08.9
- - joint M00.9
- Koch's (*see also* Tuberculosis) A16.9
- labia (majora) (minora) (acute) (*see also* Vulvitis) N76.2
- lacrimal
- - gland H04.0
- - passages (duct) (sac) H04.3
- lancet fluke B66.2
- larynx NEC J38.7
- leg (skin) NEC L08.9
- Legionella pneumophila A48.1
- - nonpneumonic A48.2

Infection, infected—*continued*
- Leishmania (*see also* Leishmaniasis) B55.9
- - aethiopica B55.1
- - braziliensis B55.2
- - chagasi B55.0
- - donovani B55.0
- - infantum B55.0
- - major B55.1
- - mexicana B55.1
- - tropica B55.1
- lentivirus, as cause of disease classified elsewhere B97.3
- Leptosphaeria senegalensis B47.0
- Leptospira interrogans A27.9
- - autumnalis A27.8
- - canicola A27.8
- - hebdomadis A27.8
- - icterohaemorrhagiae A27.0
- - pomona A27.8
- - specified type NEC A27.8
- leptospirochetal NEC (*see also* Leptospirosis) A27.9
- Listeria monocytogenes (*see also* Listeriosis) A32.9
- - congenital P37.2
- Loa loa B74.3
- - with conjunctival infestation B74.3† H13.0*
- Loboa loboi B48.0
- local, skin (staphylococcal) (streptococcal) L08.9
- - abscess – *see* Abscess, by site
- - cellulitis – *see* Cellulitis, by site
- - specified NEC L08.8
- - ulcer (*see also* Ulcer, skin) L98.4
- lung NEC (*see also* Pneumonia) J18.9
- - atypical mycobacterium A31.0
- - tuberculous (*see also* Tuberculosis, pulmonary) A16.2
- - virus – *see* Pneumonia, viral
- lymph gland (*see also* Lymphadenitis, acute) L04.9
- - mesenteric I88.0
- lymphoid tissue, base of tongue or posterior pharynx, NEC (chronic) J35.0
- Madurella (grisea) (mycetomatis) B47.0
- major
- - following
- - - abortion (subsequent episode) O08.0
- - - - current episode – *see* Abortion
- - - ectopic or molar pregnancy O08.0
- - puerperal, postpartum, childbirth O85
- Malassezia furfur B36.0

Infection, infected—*continued*
- Malleomyces pseudomallei (*see also* Melioidosis) A24.4
- mammary gland (*see also* Mastitis) N61
- Mansonella (ozzardi) (perstans) (streptocerca) B74.4
- mastoid – *see* Mastoiditis
- maxilla, maxillary K10.2
- – sinus (chronic) (*see also* Sinusitis, maxillary) J32.0
- mediastinum J98.5
- Medina (worm) B72
- meibomian cyst or gland H00.0
- meninges (*see also* Meningitis) G00.9
- meningococcal (*see also condition*) A39.9
- – brain A39.8† G05.0*
- – cerebrospinal A39.0† G01*
- – endocardium A39.5† I39.8*
- – meninges A39.0† G01*
- – myocardium A39.5† I41.0*
- – pericardium A39.5† I32.0*
- – specified site NEC A39.8
- mesenteric lymph nodes or glands NEC I88.0
- Metagonimus B66.8
- metatarsophalangeal M00.9
- Microsporum, microsporic – *see* Dermatophytosis
- mixed flora (bacterial) NEC A49.8
- Monilia (*see also* Candidiasis) B37.9
- – neonatal P37.5
- Mucor (*see also* Mucormycosis) B46.5
- multiple, resulting from HIV disease B20.7
- muscle NEC M60.0
- mycelium NEC B49
- mycetoma
- – actinomycotic NEC B47.1
- – mycotic NEC B47.0
- Mycobacterium, mycobacterial (*see also* Mycobacterium) A31.9
- – extrapulmonary systemic A31.8
- – resulting from HIV disease B20.0
- Mycoplasma NEC A49.3
- – pneumoniae, as cause of disease classified elsewhere B96.0
- – unspecified nature or site A49.2
- mycotic NEC B49
- – pathogenic to compromised host only B48.7
- – resulting from HIV disease B20.5
- – skin NEC B36.9
- myocardium NEC I40.0

Infection, infected—*continued*
- nail (chronic) (with lymphangitis) L03.0
- – ingrowing L60.0
- nasal sinus (chronic) (*see also* Sinusitis) J32.9
- nasopharynx – *see* Nasopharyngitis
- navel L08.9
- – newborn P38
- Necator americanus B76.1
- Neisseria – *see* Gonococcus
- Neotestudina rosatii B47.0
- newborn P39.9
- – skin P39.4
- – specified type NEC P39.8
- nipple N61
- – puerperal, postpartum or gestational O91.0
- Nocardia (*see also* Nocardiosis) A43.9
- obstetric surgical wound (puerperal) O86.0
- Oesophagostomum (apiostomum) B81.8
- Oestrus ovis (*see also* Myiasis) B87.9
- Onchocerca (volvulus) B73
- oncovirus, as cause of disease classified elsewhere B97.3
- operation wound T81.4
- Opisthorchis (felineus) (viverrini) B66.0
- orbit, orbital H05.0
- orthopoxvirus NEC B08.0
- ovary (*see also* Salpingo-oophoritis) N70.9
- Oxyuris vermicularis B80
- pancreas (acute) K85.-
- papillomavirus, as cause of disease classified elsewhere B97.7
- papovavirus NEC B34.4
- – resulting from HIV disease B20.3
- – unspecified nature or site B34.4
- Paracoccidioides brasiliensis (*see also* Paracoccidioidomycosis) B41.9
- Paragonimus (westermani) B66.4
- parainfluenza virus B34.8
- parasitic B89
- – resulting from HIV disease B20.8
- Parastrongylus
- – cantonensis B83.2
- – costaricensis B81.3
- paraurethral ducts N34.2
- parotid gland K11.2
- parvovirus NEC B34.3
- – as cause of disease classified elsewhere B97.6
- – unspecified nature or site B34.3
- Pasteurella NEC A28.0

Infection, infected—*continued*
– Pasteurella NEC—*continued*
– – multocida A28.0
– – pestis (*see also* Plague) A20.9
– – tularensis (*see also* Tularemia) A21.9
– pelvic, female (*see also* Disease, pelvis, inflammatory) N73.9
– Penicillium (marneffei) B48.4
– penis (glans) (retention) NEC N48.2
– periapical K04.5
– peridental K05.2
– perinatal period P39.9
– – specified type NEC P39.8
– perineal repair (puerperal) O86.0
– periodontal K05.2
– periorbital H05.0
– perirectal K62.8
– perirenal (*see also* Infection, kidney) N15.9
– peritoneal (*see also* Peritonitis) K65.9
– periureteral N28.8
– Petriellidium boydii B48.2
– pharynx (*see also* Pharyngitis) J02.9
– – coxsackievirus B08.5
– – posterior, lymphoid (chronic) J35.0
– Phialophora
– – gougerotii (subcutaneous abscess or cyst) B43.2† L99.8*
– – jeanselmei (subcutaneous abscess or cyst) B43.2† L99.8*
– – verrucosa (skin) B43.0† L99.8*
– Piedraia hortae B36.3
– pinworm B80
– pleuro-pneumonia-like organism (PPLO) NEC A49.3
– – as cause of disease classified elsewhere B96.0
– pneumococcus, pneumococcal NEC A49.1
– – as cause of disease classified elsewhere B95.3
– – generalized (purulent) A40.3
– – – with pneumonia J13
– – unspecified nature or site A49.1
– Pneumocystis carinii (pneumonia) B59† J17.3*
– – resulting from HIV disease B20.6
– Pneumocystis jirovecii (pneumonia) B59† J17.3*
– – resulting from HIV disease B20.6
– postoperative wound T81.4
– post-traumatic NEC T79.3
– postvaccinal T88.0
– prepuce NEC N48.1

Infection, infected—*continued*
– prion – *see* Disease, prion, central nervous system
– prostate (capsule) (*see also* Prostatitis) N41.9
– Proteus (mirabilis) (morganii) (vulgaris) NEC A49.8
– – as cause of disease classified elsewhere B96.4
– protozoal NEC B64
– – intestinal A07.9
– – – specified NEC A07.8
– – specified NEC B60.8
– Pseudallescheria boydii B48.2
– Pseudomonas, pseudomonad NEC A49.8
– – as cause of disease classified elsewhere B96.5
– – mallei – *see* Infection, Burkholderia, mallei
– – pseudomallei – *see* Infection, Burkholderia, pseudomallei
– pseudotuberculosis (extra-intestinal) A28.2
– puerperal O86.4
– – genitourinary tract NEC O86.3
– – major or generalized O85
– – minor O86.4
– – specified NEC O86.8
– pulmonary – *see* Infection, lung
– purulent – *see* Abscess
– pyemic – *see* Sepsis
– Pyrenochaeta romeroi B47.0
– rectum (sphincter) K62.8
– renal (*see also* Infection, kidney) N15.9
– – pelvis and ureter (cystic) N28.8
– reovirus, as cause of disease classified elsewhere B97.5
– respiratory (tract) NEC J98.8
– – acute J22
– – chronic J98.8
– – influenzal (*see also* Influenza, with, respiratory manifestations) J11.1
– – lower (acute) J22
– – – chronic (*see also* Bronchitis, chronic) J42
– – rhinovirus J00
– – syncytial virus, as cause of disease classified elsewhere B97.4
– – upper (acute) NEC J06.9
– – – chronic J39.8
– – – multiple sites NEC J06.8
– – – streptococcal J06.9
– – – viral NEC J06.9   + B97.8

355

Infection, infected—*continued*
- resulting from
- – HIV disease B20.9
- – presence of internal prosthetic device, implant or graft – *see* Complications, by site and type
- retortamoniasis A07.8
- retrovirus NEC B33.3
- – as cause of disease classified elsewhere B97.3
- Rhinosporidium seeberi B48.1
- rhinovirus
- – as cause of disease classified elsewhere B97.8
- – unspecified nature or site B34.8
- Rhizopus (*see also* Mucormycosis) B46.5
- rickettsial NEC A79.9
- roundworm (large) NEC B82.0
- – ascariasis B77.-
- rubella (*see also* Rubella) B06.9
- – congenital P35.0
- salivary duct or gland (any) K11.2
- Salmonella (arizonae) (cholerae-suis) (enteritidis) (typhimurium) A02.9
- – with
- – – (gastro)enteritis A02.0
- – – sepsis A02.1
- – – specified manifestation NEC A02.8
- – congenital P39.8
- – due to food (poisoning) A02.9
- – hirschfeldii A01.3
- – localized NEC A02.2
- – paratyphi A01.4
- – – A A01.1
- – – B A01.2
- – – C A01.3
- – schottmuelleri A01.2
- – typhi A01.0
- Sarcocystis A07.8
- Schistosoma – *see* Infestation, Schistosoma
- scrotum (acute) NEC N49.2
- seminal vesicle (*see also* Vesiculitis) N49.0
- septic
- – generalized – *see* Sepsis
- – localized, skin (*see also* Abscess) L02.9
- septicemic – *see* Sepsis
- sheep liver fluke B66.3
- Shigella A03.9
- – boydii A03.2
- – dysenteriae A03.0
- – flexneri A03.1

Infection, infected—*continued*
- Shigella—*continued*
- – group
- – – A A03.0
- – – B A03.1
- – – C A03.2
- – – D A03.3
- – schmitzii A03.0
- – shigae A03.0
- – sonnei A03.3
- – specified NEC A03.8
- sinus (accessory) (chronic) (nasal) (*see also* Sinusitis) J32.9
- – pilonidal L05.9
- – – with abscess L05.0
- – skin NEC L08.8
- Skene's duct or gland (*see also* Urethritis) N34.2
- skin (local) (staphylococcal) (streptococcal) L08.9
- – abscess – *see* Abscess, by site
- – cellulitis – *see* Cellulitis, by site
- – due to fungus B36.9
- – – specified type NEC B36.8
- – mycotic B36.9
- – – specified type NEC B36.8
- – newborn P39.4
- – ulcer (*see also* Ulcer, skin) L98.4
- slow virus A81.9
- – specified NEC A81.8
- Sparganum (baxteri) (mansoni) (proliferum) B70.1
- specified NEC, resulting from HIV disease B20.8
- spermatic cord NEC N49.1
- sphenoidal (sinus) (*see also* Sinusitis, sphenoidal) J32.3
- spinal cord NEC (*see also* Encephalitis) G04.9
- – abscess G06.1
- – meninges – *see* Meningitis
- – streptococcal G04.8
- Spirillum A25.0
- spirochetal NEC A69.9
- – specified NEC A69.8
- Spirometra larvae B70.1
- spleen D73.8
- Sporotrichum, Sporothrix (schenckii) (*see also* Sporotrichosis) B42.9
- staphylococcal NEC A49.0
- – as cause of disease classified elsewhere B95.8
- – generalized (purulent) A41.2

Infection, infected—*continued*
- staphylococcal NEC—*continued*
-   – unspecified nature or site A49.0
- Stellantchasmus falcatus B66.8
- streptococcal NEC A49.1
-   – as cause of disease classified elsewhere B95.5
-   – congenital P39.8
-   – – sepsis P36.1
-   – – – group B P36.0
-   – generalized (purulent) A40.9
-   – unspecified nature or site A49.1
- Streptomyces B47.1
- Strongyloides (stercoralis) (*see also* Strongyloidiasis) B78.9
- stump (amputation) (surgical) T87.4
- subcutaneous tissue, local L08.9
- systemic – *see* Sepsis
- Taenia – *see* Infestation, Taenia
- tapeworm – *see* Infestation, tapeworm
- tendon (sheath) M65.1
- Ternidens deminutus B81.8
- Ternidens diminutus B81.8
- testis (*see also* Orchitis) N45.9
- threadworm B80
- throat (*see also* Pharyngitis) J02.9
- thyroglossal duct K14.8
- toe (skin) L08.9
- tongue NEC K14.0
- tonsil (faucial) (lingual) (pharyngeal) J03.9
-   – acute or subacute J03.9
-   – chronic J35.0
- tooth, teeth K04.7
-   – periapical K04.7
-   – peridental, periodontal K05.2
-   – socket K10.3
- Torula histolytica (*see also* Cryptococcosis) B45.9
- Toxocara (canis) (cati) (felis) B83.0
- Toxoplasma gondii (*see also* Toxoplasma) B58.9
-   – resulting from HIV disease B20.8
- trachea, chronic J42
- trematode NEC (*see also* Infestation, fluke) B66.9
- Treponema pallidum – *see* Syphilis
- Trichinella (spiralis) B75
- Trichomonas, trichomonad A59.9
-   – cervix A59.0† N74.8*
-   – intestine A07.8
-   – prostate A59.0† N51.0*
-   – specified site NEC A59.8
-   – urethra A59.0† N37.0*

Infection, infected—*continued*
- Trichomonas, trichomonad—*continued*
-   – urogenitalis A59.0
-   – vagina A59.0† N77.1*
-   – vulva A59.0† N77.1*
- Trichophyton, trichophytic – *see* Dermatophytosis
- Trichosporon (beigelii) cutaneum B36.2
- Trichostrongylus B81.2
- Trichuris (trichiura) B79
- Trombicula (irritans) B88.0
- Trypanosoma
-   – brucei
-   – – gambiense B56.0
-   – – rhodesiense B56.1
-   – cruzi (*see also* Chagas' disease) B57.2
- tubal (*see also* Salpingo-oophoritis) N70.9
- tuberculous NEC (*see also* Tuberculosis) A16.9
-   – resulting from HIV disease B20.0
- tubo-ovarian (*see also* Salpingo-oophoritis) N70.9
- tunica vaginalis N49.1
- tympanic membrane NEC H73.8
- typhoid (abortive) (ambulant) (bacillus) A01.0
- umbilicus L08.9
-   – newborn P38
- ureter N28.8
- urethra (*see also* Urethritis) N34.2
- urinary (tract) NEC N39.0
-   – complicating pregnancy O23.4
-   – – affecting fetus or newborn P00.1
-   – newborn P39.3
-   – puerperal (postpartum) O86.2
-   – tuberculous A18.1
- uterus, uterine (*see also* Endometritis) N71.9
- vaccination T88.0
- vagina (acute) (*see also* Vaginitis) N76.0
- varicose veins – *see* Varicose vein
- vas deferens NEC N49.1
- vesical (*see also* Cystitis) N30.9
- vibrio vulnificus, as cause of disease classified elsewhere B98.1
- Vincent's (gum) (mouth) (tonsil) A69.1
- virus NEC B34.9
-   – adenovirus
-   – – as cause of disease classified elsewhere B97.0
-   – – unspecified nature or site B34.0
-   – arborvirus, arbovirus (arthropod-borne) A94

Infection, infected—*continued*
- virus NEC—*continued*
- – as cause of disease classified elsewhere B97.8
- – central nervous system A89
- – – atypical A81.9
- – – – specified NEC A81.8
- – – enterovirus NEC A88.8
- – – – meningitis A87.0† G02.0*
- – – slow virus A81.9
- – – – specified NEC A81.8
- – – specified NEC A88.8
- – chest J98.8
- – coxsackie(virus) (*see also* Infection, coxsackie(virus)) B34.1
- – – as cause of disease classified elsewhere B97.1
- – – unspecified nature or site B34.1
- – echo(virus)
- – – as cause of disease classified elsewhere B97.1
- – – unspecified nature or site B34.1
- – enterovirus B97.1
- – – as cause of disease classified elsewhere B97.1
- – – unspecified nature or site B34.1
- – intestine (*see also* Enteritis, viral) A08.4
- – respiratory syncytial, as cause of disease classified elsewhere B97.4
- – rhinovirus
- – – as cause of disease classified elsewhere B97.8
- – – unspecified nature or site B34.8
- – slow A81.9
- – – specified NEC A81.8
- – specified type NEC B33.8
- – – as cause of disease classified elsewhere B97.8
- – – resulting from HIV disease B20.3
- – – unspecified site B34.8
- – unspecified site B34.9
- vulva (acute) (*see also* Vulvitis) N76.2
- West Nile (viral) A92.3
- whipworm B79
- worms B83.9
- – specified type NEC B83.8
- wound (local) (post-traumatic) NEC T79.3
- – open – *see* Wound, open
- – surgical T81.4
- Wuchereria (bancrofti) B74.0
- – malayi B74.1
- yeast (*see also* Candidiasis) B37.9

Infection, infected—*continued*
- Yersinia
- – enterocolitica (intestinal) A04.6
- – pestis (*see also* Plague) A20.9
- – pseudotuberculosis A28.2
- Zeis' gland H00.0
Infectious, infective – *see condition*
Infertility
- female N97.9
- – associated with
- – – anovulation N97.0
- – – cervical (mucus) disease or anomaly N97.3
- – – congenital anomaly
- – – – cervix N97.3
- – – – fallopian tube N97.1
- – – – uterus N97.2
- – – – vagina N97.8
- – – fallopian tube disease or anomaly N97.1
- – – male factors N97.4
- – – pituitary-hypothalamic origin E23.0
- – – specified origin NEC N97.8
- – – Stein-Leventhal syndrome E28.2
- – – uterine disease or anomaly N97.2
- – – vaginal disease or anomaly N97.8
- – nonimplantation N97.2
- – previous, requiring supervision of pregnancy Z35.0
- male N46
- relative N96
Infestation B88.9

Note: Parasitic diseases may be described as either "infections" or "infestations"; both lead terms should therefore be consulted.

- Acanthocheilonema (perstans) (streptocerca) B74.4
- Ancylostoma (braziliense) (caninum) (ceylanicum) (duodenal) B76.0
- anisakiasis, Anisakis larvae B81.0
- arthropod NEC B88.2
- Ascaris lumbricoides (*see also* Ascariasis) B77.9
- Balantidium coli A07.0
- beef tapeworm B68.1
- Bothriocephalus (latus) B70.0
- – larval B70.1
- broad tapeworm B70.0
- – larval B70.1
- Brugia (malayi) B74.1
- – timori B74.2
- candiru B88.8
- Capillaria – *see* Infection, Capillaria

Infestation—*continued*
- cat liver fluke B66.0
- cestodes NEC B71.9
- – specified type NEC B71.8
- chigger B88.0
- chigo, chigoe B88.1
- Clonorchis (sinensis) (liver) B66.1
- coccidial A07.3
- crab-lice B85.3
- Cysticercus cellulosae (*see also* Cysticercosis) B69.9
- Demodex (folliculorum) B88.0
- – eyelid B88.0† H03.0*
- Dermanyssus gallinae B88.0
- Dermatobia (hominis) (*see also* Myiasis) B87.9
- Dibothriocephalus (latus) B70.0
- – larval B70.1
- Dicrocoelium dendriticum B66.2
- Diphyllobothrium (adult) (intestinal) (latum) (pacificum) B70.0
- – larval B70.1
- Diplogonoporus (grandis) B71.8
- Dipylidium caninum B71.1
- Distoma hepaticum B66.3
- dog tapeworm B71.1
- Dracunculus medinensis B72
- dwarf tapeworm B71.0
- Echinococcus (*see also* Echinococcus) B67.9
- Echinostoma ilocanum B66.8
- Entamoeba (histolytica) – *see* Amebiasis
- Enterobius vermicularis B80
- eyelid
- – in (due to)
- – – leishmaniasis B55.1† H03.0*
- – – loiasis B74.3† H03.0*
- – – onchocerciasis B73† H03.0*
- – – phthiriasis B85.3† H03.0*
- – parasitic NEC B89† H03.0*
- Fasciola (gigantica) (hepatica) (indica) B66.3
- Fasciolopsis (buski) (intestine) B66.5
- filarial B74.9
- – conjunctiva B74.-† H13.0*
- – specified type NEC B74.8
- fish tapeworm B70.0
- – larval B70.1
- fluke B66.9
- – blood NEC (*see also* Schistosomiasis) B65.9
- – cat liver B66.0
- – intestinal B66.5
- – liver (sheep) B66.3

Infestation—*continued*
- fluke—*continued*
- – liver—*continued*
- – – Chinese B66.1
- – – due to Clonorchis sinensis B66.1
- – – oriental B66.1
- – lung (oriental) B66.4
- – sheep liver B66.3
- fly larvae (*see also* Myiasis) B87.9
- Gasterophilus (intestinalis) (*see also* Myiasis) B87.9
- Gastrodiscoides hominis B66.8
- Giardia lamblia A07.1
- Gongylonema B83.8
- guinea worm B72
- helminth B83.9
- – intestinal B82.0
- – – mixed (types classifiable to more than one of the rubrics B65.0-B81.3 and B81.8) B81.4
- – – specified type NEC B81.8
- – specified type NEC B83.8
- Heterophyes (heterophyes) B66.8
- hookworm B76.9
- – specified type NEC B76.8
- Hymenolepis (diminuta) (nana) B71.0
- intestinal NEC B82.9
- leeches (aquatic) (land) (*see also* Hirudiniasis) B88.3
- Leishmania – *see* Leishmaniasis
- lice, louse – *see* Infestation, Pediculus
- Linguatula B88.8
- Liponyssoides sanguineus B88.0
- Loa loa B74.3
- – conjunctival B74.3† H13.0*
- maggots (*see also* Myiasis) B87.9
- Mansonella (ozzardi) (perstans) (streptocerca) B74.4
- Medina (worm) B72
- Metagonimus (yokogawai) B66.8
- mites B88.9
- – scabic B86
- Necator americanus B76.1
- nematode NEC (intestinal) B82.0
- – Ancylostoma (species) B76.0
- – specified NEC B81.8
- Oesophagostomum (apiostomum) B81.8
- Oestrus ovis (*see also* Myiasis) B87.9
- Onchocerca (volvulus) B73
- Opisthorchis (felineus) (viverrini) B66.0
- orbit, parasitic NEC B89† H06.1*
- Oxyuris vermicularis B80
- Paragonimus (westermani) B66.4
- parasite, parasitic B89

Infestation—*continued*
- parasite, parasitic—*continued*
- - eyelid B89† H03.0*
- - intestinal NEC B82.9
- - skin B88.9
- Parastrongylus
- - cantonensis B83.2
- - costaricensis B81.3
- Pediculus B85.2
- - capitis (humanus) (any site) B85.0
- corporis (humanus) (any site) B85.1
- - mixed (classifiable to more than one of the rubrics B85.0-B85.3) B85.4
- - pubis (any site) B85.3
- Pentastoma B88.8
- Phthirus (pubis) (any site) B85.3
- - with any infestation classifiable to B85.0-B85.2 B85.4
- pinworm B80
- pork tapeworm (adult) B68.0
- protozoal NEC B64
- - intestinal A07.9
- - - specified NEC A07.8
- - specified NEC B60.8
- Pthirus – *see* Infestation, Phthirus
- rat tapeworm B71.0
- roundworm (large) NEC B82.0
- - Ascariasis B77.-
- sandflea B88.1
- Sarcoptes scabiei B86
- scabies B86
- Schistosoma, schistosome B65.9
- - bovis B65.8
- - cercariae B65.3
- - haematobium B65.0
- - intercalatum B65.8
- - japonicum B65.2
- - mansoni B65.1
- - mattheei B65.8
- - mekongi B65.8
- - specified type NEC B65.8
- - spindale B65.8
- screw worms (*see also* Myiasis) B87.9
- skin NEC B88.9
- Sparganum (baxteri) (larval) (mansoni) (proliferum) B70.1
- specified type NEC B88.8
- Spirometra larvae B70.1
- Stellantchasmus falcatus B66.8
- Strongyloides stercoralis (*see also* Strongyloidiasis) B78.9
- Taenia B68.9
- - mediocanellata B68.1
- - saginata B68.1

Infestation—*continued*
- Taenia—*continued*
- - solium (intestinal form) B68.0
- - - larval form (*see also* Cysticercosis) B69.9
- tapeworm B71.9
- - beef B68.1
- - broad B70.0
- - - larval B70.1
- - dog B71.1
- - dwarf B71.0
- - fish B70.0
- - - larval B70.1
- - pork B68.0
- - rat B71.0
- Ternidens deminutus B81.8
- Ternidens diminutus B81.8
- Tetranychus molestissimus B88.0
- threadworm B80
- Toxocara (canis) (cati) (felis) B83.0
- trematode(s) NEC (*see also* Infestation, fluke) B66.9
- Trichinella (spiralis) B75
- Trichocephalus B79
- Trichomonas – *see* Infection, Trichomonas
- Trichostrongylus B81.2
- Trichuris (trichiura) B79
- Trombicula (irritans) B88.0
- Tunga penetrans B88.1
- Uncinaria americana B76.1
- Vandellia cirrhosa B88.8
- whipworm B79
- worms B83.9
- Wuchereria (bancrofti) B74.0

Infiltrate, infiltration
- amyloid (generalized) (*see also* Amyloidosis) E85.9
- - localized E85.4
- calcareous NEC R89.7
- - localized – *see* Degeneration, by site
- calcium salt R89.7
- corneal H18.2
- eyelid H01.8
- glycogen, glycogenic (*see also* Disease, glycogen storage) E74.0
- heart, cardiac
- - fatty (*see also* Degeneration, myocardial) I51.5
- - glycogenic E74.0† I43.1*
- inflammatory, in vitreous (body) H43.8
- kidney N28.8
- leukemic – *see* Leukemia
- liver K76.8

Infiltrate, infiltration—*continued*
- liver—*continued*
- - fatty – *see* Fatty, liver NEC
- - glycogen (*see also* Disease, glycogen storage) E74.0† K77.8*
- lung (eosinophilic) J82
- lymphatic D47.9
- - gland I88.9
- muscle, fatty M62.8
- myocardium, myocardial
- - fatty (*see also* Degeneration, myocardial) I51.5
- - glycogenic E74.0† I43.1*
- thymus (gland) (fatty) E32.8
- vitreous body H43.8

Infirmity R68.8
- senile R54

Inflammation, inflamed, inflammatory (with exudation)
- abducent (nerve) H49.2
- accessory sinus (chronic) (*see also* Sinusitis) J32.9
- alveoli, teeth K10.3
- - scorbutic E54† K93.8*
- anal canal, anus K62.8
- antrum (chronic) (*see also* Sinusitis, maxillary) J32.0
- appendix (*see also* Appendicitis) K37
- arachnoid – *see* Meningitis
- areola N61
- - puerperal, postpartum or gestational O91.0
- areolar tissue NEC L08.9
- artery – *see* Arteritis
- auditory meatus (external) H60.9
- Bartholin's gland N75.8
- bile duct (common) (hepatic) or passage (*see also* Cholangitis) K83.0
- bladder (*see also* Cystitis) N30.9
- bleb
- - postprocedural H59.8
- bone – *see* Osteomyelitis
- brain (*see also* Encephalitis) G04.9
- - membrane – *see* Meningitis
- breast N61
- - puerperal, postpartum or gestational O91.2
- broad ligament (*see also* Disease, pelvis, inflammatory) N73.2
- bronchi – *see* Bronchitis
- cerebral (*see also* Encephalitis) G04.9
- - membrane – *see* Meningitis
- cerebrospinal, meningococcal A39.0† G01*

Inflammation, inflamed—*continued*
- cervix (uteri) (*see also* Cervicitis) N72
- choroid (*see also* Chorioretinitis) H30.9
- chronic, postmastoidectomy cavity H95.1
- colon – *see* Enteritis
- connective tissue (diffuse) NEC M79.8
- cornea (*see also* Keratitis) H16.9
- corpora cavernosa N48.2
- cranial nerve – *see* Disorder, nerve, cranial
- due to device, implant or graft (*see also* Complications, by site and type) T85.7
- - arterial graft NEC T82.7
- - breast (implant) T85.7
- - catheter NEC T85.7
- - - dialysis (renal) T82.7
- - - - intraperitoneal T85.7
- - - infusion NEC T82.7
- - - - spinal (epidural) (subdural) T85.7
- - - urinary (indwelling) T83.5
- - electronic (electrode) (pulse generator) (stimulator)
- - - bone T84.7
- - - cardiac T82.7
- - - nervous system (brain) (peripheral nerve) (spinal) T85.7
- - - urinary T83.5
- - fixation, internal (orthopedic) NEC T84.6
- - gastrointestinal (bile duct) (esophagus) T85.7
- - genital NEC T83.6
- - heart NEC T82.7
- - - valve (prosthesis) T82.6
- - - - graft T82.7
- - joint prosthesis T84.5
- - ocular (corneal graft) (orbital implant) NEC T85.7
- - orthopedic NEC T84.7
- - specified NEC T85.7
- - urinary NEC T83.5
- - vascular NEC T82.7
- - ventricular intracranial shunt T85.7
- duodenum K29.8
- dura mater – *see* Meningitis
- ear (middle) (*see also* Otitis, media) H66.9
- - external H60.9
- - inner H83.0
- epididymis (*see also* Epididymitis) N45.9
- esophagus K20
- ethmoidal (sinus) (chronic) (*see also* Sinusitis, ethmoidal) J32.2
- eustachian tube (catarrhal) H68.0

Inflammation, inflamed—*continued*
- eyelid H01.9
- – specified NEC H01.8
- fallopian tube (*see also* Salpingo-oophoritis) N70.9
- fascia M60.9
- gallbladder (*see also* Cholecystitis) K81.9
- gastric K29.7
- gastrointestinal – *see* Enteritis
- genital organ (internal) (diffuse)
- – female (*see also* Disease, pelvis, inflammatory) N73.9
- – male N49.9
- – – multiple sites N49.8
- – – specified NEC N49.8
- gland (lymph) (*see also* Lymphadenitis) I88.9
- glottis (*see also* Laryngitis) J04.0
- heart (*see also* Carditis) I51.8
- hepatic duct (*see also* Cholangitis) K83.0
- ileum (*see also* Enteritis) A09.9
- – infectious A09.0
- – noninfectious K52.9
- – regional or terminal K50.0
- intestine (any part) – *see* Enteritis
- jaw (acute) (bone) (chronic) (lower) (suppurative) (upper) K10.2
- joint NEC M13.9
- – sacroiliac M46.1
- knee (joint) M13.1
- – tuberculous A18.0† M01.1*
- labium (majus) (minus) (*see also* Vulvitis) N76.2
- lacrimal
- – gland H04.0
- – passages (duct) (sac) H04.3
- larynx (*see also* Laryngitis) J04.0
- – diphtheritic A36.2
- leg NEC L08.9
- lip K13.0
- lymph gland or node (*see also* Lymphadenitis) I88.9
- lymphatic vessel (*see also* Lymphangitis) I89.1
- maxilla, maxillary K10.2
- – sinus (chronic) (*see also* Sinusitis, maxillary) J32.0
- membranes of brain or spinal cord – *see* Meningitis
- meninges – *see* Meningitis
- mouth K12.1
- muscle M60.9
- myocardium (*see also* Myocarditis) I51.4

Inflammation, inflamed—*continued*
- nasal sinus (chronic) (*see also* Sinusitis) J32.9
- nasopharynx – *see* Nasopharyngitis
- navel L08.9
- – newborn P38
- nerve NEC M79.2
- nipple N61
- – puerperal, postpartum or gestational O91.0
- oculomotor (nerve) H49.0
- optic nerve H46
- orbit (chronic) H05.1
- – acute H05.0
- ovary (*see also* Salpingo-oophoritis) N70.9
- oviduct (*see also* Salpingo-oophoritis) N70.9
- pancreas (acute) – *see* Pancreatitis
- parotid region L08.9
- pelvis, female (*see also* Disease, pelvis, inflammatory) N73.9
- penis N48.2
- perianal K62.8
- pericardium (*see also* Pericarditis) I31.9
- perineum (female) (male) L08.9
- perirectal K62.8
- peritoneum (*see also* Peritonitis) K65.9
- periuterine (*see also* Disease, pelvis, inflammatory) N73.2
- perivesical (*see also* Cystitis) N30.9
- petrous bone (acute) (chronic) H70.2
- pharynx (acute) (*see also* Pharyngitis) J02.9
- pia mater – *see* Meningitis
- pleura – *see* Pleurisy
- polyp
- – colon K51.4
- prostate (*see also* Prostatitis) N41.9
- rectosigmoid – *see* Rectosigmoiditis
- rectum (*see also* Proctitis) K62.8
- respiratory, upper (*see also* Infection, respiratory, upper) J06.9
- – acute, due to radiation J70.0
- – chronic, due to external agent – *see* condition, due to specified external agent
- – due to chemicals, gases, fumes or vapors (inhalation) NEC J68.2
- retina (*see also* Chorioretinitis) H30.9
- retroperitoneal (*see also* Peritonitis) K65.9
- salivary duct or gland (any) (suppurative) K11.2

Inflammation, inflamed—*continued*
- scorbutic, gum E54† K93.8*
- scrotum N49.2
- seminal vesicle (*see also* Vesiculitis) N49.0
- sigmoid – *see* Enteritis
- sinus (*see also* Sinusitis) J32.9
- Skene's duct or gland (*see also* Urethritis) N34.2
- skin L08.9
- spermatic cord N49.1
- sphenoidal (sinus) (*see also* Sinusitis, sphenoidal) J32.3
- spinal
- – cord (*see also* Encephalitis) G04.9
- – membrane – *see* Meningitis
- – nerve – *see* Disorder, nerve
- spine (*see also* Spondylitis) M46.9
- spleen (capsule) D73.8
- stomach – *see* Gastritis
- subcutaneous tissue L08.9
- synovial (fringe) (membrane) – *see* Synovitis
- tendon (sheath) NEC M65.9
- testis (*see also* Orchitis) N45.9
- throat (acute) (*see also* Pharyngitis) J02.9
- thymus (gland) E32.8
- thyroid (gland) (*see also* Thyroiditis) E06.9
- tongue K14.0
- tonsil (*see also* Tonsillitis) J03.9
- trachea (*see also* Tracheitis) J04.1
- trochlear (nerve) H49.1
- tubal (*see also* Salpingo-oophoritis) N70.9
- tuberculous NEC (*see also* Tuberculosis) A16.9
- tubo-ovarian (*see also* Salpingo-oophoritis) N70.9
- tunica vaginalis N49.1
- tympanic membrane – *see* Tympanitis
- umbilicus L08.9
- – newborn P38
- uterine ligament (*see also* Disease, pelvis, inflammatory) N73.2
- uterus (catarrhal) (*see also* Endometritis) N71.9
- uveal tract (anterior) NEC (*see also* Iridocyclitis) H20.9
- – posterior – *see* Chorioretinitis
- vagina (*see also* Vaginitis) N76.0
- vas deferens N49.1
- vein (*see also* Phlebitis) I80.9
- – intracranial or intraspinal (septic) G08

Inflammation, inflamed—*continued*
- vein—*continued*
- – thrombotic I80.9
- – – leg I80.3
- – – – deep (vessels) NEC I80.2
- – – – superficial (vessels) I80.0
- – – lower extremity I80.3
- – – – deep (vessels) NEC I80.2
- – – – superficial (vessels) I80.0
- vocal cord J38.3
- vulva (*see also* Vulvitis) N76.2
- Wharton's duct (suppurative) K11.2

Influenza (specific virus not identified) J11.1
- with
- – digestive manifestations J11.8
- – – avian influenza virus identified J09
- – – other influenza virus identified J10.8
- – enteritis J11.8
- – – avian influenza virus identified J09
- – – other influenza virus identified J10.8
- – gastroenteritis J11.8
- – – avian influenza virus identified J09
- – – other influenza virus identified J10.8
- – involvement of
- – – gastrointestinal tract J11.8
- – – – avian influenza virus identified J09
- – – – other influenza virus identified J10.8
- – – nervous system NEC J11.8
- – – – avian influenza virus identified J09
- – – – other influenza virus identified J10.8
- – laryngitis J11.1
- – – avian influenza virus identified J09
- – – other influenza virus identified J10.1
- – manifestations NEC J11.8
- – – avian influenza virus identified J09
- – – other influenza virus identified J10.8
- – meningismus J11.8
- – – avian influenza virus identified J09
- – – other influenza virus identified J10.8
- – myocarditis J11.8† I41.1*
- – – avian influenza virus identified J09† I41.1*
- – – other influenza virus identified J10.8† I41.1*
- – pharyngitis J11.1
- – – avian influenza virus identified J09
- – – other influenza virus identified J10.1
- – pleural effusion NEC J11.1
- – – avian influenza virus identified J09

Influenza—*continued*
- with—*continued*
- - pleural effusion NEC—*continued*
- - - othcr influenza virus identified J10.1
- - pneumonia (any form in J12-J16, J18) J11.0
- - - avian influenza virus identified J09
- - - other influenza virus identified J10.0
- - respiratory manifestations NEC J11.1
- - - avian influenza virus identified J09
- - - other influenza virus identified J10.1
- - upper respiratory infection (acute) NEC J11.1
- - - avian influenza virus identified J09
- - - other influenza virus identified J10.1
- avian J09
- - other J10.1
- bronchial (*see also* Influenza, with, respiratory manifestations) J11.1
- epidemic J11.1
- maternal, affecting fetus or newborn P00.2
- respiratory (upper) (*see also* Influenza, with, respiratory manifestations) J11.1
- summer, of Italy A93.1
- virus identified J10.1
Influenza-like disease (*see also* Influenza) J11.1
Infraction, Freiberg's (metatarsal head) M92.7
Infusion complication, misadventure or reaction – *see* Complications, infusion
Ingestion
- chemical – *see* Table of drugs and chemicals
- drug or medicament
- - correct substance properly administered T88.7
- - overdose or wrong substance given or taken T50.9
- - - specified drug – *see* Table of drugs and chemicals
- foreign body (*see also* Foreign body) T18.9
Ingrowing
- hair (beard) L73.1
- nail (finger) (toe) L60.0
Inguinal – *see also condition*
- testicle Q53.9
- - bilateral Q53.2
- - unilateral Q53.1
Inhalation
- anthrax A22.1
- carbon monoxide T58

Inhalation—*continued*
- flame T27.3
- food or foreign body (*see also* Asphyxia, food) T17.9
- gas, fumes or vapor T59.9
- - specified agent – *see* Tablc of drugs and chemicals
- liquid or vomitus (*see also* Asphyxia, food) T17.9
- meconium (newborn) P24.0
- mucus (*see also* Asphyxia, mucus) T17.9
- oil (causing suffocation) (*see also* Asphyxia, food) T17.9
- smoke T59.8
- steam T59.9
- stomach contents or secretions T17.9
- - due to anesthesia (general) (local) or other sedation T88.5
- - - in labor and delivery O74.0
- - - in pregnancy O29.0
- - - postpartum, puerperal O89.0
Inhibition, orgasm (female) (male) F52.3
Inhibitor, systemic lupus erythematosus, presence D68.6
Iniencephalus, iniencephaly Q00.2
Injection, traumatic jet (air) (industrial) (paint or dye) (water) T70.4
Injury (*see also* specified injury type) T14.9
- abdomen, abdominal S39.9
- - with pelvic organs S39.6
- - specified NEC S39.8
- Achilles tendon S86.0
- acoustic, resulting in deafness S04.6
- adenoid S09.9
- adrenal (gland) S37.8
- alveolar (process) S09.9
- ankle S99.9
- - specified NEC S99.8
- anterior chamber, eye S05.8
- anus S39.9
- aorta (thoracic) S25.0
- - abdominal S35.0
- arm
- - lower – *see* Injury, forearm
- - meaning upper limb – *see* Injury, limb, upper
- - upper S49.9
- - - and shoulder (level), multiple S49.7
- - - specified NEC S49.8
- artery (complicating trauma) (*see also* Injury, blood vessel) T14.5
- - cerebral or meningeal S06.8
- auditory canal (external) (meatus) S09.9

Injury—*continued*
- auricle, auris S09.9
- axilla S49.9
- back S39.9
- bile duct S36.1
- birth (*see also* Birth injury) P15.9
- bladder (sphincter) S37.2
- – obstetric trauma O71.5
- blast (air) (hydraulic) (immersion) (underwater) NEC T14.8
- – brain S06.0
- – generalized T70.8
- – multiple body organs T70.8
- blood vessel NEC T14.5
- – abdomen S35.9
- – – and lower back, pelvis, multiple S35.7
- – – multiple S35.7
- – – specified NEC S35.8
- – ankle (level) S95.9
- – – and foot, multiple S95.7
- – – specified NEC S95.8
- – arm S45.9
- – – meaning upper limb – *see* Injury, blood vessel, limb, upper
- – – upper (level) S45.9
- – – – and shoulder, multiple S45.7
- – – – specified NEC S45.8
- – axillary S45.9
- – – artery S45.0
- – – vein S45.2
- – azygos vein S25.8
- – brachial S45.9
- – – artery S45.1
- – – vein S45.2
- – carotid artery (common) (external) (internal) S15.0
- – celiac artery S35.2
- – cerebral S06.-
- – digital (hand) S65.5
- – dorsal
- – – artery, foot S95.0
- – – vein, foot S95.2
- – due to accidental puncture or laceration during procedure T81.2
- – extremity – *see* Injury, blood vessel, limb
- – femoral S75.9
- – – artery (common) (superficial) S75.0
- – – vein (hip level) (thigh level) S75.1
- – finger S65.5
- – – thumb S65.4
- – foot (level) S95.9
- – – and ankle, multiple S95.7

Injury—*continued*
- blood vessel NEC—*continued*
- – foot—*continued*
- – – specified NEC S95.8
- – forearm S55.9
- – – multiple S55.7
- – – radial artery S55.1
- – – specified NEC S55.8
- – – ulnar artery S55.0
- – – vein S55.2
- – gastric
- – – artery S35.2
- – – vein S35.8
- – gastroduodenal artery S35.2
- – greater saphenous vein (lower leg level) S85.3
- – – hip and thigh level S75.2
- – hand (level) S65.9
- – – and wrist, multiple S65.7
- – – specified NEC S65.8
- – head S09.0
- – – intracranial S06.9
- – – multiple S09.0
- – – specified NEC S09.0
- – hepatic
- – – artery S35.2
- – – vein S35.1
- – hip (level) S75.9
- – – and thigh, multiple S75.7
- – – specified NEC S75.8
- – hypogastric (artery) (vein) S35.5
- – iliac (artery) (vein) S35.5
- – innominate
- – – artery S25.1
- – – vein S25.3
- – intercostal (artery) (vein) S25.5
- – jugular vein (external) S15.2
- – – internal S15.3
- – leg
- – – lower (level) S85.9
- – – – multiple S85.7
- – – – specified NEC S85.8
- – – meaning lower limb – *see* Injury, blood vessel, limb, lower
- – lesser saphenous vein (lower leg level) S85.4
- – limb T14.5
- – – lower T13.4
- – – – multiple T06.3
- – – upper T11.4
- – – – multiple T06.3
- – lower back S35.9
- – – and abdomen, pelvis, multiple S35.7
- – – multiple S35.7

Injury—*continued*
- blood vessel NEC—*continued*
- – lower back—*continued*
- – – specified NEC S35.8
- – mammary (artery) (vein) S25.8
- – mesenteric (inferior) (superior) S35.9
- – – artery S35.2
- – – vein S35.3
- – multiple (regions) (sites) T06.3
- – – abdomen, lower back and pelvis S35.7
- – – ankle (and foot) level S95.7
- – – arm, upper S45.7
- – – foot (and ankle) level S95.7
- – – forearm (level) S55.7
- – – hand (and wrist) level S65.7
- – – hip (and thigh) level S75.7
- – – leg
- – – – lower S85.7
- – – – upper S75.7
- – – neck S15.7
- – – shoulder (and upper arm) level S45.7
- – – thigh (and hip) level S75.7
- – – thorax S25.7
- – – wrist (and hand) level S65.7
  neck S15.9
- – – multiple S15.7
- – – specified NEC S15.8
- – ovarian (artery) (vein) S35.8
- – palmar arch (superficial) S65.2
- – – deep S65.3
- – pelvis S35.9
- – – and abdomen, lower back, multiple S35.7
- – – multiple S35.7
- – – specified NEC S35.8
- – peroneal artery S85.2
- – plantar artery (deep) (foot) S95.1
- – popliteal S85.9
- – – artery S85.0
- – – vein S85.5
- – portal vein S35.3
- – precerebral S15.-
- – pulmonary (artery) (vein) S25.4
- – radial artery (forearm (level)) S55.1
- – – hand and wrist (level) S65.1
- – renal (artery) (vein) S35.4
- – saphenous vein (greater) (lower leg level) S85.3
- – – hip and thigh level S75.2
- – – lesser S85.4
- – shoulder S45.9
- – – and upper arm level, multiple S45.7

Injury—*continued*
- blood vessel NEC—*continued*
- – shoulder—*continued*
- – – specified NEC S45.8
- – – superficial vein S45.3
- – specified NEC (*see also* Injury, blood vessel, by site) T14.5
- – splenic S35.9
- – – artery S35.2
- – – vein S35.3
- – subclavian
- – – artery S25.1
- – – vein S25.3
- – thigh (level) S75.9
- – – and hip, multiple S75.7
- – – specified NEC S75.8
- – thoracic S25.9
- – – multiple S25.7
- – – specified NEC S25.8
- – thumb S65.4
- – tibial artery (anterior) (posterior) S85.1
- – ulnar artery (forearm (level)) S55.0
- – – hand and wrist (level) S65.0
- – upper arm (level) S45.9
- – – superficial vein S45.3
- – uterine (artery) (vein) S35.5
- – vena cava (superior) S25.2
- – – inferior S35.1
- – vertebral artery S15.1
- – wrist (level) S65.9
- – – and hand, multiple S65.7
- – – specified NEC S65.8
- brachial plexus S14.3
- – newborn P14.3
- brain S06.9   *Hypoxic G93.1*
- – with
- – – cranial nerve(s) (multiple) S09.7
- – – spinal cord (neck) (multiple) T06.0
- – diffuse S06.2
- – focal S06.3
- – specified NEC S06.8
- breast NEC S29.9
- broad ligament S37.8
- bronchus, bronchi S27.4
- brow S09.9
- buttock S39.9
- canthus, eye S09.9
- cauda equina S34.3
- cavernous sinus S06.8
- cecum S36.5
- celiac ganglion or plexus S34.5
- cerebellum S06.8
- cerebral S06.9
- – diffuse S06.2

Injury—*continued*
- cerebral—*continued*
- − − focal S06.3
- − − specified NEC S06.8
- cervix (uteri) S37.6
- cheek (wall) S09.9
- childbirth (fetus or newborn) (*see also* Birth injury) P15.9
- − − maternal NEC O71.9
- chin S09.9
- choroid (eye) S05.8
- clitoris S39.9
- coccyx S39.9
- − − complicating delivery O71.6
- colon S36.5
- common bile duct S36.1
- conjunctiva (superficial) S05.0
- cord
- − − spermatic (pelvic region) S37.8
- − − − scrotal region S39.8
- − − spinal – *see* Injury, spinal cord, by region
- cornea S05.8
- − − abrasion S05.0
- cortex (cerebral) S06.8
- − − visual S04.0
- costal region NEC S29.9
- costochondral NEC S29.9
- cranial
- − − cavity S06.8
- − − nerve – *see* Injury, nerve, cranial
- crushing – *see* Crush
- cutaneous sensory nerve – *see* Injury, nerve, cutaneous sensory
- cystic duct S36.1
- delivery (fetus or newborn) P15.9
- − − maternal NEC O71.9
- Descemet's membrane – *see* Injury, eyeball, penetrating
- diaphragm S27.8
- duodenum S36.4
- ear (auricle) (external) (canal) S09.9
- elbow S59.9
- − − and forearm, multiple S59.7
- − − specified NEC S59.8
- epididymis S39.9
- epigastric region S39.9
- epiglottis NEC S19.8
- esophagus (thoracic part) S27.8
- − − cervical NEC S19.8
- eustachian tube S09.9
- eye S05.9
- eyeball S05.8
- − − penetrating S05.6

Injury—*continued*
- eyeball—*continued*
- − − penetrating—*continued*
- − − − with
- − − − − foreign body S05.5
- − − − − prolapse or loss of intraocular tissue S05.2
- − − − without prolapse or loss of intraocular tissue S05.3
- − − specified NEC S05.8
- − − superficial S05.8
- eyebrow S09.9
- eyelid S09.9
- − − superficial S00.2
- face S09.9
- fallopian tube S37.5
- fascia – *see* Injury, muscle
- finger (nail) S69.9
- foot S99.9
- − − and ankle, multiple S99.7
- − − specified NEC S99.8
- forearm S59.9
- − − and elbow, multiple S59.7
- − − specified NEC S59.8
- forehead S09.9
- gallbladder S36.1
- ganglion
- − − celiac, coeliac S34.5
- − − gasserian S04.3
- − − stellate S24.4
- − − thoracic sympathetic S24.4
- gastrointestinal tract S36.9
- genital organ(s)
- − − external S39.9
- − − internal S37.9
- − − obstetric trauma O71.9
- gland
- − − lacrimal (laceration) S05.8
- − − salivary S09.9
- − − thyroid NEC S19.8
- globe (eye) S05.9
- − − specified NEC S05.8
- groin S39.9
- gum S09.9
- hand S69.9
- − − and wrist, multiple S69.7
- − − specified NEC S69.8
- head S09.9
- − − multiple (classifiable to categories S00-S09.2) S09.7
- − − specified NEC S09.8
- heart S26.9
- − − with hemopericardium S26.0
- − − specified NEC S26.8

Injury—*continued*
- heel S99.9
- hepatic duct S36.1
- hip S79.9
- – and thigh, multiple S79.7
- – specified NEC S79.8
- hymen S39.9
- hypogastric plexus S34.5
- ileum S36.4
- iliac region S39.9
- infrared rays NEC T66
- instrumental (during surgery) T81.2
- – birth injury – *see* Birth injury
- – nonsurgical (*see also* Injury, by site)
  T14.9
- – obstetric O71.9
- – – bladder O71.5
- – – cervix O71.3
- – – high vaginal O71.4
- – – perineal NEC O70.9
- – – urethra O71.5
- – – uterus O71.5
- – – – with rupture or perforation O71.1
- internal T14.8

Note: For injury of internal organ(s) by foreign body entering through a natural orifice (e.g. inhaled, ingested or swallowed) - *see* Foreign body, entering through orifice.

- – bladder (sphincter) S37.2
- – – obstetric trauma O71.5
- – cervix (uteri) S37.6
- – – obstetric trauma O71.3
- – chest (*see also* Injury, intrathoracic
  organ) S27.9
- – multiple T06.5
- – – intra-abdominal organs S36.7
- – – – with intrathoracic organ(s) T06.5
- – – intrathoracic organs S27.7
- – – – with intra-abdominal organ(s)
    T06.5
- – – pelvic organs S37.7
- – pelvis, pelvic (organ) S37.9
- – – and abdomen, lower back, multiple
    S39.7
- – – following
- – – – abortion (subsequent episode)
    O08.6
- – – – – current episode – *see* Abortion
- – – – ectopic or molar pregnancy
    (subsequent episode) O08.6
- – – – – current episode – *see*
    Pregnancy, by site
- – – obstetric trauma NEC O71.5

Injury—*continued*
- internal—*continued*
- – pelvis, pelvic—*continued*
- – – obstetric trauma NEC—*continued*
- – – – rupture or perforation O71.1
- – – – specified NEC S39.8
- intervertebral disk T09.9
- intestine S36.9
- – large S36.5
- – small S36.4
- intra-abdominal organ S36.9
- – with intrathoracic (and pelvic) organs
    T06.5
- – multiple S36.7
- – specified NEC S36.8
- intracranial S06.9
- – with prolonged coma S06.7
- – specified NEC S06.8
- intraocular S05.6
- intrathoracic organ S27.9
- – with intra-abdominal (and pelvic)
    organs T06.5
- – multiple S27.7
- – specified NEC S27.8
- iris S05.8
- – penetrating S05.6
- jaw S09.9
- jejunum S36.4
- joint NEC T14.9
- – old or residual M25.8
- kidney S37.0
- knee S89.9
- – meniscus (lateral) (medial) S83.6
- – – with ligament (collateral) (cruciate)
    S83.7
- – – old injury or tear M23.2
- – multiple structures S83.7
- labium (majus) (minus) S39.9
- labyrinth, ear S09.9
- lacrimal duct S05.8
- larynx NEC S19.8
- leg
- – lower S89.9
- – – multiple S89.7
- – – specified NEC S89.8
- – meaning lower limb – *see* Injury, limb,
    lower
- lens (eye) S05.8
- – penetrating S05.6
- limb T14.9
- – lower T13.9
- – – specified NEC T13.8
- – upper T11.9
- – – specified NEC T11.8

Injury—*continued*
- lip S09.9
- liver S36.1
- lower back S39.9
- – specified NEC S39.8
- lumbar, lumbosacral (region) S39.9
- – plexus S34.4
- lung S27.3
- – with
- – – hemopneumothorax S27.2
- – – hemothorax S27.1
- – – pneumohemothorax S27.2
- – – pneumothorax S27.0
- – specified NEC S27.3
- lymphatic thoracic duct S27.8
- malar region S09.9
- mastoid region S09.9
- maternal, during pregnancy, affecting
  fetus or newborn P00.5
- maxilla S09.9
- mediastinum S27.8
- membrane, brain S06.8
- meningeal artery S06.5
- meninges (cerebral) S06.8
- mesenteric
- – artery (inferior) (superior) S35.2
- – plexus (inferior) (superior) S34.5
- – vein (inferior) (superior) S35.3
- mesentery S36.8
- mesosalpinx S37.8
- middle ear S09.9
- midthoracic region NEC S29.9
- mouth S09.9
- multiple sites T07

Note: Multiple injuries of sites classifiable to the same three- or four-character rubric should be classified to that rubric.

Multiple injuries classifiable to different three-character categories within the same block should be assigned to the subcategory for multiple injuries of that body region.

Multiple injuries of sites classifiable to different body regions should be coded to T00-T07.

- – abdomen, lower back and pelvis S39.7
- – ankle (and foot) S99.7
- – arm, upper (and shoulder) S49.7
- – blood vessels T06.3
- – foot (and ankle) S99.7
- – forearm S59.7
- – hand (and wrist) S69.7
- – head S09.7

Injury—*continued*
- multiple sites—*continued*
- – hip (and thigh) S79.7
- – intra-abdominal organs S36.7
- – – with pelvic organs S39.6
- – intrathoracic organs S27.7
- – knee NEC S83.7
- – – and lower leg S89.7
- – leg, lower (and knee) S89.7
- – muscle and tendons T06.4
- – neck S19.7
- – pelvic organs S37.7
- – – with intra-abdominal organs S39.6
- – shoulder (and upper arm) S49.7
- – specified NEC T06.8
- – thigh (and hip) S79.7
- – thorax, thoracic S29.7
- – – internal S27.7
- – trunk, internal T06.5
- – wrist (and hand) S69.7
- muscle (and fascia) (and tendon) T14.6
- – abdomen S39.0
- – abductor, thumb, forearm level S56.3
- – ankle (level) S96.9
- – – and foot, multiple S96.7
- – – specified NEC S96.8
- – anterior muscle group, at leg level
  (lower) S86.2
- – arm
- – – meaning upper limb T11.5
- – – upper (level) S46.9
- – – – and shoulder, multiple S46.7
- – – – specified NEC S46.8
- – biceps (parts NEC) S46.2
- – – long head S46.1
- – extensor
- – – finger(s) (other than thumb), forearm
  level S56.4
- – – – wrist and hand level S66.3
- – – forearm level, specified NEC S56.5
- – – multiple, wrist (and hand) level
  S66.7
- – – thumb, forearm level S56.3
- – – – wrist and hand level S66.2
- – – toe (large) (ankle level) (foot level)
  S96.1
- – – wrist and hand level, multiple S66.7
- – flexor
- – – finger(s) (other than thumb), forearm
  level S56.1
- – – – wrist and hand level S66.1
- – – forearm level, specified NEC S56.2
- – – multiple, wrist (and hand) level
  S66.6

Injury—*continued*
- muscle—*continued*
- – flexor—*continued*
- – – thumb, long (wrist and hand level) S66.0
- – – – forearm level S56.0
- – – toe (long) (ankle level) (foot level) S96.0
- – – wrist and hand (level), multiple S66.6
- – foot (level) S96.9
- – – and ankle, multiple S96.7
- – – specified NEC S96.8
- – forearm (level) S56.8
- – – multiple S56.7
- – hand (level) S66.9
- – – specified NEC S66.8
- – head S09.1
- – hip (level) NEC S76.0
- – – and thigh, multiple S76.7
- – intrinsic
- – – ankle and foot level S96.2
- – – finger (other than thumb), at wrist and hand level S66.5
- – – foot (level) S96.2
- – – thumb, at wrist and hand level S66.4
- – leg
- – – lower (level) S86.9
- – – – multiple S86.7
- – – – specified NEC S86.8
- – – meaning lower limb T13.5
- – limb
- – – lower T13.5
- – – upper T11.5
- – long
- – – extensor, toe, at ankle and foot level S96.1
- – – flexor, toe, at ankle and foot level S96.0
- – – head, biceps S46.1
- – lower back S39.0
- – multiple T06.4
- – – ankle and foot level S96.7
- – – arm, upper (and shoulder) level S46.7
- – – extensor, wrist (and hand) level S66.7
- – – flexor, wrist (and hand) level S66.6
- – – forearm (level) S56.7
- – – hip (and thigh) level S76.7
- – – leg
- – – – lower S86.7
- – – – upper S76.7

Injury—*continued*
- muscle—*continued*
- – multiple—*continued*
- – – shoulder (and upper arm) level S46.7
- – – thigh (and hip) level S76.7
- – neck (level) S16
- – pelvis S39.0
- – peroneal muscle group, at lower leg level S86.3
- – posterior muscle (group)
- – – leg level, lower S86.1
- – – thigh level S76.3
- – quadriceps (thigh) S76.1
- – shoulder S46.9
- – – and upper arm level, multiple S46.7
- – – rotator cuff S46.0
- – – specified NEC S46.8
- – thigh NEC (level) S76.4
- – – adductor S76.2
- – – and hip, multiple S76.7
- – – posterior muscle (group) S76.3
- – – quadriceps S76.1
- – thorax (level) S29.0
- – triceps S46.3
- – trunk T09.5
- – upper limb T11.5
- – wrist (and hand) level S66.9
- myocardium S26.9
- nasal (septum) (sinus) S09.9
- nasopharynx S09.9
- neck S19.9
- – multiple S19.7
- – specified NEC S19.8
- nerve T14.4
- – abdomen S34.8
- – – peripheral S34.6
- – abducent S04.4
- – accessory S04.7
- – acoustic S04.6
- – ankle S94.9
- – – and foot, multiple S94.7
- – – deep peroneal S94.2
- – – lateral plantar S94.0
- – – medial plantar S94.1
- – – specified NEC S94.8
- – arm
- – – meaning upper limb T11.3
- – – upper (level) S44.9
- – – – and shoulder, multiple S44.7
- – – – axillary S44.3
- – – – multiple S44.7
- – – – specified NEC S44.8
- – auditory S04.6

Injury—*continued*
- nerve—*continued*
- – axillary S44.3
- – brachial plexus S14.3
- – cervical sympathetic S14.5
- – cranial S04.9
- – – with
- – – – brain (multiple) S09.7
- – – – spinal nerves (and cord) at neck level T06.0
- – – eighth (acoustic or auditory) S04.6
- – – eleventh (accessory) S04.7
- – – fifth (trigeminal) S04.3
- – – first (olfactory) S04.8
- – – fourth (trochlear) S04.2
- – – ninth (glossopharyngeal) S04.8
- – – second (optic) S04.0
- – – seventh (facial) S04.5
- – – sixth (abducent) S04.4
- – – specified NEC S04.8
- – – tenth (pneumogastric or vagus) S04.8
- – – third (oculomotor) S04.1
- – – twelfth (hypoglossal) S04.8
- – cutaneous sensory
- – – ankle (level) S94.3
- – – arm, upper (level) S44.5
- – – foot (level) S94.3
- – – forearm (level) S54.3
- – – hip (level) S74.2
- – – leg, lower (level) S84.2
- – – shoulder (level) S44.5
- – – thigh (level) S74.2
- – deep peroneal (ankle level) (foot level) S94.2
- – digital
- – – finger S64.4
- – – thumb S64.3
- – – toe S94.8
- – eighth cranial (acoustic or auditory) S04.6
- – eleventh cranial (accessory) S04.7
- – facial S04.5
- – – newborn P11.3
- – femoral (hip level) (thigh level) S74.1
- – fifth cranial (trigeminal) S04.3
- – finger (digital) S64.4
- – first cranial (olfactory) S04.8
- – foot S94.9
- – – and ankle, multiple S94.7
- – – cutaneous sensory S94.3
- – – deep peroneal S94.2
- – – lateral plantar S94.0
- – – medial plantar S94.1

Injury—*continued*
- nerve—*continued*
- – foot—*continued*
- – – specified NEC S94.8
- – forearm (level) S54.9
- – – multiple S54.7
- – – specified NEC S54.8
- – fourth cranial (trochlear) S04.2
- – glossopharyngeal S04.8
- – hand S64.9
- – – and wrist (level), multiple S64.7
- – – median S64.1
- – – radial S64.2
- – – specified NEC S64.8
- – – ulnar S64.0
- – hip (level) S74.9
- – – and thigh (level), multiple S74.7
- – – cutaneous sensory S74.2
- – – femoral S74.1
- – – sciatic S74.0
- – – specified NEC S74.8
- – hypoglossal S04.8
- – lateral plantar (ankle level) (foot level) S94.0
- – leg
- – – lower S84.9
- – – – cutaneous sensory S84.2
- – – – multiple S84.7
- – – – specified NEC S84.8
- – – meaning lower limb T13.3
- – – upper – *see* Injury, nerve, thigh
- – lower
- – – back S34.8
- – – – peripheral S34.6
- – – limb T13.3
- – medial plantar (ankle level) (foot level) S94.1
- – median (forearm (level)) S54.1
- – – hand (level) S64.1
- – – upper arm (level) S44.1
- – – wrist (level) S64.1
- – multiple regions T06.2
- – – ankle (and foot) level S94.7
- – – arm, upper (and shoulder) (level) S44.7
- – – foot (and ankle) (level) S94.7
- – – forearm S54.7
- – – hand (and wrist) (level) S64.7
- – – hip (and thigh) (level) S74.7
- – – leg, lower S84.7
- – – not classifiable to the same three-character category T06.2
- – – shoulder (and upper arm) (level) S44.7

Injury—*continued*
- nerve—*continued*
- – multiple regions—*continued*
- – – thigh (and hip) (level) S74.7
- – – wrist (and hand) (level) S64.7
- – musculocutaneous S44.4
- – musculospiral (upper arm level) S44.2
- – neck S14.6
- – – peripheral S14.4
- – – sympathetic S14.5
- – ninth cranial (glossopharyngeal) S04.8
- – oculomotor S04.1
- – olfactory S04.8
- – optic S04.0
- – pelvic girdle S74.9
- – – specified NEC S74.8
- – pelvis S34.8
- – – peripheral S34.6
- – peripheral T14.4
- – – abdomen S34.6
- – – lower back S34.6
- – – multiple T06.2
- – – neck S14.4
- – – pelvis S34.6
- – – specified NEC T14.4
- – peroneal (lower leg level) S84.1
- – – ankle and foot (level) S94.2
- – plexus
- – – brachial S14.3
- – – celiac, coeliac S34.5
- – – mesenteric, inferior S34.5
- – – spinal T09.4
- – – – multiple sites T06.1
- – pneumogastric S04.8
- – radial (forearm (level)) S54.2
- – – hand S64.2
- – – upper arm (level) S44.2
- – – wrist (level) S64.2
- – sciatic (hip level) (thigh level) S74.0
- – second cranial (optic) S04.0
- – seventh cranial (facial) S04.5
- – shoulder S44.9
- – – and upper arm (level), multiple S44.7
- – – specified NEC S44.8
- – sixth cranial (abducent) S04.4
- – spinal T09.4
- – – plexus – *see* Injury, nerve, plexus, spinal
- – – root T09.4
- – – – with multiple body regions T06.1
- – – – cervical S14.2
- – – – dorsal S24.2
- – – – lumbar, lumbosacral S34.2

Injury—*continued*
- nerve—*continued*
- – spinal—*continued*
- – – root—*continued*
- – – – sacral S34.2
- – – – thoracic S24.2
- – – splanchnic S34.5
- – sympathetic NEC S34.5
- – – cervical S14.5
- – tenth cranial (pneumogastric or vagus) S04.8
- – thigh (level) S74.9
- – – and hip (level), multiple S74.7
- – – cutaneous sensory S74.2
- – – femoral S74.1
- – – sciatic S74.0
- – – specified NEC S74.8
- – third cranial (oculomotor) S04.1
- – thorax S24.6
- – – peripheral S24.3
- – – specified NEC S24.5
- – – sympathetic S24.4
- – thumb, digital S64.3
- – tibial (lower leg level) S84.0
- – toe S94.9
- – trigeminal S04.3
- – trochlear S04.2
- – trunk T09.4
- – twelfth cranial (hypoglossal) S04.8
- – ulnar (forearm (level)) S54.0
- – – hand (level) S64.0
- – – upper arm (level) S44.0
- – – wrist (level) S64.0
- – upper limb T11.3
- – vagus S04.8
- – wrist (level) S64.9
- – – and hand (level), multiple S64.7
- – – median S64.1
- – – radial S64.2
- – – specified NEC S64.8
- – – ulnar S64.0
- nose (septum) S09.9
- obstetric (*see also* Delivery, complicated by, injury by type) O71.9
- – specified NEC O71.8
- occipital (region) (scalp) S09.9
- – lobe (*see also* Injury, intracranial) S06.8
- optic (chiasm) (cortex) (nerve) (pathways) S04.0
- orbit, orbital (region) S05.9
- – penetrating (with foreign body) S05.4
- – specified NEC S05.8
- ovary S37.4

Injury—*continued*
- palate (hard) (soft) S09.9
- pancreas S36.2
- parietal (region) (scalp) S09.9
- – lobe (*see also* Injury, intracranial) S06.8
- pelvis, pelvic (floor) S39.9
- – complicating delivery O70.1
- – joint or ligament, complicating delivery O71.6
- – organ S37.9
- – – with
- – – – abdominal organ(s) S39.6
- – – – intrathoracic organs T06.5
- – – – complication of abortion – *code to* O03-O07 with fourth character .3 or .8
- – – obstetric trauma NEC O71.5
- – specified NEC S39.8
  penis S39.9
- perineum S39.9
- peritoneum S36.8
- periurethral tissue S37.3
- – complicating delivery O71.5
- phalanges
- – foot S99.9
- – hand S69.9
- pharynx S09.9
- pleura S27.6
- plexus
- – brachial S14.3
- – cardiac S24.4
- – celiac S34.5
- – esophageal S24.4
- – hypogastric S34.5
- – lumbar, lumbosacral S34.4
- – mesenteric S34.5
- – pulmonary S24.4
- prepuce S39.9
- prostate S37.8
- pubic region S39.9
- pudendum S39.9
- radiation NEC T66
- rectovaginal septum NEC S39.8
- rectum S36.6
- retina S05.8
- – penetrating S05.6
- retroperitoneal S36.8
- rotator cuff S46.0
- round ligament S37.8
- sacral plexus S34.4
- salivary duct or gland S09.9
- scalp S09.9
- – fetus or newborn (birth injury) P12.9

Injury—*continued*
- scalp—*continued*
- – fetus or newborn—*continued*
- – – due to monitoring (electrode) (sampling incision) P12.4
- – – specified NEC P12.8
- scapular region S49.9
- sclera S05.8
- – penetrating S05.6
- scrotum S39.9
- seminal vesicle S37.8
- shoulder S49.9
- – and upper arm level, multiple S49.7
- – specified NEC S49.8
- sinus
- – cavernous S06.8
- – nasal S09.9
- skeleton, birth injury P13.9
- – specified part NEC P13.8
- skin, alone – *see also* Injury, superficial
- – surface intact – *see* Injury, superficial
- skull NEC S09.9
- spermatic cord (pelvic region) S37.8
- – scrotal region S39.8
- spinal cord T09.3
- – with nerves involving multiple body regions T06.1
- – cervical (neck) S14.1
- – – with brain (multiple) T06.0
- – dorsal S24.1
- – lumbar S34.1
- – nerve root NEC T09.4
- – – cervical S14.2
- – – dorsal S24.2
- – – lumbar, lumbosacral S34.2
- – – sacral S34.2
- – – thoracic S24.2
- – plexus T09.4
- – – brachial S14.3
- – – lumbosacral S34.4
- – – multiple sites T06.1
- – – trunk T09.4
- – thoracic S24.1
- spleen S36.0
- stellate ganglion S24.4
- sternal region S29.9
- stomach S36.3
- subconjunctival S05.0
- subcutaneous NEC T14.0
- submaxillary region S09.9
- submental region S09.9
- subungual
- – fingers S69.9
- – toes S90.9

373

Injury—*continued*
- superficial (for contusions, see first Contusion)
- – – abdomen, abdominal S30.9
- – – – with lower back and pelvic regions, multiple S30.7
- – – – specified NEC S30.8
- – – – wall S30.8
- – – adnexa, eye NEC S05.8
- – – alveolar process S00.5
- – – ankle S90.9
- – – – and foot, multiple S90.7
- – – – specified NEC S90.8
- – – anus S30.8
- – – arm
- – – – meaning upper limb – *see* Injury, superficial, limb, upper
- – – – upper S40.9
- – – – – and shoulder, multiple S40.7
- – – – – specified NEC S40.8
- – – auditory canal (external) (meatus) S00.4
- – – auricle S00.4
- – – axilla S40.9
- – – back, lower S30.89
- – – breast S20.1
- – brow S00.1
- – – buttock S30.8
- – – canthus, eye S00.2
- – – cheek (external) S00.8
- – – – internal S00.5
- – – chest wall S20.8
- – – chin S00.8
- – – clitoris S30.8
- – – conjunctiva S05.0
- – – – with foreign body (in conjunctival sac) T15.1
- – – cornea S05.0
- – – – with foreign body T15.0
- – – costal region S20.8
- – – – back S20.4
- – – – front S20.3
- – – – multiple S20.7
- – – ear (auricle) (canal) (external) S00.4
- – – elbow S50.9
- – – – and forearm (level), multiple S50.7
- – – epididymis S30.8
- – – epigastric region S30.8
- – – epiglottis S10.8
- – – esophagus (thoracic) S27.8
- – – – cervical S10.1
- – – extremity – *see* Injury, superficial, limb
- – – eyeball NEC S05.8
- – – eyebrow S00.1

Injury—*continued*
- superficial—*continued*
- – – eyelid S00.2
- – face NEC S00.8
- – – finger(s) S60.9
- – – flank S30.8
- – foot S90.9
- – – foot S90.9
- – – – and ankle, multiple S90.7
- – – – specified NEC S90.8
- – – forearm S50.9
- – – – and elbow (level), multiple S50.7
- – – – specified NEC S50.8
- – – forehead S00.8
- – – genital organs, external S30.8
- – – globe (eye) S05.8
- – – groin S30.8
- – – gum S00.5
- – – hand S60.9
- – – – and wrist, multiple S60.7
- – – – specified NEC S60.8
- – – head S00.9
- – – – multiple S00.7
- – – – scalp S00.0
- – – – specified NEC S00.8
- – – heel S90.9
- – – hip S70.9
- – – – and thigh, multiple S70.7
- – – – specified NEC S70.8
- – – iliac region S30.8
- – – inguinal region S30.8
- – – interscapular region S20.4
- – – jaw S00.8
- – – knee S80.9
- – – – and lower leg, multiple S80.7
- – – labium (majus) (minus) S30.8
- – – lacrimal (apparatus) (gland) (sac) S05.8
- – – larynx S10.1
- – – leg
- – – – lower S80.9
- – – – – and knee, multiple S80.7
- – – – – multiple S80.7
- – – – – specified NEC S80.8
- – – – meaning lower limb – *see* Injury, superficial, limb, lower
- – – limb T14.0
- – – – lower NEC (with) T13.0
- – – – – other body region(s) T00.8
- – – – – upper limb(s) T00.6
- – – – upper NEC (with) T11.0
- – – – – lower limb(s) T00.6
- – – – – other body region(s) T00.8
- – – lip S00.5
- – – lower back S30.9

Injury—*continued*
– superficial—*continued*
– – lower back—*continued*
– – – with abdominal and pelvic regions,
    multiple S30.7
– – – specified NEC S30.8
– – lumbar region S30.8
– – malar region S00.8
– – mammary S20.1
– – mastoid region S00.8
– – mouth S00.5
– – multiple T00.9
– – – abdominal, lower back and pelvic
    regions (with) S30.7
– – – – other body regions T00.8
– – – – thorax T00.1
– – – ankle (and foot) S90.7
– – – arm
– – – – meaning upper limb – *see* Injury,
    superficial, multiple, limb, upper
– – – – upper (and shoulder) S40.7
– – – body regions NEC T00.8
– – – calf S80.7
– – – foot (and ankle) S90.7
– – – forearm (and elbow) S50.7
– – – hand (and wrist) S60.7
– – – head (with) S00.7
– – – – neck T00.0
– – – – other body regions T00.8
– – – hip (and thigh) S70.7
– – – knee (and lower leg) S80.7
– – – leg
– – – – lower (and knee) S80.7
– – – – meaning lower limb – *see* Injury,
    superficial, multiple, limb, lower
– – – limb
– – – – lower (with) T00.3
– – – – – abdominal, lower back and
    pelvic regions T00.8
– – – – – thorax T00.8
– – – – – upper limb(s) T00.6
– – – – upper (with) T00.2
– – – – – abdominal, lower back and
    pelvic regions T00.8
– – – – – lower limb(s) T00.6
– – – – – thorax T00.8
– – – neck (with) S10.7
– – – – head T00.0
– – – – other body regions T00.8
– – – shoulder (and upper arm) S40.7
– – – specified NEC T00.8
– – – thigh (and hip) S70.7
– – – thorax (with) S20.7

Injury—*continued*
– superficial—*continued*
– – multiple—*continued*
– – – thorax—*continued*
– – – – abdominal, lower back and pelvic
    regions T00.1
– – – – other body regions T00.8
– – – trunk T09.0
– – – wrist (and hand) S60.7
– – muscle T14.6
– – nail
– – – finger S60.9
– – – toe S90.9
– – nasal (septum) S00.3
– – neck S10.9
– – – multiple S10.7
– – – specified part NEC S10.8
– – nose (septum) S00.3
– – occipital region S00.0
– – oral cavity S00.5
– – orbital region S00.2
– – palate S00.5
– – parietal region S00.0
– – pelvis S30.9
– – – with abdominal and lower back
    regions, multiple S30.7
– – – specified NEC S30.8
– – penis S30.8
– – perineum S30.8
– – periocular area S00.2
– – phalanges
– – – finger S60.9
– – – toe S90.9
– – pharynx S10.1
– – pinna S00.4
– – popliteal space S80.9
– – prepuce S30.8
– – pubic region S30.8
– – pudendum S30.8
– – sacral region S30.8
– – scalp S00.0
– – scapular region S40.9
– – sclera S05.8
– – scrotum S30.8
– – shoulder (and upper arm) S40.9
– – – multiple S40.7
– – – specified NEC S40.8
– – skin NEC T14.0
– – sternal region S20.3
– – subconjunctival S05.8
– – subcutaneous NEC T14.0
– – submaxillary region S00.8
– – submental region S00.8

Injury—*continued*
- superficial—*continued*
- - subungual
- - - finger(s) S60.9
- - - toe(s) S90.9
- - supraclavicular fossa S10.8
- - supraorbital S00.8
- - temple S00.8
- - temporal region S00.8
- - testis S30.8
- - thigh S70.9
- - - and hip, multiple S70.7
- - - specified NEC S70.8
- - thorax, thoracic (wall) S20.8
- - - back S20.4
- - - front S20.3
- - - multiple S20.7
- - throat S10.1
- - thumb S60.9
- - toe(s) S90.9
- - tongue S00.5
- - tooth, teeth S00.5
- - trachea (cervical) S10.1
- - - thoracic S27.5
- - trunk NEC T09.0
- - tunica vaginalis S30.8
- - tympanum, tympanic membrane S00.4
- - upper limb NEC T11.0
- - - with other body regions T00.8
- - uvula S00.5
- - vagina S30.8
- - vocal cord(s) S10.1
- - vulva S30.8
- - wrist S60.9
- - - and hand, multiple S60.7
- - - specified NEC S60.8
- supraclavicular fossa NEC S19.9
- supraorbital S09.9
- suprarenal gland (multiple) S37.8
- surgical complication (external or internal site) T81.2
- temple S09.9
- temporal region S09.9
- tendon (*see also* Injury, muscle, by site) T14.6
- - abdomen S39.0
- - Achilles S86.0
- - lower back S39.0
- - pelvic organs S39.0
- testis S39.9
- thigh S79.9
- - and hip, multiple S79.7
- - specified NEC S79.8
- thorax, thoracic S29.9

Injury—*continued*
- thorax, thoracic—*continued*
- - cavity S27.9
- - - multiple S27.7
- - external S29.9
- - - specified NEC S29.8
- - internal S27.9
- - - specified NEC S27.8
- - intrathoracic organ S27.9
- - - multiple S27.7
- - - specified NEC S27.8
- - multiple S29.7
- throat NEC S19.8
- thumb S69.9
- thymus (gland) S27.8
- thyroid (gland) NEC S19.8
- toe S99.9
- tongue S09.9
- tonsil S09.9
- tooth S09.9
- trachea (cervical) NEC S19.8
- - thoracic S27.5
- trunk T09.9
- - internal, multiple T06.5
- - specified type NEC T09.8
- tunica vaginalis S39.9
- ultraviolet rays NEC T66
- ureter S37.1
- urethra (sphincter) S37.3
- uterus S37.6
- uvula S09.9
- vagina S39.9
- vas deferens S37.8
- vein (*see also* Injury, blood vessel) T14.5
- vena cava (superior) S25.2
- - inferior S35.1
- vesical (sphincter) S37.2
- viscera (abdominal), multiple S36.7
- - thoracic NEC S27.7
- visual cortex S04.0
- vitreous (humor) S05.9
- - specified NEC S05.8
- vulva S39.9
- whiplash (cervical spine) S13.4
- wrist S69.9
- - and hand, multiple S69.7
- - specified NEC S69.8
- X-ray NEC T66

Inoculation – *see also* Vaccination
- complication or reaction – *see* Complications, vaccination

Insanity, insane (*see also condition*) F99

Insect
- bite – *see* Injury, superficial

Insect—*continued*
– venomous, poisoning NEC T63.4
Insemination, artificial Z31.1
Insertion
– cord (umbilical) lateral or velamentous O43.1
– intrauterine contraceptive device Z30.1
– placenta, vicious – *see* Placenta, previa
Insolation (sunstroke) T67.0
Insomnia (organic) G47.0
– nonorganic origin F51.0
– primary F51.0
Inspiration
– food or foreign body (*see also* Asphyxia, food) T17.9
– mucus (*see also* Asphyxia, mucus) T17.9
Inspissated bile syndrome (newborn) P59.1
Instability
– emotional (excessive) F60.3
– joint (post-traumatic) M25.3
– – due to old ligament injury M24.2
– – lumbosacral M53.2
– – sacroiliac M53.2
– – secondary to removal of joint prosthesis M96.8
– – specified NEC M25.3
– knee (chronic) M23.5
– lumbosacral M53.2
– nervous F48.8
– personality (emotional) F60.3
– spine M53.2
– vasomotor R55
Institutional syndrome (childhood) F94.2
Institutionalization, affecting child Z62.2
– disinhibited attachment F94.2
Insufficiency, insufficient
– accommodation H52.5
– – old age H52.4
– adrenal (gland) E27.4
– – primary E27.1
– adrenocortical E27.4
– – drug-induced E27.3
– – iatrogenic E27.3
– – primary E27.1
– anus K62.8
– aortic (valve) I35.1
– – with
– – – mitral (valve) disease (unspecified origin) I08.0
– – – – with tricuspid (valve) disease (unspecified origin) I08.3
– – – stenosis I35.2

Insufficiency, insufficient—*continued*
– aortic—*continued*
– – with—*continued*
– – – tricuspid (valve) disease (unspecified origin) I08.2
– – – – with mitral (valve) disease (unspecified origin) I08.3
– – congenital Q23.1
– – rheumatic (with) I06.1
– – – mitral (valve) disease I08.0
– – – – with tricuspid (valve) disease I08.3
– – – stenosis I06.2
– – – – with mitral (valve) disease I08.0
– – – – – with tricuspid (valve) disease I08.3
– – – tricuspid (valve) disease I08.2
– – – – with mitral (valve) disease I08.3
– – specified cause NEC I35.1
– – syphilitic A52.0† I39.1*
– arterial I77.1
– – basilar G45.0
– – carotid (hemispheric) G45.1
– – cerebral I67.8
– – mesenteric (chronic) K55.1
– – – acute K55.0
– – peripheral I73.9
– – precerebral (bilateral) (multiple) G45.2
– – vertebral G45.0
– arteriovenous I99
– biliary K83.8
– cardiac (*see also* Insufficiency, myocardial) I50.9
– – complicating surgery T81.8
– – due to presence of (cardiac) prosthesis I97.1
– – postoperative I97.8
– – – long term effect of cardiac surgery I97.1
– – specified during or due to a procedure T81.8
– cardiorenal, hypertensive (*see also* Hypertension, cardiorenal) I13.2
– cardiovascular (*see also* Disease, cardiovascular) I51.6
– – renal (hypertensive) (*see also* Hypertension, cardiorenal) I13.2
– cerebrovascular (acute) I67.8
– – with transient focal neurological signs and symptoms G45.8
– circulatory NEC I99
– – fetus or newborn P29.8
– convergence H51.1
– coronary (acute) (subacute) I24.8

Insufficiency, insufficient—*continued*
- coronary—*continued*
- – – chronic or with a stated duration of over
 4 weeks I25.8
- corticoadrenal E27.4
- – primary E27.1
 dietary E63.9
- divergence H51.8
- food T73.0
- gonadal
- – ovary E28.3
- – testis E29.1
- heart (*see also* Insufficiency, myocardial)
 I50.9
- – newborn P29.0
- – valve (*see also* Endocarditis) I38
- hepatic – *see* Failure, hepatic
- idiopathic autonomic G90.0
- kidney (*see also* Failure, kidney) N19
- lacrimal (secretion) H04.1
- – passages H04.5
- liver (*see also* Failure, hepatic) K72.9
- lung (*see also* Insufficiency, pulmonary)
 J98.4
- – newborn P28.5
- mental (congenital) (*see also* Retardation,
 mental) F79.-
- mitral I34.0
- – with
- – – aortic valve disease (unspecified
 origin) I08.0
- – – – with tricuspid (valve) disease
 (unspecified origin) I08.3
- – – obstruction or stenosis I05.2
- – – – with aortic valve disease
 (unspecified origin) I08.0
- – – tricuspid (valve) disease (unspecified
 origin) I08.1
- – – – with aortic (valve) disease
 (unspecified origin) I08.3
- – congenital Q23.3
- – rheumatic I05.1
- – – with
- – – – aortic valve disease I08.0
- – – – – with tricuspid (valve) disease
 I08.3
- – – – obstruction or stenosis I05.2
- – – – – with aortic valve disease I08.0
- – – – – – with tricuspid (valve) disease
 I08.3
- – – – tricuspid (valve) disease I08.1
- – – – – with aortic (valve) disease I08.3
- – – active or acute I01.1

Insufficiency, insufficient—*continued*
- mitral—*continued*
- – rheumatic—*continued*
- – – active or acute—*continued*
- – – – with chorea, rheumatic
 (Sydenham's) I02.0
- specified cause, except rheumatic I34.0
- muscle (*see also* Disease, muscle)
- – heart – *see* Insufficiency, myocardial
- – ocular NEC H50.9
- myocardial, myocardium I50.9
- – with
- – – rheumatic fever (conditions in I00)
 I09.0
- – – – active, acute or subacute I01.2
- – – – – with chorea I02.0
- – – – inactive or quiescent (with chorea)
 I09.0
- – congenital Q24.8
- – hypertensive (*see also* Hypertension,
 heart) I11.9
- – newborn P29.0
- – rheumatic I09.0
- – – active, acute or subacute I01.2
- – syphilitic A52.0† I52.0*
- nourishment T73.0
- organic R68.8
- ovary E28.3
- pancreatic K86.8
- parathyroid (gland) E20.9
- peripheral vascular I73.9
- pituitary E23.0
- placental (mother) O36.5
- – affecting fetus or newborn P02.2
- prenatal care affecting management of
 pregnancy Z35.3
- progressive pluriglandular E31.0
- pulmonary J98.4
- – acute, following surgery (nonthoracic)
 J95.2
- – – thoracic J95.1
- – chronic, following surgery J95.3
- – following
- – – shock J80
- – – trauma J80
- – newborn P28.5
- – valve I37.1
- – – with stenosis I37.2
- – – congenital Q22.2
- – – rheumatic I09.8
- – – – with aortic, mitral or tricuspid
 (valve) disease I08.8
- pyloric K31.8
- renal (*see also* Failure, kidney) N19

Insufficiency, insufficient—*continued*
- renal—*continued*
- – – postprocedural N99.0
- – respiratory R06.8
- – – newborn P28.5
- – rotation – *see* Malrotation
- – social insurance Z59.7
- – suprarenal E27.4
- – – primary E27.1
- – tarso-orbital fascia, congenital Q10.3
- – testis E29.1
- – thyroid (gland) (acquired) E03.9
- – – congenital E03.1
- – tricuspid (valve) (rheumatic) I07.1
- – – with
- – – – aortic (valve) disease (unspecified origin) I08.2
- – – – – with mitral (valve) disease (unspecified origin) I08.3
- – – – mitral (valve) disease (unspecified origin) I08.1
- – – – – with aortic (valve) disease (unspecified origin) I08.3
- – – – obstruction or stenosis I07.2
- – – – – with aortic (valve) disease (unspecified origin) I08.2
- – – – – – with mitral (valve) disease (unspecified origin) I08.3
- – – congenital Q22.8
- – – nonrheumatic I36.1
- – – – with stenosis I36.2
- – urethral sphincter R32
- – valve, valvular (heart) (*see also* Endocarditis) I38
- – – congenital Q24.8
- – vascular I99
- – – intestine K55.9
- – – mesenteric (chronic) K55.1
- – – – acute K55.0
- – – peripheral I73.9
- – – renal (*see also* Hypertension, kidney) I12.9
- – venous (chronic) (peripheral) I87.2
- – ventricular – *see* Insufficiency, myocardial
- – welfare support Z59.7

Insufflation, fallopian Z31.4
Insular – *see condition*
Insulinoma
- malignant (M8151/3)
- – pancreas C25.4
- – specified site NEC – *see* Neoplasm, malignant
- – unspecified site C25.4

Insulinoma—*continued*
- pancreas
- – benign (M8152/0) D13.7
- – uncertain or unknown behavior (M8152/1) D37.7
- – malignant (M8152/3) C25.4
- specified site NEC
- – benign (M8152/0) – *see* Neoplasm benign
- – uncertain or unknown behavior (M8152/1) – *see* Neoplasm uncertain or unknown behavior
- – malignant (M8152/3) – *see* Neoplasm malignant
- unspecified site
- – benign (M8152/0) D13.7
- – uncertain or unknown behavior (M8152/1) D37.7
- – malignant (M8152/3) C25.4

Insuloma (M8151/0) – *see* Insulinoma
Interception of pregnancy Z30.3
Intermenstrual – *see condition*
Intermittent – *see condition*
Internal – *see condition*
Interruption
- bundle of His I44.3
- fallopian tube Z30.2
- vas deferens Z30.2
Interstitial – *see condition*
Intertrigo L30.4
Intervertebral disk – *see condition*
Intestine, intestinal – *see condition*
Intolerance
- carbohydrate K90.4
- disaccharide, hereditary E73.0
- fat NEC K90.4
- – pancreatic K90.3
- food K90.4
- – dietary counseling and surveillance Z71.3
- fructose (hereditary) E74.1
- glucose(-galactose) E74.3
- lactose E73.9
- – specified NEC E73.8
- lysine E72.3
- milk NEC K90.4
- – lactose E73.9
- protein K90.4
- starch NEC K90.4
- sucrose(-isomaltose) E74.3
Intoxicated NEC F10.0
Intoxication
- alcoholic (acute) (with) F10.0
- – delirium F10.0

Intoxication—*continued*
- alcoholic—*continued*
- - - hangover effects F10.0
- - - idiosyncratic F10.0
- - - pathological F10.0
- - - withdrawal state F10.3
- - - - with delirium F10.4
- amfetamine (or related substnace) (acute) F15.0
- anxiolytic (acute) F13.0
- caffeine (acute) F15.0
- cannabinoids (acute) F12.0
- chemical (*see also* Table of drugs and chemicals) T65.9
- - - via placenta or breast milk – *see* Absorption, chemical, through placenta
- cocaine (acute) F14.0
- drug
- - addictive
- - - acute – *code to* F10-F19 with fourth character .0
- - - via placenta or breast milk – *see* Absorption, drug, addictive, through placenta
- - correct substance properly administered (*see also* Allergy, drug) T88.7
- - newborn P93
- - overdose or wrong substance given or taken – *see* Table of drugs and chemicals
- enteric – *see* Intoxication, intestinal
- fetus or newborn, via placenta or breast milk – *see* Absorption, chemical, through placenta
- foodborne A05.9
- - bacterial A05.9
- - classical, due to Clostridium botulinum A05.1
- - due to
- - - Bacillus cereus A05.4
- - - bacterium A05.9
- - - - specified NEC A05.8
- - - Clostridium
- - - - botulinum A05.1
- - - - difficile A04.7
- - - - perfringens A05.2
- - - - welchii A05.2
- - - salmonella A02.9
- - - - with
- - - - - (gastro)enteritis A02.0
- - - - - localized infection(s) A02.2
- - - - - sepsis A02.1

Intoxication—*continued*
- foodborne—*continued*
- - due to—*continued*
- - - salmonella—*continued*
- - - - with—*continued*
- - - - - specified manifestation NEC A02.8
- - - Staphylococcus A05.0
- - - Vibrio parahaemolyticus A05.3
- - enterotoxin, staphylococcal A05.0
- - noxious – *see* Poisoning, food, noxious
- hallucinogenic (acute) F16.0
- hypnotic (acute) F13.0
- inhalant (acute) F18.0
- intestinal K63.8
- maternal medication, via placenta or breast milk – *see* Absorption, maternal medication, through placenta
- meaning
- - inebriation – *code to* F10-F19 with fourth character .0
- - poisoning – *see* Table of drugs and chemicals
- methyl alcohol (acute) F10.0
- opioid (acute) F11.0
- pathologic NEC F10.0
- phencyclidine (or related substance) (acute) F19.0
- psychoactive substance NEC F19.0
- sedative (acute) F13.0
- septic (*see also* Shock, septic) A41.9
- - during labor O75.3
- - following
- - - abortion (subsequent episode) O08.0
- - - - current episode – *see* Abortion
- - - ectopic gestation O08.0
- - general A41.9
- - puerperal, postpartum, childbirth O85
- serum (prophylactic) (therapeutic) T80.6
- uremic – *see* Uremia
- volatile solvents (acute) F18.0
- water E87.7
Intracranial – *see condition*
Intrahepatic gallbladder Q44.1
Intraligamentous – *see condition*
Intrathoracic – *see also condition*
- kidney Q63.2
Intrauterine contraceptive device
- checking, reinsertion, removal Z30.5
- in situ Z97.5
- insertion Z30.1
- retention in pregnancy O26.3
Intraventricular – *see condition*
Intubation, difficult or failed T88.4

Intumescence, lens (eye) (cataract) H26.9
Intussusception (bowel) (colon) (intestine) (rectum) K56.1
– appendix K38.8
– congenital Q43.8
– ureter (with obstruction) N13.5
Invagination (bowel) (colon) (intestine) (rectum) K56.1
Invalid, invalidism (chronic) (since birth) R68.8
Inversion
– albumin-globulin (A-G) ratio E88.0
– bladder N32.8
– cervix N88.8
– chromosome in normal individual Q95.1
– circadian rhythm G47.2
– – psychogenic F51.2
– nipple N64.5
– – congenital Q83.8
– – gestational O92.0
– – puerperal, postpartum O92.0
– nyctohemeral rhythm G47.2
– – psychogenic F51.2
– optic papilla Q14.2
– organ or site, congenital NEC – *see* Anomaly, by site
– sleep rhythm G47.2
– – nonorganic origin F51.2
– testis (congenital) Q55.2
– uterus (chronic) N85.5
– – postpartum O71.2
– vagina (posthysterectomy) N99.3
– ventricular Q20.5
Investigation (*see also* Examination) Z04.9
– allergens Z01.5
– clinical research subject (control) Z00.6
Involuntary movement, abnormal R25.8
Involution, involutional – *see also* condition
– breast, cystic N60.8
– ovary, senile N83.3
I.Q.
– under 20 F73.-
– 20-34 F72.-
– 35-49 F71.-
– 50-69 F70.-
Irideremia Q13.1
Iridis rubeosis H21.1
Iridochoroiditis (panuveitis) H44.1
Iridocyclitis H20.9
– acute H20.0
– chronic H20.1
– due to allergy H20.0
– endogenous H20.0

Iridocyclitis—*continued*
– gonococcal A54.3† H22.0*
– granulomatous H20.1
– herpes, herpetic (simplex) B00.5† H22.0*
– – zoster B02.3† H22.0*
– hypopyon H20.0
– in (due to)
– – ankylosing spondylitis M45† H22.1*
– – gonococcal infection A54.3† H22.0*
– – herpes (simplex) virus B00.5† H22.0*
– – – zoster B02.3† H22.0*
– – infectious disease NEC B99† H22.0*
– – parasitic disease NEC B89† H22.0*
– – sarcoidosis D86.8† H22.1*
– – syphilis A51.4† H22.0*
– – tuberculosis A18.5† H22.0*
– – zoster B02.3† H22.0*
– lens-induced H20.2
– nongranulomatous H20.0
– recurrent H20.0
– specified NEC H20.8
– subacute H20.0
– sympathetic H44.1
– syphilitic (early) (secondary) A51.4† H22.0*
– – congenital (early) A50.0† H22.0*
– – – late A50.3† H22.0*
– – late A52.7† H22.0*
– tuberculous (chronic) A18.5† H22.0*
Iridocyclochoroiditis (panuveitis) H44.1
Iridodialysis H21.5
Iridodonesis H21.8
Iridoplegia (complete) (partial) (reflex) H57.0
Iridoschisis H21.2
Iris – *see also* condition
– bombé H21.4
Iritis (*see also* Iridocyclitis) H20.9
– diabetic (*see also* E10-E14 with fourth character .3) E14.3† H22.1*
– due to
– – herpes simplex B00.5† H22.0*
– – leprosy A30.-† H22.0*
– gonococcal A54.3† H22.0*
– gouty M10.9† H22.1*
– papulosa (syphilitic) A52.7† H22.0*
– syphilitic (early) (secondary) A51.4† H22.0*
– – congenital (early) A50.0† H22.0*
– – – late A50.3† H22.0*
– – late A52.7† H22.0*
– tuberculous A18.5† H22.0*
Iron – *see condition*
Iron-miner's lung J63.4

Irradiated enamel (tooth, teeth) K03.8
Irradiation effects, adverse NEC T66
Irreducible, irreducibility – *see condition*
Irregular, irregularity
– action, heart I49.9
– alveolar process K08.8
– bleeding N92.6
– breathing R06.8
– contour of cornea (acquired) H18.7
– – congenital Q13.4
– dentin (in pulp) K04.3
– menstruation (cause unknown) N92.6
– periods N92.6
– pupil H21.5
– respiratory R06.8
– septum (nasal) J34.2
– shape, organ or site, congenital NEC – *see* Distortion
Irritable, irritability R45.4
– bladder N32.8
– bowel (syndrome) K58.9
– – with diarrhea K58.0
– – psychogenic F45.3
– cerebral, in newborn P91.3
– colon K58.9
– – with diarrhea K58.0
– – psychogenic F45.3
– duodenum K59.8
– heart (psychogenic) F45.3
– hip M65.8
– ileum K59.8
– infant R68.1
– jejunum K59.8
– rectum K59.8
– stomach K31.8
– – psychogenic F45.3
– sympathetic G90.8
– urethra N36.8
Irritation
– anus K62.8
– bladder N32.8
– brachial plexus G54.0
– cervix (*see also* Cervicitis) N72
– choroid, sympathetic H44.1
– cranial nerve – *see* Disorder, nerve, cranial
– gastric K31.8
– – psychogenic F45.3
– globe, sympathetic H44.1
– labyrinth H83.2
– lumbosacral plexus G54.1
– meninges (traumatic) (*see also* Injury, intracranial) S06.0
– – nontraumatic – *see* Meningismus

Irritation—*continued*
– nerve – *see* Disorder, nerve
– nervous R45.0
– penis N48.8
– perineum NEC L29.3
– peripheral autonomic nervous system G90.8
– pharynx J39.2
– spinal (cord) – *see* Myelopathy
– stomach K31.8
– – psychogenic F45.3
– sympathetic nerve NEC G90.8
– vagina N89.8
Ischemia, ischemic I99
– brain (*see also* Ischemia, cerebral) I67.8
– cardiac – *see* Disease, heart, ischemic
– cardiomyopathy I25.5
– cerebral (chronic) (generalized) I67.8
– – arteriosclerotic I67.2
– – intermittent G45.9
– – newborn P91.0
– – puerperal, postpartum, childbirth O99.4
– – recurrent focal G45.8
– – transient G45.9
– coronary (*see also* Ischemia, heart) I25.9
– heart (chronic or with a stated duration of over 4 weeks) I25.9
– – acute or with a stated duration of 4 weeks or less I24.9
– – failure I25.5
– infarction, muscle M62.2
– intestine (large) (small) K55.9
– – acute K55.0
– – chronic K55.1
– kidney N28.0
– mesenteric, acute K55.0
– – chronic K55.1
– muscle, traumatic T79.6
– myocardium, myocardial (chronic or with a stated duration of over 4 weeks) I25.9
– – silent (asymptomatic) I25.6
– – transient, of newborn P29.4
– retina, retinal H34.2
– spinal cord G95.1
– subendocardial (*see also* Insufficiency, coronary) I24.8
Ischial spine – *see condition*
Ischialgia (*see also* Sciatica) M54.3
Ischiopagus Q89.4
Ischium, ischial – *see condition*
Ischuria R34
Iselin's disease or osteochondrosis M92.7

Islands of
- parotid tissue in
- - lymph nodes Q38.6
- - neck structures Q38.6
- submaxillary glands in
- - fascia Q38.6
- - lymph nodes Q38.6
- - neck muscles Q38.6

Islet cell tumor, pancreas (M8150/0)
D13.7

Isoimmunization NEC (*see also*
Incompatibility)
- fetus or newborn P55.9
- - with
- - - hydrops fetalis P56.0
- - - kernicterus P57.0
- - ABO P55.1
- - Rh P55.0
- - specified type NEC P55.8

Isolation, isolated Z29.0
- dwelling Z59.8
- family Z63.7
- social Z60.4

Isoleucinosis E71.1

**Isomerism, atrial appendages (with
asplenia or polysplenia)** Q20.6

Isosporiasis, isosporosis A07.3

Isovaleric acidemia E71.1

Issue of
- medical certificate (cause of death)
(fitness) (incapacity) (invalidity) Z02.7
- repeat prescription (appliance) (glasses)
(medicament) Z76.0
- - contraceptive (pill) Z30.4

Issue of—*continued*
- repeat prescription—*continued*
- - contraceptive—*continued*
- - - device (intrauterine) Z30.5

Itch, itching (*see also* Pruritus) L29.9
- baker's L25.4
- - allergic L23.6
- - irritant L24.6
- barber's B35.0
- bricklayer's L25.3
- - allergic L23.5
- - irritant L24.5
- cheese B88.0
- clam digger's B65.3
- coolie B76.9
- copra B88.0
- dew B76.9
- dhobi B35.6
- filarial (*see also* Filaria, filarial, filariasis)
B74.9
- grain B88.0
- grocer's B88.0
- ground B76.9
- harvest B88.0
- jock B35.6
- Malabar (any site) B35.5
- meaning scabies B86
- Norwegian B86
- poultryman's B88.0
- sarcoptic B86
- scrub B88.0
- straw B88.0
- swimmer's B65.3
- water B76.9
- winter L29.8

Ixodiasis NEC B88.8

383

If breast milk, or any neonatal jaundice after 28 days, can code to the P code so long as it first appeared within the first 28 days

J

Jaccoud's syndrome M12.0
Jacksonian epilepsy or seizures (focal) G40.1
Jackson's
− membrane or veil Q43.3
− paralysis (syndrome) G83.8
Jacquet's dermatitis L22
Jadassohn-Pellizari's disease or anetoderma L90.2
Jadassohn's
− blue nevus (M8780/0) (*see also* Nevus, by site) D22.9
− intraepidermal epithelioma (M8096/0) − *see* Neoplasm, skin, benign
Jaffe-Lichtenstein(-Uehlinger) syndrome M85.0
Jakob-Creutzfeldt disease or syndrome A81.0
− with dementia A81.0† F02.1*
Jaksch-Luzet disease D64.8
Janet's disease F48.8
Janiceps Q89.4
Jansky-Bielschowsky amaurotic idiocy E75.4
Jaundice (yellow) R17
− acholuric (familial) (splenomegalic) (*see also* Spherocytosis) D58.0
− − acquired D59.8
− breast-milk (inhibitor) P59.3
− due to or associated with
− − delayed conjugation P59.8
− − − associated with preterm delivery P59.0
− − preterm delivery P59.0
− epidemic (catarrhal)
− − leptospiral A27.0
− − spirochetal A27.0
− familial nonhemolytic E80.4
− − congenital E80.5
− fetus or newborn (physiological) P59.9
− − due to or associated with
− − − ABO
− − − − antibodies P55.1
− − − − incompatibility, maternal/fetal P55.1
− − − − isoimmunization P55.1

Jaundice—*continued*
− fetus or newborn—*continued*
− − due to or associated with—*continued*
− − − absence or deficiency of enzyme system for bilirubin conjugation (congenital) P59.8
− − − bleeding P58.1
− − − breast milk inhibitors to conjugation P59.3
− − − bruising P58.0
− − − Crigler-Najjar syndrome E80.5
− − − delayed conjugation P59.8
− − − − associated with preterm delivery P59.0
− − − drugs or toxins
− − − − given to newborn P58.4
− − − − transmitted from mother P58.4
− − − excessive hemolysis NEC P58.9
− − − − specified type NEC P58.8
− − − galactosemia E74.2
− − − Gilbert's syndrome E80.4
− − − hepatocellular damage P59.2
− − − hereditary hemolytic anemia D58.9
− − − hypothyroidism, congenital E03.1
− − − incompatibility, maternal/fetal NEC P55.9
− − − infection P58.2
− − − inspissated bile syndrome P59.1
− − − isoimmunization NEC P55.9
− − − mucoviscidosis E84.8
− − − polycythemia P58.3
− − − preterm delivery P59.0
− − − Rh
− − − − antibodies P55.0
− − − − incompatibility, maternal/fetal P55.0
− − − − isoimmunization P55.0
− − − swallowed maternal blood P58.5
− − specified cause NEC P59.8
− hematogenous D59.9
− hemolytic (acquired) D59.9
− − congenital (*see also* Spherocytosis) D58.0
− hemorrhagic leptosprial (acute) (spirochetal) A27.0
− leptospiral (hemorrhagic) A27.0
− malignant (*see also* Failure, hepatic) K72.9
− neonatal − *see* Jaundice, fetus or newborn

Jaundice—*continued*
- nonhemolytic congenital familial (Gilbert)
  E80.4
- nuclear, newborn (*see also* Kernicterus of
  newborn) P57.9
- obstructive (*see also* Obstruction, bile
  duct) K83.1
- post-immunization – *see* Hepatitis, viral,
  type B
- post-transfusion – *see* Hepatitis, viral,
  type B
- regurgitation (*see also* Obstruction, bile
  duct) K83.1
- serum (homologous) (prophylactic)
  (therapeutic) – *see* Hepatitis, viral, type B
- spirochetal (hemorrhagic) A27.0
Jaw – *see condition*
Jaw-winking phenomenon or syndrome
  Q07.8

Jealousy
- alcoholic F10.5
- childhood F93.8
- sibling F93.3
Jejunitis (*see also* Enteritis) A09.9
- infectious A09.0
- noninfectious K52.9
Jejunum, jejunal – *see condition*
Jensen's disease H30.0
Jerks, myoclonic G25.3
Jervell and Lange-Nielsen syndrome
  I45.8
Jeune's disease Q77.2
Jigger disease B88.1
Joint – *see also condition*
- mice M24.0
- – knee M23.4
Jüngling's disease (*see also* Sarcoidosis)
  D86.9
Juvenile – *see condition*

Jittery Baby R25.8

K

Kahler disease C90.0
Kakke E51.1
Kala-azar B55.0
Kallmann's syndrome E23.0
Kanner's syndrome F84.0
Kaposi's
– sarcoma (M9140/3)
– – connective tissue C46.1
– – lymph node (multiple) C46.3
– – multiple organs C46.8
– – palate (hard) (soft) C46.2
– – resulting from HIV disease B21.0
– – skin (multiple sites) C46.0
– – specified site NEC C46.7
– – unspecified site C46.9
– varicelliform eruption B00.0
Kartagener's syndrome or triad Q89.3
Karyotype – *see also condition*
– 45,X Q96.0
– 46,X
– – with abnormality except iso (Xq)
 Q96.2
– – iso (Xq) Q96.1
– 46,XX
– – with streak gonads Q99.1
– – hermaphrodite (true) Q99.1
– – male Q98.3
– – – in Klinefelter's syndrome Q98.2
– 46,XY
– – with streak gonads Q99.1
– – female Q97.3
– 47,XXX Q97.0
– 47,XXY, with Klinefelter's syndrome
 Q98.0
– 47,XYY Q98.5
Kaschin-Beck disease M12.1
Katayama's disease or fever B65.2
Kawasaki's syndrome M30.3
Kayser-Fleischer ring (cornea) H18.0
Kearns-Sayre syndrome H49.8
Kelis L91.0
Kelly-Paterson syndrome D50.1
Keloid, cheloid L91.0
– acne L73.0
– Addison's L94.0
– cornea H17.8
– scar L91.0
Keratectasia H18.7
– congenital Q13.4

Keratitis (nonulcerative) H16.9
– with ulceration (central) (marginal)
 (perforated) (ring) H16.0
– actinic H16.1
– arborescens (herpes simplex) B00.5†
 H19.1*
– areolar H16.1
– bullosa H16.8
– deep H16.3
– dendritic(a) (herpes simplex) B00.5†
 H19.1*
– disciform(is) (herpes simplex) B00.5†
 H19.1*
– – varicella B01.8† H19.2*
– filamentary H16.1
– gonococcal (congenital) (prenatal)
 A54.3† H19.2*
– herpes, herpetic (simplex) NEC B00.5†
 H19.1*
– – zoster B02.3† H19.2*
– in (due to)
– – acanthamebiasis B60.1† H19.2*
– – adenovirus B30.0† H19.2*
– – herpes (simplex) virus B00.5† H19.1*
– – infectious disease NEC B99† H19.2*
– – measles B05.8† H19.2*
– – parasitic disease NEC B89† H19.2*
– – syphilis A50.3† H19.2*
– – tuberculosis A18.5† H19.2*
– – zoster B02.3† H19.2*
– interstitial (nonsyphilitic) H16.3
– – herpes, herpetic (simplex) B00.5†
 H19.1*
– – – zoster B02.3† H19.2*
– – syphilitic (congenital) (late) A50.3†
 H19.2*
– – tuberculous A18.5† H19.2*
– nummular H16.1
– parenchymatous – *see* Keratitis, interstitial
– petrificans H16.8
– postmeasles B05.8† H19.2*
– punctata
– – leprosa A30.-† H19.2*
– – syphilitic (profunda) A50.3† H19.2*
– purulent H16.8
– rosacea L71.8† H19.3*
– sclerosing H16.3
– specified NEC H16.8
– stellate H16.1

Keratitis—*continued*
- striate H16.1
- superficial (punctate) H16.1
- – with conjunctivitis H16.2
- suppurative H16.8
- syphilitic (congenital) (prenatal) A50.3†
  H19.2∗
- trachomatous A71.1
- tuberculous A18.5† H19.2∗
- vesicular H16.8
- xerotic H16.8
- – vitamin A deficiency E50.4† H19.8∗
Keratoacanthoma L85.8
Keratocele H18.7
Keratoconjunctivitis H16.2
- Acanthamoeba B60.1† H19.2∗
- adenoviral B30.0† H19.2∗
- epidemic B30.0† H19.2∗
- exposure H16.2
- herpes, herpetic (simplex) B00.5† H19.1∗
- – zoster B02.3† H19.2∗
- infectious B30.0† H19.2∗
- lagophthalmic H16.2
- neurotrophic H16.2
- phlyctenular H16.2
- postmeasles B05.8† H19.2∗
- shipyard B30.0† H19.2∗
- sicca (Sjögren's) M35.0† H19.3∗
- tuberculous (phlyctenular) A18.5†
  H19.2∗
Keratoconus H18.6
- congenital Q13.4
- in Down's syndrome Q90.-† H19.8∗
Keratocyst (odontogenic) D16.4
Keratoderma, keratodermia (congenital)
  (palmaris et plantaris) (symmetrical)
  Q82.8
- acquired L85.1
- climactericum L85.1
- gonococcal A54.8† L86∗
- gonorrheal A54.8† L86∗
- punctata L85.2
- Reiter's M02.3† L86∗
Keratodermatocele H18.7
Keratoglobus H18.7
- congenital Q15.8
- – with glaucoma Q15.0
Keratohemia H18.0
Keratoiritis (*see also* Iridocyclitis) H20.9
- syphilitic (congenital late) (*see also* Iritis,
  syphilitic)) A50.3† H22.0∗
- tuberculous A18.5† H22.0∗
Keratoma L57.0
- palmaris et plantaris hereditarium Q82.8

Keratoma—*continued*
- senile L57.0
Keratomalacia H18.4
- vitamin A deficiency E50.4† H19.8∗
Keratomegaly Q13.4
Keratomycosis B49† H19.2∗
- nigrans, nigricans (palmaris) B36.1
Keratopathy H18.9
- band H18.4
- bullous H18.1
- – following cataract surgery H59.0
Keratoscleritis, tuberculous A18.5†
  H19.2∗
Keratosis L57.0
- actinic L57.0
- arsenical L85.8
- congenital, specified NEC Q80.8
- female genital NEC N94.8
- follicularis Q82.8
- – acquired L11.0
- – congenital Q82.8
- – et parafollicularis in cutem penetrans
  L87.0
- – spinulosa (decalvans) Q82.8
- – vitamin A deficiency E50.8† L86∗
- gonococcal A54.8† L86∗
- male genital (external) N50.8
- nigricans L83
- obturans, external ear (canal) H60.4
- palmaris et plantaris (inherited)
  (symmetrical) Q82.8
- – acquired L85.1
- penile N48.8
- pharynx J39.2
- pilaris, acquired L85.8
- punctata (palmaris et plantaris) L85.2
- scrotal N50.8
- seborrheic L82
- senile L57.0
- solar L57.0
- tonsillaris J35.8
- vegetans Q82.8
- vitamin A deficiency E50.8† L86∗
- vocal cord J38.3
Kerato-uveitis (*see also* Iridocyclitis)
  H20.9
Kerion (celsi) B35.0
Kernicterus of newborn P57.9
- due to isoimmunization (conditions in
  P55.-) P57.0
- specified type NEC P57.8
Keshan disease E59

Ketoacidosis NEC E87.2
– diabetic – *code to* E10-E14 with fourth
character .1
Ketonuria R82.4
Ketosis NEC E88.8
– diabetic – *code to* E10-E14 with fourth
character .1
Kew Garden fever A79.1
Kidney – *see condition*
Kienböck's disease or osteochondrosis
M92.2
– adult M93.1
**Kimmelstiel(-Wilson) disease or syndrome
(diabetic glomerulosclerosis)** – *code to*
E10-E14 with fourth character .2
Kink
– artery I77.1
– ileum or intestine (*see also* Obstruction,
intestine) K56.6
– Lane's (*see also* Obstruction, intestine)
K56.6
– organ or site, congenital NEC – *see*
Anomaly, by site
– ureter (pelvic junction) N13.5
– – with
– – – hydronephrosis N13.1
– – – – with infection N13.6
– – – pyelonephritis (chronic) N11.1
– – congenital Q62.3
– vein(s) I87.8
Kinking hair (acquired) L67.8
Kissing spine M48.2
Klatskin's tumor (M8162/3) C22.1
Klauder's disease A26.8
Klebs' disease (*see also*
Glomerulonephritis) N05.-
**Klebsiella (K.) pneumoniae, as cause of
disease classified elsewhere** B96.1
Kleine-Levin syndrome G47.8
Kleptomania F63.2
Klinefelter's syndrome Q98.4
– karyotype 47,XXY Q98.0
– male with
– – karyotype 46,XX Q98.2
– – more than two X chromosomes Q98.1
Klippel-Feil deficiency or syndrome
Q76.1
Klippel's disease I67.2
Klippel-Trenaunay(-Weber) syndrome
Q87.2
**Klumpke(-Déjerine) palsy, paralysis
(birth) (newborn)** P14.1
Knee – *see condition*

Knock knee (acquired) M21.0
– congenital Q74.1
Knot (true), umbilical cord O69.2
affecting fetus or newborn P02.5
Knotting of hair L67.8
Knuckle pad (Garrod's) M72.1
Koch's infection (*see also* Tuberculosis)
A16.9
Koch-Weeks' conjunctivitis H10.0
Koebner's syndrome Q81.8
Köhler's disease
– patellar M92.4
– tarsal navicular M92.6
Koilonychia L60.3
– congenital Q84.6
Kojevnikov's, Kozhevnikof's epilepsy
G40.5
Koplik's spots B05.9
**Korsakov's disease, psychosis or
syndrome (alcoholic)** F10.6
– drug-induced – *see* F11-F19 with fourth
character .6
– nonalcoholic F04
Kostmann's disease D70
Krabbe's disease E75.2
Kraepelin-Morel disease (*see also*
Schizophrenia) F20.9
Kraft-Weber-Dimitri disease Q85.8
Kraurosis
– anus K62.8
– penis N48.0
– vagina N89.8
– vulva N90.4
Krukenberg's
– spindle H18.0
– tumor (M8490/6) C79.6
Kufs' disease E75.4
Kugelberg-Welander disease G12.1
Kuhnt-Junius degeneration H35.3
Kümmell's disease or spondylitis M48.3
Kupffer cell sarcoma (M9124/3) C22.3
Kuru A81.8
Kussmaul's
– disease M30.0
– respiration E87.2
– – in diabetic acidosis – *code to* E10-E14
with fourth character .1
Kwashiorkor E40
– marasmic, marasmus type E42
Kyasanur Forest disease A98.2
**Kyphoscoliosis, kyphoscoliotic
(acquired)** (*see also* Scoliosis) M41.9
– congenital Q67.5
– heart (disease) I27.1

Kyphoscoliosis, kyphoscoliotic—*continued*
- late effect of rickets E64.3
- tuberculous A18.0† M49.0∗

Kyphosis, kyphotic (acquired) M40.2
- congenital Q76.4
- late effect of rickets E64.3
- Morquio-Brailsford type (spinal) E76.2†
  M49.8∗

Kyphosis, kyphotic—*continued*
- postlaminectomy M96.3
- postradiation therapy M96.2
- postural (adolescent) M40.0
- secondary NEC M40.1
- syphilitic, congenital A50.5† M49.3∗
- tuberculous A18.0† M49.0∗

Kyrle's disease L87.0

L

Labia, labium – *see condition*
Labile
– blood pressure R09.8
– vasomotor system I73.9
Labioglossal paralysis G12.2
Labium leporinum (*see also* Cleft, lip)
    Q36.9
Labor (*see also* Delivery)
– abnormal NEC O75.8
– – affecting fetus or newborn P03.6
– arrested active phase O62.1
– – affecting fetus or newborn P03.6
– desultory O62.2
– – affecting fetus or newborn P03.6
– dyscoordinate O62.4
– – affecting fetus or newborn P03.6
– early onset (before 37 completed weeks of
    gestation)
– – with
– – – pre-term delivery O60.1
– – – term delivery O60.2
– – induced
– – – with delivery O60.3
– – – without delivery O60.0
– – spontaneous
– – – with delivery
– – – – preterm O60.1
– – – – term O60.2
– – – without delivery O60.0
– – without delivery O60.0
– false O47.9
– – at or after 37 completed weeks of
    gestation O47.1
– – before 37 completed weeks of gestation
    O47.0
– forced or induced, affecting fetus or
    newborn P03.8
– hypertonic O62.4
– – affecting fetus or newborn P03.6
– hypotonic O62.2
– – affecting fetus or newborn P03.6
– – primary O62.0
– – secondary O62.1
– incoordinate O62.4
– – affecting fetus or newborn P03.6
– irregular O62.2
– – affecting fetus or newborn P03.6
– long – *see* Labor, prolonged
– missed O36.4

Labor—*continued*
– obstructed O66.9
– – affecting fetus or newborn P03.1
– – by or due to
– – – abnormal
– – – – cervix O65.5
– – – – pelvic organs or tissues O65.5
– – – – pelvis (bony) O65.9
– – – – – affecting fetus or newborn
        P03.1
– – – – – specified NEC O65.8
– – – – presentation or postition O64.9
– – – – – affecting fetus or newborn
        P03.1
– – – – size, fetus O66.2
– – – – – affecting fetus or newborn
        P03.1
– – – – soft parts (of pelvis) O65.5
– – – – uterus O65.5
– – – – vagina O65.5
– – – acromion presentation O64.4
– – – anteversion, cervix or uterus O65.5
– – – bicornis or bicornate uterus O65.5
– – – breech presentation O64.1
– – – brow presentation O64.3
– – – cephalopelvic disproportion
        (normally formed fetus) O65.4
– – – – affecting fetus or newborn P03.1
– – – chin presentation O64.2
– – – cicatrix of cervix O65.5
– – – compound presentation O64.5
– – – conditions in O32.- O64.9
– – – conditions in O34.- O65.5
– – – contracted pelvis (general) O65.1
– – – – inlet O65.2
– – – – mid-cavity O65.3
– – – – outlet O65.3
– – – cystocele O65.5
– – – deep transverse arrest O64.0
– – – deformity (acquired) (congenital)
– – – – pelvic organs or tissues NEC
        O65.5
– – – – pelvis (bony) NEC O65.0
– – – displacement, uterus NEC O65.5
– – – disproportion, fetopelvic NEC O65.4
– – – – affecting fetus or newborn P03.1
– – – double uterus (congenital) O65.5
– – – face presentation O64.2
– – – – to pubes O64.0

Labor—*continued*
- obstructed—*continued*
- − by or due to—*continued*
- − − failure, fetal head to enter pelvic brim O64.8
- − − fibroid (tumor) (uterus) O65.5
- − − hydrocephalic fetus O66.3
- − − − affecting fetus or newborn P03.1
- − − impacted shoulders O66.0
- − − incarceration of uterus O65.5
- − − lateroversion, uterus or cervix O65.5
- − − locked twins O66.1
- − − mal lie O64.9
- − − malposition
- − − − fetus NEC O64.9
- − − − pelvic organs or tissues NEC O65.5
- − − malpresentation O64.9
- − − − affecting fetus or newborn P03.1
- − − − specified NEC O64.8
- − − nonengagement of fetal head O64.8
- − − oblique presentation O64.4
- − − oversize fetus O66.2
- − − pelvic tumor NEC O65.5
- − − persistent occipitoposterior or occipitotransverse (position) O64.0
- − − prolapse
- − − − arm or hand O64.4
- − − − foot or leg O64.8
- − − − uterus O65.5
- − − rectocele O65.5
- − − retroversion, uterus or cervix O65.5
- − − rigid
- − − − cervix O65.5
- − − − pelvic floor O65.5
- − − − perineum or vulva O65.5
- − − − vagina O65.5
- − − shoulder
- − − − distocia or impaction O66.0
- − − − presentation O64.4
- − − stenosis O65.5
- − − transverse
- − − − arrest (deep) O64.0
- − − − presentation or lie O64.8
- − specified NEC O66.8
- precipitate O62.3
- − affecting fetus or newborn P03.5
- premature or preterm
- − with
- − − pre-term delivery O60.1
- − − term delivery O60.2
- − induced
- − − with delivery O60.3
- − − without delivery O60.0

Labor—*continued*
- premature or preterm—*continued*
- − spontaneous
- − − with
- − − − preterm delivery O60.1
- − − − term delivery O60.2
- − − without delivery O60.0
- − without delivery O60.0
- prolonged or protracted O63.9
- − affecting fetus or newborn P03.8
- − first stage O63.0
- − second stage O63.1

Labored breathing (*see also* Hyperventilation) R06.4

Labyrinthitis (circumscribed) (destructive) (diffuse) (inner ear) (latent) (purulent) (suppurative) H83.0
- syphilitic A52.7† H94.8*

Laceration (*see also* Wound, open) T14.1
- with abortion (subsequent episode) O08.6
- − current episode – *see* Abortion
- accidental, complicating surgery T81.2
- Achilles tendon S86.0
- anus (sphincter) S31.8
- − complicating delivery O70.2
- − − with laceration of anal or rectal mucosa O70.3
- − nontraumatic, nonpuerperal (*see also* Fissure, anus) K60.2
- bladder (urinary) S37.2
- − obstetric trauma O71.5
- blood vessel – *see* Injury, blood vessel
- bowel
- − complicating abortion – *code to* O03-O07 with fourth character .3 or .8
- − obstetric trauma O71.5
- brain (any part) (cortex) (diffuse) (membrane) S06.2
- − during birth P10.8
- − − with hemorrhage P10.1
- − focal S06.3
- broad ligament
- − laceration syndrome N83.8
- − obstetric trauma O71.6
- − syndrome (laceration) N83.8
- capsule, joint – *see* Sprain
- causing eversion of cervix uteri (old) N86
- central (perineal), complicating delivery O70.9
- cerebellum S06.2
- cerebral (diffuse) S06.2
- − during birth P10.8
- − − with hemorrhage P10.1
- − focal S06.3

Laceration—*continued*
- cervix (uteri)
-   – nonpuerperal, nontraumatic N88.1
-   – obstetric trauma (current) O71.3
-   – old (postpartal) N88.1
-   – traumatic S37.6
- chordae tendineae NEC I51.1
-   – concurrent with acute myocardial
  infarction – *see* Infarct, myocardium
-   – following acute myocardial infarction
  (current complication) I23.4
- cortex (cerebral) S06.2
- eye(ball) (without prolapse or loss of
  intraocular tissue) S05.3
-   – with prolapse or loss of intraocular
  tissue S05.2
-   – penetrating S05.6
- eyelid S01.1
- fourchette, complicating delivery O70.0
- heart S26.8
-   – with hemopericardium S26.0
- internal organ – *see* Injury, by site
- intracranial NEC S06.2
-   – birth injury P10.9
- labia, complicating delivery O70.0
- ligament (*see also* Sprain) T14.3
- meninges S06.2
- meniscus (*see also* Tear, meniscus) S83.2
-   – old (tear) M23.2
-   – site other than knee – *see* Sprain, by site
- multiple T01.9
- muscle – *see* Injury, muscle
- nerve – *see* Injury, nerve
- ocular NEC S05.3
-   – adnexa NEC S01.1
- pelvic
-   – floor S31.0
-   – – complicating delivery O70.1
-   – – nonpuerperal S31.0
-   – – old (postpartal) N81.8
-   – organ NEC, obstetric trauma O71.5
- perineum, perineal S31.0
-   – complicating delivery O70.9
-   – – central O70.9
-   – – first degree O70.0
-   – – fourth degree O70.3
-   – – involving
-   – – – anus (sphincter) O70.2
-   – – – fourchette O70.0
-   – – – hymen O70.0
-   – – – labia O70.0
-   – – – pelvic floor O70.1
-   – – – perineal muscles O70.1
-   – – – rectovaginal septum O70.2

Laceration—*continued*
-   perineum, perineal—*continued*
-   – complicating delivery—*continued*
-   – – involving—*continued*
-   – – – rectovaginal septum—*continued*
-   – – – – with anal or rectal mucosa
  O70.3
-   – – – skin O70.0
-   – – – sphincter (anal) O70.2
-   – – – – with anal or rectal mucosa
  O70.3
-   – – – vagina O70.0
-   – – – vaginal muscles O70.1
-   – – – vulva O70.0
-   – – second degree O70.1
-   – – secondary O90.1
-   – – third degree O70.2
-   – male S31.0
-   – muscles, complicating delivery O70.1
-   – old (postpartal) N81.8
-   – secondary (postpartal) O90.1
- peritoneum, obstetric trauma O71.5
- periurethral tissue S37.8
-   – obstetric trauma O71.5
- rectovaginal (septum) S31.8
-   – complicating delivery O71.4
-   – – with perineum O70.2
-   – – – involving anal or rectal mucosa
  O70.3
-   – nonpuerperal, nontraumatic N89.8
-   – old (postpartal) N89.8
- spinal cord (meninges) (*see also* Injury,
  spinal cord, by region) T09.3
-   – fetus or newborn (birth injury) P11.5
- tendon (*see also* Injury, muscle or tendon)
  T14.6
-   – Achilles S86.0
- tentorium cerebelli S06.2
- urethra, obstetric trauma O71.5
- uterus S37.6
-   – nonpuerperal, nontraumatic N85.8
-   – obstetric trauma NEC O71.1
-   – old (postpartal) N85.8
- vagina (high) S31.4
-   – complicating delivery O71.4
-   – – with perineum O70.0
-   – – – muscles O70.1
-   – nonpuerperal, nontraumatic N89.8
-   – old (postpartal) N89.8
- vulva S31.4
-   – complicating delivery O70.0
-   – nonpuerperal, nontraumatic N90.8
-   – old (postpartal) N90.8

Lack of
- achievement in school Z55.3
- adequate food NEC Z59.4
- appetite (*see also* Anorexia) R63.0
- care
- – in home Z74.2
- – of infant (at or after birth) T74.0
- coordination R27.8
- financial resources Z59.6
- food T73.0
- growth R62.8
- heating Z59.1
- housing (permanent) (temporary) Z59.0
- – adequate Z59.1
- learning experiences in childhood Z62.5
- leisure time (affecting lifestyle) Z73.2
- material resources Z59.6
- memory (*see also* Amnesia) R41.3
- – mild, following organic brain damage F06.7
- ovulation N97.0
- parental supervision or control of child Z62.0
- person able to render necessary care Z74.2
- physical exercise Z72.3
- play experience in childhood Z62.5
- prenatal care, affecting management of pregnancy Z35.3
- relaxation (affecting lifestyle) Z73.2
- sexual
- – desire F52.0
- – enjoyment F52.1
- shelter Z59.0
- supervision of child by parent Z62.0
- water T73.1

Lacrimal – *see condition*
Lacrimation, abnormal H04.2
Lacrimonasal duct – *see condition*
Lactation, lactating (breast) (puerperal, postpartum)
- defective O92.4
- disorder NEC O92.7
- excessive O92.6
- failed (complete) O92.3
- – partial O92.4
- mastitis NEC O91.2
- mother (care and/or examination) Z39.1
- nonpuerperal N64.3

Lacunar skull Q75.8
Laennec's cirrhosis K74.6 K70.3
— nonalcoholic K70.3 K74.6
Lafora's disease G40.3
Lag, lid (nervous) H02.5

Lagophthalmos (eyelid) (nervous) H02.2
- keratoconjunctivitis H16.2
Lalling F80.0
Lambert-Eaton syndrome (*see also* Neoplasm) C80.-† G73.1*
- unassociated with neoplasm G70.8
Lambliasis, lambliosis A07.1
Lancereaux's diabetes E14.6
Landau-Kleffner syndrome F80.3
Landouzy-Déjerine dystrophy or facioscapulohumeral atrophy G71.0
Landouzy's disease (icterohemorrhagic leptospirosis) A27.0
Landry-Guillain-Barré syndrome or paralysis G61.0
Lane's
- kink (*see also* Obstruction, intestine) K56.6
- syndrome K90.2
Langdon Down's syndrome (*see also* Trisomy, 21) Q90.9
Large
- ear, congenital Q17.1
- fetus – *see* Oversize fetus
Large-for-dates NEC (fetus or infant) P08.1
- affecting management of pregnancy O36.6
- exceptionally (4500 g or more) P08.0
Larsen-Johansson disease or osteochondrosis M92.4
Larsen's syndrome Q74.8
Larva migrans
- cutaneous NEC B76.9
- – Ancylostoma (species) B76.0
- visceral NEC B83.0
Laryngismus (stridulus) J38.5
- congenital P28.8
- diphtheritic A36.2
Laryngitis (acute) (edematous) (subglottic) (suppurative) (ulcerative) J04.0
- with
- – influenza, flu, or grippe (*see also* Influenza, with, respiratory manifestations) J11.1
- – tracheitis (acute) (*see also* Laryngotracheitis) J04.2
- – – chronic J37.1
- – – obstructive J05.0
- atrophic J37.0
- catarrhal J37.0
- chronic J37.0
- – with tracheitis (chronic) J37.1

Laryngitis—*continued*
– diphtheritic A36.2
– due to external agent (chronic) J37.0
– Haemophilus influenzae J04.0
– hypertrophic J37.0
– influenzal (*see also* Influenza, with, respiratory manifestations) J11.1
– obstructive J05.0
– sicca J37.0
– spasmodic J05.0
– – acute J04.0
– streptococcal J04.0
– stridulous J05.0
– syphilitic (late) A52.7† J99.8∗
– – congenital A50.5† J99.8∗
– – – early A50.0† J99.8∗
– tuberculous A16.4
– – with bacteriological and histological confirmation A15.5
– Vincent's A69.1
Laryngocele (congenital) (ventricular) Q31.3
Laryngofissure J38.7
Laryngomalacia (congenital) Q31.5
Laryngopharyngitis (acute) J06.0
– chronic J37.0
Laryngoplegia J38.0
Laryngoptosis J38.7
Laryngospasm J38.5
Laryngostenosis J38.6
Laryngotracheitis (acute) (infective) J04.2
– atrophic J37.1
– catarrhal J37.1
– chronic J37.1
– diphtheritic A36.2
– due to external agent (chronic) J37.1
– Haemophilus influenzae J04.2
– hypertrophic J37.1
– influenzal (*see also* Influenza, with, respiratory manifestations) J11.1
– pachydermic J38.7
– sicca J37.1
– spasmodic J38.5
– – acute J05.0
– streptoccocal J04.2
– stridulous J38.5
– syphilitic (late) A52.7† J99.8∗
– – congenital A50.5† J99.8∗
– – – early A50.0† J99.8∗
– tuberculous A16.4
– Vincent's A69.1
Laryngotracheobronchitis (*see also* Bronchitis) J40
– acute (*see also* Bronchitis, acute) J20.9

Laryngotracheobronchitis—*continued*
– chronic J42
Larynx, laryngeal – *see condition*
Lassa fever A96.2
Lassitude – *see* Weak, weakness
Late
– talker R62.0
– walker R62.0
Late effect(s) – *see* Sequelae
Latent – *see condition*
Laterocession – *see* Lateroversion
Lateroflexion – *see* Lateroversion
Lateroversion
– cervix – *see* Lateroversion, uterus
– uterus, uterine (cervix) (postinfectional) (postpartal, old) N85.4
– – congenital Q51.8
– – in pregnancy or childbirth O34.5
– – – affecting fetus or newborn P03.8
Lathyrism T62.2
Launois' syndrome E22.0
Launois-Bensaude adenolipomatosis E88.8
Laurence-Moon(-Bardet)-Biedl syndrome Q87.8
Lax, laxity – *see also* Relaxation
– ligament(ous) M24.2
– – familial M35.7
– – knee M23.8
– skin (acquired) L57.4
– – congenital Q82.8
Laxative habit F55
Lead miner's lung J63.8
Leak, leakage
– amniotic fluid (*see also* Rupture, membranes, premature) O42.9
– – with delayed delivery O75.6
– blood (microscopic), fetal, into maternal circulation. affecting management of pregnancy or puerperium O43.0
– cerebrospinal fluid G96.0
– – from spinal (lumbar) puncture G97.0
– device, implant or graft (*see also* Complications, by site and type) T85.6
– – arterial graft NEC T82.3
– – – coronary (bypass) T82.2
– – breast (implant) T85.4
– – catheter NEC T85.6
– – – dialysis (renal) T82.4
– – – – intraperitoneal T85.6
– – – infusion NEC T82.5
– – – – spinal (epidural) (subdural) T85.6
– – – urinary (indwelling) T83.0

Leak, leakage—*continued*
- device, implant or graft—*continued*
- – gastrointestinal (bile duct) (esophagus) T85.5
- – genital NEC T83.4
- – heart NEC T82.5
- – – valve (prosthesis) T82.0
- – – – graft T82.2
- – ocular (corneal graft) (orbital implant) NEC T85.3
- – – intraocular lens T85.2
- – orthopedic NEC T84.4
- – specified NEC T85.6
- – urinary NEC T83.1
- – – graft T83.2
- – vascular NEC T82.5
- – ventricular intracranial shunt T85.0
Leaky heart – *see* Endocarditis
Learning defect (specific) F81.9
Leather bottle stomach (M8142/3) C16.9
Leber's
- congenital amaurosis H35.5
- optic atrophy (hereditary) H47.2
Lederer's anemia D59.1
Leeches (external) (*see also* Hirudiniasis) B88.3
- internal B83.4
Leg – *see condition*
Legg(-Calvé)-Perthes disease, syndrome or osteochondrosis M91.1
Legionellosis A48.1
- nonpneumonic A48.2
Legionnaire's
- disease A48.1
- – nonpneumonic A48.2
- pneumonia A48.1
Leigh's disease G31.8
Leiner's disease L21.1
Leiofibromyoma (M8890/0) – *see also* Leiomyoma
- uterus (cervix) (corpus) – *see* Leiomyoma, uterus
Leiomyoblastoma (M8891/0) – *see* Neoplasm, connective tissue, benign
Leiomyofibroma (M8890/0) – *see also* Neoplasm, connective tissue, benign
- uterus (cervix) (corpus) D25.9
Leiomyoma (M8890/0) – *see also* Neoplasm, connective tissue, benign
- bizarre (M8893/0) – *see* Neoplasm, connective tissue, benign
- cellular (M8892/0) – *see* Neoplasm, connective tissue, benign

Leiomyoma—*continued*
- epithelioid (M8891/0) – *see* Neoplasm, connective tissue, benign
- uterus (cervix) (corpus) D25.9
- – intramural D25.1
- – submucous D25.0
- – subserosal D25.2
- vascular (M8894/0) – *see* Neoplasm, connective tissue, benign
Leiomyomatosis (intravascular) (M8890/1) – *see* Neoplasm, connective tissue, uncertain behavior
Leiomyosarcoma (M8890/3) – *see also* Neoplasm, connective tissue, malignant
- epithelioid (M8891/3) – *see* Neoplasm, connective tissue, malignant
- myxoid (M8896/3) – *see* Neoplasm, connective tissue, malignant
Leishmaniasis B55.9
- American (mucocutancous) B55.2
- – cutaneous B55.1
- Asian desert B55.1
- Brazilian B55.2
- cutaneous (any type) B55.1
- – eyelid B55.1† H03.0*
- dermal (*see also* Leishmaniasis, cutaneous) B55.1
- – post-kala-azar B55.0
- eyelid B55.1† H03.0*
- infantile B55.0
- mucocutaneous (American) (New World) B55.2
- naso-oral B55.2
- nasopharyngeal B55.2
- Old World B55.1
- tegumentaria diffusa B55.1
- visceral B55.0
Leishmanoid, dermal (*see also* Leishmaniasis, cutaneous) B55.1
- post-kala-azar B55.0
Lengthening, leg M21.7
Lennert's lymphoma C84.4
Lennox-Gastaut syndrome G40.4
Lens – *see condition*
Lenticonus (anterior) (congenital) (posterior) Q12.8
Lenticular degeneration, progressive E83.0
Lentiglobus (congenital) (posterior) Q12.8
Lentigo (congenital) L81.4
- maligna (M8742/2) – *see also* Melanoma, in situ
- – melanoma (M8742/3) – *see* Melanoma

Lentivirus, as cause of disease classified elsewhere B97.3
Leontiasis
– ossium M85.2
– syphilitic (late) A52.7
– – congenital A50.5
Lepothrix A48.8
Lepra – *see* Leprosy
Leprechaunism E34.8
Leprosy A30.9
– anesthetic A30.9
– BB A30.3
– BL A30.4
– borderline (infiltrated) (neuritic) A30.3
– – lepromatous A30.4
– – tuberculoid A30.2
– BT A30.2
– cornea A30.-† H19.2*
– dimorphous (infiltrated) (neuritic) A30.3
– eyelid A30.-† H03.1*
– I A30.0
– indeterminate (macular) (neuritic) A30.0
– lepromatous (diffuse) (infiltrated) (macular) (neuritic) (nodular) A30.5
– LL A30.5
– macular A30.9
– maculoanesthetic A30.9
– mixed A30.3
– neural A30.9
– nodular A30.5
– specified type NEC A30.8
– TT A30.1
– tuberculoid (major) (minor) A30.1
Leptocytosis, hereditary D56.9
Leptomeningitis (chronic) (circumscribed) (hemorrhagic) (nonsuppurative) (*see also* Meningitis) G03.9
– tuberculous A17.0† G01*
Leptomeningopathy NEC G96.1
Leptospiral – *see condition*
Leptospirochetal – *see condition*
Leptospirosis A27.9
– canicola A27.8
– due to Leptospira interrogans serovar icterohaemorrhagiae A27.0
– icterohemorrhagica A27.0
– pomona A27.8
Lequesne's osteoporosis (localized) M81.6
Leriche's syndrome I74.0
Leri's pleonosteosis Q78.8
Leri-Weill syndrome Q77.8
Lermoyez' syndrome H81.3
Lesch-Nyhan syndrome E79.1

Leser-Trélat disease L82
Lesion (nontraumatic)
– alveolar process K08.9
– angiocentric immunoproliferative C83.8
– anorectal K62.9
– aortic (valve) I35.9
– auditory nerve H93.3
– basal ganglion G25.9
– bile duct (*see also* Disease, bile duct) K83.9
– biomechanical M99.9
– – specified NEC M99.8
– bone M89.9
– brachial plexus G54.0
– brain G93.9
– – congenital Q04.9
– – vascular I67.9
– – – degenerative I67.9
– buccal cavity K13.7
– calcified – *see* Calcification
– canthus H02.9
– carate – *see* Pinta, lesions
– cardia K22.9
– cardiac – *see also* Disease, heart
– – congenital Q24.9
– – valvular – *see* Endocarditis
– cauda equina G83.4
– cecum K63.9
– cerebral – *see* Lesion, brain
– cerebrovascular I67.9
– cervical (nerve) root NEC G54.2
– chiasmal H47.4
– chorda tympani G51.8
– coin, lung R91
– colon K63.9
– congenital – *see* Anomaly, by site
– conjunctiva H11.9
– coronary artery (*see also* Ischemia, heart) I25.9
– cystic – *see* Cyst
– degenerative – *see* Degeneration
– duodenum K31.9
– edentulous (alveolar) ridge, associated with trauma, due to traumatic occlusion K06.2
– en coup de sabre L94.1
– eyelid H02.9
– gasserian ganglion G50.8
– gastric K31.9
– gastroduodenal K31.9
– gastrointestinal K63.9
– gingiva, associated with trauma K06.2

Lesion—*continued*
- glomerular
- - focal and segmental – *code to* N00-N07 with fourth character .1
- - minimal change – *code to* N00-N07 with fourth character .0
- heart (organic) – *see* Disease, heart
- hyperkeratotic (*see also* Hyperkeratosis) L85.9
- hypothalamic E23.7
- ileocecal K63.9
- ileum K63.9
- inflammatory – *see* Inflammation
- intestine K63.9
- intracerebral – *see* Lesion, brain
- intrachiasmal (optic) H47.4
- intracranial, space-occupying NEC R90.0
- joint M25.9
- - sacroiliac (old) M53.3
- keratotic – *see* Keratosis
- kidney (*see also* Disease, renal) N28.9
- laryngeal nerve (recurrent) G52.2
- lip K13.0
- liver K76.9
- lumbosacral
- - plexus G54.1
- - root (nerve) NEC G54.4
- lung (coin) R91
- mitral I05.9
- motor cortex NEC G93.8
- mouth K13.7
- nerve (*see also* Disorder, nerve) G58.9
- nervous system, congenital Q07.9
- nonallopathic – *see* Lesion, biomechanical
- nose (internal) J34.8
- obstructive – *see* Obstruction
- oral mucosa K13.7
- organ or site NEC – *see* Disease, by site
- osteolytic M89.5
- peptic NEC K27.9
- periodontal, due to traumatic occlusion K05.5
- pharynx J39.2 – *Myu29*
- pigment (skin) L81.9
- pinta – *see* Pinta, lesions
- polypoid – *see* Polyp
- prechiasmal (optic) H47.4
- primary A51.0
- - carate A67.0
- - pinta A67.0
- - syphilis A51.0
- - yaws A66.0
- pulmonary J98.4
- - valve I37.9

Lesion—*continued*
- pylorus K31.9
- radiation NEC T66
- radium NEC T66
- rectosigmoid K63.9
- retina, retinal H35.9
- - vascular H35.0
- sacroiliac (joint) (old) M53.3
- salivary gland K11.9
- - benign lymphoepithelial K11.8
- sciatic nerve G57.0
- secondary – *see* Syphilis, secondary
- shoulder M75.9
- - specified NEC M75.8
- sigmoid K63.9
- sinus (accessory) (nasal) J34.8
- skin L98.9
- - suppurative L08.0
- spinal cord G95.9
- - congenital Q06.9
- - traumatic (complete) (incomplete) (transverse) (*see also* Injury, spinal cord, by region) T09.3
- spleen D73.8
- stomach K31.9
- syphilitic – *see* Syphilis
- tertiary – *see* Syphilis, tertiary
- thoracic root (nerve) NEC G54.3
- tonsillar fossa J35.9
- tooth, teeth K08.9
- - white spot K02.0
- traumatic NEC (*see also* Injury, by site and type) T14.9
- tricuspid (valve) I07.9
- - nonrheumatic I36.9
- ulcerated or ulcerative – *see* Ulcer
- uterus N85.9
- valvular – *see* Endocarditis
- vascular I99
- - affecting central nervous system I67.9
- - retina, retinal H35.0
- - umbilical cord, complicating delivery O69.5
- - - affecting fetus or newborn P02.6
- warty – *see* Verruca
- X-ray (radiation) NEC T66
Lethargic – *see* condition
Lethargy R53
Letterer-Siwe's disease C96.0
Leuc(o) – *see* Leuk(o)
Leukemia C95.9
- acute (bilineal) (biphenotypic) (mixed lineage) NEC C95.0
- adult T-cell C91.5

Leukemia—*continued*
- aleukemic NEC C95.9
- B-cell type
- – lymphocytic, chronic C91.1
- – prolymphocytic C91.3
- basophilic C92.7
- – acute C94.7
- bilineal, acute C95.0
- biphenotypic, acute C95.0
- blast (cell) C95.0
- blastic C95.0
- – granulocytic C92.0
- chronic NEC C95.1
- eosinophilic C92.7
- – chronic (hypereosinophilic syndrome)
  D47.5
- erythroid, acute C94.0
- granulocytic C92.9
- – acute C92.0
- – aleukemic C92.9
- – blastic C92.0
- – chronic C92.1
- – subacute C92.2
- hairy cell C91.4
- histiocytic C93.9
- lymphatic C91.9
- – acute C91.0
- – aleukemic C91.9
- – chronic C91.1
- – subacute C91.9
- lymphoblastic (acute) (ALL) C91.0
- lymphocytic C91.9
- – acute C91.0
- – aleukemic C91.9
- – chronic C91.1
- – subacute C91.9
- lymphogenous – *see* Leukemia, lymphoid
- lymphoid NEC C91.9
- – acute C91.0
- – aleukemic C91.9
- – blastic C91.0
- – chronic C91.1
- – subacute C91.9
- lymphoplasmacytic C91.1
- lymphosarcoma cell C91.9
- mast cell C94.3
- megakaryoblastic (acute) C94.2
- megakaryocytic (acute) C94.2
- mixed lineage, acute C95.0
- monoblastic (acute)
  (monocytoid/monocytic) C93.0
- monocytic, monocytoid C93.9
- – acute C93.0
- – aleukemic C93.9

Leukemia—*continued*
- monocytic, monocytoid—*continued*
- – chronic C93.1
- – Naegeli-type C93.1
- – subacute C93.9
- myeloblastic (acute) C92.0
- – with
- – – maturation C92.0
- – – t(8;21) C92.0
- – 1/ETO C92.0
- – M0 C92.0
- – M1 C92.0
- – M2 C92.0
- – M3 C92.4
- – – with t(15;17) and variants C92.4
- – M4 C92.5
- – M4 Eo with inv(16) or t(16;16) C92.5
- – M5 C93.0
- – M5a C93.0
- – M5b C93.0
- – minimal differentiation C92.0
- – NEC C92.0
- myelocytic C92.9
- – acute C92.0
- – chronic C92.1
- myelogenous C92.9
- – acute C92.0
- – aleukemic C92.9
- – chronic C92.1
- – – with crisis of blast cells C92.1
- – – Philadelphia chromosome (Phl)
    positive C92.1
- – – t(9;22)(q34;q11) C92.1
- – subacute C92.2
- myeloid C92.9
- – acute C92.0
- – – with
- – – – 11q23-abnormity C92.6
- – – – multilineage dysplasia C92.8
- – – M6 (a) (b) C94.0
- – – M7 C94.2
- – aleukemic C92.9
- – chronic (BCR/ABL-positive [CML])
    C92.1
- – – atypical, BCR/ABL-negative C92.2
- – NEC (without a FAB classification)
    C92.0
- – subacute C92.2
- myelomonocytic C92.5
- – acute C92.5
- – chronic (CMML-1) (CMML-2) (with
    eosinophilia) C93.1
- juvenile C93.3
- Naegeli-type monocytic C93.1

Leukemia—*continued*
- neutrophilic, chronic D47.1
- NK-cell, aggressive C94.7
- plasma cell C90.1
- plasmacytic C90.1
- prolymphocytic (B-cell type) C91.3
- - acute (PML) C92.4
- - T-cell type C91.6
- promyelocytic, acute C92.4
- - acute (PML) C92.4
- - T-cell type C91.6
- stem cell C95.0
- - of unclear lineage C95.0
- subacute NEC C95.9
- T-cell type
- - adult (HTLV-1-associated) (acute)
    (chronic) (lymphomatoid) (smoldering)
    C91.5
- - large granular lymphocytic (associated
    with rheumatic arthritis) C91.7
- - prolymphocytic C91.6
- thrombocytic C94.2
- undifferentiated C95.0
- unspecified cell type C95.9
- - acute C95.0
- - chronic C95.1
**Leukemoid reaction (lymphocytic)
(monocytic) (myelocytic)** D72.8
Leukocytosis D72.8
Leukoderma, leukodermia NEC L81.5
- syphilitic A51.3† L99.8*
- - late A52.7† L99.8*
**Leukodystrophy (cerebral) (globoid cell)
(Krabbe's) (metachromatic)
(progressive) (sudanophilic)** E75.2
Leukoedema, oral epithelium K13.2
Leukoencephalitis (postinfectious) G04.8
- acute (subacute) hemorrhagic G36.1
- - postimmunization or postvaccinal
    G04.0
- subacute sclerosing A81.1
- van Bogaert's (sclerosing) A81.1
Leukoencephalopathy (*see also*
    Encephalopathy) G93.4
- heroin vapor G92
- metachromatic E75.2
- multifocal (progressive) A81.2
- postimmunization and postvaccinal
    G04.0
- van Bogaert's (sclerosing) A81.1
- vascular, progressive I67.3
Leukoerythroblastosis D64.8
Leukokeratosis
- nicotina palati K13.2

Leukokeratosis—*continued*
- vocal cord J38.3
Leukokraurosis vulva(e) N90.4
Leukoma (cornea) H17.8
- adherent H17.0
Leukomalacia, cerebral, newborn P91.2
Leukomelanopathy, hereditary D72.0
Leukonychia (punctata) (striata) L60.8
- congenital Q84.4
Leukopathia unguium L60.8
- congenital Q84.4
Leukopenia (malignant) D70
Leukopenic – *see condition*
Leukoplakia
- anus K62.8
- bladder (postinfectional) N32.8
- buccal K13.2
- cervix (uteri) N88.0
- esophagus K22.8
- hairy (oral mucosa) (tongue) K13.3
- kidney (pelvis) N28.8
- larynx J38.7
- mouth K13.2
- oral epithelium, including tongue
    (mucosa) K13.2
- pelvis (kidney) N28.8
- penis (infectional) N48.0
- rectum K62.8
- syphilitic (late) A52.7
- tongue K13.2
- ureter (postinfectional) N28.8
- urethra (postinfectional) N36.8
- uterus N85.8
- vagina N89.4
- vocal cord J38.3
- vulva N90.4
Leukorrhea N89.8
- due to Trichomonas (vaginalis) A59.0
- trichomonal A59.0
Leukosarcoma C85.9
Levocardia (isolated) Q24.1
Levotransposition Q20.5
Levulosuria – *see* Fructosuria
Levurid L30.2
Lewy body (ies) (dementia) (disease)
    G31.8
Leyden-Moebius dystrophy G71.0
Leydig cell
- carcinoma (M8650/3)
- - specified site – *see* Neoplasm,
    malignant
- - unspecified site
- - - female C56
- - - male C62.9

Leydig cell—*continued*
– tumor (M8650/1)
– – benign (M8650/0)
– – – specified site – *see* Neoplasm, benign
– – – unspecified site
– – – – female D27
– – – – male D29.2
– – malignant (M8650/3)
– – – specified site – *see* Neoplasm, malignant
– – – unspecified site
– – – – female C56
– – – – male C62.9
– – specified site – *see* Neoplasm, uncertain behavior
– – unspecified site
– – – female D39.1
– – – male D40.1
Leydig-Sertoli cell tumor (M8631/0)
– specified site – *see* Neoplasm, benign
– unspecified site
– – female D27
– – male D29.2
Liar, pathologic F60.2
Libman-Sacks disease M32.1† I39.8*
Lice (infestation) B85.2
– body (Pediculus corporis) B85.1
– crab B85.3
– head (Pediculus capitis) B85.0
– mixed (classifiable to more than one of the subcategories B85.0-B85.3) B85.4
– pubic (Phthirus pubis) B85.3
Lichen L28.0
– albus L90.0
– – penis N48.0
– – vulva N90.4
– amyloidosis E85.4† L99.0*
– atrophicus L90.0
– – penis N48.0
– – vulva N90.4
– congenital Q82.8
– myxedematosus L98.5
– nitidus L44.1
– pilaris Q82.8
– – acquired L85.8
– planopilaris L66.1
– planus (chronicus) L43.9
– – annularis L43.8
– – bullous L43.1
– – follicular L66.1
– – hypertrophic L43.0
– – moniliformis L44.3
– – of Wilson L43.9
– – specified NEC L43.8

Lichen—*continued*
– planus—*continued*
– – subacute (active) L43.3
– – tropicus L43.3
– ruber
– – moniliformis L44.3
– – planus L43.9
– sclerosus (et atrophicus) L90.0
– – penis N48.0
– – vulva N90.4
– scrofulosus (primary) (tuberculous) A18.4
– simplex (chronicus) (circumscriptus) L28.0
– striatus L44.2
– urticatus L28.2
Lichenification L28.0
Lichenoides tuberculosis (primary) A18.4
Lichtheim's disease or syndrome – *see* Degeneration, combined
Lie, abnormal (maternal care) (*see also* Presentation, fetal, abnormal) O32.9
– before labor, affecting fetus or newborn P01.7
Lien migrans D73.8
Ligament – *see condition*
Light
– fetus or newborn, for gestational age P05.0
– headedness R42
Light-for-dates (infant) P05.0
– affecting management of pregnancy O36.5
– and small-for-dates P05.1
Lightning (effects) (shock) (stroke) (struck by) T75.0
– burn – *see* Burn
Lightwood-Albright syndrome N25.8
Lignac(-de Toni-Fanconi-Debré) syndrome E72.0
Ligneous thyroiditis E06.5
Limb – *see condition*
Limbic epilepsy personality syndrome F07.0
Limitation, limited
– activities due to disability Z73.6
– cardiac reserve – *see* Disease, heart
Lindau(-von Hippel) disease Q85.8
Line(s)
– Beau's L60.4
– Harris' M89.1
– Hudson's (cornea) H18.0
– Stähli's (cornea) H18.0
Linea corneae senilis H18.4

Lingua
- geographica K14.1
- nigra (villosa) K14.3
- plicata K14.5
- tylosis K13.2

Lingual – *see condition*
Linguatulosis B88.8
Linitis (gastric) plastica (M8142/3) C16.9
Lip – *see condition*
Lipedema – *see* Edema
Lipemia (*see also* Hyperlipemia) E78.5
Lipidosis E75.6
- cerebral (infantile) (juvenile) (late) E75.4
- cerebroretinal E75.4
- cerebroside E75.2
- cholesterol (cerebral) E75.5
- glycolipid E75.2
- sulfatide E75.2

Lipoadenoma (M8324/0) – *see* Neoplasm, benign
Lipoblastoma (M8881/0) – *see* Lipoma
Lipoblastomatosis (M8881/0) – *see* Lipoma
Lipochondrodystrophy E76.0
Lipodermatosclerosis I83.1
- ulcerated I83.2

Lipodystrophy E88.1
- intestinal K90.8

Lipofibroma (M8851/0) – *see* Lipoma
Lipofuscinosis, neuronal (with ceroidosis) E75.4
Lipogranuloma, sclerosing L92.8
Lipogranulomatosis E78.8
Lipoid – *see also condition*
- histiocytosis (essential) E75.2
- nephrosis (*see also* Nephrosis) N04.-
- proteinosis of Urbach E78.8

Lipoidemia (*see also* Hyperlipemia) E78.5
Lipoidosis (*see also* Lipidosis) E75.6
Lipoma (M8850/0) D17.9
- fetal (M8881/0) D17.9
- – fat cell (M8880/0) D17.9
- infiltrating (M8856/0) D17.9
- intramuscular (M8856/0) D17.9
- pleomorphic (M8854/0) D17.9
- site classification
- – connective tissue NEC D17.3
- – – intra-abdominal D17.5
- – – intrathoracic D17.4
- – – peritoneum D17.7
- – – retroperitoneum D17.7
- – – spermatic cord D17.6
- – face (skin) (subcutaneous) D17.0
- – head (skin) (subcutaneous) D17.0
- – intra-abdominal D17.5

Lipoma—*continued*
- site classification—*continued*
- – intrathoracic D17.4
- – limbs (skin) (subcutaneous) D17.2
- – neck (skin) (subcutaneous) D17.0
- – peritoneum D17.7
- – retroperitoneum D17.7
- – skin NEC D17.3
- – specified site NEC D17.7
- – spermatic cord D17.6
- – subcutaneous NEC D17.3
- – trunk (skin) (subcutaneous) D17.1
- – unspecified D17.9
- spindle cell (M8857/0) D17.9

Lipomatosis E88.2
- dolorosa (Dercum) E88.2
- fetal (M8881/0) – *see* Lipoma
- Launois-Bensaude E88.8

Lipomyoma (M8860/0) – *see* Lipoma
Lipomyxoma (M8852/0) – *see* Lipoma
Lipomyxosarcoma (M8852/3) – *see* Neoplasm, connective tissue, malignant
Lipoprotein metabolism disorder E78.9
Lipoproteinemia E78.5
- broad-beta- E78.2
- floating-beta- E78.2
- hyperprebeta- E78.1

Liposarcoma (M8850/3) – *see also* Neoplasm, connective tissue, malignant
- dedifferentiated (M8858/3) C49.9
- differentiated type (M8851/3) C49.9
- embryonal (M8852/3) C49.9
- mixed type (M8855/3) C49.9
- myxoid (M8852/3) C49.9
- pleomorphic (M8854/3) C49.9
- round cell (M8853/3) C49.9
- well differentiated type (M8851/3) C49.9

Liposynovitis prepatellaris E88.8
Lipping, cervix N86
Lipuria R82.0
- schistosomiasis (bilharziasis) B65.0

Lisping F80.8
Lissauer's paralysis A52.1
Lissencephalia, lissencephaly Q04.3
Listeriosis, listerellosis A32.9
- congenital (disseminated) P37.2
- cutaneous A32.0
- fetal P37.2
- neonatal (disseminated) P37.2
- oculoglandular A32.8
- specified NEC A32.8
- suspected damage to fetus affecting management of pregnancy O35.8

Lithemia E79.0

Lithiasis – *see* Calculus
Lithopedion P95
Lithosis J62.8
Lithuria R82.9
Litigation, anxiety concerning Z65.3
Little leaguer's elbow M77.0
Little's disease G80.9
Littre's
– gland – *see condition*
– hernia – *see* Hernia, abdomen
Littritis (*see also* Urethritis) N34.2
**Livedo (annularis) (racemosa)
  (reticularis)** R23.1
Liver – *see condition*
Lloyd's syndrome (M8360/1) – *see*
  Adenomatosis, endocrine
Loa loa, loaiasis, loasis – *see* Loiasis
Lobar – *see condition*
Lobomycosis B48.0
Lobo's disease B48.0
Lobotomy syndrome F07.0
Lobstein(-Ekman) syndrome Q78.0
Lobster-claw hand Q71.6
Lobulation (congenital) – *see also*
  Anomaly, by site
– kidney, fetal Q63.1
– liver, abnormal Q44.7
– spleen Q89.0
Lobule, lobular – *see condition*
Local, localized – *see condition*
Locked twins causing obstructed labor
  O66.1
– affecting fetus or newborn P03.1
Locking
– joint (*see also* Derangement, joint) M24.8
– – knee M23.8
Lockjaw (*see also* Tetanus) A35
Löffler's
– endocarditis I42.3
– pneumonia or syndrome J82
Loiasis B74.3
– with conjunctival infestation B74.3†
  H13.0*
– eyelid B74.3† H03.0*
Lone Star fever A77.0
Long
– labor O63.9
– – affecting fetus or newborn P03.8
– – first stage O63.0
– – second stage O63.1
– term use (current) of
– – anticoagulants Z92.1
– – aspirin Z92.2
– – medicaments NEC Z92.2

Longitudinal stripes or grooves, nails
  L60.8
– congenital Q84.6
Loop
– intestine (*see also* Volvulus) K56.2
– vascular, on papilla (optic) Q14.2
Loose – *see also condition*
– body
– – joint, except knee M24.0
– – knee M23.4
– – sheath, tendon M67.8
– tooth, teeth K08.8
Looser-Milkman(-Debray) syndrome
  M83.8
Lop ear (deformity) Q17.3
Lorain(-Levi) short stature syndrome
  E23.0
Lordosis M40.5
– acquired M40.4
– congenital Q76.4
– late effect of rickets E64.3
– postsurgical M96.4
– postural M40.4
– rachitic (late effect) E64.3
– tuberculous A18.0† M49.0*
Loss (of)
– appetite R63.0
– – hysterical F50.8
– – nonorganic origin F50.8
– – psychogenic F50.8
– blood – *see* Hemorrhage
– control, sphincter, rectum R15
– – nonorganic origin F98.1
– family (member) in childhood Z61.0
– fluid (acute) E86
– – fetus or newborn P74.1
– function of labyrinth H83.2
– hair, nonscarring (*see also* Alopecia)
  L65.9
– hearing (*see also* Deafness) H91.9
– – noise-induced H83.3
– limb or member, traumatic, current – *see*
  Amputation, traumatic
– love relationship in childhood Z61.0
– memory (*see also* Amnesia) R41.3
– – mild, following organic brain damage
  F06.7
– mind (*see also* Psychosis) F29
– organ or part – *see* Absence, by site,
  acquired
– ossicles, ear (partial) H74.3
– parent in childhood Z61.0
– self-esteem, in childhood Z61.3

Loss—*continued*
- sense of
- – – smell R43.1
- – – taste R43.2
- – – – and smell, mixed R43.8
- – – touch R20.8
- – sensory R44.8
- – – dissociative F44.6
- – sexual desire F52.0
- – sight (acquired) (complete) (congenital) – *see* Blindness
- – substance of
- – – bone M85.8
- – – cartilage M94.8
- – – – auricle (ear) H61.1
- – – vitreous (humor) H15.8
- – tooth, teeth due to accident, extraction or local periodontal disease K08.1
- – vision, sudden H53.1
- – voice (*see also* Aphonia) R49.1
- – weight (abnormal) (cause unknown) R63.4

Louis-Bar syndrome G11.3
Louping ill (encephalitis) A84.8
Louse, lousiness – *see* Lice
Low
- – achiever, school Z55.3
- – basal metabolic rate R94.8
- – birthweight (2499 grams or less) P07.1
- – – extreme (999 grams or less) P07.0
- – – for gestational age P05.0
- – blood pressure (*see also* Hypotension) I95.9
- – – reading (incidental) (isolated) (nonspecific) R03.1
- – cardiac reserve – *see* Disease, heart
- – function – *see also* Hypofunction
- – – kidney (*see also* Failure, kidney) N19
- – hemoglobin D64.9
- – implantation, placenta (*see also* Placenta, previa) O44.1
- – income Z59.6
- – insertion, placenta (*see also* Placenta, previa) O44.1
- – level of literacy Z55.0
- – lying
- – – kidney N28.8
- – – organ or site, congenital – *see* Malposition, congenital
- – – placenta (*see also* Placenta, previa) O44.1
- – platelets (blood) (*see also* Thrombocytopenia) D69.6
- – reserve, kidney N28.8

Low—*continued*
- – salt syndrome E87.1
- – set ears Q17.4
- – white blood cell count R72
Low-density-lipoprotein-type (LDL) hyperlipoproteinemia E78.0
Lowe's syndrome (with Fanconi's syndrome) E72.0
Lown-Ganong-Levine syndrome I45.6
LSD reaction (acute) F16.0
L-shaped kidney Q63.8
Ludwig's angina or disease K12.2
Lues (venerea), luetic – *see* Syphilis
Lumbago, lumbalgia M54.5
- – with sciatica M54.4
- – due to intervertebral disk disorder M51.1† G55.1*
- – due to displacement, intervertebral disk M51.2
- – – with sciatica M51.1† G55.1*
Lumbar – *see condition*
Lumbarization, vertebra, congenital Q76.4
Lump – *see also* Mass
- – breast N63
- – intra-abdominal R19.0
- – pelvic R19.0
Lunacy (*see also* Psychosis) F29
Lung – *see condition*
Lupoid (miliary) of Boeck D86.3
Lupus
- – discoid (local) L93.0
- – erythematosus (discoid) (local) L93.0
- – – disseminated – *see* Lupus, erythematosus, systemic
- – – eyelid H01.1
- – – profundus L93.2
- – – specified NEC L93.2
- – – subacute cutaneous L93.1
- – – systemic M32.9
- – – – with
- – – – – lung involvement M32.1† J99.1*
- – – – – renal tubulo-interstitial disease M32.1† N16.4*
- – – – drug-induced M32.0
- – – – inhibitor (presence of) D68.6
- – – – maternal, affecting fetus or newborn P00.8
- – – – specified NEC M32.8
- – exedens A18.4
- – hydralazine
- – – correct substance properly administered M32.0

Lupus—*continued*
- hydralazine—*continued*
- − − overdose or wrong substance given or taken T46.5
- nephritis (chronic) M32.1† N08.5∗
- nontuberculous, not disseminated L93.0
- panniculitis L93.2
- pernio (Besnier) D86.3
- systemic – *see* Lupus, erythematosus, systemic
- tuberculous A18.4
- − − eyelid A18.4† H03.1∗
- vulgaris A18.4
- − − eyelid A18.4† H03.1∗

Luteinoma (M8610/0) D27

Lutembacher's disease or syndrome Q21.1

Luteoma (M8610/0) D27

Lutz(-Splendore-de Almeida) disease (*see also* Paracoccidioidomycosis) B41.9

Luxation – *see also* Dislocation
- eyeball (nontraumatic) H44.8
- − − birth injury P15.3
- globe, nontraumatic H44.8
- lacrimal gland H04.1
- lens (old) (partial) (spontaneous) H27.1
- − − congenital Q12.1
- − − − syphilitic A50.3† H28.8∗

Lycanthropy F22.8

Lyell's syndrome L51.2
- due to drug
- − − correct substance properly administered L51.2
- − − overdose or wrong substance given or taken T50.9
- − − − specified drug – *see* Table of drugs and chemicals

Lyme disease A69.2

Lymph gland or node – *see condition*

Lymphadenitis I88.9
- acute L04.9
- − − axilla L04.2
- − − face L04.0
- − − head L04.0
- − − hip L04.3
- − − limb
- − − − lower L04.3
- − − − upper L04.2
- − − neck L04.0
- − − shoulder L04.2
- − − specified site NEC L04.8
- − − trunk L04.1

Lymphadenitis—*continued*
- breast
- − − gestational (nonpurulent) O91.2
- − − − purulent O91.1
- − − puerperal, postpartum (nonpurulent) O91.2
- − − − purulent O91.1
- chancroidal (congenital) A57
- chronic I88.1
- − − mesenteric I88.0
- − − nonspecific, specified site NEC I88.1
- due to
- − − Brugia (malayi) B74.1
- − − − timori B74.2
- − − chlamydial lymphogranuloma A55
- − − diphtheria (toxin) A36.8
- − − Wuchereria bancrofti B74.0
- gonorrheal A54.8
- infective (*see also* Lymphadenitis, acute) L04.9
- mesenteric (acute) (chronic) (nonspecific) (subacute) I88.0
- − − due to Salmonella typhi A01.0
- − − tuberculous A18.3† K93.0∗
- purulent (*see also* Lymphadenitis, acute) L04.9
- pyogenic (*see also* Lymphadenitis, acute) L04.9
- regional, nonbacterial I88.8
- septic (*see also* Lymphadenitis, acute) L04.9
- subacute, unspecified site I88.1
- suppurative (*see also* Lymphadenitis, acute) L04.9
- syphilitic (early) (secondary) A51.4
- − − late A52.7† I98.8∗
- tuberculous (*see also* Tuberculosis, lymph gland) A18.2
- venereal (chlamydial) A55

Lymphadenoid goiter E06.3

Lymphadenopathy (generalized) R59.1
- angioimmunoblastic (with dysproteinemia) C86.5
- due to toxoplasmosis (acquired) B58.8
- − − congenital (acute) (chronic) (subacute) P37.1
- localized R59.0
- resulting from HIV disease B23.1
- syphilitic (early) (secondary) A51.4

Lymphadenosis R59.1

Lymphangiectasis I89.0
- conjunctiva H11.8
- postinfectional I89.0
- scrotum I89.0

Lymphangioendothelioma (M9170/0)
D18.1
- malignant (M9170/3) – *see* Neoplasm,
connective tissue, malignant
Lymphangioma (M9170/0) D18.1
- capillary (M9171/0) D18.1
- cavernous (M9172/0) D18.1
- cystic (M9173/0) D18.1
- malignant (M9170/3) – *see* Neoplasm,
connective tissue, malignant
Lymphangiomyoma (M9174/0) D18.1
Lymphangiomyomatosis (M9174/1) – *see*
Neoplasm, connective tissue, uncertain
behavior
Lymphangiosarcoma (M9170/3) – *see*
Neoplasm, connective tissue, malignant
Lymphangitis I89.1
- with
- - abscess – *see* Abscess, by site
- - cellulitis – *see* Abscess, by site
- acute – *see* Cellulitis
- breast
- - gestational O91.2
- - puerperal, postpartum (nonpurulent)
O91.2
- - - purulent O91.1
- chancroidal A57
- chronic (any site) I89.1
- due to
- - Brugia (malayi) B74.1
- - - timori B74.2
- - Wuchereria bancrofti B74.0
- following
- - abortion (subsequent episode) O08.8
- - - current episode – *see* Abortion
- - ectopic or molar pregnancy O08.8
- gangrenous I89.1
- penis
- - acute N48.2
- - gonococcal (acute) (chronic) A54.0
- puerperal, postpartum, childbirth O86.8
- strumous, tuberculous A18.2
- subacute (any site) I89.1
- tuberculous (*see also* Tuberculosis, lymph
gland) A18.2
Lymphatic (vessel) – *see condition*
Lymphectasia I89.0
Lymphedema (*see also* Elephantiasis)
I89.0
- hereditary Q82.0
- postmastectomy I97.2
- precox I89.0
- secondary I89.0
- surgical NEC I97.8

Lymphedema—*continued*
- surgical NEC—*continued*
- - postmastectomy (syndrome) I97.2
Lymphoblastic – *see condition*
Lymphoblastoma (diffuse) C85.9
Lymphocele I89.8
Lymphocytic
- chorioencephalitis (acute) (serous)
A87.2† G05.1∗
- choriomeningitis (acute) (serous) A87.2†
G02.0∗
- colitis K52.8
- meningoencephalitis A87.2† G05.1∗
Lymphocytoma, benign cutis L98.8
Lymphocytosis (symptomatic) D72.8
- infectious (acute) B33.8
Lymphoepithelioma (M8082/3) – *see*
Neoplasm, malignant
Lymphogranuloma (malignant) C81.9
- chlamydial A55
- inguinale A55
- venereum (any site) (chlamydial) A55
Lymphogranulomatosis (malignant)
C81.9
- benign (Boeck's sarcoid) (Schaumann's)
D86.1
Lymphohistiocytosis, hemophagocytic
D76.1
Lymphoid – *see condition*
Lymphoma (malignant) C85.9
- adult T-cell C91.5
- AILD C86.5
- angiocentric T-cell C86.0
- angioimmunoblastic C86.5
- B-cell NEC C85.1
- - diffuse large (ALK-positive)
(anaplastic) (centroblastic)
(immunoblastic) (plasmablastic) (T-cell
rich) C83.3
- - extranodal, marginal zone of mucosa-
associated lymphoid tissue (MALT-
lymphoma) C88.4
- - large
- - - cell, mediastinal (thymic) C85.2
- - - intravascular C83.8
- - monocytoid C85.9
- - primary effusion C83.8
- - small cell C83.0
- B-CLL, non-leukemic variant C83.0
- B-precursor NEC C83.5
- Burkitt (atypical) (-like) (small
noncleaved, diffuse) (undifferentiated)
C83.7
- - resulting from HIV disease B21.1

marginal zone B-cell lymphoma - slow growing
NHL B-cell lymphomas

Lymphoma—_continued_
- centroblastic (diffuse) C83.3
- – follicular C82.2
- centroblastic-centrocytic (diffuse) C83.9
- – follicular C82.5
- centrocytic C83.1
- cleaved cell (diffuse) C83.1
- – with
-   – – large cell, follicular C82.1
-   – – noncleaved, large cell C83.9
- – follicular C82.9
- – large (diffuse) C83.3
-   – – follicular C82.2
- – small (diffuse) C83.1
- convoluted cell C83.5
- cutaneous NEC C84.8
- diffuse C83.9
- – histiocytic C83.9
- – large cell C83.3
-   – – noncleaved C83.3
- – lymphocytic (well differentiated) C83.0
-   – – intermediate differentiation C83.0
-   – – poorly differentiated C85.9
- – mixed cell type C85.9
-   – – lymphocytic-histiocytic C85.9
-   – – small and large cell C85.9
- – noncleaved C83.9
-   – – large cell C83.3
-   – – small cell C83.0
- – reticulum cell sarcoma C83.3
- – small cell C83.0
-   – – cleaved C83.1
-   – – lymphocytic C83.0
-   – – noncleaved, Burkitt C83.7
- follicle centre (centroblastic-centrocytic)
- – cutaneous C82.6
- – diffuse C82.5
- follicular (centroblastic-centrocytic) (nodular) (with or without diffuse areas) C82.9
- – grade
-   – – I C82.0
-   – – II C82.1
-   – – III NEC C82.2
-   – – IIIa C82.3
-   – – IIIb C82.4
- – histiocytic C82.2
- – large cell (cleaved) (noncleaved) C82.2
- – mixed cell type C82.1
- – noncleaved (large cell) C82.3
- – small cleaved cell C82.0
-   – – and large cell C82.1
- histiocytic C85.9

Lymphoma—_continued_
- histiocytic—_continued_
- – true C96.8
- Hodgkin C81.9
- immunoblastic (diffuse) (large type) C83.3
- large cell
- – anaplastic
-   – – ALK-negative C84.7
-   – – ALK-positive C84.6
-   – – CD30-positive C84.6
-   – – primary cutaneous C86.6
- – diffuse C83.3
-   – – with
-    – – – small cell, mixed diffuse C85.9
-    – – – small cleaved, mixed, follicular C82.1
-   – – Ki-1+ 7 C84.6
-   – – noncleaved and cleaved C83.3
- Lennert C84.4
- leukemia, adult T-cell C91.5
- lymphoblastic (diffuse) C83.5
- lymphocytic (diffuse) C83.0
- – intermediate differentiation, nodular C82.9
- – nodular (intermediate differentiation) (poorly differentiated) (well differentiated) C82.9
- – small C83.0 B6273
- lymphoepithelioid C84.4
- lymphoid tissue
- – bronchial-associated (BALT-lymphoma) C88.4
- – skin-associated (SALT- lymphoma) C88.4
- lymphoplasmacytic C83.0
- – with, IgM-production C88.0
- lymphoplasmacytoid C83.0
- lymphoplasmatic C83.0
- mantle
- – cell C83.1
- – zone C83.1
- Mediterranean C88.3
- mixed cell type
- – diffuse C85.9
- – follicular C82.1
- – lymphocytic-histiocytic (diffuse) C85.9
-   – – nodular C82.1
- – small and large cell (diffuse) C85.9
- – small cleaved and large cell, follicular C82.1
- monocytoid B-cell C85.9
- NK-cell, blastic C86.4
- nodal marginal C83.0

406

Lymphoma—*continued*
- nodular (with or without diffuse areas) C82.9
- − histiocytic C82.2
- − lymphocytic C82.9
- − − intermediate differentiation C82.9
- − − poorly differentiated C82.9
- − − well differentiated C82.9
- − mixed (cell type) C82.1
- − mixed lymphocytic-histiocytic C82.1
- non-Burkitt, undifferentiated cell C83.3
- noncleaved (diffuse) C83.9
- − follicular C82.2
- − large cell (diffuse) C83.3
- − − follicular C82.2
- − small cell (diffuse) C83.0 ʹ
- non-Hodgkin (type) NEC C85.9
- − non-follicular (diffuse) NEC C83.9
- − resulting from HIV disease B21.2
- − − (type) NEC C85.9
- peripheral T-cell C84.4
- − AILD C86.5
- − angioimmunoblastic lymphadenopathy with dysproteinemia C86.5
- − pleomorphic
- − − medium and large cell C84.4
- − − small cell C84.4
- plasmacytic C83.0
- plasmacytic-lymphocytic C83.0
- plasmacytoid C83.0
- − small lymphocytic C83.0
- resulting from HIV disease B21.2
- small cell (diffuse) C83.0
- − with large cell, mixed (diffuse) C85.9
- − cleaved (diffuse) C83.1
- − − and large cell, mixed, follicular C82.1
- − − follicular C82.9
- − lymphocytic (diffuse) C83.0
- − noncleaved (diffuse) C83.0
- − − Burkitt C83.7
- T-cell NEC C84.4
- − adult C91.5

Lymphoma—*continued*
- T-cell NEC—*continued*
- − angiocentric C86.0
- − angioimmunoblastic C86.5
- − cutaneous C84.8
- − enteropathy associated C86.2
- − enteropathy-type (intestinal) C86.2
- − hepatosplenic (alpha-beta and gamma-delta types) C86.1
- − mature, not classified C84.4
- − panniculitis-like, subcutaneous C86.3
- − peripheral AILD C86.5
- − − angioimmunoblastic lymphadenopathy with dysproteinemia C86.5
- − − pleomorphic
- − − − medium and large cell C84.4
- − − − small cell C84.4
- − primary cutaneous, CD30-positive C86.6
- T-precursor NEC C83.5
- T/NK-cell NEC C84.5
- − extranodal, nasal type C86.0
- − mature NEC C84.9
- true histiocytic C96.8
- T-zone C84.4
- undifferentiated cell C83.9
- − − Burkitt type C83.7
Lymphomatosis – *see* Lymphoma
Lymphopathia venereum, veneris A55
Lymphopenia D72.8
Lymphoproliferation, X-linked disease D82.3
Lymphoreticulosis, benign (of inoculation) A28.1
Lymphorrhea I89.8
Lymphosarcoma (diffuse) C85.9
- cell leukemia C91.9
- follicular C82.9
- − mixed cell type C82.9
Lymphostasis I89.8
Lysine and hydroxylysine metabolism disorder E72.3
Lyssa – *see* Rabies

Macrosomia – excessive fetal growth
– O36.6 Maternal care for (known or suspected) excessive fetal growth

M

Macacus ear Q17.3
Maceration, fetus (cause not stated) P95
MacLeod's syndrome J43.0
Macrocephalia, macrocephaly Q75.3
Macrocheilia, macrochilia (congenital) Q18.6
Macrocolon (*see also* Megacolon) Q43.1
Macrocornea Q15.8
– with glaucoma Q15.0
Macrocytic – *see condition*
Macrocytosis D75.8
Macrodactylia, macrodactylism (fingers) (thumbs) Q74.0
– toes Q74.2
Macrodontia K00.2
Macrogenitosomia (adrenal) (male) (precox) E25.9
– congenital E25.0
Macroglobulinemia (idiopathic) (primary) C88.0
– Waldenström C88.0
Macroglossia (congenital) Q38.2
– acquired K14.8
Macrognathia, macrognathism (congenital) (mandibular) (maxillary) K07.0
Macrogyria (congenital) Q04.8
Macrohydrocephalus (*see also* Hydrocephalus) G91.9
Macromastia (*see also* Hypertrophy, breast) N62
Macrophthalmos Q11.3
– in congenital glaucoma Q15.0
Macropsia H53.1
Macrosigmoid K59.3
– congenital Q43.2
Macrostomia (congenital) Q18.4
Macrotia (congenital) (external ear) Q17.1
Macula
– cornea, corneal H17.8
– degeneration (atrophic) (exudative) (senile) H35.3
– – hereditary H35.5
Maculopathy, toxic H35.3
Madarosis (eyelid) H02.7
Madelung's
– deformity (radius) Q74.0

Madelung's—*continued*
– disease
– – radial deformity Q74.0
– – symmetrical lipomas, neck E88.8
Madura foot B47.9
– mycotic B47.0
Maduromycosis B47.0
Maffucci's syndrome Q78.4
Magnesium metabolism disorder E83.4
Main en griffe (acquired) M21.5
– congenital Q74.0
Maintenance
– chemotherapy NEC Z51.2
– – neoplasm Z51.1
– external fixation NEC Z47.8
– traction NEC Z47.8
Majocchi's
– disease L81.7
– granuloma B35.8
Major – *see condition*
Mal de mer T75.3
Mal lie (*see also* Presentation, fetal) O32.9
Malabar itch (any site) B35.5
Malabsorption K90.9
– calcium K90.8
– carbohydrate K90.4
– disaccharide E73.9
– fat K90.4
– galactose E74.2
– glucose(-galactose) E74.3
– intestinal K90.9
– – specified NEC K90.8
– isomaltose E74.3
– lactose E73.9
– monosaccharide E74.3
– protein K90.4
– starch K90.4
– sucrose E74.3
– syndrome K90.9
– – postsurgical K91.2
Malacia, bone (adult) M83.9
– juvenile (*see also* Rickets) E55.0
Malacoplakia
– bladder N32.8
– pelvis (kidney) N28.8
– ureter N28.8
– urethra N36.8
Maladaptation – *see* Maladjustment

Maladjustment
- conjugal Z63.0
- educational Z55.4
- marital Z63.0
- – involving divorce or estrangement
  Z63.5
- occupational NEC Z56.7
- simple, adult (*see also* Reaction,
  adjustment) F43.2
- situational (*see also* Reaction, adjustment)
  F43.2
- social (due to) Z60.9
- – acculturation difficulty Z60.3
- – discrimination and persecution
  (perceived) Z60.5
- – exclusion and isolation Z60.4
- – life-cycle (phase of life) transition
  Z60.0
- – rejection Z60.4
- – specified reason NEC Z60.8

Malaise R53

Malakoplakia – *see* Malacoplakia

Malaria, malarial (fever) B54
- with
- – blackwater fever B50.8
- – – hemoglobinuric (bilious) B50.8
- – hemoglobinuria B50.8
- accidentally induced (therapeutically) –
  see Malaria, by type
- algid B50.9
- cerebral B50.0† G94.8*
- clinically diagnosed (without
  parasitological confirmation) B54
- complicating pregnancy, childbirth or
  puerperium O98.6
- congenital NEC P37.4
- – falciparum P37.3
- continued (fever) B50.9
- estivo-autumnal B50.9
- falciparum B50.9
- – with complications NEC B50.8
- – – cerebral B50.0† G94.8*
- – severe B50.8
- malariae (with) B52.9
- – complications NEC B52.8
- – glomerular disorder B52.0† N08.0*
- malignant (tertian) (*see also* Malaria,
  falciparum) B50.9
- ovale B53.0
- parasitologically confirmed NEC B53.8
- pernicious, acute – *see* Malaria,
  falciparum

Malaria, malarial—*continued*
- Plasmodium (P.)
- – falciparum NEC (*see also* Malaria,
  falciparum) B50.9
- – – with other Plasmodium (*see also*
  Malaria, falciparum) B50.-
- – malariae NEC B52.9
- – – with Plasmodium
- – – – falciparum (and vivax) (*see also*
  Malaria, falciparum) B50.-
- – – – vivax (*see also* Malaria, vivax)
  B51.-
- – – – – and falciparum (*see also*
  Malaria, falciparum) B50.-
- – – ovale B53.0
- – – with Plasmodium malariae (*see also*
  Malaria, malariae) B52.-
- – – – and vivax (*see also* Malaria, vivax)
  B51.-
- – – – – and falciparum (*see also*
  Malaria, falciparum) B50.-
- – – simian B53.1
- – – with Plasmodium malariae (*see also*
  Malaria, malariae) B52.-
- – – – and vivax (*see also* Malaria, vivax)
  B51.-
- – – – – and falciparum (*see also*
  Malaria, falciparum) B50.-
- – – vivax NEC B51.9
- – – with Plasmodium
  falciparum (*see also* Malaria,
  falciparum) B50.-
- quartan (*see also* Malaria, malariae)
  B52.9
- quotidian (*see also* Malaria, falciparum)
  B50.9
- recurrent B54
- remittent B54
- specified type NEC (parasitologically
  confirmed) B53.8
- subtertian (fever) (*see also* Malaria,
  falciparum) B50.9
- tertian (benign) (*see also* Malaria, vivax)
  B51.9
- – malignant B50.9
- tropical B50.9
- vivax (with) B51.9
- – complications NEC B51.8
- – ruptured spleen B51.0† D77*

Malassez's disease (cystic) N50.8

Maldescent, testis Q53.9
- bilateral Q53.2
- unilateral Q53.1

AV malformation — index under fistula, congenital

Maldevelopment – *see also* Anomaly
– colon Q43.9
– hip Q74.2
– – congenital dislocation Q65.2
– – – bilateral Q65.1
– – – unilateral Q65.0
– mastoid process Q75.8
– middle ear Q16.4
– spine Q76.4
– toe Q74.2
Male type pelvis Q74.2
– with disproportion (fetopelvic) O33.3
– – affecting fetus or newborn P03.1
– – causing obstructed labor O65.3
Malformation (congenital) – *see also*
    Anomaly
– affecting multiple systems
– – with skeletal changes specified NEC
    Q87.5
– aortic valve Q23.9
– – specified NEC Q23.8
– arteriovenous, aneurysmatic (congenital)
    Q27.3
– – precerebral vessels (nonruptured)
    Q28.0
– auricle
– – ear (congenital) (*see also* Deformity,
    ear) Q17.3
– brain (multiple) Q04.9
– branchial cleft Q18.2
– cerebral Q04.9
– choroid (congenital) Q14.3
– – plexus Q07.8
– circulatory system NEC Q28.9
– corpus callosum (congenital) Q04.0
– diaphragm Q79.1
– dura Q07.9
– – brain Q04.9
– – spinal Q06.9
– eye Q15.9
– – specified NEC Q15.8
– gum Q38.6
– heart NEC Q24.9
– internal ear Q16.5
– lung Q33.9
– meninges or membrane (congenital)
    Q07.9
– – cerebral Q04.8
– – spinal (cord) Q06.9
– mitral valve Q23.9
– – specified NEC Q23.8
– mouth (congenital) NEC Q38.6
– nervous system (central) Q07.9

Malformation—*continued*
– pelvic organs or tissues NEC
– – in pregnancy or childbirth O34.8
– – – affecting fetus or newborn P03.8
– – – causing obstructed labor O65.5
– – – – affecting fetus or newborn P03.1
– placenta O43.1
– precerebral vessels Q28.1
– respiratory system Q34.9
– skin NEC Q82.9
– specified NEC Q89.8
– spinal
– – cord Q06.9
– – nerve root Q07.8
– spine Q76.4
– throat Q38.8
– tongue (congenital) Q38.3
– umbilical cord NEC (complicating
    delivery) O69.8
– – affecting fetus or newborn P02.6
– urinary system Q64.9
Malfunction – *see also* Dysfunction
– cardiac pacemaker (electrode(s)) (pulse
    generator) T82.1
– catheter device NEC T85.6
– – dialysis (renal) (vascular) T82.4
– – – intraperitoneal T85.6
– – infusion NEC T82.5
– – – spinal (epidural) (subdural) T85.6
– – urinary, indwelling T83.0
– colostomy K91.4
– cystostomy (stoma) N99.5
– – catheter T83.0
– enteric stoma K91.4
– enterostomy K91.4
– gastrostomy K91.8
– ileostomy K91.4
– jejunostomy K91.4
– pacemaker T82.1
– prosthetic device, internal – *see*
    Complications, prosthetic device, by site,
    mechanical
– tracheostomy J95.0
– urinary device NEC T83.1
– vascular graft or shunt NEC T82.3
– – coronary artery T82.2
– ventricular (communicating shunt) T85.0
Malherbe's tumor (M8110/0) – *see*
    Neoplasm, skin, benign
Malignancy (M8000/3) – *see* Neoplasm,
    malignant
Malignant – *see condition*
Malingerer, malingering Z76.5

Mallet finger (acquired) M20.0
- congenital Q74.0
- late effect of rickets E64.3
Malleus A24.0
Mallory's bodies R89.7
Mallory-Weiss syndrome K22.6
Malnutrition E46
- degree
- - first E44.1
- - mild E44.1
- - moderate E44.0
- - second E44.0
- - severe (protein-energy) E43
- - - intermediate form (with) E42
- - - - kwashiorkor (and marasmus) E42
- - - - marasmus E41
- - third E43
- in pregnancy, childbirth or puerperium O25
- intrauterine or fetal P05.2
- - light-for-dates P05.0
- - small-for-dates P05.1
- lack of care, or neglect (child) (infant) T74.8
- malignant E40
- maternal, affecting fetus or newborn P00.4
- protein E46
- - calorie E46
- - - mild E44.1
- - - moderate E44.0
- - - severe E43
- - - - intermediate form (with) E42
- - - - - kwashiorkor (and marasmus) E42
- - - - - marasmus E41
- - energy E46
- - - mild E44.1
- - - moderate E44.0
- - - severe E43
- - - - intermediate form (with) E42
- - - - - kwashiorkor (and marasmus) E42
- - - - - marasmus E41
- severe (protein-energy) (with) E43
- - kwashiorkor (and marasmus) E42
- - marasmus E41
Malocclusion (teeth) K07.4
- due to
- - abnormal swallowing K07.5
- - displaced or missing teeth K07.3
- - mouth breathing K07.5
- - tongue, lip or finger habits K07.5
- temporomandibular (joint) K07.6

Malposition
- cervix – *see* Malposition, uterus
- congenital
- - adrenal (gland) Q89.1
- - alimentary tract Q45.8
- - - lower Q43.8
- - - upper Q40.8
- - aorta Q25.4
- - appendix Q43.8
- - arterial trunk Q20.0
- - artery (peripheral) Q27.8
- - - coronary Q24.5
- - - pulmonary Q25.7
- - auditory canal Q17.8
- - - causing impairment of hearing Q16.9
- - auricle (ear) Q17.4
- - - causing impairment of hearing Q16.9
- - - cervical Q18.2
- - biliary duct or passage Q44.5
- - bladder (mucosa) Q64.1
- - - exteriorized or extroverted Q64.1
- - brachial plexus Q07.8
- - brain tissue Q04.8
- - breast Q83.8
- - bronchus Q32.4
- - cecum Q43.8
- - clavicle Q74.0
- - colon Q43.8
- - digestive organ or tract NEC Q45.8
- - - lower Q43.8
- - - upper Q40.8
- - ear (auricle) (external) Q17.4
- - - ossicles Q16.3
- - endocrine (gland) NEC Q89.2
- - epiglottis Q31.8
- - eustachian tube Q16.4
- - eye Q15.8
- - facial features Q18.8
- - fallopian tube Q50.6
- - finger(s) Q68.1
- - - supernumerary Q69.0
- - foot Q66.9
- - gallbladder Q44.1
- - gastrointestinal tract Q45.8
- - genitalia, genital organ(s) or tract
- - - female Q52.8
- - - - external Q52.7
- - - - internal NEC Q52.8
- - - male Q55.8
- - glottis Q31.8
- - hand Q68.1
- - heart Q24.8

Malposition—*continued*
- congenital—*continued*
- - heart—*continued*
- - - dextrocardia Q24.0
- - - - with complete transposition of
viscera Q89.3
- - hepatic duct Q44,5
- - hip (joint) Q65.8
- - intestine (large) (small) Q43.8
- - - with anomalous adhesions, fixation
or malrotation Q43.3
- - joint NEC Q68.8
- - kidney Q63.2
- - larynx Q31.8
- - limb Q68.8
- - - lower Q68.8
- - - upper Q68.8
- - liver Q44.7
- - lung (lobe) Q33.8
- - nail(s) Q84.6
- - nerve Q07.8
- - nervous system NEC Q07.8
- - nose, nasal (septum) Q30.8
- - organ or site not listed – *see* Anomaly,
by site
- - ovary Q50.3
- - pancreas Q45.3
- - parathyroid (gland) Q89.2
- - patella Q74.1
- - peripheral vascular system Q27.8
- - pituitary (gland) Q89.2
- - respiratory organ or system NEC
Q34.8
- - rib (cage) Q76.6
- - - supernumerary in cervical region
Q76.5
- - scapula Q74.0
- - shoulder Q74.0
- - spinal cord Q06.8
- - spleen Q89.0
- - sternum NEC Q76.7
- - stomach Q40.2
- - symphysis pubis Q74.2
- - thymus (gland) Q89.2
- - thyroid (gland) (tissue) Q89.2
- - - cartilage Q31.8
- - toe(s) Q66.9
- - - supernumerary Q69.2
- - tongue Q38.3
- - trachea Q32.1
- - uterus Q51.8
- - vein(s) (peripheral) Q27.8
- - - great Q26.8
- - vena cava (inferior) (superior) Q26.8

Malposition—*continued*
- device, implant or graft (*see also*
Complications, by site and type,
mechanical) T85.6
- - arterial graft NEC T82.3
- - - coronary (bypass) T82.2
- - breast (implant) T85.4
- - catheter NEC T85.6
- - - dialysis (renal) T82.4
- - - - intraperitoneal T85.6
- - - infusion NEC T82.5
- - - - spinal (epidural) (subdural) T85.6
- - - urinary (indwelling) T83.0
- - electronic (electrode) (pulse generator)
(stimulator)
- - - bone T84.3
- - - cardiac T82.1
- - - nervous system (brain) (peripheral
nerve) (spinal) T85.1
- - - urinary T83.1
- - fixation, internal (orthopedic) NEC
T84.2
- - - bones of limb T84.1
- - gastrointestinal (bile duct) (esophagus)
T85.5
- - genital NEC T83.4
- - - intrauterine contraceptive device
T83.3
- - heart NEC T82.5
- - - valve (prosthesis) T82.0
- - - - graft T82.2
- - joint prosthesis T84.0
- - ocular (canal graft) (orbital implant)
NEC T85.3
- - - intraocular lens T85.2
- - orthopedic NEC T84.4
- - - bone graft T84.3
- - specified NEC T85.6
- - urinary NEC T83.1
- - - graft T83.2
- - vascular NEC T82.5
- - ventricular intracranial shunt T85.0
- fetus NEC (*see also* Presentation, fetal)
O32.9
- - causing obstructed labor O64.9
- - in multiple gestation (of one fetus or
more) O32.5
- - - causing obstructed labor O64.8
- gallbladder K82.8
- heart, congenital NEC Q24.8
- pelvic organs or tissues NEC, in
pregnancy or childbirth O34.8
- - causing obstructed labor O65.5
- placenta (*see also* Placenta, previa) O44.1

Malposition—*continued*
- stomach K31.8
- tooth, teeth (with impaction) K07.3
- uterus (acquired) (acute) (adherent) (any degree) (asymptomatic) (postinfectional) (postpartal, old) N85.4
- - anteflexion or anteversion (*see also* Anteversion, uterus) N85.4
- - flexion N85.4
- - - lateral (*see also* Lateroversion, uterus) N85.4
- - in pregnancy or childbirth O34.5
- - - causing obstructed labor O65.5
- - inversion N85.5
- - lateral (flexion) (version) (*see also* Lateroversion, uterus) N85.4
- - retroflexion or retroversion (*see also* Retroversion, uterus) N85.4
Malposture R29.3
Malpresentation, fetus (*see also* Presentation, fetal) O32.9
Malrotation
- cecum Q43.3
- colon Q43.3
- intestine Q43.3
- kidney Q63.2
Maltreatment (of)
- child NEC T74.9
- personal history of Z91.8
- syndrome
- - abuse of adult (effects of) T74.9
- - child abuse (effects of) T74.9
Maltworker's lung J67.4
Malunion, fracture M84.0
Mammillitis N61
- puerperal, postpartum O91.0
Mammitis – *see* Mastitis
Mammogram (examination) Z12.3
- routine Z01.6
Management (of)
- bone conduction device (implanted) Z45.3
- cardiac pacemaker NEC Z45.0
- cochlear device (implanted) Z45.3
- contraceptive Z30.9
- - specified NEC Z30.8
- implanted device Z45.9
- - specified NEC Z45.8
- infusion pump Z45.1
- procreative Z31.9
- - specified NEC Z31.8
- prosthesis (external) (*see also* Fitting) Z44.9
- - implanted Z45.9

Management—*continued*
- prosthesis—*continued*
- - implanted—*continued*
- - - specified NEC Z45.8
- vascular access device Z45.2
Mania (monopolar) F30.9
- with psychotic symptoms F30.2
- alcoholic (acute) (chronic) F10.5
- Bell's F30.8
- chronic (recurrent) F31.8
- hysterical F44.8
- puerperal F30.8
- recurrent F31.8
- without psychotic symptoms F30.1
Mannosidosis E77.1
Mansonelliasis, mansonellosis B74.4
Manson's
- disease B65.1
- pyosis L00
- schistosomiasis B65.1
Manual – *see* condition
Maple-bark-stripper's lung J67.6
Maple-syrup-urine disease E71.0
Marasmus E41
- due to malnutrition E41
- intestinal E41
- nutritional E41
- senile R54
- tuberculous NEC (*see also* Tuberculosis) A16.9
Marble
- bones Q78.2
- skin R23.8
Marburg virus disease A98.3
March
- fracture S92.3
- hemoglobinuria D59.6
Marchesani(-Weill) syndrome Q87.0
Marchiafava(-Bignami) syndrome or disease G37.1
Marchiafava-Micheli syndrome D59.5
Marcus Gunn's syndrome Q07.8
Marfan's syndrome Q87.4
Marginal implantation, placenta – *see* Placenta, previa
Marie-Bamberger disease M89.4
Marie-Charcot-Tooth neuropathic muscular atrophy G60.0
Marie's
- cerebellar ataxia (late-onset) G11.2
- disease or syndrome (acromegaly) E22.0
Marie-Strümpell arthritis, disease or spondylitis M45
Marion's disease N32.0

MALToma –
Code to B-Cell lymphoma
C851

Marital conflict Z63.0
Mark
– port wine Q82.5
– raspberry Q82.5
– strawberry Q82.5
– stretch L90.6
– tattoo L81.8
Marker heterochromatin Q95.4
Maroteaux-Lamy syndrome (mild)
(severe) E76.2
Marrow (bone)
– arrest D61.9
– poor function D61.9
Masculinization (female) with adrenal
hyperplasia E25.9
– congenital E25.0
Masochism (sexual) F65.5
Mason's lung J62.8
Mass
– abdominal R19.0
– breast N63
– chest R22.2
– cystic – *see* Cyst
– head R22.0
– intra-abdominal (diffuse) (generalized)
  R19.0
– kidney N28.8
– localized (skin) R22.9
– – chest R22.2
– – head R22.0
– – limb
– – – lower R22.4
– – – upper R22.3
– – multiple sites R22.7
– – neck R22.1
– – trunk R22.2
– lung R91
– malignant (M8000/3) – *see* Neoplasm,
  malignant
– neck R22.1
– pelvic (diffuse) (generalized) R19.0
– specified organ NEC – *see* Disease, by
  site
– substernal thyroid (*see also* Goiter) E04.9
– superficial (localized) R22.9
– umbilical (diffuse) (generalized) R19.0
Massive – *see condition*
Mast cell
– disease, systemic tissue D47.0
– leukemia C94.3
– sarcoma C96.2
– tumor D47.0
– – malignant C96.2

Mastalgia N64.4
– psychogenic F45.4
Masters-Allen syndrome N83.8
Mastitis (acute) (infective) (nonpuerperal)
(subacute) N61
– chronic (cystic) N60.1
– – with epithelial proliferation N60.3
– cystic (Schimmelbusch's type) N60.1
– – with epithelial proliferation N60.3
– infective N61
– – newborn P39.0
– interstitial, gestational or puerperal O91.2
– neonatal (noninfective) P83.4
– – infective P39.0
– puerperal, postpartum or gestational
  (interstitial) (nonpurulent)
  (parenchymatous) O91.2
– – purulent O91.1
Mastocytoma D47.0
– malignant C96.2
Mastocytosis Q82.2
– malignant C96.2
– – aggressive C96.2
– systemic (associated with clonal
  haematopoietic non-mast-cell disease)
  (indolent) (SM-AHNMD) D47.0
Mastodynia N64.4
– psychogenic F45.4
Mastoid – *see condition*
Mastoidalgia H92.0
Mastoiditis (coalescent) (hemorrhagic)
(suppurative) H70.9
– acute, subacute H70.0
– chronic (necrotic) (recurrent) H70.1
– in (due to)
– – infectious disease NEC B99† H75.0*
– – parasitic disease NEC B89† H75.0*
– – tuberculosis A18.0† H75.0*
– specified NEC H70.8
– tuberculous A18.0† H75.0*
Mastopathy, mastopathia N64.9
– chronica cystica N60.1
– – with epithelial proliferation N60.3
– cystic (chronic) (diffuse) N60.1
– – with epithelial proliferation N60.3
– diffuse cystic N60.1
– – with epithelial proliferation N60.3
– estrogenic, oestrogenica N64.8
– ovarian origin N64.8
Mastoplastia N62
Masturbation (excessive) F98.8
Maternal care (for) (known) (suspected)
– abnormality – *see also condition*
– – cervix uteri NEC O34.4

Maternal care—*continued*
- abnormality—*continued*
- - - gravid uterus NEC O34.5
- - pelvic organs O34.9
- - - specified NEC O34.8
- - vagina O34.6
- - vulva and perineum O34.7
- breech presentation O32.1
- central nervous system malformation, fetus O35.0
- cervical incompetence O34.3
- chromosomal abnormality, fetus O35.1
- compound presentation O32.6
- congenital malformation, uterus O34.0
- damage to fetus from
- - alcohol O35.4
- - drugs O35.5
- - maternal
- - - alcohol addiction O35.4
- - - cytomegalovirus infection O35.3
- - - drug addiction O35.5
- - - listeriosis O35.8
- - - rubella O35.3
- - - toxoplasmosis O35.8
- - - viral disease O35.3
- - medical procedure NEC O35.7
- - radiation O35.6
- disproportion (fetopelvic) (due to) O33.9
- - deformity of maternal pelvic bones O33.0
- - fetal deformity NEC O33.7
- - generally contracted maternal pelvis O33.1
- - hydrocephalic fetus O33.6
- - inlet contraction, maternal pelvis O33.2
- - mixed maternal and fetal origin O33.4
- - origin NEC O33.8
- - outlet contraction, maternal pelvis O33.3
- - unusually large fetus O33.5
- excessive fetal growth O36.6
- face, brow and chin presentation O32.3
- fetal
- - abnormality O35.9
- - - specified NEC O35.8
- - anencephaly O35.0
- - damage O35.9
- - - specified NEC O35.8
- - hypoxia (unrelated to labor and delivery) O36.3
- - problem O36.9
- - - specified NEC O36.8
- - spina bifida O35.0

Maternal care—*continued*
- habitual aborter (during pregnancy) O26.2
- hereditary disease, fetus O35.2
- high head at term (pregnancy) O32.4
- hydrops fetalis NEC (not due to isoimmunization) O36.2
- intrauterine death (late) O36.4
- isoimmunization (ABO) O36.1
- - Rh (rhesus) (anti-D) O36.0
- malpresentation (fetus) O32.9
- - specified NEC O32.8
- multiple gestation with malpresentation of one fetus or more O32.5
- placental insufficiency O36.5
- poor fetal growth O36.5
- transverse and oblique lie O32.2
- tumor, corpus uteri O34.1
- unstable lie O32.0
- uterine scar from previous surgery O34.2
- viable fetus in abdominal pregnancy O36.7

Maternal condition, affecting fetus or newborn P00.9
- acute yellow atrophy of liver P00.8
- alcohol use P04.3
- anesthesia or analgesia P04.0
- blood loss (gestational) P02.1
- cancer chemotherapy P04.1
- chorioamnionitis P02.7
- circulatory disease (conditions in I00-I99, Q20-Q28) P00.3
- complication of pregnancy NEC P01.9
- congenital heart disease (conditions in Q20-Q24) P00.3
- cortical necrosis of kidney P00.1
- cytotoxic drug P04.1
- death P01.6
- diabetes mellitus (conditions in E10-E14) P70.1
- disease NEC P00.9
- eclampsia P00.0
- exposure to environmental chemical substances P04.6
- genital tract infections NEC P00.8
- glomerular diseases (conditions in N00-N08) P00.1
- hemorrhage, gestational P02.1
- hepatitis, acute, malignant or subacute P00.8
- hyperemesis (gravidarum) P01.8
- hypertension (conditions in O10-O11, O13-O16) P00.0

415

MCADD —Medium-chain acyl-coenzyme A dehydrogenase
deficiency   E71.3   (Underdiagnosed cause of
Newborn screening   SID)

INTERNATIONAL CLASSIFICATION OF DISEASES

**Maternal condition, affecting fetus or
newborn**—*continued*
- infectious and parasitic diseases
  (conditions in A00-B99, J09-J11) P00.2
- influenza P00.2
- – manifest influenza in the infant P35.8
- injury (conditions in S00-T79) P00.5
- malaria P00.2
- – manifest malaria NEC in infant or fetus
  P37.4
- – – falciparum P37.3
- malnutrition P00.4
- necrosis of liver P00.8
- nephritis, nephrotic syndrome and
  nephrosis (conditions in N00-N08) P00.1
- noxious influence transmitted via breast
  milk or placenta P04.9
- – specified NEC P04.8
- nutritional disorder (conditions in E40-
  E64) P00.4
- operation unrelated to current pregnancy
  P00.6
- pre-eclampsia P00.0
- previous surgery, uterus or pelvic organs
  P03.8
- proteinuria P00.1
- pyelitis or pyelonephritis P00.1
- renal disease or failure P00.1
- respiratory disease (conditions in J00-J99,
  Q30-Q34) P00.3
- rheumatic heart disease (chronic)
  (conditions in I05-I09) P00.3
- rubella (conditions in B06) P00.2
- – manifest rubella in the infant or fetus
  P35.0
- septate vagina P03.8
- stenosis or stricture of vagina P03.8
- surgery unrelated to current pregnancy
  P00.6
- – to uterus or pelvic organs P03.8
- syphilis (conditions in A50-A53) P00.2
- – manifest syphilis in the infant or fetus
  A50.0
- thrombophlebitis P00.3
- tobacco use P04.2
- toxemia (of pregnancy) P00.0
- toxoplasmosis (conditions in B58.-)
  P00.2
- – manifest toxoplasmosis (acute)
  (chronic) (subacute) in the infant or
  fetus P37.1
- transmission of chemical substance
  through the placenta (*see also* Absorption,
  chemical, through placenta) P04.8

**Maternal condition, affecting fetus or
newborn**—*continued*
- tumor, vagina O34.6
- uremia P00.1
- urinary tract conditions (conditions in
  N00-N39) P00.1
- vomiting (pernicious) (persistent)
  (vicious) P01.8
Mauclaire's disease or osteochondrosis
  M92.2
Maxilla, maxillary – *see condition*
May(-Hegglin) anomaly or syndrome
  D72.0
**McArdle (-Schmid) (-Pearson) disease
  (glycogen storage)** E74.0
McCune-Albright syndrome Q78.1
Meadow's syndrome Q86.1
**Measles (black) (hemorrhagic)
  (suppressed)** B05.9
- with
- – complications NEC B05.8
- – encephalitis B05.0† G05.1∗
- – intestinal complications B05.4†
  K93.8∗
- – keratitis (keratoconjunctivitis) B05.8†
  H19.2∗
- – meningitis B05.1† G02.0∗
- – otitis media B05.3† H67.1∗
- – pneumonia B05.2† J17.1∗
- German (*see also* Rubella) B06.9
Meatitis, urethral (*see also* Urethritis)
  N34.2
Meatus, meatal – *see condition*
Meckel-Gruber syndrome Q61.9
**Meckel's diverticulitis, diverticulum
  (displaced) (hypertrophic)** Q43.0
Meconium
- ileus (with cystic fibrosis), fetus or
  newborn E84.1† P75∗
- – meaning meconium plug P76.0
- – without cystic fibrosis P76.0
- in liquor – *see also* Distress, fetal
- – complicating labor and delivery O68.1
- obstruction, fetus or newborn P76.0
- – in mucoviscidosis E84.1† P75∗
- passage of – *see* Distress, fetal
- peritonitis P78.0
- plug syndrome (newborn) NEC P76.0
Median – *see also* condition
- bar (prostate) (vesical orifice) N40
Mediastinitis (acute) (chronic) J98.5
- syphilitic A52.7† J99.8∗
- tuberculous A16.8

416

Mediastinitis—*continued*
- tuberculous—*continued*
- – with bacteriological and histological confirmation A15.8
Mediastinopericarditis (*see also* Pericarditis) I31.9
- chronic rheumatic I09.2
Mediastinum, mediastinal – *see condition*
Medicine poisoning (by overdose) (wrong substance given or taken in error) T50.9
- specified drug or substance – *see* Table of drugs and chemicals
Mediterranean
- disease or syndrome (hemipathic) D56.9
- fever A23.9
- – familial E85.0
Medulla – *see condition*
Medullary cystic kidney Q61.5
Medullated fibers
- optic (nerve) Q14.8
- retina Q14.1
Medulloblastoma (M9470/3)
- desmoplastic (M9471/3) C71.6
- specified site – *see* Neoplasm, malignant
- unspecified site C71.6
Medulloepithelioma (M9501/3) – *see also* Neoplasm, malignant
- teratoid (M9502/3) – *see* Neoplasm, malignant
Medullomyoblastoma (M9472/3)
- specified site – *see* Neoplasm, malignant
- unspecified site C71.6
Megacolon (acquired) (functional) (not Hirschsprung's disease) (in) K59.3
- Chagas' disease B57.3† K93.1∗
- congenital, congenitum (aganglionic) Q43.1
- Hirschsprung's (disease) Q43.1
- toxic K59.3
Megaesophagus (functional) K22.0
- congenital Q39.5
- in (due to) Chagas' disease B57.3† K23.1∗
Megalencephaly Q04.5
Megalerythema (epidemic) B08.3
Megaloappendix Q43.8
Megalocephalus, megalocephaly NEC Q75.3
Megalocornea Q15.8
- with glaucoma Q15.0
Megalodactylia (congenital) (fingers) (thumbs) Q74.0
- toes Q74.2

Megaloduodenum Q43.8
Megaloesophagus (functional) K22.0
- congenital Q39.5
Megalogastria (acquired) K31.8
- congenital Q40.2
Megalophthalmos Q11.3
Megalopsia H53.1
Megalosplenia – *see* Splenomegaly
Megaloureter N28.8
- congenital Q62.2
Megarectum K62.8
Megasigmoid K59.3
- congenital Q43.2
Megaureter N28.8
- congenital Q62.2
Megavitamin-B₆ syndrome E67.2
Megrim – *see* Migraine
Meibomian
- cyst, infected H00.0
- gland – *see condition*
- sty, stye H00.0
Meibomitis H00.0
Meige's syndrome Q82.0
Melancholia F32.9
- senile F03
Melanemia R79.8
Melanoameloblastoma (M9363/0) – *see* Neoplasm, bone, benign
Melanoblastoma (M8720/3) – *see* Melanoma
Melanocarcinoma (M8720/3) – *see* Melanoma
Melanocytoma, eyeball (M8726/0) D31.4
Melanoderma, melanodermia L81.4
Melanodontia, infantile K02.4
Melanodontoclasia K02.4
Melanoepithelioma (M8720/3) – *see* Melanoma
Melanoma (malignant) (M8720/3) C43.9

Note: Except where otherwise indicated, the morphological varieties of melanoma in the list below should be coded by site as for "Melanoma (malignant)", i.e. according to the list under "site classification" below. Internal sites should be coded to malignant neoplasm of those sites.

- acral lentiginous, malignant (M8744/3)
- amelanotic (M8730/3)
- balloon cell (M8722/3)
- benign (M8720/0) – *see* Nevus
- desmoplastic, malignant (M8745/3)
- epithelioid cell (M8771/3)
- – with spindle cell, mixed (M8770/3)

Melanoma—*continued*
- in
- – – giant pigmented nevus (M8761/3)
- – – Hutchinson's melanotic freckle (M8742/3)
- – – junctional nevus (M8740/3)
- – – precancerous melanosis (M8741/3)
- in situ (M8720/2)
- – – abdominal wall D03.5
- – – ala nasi D03.3
- – – ankle D03.7
- – – anus, anal (margin) (skin) D03.5
- – – arm D03.6
- – – auditory canal D03.2
- – – auricle (ear) D03.2
- – – auricular canal (external) D03.2
- – – axilla, axillary fold D03.5
- – – back D03.5
- – – breast D03.5
- – – brow D03.3
- – – buttock D03.5
- – – canthus (eye) D03.1
- – – cheek (external) D03.3
- – – chest wall D03.5
- – – chin D03.3
- – – choroid D03.8
- – – conjunctiva D03.8
- – – ear (external) D03.2
- – – external meatus (ear) D03.2
- – – eye D03.8
- – – eyebrow D03.3
- – – eyelid (lower) (upper) D03.1
- – – face NEC D03.3
- – – female genital organ (external) NEC D03.8
- – – finger D03.6
- – – flank D03.5
- – – foot D03.7
- – – forearm D03.6
- – – forehead D03.3
- – – foreskin D03.8
- – – gluteal region D03.5
- – – groin D03.5
- – – hand D03.6
- – – heel D03.7
- – – helix D03.2
- – – hip D03.7
- – – interscapular region D03.5
- – – iris D03.8
- – – jaw D03.3
- – – knee D03.7
- – – labium (majus) (minus) D03.8
- – – lacrimal gland D03.8
- – – leg D03.7

Melanoma—*continued*
- in situ—*continued*
- – – lip (lower) (upper) D03.0
- – – lower limb NEC D03.7
- – – male genital organ (external) NEC D03.8
- – – nail D03.9
- – – – finger D03.6
- – – – toe D03.7
- – – neck D03.4
- – – nose (external) D03.3
- – – orbit D03.8
- – – penis D03.8
- – – perianal skin D03.5
- – – perineum D03.5
- – – pinna D03.2
- – – popliteal fossa or space D03.7
- – – prepuce D03.8
- – – pubes D03.5
- – – pudendum D03.8
- – – retina D03.8
- – – retrobulbar D03.8
- – – scalp D03.4
- – – scrotum D03.8
- – – shoulder D03.6
- – – skin NEC D03.9
- – – specified site NEC D03.8
- – – submammary fold D03.5
- – – temple D03.3
- – – thigh D03.7
- – – toe D03.7
- – – trunk NEC D03.5
- – – umbilicus D03.5
- – – upper limb NEC D03.6
- – – vulva D03.8
- juvenile (M8770/0) – *see* Nevus
- malignant, of soft parts (M9044/3) – *see* Neoplasm, connective tissue, malignant
- metastatic
- – specified site NEC (M8720/6) C79.8
- – unspecified site (M8720/6) C79.9
- neurotropic, malignant (M8745/3)
- nodular (M8721/3)
- regressing, malignant (M8723/3)
- site classification
- – abdominal wall C43.5
- – ala nasi C43.3
- – ankle C43.7
- – anus, anal C21.0
- – – margin (skin) C43.5
- – arm C43.6
- – auditory canal (external) C43.2
- – auricle (ear) C43.2
- – auricular canal (external) C43.2

Melanoma—*continued*
- site classification—*continued*
- – axilla, axillary fold C43.5
- – back C43.5
- – breast (female) (male) C43.5
- – brow C43.3
- – buttock C43.5
- – canthus (eye) C43.1
- – cheek (external) C43.3
- – chest wall C43.5
- – chin C43.3
- – choroid C69.3
- – conjunctiva C69.0
- – ear (external) C43.2
- – elbow C43.6
- – external meatus (ear) C43.2
- – eye C69.9
- – eyebrow C43.3
- – eyelid (lower) (upper) C43.1
- – face NEC C43.3
- – female genital organ (external) NEC C51.9
- – finger C43.6
- – flank C43.5
- – foot C43.7
- – forearm C43.6
- – forehead C43.3
- – foreskin C60.0
- – glabella C43.3
- – gluteal region C43.5
- – groin C43.5
- – hand C43.6
- – heel C43.7
- – helix C43.2
- – hip C43.7
- – interscapular region C43.5
- – iris C69.4
- – jaw (external) C43.3
- – knee C43.7
- – labium C51.9
- – – majus C51.0
- – – minus C51.1
- – lacrimal gland C69.5
- – leg C43.7
- – lip (lower) (upper) C43.0
- – liver (primary) C22.9
- – lower limb NEC C43.7
- – male genital organ (external) NEC C63.9
- – nail C43.9
- – – finger C43.6
- – – toe C43.7
- – nasolabial groove C43.3
- – nates C43.5

Melanoma—*continued*
- site classification—*continued*
- – neck C43.4
- – nose (external) C43.3
- – orbit C69.6
- – palpebra C43.1
- – penis C60.9
- – perianal skin C43.5
- – perineum C43.5
- – pinna C43.2
- – popliteal fossa or space C43.7
- – prepuce C60.0
- – pubes C43.5
- – pudendum C51.9
- – retina C69.2
- – retrobulbar C69.6
- – scalp C43.4
- – scrotum C63.2
- – shoulder C43.6
- – skin NEC C43.9
- – specified site NEC – *see* Neoplasm, malignant
- – submammary fold C43.5
- – temple C43.3
- – thigh C43.7
- – toe C43.7
- – trunk NEC C43.5
- – umbilicus C43.5
- – upper limb NEC C43.6
- – vulva C51.9
- spindle cell (M8772/3)
- – with epithelioid, mixed (M8770/3)
- – type A (M8773/3) C69.4
- – type B (M8774/3) C69.4
- superficial spreading (M8743/3)

Melanosarcoma (M8720/3) – *see also* Melanoma
- epithelioid cell (M8771/3) – *see* Melanoma

Melanosis L81.4
- addisonian E27.1
- – tuberculous A18.7† E35.1*
- adrenal E27.1
- colon K63.8
- conjunctiva H11.1
- – congenital Q13.8
- cornea (presenile) (senile) H18.0
- – congenital Q13.4
- eye NEC H57.8
- – congenital Q15.8
- lenticularis progressiva Q82.1
- liver K76.8
- precancerous (M8741/2) – *see also* Melanoma, in situ

Melanosis—*continued*
– precancerous—*continued*
– – malignant melanoma in (M8741/3) –
  see Melanoma
– Riehl's L81.4
– sclera H15.8
– – congenital Q13.8
– suprarenal E27.1
– tar L81.4
– toxic L81.4
Melanuria R82.9
Melasma L81.1
– adrenal (gland) E27.1
– suprarenal (gland) E27.1
Melena K92.1
– with ulcer (*see also* Ulcer, by site, with
  hemorrhage) K27.4
– newborn, neonatal P54.1
– – due to swallowed maternal blood P78.2
Meleney's
– gangrene (cutaneous) L98.4
– ulcer (chronic undermining) L98.4
Melioidosis A24.4
– acute A24.1
– chronic A24.2
– fulminating A24.1
– pneumonia A24.1
– pulmonary (chronic) A24.2
– – acute A24.1
– – subacute A24.2
– sepsis A24.1
– specified NEC A24.3
– subacute A24.2
Melkersson(-Rosenthal) syndrome G51.2
Mellitus, diabetes – *see* Diabetes
Melorheostosis (bone) M85.8
Melotia Q17.4
Membrana capsularis lentis posterior
  Q13.8
Membranacea placenta O43.1
Membranaceous uterus N85.8
Membrane(s), membranous – *see also*
  condition
– cyclitic H21.4
– folds, congenital – *see* Web
– Jackson's Q43.3
– premature rupture – *see* Rupture,
  membranes, premature
– pupillary H21.4
– – persistent Q13.8
– retained (complicating delivery) (with
  hemorrhage) O72.2
– – without hemorrhage O73.1
– secondary cataract H26.4

Membrane(s), membranous—*continued*
– unruptured (causing asphyxia) – *see*
  Asphyxia, newborn
– vitreous H43.3
Membranitis O41.1
– affecting fetus or newborn P02.7
Memory disturbance, lack or loss (*see also*
  Amnesia) R41.3
– mild, following organic brain damage
  F06.7
Menarche
– delayed E30.0
– precocious E30.1
Mendacity, pathologic F60.2
Mendelson's syndrome (due to anesthesia)
  J95.4
– in labor and delivery O74.0
– in pregnancy O29.0
– postpartum, puerperal O89.0
Ménétrier's disease or syndrome K29.6
Ménière's disease, syndrome or vertigo
  H81.0
Meninges, meningeal – *see condition*
Meningioma (M9530/0) – *see also*
  Neoplasm, meninges, benign
– angioblastic (M9535/0) D32.9
– angiomatous (M9534/0) D32.9
– endotheliomatous (M9531/0) D32.9
– fibroblastic (M9532/0) D32.9
– fibrous (M9532/0) D32.9
– hemangioblastic (M9535/0) D32.9
– hemangiopericytic (M9536/0) D32.9
– malignant (M9530/3) – *see* Neoplasm,
  meninges, malignant
– meningiothelial (M9531/0) D32.9
– meningotheliomatous (M9531/0) D32.9
– mixed (M9537/0) D32.9
– multiple (M9530/1) – *see* Neoplasm,
  meninges, uncertain behavior
– papillary (M9538/1) – *see* Neoplasm,
  meninges, uncertain behavior
– psammomatous (M9533/0) D32.9
– syncytial (M9531/0) D32.9
– transitional (M9537/0) D32.9
Meningiomatosis (diffuse) (M9530/1) – *see*
  Neoplasm, meninges, uncertain behavior
Meningismus R29.1
– due to serum or vaccine R29.1
– influenzal (specific virus not identified)
  J11.8
– – avian influenza virus identified J09
– – other influenza virus identified J10.8

Meningitis (basal) (cerebral) (spinal)
G03.9
- abacterial NEC G03.0
- actinomycotic A42.8† G01∗
- adenoviral A87.1† G02.0∗
- arbovirus A87.8† G02.0∗
- aseptic (acute) NEC G03.0
- bacterial G00.9
- – Gram-negative NEC G00.9
- – specified organism NEC G00.8
- benign recurrent (Mollaret) G03.2
- candidal B37.5† G02.1∗
- caseous (tuberculous) A17.0† G01∗
- cerebrospinal A39.0† G01∗
- chronic NEC G03.1
- clear cerebrospinal fluid NEC G03.0
- coxsackievirus A87.0† G02.0∗
- cryptococcal B45.1† G02.1∗
- diplococcal A39.0† G01∗
- echovirus A87.0† G02.0∗
- enteroviral A87.0† G02.0∗
- eosinophilic B83.2† G05.2∗
- epidemic NEC A39.0† G01∗
- Escherichia coli (E. coli) G00.8
- fibrinopurulent G00.9
- – specified organism NEC G00.8
- Friedländer (bacillus) G00.8
- gonococcal A54.8† G01∗
- Gram-negative cocci NEC G00.9
- Gram-positive cocci NEC G00.9
- Haemophilus (influenzae) G00.0
- in (due to)
- – adenovirus A87.1† G02.0∗
- – African trypanosomiasis B56.-†
   G02.8∗
- – anthrax A22.8† G01∗
- – Chagas' disease (chronic) B57.4†
   G02.8∗
- – chickenpox B01.0† G02.0∗
- – coccidioidomycosis B38.4† G02.1∗
- – enterovirus A87.0† G02.0∗
- – herpes (simplex) virus B00.3† G02.0∗
- – – zoster B02.1† G02.0∗
- – infectious mononucleosis B27.-†
   G02.0∗
- – leptospirosis A27.-† G01∗
- – Listeria monocytogenes A32.1† G01∗
- – Lyme disease A69.2† G01∗
- – measles B05.1† G02.0∗
- – mumps (virus) B26.1† G02.0∗
- – neurosyphilis (late) A52.1† G01∗
- – parasitic disease NEC B89† G02.8∗
- – poliovirus A80.9† G02.0∗

Meningitis—*continued*
- in—*continued*
- – preventive immunization, inoculation or
   vaccination G03.8
- – rubella B06.0† G02.0∗
- – salmonella infection A02.2† G01∗
- – specified cause NEC G03.8
- – typhoid fever A01.0† G01∗
- – varicella B01.0† G02.0∗
- – viral disease NEC A87.8
- – zoster B02.1† G02.0∗
- influenzal (Haemophilus influenzae)
   G00.0
- Klebsiella G00.8
- leptospiral (aseptic) A27.-† G01∗
- lymphocytic (acute) (benign) (serous)
   A87.2† G02.0∗
- meningococcal A39.0† G01∗
- Mollaret (benign recurrent) G03.2
- monilial B37.5† G02.1∗
- mycotic NEC B49† G02.1∗
- Neisseria meningitidis A39.0† G01∗
- nonbacterial G03.0
- nonpyogenic NEC G03.0
- nonspecific G03.9
- ossificans G96.1
- pneumococcal G00.1
- poliovirus A80.9† G01∗
- postmeasles B05.1† G02.0∗
- purulent G00.9
- – specified organism NEC G00.8
- pyogenic G00.9
- – specified organism NEC G00.8
- Salmonella (arizonae) (cholerae-suis)
   (enteritidis) (typhimurium) A02.2† G01∗
- septic G00.9
- – specified organism NEC G00.8
- serosa circumscripta NEC G03.0
- specified organism NEC G00.8
- sporotrichosis B42.8† G02.1∗
- staphylococcal G00.3
- sterile G03.0
- streptococcal (acute) G00.2
- suppurative G00.9
- – specified organism NEC G00.8
- syphilitic (late) (tertiary) A52.1† G01∗
- – acute A51.4† G01∗
- – congenital A50.4† G01∗
- – secondary A51.4† G01∗
- Torula histolytica (cryptococcal) B45.1†
   G02.1∗
- traumatic (complication of injury) T79.8
- tuberculous A17.0† G01∗
- viral NEC A87.9

Meningitis—*continued*
- Yersinia pestis A20.3† G01*
Meningocele (spinal) (*see also* Spina bifida)
  Q05.9
- with hydrocephalus (*see also* Spina bifida,
  with hydrocephalus) Q05.4
- cerebral (*see also* Encephalocele) Q01.9
Meningocerebritis – *see*
  Meningoencephalitis
Meningococcemia A39.4
- acute A39.2
- chronic A39.3
Meningococcus, meningococcal (*see also*
  condition) A39.9
Meningoencephalitis (*see also*
  Encephalitis) G04.9
- acute NEC (*see also* Encephalitis, viral)
  A86
- bacterial NEC G04.2
- California A83.5
- diphasic A84.1
- eosinophilic B83.2† G05.2*
- epidemic A39.8† G05.0*
- herpesviral B00.4† G05.1*
- in (due to)
- – Angiostrongylus cantonensis B83.2†
  G05.2*
- – blastomycosis NEC B40.8† G05.2*
- – free-living amebae B60.2† G05.2*
- – Haemophilus influenzae (H. influenzae)
  G04.2
- – mumps B26.2† G05.1*
- – Naegleria (amebae) (organisms)
  (fowleri) B60.2† G05.2*
- – Parastrongylus cantonensis B83.2†
  G05.2*
- – toxoplasmosis (acquired) B58.2†
  G05.2*
- – – congenital P37.1† G05.2*
- infectious (acute) (viral) A86
- influenzal (Haemophilus influenzae)
  G04.2
- Listeria monocytogenes A32.1† G05.0*
- lymphocytic (serous) A87.2† G05.1*
- mumps B26.2† G05.1*
- parasitic NEC B89† G05.2*
- pneumococcal G04.2
- primary amebic B60.2† G05.2*
- specific (syphilitic) A52.1† G05.0*
- specified organism NEC G04.8
- staphylococcal G04.2
- streptococcal G04.2
- syphilitic A52.1† G05.0*
- toxic NEC G92

Meningoencephalitis—*continued*
- tuberculous A17.8† G05.0*
- virus NEC A86
Meningoencephalocele (*see also*
  Encephalocele) Q01.9
- syphilitic A52.1† G94.8*
- – congenital A50.4† G94.8*
Meningoencephalomyelitis (*see also*
  Meningoencephalitis) G04.9
- acute NEC (viral) A86
- – disseminated (postimmunization or
  postvaccination) (postinfectious) G04.0
- due to
- – actinomycosis A42.8† G05.0*
- – Torula (histolytica) B45.1† G05.2*
- – toxoplasma or toxoplasmosis (acquired)
  B58.2† G05.2*
- – – congenital P37.1† G05.2*
Meningoencephalomyelopathy G96.9
Meningoencephalopathy G96.9
Meningomyelitis (*see also*
  Meningoencephalitis) G04.9
- bacterial NEC G04.2
- blastomycotic NEC B40.8† G05.2*
- cryptococcal B45.1† G05.2*
- meningococcal A39.8† G05.0*
- syphilitic A52.1† G05.0*
- tuberculous A17.8† G05.0*
Meningomyelocele (*see also* Spina bifida)
  Q05.9
- with hydrocephalus (*see also* Spina bifida,
  with hydrocephalus) Q05.4
- fetal, causing obstructed labor (mother)
  O66.3
- syphilitic A52.1† G94.8*
Meningomyeloneuritis (*see also*
  Meningoencephalitis) G04.9
Meningoradiculitis – *see* Meningitis
Meningovascular – *see condition*
Menkes' disease or syndrome E83.0
- meaning maple-syrup-urine disease E71.0
Menometrorrhagia N92.1
**Menopause, menopausal (symptoms)
  (syndrome)** N95.1
- arthritis (any site) NEC M13.8
- artificial N95.3
- crisis N95.1
- paranoid state F22.8
- premature E28.3
- psychosis NEC F28
- surgical N95.3
- toxic polyarthritis NEC M13.8
Menorrhagia (primary) N92.0
- climacteric N92.4

Menorrhagia—*continued*
– climacteric—*continued*
– – menopausal N92.4
– menopausal N92.4
– postclimacteric N95.0
– postmenopausal N95.0
– preclimacteric or premenopausal N92.4
– puberal (menses retained) N92.2
Menses, retention N94.8
Menstrual – *see also* Menstruation
– cycle, irregular N92.6
– disorder N92.6
– extraction Z30.3
– period, normal Z71.1
– regulation Z30.3
Menstruation
– absent – *see* Amenorrhea
– disorder N92.6
– – psychogenic F45.8
– during pregnancy O20.8
– excessive (with regular cycle) N92.0
– – with irregular cycle N92.1
– – at puberty N92.2
– frequent N92.0
– infrequent (*see also* Oligomenorrhea)
  N91.5
– irregular N92.6
– – specified NEC N92.5
– latent N92.5
– membranous N92.5
– painful (*see also* Dysmenorrhea) N94.6
– – primary N94.4
– – psychogenic F45.8
– – secondary N94.5
– precocious E30.1
– protracted N92.5
– rare (*see also* Oligomenorrhea) N91.5
– retained N94.8
– retrograde N92.5
– scanty (*see also* Oligomenorrhea) N91.5
– suppression N94.8
– vicarious (nasal) N94.8
Mental – *see also* condition
– deficiency – *see* Retardation, mental
– deterioration (*see also* Psychosis) F29
– disorder (*see also* Disorder, mental) F99
– – suspected, observation for, without
    need for further medical care Z03.2
– exhaustion F48.0
– insufficiency (congenital) (*see also*
    Retardation, mental) F79.-
– retardation – *see* Retardation, mental
– subnormality – *see* Retardation, mental
– upset (*see also* Disorder, mental) F99

Meralgia paraesthetica G57.1
Mercurial – *see* condition
Mercurialism NEC T56.1
Merkel cell tumor (M8247/3) – *see*
  Neoplasm, skin, malignant
Merocele – *see* Hernia, femoral
Merzbacher-Pelizaeus disease E75.2
Mesaortitis – *see* Aortitis
Mesarteritis – *see* Arteritis
Mesencephalitis (*see also* Encephalitis)
  G04.9
Mesenchymoma (M8990/1) – *see also*
  Neoplasm, connective tissue, uncertain
  behavior
– benign (M8990/0) – *see* Neoplasm,
  connective tissue, benign
– malignant (M8990/3) – *see* Neoplasm,
  connective tissue, malignant
Mesenteritis K65.9
– sclerosing K65.8
Mesentery, mesenteric – *see* condition
Mesiodens, mesiodentes K00.1
– causing crowding K07.3
Mesio-occlusion K07.2
Mesocolon – *see* condition
Mesonephroma (malignant) (M9110/3) –
  see also Neoplasm, malignant
– benign (M9110/0) – *see* Neoplasm, benign
Mesophlebitis – *see* Phlebitis
Mesostromal dysgenesia Q13.8
Mesothelioma (malignant) (M9050/3)
  C45.9
– benign (M9050/0)
– – mesentery D19.1
– – mesocolon D19.1
– – omentum D19.1
– – peritoneum D19.1
– – pleura D19.0
– – specified site NEC D19.7
– – unspecified site D19.9
– biphasic (M9053/3) C45.9
– – benign (M9053/0)
– – – mesentery D19.1
– – – mesocolon D19.1
– – – omentum D19.1
– – – peritoneum D19.1
– – – pleura D19.0
– – – specified site NEC D19.7
– – – unspecified site D19.9
– cystic (M9055/1) D48.4
– epithelioid (M9052/3) C45.9
– – benign (M9052/0)
– – – mesentery D19.1
– – – mesocolon D19.1

Mesothelioma—*continued*
– epithelioid—*continued*
– – benign—*continued*
– – – omentum D19.1
– – – peritoneum D19.1
– – – pleura D19.0
– – – specified site NEC D19.7
– – – unspecified site D19.9
– fibrous (M9051/3) C45.9
– – benign (M9051/0)
– – – mesentery D19.1
– – – mesocolon D19.1
– – – omentum D19.1
– – – peritoneum D19.1
– – – pleura D19.0
– – – specified site NEC D19.7
– – – unspecified site D19.9
– site classification
– – liver C45.7
– – lung C45.7
– – mediastinum C45.7
– – mesentery C45.1
– – mesocolon C45.1
– – omentum C45.1
– – pericardium C45.2
– – peritoneum C45.1
– – pleura C45.0
– – – parietal C45.0
– – retroperitoneum C45.7
– – specified site NEC C45.7
– – unspecified C45.9
Metagonimiasis B66.8
Metagonimus infestation (intestine) B66.8
Metal
– pigmentation L81.8
– polisher's disease J62.8
Metamorphopsia H53.1
Metaplasia
– apocrine (breast) ~~R87.7~~ N60.8
– cervix (squamous) R87.~~7~~
– endometrium (squamous) (uterus) N85.8
– kidney (pelvis) (squamous) N28.8
– myelogenous D73.1
– myeloid (agnogenic) (megakaryocytic) D73.1
– spleen D73.1
– squamous cell, bladder N32.8
Metastasis, metastatic
– abscess – *see* Abscess
– calcification E83.5
– cancer or neoplasm (M8000/6) C79.9
– – from specified site (M8000/3) – *see* Neoplasm, malignant, by site

Metastasis, metastatic—*continued*
– cancer or neoplasm—*continued*
– – to specified site (M8000/6) – *see* Neoplasm, secondary, by site
– deposits (in) (M8000/6) – *see* Neoplasm, secondary, by site
– spread (to) (M8000/6) – *see* Neoplasm, secondary, by site
Metastrongyliasis B83.8
Metatarsalgia M77.4
– Morton's G57.6
Metatarsus, metatarsal – *see also* condition
– valgus (abductus), congenital Q66.6
– varus (adductus) (congenital) Q66.2
Methemoglobinemia D74.9
– acquired (with sulfhemoglobinemia) D74.8
– congenital D74.0
– enzymatic (congenital) D74.0
– Hb-M disease D74.0
– hereditary D74.0
– toxic D74.8
Methemoglobinuria (*see also* Hemoglobinuria) R82.3
Methioninemia E72.1
Methylmalonic acidemia E71.1
Metritis (catarrhal) (hemorrhagic) (septic) (suppurative) (*see also* Endometritis) N71.9
– cervical (*see also* Cervicitis) N72
Metropathia hemorrhagica N93.8
Metroperitonitis (*see also* Peritonitis, pelvic, female) N73.5
Metrorrhagia N92.1
– climacteric N92.4
– menopausal N92.4
– postpartum NEC (atonic) (following delivery of placenta) O72.1
– – delayed or secondary O72.2
– preclimacteric or premenopausal N92.4
– psychogenic F45.8
Metrorrhexis – *see* Rupture, uterus
Metrosalpingitis (*see also* Salpingo-oophoritis) N70.9
Metrostaxis N93.8
Metrovaginitis (*see also* Endometritis) N71.9
Meyer-Schwickerath and Weyer's syndrome Q87.0
Mibelli's disease (porokeratosis) Q82.8
Mice, joint M24.0
– knee M23.4
Micrencephalon Q02

Microaneurysm, retinal H35.0
– diabetic (*see also* E10-E14 with fourth
   character .3) E14.3† H36.0*
Microangiopathy, thrombotic M31.1
**Microcephalus, microcephalic,
   microcephaly** Q02
– due to toxoplasmosis (congenital) P37.1
Microcheilia Q18.7
Microcolon (congenital) Q43.8
Microcornea (congenital) Q13.4
Microcytic – *see condition*
Microdontia K00.2
Microdrepanocytosis D56.8
Microembolism, retinal H34.2
Microgastria (congenital) Q40.2
Microgenia K07.0
Microgenitalia, congenital
– female Q52.8
– male Q55.8
Microglioma C85.7
Microglossia (congenital) Q38.3
**Micrognathia, micrognathism (congenital)
   (mandibular) (maxillary)** K07.0
Microgyria (congenital) Q04.3
Microinfarct of heart (*see also*
   Insufficiency, coronary) I24.8
Microlentia (congenital) Q12.8
Microlithiasis, alveolar, pulmonary J84.0
Micromyelia (congenital) Q06.8
Microphakia (congenital) Q12.8
**Microphthalmos, microphthalmia
   (congenital)** Q11.2
– due to toxoplasmosis P37.1
Micropsia H53.1
Microscopic polyangiitis M31.7
Microsporidiosis B60.8
– intestinal A07.8
Microsporosis (*see also* Dermatophytosis)
   B35.9
– nigra B36.1
Microstomia (congenital) Q18.5
Microtia (congenital) (external ear) Q17.2
Microtropia H50.4
Micturition
– disorder NEC R39.1
– – psychogenic F45.3
– frequency (nocturnal) R35
– – psychogenic F45.3
– hesitancy R39.1
– painful R30.9
– – psychogenic F45.3
Middle
– ear – *see condition*
– lobe syndrome J98.1

Miescher's elastoma L87.2
Mietens' syndrome Q87.2
Migraine (idiopathic) G43.9
– with aura (acute-onset) (prolonged)
   (typical) G43.1
– abdominal G43.8
– basilar G43.1
– classical G43.1
– common G43.0
– complicated G43.3
– equivalent(s) G43.1
– hemiplegic (familial) G43.1
– menstrual N94.3
– ophthalmoplegic G43.8
– retinal G43.8
– specified NEC G43.8
– status G43.2
– without aura G43.0
Migration, anxiety concerning Z60.3
Migratory, migrating – *see also condition*
– testis Q55.2
Mikity-Wilson disease or syndrome P27.0
Mikulicz' disease or syndrome K11.8
Miliaria L74.3
– alba L74.1
– apocrine L75.2
– crystallina L74.1
– profunda L74.2
– rubra L74.0
– tropicalis L74.2
Miliary – *see condition*
Milium L72.0
– colloid L57.8
Milk
– crust L21.0
– excessive secretion O92.6
– poisoning T62.8
– retention O92.7
– sickness T62.8
Milk-alkali disease or syndrome E83.5
**Milk leg (puerperal, postpartum,
   childbirth)** O87.1
– complicating pregnancy O22.3
– nonpuerperal I80.1
Milkman's disease or syndrome M83.8
Milky urine – *see* Chyluria
**Millard-Gubler(-Foville) paralysis or
   syndrome** I67.9† G46.3*
Millar's asthma J38.5
Miller Fisher syndrome G61.0
Mills' disease G81.9
Millstone maker's pneumoconiosis J62.8
Milroy's disease Q82.0
Minamata disease T56.1

Minkowski-Chauffard syndrome (*see also*
Spherocytosis) D58.0
Minor – *see condition*
Minor's disease (hematomyelia) G95.1
Minot-von Willebrand-Jurgens disease
D68.0
Miosis (pupil) H57.0
Mirror writing F81.0
Misadventure (prophylactic)
(therapeutic) (*see also* Complications)
T88.9
– administration of insulin T38.3
– infusion – *see* Complications, infusion
– local applications (of fomentations,
plasters, etc.) T88.9
– – burn or scald – *see* Burn
– – specified NEC T88.8
– medical care (early) (late) T88.9
– – adverse effect of drugs or chemicals –
see Table of drugs and chemicals
– – burn or scald – *see* Burn
– – specified NEC T88.8
– radiation NEC T66
– radiotherapy NEC T66
– specified NEC T88.8
– surgical procedure (early) (late) – *see*
Complications, surgical procedure
– transfusion – *see* Complications,
transfusion
– vaccination or other immunological
procedure – *see* Complications,
vaccination
Miscarriage O03.-
Mismanagement of feeding R63.3
Misplaced, misplacement
– ear Q17.4
– kidney (acquired) N28.8
– – congenital Q63.2
– organ or site, congenital NEC – *see*
Malposition, congenital
Missed
– abortion O02.1
– delivery O36.4
Missing – *see* Absence
Misuse of drugs NEC F19.1
Mitchell's disease I73.8
Mite(s) (infestation) B88.9
Mitral – *see condition*
Mittelschmerz N94.0
Mixed – *see condition*
Mobile, mobility
– excessive – *see* Hypermobility
– gallbladder, congenital Q44.1
– kidney N28.8

Mobile, mobility—*continued*
– organ or site, congenital NEC – *see*
Malposition, congenital
Moebius
– disease (ophthalmoplegic migraine)
G43.8
– syndrome Q87.0
– – congenital oculofacial paralysis (with
other anomalies) Q87.0
– – ophthalmoplegic migraine G43.8
Moeller's glossitis K14.0
Mohr's syndrome (types I and II) Q87.0
Mola destruens (M9100/1) D39.2
Molar pregnancy NEC (M9100/0) O02.0
Molarization of premolars K00.2
Molding, head (during birth) P13.1
Mole (pigmented) (M8720/0) – *see also*
Nevus
– blood O02.0
– Breus' O02.0
– cancerous (M8720/3) – *see* Melanoma
– carneous O02.0
– destructive (M9100/1) D39.2
– fleshy O02.0
– hydatid, hydatidiform (benign)
(complicating pregnancy) (delivered)
(undelivered) (M9100/0) O01.9
– – classical (M9100/0) O01.0
– – complete (M9100/0) O01.0
– – incomplete (M9103/0) O01.1
– – invasive (M9100/1) D39.2
– – malignant (M9100/1) D39.2
– – partial (M9103/0) O01.1
– – previous, affecting management of
pregnancy Z35.1
– invasive (hydatidiform) (M9100/1) D39.2
– malignant, meaning
– – malignant hydatidiform mole
(M9100/1) D39.2
– – melanoma (M8720/3) – *see* Melanoma
– nonhydatidiform O02.0
– nonpigmented (M8730/0) – *see* Nevus
– pregnancy NEC O02.0
– skin (M8720/0) – *see* Nevus
– tubal O00.1
– vesicular (M9100/0) (*see also* Mole,
hydatidiform) O01.9
– – previous, affecting management of
pregnancy Z35.1
Molluscum contagiosum (epitheliale)
B08.1
– eyelid B08.1† H03.1*
Mönckeberg's arteriosclerosis,
degeneration, disease or sclerosis I70.2

Mongolia Blue Spot D22

Mondor's disease I80.8
Monge's disease T70.2
Monilethrix (congenital) Q84.1
Moniliasis *(see also* Candidiasis) B37.9
– neonatal P37.5
Monkey malaria B53.1
Monkeypox B04
Monoarthritis NEC M13.1
Monoblastic – *see condition*
Monochromat(ism), monochromatopsia
  (acquired) (congenital) H53.5
Monocytic – *see condition*
Monocytosis (symptomatic) D72.8
Monomania *(see also* Psychosis) F28
Mononeuritis G58.9
– cranial nerve – *see* Disorder, nerve,
  cranial
– femoral nerve G57.2
– lateral
– – cutaneous nerve of thigh G57.1
– – popliteal nerve G57.3
– lower limb G57.9
– – specified nerve NEC G57.8
– medial popliteal nerve G57.4
– median nerve G56.1
– multiplex G58.7
– plantar nerve G57.6
– radial nerve G56.3
– sciatic nerve G57.0
– specified NEC G58.8
– tibial nerve G57.4
– ulnar nerve G56.2
– upper limb G56.9
– – specified nerve NEC G56.8
Mononeuropathy *(see also* Mononeuritis)
  G58.9
– diabetic NEC *(see also* E10-E14 with
  fourth character .4) E14.4† G59.0*
Mononucleosis, infectious NEC B27.9
– cytomegaloviral B27.1
– Epstein-Barr (virus) B27.0
– gammaherpesviral B27.0
– specified NEC B27.8
Monoplegia G83.3
– congenital (cerebral) G80.8
– – spastic G80.1
– embolic (current episode) I63.4
– hysterical (transient) F44.4
– infantile (cerebral) (spinal) G80.8
– lower limb G83.1
– psychogenic (conversion reaction) F44.4
– thrombotic (current episode) I63.3
– transient R29.8
– upper limb G83.2

Monorchism, monorchidism Q55.0
Monosomy *(see also* Deletion,
  chromosome) Q93.9
– specified NEC Q93.8
– whole chromosome
– – meiotic nondisjunction Q93.0
– – mitotic nondisjunction Q93.1
– – mosaicism Q93.1
– X Q96.9
Monster, monstrosity (single) Q89.7
– acephalic Q00.0
– twin Q89.4
Monteggia's fracture(-dislocation) S52.0
Mooren's ulcer (cornea) H16.0
Moore's syndrome G40.8
Mooser's bodies A75.2
Morax-Axenfeld conjunctivitis H10.2
Morbidity, unknown cause R69
Morbilli – *see* Measles
Morbus *(see also* Disease)
– caducus *(see also* Epilepsy) G40.9
– comitialis *(see also* Epilepsy) G40.9
– cordis *(see also* Disease, heart) I51.9
– – valvulorum – *see* Endocarditis
– coxae senilis M16.9
– – tuberculous A18.0† M01.1*
Morel (-Stewart) (-Morgagni) syndrome
  M85.2
Morel-Kraepelin disease *(see also*
  Schizophrenia) F20.9
Morgagni's
– cyst, organ, hydatid or appendage
– – female Q50.5
– – male (epididymal) Q55.4
– – – testicular Q55.2
– syndrome M85.2
Morgagni-Stokes-Adams syndrome I45.9
Morgagni-Turner(-Albright) syndrome
  Q96.9
Moria F07.0
Moron (I.Q. 50-69) F70.-
Morphea L94.0
Morphinism F11.2
Morphinomania F11.2
Morquio (-Ullrich) (-Brailsford) disease or
  syndrome E76.2
Mortality, unknown cause R99
Mortification (dry) (moist) *(see also*
  Gangrene) R02
Morton's metatarsalgia (neuralgia)
  (neuroma) G57.6
Morvan's disease or syndrome G60.8

Mosaicism, mosaic (autosomal)
(chromosomal)
– sex chromosome
– – female NEC Q97.8
– – – lines with various numbers of X
   chromosomes Q97.2
– – male NEC Q98.7
– 45,X/
– – cell lines NEC with abnormal sex
   chromosome Q96.4
– – 46,XX Q96.3
– – 46,XY Q96.3
Moschowitz' disease M31.1
Motion sickness (from any vehicle) T75.3
Mottled, mottling, teeth (enamel) K00.3
Mountain sickness T70.2
Mouse, joint M24.0
– knee M23.4
Mouth – *see condition*
Movable
– coccyx M53.2
– kidney N28.8
– – congenital Q63.8
– spleen D73.8
Movements, dystonic R25.8
Moyamoya disease I67.5
Mucha-Habermann disease L41.0
Mucinosis (cutaneous) (focal) (papular)
(skin) L98.5
– oral K13.7
Mucocele
– appendix K38.8
– buccal cavity K13.7
– gallbladder K82.1
– lacrimal sac H04.4
– nasal sinus J34.1
– salivary gland (any) K11.6
– sinus (accessory) (nasal) J34.1
– turbinate (bone) (middle) (nasal) J34.1
Mucolipidosis
– I E77.1
– II, III E77.0
– IV E75.1
Mucopolysaccharidosis E76.3
– cardiopathy E76.3† I52.8*
– specified NEC E76.2
– type
– – I E76.0
– – II E76.1
– – III, IV, VI, VII E76.2
Mucormycosis B46.5
– cutaneous B46.3† L99.8*
– disseminated B46.4
– gastrointestinal B46.2† K93.8*

Mucormycosis—*continued*
– generalized B46.4
– pulmonary B46.0† J99.8*
– rhinocerebral B46.1† G99.8*
– skin B46.3† L99.8*
– subcutaneous B46.3† L99.8*
Mucositis (drug induced) (radiation
induced) (ulcerative) (*see also*
Inflammation, by site) K12.3
– anus, anal canal K92.8
– colon K92.8
– duodenum K92.8
– esophagus K92.8
– gastric K92.8
– gastrointestinal (ulcerative) K92.8
– ileum K92.8
– intestine (any part) K92.8
– mouth K12.3
– nasal (ulcerative) J34.8
– necroticans agranulocytica D70
– oral K12.3
– oropharyngeal K12.3
– perianal K92.8
– perirectal K92.8
– rectum K92.8
– sigmoid K92.8
– stomach K92.8
– vagina N76.8
– vulva N76.8
Mucous – *see also condition*
– patches (syphilitic) A51.3
– – congenital A50.0
Mucoviscidosis E84.9
– with meconium obstruction E84.1† P75*
Mucus
– asphyxia or suffocation (*see also*
Asphyxia, mucus) T17.9
– – newborn P24.1
– in stool R19.5
– plug (*see also* Asphyxia, mucus) T17.9
– – aspiration, newborn P24.1
– – tracheobronchial T17.8
– – – newborn P24.1
Muguet B37.0
Mulberry molars (congenital syphilis)
A50.5
Mullerian mixed tumor (M8950/3)
– specified site – *see* Neoplasm, malignant
– unspecified site C54.9
Multiparity (grand) Z64.1
– affecting management of pregnancy, labor
and delivery (supervision only) Z35.4
– requiring contraceptive management – *see*
Contraception

Multipartita placenta O43.1
Multiple, multiplex – *see also condition*
– birth, affecting fetus or newborn P01.5
– delivery – *see* Delivery, multiple
– digits (congenital) Q69.9
– diseases NEC, resulting from HIV disease
  B22.7
– infections, resulting from HIV disease
  B20.7
– malignant neoplasms, resulting from HIV
  disease B21.7
– personality F44.8
Mumps (parotitis) B26.9
– arthritis B26.8† M01.5*
– complication NEC B26.8
– encephalitis B26.2† G05.1*
– hepatitis B26.8† K77.0*
– meningitis (aseptic) B26.1† G02.0*
– meningoencephalitis B26.2† G05.1*
– myocarditis B26.8† I41.1*
– oophoritis B26.8† N74.8*
– orchitis B26.0† N51.1*
– pancreatitis B26.3† K87.1*
– polyneuropathy B26.8† G63.0*
Mumu (*see also* Infestation, filarial) B74.-†
  N51.8*
Münchhausen's syndrome F68.1
Münchmeyer's syndrome M61.1
Mural – *see condition*
Murmur (cardiac) (heart) (organic) R01.1
– aortic (valve) (*see also* Endocarditis,
  aortic) I35.8
– benign R01.0
– diastolic – *see* Endocarditis
– Flint I35.1
– functional R01.0
– Graham Steell I37.1
– innocent R01.0
– mitral (valve) – *see* Insufficiency, mitral
– nonorganic R01.0
– presystolic, mitral – *see* Insufficiency,
  mitral
– pulmonic (valve) I37.8
– systolic (valvular) – *see* Endocarditis
– tricuspid (valve) I07.9
– valvular – *see* Endocarditis
**Murri's disease (intermittent
  hemoglobinuria)** D59.6
Muscle, muscular – *see also condition*
– carnitine (palmityltransferase) deficiency
  E71.3
Musculoneuralgia M79.2
Mushroom-worker's disease or lung J67.5

Mutation
– prothrombin gene (factor V Leiden
  mutation) D68.5
Mutism (*see also* Aphasia) R47.0
– deaf (acquired) (congenital) NEC H91.3
– elective (adjustment reaction) (childhood)
  F94.0
– hysterical F44.4
– selective (childhood) F94.0
Myalgia (intercostal) M79.1
– epidemic (cervical) B33.0
– psychogenic F45.4
– traumatic NEC T14.9
Myasthenia, myasthenic G70.9
– congenital G70.2
– cordis – *see* Failure, heart
– developmental G70.2
– gravis G70.0
– – neonatal, transient P94.0
– stomach, psychogenic F45.3
– syndrome in
– – diabetes mellitus (*see also* E10-E14
  with fourth character .4) E14.4†
  G73.0*
– – malignant neoplasm NEC
  (M8000/3) (*see also* Neoplasm,
  malignant) C80.-† G73.2*
– – thyrotoxicosis E05.9† G73.0*
Mycelium infection NEC B49
Mycetismus T62.0
Mycetoma B47.9
– actinomycotic B47.1
– bone (mycotic) B47.9† M90.2*
– eumycotic B47.0
– foot B47.9
– – actinomycotic B47.1
– – mycotic B47.0
– madurae NEC B47.9
– – mycotic B47.0
– maduromycotic B47.0
– mycotic B47.0
– nocardial B47.1
Mycobacteriosis – *see* Mycobacterium
Mycobacterium, mycobacterial (infection)
  A31.9
– africanum – *see* Tuberculosis
– atypical A31.9
– – cutaneous A31.1
– – pulmonary A31.0
– – – tuberculous (*see also* Tuberculosis,
  pulmonary) A16.2
– – specified site NEC A31.8
– avium (intracellulare complex) A31.0
– Battey A31.0

Mycobacterium, mycobacterial—
continued
– bovis – *see* Tuberculosis
– chelonei A31.8
– cutaneous A31.1
– extrapulmonary systemic A31.8
– fortuitum A31.8
– intracellulare (Battey bacillus) A31.0
– kansasii (yellow bacillus) A31.0
– leprae (*see also* Leprosy) A30.9
– marinum (M. balnei) A31.1
– nonspecific (*see also* Mycobacterium, atypical) A31.9
– pulmonary (atypical) A31.0
– – tuberculous (*see also* Tuberculosis, pulmonary) A16.2
– resulting from HIV disease B20.0
– scrofulaceum A31.8
– simiae A31.8
– systemic, extrapulmonary A31.8
– szulgai A31.8
– terrae A31.8
– triviale A31.8
– tuberculosis – *see* Tuberculosis
– ulcerans A31.1
– xenopi A31.8
Mycoplasma (M.) pneumoniae, as cause of disease classified elsewhere B96.0
Mycosis, mycotic NEC B49
– cutaneous NEC B36.9
– fungoides C84.0
– mouth B37.0
– opportunistic B48.7
– resulting from HIV disease B20.5
– skin NEC B36.9
– specified NEC B48.8
– stomatitis B37.0
– vagina, vaginitis (candidal) B37.3†
  N77.1*
Mydriasis (pupil) H57.0
Myelatelia Q06.1
Myelinolysis, pontine, central G37.2
Myelitis (acute) (ascending) (*see also* Encephalitis) G04.9
– necrotizing, subacute G37.4
– postimmunization G04.0
– postinfectious NEC G04.8
– specified NEC G04.8
– syphilitic (transverse) A52.1† G05.0*
– transverse, acute (in demyelinating diseases of central nervous system) G37.3
– tuberculous A17.8† G05.0*
Myeloblastic – *see condition*

Myelocele (*see also* Spina bifida) Q05.9
– with hydrocephalus (*see also* Spina bifida, with hydrocephalus) Q05.4
Myelocystocele (*see also* Spina bifida) Q05.9
– with hydrocephalus (*see also* Spina bifida, with hydrocephalus) Q05.4
Myelocytic – *see condition*
Myelodysplasia (related to alkylating agent) (related to Epipodophyllotoxin) (related to therapy) D46.9
– specified NEC D46.7
– spinal cord (congenital) Q06.1
Myeloencephalitis – *see* Encephalitis
Myelofibrosis (chronic)(idiopathic) (with myeloid metaplasia) D47.4
– acute C94.4
– secondary, in myeloproliferative disease D47.4
Myelogenous – *see condition*
Myeloid – *see condition*
Myeloleukodystrophy E75.2
Myelolipoma (M8870/0) – *see* Lipoma
Myeloma (multiple) C90.0
– monostotic C90.3
– – plasma cell C90.3 -0
– plasma cell C90.3 -0
– solitary C90.3
Myelomalacia G95.8
Myelomata, multiple C90.0
Myelomatosis C90.0
Myelomeningitis – *see* Meningoencephalitis
Myelomeningocele (spinal cord) (*see also* Spina bifida) Q05.9
– with hydrocephalus (*see also* Spina bifida, with hydrocephalus) Q05.4
Myelopathic – *see condition*
Myelopathy (spinal cord) G95.9
– drug-induced G95.8
– in (due to)
– – degeneration or displacement, intervertebral disk NEC M51.0†
  G99.2*
– – infection – *see* Encephalitis
– – intervertebral disk disorder M51.0†
  G99.2*
– – – cervical, cervicothoracic M50.0†
    G99.2*
– – neoplastic disease NEC (M8000/1) (*see also* Neoplasm) D48.9† G99.2*
– – spondylosis M47.1† G99.2*
– necrotic (subacute) (vascular) G95.1
– radiation-induced G95.8

Myelopathy—*continued*
- spondylogenic NEC M47.1† G99.2∗
- toxic G95.8
- transverse, acute G37.3
- traumatic – *see* Injury, spinal cord, by site and type
- vascular G95.1
- vitamin B₁₂ E53.8† G32.0∗

Myeloradiculitis G04.9
Myeloradiculodysplasia (spinal) Q06.1
Myelosarcoma C92.3
Myelosclerosis D47.4
- with myeloid metaplasia D47.4
- disseminated, of nervous system G35
- megakaryocytic (with myeloid metaplasia) D47.4

Myelosis
- acute C92.0
- aleukemic C92.9
- chronic D47.1
- erythremic C94.0
- – acute C94.0
- megakaryocytic C94.2
- nonleukemic D72.8
- subacute C92.9

Myiasis (cavernous) B87.9
- aural B87.4† H94.8∗
- creeping B87.0† L99.8∗
- cutaneous B87.0† L99.8∗
- dermal B87.0† L99.8∗
- ear (external) (middle) B87.4† H94.8∗
- eye B87.2† H58.8∗
- genitourinary B87.8
- intestinal B87.8† K93.8∗
- laryngeal B87.3† J99.8∗
- nasopharyngeal B87.3† J99.8∗
- ocular B87.2† H58.8∗
- orbit B87.2† H06.1∗
- skin B87.0† L99.8∗
- specified site NEC B87.8
- traumatic B87.1
- wound B87.1

Myoadenoma, prostate N40
Myoblastoma, granular cell (M9580/0) – *see also* Neoplasm, connective tissue, benign
- malignant (M9580/3) – *see* Neoplasm, connective tissue, malignant
- tongue (M9580/0) D10.1

Myocardial – *see condition*
Myocardiopathy (*see also* Cardiomyopathy) I42.9

Myocarditis (chronic) (fibroid) (interstitial) (old) (progressive) (senile) (with arteriosclerosis) I51.4
- active I40.9
- – rheumatic (fever) I01.2
- – – with chorea (acute) (rheumatic) (Sydenham's) I02.0
- acute or subacute (interstitial) I40.9
- – rheumatic I01.2
- – – with chorea (acute) (rheumatic) (Sydenham's) I02.0
- – specified NEC I40.8
- aseptic, of newborn B33.2† I41.1∗
- bacterial (acute) I40.0
- coxsackie (virus) B33.2† I41.1∗
- diphtheritic A36.8† I41.0∗
- epidemic of newborn (coxsackie(virus)) B33.2† I41.1∗
- Fiedler's (acute) (isolated) I40.1
- gonococcal A54.8† I41.0∗
- hypertensive (*see also* Hypertension, heart) I11.9
- idiopathic I40.1
- in (due to)
- – diphtheria A36.8† I41.0∗
- – epidemic louse-borne typhus A75.0† I41.0∗
- – sarcoidosis D86.8† I41.8∗
- – scarlet fever A38† I41.0∗
- – toxoplasmosis (acquired) B58.8† I41.2∗
- – typhus NEC A75.9† I41.0∗
- infective I40.0
- influenzal (specific virus not identified) J11.8† I41.1∗
- – avian influenza virus identified J09† I41.1∗
- – other influenza virus identified J10.8† I41.1∗
- isolated (acute) I40.1
- meningococcal A39.5† I41.0∗
- mumps B26.8† I41.1∗
- rheumatic (chronic) (inactive) (with chorea) I09.0
- – active or acute I01.2
- – – with chorea (acute) (rheumatic) (Sydenham's) I02.0
- septic I40.0
- syphilitic (chronic) A52.0† I41.0∗
- toxic I40.8
- – rheumatic (*see also* Myocarditis, acute, rheumatic) I01.2
- tuberculous A18.8† I41.0∗
- typhoid A01.0† I41.0∗

Myocarditis—*continued*
– valvular – *see* Endocarditis
– virus, viral NEC I40.0
– – of newborn (coxsackie(virus)) B33.2†
   I41.1*
Myocardium, myocardial – *see condition*
Myocardosis (*see also* Cardiomyopathy)
   I42.9
**Myoclonus, myoclonic (essential)
   (familial) (multifocal) (simplex)** G25.3
– drug-induced G25.3
– epileptica G40.3
– facial G51.3
– jerks G25.3
– massive G25.3
– pharyngeal J39.2
Myodiastasis M62.0
Myoendocarditis – *see* Endocarditis
Myoepithelioma (M8982/0) – *see*
   Neoplasm, benign
Myofasciitis (acute) M60.9
– low back M54.5
Myofibroma (M8890/0) – *see also*
   Neoplasm, connective tissue, benign
– uterus (cervix) (corpus) – *see* Leiomyoma
Myofibromatosis (M8824/1) D48.1
Myofibrosis M62.8
– heart (*see also* Myocarditis) I51.4
– scapulohumeral M75.8
Myofibrositis M79.7
– scapulohumeral M75.8
**Myoglobinuria, myoglobulinuria
   (primary)** R82.1
Myokymia, facial G51.4
Myolipoma (M8860/0) – *see* Lipoma
Myoma (M8895/0) – *see also* Neoplasm,
   connective tissue, benign
– malignant (M8895/3) – *see* Neoplasm,
   connective tissue, malignant
– prostate D29.1
– uterus (cervix) (corpus) – *see* Leiomyoma
Myomalacia M62.8
Myometritis (*see also* Endometritis) N71.9
Myometrium – *see condition*
Myonecrosis, clostridial A48.0
Myopathy G72.9
– alcoholic G72.1
– centronuclear G71.2
– congenital (benign) G71.2
– distal G71.0
– drug-induced G72.0
– endocrine NEC E34.9† G73.5*
– extraocular muscles H05.8
– facioscapulohumeral G71.0

Myopathy—*continued*
– hereditary G71.9
– – specified NEC G71.8
– in (due to)
– – Addison's disease E27.1† G73.5*
– – alcohol G72.1
– – amyloidosis E85.4† G73.6*
– – cretinism E00.9† G73.5*
– – Cushing's syndrome E24.9† G73.5*
– – drugs G72.0
– – endocrine disease NEC E34.9† G73.5*
– – giant cell arteritis M31.6† G73.7*
– – glycogen storage disease E74.0†
     G73.6*
– – hyperadrenocorticism E24.9† G73.5*
– – hyperparathyroidism NEC E21.3†
     G73.5*
– – hypoparathyroidism E20.-† G73.5*
– – hypopituitarism E23.0† G73.5*
– – hypothyroidism E03.9† G73.5*
– – infectious disease NEC B99† G73.4*
– – lipid storage disease E75.-† G73.6*
– – malignant neoplasm NEC
     (M8000/3) (*see also* Neoplasm,
     malignant) C80.-† M63.8*
– – metabolic disease NEC E88.9† G73.6*
– – myxedema E03.9† G73.5*
– – parasitic disease NEC B89† G73.4*
– – polyarteritis nodosa M30.0† G73.7*
– – rheumatoid arthritis M05.3† G73.7*
– – sarcoidosis D86.8† G73.7*
– – scleroderma M34.8† G73.7*
– – sicca syndrome M35.0† G73.7*
– – Sjögren's syndrome M35.0† G73.7*
– – systemic lupus erythematosus M32.1†
     G73.7*
– – thyrotoxicosis (hyperthyroidism)
     E05.9† G73.5*
– – toxic agent NEC G72.2
– inflammatory NEC G72.4
– limb-girdle G71.0
– mitochondrial NEC G71.3
– myotubular G71.2
– nemaline G71.2
– ocular G71.0
– oculopharyngeal G71.0
– primary G71.9
– – specified NEC G71.8
– progressive NEC G72.8
– rod G71.2
– scapulohumeral G71.0
– specified NEC G72.8
– toxic G72.2

Myopericarditis (*see also* Pericarditis)
I31.9
– chronic rheumatic I09.2
Myopia (axial) (congenital) (progressive)
H52.1
– degenerative H44.2
– malignant H44.2
– pernicious H44.2
Myosarcoma (M8895/3) – *see* Neoplasm,
connective tissue, malignant
Myosis (pupil) H57.0
– stromal (endolymphatic) (M8931/1)
D39.0
Myositis M60.9
– clostridial A48.0
– due to posture M60.8
– epidemic B33.0
– in (due to)
– – bilharziasis B65.-† M63.1*
– – cysticercosis B69.8† M63.1*
– – leprosy A30.-† M63.0*
– – mycosis B49† M63.2*
– – sarcoidosis D86.8† M63.3*
– – schistosomiasis B65.-† M63.1*
– – syphilis
– – – late A52.7† M63.0*
– – – secondary A51.4† M63.0*
– – toxoplasmosis (acquired) B58.8†
M63.1*
– – trichinellosis B75† M63.1*
– inclusion body (IBM) G72.4
– infective M60.0
– interstitial M60.1
– juvenile M33.0
– multiple – *see* Polymyositis
– mycotic B49† M63.2*
– orbital, chronic H05.1
– ossificans or ossifying (circumscripta)
M61.5
– – in (due to)
– – – burns M61.3
– – – quadriplegia or paraplegia M61.2
– – progressiva M61.1
– – traumatica M61.0
– purulent M60.0

Myositis—*continued*
– specified NEC M60.8
– suppurative M60.0
– traumatic (old) M60.8
Myotonia (acquisita) (intermittens)
M62.8
– atrophica G71.1
– chondrodystrophic G71.1
– congenita G71.1
– drug-induced G71.1
– dystrophica G71.1
– symptomatic G71.1
Myotonic pupil H57.0
Myriapodiasis B88.2
Myringitis H73.8
– with otitis media – *see* Otitis, media
– acute H73.0
– bullous H73.0
– chronic H73.1
Mysophobia F40.2
Mytilotoxism T61.2
Myxedema (infantile) (*see also*
Hypothyroidism) E03.9
– coma E03.5
– congenital E00.1
– cutis L98.5
– papular L98.5
Myxochondrosarcoma (M9220/3) – *see*
Neoplasm, cartilage, malignant
Myxofibroma (M8811/0) – *see* Neoplasm,
connective tissue, benign
– odontogenic (M9320/0) D16.5
– – upper jaw (bone) D16.4
Myxofibrosarcoma (M8811/3) – *see*
Neoplasm, connective tissue, malignant
Myxolipoma (M8852/0) D17.9
Myxoliposarcoma (M8852/3) – *see*
Neoplasm, connective tissue, malignant
Myxoma (M8840/0) – *see also* Neoplasm,
connective tissue, benign
– nerve sheath (M9562/0) – *see* Neoplasm,
nerve, benign
– odontogenic (M9320/0) D16.5
– – upper jaw (bone) D16.4
Myxosarcoma (M8840/3) – *see* Neoplasm,
connective tissue, malignant

N

Naegeli's
– disease Q82.8
– leukemia, monocytic C93.1
Naegleriasis (with) B60.2
– meningoencephalitis B60.2† G05.2*
Naffziger's syndrome G54.0
Naga sore (*see also* Ulcer, skin) L98.4
Nägele's pelvis M95.5
– with disproportion (fetopelvic) O33.0
– – causing obstructed labor O65.0
Nail – *see also condition*
– biting F98.8
– patella syndrome Q87.2
Nanism, nanosomia (*see also* Dwarfism) E34.3
– renis, renalis N25.0
Nanophyetiasis B66.8
Nanukayami A27.8
Narcolepsy G47.4
Narcosis
– carbon dioxide (respiratory) R06.8
– due to drug
– – correct substance properly administered R41.8
– – overdose or wrong substance given or taken T40.6
– – – specified drug – *see* Table of drugs and chemicals
Narcotism – *see* Dependence, by drug
– overdose or wrong substance given or taken T40.6
– – specified drug – *see* Table of drugs and chemicals
Narrow
– anterior chamber angle H40.0
– pelvis – *see* Contraction, pelvis
Narrowing
– artery NEC I77.1
– – auditory, internal I65.8
– – basilar (*see also* Occlusion, artery, basilar) I65.1
– – – with other precerebral artery I65.3
– – carotid (*see also* Occlusion, artery, carotid) I65.2
– – – with other precerebral artery I65.3
– – – bilateral I65.3
– – cerebellar I66.3
– – cerebral I66.9
– – choroidal I66.8

Narrowing—*continued*
– artery NEC—*continued*
– – communicating posterior I66.8
– – coronary I25.1
– – – congenital (syphilitic) A50.5† I52.0*
– – – due to syphilis NEC A52.0† I52.0*
– – hypophyseal I66.8
– – pontine I66.8
– – precerebral (*see also* Occlusion, artery, precerebral) I65.9
– – – multiple or bilateral I65.3
– – vertebral (*see also* Occlusion, artery, vertebral) I65.0
– – – with other precerebral artery I65.3
– – – bilateral I65.3
– auditory canal (external) H61.3
– eustachian tube H68.1
– eyelid H02.5
– larynx J38.6
– palate K07.8
– palpebral fissure H02.5
– ureter N13.5
– – with infection N13.6
– urethra (*see also* Stricture, urethra) N35.9
Narrowness, abnormal, eyelid Q10.3
Nasal – *see condition*
Nasolachrymal, nasolacrimal – *see condition*
Nasopharyngeal – *see also condition*
– pituitary gland Q89.2
Nasopharyngitis (acute) (infective) (subacute) J00
– chronic (suppurative) (ulcerative) J31.1
– septic J00
– streptococcal J00
Nasopharynx, nasopharyngeal – *see condition*
Natal tooth, teeth K00.6
Nausea (*see also* Vomiting) R11
– epidemic A08.1
– gravidarum – *see* Hyperemesis, gravidarum
– marina T75.3
Navel – *see condition*
Nearsightedness H52.1
Nebula, cornea H17.8
Necator americanus infection or infestation B76.1
Necatoriasis B76.1

Neck – *see condition*
Necrobiosis R68.8
– lipoidica NEC L92.1
– – with diabetes (*see also* E10-E14 with fourth character .6) E14.6† L99.8*
Necrolysis, toxic epidermal L51.2
– due to drug
– – correct substance properly administered L51.2
– – overdose or wrong substance given or taken T50.9
– – – specified drug – *see* Table of drugs and chemicals
Necrophilia F65.8
Necrosis, necrotic (ischemic) (*see also* Gangrene) R02
– adrenal (capsule) (gland) E27.4
– amputation stump (late) (surgical) T87.5
– antrum J32.0
– aorta (hyaline) (*see also* Aneurysm, aorta) I71.9
– – cystic medial I71.0
– – ruptured I71.8
– artery I77.5
– bladder (aseptic) (sphincter) N32.8
– bone (*see also* Osteonecrosis) M87.9
– – aseptic or avascular M87.9
– – – idiopathic M87.0
– – ethmoid J32.2
– – jaw K10.2
– – specified NEC M87.8
– – tuberculous – *see* Tuberculosis, bone
– brain I67.8
– breast (aseptic) (fat) (segmental) N64.1
– bronchus J98.0
– central nervous system NEC I67.8
– cerebellar I67.8
– cerebral I67.8
– cornea H18.4
– cortical (acute) (renal) N17.1
– cystic medial (aorta) I71.0
– esophagus K22.8
– ethmoid (bone) J32.2
– eyelid H02.7
– fat (generalized) M79.8
– – breast (aseptic) N64.1
– – localized – *see* Degeneration, by site, fatty
– – subcutaneous, due to birth injury P15.6
– gallbladder K81.0
– heart – *see* Infarct, myocardium
– hip, aseptic or avascular (*see also* Osteonecrosis) M87.9

Necrosis, necrotic—*continued*
– intestine (acute) (hemorrhagic) (massive) K55.0
– jaw K10.2
– kidney (bilateral) N28.0
– – acute N17.9
– – cortical (acute) N17.1
– – medullary (papillary) N17.2
– – papillary N17.2
– – tubular N17.0
– – – complicating pregnancy O99.8
– – – – affecting fetus or newborn P00.1
– – – following
– – – – abortion (subsequent episode) O08.4
– – – – – current episode – *see* Abortion
– – – – ectopic or molar pregnancy O08.4
– larynx J38.7
– liver (cell) K72.9
– – with hepatic failure (*see also* Failure, hepatic) K72.9
– – complicating pregnancy, childbirth or puerperium O26.6
– – – affecting fetus or newborn P00.8
– – hemorrhagic, central K76.2
– lung J85.0
– lymphatic gland (*see also* Lymphadenitis, acute) L04.9
– mammary gland (fat) (segmental) N64.1
– mastoid (chronic) H70.1
– medullary (acute) (renal) N17.2
– mesentery K55.0
– – fat K65.8
– mitral valve – *see* Insufficiency, mitral
– myocardium, myocardial – *see* Infarct, myocardium
– nose J34.0
– omentum K55.0
– – fat K65.8
– orbit, orbital H05.1
– ossicles, ear H74.3
– ovary (*see also* Salpingo-oophoritis) N70.9
– pancreas (aseptic) (duct) (fat) K86.8
– – acute (infective) K85.-
– papillary (acute) (renal) N17.2
– peritoneum K55.0
– – fat K65.8
– pharynx J02.9
– – Vincent's A69.1
– phosphorus T54.2
– pituitary (gland) (postpartum) (Sheehan) E23.0
– placenta O43.8

435

Necrosis, necrotic—*continued*
- pressure L89.-
- – stage
- – – III L89.2
- – – IV L89.3
- pulmonary J85.0
- pulp (dental) K04.1
- radiation – *see* Necrosis, by site
- radium – *see* Necrosis, by site
- renal N28.0
- sclera H15.8
- scrotum N50.8
- skin or subcutaneous tissue NEC R02
- spine, spinal (column) M87.9
- – cord G95.1
- spleen D73.5
- stomach K31.8
- stomatitis (ulcerative) A69.0
- subcutaneous fat, fetus or newborn P83.8
- subendocardial (acute) I21.4
- – chronic I25.8
- suprarenal (capsule) (gland) E27.4
- testis N50.8
- thymus (gland) E32.8
- tonsil J35.8
- trachea J39.8
- tuberculous NEC – *see* Tuberculosis
- tubular (acute) (anoxic) (renal) (toxic) N17.0
- – postprocedural N99.0
- umbilical cord, affecting fetus or newborn P02.6
- vagina N89.8
- vertebra M87.9
- – tuberculous A18.0† M49.0∗
- X-ray – *see* Necrosis, by site

Necrospermia N46

Need for
- care provider because (of)
- – assistance with personal care Z74.1
- – continuous supervision required Z74.3
- – impaired mobility Z74.0

Need for—*continued*
- care provider—*continued*
- – no other household member able to render care Z74.2
- – specified reason NEC Z74.8
- immunization – *see* Vaccination
- vaccination – *see* Vaccination

Neglect (newborn) T74.0
- emotional, in childhood Z62.4
- - self R46.8
- – causing insufficient intake of food and water R63.6

Neisserian infection NEC – *see* Gonococcus

Nelaton's syndrome G60.8

Nelson's syndrome E24.1

Nematodiasis (intestinal) NEC B82.0
- ancylostomiasis B76.0

Neonatal – *see also* condition
- abstinence syndrome P96.1
- tooth, teeth K00.6

Neonatorum – *see* condition

Neoplasia
- endocrine, multiple (MEN) (M8360/1) (*see also* Adenomatosis, endocrine) D44.8
- intraepithelial
- – cervix (uteri) (CIN) N87.9
- – – grade I N87.0
- – – grade II N87.1
- – – grade III (severe dysplasia) (M8077/2) D06.9
- – vagina (VAIN) N89.3
- – – grade I N89.0
- – – grade II N89.1
- – – grade III (severe dysplasia) (M8077/2) D07.2
- – vulva (VIN) N90.3
- – – grade I N90.0
- – – grade II N90.1
- – – grade III (severe dysplasia) (M8077/2) D07.1
- – – Prostate
- – – – grade I N42.3
- – – – grade II N42.3
- – – – grade III 307.5

Neoplasm, neoplastic .... *unspecified* C80.9   C79.9   D09.9   D36.9   D48.9

Note: 1. The list below gives the code numbers for neoplasms by anatomical site. For each site there are five possible code numbers according to whether the neoplasm in question is malignant (primary); malignant, secondary; in situ; benign; or of uncertain behavior or unspecified nature. The description of the neoplasm will often indicate which of the five columns is appropriate, e.g. malignant melanoma of skin, carcinoma in situ of cervix uteri, benign fibroademona of breast.

Where such descriptors are not present, the remainder of the Index should be consulted, where guidance is given to the approriate columns for each morphological (histological) variety listed, e.g. Mesonephroma - *see* Neoplasm, malignant, Embryoma - *see also* Neoplasm, uncertain behavior, Bowen's disease - *see* Neoplasm, skin, in situ. However, the guidance in the Index can be overridden if one of the descriptors mentioned above is present, e.g. malignant adenoma of colon is coded to C18.9 and not to D12.6, as the adjective "malignant" overrides the Index entry "Adenoma - *see also* Neoplasm, benign".

2. Sites marked with the sign # (e.g. face NEC #) should be classified to malignant neoplasm of *skin* of these sites if the variety of neoplasm is a squamous cell carcinoma or an epidermoid carcinoma and to benign neoplasm of *skin* of these sites if the variety of neoplasm is a papilloma (any type).

3. Carcinomas and adenocarcinomas, of any type other than intraosseous or odontogenic, of sites marked with the sign ◇ (e.g. ischium ◇) should be considered as metastatic from an unspecified primary site and coded to C79.5.

	Malignant				Uncertain
	Primary	Secondary	In situ	Benign	or unknown behavior
- abdomen, abdominal..........................	C76.2	C79.8	D09.7	D36.7	D48.7
- - cavity.......................	C76.2	C79.8	D09.7	D36.7	D48.7
- - organ....................	C76.2	C79.8		D36.7	D48.7
- - viscera	C76.2	C79.8		D36.7	D48.7
- - wall.....................	C44.5	C79.2	D04.5	D23.5	D48.5
- abdominopelvic	C76.8	C79.8		D36.7	D48.7
- accessory sinus - *see* Neoplasm, sinus					
- acromion (process) ◇.................................	C40.0	C79.5		D16.0	D48.0
- adenoid (tissue)............................	C11.1	C79.8	D00.0	D10.6	D37.0
- adipose tissue - *see* Neoplasm, connective tissue					
- adnexa (uterine)............................	C57.4	C79.8	D07.3	D28.7	D39.7
- adrenal (gland)............................	C74.9	C79.7	D09.3	D35.0	D44.1
- - cortex..............................	C74.0	C79.7	D09.3	D35.0	D44.1
- - medulla................................	C74.1	C79.7	D09.3	D35.0	D44.1
- ala nasi (external)	C44.3	C79.2	D04.3	D23.3	D48.5
- alimentary canal or tract NEC	C26.9	C78.8	D01.9	D13.9	D37.9
- alveolar................................					
- - mucosa...............................	C03.9	C79.8	D00.0	D10.3	D37.0
- - - lower..............................	C03.1	C79.8	D00.0	D10.3	D37.0
- - - upper..............................	C03.0	C79.8	D00.0	D10.3	D37.0
- - ridge or process ◇	C41.1	C79.5		D16.5	D48.0
- - - carcinoma	C03.9	C79.8			
- - - - lower..............................	C03.1	C79.8			
- - - - upper..............................	C03.0	C79.8			
- - - lower ◇	C41.1	C79.5		D16.5	D48.0
- - - mucosa.............................	C03.9	C79.8	D00.0	D10.3	D37.0
- - - - lower..............................	C03.1	C79.8	D00.0	D10.3	D37.0
- - - - upper..............................	C03.0	C79.8	D00.0	D10.3	D37.0

| | Malignant | | | | Uncertain |
	Primary /3	Secondary /6	In situ	Benign	or unknown behavior
Neoplasm, neoplastic—*continued*					
– alveolar—*continued*					
– – ridge or process—*continued*					
– – upper ✧	C41.0	C79.5		D16.4	D48.0
– – sulcus	C06.1	C79.8	D00.0	D10.3	D37.0
– alveolus	C03.9	C79.8	D00.0	D10.3	D37.0
– – lower	C03.1	C79.8	D00.0	D10.3	D37.0
– – upper	C03.0	C79.8	D00.0	D10.3	D37.0
– ampulla of Vater	C24.1	C78.8	D01.5	D13.5	D37.6
– ankle NEC #	C76.5	C79.8	D04.7	D36.7	D48.7
– anorectum, anorectal (junction)	C21.8	C78.5	D01.3	D12.9	D37.7
– antecubital fossa or space #	C76.4	C79.8	D04.6	D36.7	D48.7
– antrum (Highmore) (maxillary)	C31.0	C78.3	D02.3	D14.0	D38.5
– – pyloric	C16.3	C78.8	D00.2	D13.1	D37.1
– – tympanicum	C30.1	C78.3	D02.3	D14.0	D38.5
– anus, anal	C21.0	C78.5	D01.3	D12.9	D37.7
– – canal	C21.1	C78.5	D01.3	D12.9	D37.7
– – margin	C44.5	C79.2	D04.5	D23.5	D48.5
– – skin	C44.5	C79.2	D04.5	D23.5	D48.5
– – sphincter	C21.1	C78.5	D01.3	D12.9	D37.7
– aorta (thoracic)	C49.3	C79.8		D21.3	D48.1
– – abdominal	C49.4	C79.8		D21.4	D48.1
– aortic body	C75.5	C79.8		D35.6	D44.7
– aponeurosis – *see also* Neoplasm, connective tissue					
– – palmar	C49.1	C79.8		D21.1	D48.1
– – plantar	C49.2	C79.8		D21.2	D48.1
– appendix	C18.1	C78.5	D01.0	D12.1	D37.3
– arachnoid	C70.9	C79.4		D32.9	D42.9
– – cerebral	C70.0	C79.3		D32.0	D42.0
– – spinal	C70.1	C79.4		D32.1	D42.1
– areola	C50.0	C79.8	D05.9	D24	D48.6
– arm NEC #	C76.4	C79.8	D04.6	D36.7	D48.7
– artery – *see* Neoplasm, connective tissue					
– aryepiglottic fold	C13.1	C79.8	D00.0	D10.7	D37.0
– – hypopharyngeal aspect	C13.1	C79.8	D00.0	D10.7	D37.0
– – laryngeal aspect	C32.1	C78.3	D02.0	D14.1	D38.0
– – marginal zone	C13.1	C79.8	D00.0	D10.7	D37.0
– arytenoid (cartilage)	C32.3	C78.3	D02.0	D14.1	D38.0
– – fold – *see* Neoplasm, aryepiglottic fold					
– atlas ✧	C41.2	C79.5		D16.6	D48.0
– atrium, cardiac	C38.0	C79.8		D15.1	D48.7
– auditory					
– – canal (external)	C44.2	C79.2	D04.2	D23.2	D48.5
– – – internal	C30.1	C78.3	D02.3	D14.0	D38.5
– – nerve	C72.4	C79.4		D33.3	D43.3
– – tube	C30.1	C78.3	D02.3	D14.0	D38.5
– – – opening	C11.2	C79.8	D00.0	D10.6	D37.0
– auricle, ear	C44.2	C79.2	D04.2	D23.2	D48.5
– – cartilage	C49.0	C79.8		D21.0	D48.1
– auricular canal (external)	C44.2	C79.2	D04.2	D23.2	D48.5
– – internal	C30.1	C78.3	D02.3	D14.0	D38.5

| | Malignant | | | | Uncertain |
	Primary	Secondary	In situ	Benign	or unknown behavior
Neoplasm, neoplastic—*continued*					
– autonomic nerve or nervous system – *see* Neoplasm, nerve, peripheral					
– axilla, axillary	C76.1	C79.8	D09.7	D36.7	D48.7
– – fold	C44.5	C79.2	D04.5	D23.5	D48.5
– back NEC #	C76.7	C79.8	D04.5	D36.7	D48.7
– Bartholin's gland	C51.0	C79.8	D07.1	D28.0	D39.7
– basal ganglia	C71.0	C79.3		D33.0	D43.0
– basis pedunculi	C71.7	C79.3		D33.1	D43.1
– bile or biliary (tract)	C24.9	C78.8	D01.5	D13.5	D37.6
– – canals, interlobular	C22.1	C78.8	D01.5	D13.4	D37.6
– – duct or passage (common) (cystic) (extrahepatic)	C24.0	C78.8	D01.5	D13.5	D37.6
– – – interlobular	C22.1	C78.8	D01.5	D13.4	D37.6
– – – intrahepatic	C22.1	C78.8	D01.5	D13.4	D37.6
– – – – with extrahepatic	C24.8	C78.8	D01.5	D13.5	D37.6
– bladder (urinary)	C67.9	C79.1	D09.0	D30.3	D41.4
– – dome	C67.1	C79.1	D09.0	D30.3	D41.4
– – neck	C67.5	C79.1	D09.0	D30.3	D41.4
– – orifice	C67.9	C79.1	D09.0	D30.3	D41.4
– – – ureteric	C67.6	C79.1	D09.0	D30.3	D41.4
– – – urethral	C67.5	C79.1	D09.0	D30.3	D41.4
– – sphincter	C67.8	C79.1	D09.0	D30.3	D41.4
– – trigone	C67.0	C79.1	D09.0	D30.3	D41.4
– – urachus	C67.7	C79.1	D09.0	D30.3	D41.4
– – wall	C67.9	C79.1	D09.0	D30.3	D41.4
– – – anterior	C67.3	C79.1	D09.0	D30.3	D41.4
– – – lateral	C67.2	C79.1	D09.0	D30.3	D41.4
– – – posterior	C67.4	C79.1	D09.0	D30.3	D41.4
– blood vessel – *see* Neoplasm, connective tissue					
– bone (periosteum) ◇	C41.9	C79.5		D16.9	D48.0

Note: Carcinomas and adenocarcinomas, of any type other than intraosseous or odontogenic, of the sites listed under "Neoplasm, bone" should be considered as metastatic from an unspecified primary site and coded to C79.5.

– – acetabulum	C41.4	C79.5		D16.8	D48.0
– – acromion (process)	C40.0	C79.5		D16.0	D48.0
– – ankle	C40.3	C79.5		D16.3	D48.0
– – arm NEC	C40.0	C79.5		D16.0	D48.0
– – astragalus	C40.3	C79.5		D16.3	D48.0
– – atlas	C41.2	C79.5		D16.6	D48.0
– – axis	C41.2	C79.5		D16.6	D48.0
– – back NEC	C41.2	C79.5		D16.6	D48.0
– – calcaneus	C40.3	C79.5		D16.3	D48.0
– – calvarium	C41.0	C79.5		D16.4	D48.0
– – carpus (any)	C40.1	C79.5		D16.1	D48.0
– – cartilage NEC	C41.9	C79.5		D16.9	D48.0
– – clavicle	C41.3	C79.5		D16.7	D48.0
– – clivus	C41.0	C79.5		D16.4	D48.0
– – coccygeal vertebra	C41.4	C79.5		D16.8	D48.0
– – coccyx	C41.4	C79.5		D16.8	D48.0

	Malignant				Uncertain or unknown behavior
	Primary	Secondary	In situ	Benign	

Neoplasm, neoplastic—*continued*
– bone—*continued*

– – costal cartilage	C41.3	C79.5		D16.7	D48.0
– – cranial	C41.0	C79.5		D16.4	D48.0
– – digital	C40.9	C79.5		D16.9	D48.0
– – – finger	C40.1	C79.5		D16.1	D48.0
– – – toe	C40.3	C79.5		D16.3	D48.0
– – elbow	C40.0	C79.5		D16.0	D48.0
– – ethmoid (labyrinth)	C41.0	C79.5		D16.4	D48.0
– – face	C41.0	C79.5		D16.4	D48.0
– – femur (any part)	C40.2	C79.5		D16.2	D48.0
– – fibula (any part)	C40.2	C79.5		D16.2	D48.0
– – finger (any)	C40.1	C79.5		D16.1	D48.0
– – foot	C40.3	C79.5		D16.3	D48.0
– – forearm	C40.0	C79.5		D16.0	D48.0
– – frontal	C41.0	C79.5		D16.4	D48.0
– – hand	C40.1	C79.5		D16.1	D48.0
– – heel	C40.3	C79.5		D16.3	D48.0
– – hip	C41.4	C79.5		D16.8	D48.0
– – humerus (any part)	C40.0	C79.5		D16.0	D48.0
– – hyoid	C41.0	C79.5		D16.4	D48.0
– – ilium	C41.4	C79.5		D16.8	D48.0
– – innominate	C41.4	C79.5		D16.8	D48.0
– – intervertebral cartilage or disc	C41.2	C79.5		D16.6	D48.0
– – ischium	C41.4	C79.5		D16.8	D48.0
– – jaw – *see* Neoplasm, jaw, bone					
– – knee	C40.2	C79.5		D16.2	D48.0
– – leg NEC	C40.2	C79.5		D16.2	D48.0
– – limb NEC	C40.9	C79.5		D16.9	D48.0
– – – lower (long bones)	C40.2	C79.5		D16.2	D48.0
– – – – short bones	C40.3	C79.5		D16.3	D48.0
– – – upper (long bones)	C40.0	C79.5		D16.0	D48.0
– – – – short bones	C40.1	C79.5		D16.1	D48.0
– – long	C40.9	C79.5		D16.9	D48.0
– – – lower limbs NEC	C40.2	C79.5		D16.2	D48.0
– – – upper limbs NEC	C40.0	C79.5		D16.0	D48.0
– – mandible	C41.1	C79.5		D16.5	D48.0
– – marrow NEC	C96.9	C79.5			D47.9
– – maxilla, maxillary (superior)	C41.0	C79.5		D16.4	D48.0
– – – inferior	C41.1	C79.5		D16.5	D48.0
– – metacarpus (any)	C40.1	C79.5		D16.1	D48.0
– – metatarsus (any)	C40.3	C79.5		D16.3	D48.0
– – nose, nasal	C41.0	C79.5		D16.4	D48.0
– – occipital	C41.0	C79.5		D16.4	D48.0
– – orbit	C41.0	C79.5		D16.4	D48.0
– – parietal	C41.0	C79.5		D16.4	D48.0
– – patella	C40.3	C79.5		D16.3	D48.0
– – pelvic	C41.4	C79.5		D16.8	D48.0
– – phalanges	C40.9	C79.5		D16.9	D48.0
– – – foot	C40.3	C79.5		D16.3	D48.0
– – – hand	C40.1	C79.5		D16.1	D48.0
– – pubic	C41.4	C79.5		D16.8	D48.0

ALPHABETICAL INDEX TO DISEASES AND NATURE OF INJURY

	Malignant				Uncertain
	Primary **3**	Secondary **6**	In situ **2**	Benign **O**	or unknown behavior **1**
Neoplasm, neoplastic—*continued*					
– bone—*continued*					
– – radius (any part)	C40.0	C79.5		D16.0	D48.0
– – rib	C41.3	C79.5		D16.7	D48.0
– – sacral vertebra	C41.4	C79.5		D16.8	D48.0
– – sacrum	C41.4	C79.5		D16.8	D48.0
– – scapula (any part)	C40.0	C79.5		D16.0	D48.0
– – sella turcica	C41.0	C79.5		D16.4	D48.0
– – short	C40.9	C79.5		D16.9	D48.0
– – – lower limbs	C40.3	C79.5		D16.3	D48.0
– – – upper limbs	C40.1	C79.5		D16.1	D48.0
– – shoulder	C40.0	C79.5		D16.0	D48.0
– – skeleton, skeletal NEC	C41.9	C79.5		D16.9	D48.0
– – skull	C41.0	C79.5		D16.4	D48.0
– – sphenoid	C41.0	C79.5		D16.4	D48.0
– – spine, spinal (column)	C41.2	C79.5		D16.6	D48.0
– – – coccyx	C41.4	C79.5		D16.8	D48.0
– – – sacrum	C41.4	C79.5		D16.8	D48.0
– – sternum	C41.3	C79.5		D16.7	D48.0
– – tarsus (any)	C40.3	C79.5		D16.3	D48.0
– – temporal	C41.0	C79.5		D16.4	D48.0
– – thumb	C40.1	C79.5		D16.1	D48.0
– – tibia (any part)	C40.2	C79.5		D16.2	D48.0
– – toe (any)	C40.3	C79.5		D16.3	D48.0
– – turbinate	C41.0	C79.5		D16.4	D48.0
– – ulna (any part)	C40.0	C79.5		D16.0	D48.0
– – vertebra (column)	C41.2	C79.5		D16.6	D48.0
– – – coccyx	C41.4	C79.5		D16.8	D48.0
– – – sacrum	C41.4	C79.5		D16.8	D48.0
– – vomer	C41.0	C79.5		D16.4	D48.0
– – wrist	C40.1	C79.5		D16.1	D48.0
– – xiphoid process	C41.3	C79.5		D16.7	D48.0
– – zygomatic	C41.0	C79.5		D16.4	D48.0
– book leaf (mouth)	C06.8	C79.8	D00.0	D10.3	D37.0
– bowel – *see* Neoplasm, intestine					
– brachial plexus	C47.1	C79.8		D36.1	D48.2
– brain NEC	C71.9	C79.3		D33.2	D43.2
– – meninges	C70.0	C79.3		D32.0	D42.0
– – stem	C71.7	C79.3		D33.1	D43.1
– branchial (cleft) (vestiges)	C10.4	C79.8	D00.0	D10.5	D37.0
– breast (connective tissue) (glandular tissue) (soft parts)	C50.9	C79.8	D05.9	D24	D48.6
– – areola	C50.0	C79.8	D05.9	D24	D48.6
– – axillary tail	C50.6	C79.8	D05.9	D24	D48.6
– – central portion	C50.1	C79.8	D05.9	D24	D48.6
– – ectopic site	C50.8	C79.8	D05.9	D24	D48.6
– – inner	C50.8	C79.8	D05.9	D24	D48.6
– – lower	C50.8	C79.8	D05.9	D24	D48.6
– – lower-inner quadrant	C50.3	C79.8	D05.9	D24	D48.6
– – lower-outer quadrant	C50.5	C79.8	D05.9	D24	D48.6
– – midline	C50.8	C79.8	D05.9	D24	D48.6
– – outer	C50.8	C79.8	D05.9	D24	D48.6

Ductal

Radial Scar – benign

441

| | Malignant | | | | Uncertain |
	Primary	Secondary	In situ	Benign	or unknown behavior
Neoplasm, neoplastic—*continued*					
– breast—*continued*					
– – skin	C44.5	C79.2	D04.5	D23.5	D48.5
– – tail (axillary)	C50.6	C79.8	D05.9	D24	D48.6
– – upper	C50.8	C79.8	D05.9	D24	D48.6
– – upper-inner quadrant	C50.2	C79.8	D05.9	D24	D48.6
– – upper-outer quadrant	C50.4	C79.8	D05.9	D24	D48.6
– broad ligament	C57.1	C79.8		D28.2	D39.7
– bronchiogenic, bronchogenic (lung)	C34.9	C78.0	D02.2	D14.3	D38.1
– bronchiole	C34.9	C78.0	D02.2	D14.3	D38.1
– bronchus	C34.9	C78.0	D02.2	D14.3	D38.1
– – carina	C34.0	C78.0	D02.2	D14.3	D38.1
– – lower lobe of lung	C34.3	C78.0	D02.2	D14.3	D38.1
– – main	C34.0	C78.0	D02.2	D14.3	D38.1
– – middle lobe of lung	C34.2	C78.0	D02.2	D14.3	D38.1
– – upper lobe of lung	C34.1	C78.0	D02.2	D14.3	D38.1
– brow	C44.3	C79.2	D04.3	D23.3	D48.5
– buccal (cavity)	C06.9	C79.8	D00.0	D10.3	D37.0
– – mucosa	C06.0	C79.8	D00.0	D10.3	D37.0
– – sulcus (lower) (upper)	C06.1	C79.8	D00.0	D10.3	D37.0
– bulbourethral gland	C68.0	C79.1	D09.1	D30.4	D41.3
– bursa – *see* Neoplasm, connective tissue					
– buttock NEC #	C76.3	C79.8	D04.5	D36.7	D48.7
– caecum – *see* Neoplasm, cecum					
– calf #	C76.5	C79.8	D04.7	D36.7	D48.7
– calvarium ✧	C41.0	C79.5		D16.4	D48.0
– calyx, renal	C65	C79.0	D09.1	D30.1	D41.1
– canal					
– – anal	C21.1	C78.5	D01.3	D12.9	D37.7
– – auditory (external)	C44.2	C79.2	D04.2	D23.2	D48.5
– – auricular (external)	C44.2	C79.2	D04.2	D23.2	D48.5
– canaliculi					
– – biliferi	C22.1	C78.8	D01.5	D13.4	D37.6
– – intrahepatic	C22.1	C78.8	D01.5	D13.4	D37.6
– canthus (eye) (inner) (outer)	C44.1	C79.2	D04.1	D23.1	D48.5
– capillary – *see* Neoplasm, connective tissue					
– capsule, internal	C71.0	C79.3		D33.0	D43.0
– cardia (gastric)	C16.0	C78.8	D00.2	D13.1	D37.1
– cardiac orifice (stomach)	C16.0	C78.8	D00.2	D13.1	D37.1
– cardioesophageal junction	C16.0	C78.8	D00.2	D13.1	D37.1
– cardioesophagus	C16.0	C78.8	D00.2	D13.1	D37.1
– carina (tracheal)	C34.0	C78.0	D02.2	D14.3	D38.1
– carotid (artery)	C49.0	C79.8		D21.0	D48.1
– – body	C75.4	C79.8		D35.5	D44.6
– cartilage (articular) (joint) (*see also* Neoplasm, bone)	C41.9	C79.5		D16.9	D48.0
– – arytenoid	C32.3	C78.3	D02.0	D14.1	D38.0
– – auricular	C49.0	C79.8		D21.0	D48.1
– – bronchi	C34.0	C78.0	D02.2	D14.3	D38.1
– – costal ✧	C41.3	C79.5		D16.7	D48.0
– – cricoid	C32.3	C78.3	D02.0	D14.1	D38.0
– – cuneiform	C32.3	C78.3	D02.0	D14.1	D38.0

| | Malignant | | | | Uncertain or unknown behavior |
	Primary 3	Secondary 6	In situ 2	Benign 0	
Neoplasm, neoplastic—*continued*					
− cartilage—*continued*					
− − ear (external)	C49.0	C79.8		D21.0	D48.1
− − epiglottis	C32.1	C78.3	D02.0	D14.1	D38.0
− − eyelid	C49.0	C79.8		D21.0	D48.1
− − larynx, laryngeal	C32.3	C78.3	D02.0	D14.1	D38.0
− − nose, nasal	C30.0	C78.3	D02.3	D14.0	D38.5
− − rib ◇	C41.3	C79.5		D16.7	D48.0
− − semilunar (knee) ◇	C40.2	C79.5		D16.2	D48.0
− − thyroid	C32.3	C78.3	D02.0	D14.1	D38.0
− − trachea	C33	C78.3	D02.1	D14.2	D38.1
− cauda equina	C72.1	C79.4		D33.4	D43.4
− cavity					
− − buccal	C06.9	C79.8	D00.0	D10.3	D37.0
− − nasal	C30.0	C78.3	D02.3	D14.0	D38.5
− − oral	C06.9	C79.8	D00.0	D10.3	D37.0
− − peritoneal	C48.2	C78.6		D20.1	D48.4
− − tympanic	C30.1	C78.3	D02.3	D14.0	D38.5
− cecum	C18.0	C78.5	D01.0	D12.0	D37.4
− central					
− − nervous system – *see* Neoplasm, nervous system					
− − white matter	C71.0	C79.3		D33.0	D43.0
− cerebellopontine	C71.6	C79.3		D33.1	D43.1
− cerebellum, cerebellar	C71.6	C79.3		D33.1	D43.1
− cerebrum, cerebral (cortex) (hemisphere) (white matter)	C71.0	C79.3		D33.0	D43.0
− − meninges	C70.0	C79.3		D32.0	D42.0
− − peduncle	C71.7	C79.3		D33.1	D43.1
− − ventricle (cerebral) (lateral) (third)	C71.5	C79.3		D33.0	D43.0
− − − fourth	C71.7	C79.3		D33.1	D43.1
− cervical region	C76.0	C79.8	D09.7	D36.7	D48.7
− cervix (uteri)	C53.9	C79.8	D06.9	D26.0	D39.0
− − canal	C53.0	C79.8	D06.0	D26.0	D39.0
− − squamocolumnar junction	C53.8	C79.8	D06.7	D26.0	D39.0
− − stump	C53.8	C79.8	D06.7	D26.0	D39.0
− cheek	C76.0	C79.8	D09.7	D36.7	D48.7
− − external	C44.3	C79.2	D04.3	D23.3	D48.5
− − inner aspect	C06.0	C79.8	D00.0	D10.3	D37.0
− − internal	C06.0	C79.8	D00.0	D10.3	D37.0
− − mucosa	C06.0	C79.8	D00.0	D10.3	D37.0
− chest (wall) NEC	C76.1	C79.8	D09.7	D36.7	D48.7
− chiasma opticum	C72.3	C79.4		D33.3	D43.3
− chin	C44.3	C79.2	D04.3	D23.3	D48.5
− choana	C11.3	C79.8	D00.0	D10.6	D37.0
− cholangiole	C22.1	C78.8	D01.5	D13.4	D37.6
− choledochal duct	C24.0	C78.8	D01.5	D13.5	D37.6
− choroid	C69.3	C79.4	D09.2	D31.3	D48.7
− − plexus (lateral ventricle) (third ventricle)	C71.5	C79.3		D33.0	D43.0
− − − fourth ventricle	C71.7	C79.3		D33.1	D43.1
− ciliary body	C69.4	C79.4	D09.2	D31.4	D48.7
− clavicle ◇	C41.3	C79.5		D16.7	D48.0

	Malignant		In situ	Benign	Uncertain or unknown behavior
	Primary	Secondary			

Neoplasm, neoplastic—*continued*

– clitoris	C51.2	C79.8	D07.1	D28.0	D39.7
– clivus ✧	C41.0	C79.5		D16.4	D48.0
– cloacogenic zone	C21.2	C78.5	D01.3	D12.9	D37.7
– coccygeal					
– – body or glomus	C75.5	C79.8		D35.6	D44.7
– – vertebra ✧	C41.4	C79.5		D16.8	D48.0
– coccyx ✧	C41.4	C79.5		D16.8	D48.0
– colon (*see also* Neoplasm, intestine, large)	C18.9	C78.5	D01.0	D12.6	D37.4
– – with rectum	C19	C78.5	D01.1	D12.7	D37.5
– column, spinal – *see* Neoplasm, spine					
– columnella	C44.3	C79.2	D04.3	D23.3	D48.5
– commissure					
– – labial, lip	C00.6	C79.8	D00.0	D10.0	D37.0
– – laryngeal	C32.0	C78.3	D02.0	D14.1	D38.0
– common (bile) duct	C24.0	C78.8	D01.5	D13.5	D37.6
– concha	C44.2	C79.2	D04.2	D23.2	D48.5
– – nose	C30.0	C78.3	D02.3	D14.0	D38.5
– conjunctiva	C69.0	C79.4	D09.2	D31.0	D48.7
– connective tissue NEC	C49.9	C79.8		D21.9	D48.1

Note: For neoplasms of connective tissue (blood vessels, bursa, fascia, ligament, muscle, peripheral nerves, sympathetic and parasympathetic nerves and ganglia, synovia, tendon, etc.) or of morphological types that indicate connective tissue, code according to the list under "Neoplasm, connective tissue"; for sites that do not appear in this list, code to neoplasm of that site, e.g.

> fibrosarcoma, pancreas C25.9
> leiomyosarcoma, stomach C16.9

Morphological types that indicate connective tissue appear in their proper place in the alphabetical index with the instruction "*see* Neoplasm, connective tissue, . . .".

– – abdomen	C49.4	C79.8		D21.4	D48.1
– – abdominal wall	C49.4	C79.8		D21.4	D48.1
– – ankle	C49.2	C79.8		D21.2	D48.1
– – antecubital fossa or space	C49.1	C79.8		D21.1	D48.1
– – arm	C49.1	C79.8		D21.1	D48.1
– – auricle (ear)	C49.0	C79.8		D21.0	D48.1
– – axilla	C49.3	C79.8		D21.3	D48.1
– – back	C49.6	C79.8		D21.6	D48.1
– – buttock	C49.5	C79.8		D21.5	D48.1
– – calf	C49.2	C79.8		D21.2	D48.1
– – cervical region	C49.0	C79.8		D21.0	D48.1
– – cheek	C49.0	C79.8		D21.0	D48.1
– – chest (wall)	C49.3	C79.8		D21.3	D48.1
– – chin	C49.0	C79.8		D21.0	D48.1
– – diaphragm	C49.3	C79.8		D21.3	D48.1
– – ear (external)	C49.0	C79.8		D21.0	D48.1
– – elbow	C49.1	C79.8		D21.1	D48.1
– – extrarectal	C49.5	C79.8		D21.5	D48.1
– – extremity	C49.9	C79.8		D21.9	D48.1
– – – lower	C49.2	C79.8		D21.2	D48.1
– – – upper	C49.1	C79.8		D21.1	D48.1
– – eyelid	C49.0	C79.8		D21.0	D48.1

| | Malignant | | | | Uncertain |
	Primary 3	Secondary 6	In situ 2	Benign 0	or unknown behavior 1
Neoplasm, neoplastic—*continued*					
− connective tissue—*continued*					
− − face	C49.0	C79.8		D21.0	D48.1
− − finger	C49.1	C79.8		D21.1	D48.1
− − flank	C49.6	C79.8		D21.6	D48.1
− − foot	C49.2	C79.8		D21.2	D48.1
− − forearm	C49.1	C79.8		D21.1	D48.1
− − forehead	C49.0	C79.8		D21.0	D48.1
− − gluteal region	C49.5	C79.8		D21.5	D48.1
− − great vessels NEC	C49.3	C79.8		D21.3	D48.1
− − groin	C49.5	C79.8		D21.5	D48.1
− − hand	C49.1	C79.8		D21.1	D48.1
− − head	C49.0	C79.8		D21.0	D48.1
− − heel	C49.2	C79.8		D21.2	D48.1
− − hip	C49.2	C79.8		D21.2	D48.1
− − iliopsoas muscle	C49.4	C79.8		D21.4	D48.1
− − infraclavicular region	C49.3	C79.8		D21.3	D48.1
− − inguinal (canal) (region)	C49.5	C79.8		D21.5	D48.1
− − intrathoracic	C49.3	C79.8		D21.3	D48.1
− − ischiorectal fossa	C49.5	C79.8		D21.5	D48.1
− − jaw	C03.9	C79.8		D10.3	D37.0
− − knee	C49.2	C79.8		D21.2	D48.1
− − leg	C49.2	C79.8		D21.2	D48.1
− − limb NEC	C49.9	C79.8		D21.9	D48.1
− − − lower	C49.2	C79.8		D21.2	D48.1
− − − upper	C49.1	C79.8		D21.1	D48.1
− − nates	C49.5	C79.8		D21.5	D48.1
− − neck	C49.0	C79.8		D21.0	D48.1
− − orbit	C69.6	C79.4		D31.6	D48.1
− − pararectal	C49.5	C79.8		D21.5	D48.1
− − paraurethral	C49.5	C79.8		D21.5	D48.1
− − paravaginal	C49.5	C79.8		D21.5	D48.1
− − pelvis (floor)	C49.5	C79.8		D21.5	D48.1
− − pelvoabdominal	C49.8	C79.8		D21.9	D48.1
− − perineum	C49.5	C79.8		D21.5	D48.1
− − perirectal (tissue)	C49.5	C79.8		D21.5	D48.1
− − periurethral (tissue)	C49.5	C79.8		D21.5	D48.1
− − popliteal fossa or space	C49.2	C79.8		D21.2	D48.1
− − presacral	C49.5	C79.8		D21.5	D48.1
− − psoas muscle	C49.4	C79.8		D21.4	D48.1
− − pterygoid fossa	C49.0	C79.8		D21.0	D48.1
− − rectovaginal septum or wall	C49.5	C79.8		D21.5	D48.1
− − rectovesical	C49.5	C79.8		D21.5	D48.1
− − retroperitoneal	C48.0	C78.6		D20.0	D48.3
− − sacrococcygeal region	C49.5	C79.8		D21.5	D48.1
− − scalp	C49.0	C79.8		D21.0	D48.1
− − scapular region	C49.3	C79.8		D21.3	D48.1
− − shoulder	C49.1	C79.8		D21.1	D48.1
− − submental	C49.0	C79.8		D21.0	D48.1
− − supraclavicular region	C49.0	C79.8		D21.0	D48.1
− − temple	C49.0	C79.8		D21.0	D48.1
− − temporal region	C49.0	C79.8		D21.0	D48.1

| | Malignant | | | | Uncertain or unknown behavior |
	Primary	Secondary	In situ	Benign	
Neoplasm, neoplastic—*continued*					
– connective tissue—*continued*					
– – thigh	C49.2	C79.8		D21.2	D48.1
– – thoracic (duct) (wall)	C49.3	C79.8		D21.3	D48.1
– – thorax	C49.3	C79.8		D21.3	D48.1
– – thumb	C49.1	C79.8		D21.1	D48.1
– – toe	C49.2	C79.8		D21.2	D48.1
– – trunk	C49.6	C79.8		D21.6	D48.1
– – umbilicus	C49.4	C79.8		D21.4	D48.1
– – vesicorectal	C49.5	C79.8		D21.5	D48.1
– – wrist	C49.1	C79.8		D21.1	D48.1
– conus medullaris	C72.0	C79.4		D33.4	D43.4
– cord (true) (vocal)	C32.0	C78.3	D02.0	D14.1	D38.0
– – false	C32.1	C78.3	D02.0	D14.1	D38.0
– – spermatic	C63.1	C79.8	D07.6	D29.7	D40.7
– – spinal (cervical) (lumbar) (sacral)(thoracic)	C72.0	C79.4		D33.4	D43.4
– cornea (limbus)	C69.1	C79.4	D09.2	D31.1	D48.7
– corpus					
– – callosum	C71.8	C79.3		D33.2	D43.2
– – cavernosum	C60.2	C79.8	D07.4	D29.0	D40.7
– – gastric	C16.2	C78.8	D00.2	D13.1	D37.1
– – penis	C60.2	C79.8	D07.4	D29.0	D40.7
– – striatum	C71.0	C79.3		D33.0	D43.0
– – uteri	C54.9	C79.8	D07.3	D26.1	D39.0
– – – isthmus	C54.0	C79.8	D07.3	D26.1	D39.0
– cortex					
– – adrenal	C74.0	C79.7	D09.3	D35.0	D44.1
– – cerebral	C71.0	C79.3		D33.0	D43.0
– costal cartilage ◇	C41.3	C79.5		D16.7	D48.0
– Cowper's gland	C68.0	C79.1	D09.1	D30.4	D41.3
– cranial (fossa, any)	C71.9	C79.3		D33.2	D43.2
– – meninges	C70.0	C79.3		D32.0	D42.0
– – nerve, NEC	C72.5	C79.4		D33.3	D43.3
– craniopharyngeal (duct) (pouch)	C75.2	C79.8	D09.3	D35.3	D44.4
– cricoid	C13.0	C79.8	D00.0	D10.7	D37.0
– – cartilage	C32.3	C78.3	D02.0	D14.1	D38.0
– cricopharynx	C13.0	C79.8	D00.0	D10.7	D37.0
– crypt of Morgagni	C21.8	C78.5	D01.3	D12.9	D37.7
– cutaneous – *see* Neoplasm, skin					
– cutis – *see* Neoplasm, skin					
– cystic (bile) duct	C24.0	C78.8	D01.5	D13.5	D37.6
– dermis – *see* Neoplasm, skin					
– diaphragm	C49.3	C79.8		D21.3	D48.1
– digestive organs, system, tube or tract NEC.	C26.9	C78.8	D01.9	D13.9	D37.9
– disk, intervertebral ◇	C41.2	C79.5		D16.6	D48.0
– disease, generalized		C79.9			
– – primary site not indicated	C80.9	C79.9			
– – primary site unknown, so stated	C80.0	C79.9			
– disseminated		C79.9			
– – primary site not indicated	C80.9	C79.9			
– – primary site unknown, so stated	C80.0	C79.9			

446

| | Malignant | | | | Uncertain |
	Primary 3	Secondary 6	In situ 2	Benign 0	or unknown behavior
Neoplasm, neoplastic—*continued*					
– Douglas' cul de sac or pouch	C48.1	C78.6		D20.1	D48.4
– duodenojejunal junction	C17.8	C78.4	D01.4	D13.3	D37.2
– duodenum...	C17.0	C78.4	D01.4	D13.2	D37.2
– dura (mater)...	C70.9	C79.4		D32.9	D42.9
– – cerebral..	C70.0	C79.3		D32.0	D42.0
– – cranial..	C70.0	C79.3		D32.0	D42.0
– – spinal	C70.1	C79.4		D32.1	D42.1
– ear (external)	C44.2	C79.2	D04.2	D23.2	D48.5
– – auricle	C44.2	C79.2	D04.2	D23.2	D48.5
– – canal	C44.2	C79.2	D04.2	D23.2	D48.5
– – cartilage...	C49.0	C79.8		D21.0	D48.1
– – external meatus.......................................	C44.2	C79.2	D04.2	D23.2	D48.5
– – inner..	C30.1	C78.3	D02.3	D14.0	D38.5
– – lobule...	C44.2	C79.2	D04.2	D23.2	D48.5
– – middle..	C30.1	C78.3	D02.3	D14.0	D38.5
– – skin	C44.2	C79.2	D04.2	D23.2	D48.5
– earlobe...	C44.2	C79.2	D04.2	D23.2	D48.5
– ejaculatory duct	C63.7	C79.8	D07.6	D29.7	D40.7
– elbow NEC #	C76.4	C79.8	D04.6	D36.7	D48.7
– endocardium...	C38.0	C79.8		D15.1	D48.7
– endocervix (canal) (gland)............................	C53.0	C79.8	D06.0	D26.0	D39.0
– endocrine gland NEC	C75.9	C79.8	D09.3	D35.9	D44.9
– – pluriglandular	C75.8	C79.8	D09.3	D35.8	D44.8
– endometrium (gland) (stroma).......................	C54.1	C79.8	D07.0	D26.1	D39.0
– enteric – *see* Neoplasm, intestine					
– ependyma (brain)..	C71.5	C79.3		D33.0	D43.0
– epicardium...	C38.0	C79.8		D15.1	D48.7
– epididymis	C63.0	C79.8	D07.6	D29.3	D40.7
– epidural..	C72.9	C79.4		D33.9	D43.9
– epiglottis..	C32.1	C78.3	D02.0	D14.1	D38.0
– – anterior aspect or surface..........................	C10.1	C79.8	D00.0	D10.5	D37.0
– – cartilage...	C32.1	C78.3	D02.0	D14.1	D38.0
– – free border (margin)	C10.1	C79.8	D00.0	D10.5	D37.0
– – posterior (laryngeal) surface.....................	C32.1	C78.3	D02.0	D14.1	D38.0
– – suprahyoid portion...................................	C32.1	C78.3	D02.0	D14.1	D38.0
– esophagogastric junction	C16.0	C78.8	D00.2	D13.1	D37.1
– esophagus	C15.9	C78.8	D00.1	D13.0	D37.7
– – abdominal...	C15.2	C78.8	D00.1	D13.0	D37.7
– – cervical..	C15.0	C78.8	D00.1	D13.0	D37.7
– – distal (third)...	C15.5	C78.8	D00.1	D13.0	D37.7
– – lower (third)..	C15.5	C78.8	D00.1	D13.0	D37.7
– – middle (third)..	C15.4	C78.8	D00.1	D13.0	D37.7
– – proximal (third)	C15.3	C78.8	D00.1	D13.0	D37.7
– – thoracic..	C15.1	C78.8	D00.1	D13.0	D37.7
– – upper (third)..	C15.3	C78.8	D00.1	D13.0	D37.7
– ethmoid (sinus)...	C31.1	C78.3	D02.3	D14.0	D38.5
– – bone or labyrinth ◇	C41.0	C79.5		D16.4	D48.0
– eustachian tube	C30.1	C78.3	D02.3	D14.0	D38.5
– exocervix...	C53.1	C79.8	D06.1	D26.0	D39.0

	Malignant				Uncertain or unknown behavior
	Primary	Secondary	In situ	Benign	

Neoplasm, neoplastic—*continued*
– external					
– – meatus (ear)..	C44.2	C79.2	D04.2	D23.2	D48.5
– – os uteri	C53.1	C79.8	D06.1	D26.0	D39.0
– extradural	C72.9	C79.4		D33.9	D43.9
– extraocular muscle	C69.6	C79.4		D31.6	D48.7
– extrarectal	C76.3	C79.8		D36.7	D48.7
– extremity #	C76.7	C79.8	D04.8	D36.7	D48.7
– – lower #	C76.5	C79.8	D04.7	D36.7	D48.7
– – upper #	C76.4	C79.8	D04.6	D36.7	D48.7
– eye NEC	C69.9	C79.4	D09.2	D31.9	D48.7
– eyeball..	C69.4	C79.4	D09.2	D31.4	D48.7
– eyebrow..	C44.3	C79.2	D04.3	D23.3	D48.5
– eyelid (lower) (upper) (skin)	C44.1	C79.2	D04.1	D23.1	D48.5
– – cartilage...	C49.0	C79.8		D21.0	D48.1
– face NEC #	C76.0	C79.8	D04.3	D36.7	D48.7
– fallopian tube	C57.0	C79.8	D07.3	D28.2	D39.7
– falx (cerebelli) (cerebri)	C70.0	C79.3		D32.0	D42.0
– fascia (*see also* Neoplasm, connective tissue)...	C49.9	C79.8		D21.9	D48.1
– – palmar..	C49.1	C79.8		D21.1	D48.1
– – plantar..	C49.2	C79.8		D21.2	D48.1
– fatty tissue – *see* Neoplasm, connective tissue					
– fauces, faucial NEC	C10.9	C79.8	D00.0	D10.5	D37.0
– – pillars	C09.1	C79.8	D00.0	D10.5	D37.0
– – tonsil	C09.9	C79.8	D00.0	D10.4	D37.0
– femur (any part) ◇..	C40.2	C79.5		D16.2	D48.0
– fetal membrane	C58	C79.8	D07.3	D26.7	D39.2
– fibrous tissue – *see* Neoplasm, connective tissue					
– fibula (any part) ◇	C40.2	C79.5		D16.2	D48.0
– filum terminale..	C72.0	C79.4		D33.4	D43.4
– finger NEC #	C76.4	C79.8	D04.6	D36.7	D48.7
– flank NEC #	C76.7	C79.8	D04.5	D36.7	D48.7
– foot NEC #	C76.5	C79.8	D04.7	D36.7	D48.7
– forearm NEC #	C76.4	C79.8	D04.6	D36.7	D48.7
– forehead	C44.3	C79.2	D04.3	D23.3	D48.5
– foreskin	C60.0	C79.8	D07.4	D29.0	D40.7
– fornix					
– – pharyngeal..	C11.3	C79.8	D00.0	D10.6	D37.0
– – vagina...	C52	C79.8	D07.2	D28.1	D39.7
– fossa...					
– – anterior (cranial)...	C71.9	C79.3		D33.2	D43.2
– – cranial	C71.9	C79.3		D33.2	D43.2
– – ischiorectal..	C76.3	C79.8		D36.7	D48.7
– – middle (cranial)...	C71.9	C79.3		D33.2	D43.2
– – piriform	C12	C79.8	D00.0	D10.7	D37.0
– – pituitary..	C75.1	C79.8	D09.3	D35.2	D44.3
– – posterior (cranial)..	C71.9	C79.3		D33.2	D43.2
– – pterygoid	C49.0	C79.8		D21.0	D48.1
– – Rosenmüller	C11.2	C79.8	D00.0	D10.6	D37.0

	Malignant				Uncertain or unknown behavior
	Primary 3	Secondary 6	In situ 2	Benign 0	1

Neoplasm, neoplastic—*continued*
- fossa—*continued*
-   – tonsillar.................................... C09.0 C79.8 D00.0 D10.5 D37.0
- fourchette...................................... C51.9 C79.8 D07.1 D28.0 D39.7
- frenulum ....
-   – labii – *see* Neoplasm, lip, internal
-   – linguae...................................... C02.2 C79.8 D00.0 D10.1 D37.0
- frontal ....
-   – bone ✧ C41.0 C79.5   D16.4 D48.0
-   – lobe.. C71.1 C79.3   D33.0 D43.0
-   – pole.. C71.1 C79.3   D33.0 D43.0
-   – sinus... C31.2 C78.3 D02.3 D14.0 D38.5
- fundus..
-   – stomach...................................... C16.1 C78.8 D00.2 D13.1 D37.1
-   – uterus C54.3 C79.8 D07.3 D26.1 D39.0
- gall duct (extrahepatic)................... C24.0 C78.8 D01.5 D13.5 D37.6
-   – intrahepatic............................. C22.1 C78.7 D01.5 D13.4 D37.6
- gallbladder.................................... C23 C78.8 D01.5 D13.5 D37.6
- ganglia (*see also* Neoplasm, nerve, peripheral) C47.9 C79.8   D36.1 D48.2
-   – basal... C71.0 C79.3   D33.0 D43.0
- Gartner's duct................................ C52 C79.8 D07.2 D28.1 D39.7
- gastric – *see* Neoplasm, stomach
- gastroesophageal junction............... C16.0 C78.8 D00.2 D13.1 D37.1
- gastrointestinal (tract) NEC............ C26.9 C78.8 D01.9 D13.9 D37.9
- generalized ....   ←79.9
- ~~– primary site not indicated~~............ ~~C80.9~~ ~~C79.9~~
- ~~– primary site unknown, so stated~~...... ~~C80.0~~ ~~C79.9~~
- genital organ or tract......................
-   – female NEC C57.9 C79.8 D07.3 D28.9 D39.9
-     – specified site NEC C57.7 C79.8 D07.3 D28.7 D39.7
-   – male NEC C63.9 C79.8 D07.6 D29.9 D40.9
-     – specified site NEC C63.7 C79.8 D07.6 D29.7 D40.7
- genitourinary tract ....
-   – female C57.9 C79.8 D07.3 D28.9 D39.9
-   – male C63.9 C79.8 D07.6 D29.9 D40.9
- gingiva (alveolar) (marginal)........... C03.9 C79.8 D00.0 D10.3 D37.0
-   – lower.. C03.1 C79.8 D00.0 D10.3 D37.0
-   – mandibular................................ C03.1 C79.8 D00.0 D10.3 D37.0
-   – maxillary.................................. C03.0 C79.8 D00.0 D10.3 D37.0
-   – upper.. C03.0 C79.8 D00.0 D10.3 D37.0
- gland, glandular (lymphatic) (system) – see also Neoplasm, lymph gland
-   – endocrine NEC C75.9 C79.8 D09.3 D35.9 D44.9
-   – salivary – *see* Neoplasm, salivary gland
- glans penis.................................... C60.1 C79.8 D07.4 D29.0 D40.7
- globus pallidus.............................. C71.0 C79.3   D33.0 D43.0
- glomus ....
-   – coccygeal.................................. C75.5 C79.8   D35.6 D44.7
-   – jugularis................................... C75.5 C79.8   D35.6 D44.7
- glossoepiglottic fold(s) C10.1 C79.8 D00.0 D10.5 D37.0
- glossopalatine fold........................ C09.1 C79.8 D00.0 D10.5 D37.0

| | Malignant | | | | Uncertain or unknown behavior |
	Primary	Secondary	In situ	Benign	
Neoplasm, neoplastic—*continued*					
– glossopharyngeal sulcus	C09.0	C79.8	D00.0	D10.5	D37.0
– glottis	C32.0	C78.3	D02.0	D14.1	D38.0
– gluteal region #	C76.3	C79.8	D04.5	D36.7	D48.7
– great vessels NEC	C49.3	C79.8		D21.3	D48.1
– groin NEC #	C76.3	C79.8	D04.5	D36.7	D48.7
– gum	C03.9	C79.8	D00.0	D10.3	D37.0
– – lower	C03.1	C79.8	D00.0	D10.3	D37.0
– – upper	C03.0	C79.8	D00.0	D10.3	D37.0
– hand NEC #	C76.4	C79.8	D04.6	D36.7	D48.7
– head NEC #	C76.0	C79.8	D04.4	D36.7	D48.7
– heart	C38.0	C79.8		D15.1	D48.7
– heel NEC #	C76.5	C79.8	D04.7	D36.7	D48.7
– helix	C44.2	C79.2	D04.2	D23.2	D48.5
– hematopoietic, hemopoietic tissue NEC	C96.9				D47.9
– hemisphere, cerebral	C71.0	C79.3		D33.0	D43.0
– hemorrhoidal zone	C21.1	C78.5	D01.3	D12.9	D37.7
– hepatic	C22.9	C78.7	D01.5	D13.4	D37.6
– – duct (bile)	C24.0	C78.8	D01.5	D13.5	D37.6
– – flexure (colon)	C18.3	C78.5	D01.0	D12.3	D37.4
– – primary	C22.9		D01.5	D13.4	D37.6
– hilus of lung	C34.0	C78.0	D02.2	D14.3	D38.1
– hip NEC #	C76.5	C79.8	D04.7	D36.7	D48.7
– hippocampus	C71.2	C79.3		D33.0	D43.0
– humerus (any part) ✧	C40.0	C79.5		D16.0	D48.0
– hymen	C52	C79.8	D07.2	D28.1	D39.7
– hypopharynx, hypopharyngeal NEC	C13.9	C79.8	D00.0	D10.7	D37.0
– – posterior wall	C13.2	C79.8	D00.0	D10.7	D37.0
– hypophysis	C75.1	C79.8	D09.3	D35.2	D44.3
– hypothalamus	C71.0	C79.3		D33.0	D43.0
– ileocecum, ileocecal (coil) (junction) (valve)	C18.0	C78.5	D01.0	D12.0	D37.4
– ileum	C17.2	C78.4	D01.4	D13.3	D37.2
– ilium ✧	C41.4	C79.5		D16.8	D48.0
– immunoproliferative NEC	C88.9				D47.9
– infraclavicular (region) #	C76.1	C79.8	D04.5	D36.7	D48.7
– inguinal (region) #	C76.3	C79.8	D04.5	D36.7	D48.7
– insula	C71.0	C79.3		D33.0	D43.0
– insular tissue (pancreas)	C25.4	C78.8	D01.7	D13.7	D37.7
– – brain	C71.0	C79.3		D33.0	D43.0
– interarytenoid fold	C13.1	C79.8	D00.0	D10.7	D37.0
– – hypopharyngeal aspect	C13.1	C79.8	D00.0	D10.7	D37.0
– – laryngeal aspect	C32.1	C78.3	D02.0	D14.1	D38.0
– – marginal zone	C13.1	C79.8	D00.0	D10.7	D37.0
– internal					
– – capsule	C71.0	C79.3		D33.0	D43.0
– – os	C53.0	C79.8	D06.0	D26.0	D39.0
– intervertebral cartilage or disk ✧	C41.2	C79.5		D16.6	D48.0
– intestine, intestinal	C26.0	C78.5	D01.4	D13.9	D37.7
– – large	C18.9	C78.5	D01.0	D12.6	D37.4

Neoplasm, neoplastic—*continued*
- intestine, intestinal—*continued*
- - large—*continued*

| | Malignant | | | | Uncertain |
	Primary 3	Secondary 6	In situ 2	Benign 0	or unknown behavior 1
- - - appendix	C18.1	C78.5	D01.0	D12.1	D37.3
- - - cecum	C18.0	C78.5	D01.0	D12.0	D37.4
- - - colon	C18.9	C78.5	D01.0	D12.6	D37.4
- - - - with rectum	C19	C78.5	D01.1	D12.7	D37.5
- - - - ascending	C18.2	C78.5	D01.0	D12.2	D37.4
- - - - caput	C18.0	C78.5	D01.0	D12.0	D37.4
- - - - descending	C18.6	C78.5	D01.0	D12.4	D37.4
- - - - distal	C18.7	C78.5	D01.0	D12.5	D37.4
- - - - left	C18.6	C78.5	D01.0	D12.4	D37.4
- - - - pelvic	C18.7	C78.5	D01.0	D12.5	D37.4
- - - - right	C18.2	C78.5	D01.0	D12.2	D37.4
- - - - sigmoid (flexure)	C18.7	C78.5	D01.0	D12.5	D37.4
- - - - transverse	C18.4	C78.5	D01.0	D12.3	D37.4
- - - hepatic flexure	C18.3	C78.5	D01.0	D12.3	D37.4
- - - ileocecum	C18.0	C78.5	D01.0	D12.0	D37.4
- - - sigmoid flexure	C18.7	C78.5	D01.0	D12.5	D37.4
- - - splenic flexure	C18.5	C78.5	D01.0	D12.3	D37.4
- - small	C17.9	C78.4	D01.4	D13.3	D37.2
- - - duodenum	C17.0	C78.4	D01.4	D13.2	D37.2
- - - ileum	C17.2	C78.4	D01.4	D13.3	D37.2
- - - jejunum	C17.1	C78.4	D01.4	D13.3	D37.2
- - tract NEC	C26.0	C78.5	D01.4	D13.9	D37.7
- intra-abdominal	C76.2	C79.8		D36.7	D48.7
- intracranial NEC	C71.9	C79.3		D33.2	D43.2
- intraocular	C69.4	C79.4	D09.2	D31.4	D48.7
- intraorbital	C69.6	C79.4	D09.2	D31.6	D48.7
- intrasellar	C75.1	C79.8	D09.3	D35.2	D44.3
- intrathoracic (cavity) (organs NEC)	C76.1	C79.8		D36.7	D48.7
- iris	C69.4	C79.4	D09.2	D31.4	D48.7
- ischiorectal (fossa)	C76.3	C79.8		D36.7	D48.7
- ischium ◇	C41.4	C79.5		D16.8	D48.0
- island of Reil	C71.0	C79.3		D33.0	D43.0
- islands or islets of Langerhans	C25.4	C78.8	D01.7	D13.7	D37.7
- isthmus uteri	C54.0	C79.8	D07.3	D26.1	D39.0
- jaw	C76.0	C79.8	D09.7	D36.7	D48.7
- - bone	C41.1	C79.5		D16.5	D48.0
- - - lower	C41.1	C79.5		D16.5	D48.0
- - - upper	C41.0	C79.5		D16.4	D48.0
- - carcinoma (any type) (lower) (upper)	C76.0	C79.8			
- - skin	C44.3	C79.2	D04.3	D23.3	D48.5
- - soft tissues	C03.9	C79.8		D10.3	D37.0
- - - lower	C03.1	C79.8		D10.3	D37.0
- - - upper	C03.0	C79.8		D10.3	D37.0
- jejunum	C17.1	C78.4	D01.4	D13.3	D37.2
- joint NEC ◇ (*see also* Neoplasm, bone)	C41.9	C79.5		D16.9	D48.0
- - acromioclavicular ◇	C40.0	C79.5		D16.0	D48.0
- - bursa or synovial membrane – *see* Neoplasm, connective tissue					
- - costovertebral ◇	C41.3	C79.5		D16.7	D48.0

	Malignant			Benign	Uncertain or unknown behavior
	Primary	Secondary	In situ		

Neoplasm, neoplastic—*continued*
- joint—*continued*
- - sternocostal ✧ .... C41.3 | C79.5 | | | D16.7 | D48.0
- - temporomandibular ✧ .... C41.1 | C79.5 | | | D16.5 | D48.0
- junction ....
- - anorectal................................... C21.8 | C78.5 | D01.3 | | D12.9 | D37.7
- - cardioesophageal............................. C16.0 | C78.8 | D00.2 | | D13.1 | D37.1
- - esophagogastric............................. C16.0 | C78.8 | D00.2 | | D13.1 | D37.1
- - gastroesophageal............................. C16.0 | C78.8 | D00.2 | | D13.1 | D37.1
- - hard and soft palate .... C05.8 | C79.8 | D00.0 | | D10.3 | D37.0
- - ileocecal .... C18.0 | C78.5 | D01.0 | | D12.0 | D37.4
- - pelvirectal.................................. C19 | C78.5 | D01.1 | | D12.7 | D37.5
- - pelviureteric .... C65 | C79.0 | D09.1 | | D30.1 | D41.1
- - rectosigmoid.............................. C19 | C78.5 | D01.1 | | D12.7 | D37.5
- - squamocolumnar, of cervix.............. C53.8 | C79.8 | D06.7 | | D26.0 | D39.0
- kidney (parenchyma) .... C64 | C79.0 | D09.1 | | D30.0 | D41.0
- - calyx.................................... C65 | C79.0 | D09.1 | | D30.1 | D41.1
- - hilus..................................... C65 | C79.0 | D09.1 | | D30.1 | D41.1
- - pelvis..................................... C65 | C79.0 | D09.1 | | D30.1 | D41.1
- knee NEC #.................................. C76.5 | C79.8 | D04.7 | | D36.7 | D48.7
- labia (skin) .... C51.9 | C79.8 | D07.1 | | D28.0 | D39.7
- - majora .... C51.0 | C79.8 | D07.1 | | D28.0 | D39.7
- - minora .... C51.1 | C79.8 | D07.1 | | D28.0 | D39.7
- labial (*see also* Neoplasm, lip)............ C00.9 | C79.8 | D00.0 | | D10.0 | D37.0
- - sulcus (lower) (upper) .... C06.1 | C79.8 | D00.0 | | D10.3 | D37.0
- labium (skin)............................... C51.9 | C79.8 | D07.1 | | D28.0 | D39.7
- - majus..................................... C51.0 | C79.8 | D07.1 | | D28.0 | D39.7
- - minus..................................... C51.1 | C79.8 | D07.1 | | D28.0 | D39.7
- lacrimal
- - canaliculi .... C69.5 | C79.4 | D09.2 | | D31.5 | D48.7
- - duct (nasal)............................. C69.5 | C79.4 | D09.2 | | D31.5 | D48.7
- - gland .... C69.5 | C79.4 | D09.2 | | D31.5 | D48.7
- - punctum .... C69.5 | C79.4 | D09.2 | | D31.5 | D48.7
- - sac .... C69.5 | C79.4 | D09.2 | | D31.5 | D48.7
- Langerhans, islands or islets .... C25.4 | C78.8 | D01.7 | | D13.7 | D37.7
- laryngopharynx .... C13.9 | C79.8 | D00.0 | | D10.9 | D37.0
- larynx NEC .... C32.9 | C78.3 | D02.0 | | D14.1 | D38.0
- - cartilage (arytenoid) (cricoid) (cuneiform) (thyroid) .... C32.3 | C78.3 | D02.0 | | D14.1 | D38.0
- - commissure (anterior) (posterior)........... C32.0 | C78.3 | D02.0 | | D14.1 | D38.0
- - extrinsic NEC............................ C32.1 | C78.3 | D02.0 | | D14.1 | D38.0
- - - meaning hypopharynx.................. C13.9 | C79.8 | D00.0 | | D10.7 | D37.0
- - intrinsic .... C32.0 | C78.3 | D02.0 | | D14.1 | D38.0
- - ventricular bands...................... C32.1 | C78.3 | D02.0 | | D14.1 | D38.0
- leg NEC # .... C76.5 | C79.8 | D04.7 | | D36.7 | D48.7
- lens, crystalline .... C69.4 | C79.4 | D09.2 | | D31.4 | D48.7
- lid (lower) (upper)........................ C44.1 | C79.2 | D04.1 | | D23.1 | D48.5

| | Malignant | | | | Uncertain |
	Primary ‹3›	Secondary ‹6›	In situ ‹2›	Benign ‹0›	or unknown behavior ‹1›
Neoplasm, neoplastic—*continued*					
– ligament (*see also* Neoplasm, connective tissue)	C49.9	C79.8		D21.9	D48.1
– – broad	C57.1	C79.8		D28.2	D39.7
– – nonuterine – *see* Neoplasm, connective tissue					
– – round	C57.2	C79.8		D28.2	D39.7
– – sacrouterine	C57.3	C79.8		D28.2	D39.7
– – uterine	C57.3	C79.8		D28.2	D39.7
– – utero-ovarian	C57.1	C79.8		D28.2	D39.7
– – uterosacral	C57.3	C79.8		D28.2	D39.7
– limb #	C76.7	C79.8	D04.8	D36.7	D48.7
– – lower #	C76.5	C79.8	D04.7	D36.7	D48.7
– – upper #	C76.4	C79.8	D04.6	D36.7	D48.7
– limbus of cornea	C69.1	C79.4	D09.2	D31.1	D48.7
– lingual NEC (*see also* Neoplasm, tongue)	C02.9	C79.8	D00.0	D10.1	D37.0
– lingula, lung	C34.1	C78.0	D02.2	D14.3	D38.1
– lip	C00.9	C79.8	D00.0	D10.0	D37.0
– – buccal aspect – *see* Neoplasm, lip, internal					
– – commissure	C00.6	C79.8	D00.0	D10.0	D37.0
– – external	C00.2	C79.8	D00.0	D10.0	D37.0
– – – lower	C00.1	C79.8	D00.0	D10.0	D37.0
– – – upper	C00.0	C79.8	D00.0	D10.0	D37.0
– – frenulum – *see* Neoplasm, lip, internal					
– – inner aspect – *see* Neoplasm, lip, internal					
– – internal	C00.5	C79.8	D00.0	D10.0	D37.0
– – – lower	C00.4	C79.8	D00.0	D10.0	D37.0
– – – upper	C00.3	C79.8	D00.0	D10.0	D37.0
– – lipstick area	C00.2	C79.8	D00.0	D10.0	D37.0
– – – lower	C00.1	C79.8	D00.0	D10.0	D37.0
– – – upper	C00.0	C79.8	D00.0	D10.0	D37.0
– – lower	C00.1	C79.8	D00.0	D10.0	D37.0
– – – internal	C00.4	C79.8	D00.0	D10.0	D37.0
– – mucosa – *see* Neoplasm, lip, internal					
– – oral aspect – *see* Neoplasm, lip, internal					
– – skin (commissure) (lower) (upper)	C44.0	C79.2	D04.0	D23.0	D48.5
– – upper	C00.0	C79.8	D00.0	D10.0	D37.0
– – – internal	C00.3	C79.8	D00.0	D10.0	D37.0
– – vermilion border	C00.2	C79.8	D00.0	D10.0	D37.0
– – – lower	C00.1	C79.8	D00.0	D10.0	D37.0
– – – upper	C00.0	C79.8	D00.0	D10.0	D37.0
– liver	C22.9	C78.7	D01.5	D13.4	D37.6
– – primary	C22.9		D01.5	D13.4	D37.6
– lobe (lung)					
– – azygos	C34.1	C78.0	D02.2	D14.3	D38.1
– – frontal	C71.1	C79.3		D33.0	D43.0
– – lower	C34.3	C78.0	D02.2	D14.3	D38.1
– – middle	C34.2	C78.0	D02.2	D14.3	D38.1
– – occipital	C71.4	C79.3		D33.0	D43.0
– – parietal	C71.3	C79.3		D33.0	D43.0
– – temporal	C71.2	C79.3		D33.0	D43.0

NSCL — Non small cell carcinoma of lung — adenocarcinoma
— Squamous cell ca
— Large cell ca
Small Cell Carcinoma Lung — More rapid growing & spreading forming cancer

INTERNATIONAL CLASSIFICATION OF DISEASES

	Malignant				Uncertain
	Primary	Secondary	In situ	Benign	or unknown behavior
Neoplasm, neoplastic—*continued*					
− lobe (lung) —*continued*					
− − upper	C34.1	C78.0	D02.2	D14.3	D38.1
− lumbosacral plexus	C47.5	C79.8		D36.1	D48.2
− lung	C34.9	C78.0	D02.2	D14.3	D38.1
− − azygos lobe	C34.1	C78.0	D02.2	D14.3	D38.1
− − carina	C34.0	C78.0	D02.2	D14.3	D38.1
− − hilus	C34.0	C78.0	D02.2	D14.3	D38.1
− − lingula	C34.1	C78.0	D02.2	D14.3	D38.1
− − lower lobe	C34.3	C78.0	D02.2	D14.3	D38.1
− − main bronchus	C34.0	C78.0	D02.2	D14.3	D38.1
− − middle lobe	C34.2	C78.0	D02.2	D14.3	D38.1
− − upper lobe	C34.1	C78.0	D02.2	D14.3	D38.1
− lymph, lymphatic					
− − channel NEC (*see also* Neoplasm, connective tissue)	C49.9	C79.8		D21.9	D48.1
− − gland (secondary)		C77.9		D36.0	D48.7
− − − abdominal		C77.2		D36.0	D48.7
− − − aortic		C77.2		D36.0	D48.7
− − − arm		C77.3		D36.0	D48.7
− − − auricular (anterior) (posterior)		C77.0		D36.0	D48.7
− − − axilla, axillary		C77.3		D36.0	D48.7
− − − brachial		C77.3		D36.0	D48.7
− − − bronchial		C77.1		D36.0	D48.7
− − − bronchopulmonary		C77.1		D36.0	D48.7
− − − celiac		C77.2		D36.0	D48.7
− − − cervical		C77.0		D36.0	D48.7
− − − cervicofacial		C77.0		D36.0	D48.7
− − − Cloquet		C77.4		D36.0	D48.7
− − − colic		C77.2		D36.0	D48.7
− − − common duct		C77.2		D36.0	D48.7
− − − cubital		C77.3		D36.0	D48.7
− − − diaphragmatic		C77.1		D36.0	D48.7
− − − epigastric, inferior		C77.5		D36.0	D48.7
− − − epitrochlear		C77.3		D36.0	D48.7
− − − esophageal		C77.1		D36.0	D48.7
− − − face		C77.0		D36.0	D48.7
− − − femoral		C77.4		D36.0	D48.7
− − − gastric		C77.2		D36.0	D48.7
− − − groin		C77.4		D36.0	D48.7
− − − head		C77.0		D36.0	D48.7
− − − hepatic		C77.2		D36.0	D48.7
− − − hilar (pulmonary)		C77.1		D36.0	D48.7
− − − − splenic		C77.2		D36.0	D48.7
− − − hypogastric		C77.5		D36.0	D48.7
− − − ileocolic		C77.2		D36.0	D48.7
− − − iliac		C77.5		D36.0	D48.7
− − − infraclavicular		C77.3		D36.0	D48.7
− − − inguina, inguinal		C77.4		D36.0	D48.7
− − − innominate		C77.1		D36.0	D48.7
− − − intercostal		C77.1		D36.0	D48.7
− − − intestinal		C77.2		D36.0	D48.7

ALPHABETICAL INDEX TO DISEASES AND NATURE OF INJURY

| | Malignant | | | | Uncertain |
	Primary 3	Secondary 6	In situ 2	Benign 0	or unknown behavior
Neoplasm, neoplastic—*continued*					
– lymph, lymphatic—*continued*					
– – gland (secondary) —*continued*					
– – – intra-abdominal	C77.2			D36.0	D48.7
– – – intrapelvic	C77.5			D36.0	D48.7
– – – intrathoracic	C77.1			D36.0	D48.7
– – – jugular	C77.0			D36.0	D48.7
– – – leg	C77.4			D36.0	D48.7
– – – limb					
– – – – lower	C77.4			D36.0	D48.7
– – – – upper	C77.3			D36.0	D48.7
– – – lower limb	C77.4			D36.0	D48.7
– – – lumbar	C77.2			D36.0	D48.7
– – – mandibular	C77.0			D36.0	D48.7
– – – mediastinal	C77.1			D36.0	D48.7
– – – mesenteric (inferior) (superior)	C77.2			D36.0	D48.7
– – – midcolic	C77.2			D36.0	D48.7
– – – multiple sites in categories C77.0-C77.5	C77.8			D36.0	D48.7
– – – neck	C77.0			D36.0	D48.7
– – – obturator	C77.5			D36.0	D48.7
– – – occipital	C77.0			D36.0	D48.7
– – – pancreatic	C77.2			D36.0	D48.7
– – – para-aortic	C77.2			D36.0	D48.7
– – – paracervical	C77.5			D36.0	D48.7
– – – parametrial	C77.5			D36.0	D48.7
– – – parasternal	C77.1			D36.0	D48.7
– – – parotid	C77.0			D36.0	D48.7
– – – pectoral	C77.3			D36.0	D48.7
– – – pelvic	C77.5			D36.0	D48.7
– – – periaortic	C77.2			D36.0	D48.7
– – – peripancreatic	C77.2			D36.0	D48.7
– – – popliteal	C77.4			D36.0	D48.7
– – – porta hepatis	C77.2			D36.0	D48.7
– – – portal	C77.2			D36.0	D48.7
– – – preauricular	C77.0			D36.0	D48.7
– – – prelaryngeal	C77.0			D36.0	D48.7
– – – presymphysial	C77.5			D36.0	D48.7
– – – pretracheal	C77.0			D36.0	D48.7
– – – primary NEC	C96.9				
– – – pulmonary (hilar)	C77.1			D36.0	D48.7
– – – pyloric	C77.2			D36.0	D48.7
– – – retroperitoneal	C77.2			D36.0	D48.7
– – – retropharyngeal	C77.0			D36.0	D48.7
– – – Rosenmüller's	C77.4			D36.0	D48.7
– – – sacral	C77.5			D36.0	D48.7
– – – scalene	C77.0			D36.0	D48.7
– – – splenic (hilar)	C77.2			D36.0	D48.7
– – – subclavicular	C77.3			D36.0	D48.7
– – – subinguinal	C77.4			D36.0	D48.7
– – – sublingual	C77.0			D36.0	D48.7
– – – submandibular	C77.0			D36.0	D48.7

| | Malignant | | | | Uncertain |
	Primary	Secondary	In situ	Benign	or unknown behavior
Neoplasm, neoplastic—*continued*					
– lymph, lymphatic—*continued*					
– – gland (secondary) —*continued*					
– – – submaxillary...		C77.0		D36.0	D48.7
– – – submental		C77.0		D36.0	D48.7
– – – subscapular...		C77.3		D36.0	D48.7
– – – supraclavicular		C77.0		D36.0	D48.7
– – – thoracic...		C77.1		D36.0	D48.7
– – – tibial		C77.4		D36.0	D48.7
– – – tracheal...		C77.1		D36.0	D48.7
– – – tracheobronchial....................................		C77.1		D36.0	D48.7
– – – upper limb		C77.3		D36.0	D48.7
– – – Virchow's		C77.0		D36.0	D48.7
– – node – *see also* Neoplasm, lymph gland					
– – – primary – code morphological type, behavior and site	C96.9				
– – vessel (*see also* Neoplasm, connective tissue)..	C49.9	C79.8		D21.9	D48.1
– mammary gland – *see* Neoplasm, breast					
– mandible	C41.1	C79.5		D16.5	D48.0
– – alveolar					
– – – carcinoma (mucosa)	C03.1	C79.8			
– – – mucosa	C03.1	C79.8	D00.0	D10.3	D37.0
– – – ridge or process	C41.1	C79.5		D16.5	D48.0
– marrow (bone)...	C96.9	C79.5			D47.9
– mastoid (air cell) (antrum) (cavity)	C30.1	C78.3	D02.3	D14.0	D38.5
– – bone or process ✧	C41.0	C79.5		D16.4	D48.0
– maxilla, maxillary (superior).......................	C41.0	C79.5		D16.4	D48.0
– – alveolar					
– – – carcinoma (mucosa)	C03.0	C79.8			
– – – mucosa	C03.0	C79.8	D00.0	D10.3	D37.0
– – – ridge or process	C41.0	C79.5		D16.4	D48.0
– – antrum	C31.0	C78.3	D02.3	D14.0	D38.5
– – carcinoma...	C03.0	C79.8			
– – inferior – *see* Neoplasm, mandible					
– – sinus..	C31.0	C78.3	D02.3	D14.0	D38.5
– meatus, external (ear).................................	C44.2	C79.2	D04.2	D23.2	D48.5
– Meckel's diverticulum................................	C17.3	C78.4	D01.4	D13.3	D37.2
– mediastinum, mediastinal............................	C38.3	C78.1		D15.2	D38.3
– – anterior...	C38.1	C78.1		D15.2	D38.3
– – posterior	C38.2	C78.1		D15.2	D38.3
– medulla					
– – adrenal..	C74.1	C79.7	D09.3	D35.0	D44.1
– – oblongata..	C71.7	C79.3		D33.1	D43.1
– meibomian gland..	C44.1	C79.2	D04.1	D23.1	D48.5
– meninges	C70.9	C79.4		D32.9	D42.9
– – brain	C70.0	C79.3		D32.0	D42.0
– – cerebral	C70.0	C79.3		D32.0	D42.0
– – cranial	C70.0	C79.3		D32.0	D42.0
– – intracranial	C70.0	C79.3		D32.0	D42.0
– – spinal (cord)...	C70.1	C79.4		D32.1	D42.1
– meniscus, knee joint (lateral) (medial) ✧	C40.2	C79.5		D16.2	D48.0

	Malignant				Uncertain
	Primary *3*	Secondary *6*	In situ *2*	Benign *O*	or unknown behavior *|*

Neoplasm, neoplastic—*continued*

	Primary	Secondary	In situ	Benign	Uncertain or unknown behavior
– mesentery, mesenteric	C48.1	C78.6		D20.1	D48.4
– mesoappendix	C48.1	C78.6		D20.1	D48.4
– mesocolon	C48.1	C78.6		D20.1	D48.4
– mesopharynx – *see* Neoplasm, oropharynx					
– mesosalpinx	C57.1	C79.8		D28.2	D39.7
– mesovarium	C57.1	C79.8	D07.3	D28.2	D39.7
– metacarpus (any bone) ✧	C40.1	C79.5		D16.1	D48.0
– metastatic (multiple)		*C79.9*			
– – primary site not indicated	~~C80.9~~	~~C79.9~~			
– – primary site unknown, so stated	~~C80.0~~	~~C79.9~~			
– metatarsus (any bone) ✧	C40.3	C79.5		D16.3	D48.0
– midbrain	C71.7	C79.3		D33.1	D43.1
– mons					
– – pubis	C51.9	C79.8	D07.1	D28.0	D39.7
– – veneris	C51.9	C79.8	D07.1	D28.0	D39.7
– mouth	C06.9	C79.8	D00.0	D10.3	D37.0
– – floor	C04.9	C79.8	D00.0	D10.2	D37.0
– – – anterior	C04.0	C79.8	D00.0	D10.2	D37.0
– – – lateral	C04.1	C79.8	D00.0	D10.2	D37.0
– – roof	C05.9	C79.8	D00.0	D10.3	D37.0
– – specified part NEC	C06.8	C79.8	D00.0	D10.3	D37.0
– – vestibule	C06.1	C79.8	D00.0	D10.3	D37.0
– mucosa					
– – alveolar (ridge or process)	C03.9	C79.8	D00.0	D10.3	D37.0
– – – lower	C03.1	C79.8	D00.0	D10.3	D37.0
– – – upper	C03.0	C79.8	D00.0	D10.3	D37.0
– – buccal	C06.0	C79.8	D00.0	D10.3	D37.0
– – cheek	C06.0	C79.8	D00.0	D10.3	D37.0
– – lip – *see* Neoplasm, lip, internal					
– – nasal	C30.0	C78.3	D02.3	D14.0	D38.5
– – oral NEC	C06.9	C79.8	D00.0	D10.3	D37.0
– Müllerian duct					
– – female	C57.7	C79.8	D07.3	D28.7	D39.7
– – male	C63.7	C79.8	D07.6	D29.7	D40.7
– multiple, malignant (independent primary sites) – – *independent primary sites* C97	*C97* NEC / *secondary NEC*	*C79.9*			
– muscle – *see also* Neoplasm, connective tissue	C49.9	C79.8		D21.9	D48.1
– – extraocular	C69.6	C79.4	D09.2	D31.6	D48.7
– myocardium	C38.0	C79.8		D15.1	D48.7
– myometrium	C54.2	C79.8		D26.1	D39.0
– Nabothian gland (follicle)	C53.0	C79.8	D06.0	D26.0	D39.0
– nares, naris (anterior) (posterior)	C30.0	C78.3	D02.3	D14.0	D38.5
– nasal – *see* Neoplasm, nose					
– nasolabial groove	C44.3	C79.2	D04.3	D23.3	D48.5
– nasolacrimal duct	C69.5	C79.4	D09.2	D31.5	D48.7
– nasopharynx	C11.9	C79.8	D00.0	D10.6	D37.0
– – floor	C11.3	C79.8	D00.0	D10.6	D37.0
– – roof	C11.0	C79.8	D00.0	D10.6	D37.0

| | Malignant | | | | Uncertain |
	Primary	Secondary	In situ	Benign	or unknown behavior
Neoplasm, neoplastic—*continued*					
– nasopharynx—*continued*					
– – wall	C11.9	C79.8	D00.0	D10.6	D37.0
– – – anterior	C11.3	C79.8	D00.0	D10.6	D37.0
– – – lateral ,,....	C11.2	C79.8	D00.0	D10.6	D37.0
– – – posterior	C11.1	C79.8	D00.0	D10.6	D37.0
– – – superior	C11.0	C79.8	D00.0	D10.6	D37.0
– neck NEC #	C76.0	C79.8	D09.7	D36.7	D48.7
– nerve (ganglion)	C47.9	C79.8		D36.1	D48.2
– – abducens	C72.5	C79.4		D33.3	D43.3
– – accessory (spinal)	C72.5	C79.4		D33.3	D43.3
– – acoustic	C72.4	C79.4		D33.3	D43.3
– – auditory	C72.4	C79.4		D33.3	D43.3
– – autonomic NEC (*see also* Neoplasm, nerve, peripheral)	C47.9	C79.8		D36.1	D48.2
– – brachial	C47.1	C79.8		D36.1	D48.2
– – cranial, NEC	C72.5	C79.4		D33.3	D43.3
– – facial	C72.5	C79.4		D33.3	D43.3
– – femoral	C47.2	C79.8		D36.1	D48.2
– – ganglion NEC (*see also* Neoplasm, nerve, peripheral)	C47.9	C79.8		D36.1	D48.2
– – glossopharyngeal	C72.5	C79.4		D33.3	D43.3
– – hypoglossal	C72.5	C79.4		D33.3	D43.3
– – intercostal	C47.3	C79.8		D36.1	D48.2
– – lumbar	C47.6	C79.8		D36.1	D48.2
– – median	C47.1	C79.8		D36.1	D48.2
– – obturator	C47.2	C79.8		D36.1	D48.2
– – oculomotor	C72.5	C79.4		D33.3	D43.3
– – olfactory	C72.2	C79.4		D33.3	D43.3
– – optic	C72.3	C79.4		D33.3	D43.3
– – parasympathetic NEC (*see also* Neoplasm, nerve, peripheral)	C47.9	C79.8		D36.1	D48.2
– – peripheral NEC	C47.9	C79.8		D36.1	D48.2
– – – abdomen	C47.4	C79.8		D36.1	D48.2
– – – abdominal wall	C47.4	C79.8		D36.1	D48.2
– – – ankle	C47.2	C79.8		D36.1	D48.2
– – – antecubital fossa or space	C47.1	C79.8		D36.1	D48.2
– – – arm	C47.1	C79.8		D36.1	D48.2
– – – auricle (ear)	C47.0	C79.8		D36.1	D48.2
– – – axilla	C47.3	C79.8		D36.1	D48.2
– – – back	C47.6	C79.8		D36.1	D48.2
– – – buttock	C47.5	C79.8		D36.1	D48.2
– – – calf	C47.2	C79.8		D36.1	D48.2
– – – cervical region	C47.0	C79.8		D36.1	D48.2
– – – cheek	C47.0	C79.8		D36.1	D48.2
– – – chest (wall)	C47.3	C79.8		D36.1	D48.2
– – – chin	C47.0	C79.8		D36.1	D48.2
– – – ear (external)	C47.0	C79.8		D36.1	D48.2
– – – elbow	C47.1	C79.8		D36.1	D48.2
– – – extrarectal	C47.5	C79.8		D36.1	D48.2

| | Malignant | | | | Uncertain |
	Primary 3	Secondary 6	In situ 0	Benign 2	or unknown behavior 1
Neoplasm, neoplastic—*continued*					
– nerve (ganglion) —*continued*					
– – peripheral—*continued*					
– – – extremity	C47.9	C79.8		D36.1	D48.2
– – – – lower	C47.2	C79.8		D36.1	D48.2
– – – – upper	C47.1	C79.8		D36.1	D48.2
– – – eyelid	C47.0	C79.8		D36.1	D48.2
– – – face	C47.0	C79.8		D36.1	D48.2
– – – finger	C47.1	C79.8		D36.1	D48.2
– – – flank	C47.6	C79.8		D36.1	D48.2
– – – foot	C47.2	C79.8		D36.1	D48.2
– – – forearm	C47.1	C79.8		D36.1	D48.2
– – – forehead	C47.0	C79.8		D36.1	D48.2
– – – gluteal region	C47.5	C79.8		D36.1	D48.2
– – – groin	C47.5	C79.8		D36.1	D48.2
– – – hand	C47.1	C79.8		D36.1	D48.2
– – – head	C47.0	C79.8		D36.1	D48.2
– – – heel	C47.2	C79.8		D36.1	D48.2
– – – hip	C47.2	C79.8		D36.1	D48.2
– – – infraclavicular region	C47.3	C79.8		D36.1	D48.2
– – – inguinal (canal) (region)	C47.5	C79.8		D36.1	D48.2
– – – intrathoracic	C47.3	C79.8		D36.1	D48.2
– – – ischiorectal fossa	C47.5	C79.8		D36.1	D48.2
– – – knee	C47.2	C79.8		D36.1	D48.2
– – – leg	C47.2	C79.8		D36.1	D48.2
– – – limb NEC	C47.9	C79.8		D36.1	D48.2
– – – – lower	C47.2	C79.8		D36.1	D48.2
– – – – upper	C47.1	C79.8		D36.1	D48.2
– – – nates	C47.5	C79.8		D36.1	D48.2
– – – neck	C47.0	C79.8		D36.1	D48.2
– – – orbit	C69.6	C79.4		D31.6	D48.7
– – – pararectal	C47.5	C79.8		D36.1	D48.2
– – – paraurethral	C47.5	C79.8		D36.1	D48.2
– – – paravaginal	C47.5	C79.8		D36.1	D48.2
– – – pelvis (floor)	C47.5	C79.8		D36.1	D48.2
– – – pelvoabdominal	C47.8	C79.8		D36.1	D48.2
– – – perineum	C47.5	C79.8		D36.1	D48.2
– – – perirectal (tissue)	C47.5	C79.8		D36.1	D48.2
– – – periurethral (tissue)	C47.5	C79.8		D36.1	D48.2
– – – popliteal fossa or space	C47.2	C79.8		D36.1	D48.2
– – – presacral	C47.5	C79.8		D36.1	D48.2
– – – pterygoid fossa	C47.0	C79.8		D36.1	D48.2
– – – rectovaginal septum or wall	C47.5	C79.8		D36.1	D48.2
– – – rectovesical	C47.5	C79.8		D36.1	D48.2
– – – sacrococcygeal region	C47.5	C79.8		D36.1	D48.2
– – – scalp	C47.0	C79.8		D36.1	D48.2
– – – scapular region	C47.3	C79.8		D36.1	D48.2
– – – shoulder	C47.1	C79.8		D36.1	D48.2
– – – submental	C47.0	C79.8		D36.1	D48.2
– – – supraclavicular region	C47.0	C79.8		D36.1	D48.2
– – – temple	C47.0	C79.8		D36.1	D48.2
– – – temporal region	C47.0	C79.8		D36.1	D48.2

	Malignant				Uncertain
	Primary	Secondary	In situ	Benign	or unknown behavior

Neoplasm, neoplastic—*continued*
- nerve (ganglion) —*continued*
-   - peripheral—*continued*

- - - thigh	C47.2	C79.8		D36.1	D48.2
- - - thoracic (duct) (wall)	C47.3	C79.8		D36.1	D48.2
- - - thorax	C47.3	C79.8		D36.1	D48.2
- - - thumb	C47.1	C79.8		D36.1	D48.2
- - - toe	C47.2	C79.8		D36.1	D48.2
- - - trunk	C47.6	C79.8		D36.1	D48.2
- - - umbilicus	C47.4	C79.8		D36.1	D48.2
- - - vesicorectal	C47.5	C79.8		D36.1	D48.2
- - - wrist	C47.1	C79.8		D36.1	D48.2
- - radial	C47.1	C79.8		D36.1	D48.2
- - sacral	C47.5	C79.8		D36.1	D48.2
- - sciatic	C47.2	C79.8		D36.1	D48.2
- - spinal NEC	C47.9	C79.8		D36.1	D48.2
- - - accessory	C72.5	C79.4		D33.3	D43.3
- - sympathetic NEC (*see also* Neoplasm, nerve, peripheral)	C47.9	C79.8		D36.1	D48.2
- - trigeminal	C72.5	C79.4		D33.3	D43.3
- - trochlear	C72.5	C79.4		D33.3	D43.3
- - ulnar	C47.1	C79.8		D36.1	D48.2
- - vagus	C72.5	C79.4		D33.3	D43.3
- nervous system (central) NEC	C72.9	C79.4		D33.9	D43.9
- - autonomic – *see* Neoplasm, nerve, peripheral					
- - parasympathetic – *see* Neoplasm, nerve, peripheral					
- - sympathetic – *see* Neoplasm, nerve, peripheral					
- nipple	C50.0	C79.8	D05.9	D24	D48.6
- nose, nasal	C76.0	C79.8	D04.3	D36.7	D48.7
- - ala (external)	C44.3	C79.2	D04.3	D23.3	D48.5
- - bone ◇	C41.0	C79.5		D16.4	D48.0
- - cartilage	C30.0	C78.3	D02.3	D14.0	D38.5
- - cavity	C30.0	C78.3	D02.3	D14.0	D38.5
- - choana	C11.3	C79.8	D00.0	D10.6	D37.0
- - external (skin)	C44.3	C79.2	D04.3	D23.3	D48.5
- - fossa	C30.0	C78.3	D02.3	D14.0	D38.5
- - internal	C30.0	C78.3	D02.3	D14.0	D38.5
- - mucosa	C30.0	C78.3	D02.3	D14.0	D38.5
- - septum	C30.0	C78.3	D02.3	D14.0	D38.5
- - - posterior margin	C11.3	C79.8	D00.0	D10.6	D37.0
- - sinus – *see* Neoplasm, sinus					
- - skin	C44.3	C79.2	D04.3	D23.3	D48.5
- - turbinate (mucosa)	C30.0	C78.3	D02.3	D14.0	D38.5
- - - bone ◇	C41.0	C79.5		D16.4	D48.0
- - vestibule	C30.0	C78.3	D02.3	D14.0	D38.5
- nostril	C30.0	C78.3	D02.3	D14.0	D38.5
- nucleus pulposus ◇	C41.2	C79.5		D16.6	D48.0
- occipital lobe or pole	C71.4	C79.3		D33.0	D43.0
- odontogenic – *see* Neoplasm, jaw, bone					

| | Malignant | | | | Uncertain |
	Primary 3	Secondary 6	In situ 0	Benign 2	or unknown behavior 1
Neoplasm, neoplastic—*continued*					
– oesophagus – *see* Neoplasm, esophagus					
– olfactory nerve or bulb	C72.2	C79.4		D33.3	D43.3
– olive (brain)	C71.7	C79.3		D33.1	D43.1
– omentum	C48.1	C78.6		D20.1	D48.4
– operculum (brain)	C71.0	C79.3		D33.0	D43.0
– optic nerve, chiasm or tract	C72.3	C79.4		D33.3	D43.3
– oral (cavity)	C06.9	C79.8	D00.0	D10.3	D37.0
– – mucosa NEC	C06.9	C79.8	D00.0	D10.3	D37.0
– orbit	C69.6	C79.4	D09.2	D31.6	D48.7
– – autonomic nerve	C69.6	C79.4		D31.6	D48.7
– – bone ✧	C41.0	C79.5		D16.4	D48.0
– – peripheral nerves	C69.6	C79.4		D31.6	D48.7
– – soft parts	C69.6	C79.4		D31.6	D48.7
– organ of Zuckerkandl	C75.5	C79.8		D35.6	D44.7
– oropharynx	C10.9	C79.8	D00.0	D10.5	D37.0
– – junctional region	C10.8	C79.8	D00.0	D10.5	D37.0
– – lateral wall	C10.2	C79.8	D00.0	D10.5	D37.0
– – posterior wall	C10.3	C79.8	D00.0	D10.5	D37.0
– os					
– – external	C53.1	C79.8	D06.1	D26.0	D39.0
– – internal	C53.0	C79.8	D06.0	D26.0	D39.0
– ovary	C56	C79.6	D07.3	D27	D39.1
– oviduct	C57.0	C79.8	D07.3	D28.2	D39.7
– palate	C05.9	C79.8	D00.0	D10.3	D37.0
– – hard	C05.0	C79.8	D00.0	D10.3	D37.0
– – junction of hard and soft	C05.8	C79.8	D00.0	D10.3	D37.0
– – soft	C05.1	C79.8	D00.0	D10.3	D37.0
– – – nasopharyngeal surface	C11.3	C79.8	D00.0	D10.6	D37.0
– – – posterior surface	C11.3	C79.8	D00.0	D10.6	D37.0
– – – superior surface	C11.3	C79.8	D00.0	D10.6	D37.0
– palatoglossal arch	C09.1	C79.8	D00.0	D10.5	D37.0
– palatopharyngeal arch	C09.1	C79.8	D00.0	D10.5	D37.0
– pallium (brain)	C71.0	C79.3		D33.0	D43.0
– palpebra	C44.1	C79.2	D04.1	D23.1	D48.5
– pancreas	C25.9	C78.8	D01.7	D13.6	D37.7
– – body	C25.1	C78.8	D01.7	D13.6	D37.7
– – duct (of Santorini) (of Wirsung)	C25.3	C78.8	D01.7	D13.6	D37.7
– – head	C25.0	C78.8	D01.7	D13.6	D37.7
– – islet cells	C25.4	C78.8	D01.7	D13.7	D37.7
– – neck	C25.7	C78.8	D01.7	D13.6	D37.7
– – tail	C25.2	C78.8	D01.7	D13.6	D37.7
– para-aortic body	C75.5	C79.8		D35.6	D44.7
– paraganglion NEC	C75.5	C79.8		D35.6	D44.7
– parametrium	C57.3	C79.8		D28.2	D39.7
– paranephric	C48.0	C78.6		D20.0	D48.3
– pararectal	C76.3	C79.8		D36.7	D48.7
– parasellar	C71.9	C79.3		D33.2	D43.2
– parathyroid (gland)	C75.0	C79.8	D09.3	D35.1	D44.2
– paraurethral	C76.3	C79.8		D36.7	D48.7
– – gland	C68.1	C79.1	D09.1	D30.7	D41.7
– paravaginal	C76.3	C79.8		D36.7	D48.7

461

Malignant neoplasm of pharynx + cervical oesophagus (point of origin cannot be determined)- C76.8

| | Malignant | | | | Uncertain |
	Primary	Secondary	In situ	Benign	or unknown behaviour
Neoplasm, neoplastic—*continued*					
− parenchyma, kidney	C64	C79.0	D09.1	D30.0	D41.0
− parietal lobe	C71.3	C79.3		D33.0	D43.0
− parotid (duct) (gland)	C07	C79.8	D00.0	D11.0	D37.0
− parovarium	C57.1	C79.8	D07.3	D28.2	D39.7
− patella ✧	C40.3	C79.5		D16.3	D48.0
− peduncle, cerebral	C71.7	C79.3		D33.1	D43.1
− pelvirectal junction	C19	C78.5	D01.1	D12.7	D37.5
− pelvis, pelvic	C76.3	C79.8	D09.7	D36.7	D48.7
− − bone ✧	C41.4	C79.5		D16.8	D48.0
− − floor	C76.3	C79.8	D09.7	D36.7	D48.7
− − renal	C65	C79.0	D09.1	D30.1	D41.1
− − viscera	C76.3	C79.8		D36.7	D48.7
− − wall	C76.3	C79.8	D09.7	D36.7	D48.7
− pelvoabdominal	C76.8	C79.8	D09.7	D36.7	D48.7
− penis	C60.9	C79.8	D07.4	D29.0	D40.7
− − body	C60.2	C79.8	D07.4	D29.0	D40.7
− − corpus (cavernosum)	C60.2	C79.8	D07.4	D29.0	D40.7
− − glans	C60.1	C79.8	D07.4	D29.0	D40.7
− − skin NEC	C60.9	C79.8	D07.4	D29.0	D40.7
− periadrenal	C48.0	C78.6		D20.0	D48.3
− periampullary	C24.1	C78.8	D01.5	D13.5	D37.6
− perianal (skin)	C44.5	C79.2	D04.5	D23.5	D48.5
− pericardium	C38.0	C79.8		D15.1	D48.7
− perinephric	C48.0	C78.6		D20.0	D48.3
− perineum	C76.3	C79.8	D09.7	D36.7	D48.7
− periodontal tissue NEC	C03.9	C79.8	D00.0	D10.3	D37.0
− periosteum – *see* Neoplasm, bone					
− peripancreatic	C48.0	C78.6		D20.0	D48.3
− peripheral nerve NEC	C47.9	C79.8		D36.1	D48.2
− perirectal (tissue)	C76.3	C79.8		D36.7	D48.7
− perirenal (tissue)	C48.0	C78.6		D20.0	D48.3
− peritoneal cavity	C48.2	C78.6		D20.1	D48.4
− peritoneum	C48.2	C78.6		D20.1	D48.4
− − parietal	C48.1	C78.6		D20.1	D48.4
− − pelvic	C48.1	C78.6		D20.1	D48.4
− − specified part NEC	C48.1	C78.6		D20.1	D48.4
− periurethral tissue	C76.3	C79.8		D36.7	D48.7
− phalanges ✧	C40.9	C79.5		D16.9	D48.0
− − foot ✧	C40.3	C79.5		D16.3	D48.0
− − hand ✧	C40.1	C79.5		D16.1	D48.0
− pharynx, pharyngeal	C14.0	C79.8	D00.0	D10.9	D37.0
− − fornix	C11.3	C79.8	D00.0	D10.6	D37.0
− − recess	C11.2	C79.8	D00.0	D10.6	D37.0
− − region	C14.0	C79.8	D00.0	D10.9	D37.0
− − tonsil	C11.1	C79.8	D00.0	D10.6	D37.0
− − wall (lateral) (posterior)	C14.0	C79.8	D00.0	D10.9	D37.0
− pia mater	C70.9	C79.4		D32.9	D42.9
− − cerebral	C70.0	C79.3		D32.0	D42.0
− − cranial	C70.0	C79.3		D32.0	D42.0
− − spinal	C70.1	C79.4		D32.1	D42.1
− pillars of fauces	C09.1	C79.8	D00.0	D10.5	D37.0

462

	Malignant		In situ	Benign	Uncertain or unknown behavior
	Primary 3	Secondary 6	2	0	1

Neoplasm, neoplastic—*continued*

– pineal (body) (gland)	C75.3	C79.8		D35.4	D44.5
– pinna (ear) NEC	C44.2	C79.2	D04.2	D23.2	D48.5
– piriform fossa or sinus	C12	C79.8	D00.0	D10.7	D37.0
– pituitary (body) (fossa) (gland) (lobe)	C75.1	C79.8	D09.3	D35.2	D44.3
– placenta	C58	C79.8	D07.3	D26.7	D39.2
– pleura, pleural (cavity)	C38.4	C78.2		D15.7	D38.2
– – parietal	C38.4	C78.2		D15.7	D38.2
– – visceral	C38.4	C78.2		D15.7	D38.2
– plexus					
– – brachial	C47.1	C79.8		D36.1	D48.2
– – cervical	C47.0	C79.8		D36.1	D48.2
– – choroid	C71.5	C79.3		D33.0	D43.0
– – lumbosacral	C47.5	C79.8		D36.1	D48.2
– – sacral	C47.5	C79.8		D36.1	D48.2
– pluriendocrine	C75.8	C79.8	D09.3	D35.8	D44.8
– pole					
– – frontal	C71.1	C79.3		D33.0	D43.0
– – occipital	C71.4	C79.3		D33.0	D43.0
– pons (varolii)	C71.7	C79.3		D33.1	D43.1
– popliteal fossa or space #	C76.5	C79.8	D04.7	D36.7	D48.7
– postcricoid (region)	C13.0	C79.8	D00.0	D10.7	D37.0
– posterior fossa (cranial)	C71.9	C79.3		D33.2	D43.2
– postnasal space	C11.9	C79.8	D00.0	D10.6	D37.0
– prepuce	C60.0	C79.8	D07.4	D29.0	D40.7
– prepylorus	C16.4	C78.8	D00.2	D13.1	D37.1
– presacral (region)	C76.3	C79.8		D36.7	D48.7
– ✓ primary site unknown, so stated	C80.0	C79.9			
– prostate (gland)	C61	C79.8	D07.5	D29.1	D40.0
– pterygoid fossa NEC	C49.0	C79.8		D21.0	D48.1
– – autonomic nervous system	C47.0	C79.8		D36.1	D48.2
– – connective tissue	C49.0	C79.8		D21.0	D48.1
– – fibrous tissue	C49.0	C79.8		D21.0	D48.1
– – peripheral nerve	C47.0	C79.8		D36.1	D48.2
– – soft tissue	C49.0	C79.8		D21.0	D48.1
– pubic bone ✧	C41.4	C79.5		D16.8	D48.0
– pudenda, pudendum (female)	C51.9	C79.8	D07.1	D28.0	D39.7
– pulmonary (*see also* Neoplasm, lung)	C34.9	C78.0	D02.2	D14.3	D38.1
– putamen	C71.0	C79.3		D33.0	D43.0
– pyloric					
– – antrum	C16.3	C78.8	D00.2	D13.1	D37.1
– – canal	C16.4	C78.8	D00.2	D13.1	D37.1
– pylorus	C16.4	C78.8	D00.2	D13.1	D37.1
– pyramid (brain)	C71.7	C79.3		D33.1	D43.1
– pyriform fossa or sinus	C12	C79.8	D00.0	D10.7	D37.0
– radius (any part) ✧	C40.0	C79.5		D16.0	D48.0
– Rathke's pouch	C75.1	C79.8	D09.3	D35.2	D44.3
– rectosigmoid (colon) (junction)	C19	C78.5	D01.1	D12.7	D37.5
– rectouterine pouch	C48.1	C78.6		D20.1	D48.4
– rectovaginal septum or wall	C76.3	C79.8	D09.7	D36.7	D48.7
– rectovesical septum	C76.3	C79.8	D09.7	D36.7	D48.7

| | Malignant | | | | Uncertain |
	Primary	Secondary	In situ	Benign	or unknown behavior
Neoplasm, neoplastic—*continued*					
– rectum (ampulla)	C20	C78.5	D01.2	D12.8	D37.5
– – with colon	C19	C78.5	D01.1	D12.7	D37.5
– renal	C64	C79.0	D09.1	D30.0	D41.0
– – calyx	C65	C79.0	D09.1	D30.1	D41.1
hilus	C65	C79.0	D09.1	D30.1	D41.1
– – pelvis	C65	C79.0	D09.1	D30.1	D41.1
– respiratory					
– – organs or system NEC	C39.9	C78.3	D02.4	D14.4	D38.6
– – tract NEC	C39.9	C78.3	D02.4	D14.4	D38.6
– – – upper	C39.0	C78.3	D02.4	D14.4	D38.6
– retina	C69.2	C79.4	D09.2	D31.2	D48.7
– retrobulbar	C69.6	C79.4		D31.6	D48.7
– retrocecal	C48.0	C78.6		D20.0	D48.3
– retromolar (area) (triangle) (trigone)	C06.2	C79.8	D00.0	D10.3	D37.0
– retroperitoneal (space) (tissue)	C48.0	C78.6		D20.0	D48.3
– retroperitoneum	C48.0	C78.6		D20.0	D48.3
– retropharyngeal	C14.0	C79.8	D00.0	D10.9	D37.0
– retrovesical	C76.3	C79.8		D36.7	D48.7
– rhinencephalon	C71.0	C79.3		D33.0	D43.0
– rib ✧	C41.3	C79.5		D16.7	D48.0
– Rosenmüller's fossa	C11.2	C79.8	D00.0	D10.6	D37.0
– round ligament	C57.2	C79.8		D28.2	D39.7
– sacrococcyx, sacrococcygeal ✧	C41.4	C79.5		D16.8	D48.0
– – region	C76.3	C79.8	D09.7	D36.7	D48.7
– sacrouterine ligament	C57.3	C79.8		D28.2	D39.7
– sacrum, sacral (vertebra) ✧	C41.4	C79.5		D16.8	D48.0
– salivary gland or duct (major)	C08.9	C79.8	D00.0	D11.9	D37.0
– – minor NEC	C06.9	C79.8	D00.0	D10.3	D37.0
– – parotid	C07	C79.8	D00.0	D11.0	D37.0
– – sublingual	C08.1	C79.8	D00.0	D11.7	D37.0
– – submandibular	C08.0	C79.8	D00.0	D11.7	D37.0
– – submaxillary	C08.0	C79.8	D00.0	D11.7	D37.0
– salpinx	C57.0	C79.8	D07.3	D28.2	D39.7
– Santorini's duct	C25.3	C78.8	D01.7	D13.6	D37.7
– scalp	C44.4	C79.2	D04.4	D23.4	D48.5
– scapula (any part) ✧	C40.0	C79.5		D16.0	D48.0
– scapular region #	C76.1	C79.8	D04.5	D36.7	D48.7
– sclera	C69.4	C79.4	D09.2	D31.4	D48.7
– scrotum	C63.2	C79.8	D07.6	D29.4	D40.7
– sebaceous gland – *see* Neoplasm, skin					
– sella turcica, bone ✧	C41.0	C79.5		D16.4	D48.0
– seminal vesicle	C63.7	C79.8	D07.6	D29.7	D40.7
– septum					
– – nasal	C30.0	C78.3	D02.3	D14.0	D38.5
– – – posterior margin	C11.3	C79.8	D00.0	D10.6	D37.0
– – rectovaginal	C76.3	C79.8	D09.7	D36.7	D48.7
– – rectovesical	C76.3	C79.8	D09.7	D36.7	D48.7
– – urethrovaginal	C57.9	C79.8	D07.3	D28.9	D39.7
– – vesicovaginal	C57.9	C79.8	D07.3	D28.9	D39.7
– shoulder NEC #	C76.4	C79.8	D04.6	D36.7	D48.7
– sigmoid (flexure)	C18.7	C78.5	D01.0	D12.5	D37.4

	Malignant				Uncertain
	Primary 3	Secondary 6	In situ 2	Benign 0	or unknown behavior 1
Neoplasm, neoplastic—*continued*					
– sinus (accessory)	C31.9	C78.3	D02.3	D14.0	D38.5
– – bone (any) ✧	C41.0	C79.5		D16.4	D48.0
– – ethmoidal	C31.1	C78.3	D02.3	D14.0	D38.5
– – frontal	C31.2	C78.3	D02.3	D14.0	D38.5
– – maxillary	C31.0	C78.3	D02.3	D14.0	D38.5
– – nasal, paranasal NEC	C31.9	C78.3	D02.3	D14.0	D38.5
– – piriform	C12	C79.8	D00.0	D10.7	D37.0
– – sphenoidal	C31.3	C78.3	D02.3	D14.0	D38.5
– skeleton, skeletal NEC ✧	C41.9	C79.5		D16.9	D48.0
– Skene's gland	C68.1	C79.1	D09.1	D30.7	D41.7
– skin (nonmelanotic)	C44.9	C79.2	D04.9	D23.9	D48.5
– – abdominal wall	C44.5	C79.2	D04.5	D23.5	D48.5
– – ala nasi	C44.3	C79.2	D04.3	D23.3	D48.5
– – ankle	C44.7	C79.2	D04.7	D23.7	D48.5
– – antecubital space	C44.6	C79.2	D04.6	D23.6	D48.5
– – anus	C44.5	C79.2	D04.5	D23.5	D48.5
– – arm	C44.6	C79.2	D04.6	D23.6	D48.5
– – auditory canal (external)	C44.2	C79.2	D04.2	D23.2	D48.5
– – auricle (ear)	C44.2	C79.2	D04.2	D23.2	D48.5
– – auricular canal (external)	C44.2	C79.2	D04.2	D23.2	D48.5
– – axilla, axillary fold	C44.5	C79.2	D04.5	D23.5	D48.5
– – back	C44.5	C79.2	D04.5	D23.5	D48.5
– – breast	C44.5	C79.2	D04.5	D23.5	D48.5
– – brow	C44.3	C79.2	D04.3	D23.3	D48.5
– – buttock	C44.5	C79.2	D04.5	D23.5	D48.5
– – calf	C44.7	C79.2	D04.7	D23.7	D48.5
– – canthus (eye) (inner) (outer)	C44.1	C79.2	D04.1	D23.1	D48.5
– – cervical region	C44.4	C79.2	D04.4	D23.4	D48.5
– – cheek	C44.3	C79.2	D04.3	D23.3	D48.5
– – chest (wall)	C44.5	C79.2	D04.5	D23.5	D48.5
– – chin	C44.3	C79.2	D04.3	D23.3	D48.5
– – clavicular area	C44.5	C79.2	D04.5	D23.5	D48.5
– – clitoris	C51.2	C79.8	D07.1	D28.0	D39.7
– – columella	C44.3	C79.2	D04.3	D23.3	D48.5
– – concha, ear	C44.2	C79.2	D04.2	D23.2	D48.5
– – ear (external)	C44.2	C79.2	D04.2	D23.2	D48.5
– – elbow	C44.6	C79.2	D04.6	D23.6	D48.5
– – eyebrow	C44.3	C79.2	D04.3	D23.3	D48.5
– – eyelid	C44.1	C79.2	D04.1	D23.1	D48.5
– – face NEC	C44.3	C79.2	D04.3	D23.3	D48.5
– – female genital organ	C51.9	C79.8	D07.1	D28.0	D39.7
– – – clitoris	C51.2	C79.8	D07.1	D28.0	D39.7
– – – labium NEC	C51.9	C79.8	D07.1	D28.0	D39.7
– – – – majus	C51.0	C79.8	D07.1	D28.0	D39.7
– – – – minus	C51.1	C79.8	D07.1	D28.0	D39.7
– – – pudendum	C51.9	C79.8	D07.1	D28.0	D39.7
– – – vulva	C51.9	C79.8	D07.1	D28.0	D39.7
– – finger	C44.6	C79.2	D04.6	D23.6	D48.5
– – flank	C44.5	C79.2	D04.5	D23.5	D48.5
– – foot	C44.7	C79.2	D04.7	D23.7	D48.5
– – forearm	C44.6	C79.2	D04.6	D23.6	D48.5

Neoplasm type for Skin - BCC & Epidermoid

| | Malignant | | | | Uncertain |
	Primary	Secondary	In situ	Benign	or unknown behavior
Neoplasm, neoplastic—*continued*					
– skin (nonmelanotic) —*continued*					
– – forehead	C44.3	C79.2	D04.3	D23.3	D48.5
– – gluteal region	C44.5	C79.2	D04.5	D23.5	D48.5
– – groin	C44.5	C79.2	D04.5	D23.5	D48.5
– – hand	C44.6	C79.2	D04.6	D23.6	D48.5
– – head NEC	C44.4	C79.2	D04.4	D23.4	D48.5
– – heel	C44.7	C79.2	D04.7	D23.7	D48.5
– – helix	C44.2	C79.2	D04.2	D23.2	D48.5
– – hip	C44.7	C79.2	D04.7	D23.7	D48.5
– – infraclavicular region	C44.5	C79.2	D04.5	D23.5	D48.5
– – inguinal region	C44.5	C79.2	D04.5	D23.5	D48.5
– – jaw	C44.3	C79.2	D04.3	D23.3	D48.5
– – knee	C44.7	C79.2	D04.7	D23.7	D48.5
– – labia	C51.9	C79.8	D07.1	D28.0	D39.7
– – – majora	C51.0	C79.8	D07.1	D28.0	D39.7
– – – minora	C51.1	C79.8	D07.1	D28.0	D39.7
– – leg	C44.7	C79.2	D04.7	D23.7	D48.5
– – lid (lower) (upper)	C44.1	C79.2	D04.1	D23.1	D48.5
– – limb NEC	C44.9	C79.2	D04.9	D23.9	D48.5
– – – lower	C44.7	C79.2	D04.7	D23.7	D48.5
– – – upper	C44.6	C79.2	D04.6	D23.6	D48.5
– – lip (lower) (upper)	C44.0	C79.2	D04.0	D23.0	D48.5
– – male genital organ	C63.9	C79.8	D07.6	D29.9	D40.9
– – – penis NEC	C60.9	C79.8	D07.4	D29.0	D40.7
– – – prepuce	C60.0	C79.8	D07.4	D29.0	D40.7
– – – scrotum	C63.2	C79.8	D07.6	D29.4	D40.7
– – melanotic – *see* Melanoma					
– – nates	C44.5	C79.2	D04.5	D23.5	D48.5
– – neck	C44.4	C79.2	D04.4	D23.4	D48.5
– – nose (external)	C44.3	C79.2	D04.3	D23.3	D48.5
– – palm	C44.6	C79.2	D04.6	D23.6	D48.5
– – palpebra	C44.1	C79.2	D04.1	D23.1	D48.5
– – penis NEC	C60.9	C79.8	D07.4	D29.0	D40.7
– – perianal	C44.5	C79.2	D04.5	D23.5	D48.5
– – perineum	C44.5	C79.2	D04.5	D23.5	D48.5
– – pinna	C44.2	C79.2	D04.2	D23.2	D48.5
– – plantar	C44.7	C79.2	D04.7	D23.7	D48.5
– – popliteal fossa or space	C44.7	C79.2	D04.7	D23.7	D48.5
– – prepuce	C60.0	C79.8	D07.4	D29.0	D40.7
– – pubes	C44.5	C79.2	D04.5	D23.5	D48.5
– – sacrococcygeal region	C44.5	C79.2	D04.5	D23.5	D48.5
– – scalp	C44.4	C79.2	D04.4	D23.4	D48.5
– – scapular region	C44.5	C79.2	D04.5	D23.5	D48.5
– – scrotum	C63.2	C79.8	D07.6	D29.4	D40.7
– – shoulder	C44.6	C79.2	D04.6	D23.6	D48.5
– – sole (foot)	C44.7	C79.2	D04.7	D23.7	D48.5
– – submammary fold	C44.5	C79.2	D04.5	D23.5	D48.5
– – supraclavicular region	C44.4	C79.2	D04.4	D23.4	D48.5
– – temple	C44.3	C79.2	D04.3	D23.3	D48.5
– – thigh	C44.7	C79.2	D04.7	D23.7	D48.5
– – thoracic wall	C44.5	C79.2	D04.5	D23.5	D48.5

	Malignant		In situ	Benign	Uncertain or unknown behavior
	Primary	Secondary			

Neoplasm, neoplastic—*continued*
- skin (nonmelanotic) —*continued*

− − thumb	C44.6	C79.2	D04.6	D23.6	D48.5
− − toe	C44.7	C79.2	D04.7	D23.7	D48.5
− − tragus	C44.2	C79.2	D04.2	D23.2	D48.5
− − trunk	C44.5	C79.2	D04.5	D23.5	D48.5
− − umbilicus	C44.5	C79.2	D04.5	D23.5	D48.5
− − vulva	C51.9	C79.8	D07.1	D28.0	D39.7
− − wrist	C44.6	C79.2	D04.6	D23.6	D48.5
− skull ◇	C41.0	C79.5		D16.4	D48.0
− soft parts or tissues – *see* Neoplasm, connective tissue					
− specified site NEC	C76.7	C79.8	D09.7	D36.7	D48.7
− spermatic cord	C63.1	C79.8	D07.6	D29.7	D40.7
− sphenoid	C31.3	C78.3	D02.3	D14.0	D38.5
− − bone ◇	C41.0	C79.5		D16.4	D48.0
− − sinus	C31.3	C78.3	D02.3	D14.0	D38.5
− sphincter					
− − anal	C21.1	C78.5	D01.3	D21.9	D37.7
− − of Oddi	C24.0	C78.8	D01.5	D13.5	D37.6
− spine, spinal (column) ◇	C41.2	C79.5		D16.6	D48.0
− − bulb	C71.7	C79.4		D33.1	D43.1
− − coccyx ◇	C41.4	C79.5		D16.8	D48.0
− − cord	C72.0	C79.4		D33.4	D43.4
− − dura mater	C70.1	C79.4		D32.1	D42.1
− − lumbosacral ◇	C41.2	C79.5		D16.6	D48.0
− − membrane	C70.1	C79.4		D32.1	D42.1
− − meninges	C70.1	C79.4		D32.1	D42.1
− − nerve (root)	C47.9	C79.8		D36.1	D48.2
− − pia mater	C70.1	C79.4		D32.1	D42.1
− − sacrum ◇	C41.4	C79.5		D16.8	D48.0
− spleen, splenic NEC	C26.1	C78.8		D13.9	D37.7
− − flexure (colon)	C18.5	C78.5	D01.0	D12.3	D37.4
− Stensen's duct	C07	C79.8	D00.0	D11.0	D37.0
− sternum ◇	C41.3	C79.5		D16.7	D48.0
− stomach	C16.9	C78.8	D00.2	D13.1	D37.1
− − antrum	C16.3	C78.8	D00.2	D13.1	D37.1
− − body	C16.2	C78.8	D00.2	D13.1	D37.1
− − cardia	C16.0	C78.8	D00.2	D13.1	D37.1
− − cardiac orifice	C16.0	C78.8	D00.2	D13.1	D37.1
− − corpus	C16.2	C78.8	D00.2	D13.1	D37.1
− − fundus	C16.1	C78.8	D00.2	D13.1	D37.1
− − greater curvature NEC	C16.6	C78.8	D00.2	D13.1	D37.1
− − lesser curvature NEC	C16.5	C78.8	D00.2	D13.1	D37.1
− − prepylorus	C16.4	C78.8	D00.2	D13.1	D37.1
− − pylorus	C16.4	C78.8	D00.2	D13.1	D37.1
− − wall NEC	C16.9	C78.8	D00.2	D13.1	D37.1
− − − anterior NEC	C16.8	C78.8	D00.2	D13.1	D37.1
− − − posterior NEC	C16.8	C78.8	D00.2	D13.1	D37.1
− stroma, endometrial	C54.1	C79.8	D07.0	D26.1	D39.0
− stump, cervical	C53.8	C79.8	D06.7	D26.0	D39.0

467

	Malignant				Uncertain
	Primary	Secondary	In situ	Benign	or unknown behavior
Neoplasm, neoplastic—*continued*					
– subcutaneous (nodule) (tissue) NEC – *see* Neoplasm, connective tissue					
– subdural	C70.9	C79.4		D32.9	D42.9
– subglottis, subglottic	C32.2	C78.3	D02.0	D14.1	D38.0
– sublingual	C04.9	C79.8	D00.0	D10.2	D37.0
– – gland or duct	C08.1	C79.8	D00.0	D11.7	D37.0
– submandibular gland	C08.0	C79.8	D00.0	D11.7	D37.0
– submaxillary gland or duct	C08.0	C79.8	D00.0	D11.7	D37.0
– submental	C76.0	C79.8	D09.7	D36.7	D48.7
– subpleural	C34.9	C78.0	D02.2	D14.3	D38.1
– substernal	C38.1	C78.1		D15.2	D38.3
– supraclavicular region	C76.0	C79.8	D09.7	D36.7	D48.7
– supraglottis	C32.1	C78.3	D02.0	D14.1	D38.0
– suprarenal	C74.9	C79.7	D09.3	D35.0	D44.1
– – capsule	C74.9	C79.7	D09.3	D35.0	D44.1
– – cortex	C74.0	C79.7	D09.3	D35.0	D44.1
– – gland	C74.9	C79.7	D09.3	D35.0	D44.1
– – medulla	C74.1	C79.7	D09.3	D35.0	D44.1
– suprasellar (region)	C71.9	C79.3		D33.2	D43.2
– supratentorial (brain) NEC	C71.0	C79.3		D33.0	D43.0
– sweat gland (apocrine) (eccrine), site unspecified	C44.9	C79.2	D04.9	D23.9	D48.5
– sympathetic nerve or nervous system NEC	C47.9	C79.8		D36.1	D48.2
– symphysis pubis	C41.4	C79.5		D16.8	D48.0
– synovial membrane – *see* Neoplasm, connective tissue					
– tapetum	C71.8	C79.3		D33.2	D43.2
– tarsus (any bone) ✧	C40.3	C79.5		D16.3	D48.0
– temple	C44.3	C79.2	D04.3	D23.3	D48.5
– temporal					
– – pole or lobe	C71.2	C79.3		D33.0	D43.0
– – region	C76.0	C79.8	D09.7	D36.7	D48.7
– tendon (sheath) – *see* Neoplasm, connective tissue					
– tentorium (cerebelli)	C70.0	C79.3		D32.0	D42.0
– testis	C62.9	C79.8	D07.6	D29.2	D40.1
– – descended	C62.1	C79.8	D07.6	D29.2	D40.1
– – ectopic	C62.0	C79.8	D07.6	D29.2	D40.1
– – retained	C62.0	C79.8	D07.6	D29.2	D40.1
– – scrotal	C62.1	C79.8	D07.6	D29.2	D40.1
– – undescended	C62.0	C79.8	D07.6	D29.2	D40.1
– thalamus	C71.0	C79.3		D33.0	D43.0
– thigh NEC #	C76.5	C79.8	D04.7	D36.7	D48.7
– thorax, thoracic (cavity) (organs NEC)	C76.1	C79.8	D09.7	D36.7	D48.7
– – duct	C49.3	C79.8		D21.3	D48.1
– – wall NEC	C76.1	C79.8	D09.7	D36.7	D48.7
– throat	C14.0	C79.8	D00.0	D10.9	D37.0
– thumb NEC #	C76.4	C79.8	D04.6	D36.7	D48.7
– thymus (gland)	C37	C79.8	D09.3	D15.0	D38.4
– thyroglossal duct	C73	C79.8	D09.3	D34	D44.0

| | Malignant | | | | Uncertain |
| | Primary | Secondary | In situ | Benign | or unknown behavior |

Neoplasm, neoplastic—*continued*

	Primary	Secondary	In situ	Benign	Uncertain
– thyroid (gland)	C73	C79.8	D09.3	D34	D44.0
– – cartilage	C32.3	C78.3	D02.0	D14.1	D38.0
– tibia (any part) ✧	C40.2	C79.5		D16.2	D48.0
– toe NEC #	C76.5	C79.8	D04.7	D36.7	D48.7
– tongue	C02.9	C79.8	D00.0	D10.1	D37.0
– – anterior (two-thirds) NEC	C02.3	C79.8	D00.0	D10.1	D37.0
– – – dorsal surface	C02.0	C79.8	D00.0	D10.1	D37.0
– – – ventral surface	C02.2	C79.8	D00.0	D10.1	D37.0
– – base (dorsal surface)	C01	C79.8	D00.0	D10.1	D37.0
– – border (lateral)	C02.1	C79.8	D00.0	D10.1	D37.0
– – fixed part	C01	C79.8	D00.0	D10.1	D37.0
– – frenulum	C02.2	C79.8	D00.0	D10.1	D37.0
– – junctional zone	C02.8	C79.8	D00.0	D10.1	D37.0
– – margin (lateral)	C02.1	C79.8	D00.0	D10.1	D37.0
– – midline NEC	C02.0	C79.8	D00.0	D10.1	D37.0
– – mobile part NEC	C02.3	C79.8	D00.0	D10.1	D37.0
– – posterior (third)	C01	C79.8	D00.0	D10.1	D37.0
– – root	C01	C79.8	D00.0	D10.1	D37.0
– – surface (dorsal)	C02.0	C79.8	D00.0	D10.1	D37.0
– – – base	C01	C79.8	D00.0	D10.1	D37.0
– – – ventral	C02.2	C79.8	D00.0	D10.1	D37.0
– – tip	C02.1	C79.8	D00.0	D10.1	D37.0
– – tonsil	C02.4	C79.8	D00.0	D10.1	D37.0
– tonsil	C09.9	C79.8	D00.0	D10.4	D37.0
– – fauces, faucial	C09.9	C79.8	D00.0	D10.4	D37.0
– – lingual	C02.4	C79.8	D00.0	D10.1	D37.0
– – palatine	C09.9	C79.8	D00.0	D10.4	D37.0
– – pharyngeal	C11.1	C79.8	D00.0	D10.6	D37.0
– – pillar (anterior) (posterior)	C09.1	C79.8	D00.0	D10.5	D37.0
– tonsillar fossa	C09.0	C79.8	D00.0	D10.5	D37.0
– tooth socket NEC	C03.9	C79.8	D00.0	D10.3	D37.0
– trachea (cartilage) (mucosa)	C33	C78.3	D02.1	D14.2	D38.1
– tracheobronchial	C34.8	C78.0	D02.2	D14.2	D38.1
– tragus	C44.2	C79.2	D04.2	D23.2	D48.5
– trunk NEC #	C76.7	C79.8	D04.5	D36.7	D48.7
– tubo-ovarian	C57.8	C79.8	D07.3	D28.7	D39.7
– tunica vaginalis	C63.7	C79.8	D07.6	D29.7	D40.7
– turbinate (bone) ✧	C41.0	C79.5		D16.4	D48.0
– – nasal	C30.0	C78.3	D02.3	D14.0	D38.5
– tympanic cavity	C30.1	C78.3	D02.3	D14.0	D38.5
– ulna (any part) ✧	C40.0	C79.5		D16.0	D48.0
– umbilicus, umbilical	C44.5	C79.2	D04.5	D23.5	D48.5
– uncus	C71.2	C79.3		D33.0	D43.0
– unknown site, primary	C80.0				
– unknown site, so stated	C80.0	C79.9			
– unknown site, whether primary or secondary	C80.9				
– urachus	C67.7	C79.1	D09.0	D30.3	D41.4
– ureter	C66	C79.1	D09.1	D30.2	D41.2
– – orifice	C67.6	C79.1	D09.0	D30.3	D41.4
– urethra, urethral (gland)	C68.0	C79.1	D09.1	D30.4	D41.3
– – orifice, internal	C67.5	C79.1	D09.0	D30.3	D41.4
– urethrovaginal (septum)	C57.9	C79.8	D07.3	D28.9	D39.9

| | Malignant | | | | Uncertain |
	Primary	Secondary	In situ	Benign	or unknown behavior
Neoplasm, neoplastic—*continued*					
– urinary organ or system NEC	C68.9	C79.1	D09.1	D30.9	D41.9
– – bladder – *see* Neoplasm, bladder					
– utero-ovarian	C57.8	C79.8		D28.7	D39.7
– – ligament	C57.1	C79.8		D28.2	D39.7
– uterosacral ligament	C57.3	C79.8		D28.2	D39.7
– uterus, uteri, uterine	C55	C79.8	D07.3	D26.9	D39.0
– – adnexa	C57.4	C79.8	D07.3	D28.7	D39.7
– – body	C54.9	C79.8	D07.3	D26.1	D39.0
– – cervix	C53.9	C79.8	D06.9	D26.0	D39.0
– – cornu	C54.9	C79.8	D07.3	D26.1	D39.0
– – corpus	C54.9	C79.8	D07.3	D26.1	D39.0
– – endocervix (canal) (gland)	C53.0	C79.8	D06.0	D26.0	D39.0
– – exocervix	C53.1	C79.8	D06.1	D26.0	D39.0
– – external os	C53.1	C79.8	D06.1	D26.0	D39.0
– – fundus	C54.3	C79.8	D07.3	D26.1	D39.0
– – internal os	C53.0	C79.8	D06.0	D26.0	D39.0
– – isthmus	C54.0	C79.8	D07.3	D26.1	D39.0
– – ligament	C57.3	C79.8		D28.2	D39.7
– – – broad	C57.1	C79.8	D07.3	D28.2	D39.7
– – – round	C57.2	C79.8		D28.2	D39.7
– – lower segment	C54.0	C79.8	D07.3	D26.1	D39.0
– – squamocolumnar junction	C53.8	C79.8	D06.7	D26.0	D39.0
– – tube	C57.0	C79.8	D07.3	D28.2	D39.7
– utricle, prostatic	C68.0	C79.1	D09.1	D30.4	D41.3
– uveal tract	C69.4	C79.4	D09.2	D31.4	D48.7
– uvula	C05.2	C79.8	D00.0	D10.3	D37.0
– vagina, vaginal (fornix) (vault) (wall)	C52	C79.8	D07.2	D28.1	D39.7
– vaginovesical	C57.9	C79.8	D07.3	D28.9	D39.9
– – septum	C57.9	C79.8	D07.3	D28.9	D39.9
– vallecula (epiglottis)	C10.0	C79.8	D00.0	D10.5	D37.0
– vas deferens	C63.1	C79.8	D07.6	D29.7	D40.7
– vascular – *see* Neoplasm, connective tissue					
– vein, venous – *see* Neoplasm, connective tissue					
– vena cava (abdominal) (inferior)	C49.4	C79.8		D21.4	D48.1
– – superior	C49.3	C79.8		D21.3	D48.1
– ventricle	C71.5	C79.3		D33.0	D43.0
– – cardiac (left) (right)	C38.0	C79.8		D15.1	D48.7
– – cerebral	C71.5	C79.3		D33.0	D43.0
– – – floor	C71.5	C79.3		D33.0	D43.0
– – – fourth	C71.7	C79.3		D33.1	D43.1
– – – lateral	C71.5	C79.3		D33.0	D43.0
– – – third	C71.5	C79.3		D33.0	D43.0
– ventricular band of larynx	C32.1	C78.3	D02.0	D14.1	D38.0
– ventriculus – *see* Neoplasm, stomach					
– vermilion border – *see* Neoplasm, lip					
– vermis, cerebellum	C71.6	C79.3		D33.1	D43.1
– vertebral (column) ◇	C41.2	C79.5		D16.6	D48.0
– – coccyx ◇	C41.4	C79.5		D16.8	D48.0
– – sacrum ◇	C41.4	C79.5		D16.8	D48.0
– vesical – *see* Neoplasm, bladder					

| | Malignant | | | | Uncertain |
	Primary 3	Secondary 6	In situ 2	Benign 0	or unknown behavior 1
Neoplasm, neoplastic—*continued*					
– vesicle, seminal	C63.7	C79.8	D07.6	D29.7	D40.7
– vesicocervical tissue	C57.9	C79.8	D07.3	D28.9	D39.9
– vesicorectal	C76.3	C79.8	D09.7	D36.7	D48.7
– vesicovaginal	C57.9	C79.8	D07.3	D28.9	D39.9
– – septum	C57.9	C79.8	D07.3	D28.9	D39.9
– vessel (blood) – *see* Neoplasm, connective tissue					
– vestibular gland, greater	C51.0	C79.8	D07.1	D28.0	D39.7
– vestibule					
– – mouth	C06.1	C79.8	D00.0	D10.3	D37.0
– – nose	C30.0	C78.3	D02.3	D14.0	D38.5
– Virchow's gland	C77.0	C77.0		D36.0	D48.7
– viscera NEC	C76.7	C79.8		D36.7	D48.7
– vocal cord (true)	C32.0	C78.3	D02.0	D14.1	D38.0
– – false	C32.1	C78.3	D02.0	D14.1	D38.0
– vomer	C41.0	C79.5		D16.4	D48.0
– vulva	C51.9	C79.8	D07.1	D28.0	D39.7
– vulvovaginal gland	C51.0	C79.8	D07.1	D28.0	D39.7
– Waldeyer's ring	C14.2	C79.8	D00.0	D10.9	D37.0
– Wharton's duct	C08.0	C79.8	D00.0	D11.7	D37.0
– white matter (central) (cerebral)	C71.0	C79.3		D33.0	D43.0
– windpipe	C33	C78.3	D02.1	D14.2	D38.1
– Wirsung's duct	C25.3	C78.8	D01.7	D13.6	D37.7
– Wolffian (body) (duct)					
– – female	C57.7	C79.8	D07.3	D28.7	D39.7
– – male	C63.7	C79.8	D07.6	D29.7	D40.7
– womb – *see* Neoplasm, uterus					
– wrist NEC #	C76.4	C79.8	D04.6	D36.7	D48.7
– xiphoid process ✧	C41.3	C79.5		D16.7	D48.0
– Zuckerkandl's organ	C75.5	C79.8		D35.6	D44.7

Neovascularization
– ciliary body H21.1
– cornea H16.4
– iris H21.1
– retina H35.0
Nephralgia N23
Nephritis, nephritic N05.-

Note: Where a term is indexed only at the three-character level, e.g. N00.-, reference should be made to the list of fourth-character subdivisions in Volume 1 at N00-N08.

– with
– – edema – *see* Nephrosis
– – foot process disease N04.-
– – glomerular lesion
– – – diffuse sclerosing (*see also* Disease, kidney, chronic) N18.9
– – – hypocomplementemic – *see* Nephritis, membranoproliferative
– – – IgA – *see* Nephropathy, IgA
– – – lobular, lobulonodular – *see* Nephritis, membranoproliferative
– – – necrotic, necrotizing NEC – *code to* N00-N07 with fourth character .8
– – – nodular – *see* Nephritis, membranoproliferative
– – – specified pathology NEC – *code to* N00-N07 with fourth character .8
– acute N00.-
– amyloid E85.4† N08.4*
– antiglomerular basement membrane (anti-GBM) antibody, in Goodpasture's syndrome M31.0† N08.5*
– antitubular basement membrane (tubulo-interstitial) NEC N12
– – toxic – *see* Nephropathy, toxic
– arteriolar (*see also* Hypertension, kidney) I12.9
– arteriosclerotic (*see also* Hypertension, kidney) I12.9
– ascending – *see* Nephritis, tubulo-interstitial
– Balkan (endemic) N15.0
– calculous, calculus (*see also* Calculus, kidney) N20.9
– cardiac – *see* Hypertension, kidney
– cardiovascular – *see* Hypertension, kidney
– chronic N03.-
– – arteriosclerotic (*see also* Hypertension, kidney) I12.9
– cirrhotic (*see also* Sclerosis, renal) N26

Nephritis, nephritic—*continued*
– complicating pregnancy, childbirth or puerperium O99.8
– – with secondary hypertension, pre-existing O10.4
– – – affecting fetus or newborn P00.0
– – affecting fetus or newborn P00.1
– degenerative – *see* Nephrosis
– diffuse sclerosing (*see also* Disease, kidney, chronic) N18.9
– due to
– – diabetes mellitus (*see also* E10-E14 with fourth character .2) E14.2† N08.3*
– – systemic lupus erythematosus (chronic) M32.1† N08.5*
– gonococcal (acute) (chronic) A54.2† N08.0*
– hypocomplementemic – *see* Nephritis, membranoproliferative
– IgA – *see* Nephropathy, IgA
– immune complex (circulating) NEC N05.8
– infective – *see* Nephritis, tubulo-interstitial
– interstitial – *see* Nephritis, tubulo-interstitial
– lead N14.3
– membranoproliferative (diffuse) (type 1) (type 3) – *code to* N00-N07 with fourth character .5
– – type 2 – *code to* N00-N07 with fourth character .6
– necrotic, necrotizing NEC – *code to* N00-N07 with fourth character .8
– nephrotic – *see* Nephrosis
– nodular – *see* Nephritis, membranoproliferative
– poststreptococcal NEC N05.9
– – acute N00.-
– – chronic N03.-
– – rapidly progressive N01.-
– proliferative NEC – *code to* N00-N07 with fourth character .8
– puerperal (postpartum) O90.8
– purulent – *see* Nephritis, tubulo-interstitial
– rapidly progressive N01.-
– salt-losing or -wasting NEC N28.8
– saturnine N14.3
– sclerosing, diffuse (*see also* Disease, kidney, chronic) N18.9
– septic – *see* Nephritis, tubulo-interstitial
– specified pathology NEC – *code to* N00-N07 with fourth character .8
– subacute N01.-

Nephronia - an intermediate stage between acute pyelonephritis and renal abscess, and is a focal region of interstitial nephritis

Nephritis, nephritic—*continued*
- suppurative – *see* Nephritis, tubulo-interstitial
- syphilitic (late) A52.7† N08.0*
- – congenital A50.5† N08.0*
- – early (secondary) A51.4† N08.0*
- toxic – *see* Nephropathy, toxic
- tubal, tubular – *see* Nephritis, tubulo-interstitial
- tuberculous A18.1† N29.1*
- tubulo-interstitial (in) N12
- – acute (infectious) N10
- – chronic (infectious) N11.9
- – – nonobstructive N11.8
- – – – reflux-associated N11.0
- – – obstructive N11.1
- – – specified NEC N11.8
- – – Sjögren's syndrome M35.0† N16.4*
- vascular – *see* Hypertension, kidney

Nephroblastoma (epithelial) (mesenchymal) (M8960/3) C64
Nephrocalcinosis E83.5† N29.8*
Nephrocystitis, pustular (*see also* Nephritis, tubulo-interstitial) N12
Nephrolithiasis (congenital) (pelvis) (recurrent) (*see also* Calculus, kidney) N20.0
- gouty M10.0† N22.8*
- uric acid M10.0† N22.8*

Nephroma (M8960/3) C64
- mesoblastic (M8960/1) D41.0
Nephropathia epidemica (Puumala hantavirus) A98.5† N08.0*
Nephropathy (*see also* Nephritis) N28.9

Note: Where a term is indexed only at the three-character level, e.g. N07.-, reference should be made to the list of fourth-character subdivisions in Volume 1 at N00-N08.

- with
- – edema – *see* Nephrosis
- – glomerular lesion – *see* Glomerulonephritis
- amyloid, hereditary E85.0
- analgesic N14.0
- Balkan (endemic) N15.0
- chemical – *see* Nephropathy, toxic
- diabetic (*see also* E10-E14 with fourth character .2) E14.2† N08.3*
- drug-induced N14.2
- – specified NEC N14.1
- focal and segmental hyalinosis or sclerosis N02.1
- heavy metal-induced N14.3
- hereditary NEC N07.-

Nephropathy—*continued*
- hereditary NEC—*continued*
- – end-stage (failure) I12.0
- hypertensive (*see also* Hypertension, kidney) I12.9
- IgA N02.8
- – with glomerular lesion N02.-
- – – focal and segmental hyalinosis or sclerosis N02.1
- – – membranoproliferative (diffuse) N02.5
- – – membranous (diffuse) N02.2
- – – mesangial proliferative (diffuse) N02.3
- – – mesangiocapillary (diffuse) N02.5
- – – proliferative NEC N02.8
- – – specified pathology NEC N02.8
- lead N14.3
- membranoproliferative (diffuse) N02.5
- membranous (diffuse) N02.2
- mesangial (IgA/IgG) – *see* Nephropathy, IgA
- – proliferative (diffuse) N02.3
- – mesangiocapillary (diffuse) N02.5
- mesangial (IgA/IgG) – *see* Nephropathy, IgA
- obstructive N13.8
- pregnancy-related O26.8
- proliferative NEC – *code to* N00-N07 with fourth character .8
- saturnine N14.3
- sickle-cell (*see also* Disease, sickle-cell) D57.1† N08.2*
- toxic NEC (due to) N14.4
- – drugs N14.2
- – – analgesic N14.0
- – – specified NEC N14.1
- – heavy metals N14.3
Nephroptosis N28.8
Nephropyosis (*see also* Abscess, kidney) N15.1
Nephrorrhagia N28.8
Nephrosclerosis (arteriolar) (arteriosclerotic) (chronic) (hyaline) (*see also* Hypertension, kidney) I12.9
- senile (*see also* Sclerosis, renal) N26
Nephrosis, nephrotic (congenital) (Epstein's) (syndrome) N04.-

Note: Where a term is indexed only at the three-character level, e.g. N04.-, reference should be made to the list of fourth-character subdivisions in Volume 1 at N00-N08.

- with glomerular lesion N04.-

Nephrosis, nephrotic—*continued*
– with glomerular lesion—*continued*
– – foot process disease N04.-
– – hypocomplementemic N04.5
– acute N04.
– anoxic – *see* Nephrosis, tubular
– chemical – *see* Nephrosis, tubular
– complicating pregnancy O26.8
– diabetic (*see also* E10-E14 with fourth
  character .2) E14.2† N08.3*
– hemoglobinuric – *see* Nephrosis, tubular
– in
– – amyloidosis E85.4† N08.4*
– – diabetes mellitus (*see also* E10-E14
  with fourth character .2) E14.2†
  N08.3*
– – epidemic hemorrhagic fever A98.5†
  N08.0*
– – malaria (malariae) B52.0† N08.0*
– ischemic – *see* Nephrosis, tubular
– lipoid N04.-
– lower nephron – *see* Nephrosis, tubular
– malarial (malariae) B52.0† N08.0*
– necrotizing – *see* Nephrosis, tubular
– syphilitic (late) A52.7† N08.0*
– toxic – *see* Nephrosis, tubular
– tubular (acute) N17.0
– – postprocedural N99.0
**Nephrosonephritis, hemorrhagic
  (endemic)** A98.5† N08.0*
Nephrostomy
– attention to Z43.6
– status Z93.6
Nerve – *see condition*
Nervous (*see also condition*) R45.0
– heart F45.3
– stomach F45.3
– tension R45.0
Nervousness R45.0
Nesidioblastoma (M8150/0)
– pancreas D13.7
– specified site NEC – *see* Neoplasm,
  benign
– unspecified site D13.7
Nettleship's syndrome Q82.2
Neumann's disease or syndrome L10.1
Neuralgia, neuralgic (acute) (*see also*
  Neuritis) M79.2
– ciliary G44.0
– cranial
– – nerve – *see also* Disorder, nerve, cranial
– – – fifth or trigeminal (*see also*
     Neuralgia, trigeminal) G50.0
– – postherpetic, postzoster B02.2† G53.0*
– ear H92.0

Neuralgia, neuralgic—*continued*
– facialis vera G51.1
– Fothergill's (*see also* Neuralgia,
  trigeminal) G50.0
– glossopharyngeal (nerve) G52.1
– Hunt's B02.2† G53.0*
– hypoglossal (nerve) G52.3
– infraorbital (*see also* Neuralgia,
  trigeminal) G50.0
– migrainous G44.0
– Morton's G57.6
– nerve, cranial – *see* Disorder, nerve,
  cranial
– postherpetic NEC B02.2† G53.0*
– – trigeminal B02.2† G53.0*
– specified nerve NEC G58.8
– sphenopalatine (ganglion) G44.8
– trifacial (*see also* Neuralgia, trigeminal)
  G50.0
– trigeminal G50.0
– – postherpetic, postzoster B02.2† G53.0*
– writer's F48.8
– – organic G25.8
Neurapraxia – *see* Injury, nerve
Neurasthenia F48.0
– cardiac F45.3
– gastric F45.3
– heart F45.3
Neurilemmoma (M9560/0) – *see also*
  Neoplasm, nerve, benign
– acoustic (nerve) D33.3
– malignant (M9560/3) – *see also*
  Neoplasm, nerve, malignant
– – acoustic (nerve) C72.4
Neurilemmosarcoma (M9560/3) – *see*
  Neoplasm, nerve, malignant
Neurinoma (M9560/0) – *see* Neoplasm,
  nerve, benign
Neurinomatosis (M9560/1) – *see*
  Neoplasm, nerve, uncertain behavior
Neuritis M79.2
– abducens (nerve) H49.2
– acoustic (nerve) H93.3
– – in (due to)
– – – infectious disease NEC B99†
     H94.0*
– – – parasitic disease NEC B89† H94.0*
– – syphilitic A52.1† H94.0*
– amyloid, any site E85.4† G63.3*
– arising during pregnancy O26.8
– auditory (nerve) H93.3
– brachial M54.1
– – due to displacement, intervertebral disk
  M50.1† G55.1*

Neuritis—*continued*
- cranial nerve
- – eighth or acoustic or auditory H93.3
- – fourth or trochlear H49.1
- – second or optic H46
- – seventh or facial G51.8
- – – newborn (birth injury) P11.3
- – sixth or abducent H49.2
- – third or oculomotor H49.0
- Déjerine-Sottas G60.0
- diabetic (polyneuropathy) (*see also* E10-E14 with fourth character .4) E14.4† G63.2*
- – mononeuropathy E14.4† G59.0*
- due to
- – beriberi E51.1† G63.4*
- – displacement, prolapse, protrusion or rupture, intervertebral disk M51.1† G55.1*
- – – cervical M50.1† G55.1*
- – – lumbar, lumbosacral M51.1† G55.1*
- – – thoracic, thoracolumbar M51.1† G55.1*
- – herniation, nucleus pulposus M51.1† G55.1*
- – – cervical M50.1† G55.1*
- – – lumbar, lumbosacral M51.1† G55.1*
- – – thoracic, thoracolumbar M51.1† G55.1*
- endemic E51.1† G63.4*
- facial G51.8
- – newborn (birth injury) P11.3
- general – *see* Polyneuropathy
- geniculate ganglion G51.1
- – due to herpes (zoster) B02.2† G53.0*
- gouty M10.0† G63.6*
- in disease classified elsewhere – *see* Polyneuropathy
- infectious (multiple) NEC G61.0
- interstitial hypertrophic progressive G60.0
- lumbar, lumbosacral M54.1
- multiple (*see also* Polyneuropathy) G62.9
- – endemic E51.1† G63.4*
- – infective, acute G61.0
- multiplex endemica E51.1† G63.4*
- nerve root (*see also* Radiculitis) M54.1
- oculomotor (nerve) H49.0
- olfactory nerve G52.0
- optic (hereditary) (sympathetic) H46
- – with demyelination G36.0
- peripheral (nerve) G62.9
- – complicating pregnancy or puerperium O26.8

Neuritis—*continued*
- peripheral—*continued*
- – multiple (*see also* Polyneuropathy) G62.9
- – single – *see* Mononeuritis
- postherpetic, postzoster B02.2† G53.0*
- pregnancy-related O26.8
- progressive hypertrophic interstitial G60.0
- puerperal, postpartum O90.8
- retrobulbar H46
- – in (due to)
- – – late syphilis A52.1† H48.1*
- – – meningococcal infection A39.8† H48.1*
- – – multiple sclerosis G35† H48.1*
- – meningococcal A39.8† H48.1*
- – syphilitic A52.1† H48.1*
- rheumatoid (chronic) M79.2
- sciatic (nerve) M54.3
- – due to displacement of intervertebral disk M51.1† G55.1*
- shoulder-girdle G54.5
- specified nerve NEC G58.8
- spinal (nerve) root (*see also* Radiculitis) M54.1
- syphilitic A52.1† G59.8*
- thoracic M54.1
- toxic NEC G62.2
- trochlear (nerve) H49.1
Neuroastrocytoma (M9505/1) – *see* Neoplasm, uncertain behavior
Neuroavitaminosis E56.9† G99.8*
Neuroblastoma (M9500/3)
- olfactory (M9522/3) C30.0
- specified site – *see* Neoplasm, malignant
- unspecified site C74.9
Neurochorioretinitis (*see also* Chorioretinitis) H30.9
Neurocirculatory asthenia F45.3
Neurocysticercosis B69.0† G99.8*
Neurocytoma (M9506/0) – *see* Neoplasm, benign
Neurodermatitis (circumscribed) (circumscripta) (local) L28.0
- atopic L20.8
- diffuse (Brocq) L20.8
- disseminated L20.8
Neuroencephalomyelopathy, optic G36.0
Neuroepithelioma (M9503/3) – *see also* Neoplasm, malignant
- olfactory (M9523/3) C30.0

Neurofibroma (M9540/0) – *see also*
Neoplasm, nerve, benign
- melanotic (M9541/0) – *see* Neoplasm,
nerve, benign
- multiple – *see* Neurofibromatosis
- plexiform (M9550/0) – *see* Neoplasm,
nerve, benign
Neurofibromatosis (multiple)
(nonmalignant) (M9540/1) Q85.0
- malignant (M9540/3) – *see* Neoplasm,
nerve, malignant
Neurofibrosarcoma (M9540/3) – *see*
Neoplasm, nerve, malignant
Neurogenic – *see also* condition
- bladder (*see also* Dysfunction, bladder,
neuromuscular) N31.9
- – cauda equina syndrome G83.4
- bowel NEC K59.2
- heart F45.3
Neuroglioma (M9505/1) – *see* Neoplasm,
uncertain behavior
Neurolathyrism T62.2
Neuroleprosy A30.9
Neuroma (M9570/0) – *see also* Neoplasm,
nerve, benign
- acoustic (nerve) (M9560/0) D33.3
- amputation (stump) (late) (surgical
complication) (traumatic) T87.3
- interdigital G58.8
- – lower limb NEC G57.8
- – upper limb G56.8
- intermetatarsal NEC G57.8
- Morton's G57.6
- optic (nerve) D33.3
- plexiform (M9550/0) – *see* Neoplasm,
nerve, benign
Neuromyalgia M79.2
Neuromyasthenia (epidemic)
(postinfectious) G93.3
Neuromyelitis G36.9
- ascending G61.0
- optica G36.0
Neuromyopathy G70.9
- paraneoplastic D48.9† G13.0*
Neuromyotonia (Isaacs') G71.1
Neuronevus (M8725/0) – *see* Nevus
Neuronitis G58.9
- vestibular H81.2
Neuroparalytic – *see condition*
Neuropathy, neuropathic G62.9
- with hereditary ataxia (associated) G60.2
- autonomic, peripheral – *see* Neuropathy,
peripheral, autonomic
- bladder N31.9
- – atonic (motor) (sensory) N31.2

Neuropathy, neuropathic—*continued*
- bladder—*continued*
- – autonomous N31.2
- – flaccid N31.2
- – nonreflex N31.2
- – reflex N31.1
- – uninhibited N31.0
- brachial plexus G54.0
- carcinomatous C80.-† G13.0*
- chronic
- – progressive, segmentally demyelinating
G62.8
- – relapsing, demyelinating G62.8
- Déjerine-Sottas G60.0
- diabetic (*see also* E10-E14 with fourth
character .4) E14.4† G63.2*
- – mononeuropathy E14.4† G59.0*
- entrapment G58.9
- – lateral cutaneous nerve of thigh G57.1
- – median nerve G56.0
- – peroneal nerve G57.3
- – posterior tibial nerve G57.5
- – ulnar nerve G56.2
- facial nerve G51.9
- hereditary G60.9
- – motor and sensory (types I-IV) G60.0
- – sensory G60.8
specified NEC G60.8
- hypertrophic G60.0
- – Charcot-Marie-Tooth G60.0
- – Déjerine-Sottas G60.0
- – interstitial progressive G60.0
- – of infancy G60.0
- idiopathic G60.9
- – progressive G60.3
- – specified NEC G60.8
- intercostal G58.0
- ischemic – *see* Disorder, nerve
- Jamaica (ginger) G62.2
- lumbar plexus G54.1
- motor and sensory (*see also*
Polyneuropathy) G62.8
- – hereditary (types I-IV) G60.0
- multiple (acute) (chronic) G62.9
- optic (nerve) H46
- – ischemic H47.0
- paraneoplastic (sensorial) (Denny Brown)
D48.9† G13.0*
- peripheral (nerve) (*see also*
Polyneuropathy) G62.9
- – autonomic G90.9
- – – idiopathic G90.0
- – – in (due to)
- – – – amyloidosis E85.4† G99.0*

Neuropathy, neuropathic—*continued*
- peripheral—*continued*
- – autonomic—*continued*
- – – in—*continued*
- – – – diabetes mellitus (*see also* E10-E14 with fourth character .4) E14.4† G99.0*
- – – – endocrine disease NEC E34.9† G99.0*
- – – – gout M10.0† G99.1*
- – – – hyperthyroidism E05.9† G99.0*
- – – – metabolic disease NEC E88.9† G99.0*
- – – idiopathic G60.9
- radicular NEC M54.1
- – with intervertebral disk disorder (*see also* Disease, intervertebral disk, by site, with neuritis) M51.1† G55.1*
- – brachial M54.1
- – cervical NEC M54.1
- – hereditary sensory G60.8
- – lumbar, lumbosacral M54.1
- – thoracic NEC M54.1
- sacral plexus G54.1
- sciatic G57.0
- serum G61.1
- toxic NEC G62.2
- uremic N18.5† G63.8*
- vitamin B₁₂ E53.8† G63.4*
- – with anemia (pernicious) D51.0† G63.4*
- – – due to dietary deficiency D51.3† G63.4*

Neurophthisis – *see also* Disorder, nerve
- peripheral, diabetic (*see also* E10-E14 with fourth character .4) E14.4† G63.2*

Neuroretinitis (*see also* Chorioretinitis) H30.9

Neurosarcoma (M9540/3) – *see* Neoplasm, nerve, malignant

Neurosclerosis – *see* Disorder, nerve

Neurosis, neurotic F48.9
- anankastic F42.9
- anxiety (state) F41.1
- asthenic F48.0
- bladder F45.3
- cardiac (reflex) F45.3
- cardiovascular F45.3
- character F60.9
- climacteric N95.1
- colon F45.3
- compensation F68.0
- compulsive, compulsion F42.1
- conversion F44.9

Neurosis, neurotic—*continued*
- craft F48.8
- cutaneous F45.8
- depressive (reaction) (type) F34.1
- environmental F48.8
- excoriation L98.1
- fatigue F48.0
- functional (*see also* Disorder, somatoform) F45.9
- gastric F45.3
- gastrointestinal F45.3
- heart F45.3
- hypochondriacal F45.2
- hysterical F44.9
- incoordination F45.8
- – larynx F45.3
- – vocal cord F45.3
- intestine F45.3
- larynx (sensory) F45.3
- – hysterical F44.4
- menopause N95.1
- mixed NEC F48.8
- musculoskeletal F45.8
- obsessional F42.0
- obsessive-compulsive F42.9
- occupational F48.8
- ocular NEC F45.8
- organ (*see also* Disorder, somatoform) F45.9
- pharynx F45.3
- phobic F40.9
- psychasthenic (type) F48.8
- railroad F48.8
- rectum F45.3
- respiratory F45.3
- rumination F45.3
- sexual F65.9
- situational F48.8
- social F40.1
- specified type NEC F48.8
- state F48.9
- – with depersonalization episode F48.1
- stomach F45.3
- traumatic F43.1
- vasomotor F45.3
- visceral F45.3
- war F48.8

Neurosyphilis, neurosyphilitic (arrested) (late) (recurrent) A52.3
- with ataxia (cerebellar) (locomotor) (spastic) (spinal) A52.1
- aneurysm (cerebral) A52.0† I68.8*
- arachnoid (adhesive) A52.1† G01*
- arteritis (any artery) (cerebral) A52.0† I68.1*

Neurosyphilis, neurosyphilitic—*continued*
- asymptomatic A52.2
- congenital A50.4
- dura (mater) A52.1† G01*
- general paresis A52.1
- gumma A52.3
- hemorrhagic A52.3
- juvenile (asymptomatic) (meningeal) A50.4
- leptomeninges (aseptic) A52.1† G01*
- meningeal, meninges (adhesive) A52.1† G01*
- meningitis A52.1† G01*
- meningovascular (diffuse) A52.1† G01*
- optic atrophy A52.1† H48.0*
- parenchymatous (degenerative) A52.1
- paresis, paretic (*see also* Paresis, general) A52.1
- serological (without symptoms) A52.2
- specified nature or site NEC A52.1
- tabes, tabetic (dorsalis) A52.1
- – juvenile A50.4
- taboparesis A52.1
- – juvenile A50.4
- thrombosis (cerebral) A52.0† I68.8*
- vascular (cerebral) NEC A52.0† I68.8*

Neurothekeoma (M9562/0) – *see* Neoplasm, nerve, benign

Neurotic – *see* Neurosis

Neurotoxemia – *see* Toxemia

Neutropenia, neutropenic (congenital) (cyclic) (drug-induced) (periodic) (primary) (splenic) (toxic) D70
- neonatal, transitory (isoimmune) (maternal transfer) P61.5

Nevocarcinoma (M8720/3) – *see* Melanoma

Nevus (M8720/0) D22.9

Note: Except where otherwise indicated, the morphological varieties of nevus in the list below should be coded by site according to the list under "Nevus, site classification".

- achromic (M8730/0)
- amelanotic (M8730/0)
- angiomatous (M9120/0) D18.0
- araneus I78.1
- balloon cell (M8722/0)
- bathing trunk (M8761/1) D48.5
- blue (M8780/0)
- – cellular (M8790/0)
- – giant (M8790/0)
- – Jadassohn's (M8780/0)
- – malignant (M8780/3) – *see* Melanoma
- capillary (M9131/0) D18.0
- cavernous (M9121/0) D18.0

Nevus—*continued*
- cellular (M8720/0)
- – blue (M8790/0)
- comedonicus Q82.5
- compound (M8760/0)
- conjunctiva (M8720/0)
- dermal (M8750/0)
- – with epidermal nevus (M8760/0)
- dysplastic (M8727/0)
- epitheloid cell (M8771/0)
- – with spindle cell (M8770/0)
- flammeus Q82.5
- hairy (M8720/0)
- halo (M8723/0)
- hemangiomatous (M9120/0) D18.0
- intradermal (M8750/0)
- intraepidermal (M8740/0)
- involuting (M8724/0)
- Jadassohn's blue (M8780/0)
- junction, junctional (M8740/0)
- – malignant melanoma in (M8740/3) C43.9
- juvenile (M8770/0)
- lymphatic (M9170/0) D18.1
- magnocellular (M8726/0)
- – specified site – *see* Neoplasm, benign
- – unspecified site D31.4
- malignant (M8720/3) – *see* Melanoma
- meaning hemangioma (M9120/0) D18.0
- melanotic (pigmented) (M8720/0)
- non-neoplastic I78.1
- nonpigmented (M8730/0)
- nonvascular (M8720/0)
- oral mucosa, white sponge Q38.6
- papillaris (M8720/0)
- papillomatosus (M8720/0)
- pigmented (M8720/0)
- – giant (M8761/1) – *see also* Neoplasm, skin, uncertain behavior
- – – malignant melanoma in (M8761/3) – *see* Melanoma
- pilosus (M8720/0)
- portwine Q82.5
- regressing (M8723/0)
- sanguineous Q82.5
- senile I78.1
- site classification
- – abdominal wall D22.5
- – ala nasi D22.3
- – ankle D22.7
- – anus, anal D22.5
- – arm D22.6
- – auditory canal (external) D22.2
- – auricle (ear) D22.2
- – auricular canal (external) D22.2

Nevus—*continued*
- site classification—*continued*
- – axilla, axillary fold D22.5
- – back D22.5
- – breast D22.5
- – brow D22.3
- – buttock D22.5
- – canthus (eye) D22.1
- – cheek (external) D22.3
- – chest wall D22.5
- – chin D22.3
- – choroid D31.3
- – conjunctiva D31.0
- – ear (external) D22.2
- – external meatus (ear) D22.2
- – eye D31.9
- – eyebrow D22.3
- – eyelid (lower) (upper) D22.1
- – face NEC D22.3
- – female genital organ (external) NEC
  D28.0
- – finger D22.6
- – flank D22.5
- – foot D22.7
- – forearm D22.6
- – forehead D22.3
- – foreskin D29.0
- – genital organ (external) NEC
- – – female D28.0
- – – male D29.9
- – gluteal region D22.5
- – groin D22.5
- – hand D22.6
- – heel D22.7
- – helix D22.2
- – hip D22.7
- – interscapular region D22.5
- – iris D31.4
- – jaw D22.3
- – knee D22.7
- – labium (majus) (minus) D28.0
- – lacrimal gland D31.5
- – leg D22.7
- – lip (lower) (upper) D22.0
- – lower limb NEC D22.7
- – male genital organ (external) NEC
  D29.9
- – mouth (mucosa) D10.3
- – – white sponge Q38.6
- – nail D22.9
- – – finger D22.6
- – – toe D22.7
- – nasolabial groove D22.3
- – nates D22.5
- – neck D22.4

Nevus—*continued*
- site classification—*continued*
- – nose (external) D22.3
- – oral mucosa D10.3
- – – white sponge Q38.6
- – orbit D31.6
- – palpebra D22.1
- – penis D29.0
- – perianal skin D22.5
- – perineum D22.5
- – pinna D22.2
- – popliteal fossa or space D22.7
- – prepuce D29.0
- – pubes D22.5
- – pudendum D28.0
- – retina D31.2
- – retrobulbar D31.6
- – scalp D22.4
- – scrotum D29.4
- – shoulder D22.6
- – skin D22.9
- – specified site NEC – *see* Neoplasm,
  benign
- – submammary fold D22.5
- – temple D22.3
- – thigh D22.7
- – toe D22.7
- – trunk NEC D22.5
- – umbilicus D22.5
- – upper limb NEC D22.6
- – vulva D28.0
- spider I78.1
- spindle cell (M8772/0)
- – with epithelioid cell (M8770/0)
- Spitz – *see* Nevus, spindle cell
- stellar I78.1
- strawberry Q82.5
- Sutton's (M8723/0)
- unius lateris Q82.5
- vascular Q82.5
- verrucous Q82.5

Newborn (infant) (liveborn) (singleton)
  Z38.2
- born in hospital Z38.0
- born outside hospital Z38.1
- multiple (delivery) Z38.8
- – born in hospital Z38.6
- – born outside hospital Z38.7
- twin Z38.5
- – born in hospital Z38.3
- – born outside hospital Z38.4

Newcastle conjunctivitis or disease
  B30.8† H13.1*

Nezelof's syndrome D81.4

Niacin(amide) deficiency E52

Nicolas(-Durand)-Favre disease A55
Nicotine – *see* Tobacco
Nicotinic acid deficiency E52
Niemann-Pick disease or syndrome (all types) E75.2
Night
– blindness H53.6
– – congenital H53.6
– – vitamin A deficiency E50.5† H58.1*
– sweats R61.9
– terrors (child) F51.4
Nightmares F51.5
Nipple – *see condition*
Nitritoid crisis or reaction – *see* Crisis, nitritoid
Nitrosohemoglobinemia D74.8
Njovera A65
No diagnosis (feared complaint unfounded) Z71.1
No disease (found) Z03.9
Nocardiosis, nocardiasis A43.9
– cutaneous A43.1
– lung A43.0† J99.8*
– pneumonia A43.0† J17.0*
– pulmonary A43.0† J99.8*
– specified site NEC A43.8
Nocturia R35
– psychogenic F45.3
Nocturnal – *see condition*
Nodal rhythm I49.8
Node(s) – *see also* Nodule
– Bouchard's (with arthropathy) M15.2
– Haygarth's M15.8
– Heberden's (with arthropathy) M15.1
– larynx J38.7
– lymph – *see condition*
– milker's B08.0
– Osler's I33.0
– Schmorl's M51.4
– singer's J38.2
– teacher's J38.2
– tuberculous – *see* Tuberculosis, lymph gland
– vocal cord J38.2
Nodule(s), nodular
– actinomycotic (*see also* Actinomycosis) A42.9
– breast NEC N63
– colloid (cystic), thyroid E04.9
– cutaneous – *see* Swelling, localized
– endometrial (stromal) (M8930/0) D26.1
– Haygarth's M15.8
– inflammatory – *see* Inflammation
– juxta-articular
– – syphilitic A52.7† M14.8*

Nodule(s), nodular—*continued*
– juxta-articular—*continued*
– – yaws A66.7
– larynx J38.7
– milker's B08.0
– prostate N40
– rheumatoid M06.3
– scrotum (inflammatory) N49.2
– singer's J38.2
– solitary, lung J98.4
– subcutaneous – *see* Swelling, localized
– teacher's J38.2
– thyroid (gland) E04.1
– – toxic or with hyperthyroidism (multinodular) E05.2
– – – single E05.1
– vocal cord J38.2
Noise exposure Z58.0
– occupational Z57.0
Noma (gangrenous) (infective) A69.0
– auricle R02
– mouth A69.0
– pudendi N76.8
– vulvae N76.8
Nonautoimmune hemolytic anemia D59.4
– drug-induced D59.2
Nonclosure – *see also* Imperfect, closure
– ductus arteriosus (botalli) Q25.0
– foramen
– – botalli Q21.1
– – ovale Q21.1
Noncompliance with medical treatment or regimen Z91.1
Nondescent (congenital) – *see also* Malposition, congenital
– testicle Q53.9
– – bilateral Q53.2
– – unilateral Q53.1
Nondevelopment
– brain Q02
– – part of Q04.3
– heart Q24.8
– organ or site, congenital NEC – *see* Hypoplasia
Nonengagement
– head NEC O32.4
– – in labor, causing obstructed labor O64.8
Nonexpansion, lung (newborn) P28.0
Nonfunctioning
– gallbladder K82.8
– kidney (*see also* Failure, kidney) N19
– labyrinth H83.2
Non-Hodgkin lymphoma NEC C85.9
– resulting from HIV disease B21.2

Nonimplantation, ovum N97.2
Noninsufflation, fallopian tube N97.1
Nonketotic hyperglycinemia E72.5
Nonne-Milroy syndrome Q82.0
Nonovulation N97.0
Nonpatent fallopian tube N97.1
Nonretention, food R11
Nonrotation – *see* Malrotation
Nonsecretion, urine (*see also* Anuria) R34
Nonunion
– fracture M84.1
– organ or site, congenital NEC – *see*
  Imperfect, closure
– symphysis pubis, congenital Q74.2
Nonvisualization, gallbladder R93.2
Nonvital tooth K04.9
Noonan's syndrome Q87.1
Normal
– delivery O80.-
– state (feared complaint unfounded) Z71.1
North American blastomycosis B40.9
Nose, nasal – *see condition*
Nosebleed R04.0
Nose-picking F98.8
Nosomania F45.2
Nosophobia F45.2
Nostalgia F43.2
Notch of iris Q13.2
Notching nose, congenital (tip) Q30.2

Nothnagel's
– syndrome H49.0
– vasomotor acroparesthesia I73.8
Novy's relapsing fever A68.9
– louse-borne A68.0
– tick-borne A68.1
Nucleus pulposus – *see condition*
Numbness R20.8
Nun's knee M70.4
Nutmeg liver K76.1
Nutrient element deficiency E61.9
– specified NEC E61.8
Nutrition deficient or insufficient (*see also*
  Malnutrition) E46
– due to
– – insufficient food T73.0
– – lack of
– – – care T74.8
– – – food T73.0
Nutritional stunting E45
Nyctalopia (night blindness) H53.6
– vitamin A deficiency E50.5† H58.1*
Nycturia R35
– psychogenic F45.3
Nymphomania F52.7
Nystagmus (congenital) (deprivation)
  (dissociated) (latent) H55
– benign paroxysmal H81.1
– central positional H81.4
– miner's H55

O

Oast-house-urine disease E72.1
Obermeyer's relapsing fever (European)
   A68.0
Obesity (simple) E66.9
– constitutional E66.8
– dietary counseling and surveillance (for)
   Z71.3
– drug-induced E66.1
– due to
– – excess calories E66.0
– – overalimentation E66.0
– endocrine E66.8
– endogenous E66.8
– exogenous E66.0
– extreme, with alveolar hypoventilation
   E66.2
– familial E66.8
– glandular E66.8
– hypothyroid (*see also* Hypothyroidism)
   E03.9
– morbid E66.8
– nutritional E66.0
– pituitary E23.6
– specified NEC E66.8
Oblique – *see condition*
Obliteration
– appendix (lumen) K38.8
– artery I77.1
– bile duct (noncalculous) K83.1
– common duct (noncalculous) K83.1
– cystic duct (*see also* Obstruction, cystic
   duct) K82.0
– eye, anterior chamber H44.4
– fallopian tube N97.1
– lymphatic vessel I89.0
– – due to mastectomy I97.2
– organ or site, congenital NEC – *see*
   Atresia, by site
– placental blood vessels O43.8
– ureter N13.5
– – with infection N13.6
– urethra (*see also* Stricture, urethra) N35.9
– vein I87.8
Observation (for) Z04.9
– accident NEC Z04.3
– – at work Z04.2
– – transport Z04.1
– adverse effect of drug Z03.6
– cardiovascular disease Z03.5

Observation—*continued*
– cardiovascular disease—*continued*
– – myocardial infarction Z03.4
– development state
– – adolescent Z00.3
– – infant or child Z00.1
– – period of rapid growth in childhood
   Z00.2
– – puberty Z00.3
– disease Z03.9
– – cardiovascular NEC Z03.5
– – – myocardial infarction Z03.4
– – heart NEC Z03.5
– – – myocardial infarction Z03.4
– – mental (suspected) Z03.2
– – nervous system Z03.3
– – specified NEC Z03.8
– dissocial behavior, without manifest
   psychiatric disorder Z03.2
– fire-setting (behavior), without manifest
   psychiatric disorder Z03.2
– gang activity or bahavior, without
   manifest psychiatric disorder Z03.2
– growth and development state – *see*
   Observation, development state
– injuries (accidental) NEC (*see also*
   Observation, accident) Z04.3
– – inflicted NEC Z04.5
– – – during alleged rape or seduction
   Z04.4
– malignant neoplasm, suspected Z03.1
– myocardial infarction Z03.4
– rape or seduction, alleged Z04.4
– shoplifting (behavior), without manifest
   psychiatric disorder Z03.2
– suicide attempt, alleged NEC Z03.8
– – self-poisoning Z03.6
– suspected (undiagnosed) (unproven)
– – behavioral disorder Z03.2
– – cardiovascular disease NEC Z03.5
– – – myocardial infarction Z03.4
– – concussion (cerebral) Z04.5
– – condition NEC Z03.8
– – drug poisoning or adverse effect Z03.6
– – infectious disease not requiring
   isolation Z03.8
– – malignant neoplasm Z03.1
– – mental disorder Z03.2
– – myocardial infarction Z03.4

Observation—*continued*
- suspected—*continued*
- − − neoplasm (malignant) Z03.1
- − − − benign Z03.8
- − − nervous system disorder Z03.3
- − − suicide attempt, alleged Z03.8
- − − − self-poisoning Z03.6
- − − toxic effects from ingested substance (drug) (poison) Z03.6
- − − tuberculosis Z03.0
- − − victim of battering (child) (spouse) Z04.5
- toxic effects from ingested substance (drug) (poison) Z03.6
- tuberculosis, suspected Z03.0
- without need for further medical care Z04.9

Obsession, obsessional F42.0
- ideas and mental images F42.0
- neurosis F42.0
- rituals F42.1
- ruminations F42.0
- state F42.0
- − mixed with compulsive acts F42.2
- syndrome F42.0
- thoughts F42.0

Obsessive-compulsive neurosis or reaction F42.9

Obstetric trauma NEC (complicating delivery O71.9
- affecting fetus or newborn P03.8
- following abortion (subsequent episode) O08.6
- − current episode – *see* Abortion

Obstipation (*see also* Constipation) K59.0

Obstruction, obstructed, obstructive
- airway J98.8
- − with
- − − − allergic alveolitis J67.9
- − − − asthma NEC J45.9
- − − − bronchiectasis J47
- − − − bronchitis (chronic) J44.8
- − − − emphysema J43.9
- − − chronic J44.9
- aortic (heart) (valve) (*see also* Stenosis, aortic) I35.0
- − − rheumatic I06.0
- aqueduct of Sylvius G91.1
- − − congenital Q03.0
- − − − with spina bifida (*see also* Spina bifida, with hydrocephalus) Q05.4
- Arnold-Chiari Q07.0
- artery (*see also* Embolism, artery) I74.9

Obstruction, obstructed—*continued*
- artery—*continued*
- − − basilar (complete) (partial) (*see also* Occlusion, artery, basilar) I65.1
- − − carotid (complete) (partial) (*see also* Occlusion, artery, carotid) I65.2
- − − precerebral (*see also* Occlusion, artery, precerebral) I65.9
- − − renal N28.0
- − − retinal NEC H34.2
- − − − central H34.1
- − − − transient H34.0
- − − vertebral (complete) (partial) (*see also* Occlusion, artery, vertebral) I65.0
- bile duct (common) (hepatic) (noncalculous) K83.1
- − − with calculus K80.5
- − − congenital (causing jaundice) Q44.3
- bladder-neck (acquired) N32.0
- − − congenital Q64.3
- bowel (*see also* Obstruction, intestine) K56.6
- bronchus J98.0
- canal, ear H61.3
- cardia NEC K22.2
- caval veins (inferior) (superior) I87.1
- cecum (*see also* Obstruction, intestine) K56.6
- circulatory I99
- colon (*see also* Obstruction, intestine) K56.6
- common (bile) duct (noncalculous) K83.1
- coronary (artery) I25.1
- cystic duct (*see also* Obstruction, gallbladder) K82.0
- − − with calculus – *see* Cholelithiasis
- device, implant or graft (*see also* Complications, by site and type) T85.6
- − − arterial graft NEC T82.3
- − − − coronary (bypass) T82.2
- − − catheter NEC T85.6
- − − − dialysis (renal) T82.4
- − − − − intraperitoneal T85.6
- − − − infusion NEC T82.5
- − − − − spinal (epidural) (subdural) T85.6
- − − − urinary (indwelling) T83.0
- − − due to infection T85.7
- − − gastrointestinal (bile duct) (esophagus) T85.5
- − − genital NEC T83.4
- − − − intrauterine contraceptive device T83.3
- − − heart NEC T82.5
- − − − valve (prosthesis) T82.0

Obstruction, obstructed—*continued*
- device, implant or graft—*continued*
- - heart NEC—*continued*
- - - valve—*continued*
- - - - graft T82.2
- - joint prosthesis T84.0
- - orthopedic NEC T84.4
- - specified NEC T85.6
- - urinary NEC T83.1
- - - graft T83.2
- - vascular NEC T82.5
- - ventricular intracranial shunt T85.0
- due to foreign body accidentally left in operation wound T81.5
- duodenum K31.5
- ejaculatory duct N50.8
- esophagus K22.2
- eustachian tube (complete) (partial) H68.1
- fallopian tube (bilateral) N97.1
- fecal K56.4
- - with hernia (*see also* Hernia, by site, with obstruction) K46.0
- foramen of Monro (congenital) Q03.8
- - with spina bifida (*see also* Spina bifida, with hydrocephalus) Q05.4
- foreign body (causing) – *see* Foreign body
- gallbladder K82.0
- - with calculus or stone – *see* Cholelithiasis
- - congenital Q44.1
- gastric outlet K31.1
- gastrointestinal (*see also* Obstruction, intestine) K56.6
- hepatic K76.8
- - duct (noncalculous) K83.1
- ileum (*see also* Obstruction, intestine) K56.6
- intestine (mechanical) (paroxysmal) (postinfective) K56.6
- - with adhesions (intestinal) (peritoneal) K56.5
- - adynamic (*see also* Ileus) K56.0
- - congenital (small) Q41.9
- - - large Q42.9
- - - - specified part NEC Q42.8
- - distal (syndrome) E84.1
- - gallstone K56.3
- - neurogenic K56.0
- - - Hirschsprung's disease or megacolon Q43.1
- - newborn P76.9
- - - due to
- - - - fecaliths P76.8

Obstruction, obstructed—*continued*
- intestine—*continued*
- - newborn—*continued*
- - - due to—*continued*
- - - - inspissated milk P76.2
- - - - meconium (plug) P76.0
- - - - - in mucoviscidosis E84.1† P75*
- - - specified NEC P76.8
- - postoperative K91.3
- - reflex K56.0
- - volvulus K56.2
- jejunum (*see also* Obstruction, intestine) K56.6
- labor (*see also* Labor, obstructed) O66.9
- - affecting fetus or newborn P03.1
- - due to
- - - bony pelvis (conditions in O33.-) O65.0
- - - - pelvic deformity O65.0
- - - fetopelvic disproportion NEC O65.4
- - - impacted shoulder O66.0
- - - malposition (fetus) O64.9
- - - maternal pelvic abnormality O65.9
- - - - specified NEC O65.8
- - - persistent occipitoposterior or transverse position O64.0
- - - soft tissues and organs of pelvis (conditions in O34.-) O65.5
- - - specified NEC O66.8
- lacrimal (duct) (passages) H04.5
- - congenital Q10.5
- lacrimonasal duct H04.5
- - congenital Q10.5
- larynx NEC J38.6
- - congenital Q31.8
- lung J98.4
- - disease, chronic J44.9
- lymphatic I89.0
- meconium plug, newborn P76.0
- - in mucoviscidosis E84.1† P75*
- mitral – *see* Stenosis, mitral
- nasal J34.8
- nasolacrimal duct H04.5
- - congenital Q10.5
- nasopharynx J39.2
- nose J34.8
- organ or site, congenital NEC – *see* Atresia, by site
- pancreatic duct K86.8
- parotid duct K11.8
- pelviureteral junction N13.5
- pharynx J39.2
- portal (circulation) (vein) I81
- prostate N40

Obstruction, obstructed—*continued*
- pulmonary valve (heart) I37.0
- pyelonephritis (chronic) N11.1
- pylorus
- – adult K31.1
- – congenital or infantile Q40.0
- rectosigmoid (*see also* Obstruction, intestine) K56.6
- rectum K62.4
- renal
- – outflow N13.8
- – pelvis, congenital Q62.3
- repiratory, chronic J44.9
- retinal (vessels) H34.9
- – specified NEC H34.8
- salivary duct (any) K11.8
- sigmoid (*see also* Obstruction, intestine) K56.6
- sinus (accessory) (nasal) J34.8
- Stensen's duct K11.8
- stomach NEC K31.8
- – congenital Q40.2
- – due to pylorospasm K31.3
- submandibular duct K11.8
- thoracic duct I89.0
- thrombotic – *see* Thrombosis
- trachea J39.8
- tracheostomy airway J95.0
- tricuspid (valve) – *see* Stenosis, tricuspid
- upper respiratory, congenital Q34.8
- ureter (functional) NEC N13.5
- – with
- – – hydronephrosis N13.1
- – – – and infection N13.6
- – – pyelonephritis (chronic) N11.1
- – congenital Q62.3
- – due to calculus (*see also* Calculus, ureter) N20.1
- – pelvic junction (with) N13.5
- – – hydronephrosis N13.0
- – – – and infection N13.6
- – – pyelonephritis (chronic) N11.1
- urethra NEC N36.8
- – congenital Q64.3
- urinary (moderate) N13.9
- – organ or tract N13.9
- – prostatic valve N32.0
- uterus N85.8
- vagina N89.5
- valvular – *see* Endocarditis
- vein, venous I87.1
- – caval (inferior) (superior) I87.1
- – thrombotic – *see* Thrombosis
- vena cava (inferior) (superior) I87.1

Obstruction, obstructed—*continued*
- vesical NEC N32.0
- vesicourethral orifice N32.0
- vessel NEC I99
Obturator – *see condition*
Occlusio pupillae H21.4
Occlusion, occluded
- anus K62.4
- – congenital Q42.3
- – – with fistula Q42.2
- aqueduct of Sylvius G91.1
- – congenital Q03.0
- – – with spina bifida (*see also* Spina bifida, with hydrocephalus) Q05.4
- artery – *see also* Embolism, artery
- – auditory, internal I65.8
- – basilar (with) I65.1
- – – infarction (due to) I63.2
- – – – embolism I63.1
- – – – thrombosis I63.0
- – – other precerebral artery I65.3
- – brain or cerebral I66.9
- – – with infarction (due to) I63.5
- – – – embolism I63.4
- – – – thrombosis I63.3
- – carotid (with) I65.2
- – – infarction (due to) I63.2
- – – – embolism I63.1
- – – – thrombosis I63.0
- – – other precerebral artery I65.3
- – – bilateral I65.3
- – cerebellar (anterior inferior) (posterior inferior) (superior) I66.3
- – – with infarction (due to) I63.5
- – – – embolism I63.4
- – – – thrombosis I63.3
- – cerebral I66.9
- – – with infarction (due to) I63.5
- – – – embolism I63.4
- – – – thrombosis I63.3
- – – anterior I66.1
- – – – with infarction (due to) I63.5
- – – – – embolism I63.4
- – – – – thrombosis I63.3
- – – bilateral I66.4
- – – middle I66.0
- – – – with infarction (due to) I63.5
- – – – – embolism I63.4
- – – – – thrombosis I63.3
- – – multiple or bilateral I66.4
- – – – with infarction (due to) I63.5
- – – – – embolism I63.4
- – – – – thrombosis I63.3
- – – posterior I66.2

Occlusion, occluded—*continued*
- artery—*continued*
- – cerebral—*continued*
- – – posterior—*continued*
- – – – with infarction (due to) I63.5
- – – – – embolism I63.4
- – – – – thrombosis I63.3
- – – – specified NEC I66.8
- – – – – with infarction (due to) I63.5
- – – – – embolism I63.4
- – – – – thrombosis I63.3
- – – choroidal (anterior) I66.8
- – – communicating posterior I66.8
- – – mesenteric (chronic) K55.1
- – – – acute K55.0
- – – perforating I66.8
- – – – with infarction (due to) I63.5
- – – – – embolism I63.4
- – – – – thrombosis I63.3
- – – peripheral I77.9
- – – – thrombotic or embolic I74.4
- – – pontine I66.8
- – – precerebral I65.9
- – – – with infarction (due to) I63.2
- – – – – embolism I63.1
- – – – – thrombosis I63.0
- – – – multiple or bilateral I65.3
- – – – – with infarction (due to) I63.2
- – – – – – embolism I63.1
- – – – – – thrombosis I63.0
- – – – puerperal, postpartum, childbirth O88.2
- – – – – embolic O88.2
- – – – specified NEC I65.8
- – – – – with infarction (due to) I63.2
- – – – – – embolism I63.1
- – – – – – thrombosis I63.0
- – – renal N28.0
- – – retinal (branch) (partial) H34.2
- – – – central H34.1
- – – – specified NEC H34.2
- – – – transient H34.0
- – – vertebral I65.0
- – – – with
- – – – – infarction (due to) I63.2
- – – – – – embolism I63.1
- – – – – – thrombosis I63.0
- – – – – other precerebral artery I65.3
- – – – bilateral I65.3
- – basilar artery – *see* Occlusion, artery, basilar
- – bile duct (common) (hepatic) (noncalculous) K83.1

Occlusion, occluded—*continued*
- – bowel (*see also* Obstruction, intestine) K56.6
- – carotid (artery) (common) (internal) – *see* Occlusion, artery, carotid
- – cerebellar (artery) – *see* Occlusion, artery, cerebellar
- – cerebral (artery) – *see* Occlusion, artery, cerebral
- – cerebrovascular (*see also* Occlusion, artery, cerebral) I66.9
- – – with infarction I63.5
- – – diffuse (without infarction) I66.9
- – cervical canal (*see also* Stricture, cervix) N88.2
- – cervix (uteri) (*see also* Stricture, cervix) N88.2
- – colon (*see also* Obstruction, intestine) K56.6
- – coronary (artery) (*see also* Infarct, myocardium) I21.9
- – – not resulting in infarction I24.0
- – cystic duct (*see also* Obstruction, gallbladder) K82.0
- – embolic – *see* Embolism
- – fallopian tube N97.1
- – – congenital Q50.6
- – gallbladder (*see also* Obstruction, gallbladder) K82.0
- – – congenital (causing jaundice) Q44.1
- – gingiva, traumatic K06.2
- – hymen N89.6
- – – congenital Q52.3
- – intestine (*see also* Obstruction, intestine) K56.6
- – lacrimal passages H04.5
- – lung J98.4
- – lymph or lymphatic channel I89.0
- – mammary duct N64.8
- – mesenteric artery (chronic) K55.1
- – – acute K55.0
- – nose J34.8
- – organ or site, congenital NEC – *see* Atresia, by site
- – oviduct N97.1
- – – congenital Q50.6
- – posterior lingual, of mandibular teeth K07.2
- – precerebral artery – *see* Occlusion, artery, precerebral
- – punctum lacrimale H04.5
- – pupil H21.4
- – pylorus, adult (*see also* Stricture, pylorus) K31.1

Occlusion, occluded—*continued*
- renal artery N28.0
- retinal
- - artery (*see also* Occlusion, artery, retinal) H34.2
- - vein (central) (incipient) (partial) (tributary) H34.8
- - vessels H34.9
- - - specified NEC H34.8
- thoracic duct I89.0
- traumatic
- - edentulous (alveolar) ridge K06.2
- - gingiva K06.2
- - periodontal K05.5
- tubal N97.1
- ureter (complete) (partial) N13.5
- - congenital Q62.1
- ureteropelvic junction N13.5
- - congenital Q62.1
- ureterovesical orifice N13.5
- - congenital Q62.1
- urethra (*see also* Stricture, urethra) N35.9
- - congenital Q64.3
- uterus N85.8
- vagina N89.5
- vascular NEC I99
- vein – *see* Thrombosis
- vena cava I82.2
- ventricle (brain) NEC G91.1
- vertebral (artery) – *see* Occlusion, artery, vertebral
- vessel (blood) I99
- vulva N90.5
Occult
- blood in feces R19.5
Occupational
- problems NEC Z56.7
- therapy Z50.7
Ochlophobia F40.0
Ochronosis (endogenous) E70.2
- with chloasma of eyelid E70.2† H03.8*
Ocular muscle – *see* condition
Oculogyric crisis or disturbance H51.8
- psychogenic F45.8
Oculomotor syndrome H51.9
Oculopathy
- syphilitic NEC A52.7† H58.8*
- - congenital
- - - early A50.0† H58.8*
- - - late A50.3† H58.8*
- - early (secondary) A51.4† H58.8*
- - late A52.7† H58.8*
Odontalgia K08.8

Odontoameloblastoma (M9311/0) D16.5
- upper jaw (bone) D16.4
Odontoclasia K02.4
Odontodysplasia, regional K00.4
Odontogenesis imperfecta K00.5
Odontoma (M9280/0) D16.5
- ameloblastic (M9311/0) D16.5
- - upper jaw (bone) D16.4
- complex (M9282/0) D16.5
- - upper jaw (bone) D16.4
- compound (M9281/0) D16.5
- - upper jaw (bone) D16.4
- fibroameloblastic (M9290/0) D16.5
- - upper jaw (bone) D16.4
- upper jaw (bone) (M9280/0) D16.4
Odontorrhagia K08.8
Odontosarcoma, ameloblastic (M9290/3) C41.1
- upper jaw (bone) C41.0
Oedema, oedematous – *see* Edema
Oesophag(o) – *see* Esophag(o)
Oesophagus – *see* condition, esophagus
Oestriasis (*see also* Myiasis) B87.9
Oguchi's disease H53.6
Ohara's disease (*see also* Tularemia) A21.9
Old age – *see* Senile, senility
Olfactory – *see condition*
Oligemia – *see* Anemia
Oligoastrocytoma, mixed (M9382/3)
- specified site – *see* Neoplasm, malignant
- unspecified site C71.9
Oligocythemia D64.9
Oligodendroblastoma (M9460/3)
- specified site – *see* Neoplasm, malignant
- unspecified site C71.9
Oligodendroglioma (M9450/3)
- anaplastic type (M9451/3)
- - specified site – *see* Neoplasm, malignant
- - unspecified site C71.9
- specified site – *see* Neoplasm, malignant
- unspecified site C71.9
Oligodontia (*see also* Anodontia) K00.0
Oligohidrosis L74.4
Oligohydramnios O41.0
- affecting fetus or newborn P01.2
Oligomenorrhea N91.5
- primary N91.3
- secondary N91.4
Oligophrenia (*see also* Retardation, mental) F79.-
- phenylpyruvic E70.0
Oligospermia N46

Oligotrichia (*see also* Alopecia) L65.9
– congenital Q84.0
Oliguria R34
– following
– – abortion (subsequent episode) O08.4
– – – current episode – *see* Abortion
– ectopic or molar pregnancy O08.4
– postprocedural N99.0
Ollier's disease Q78.4
Omentitis (*see also* Peritonitis) K65.9
Omentum, omental – *see condition*
**Omphalitis (congenital) (newborn) (with
mild hemorrhage)** P38
– not of newborn L08.9
– tetanus A33
Omphalocele Q79.2
Omphalomesenteric duct, persistent
Q43.0
Omphalorrhagia, newborn P51.9
Onanism (excessive) F98.8
Onchocerciasis, onchocercosis B73
– eye NEC B73† H45.1*
– eyelid B73† H03.0*
Oncocytoma (M8290/0) – *see* Neoplasm,
benign
**Oncovirus, as cause of disease classified
elsewhere** B97.3
Ondine's curse G47.3
Oneirophrenia F23.2
Onychauxis L60.2
– congenital Q84.5
Onychia (with lymphangitis) L03.0
– candidal B37.2
– dermatophytic B35.1
Onychitis (with lymphangitis) L03.0
Onychocryptosis L60.0
Onychodystrophy L60.3
– congenital Q84.6
Onychogryphosis, onychogryposis L60.2
Onycholysis L60.1
Onychomadesis L60.8
Onychomalacia L60.3
Onychomycosis B35.1
Onychophagia F98.8
Onychophosis L60.8
Onychoptosis L60.8
Onychorrhexis L60.3
– congenital Q84.6
Onychoschizia L60.3
Onyxitis (with lymphangitis) L03.0
**Oophoritis (cystic) (infectional)
(interstitial)** (*see also* Salpingo-
oophoritis) N70.9
– acute N70.0

Oophoritis—*continued*
– chronic N70.1
Oophorocele N83.4
Opacity, opacities
– cornea H17.9
– – central NEC H17.1
– – congenital Q13.3
– – degenerative H18.4
– – hereditary H18.5
– – inflammatory – *see* Keratitis
– – specified NEC H17.8
– enamel (teeth) (fluoride) (nonfluoride)
K00.3
– lens (*see also* Cataract) H26.9
– vitreous (humor) NEC H43.3
– – congenital Q14.0
Open, opening
– abnormal, organ or site, congenital – *see*
Imperfect, closure
– angle with
– – borderline intraocular pressure H40.0
– – glaucoma (primary) H40.1
– false – *see* Imperfect, closure
– wound – *see* Wound, open
Openbite (anterior) (posterior) K07.2
Operation R69
– for delivery, affecting fetus or
newborn (*see also* Delivery, by type,
affecting fetus) P03.8
– maternal, unrelated to current delivery,
affecting fetus or newborn P00.6
Operational fatigue F48.8
Operative – *see condition*
Operculum H33.3
Ophiasis L63.2
Ophthalmia H10.9
– actinic rays H16.1
– allergic (acute) H10.1
– blennorrhagic (gonococcal) (neonatorum)
A54.3† H13.1*
– catarrhal H10.2
– diphtheritic A36.8† H13.1*
– Egyptian A71.1† H13.1*
– electrica H16.1
– gonococcal (neonatorum) A54.3† H13.1*
– metastatic H44.0
– neonatorum, newborn P39.1
– – gonococcal A54.3† H13.1*
– nodosa H16.2
– purulent H10.0
– spring H10.1
– sympathetic H44.1
Ophthalmitis – *see* Ophthalmia
Ophthalmocele (congenital) Q15.8

Ophthalmoneuromyelitis G36.0
Ophthalmoplegia (*see also* Strabismus, paralytic) H49.9
– diabetic (*see also* E10-E14 with fourth character .3) E14.3† H58.8∗
– external NEC H49.8
– internal (complete) (total) H52.5
– internuclear H51.2
– migraine G43.8
– Parinaud's H49.8
– progressive external H49.4
– supranuclear, progressive G23.1
– total (external) H49.3
Opioid(s)
– dependence syndrome F11.2
– harmful use F11.1
– intoxication (acute) F11.0
– withdrawal state F11.3
Opisthorchiasis (O. felineus) (O. viverrini) B66.0
Opitz' disease D73.2
Opiumism F11.2
Oppenheim's disease G70.2
Oppenheim-Urbach disease L92.1
Optic nerve – *see condition*
Orbit – *see condition*
Orchioblastoma (M9071/3) C62.9
Orchitis (nonspecific) (septic) (suppurative) N45.9
– with abscess N45.0
– blennorrhagic (acute) (chronic) (gonococcal) A54.2† N51.1∗
– chlamydial A56.1† N51.1∗
– gonococcal (acute) (chronic) A54.2† N51.1∗
– mumps B26.0† N51.1∗
– syphilitic A52.7† N51.1∗
– tuberculous A18.1† N51.1∗
Orf (virus disease) B08.0
Organ of Morgagni (persistence of)
– female Q50.5
– male (epididymal) Q55.4
– – testicular Q55.2
Organic – *see condition*
Orientation, sexual, egodystonic (bisexual) (heterosexual) (homosexual) (prepubertal) F66.1
Orifice – *see condition*
Ormond's disease (with ureteral obstruction) N13.5
– with infection N13.6
Ornithine metabolism disorder E72.4
Ornithinemia (type I) (type II) E72.4

Ornithosis A70
– with pneumonia A70† J17.8∗
Orotic aciduria (congenital) (hereditary) (pyrimidine deficiency) E79.8
– anemia D53.0
Orthodontics
– adjustment Z46.4
– fitting Z46.4
Orthopnea R06.0
Orthoptic training Z50.6
Os, uterus – *see condition*
Osgood-Schlatter disease or osteochondrosis M92.5
Osler-Rendu disease I78.0
Osler's nodes I33.0
Osmidrosis L75.0
Osseous – *see condition*
Ossification
– artery – *see* Arteriosclerosis
– auricle (ear) H61.1
– bronchial J98.0
– cardiac (*see also* Degeneration, myocardial) I51.5
– cartilage (senile) M94.8
– coronary (artery) I25.1
– diaphragm J98.6
– falx cerebri G96.1
– fontanel, premature Q75.0
– heart (*see also* Degeneration, myocardial) I51.5
– – valve – *see* Endocarditis
– larynx J38.7
– ligament M67.8
– – posterior longitudinal M48.8
– meninges (cerebral) (spinal) G96.1
– multiple, eccentric centers M89.2
– muscle M61.9
– – due to burns M61.3
– – paralytic M61.2
– – specified NEC M61.5
– myocardium, myocardial (*see also* Degeneration, myocardial) I51.5
– penis N48.8
– periarticular M25.8
– pinna H61.1
– rider's bone M61.5
– sclera H15.8
– subperiosteal, post-traumatic M89.8
– tendon M67.8
– trachea J39.8
– tympanic membrane H73.8
– vitreous (humor) H43.2
Osteitis (*see also* Osteomyelitis) M86.9
– alveolar K10.3

Osteitis—*continued*
- condensans M85.3
- deformans M88.9
- – in (due to)
- – – malignant neoplasm of bone
  (M8000/3) C41.9† M90.6∗
- – – neoplastic disease NEC
  (M8000/1) (*see also* Neoplasm)
  D48.9† M90.6∗
- – skull M88.0
- – specified NEC M88.8
- due to yaws A66.6† M90.2∗
- fibrosa NEC M85.6
- – circumscripta M85.0
- – cystica (generalisata) E21.0
- – disseminata Q78.1
- – osteoplastica E21.0
- fragilitans Q78.0
- Garré's (sclerosing) M86.8
- jaw (acute) (chronic) (lower)
  (suppurative) (upper) K10.2
- parathyroid E21.0
- petrous bone (acute) (chronic) H70.2
- sclerotic, nonsuppurative M86.8
- tuberculosa A18.0† M90.0∗
- – cystica D86.8
- – multiplex cystoides D86.8
Osteoarthritis (*see also* Arthrosis) M19.9
- generalized M15.9
- interphalangeal
- – distal (Heberden) M15.1
- – proximal (Bouchard) M15.2
Osteoarthropathy (*see also* Osteoarthrosis)
  M19.9
- hypertrophic M19.9
- – pulmonary M89.4
- – specified NEC M89.4
- secondary hypertrophic M89.4
Osteoarthrosis (degenerative)
  (hypertrophic) (*see also* Arthrosis)
  M19.9
- deformans alkaptonurica E70.2† M36.8∗
- erosive M15.4
- generalized M15.9
- – primary M15.0
- joint NEC M19.9
- – primary M19.0
- – secondary NEC M19.2
- localized M19.9
- polyarticular M15.9
- spine (*see also* Spondylosis) M47.9

Osteoblastoma (M9200/0) – *see* Neoplasm,
  bone, benign
- aggressive (M9200/1) – *see* Neoplasm,
  bone, uncertain behavior
Osteochondritis (*see also* Osteochondrosis)
  M93.9
- Brailsford's M92.1
- dissecans M93.2
- juvenile M92.9
- – patellar M92.4
- syphilitic (congenital) (early) A50.0†
  M90.2∗
Osteochondrodysplasia Q78.9
- with defects of growth of tubular bones
  and spine Q77.9
- – specified NEC Q77.8
- specified NEC Q78.8
Osteochondrodystrophy E78.9
- deformans E76.2
- familial E76.2
Osteochondroma (M9210/0) – *see*
  Neoplasm, bone, benign
Osteochondromatosis (M9210/1) D48.0
- syndrome Q78.4
Osteochondromyxosarcoma (M9180/3) –
  see Neoplasm, bone, malignant
Osteochondropathy M93.9
- specified NEC M93.8
- syphilitic, congenital
- – early A50.0† M90.2∗
- – late A50.5† M90.2∗
Osteochondrosarcoma (M9180/3) – *see*
  Neoplasm, bone, malignant
Osteochondrosis M93.9
- acetabulum (juvenile) M91.0
- adult NEC M93.8
- – carpal lunate (Kienböck's) M93.1
- astragalus (juvenile) M92.6
- Blount's M92.5
- Buchanan's M91.0
- Burns' M92.1
- calcaneus (juvenile) M92.6
- capitular epiphysis (femur) (juvenile)
  M91.1
- carpal (juvenile) (lunate) (scaphoid)
  M92.2
- coxae juvenilis M91.1
- deformans juvenilis, coxae M91.1
- Diaz's M92.6
- dissecans (knee) (shoulder) M93.2
- femoral capital epiphysis (juvenile)
  M91.1
- femur (head), juvenile M91.1
- fibula (juvenile) M92.5

Osteochondrosis—*continued*
- foot NEC (juvenile) M92.8
- Freiberg's M92.7
- Haas' (juvenile) M92.0
- Haglund's M92.6
- hip (juvenile) M91.1
- humerus (capitulum) (head) (juvenile) M92.0
- ilium, iliac crest (juvenile) M91.0
- ischiopubic synchondrosis M91.0
- Iselin's M92.7
- juvenile, juvenilis M92.9
- – after reduction of congenital dislocation of hip M91.8
- – arm M92.3
- – capitular epiphysis (femur) M91.1
- – clavicle, sternal epiphysis M92.3
- – coxae M91.1
- – deformans M92.9
- – foot NEC M92.8
- – hand M92.2
- – head of femur M91.1
- – hip and pelvis M91.9
- – – specified NEC M91.8
- – limb
- – – lower NEC M92.8
- – – upper NEC M92.3
- – medial cuneiform bone M92.6
- – specified site NEC M92.8
- – spine M42.0
- – vertebra (body) (Calvé's) M42.0
- – – epiphyseal plates (Scheuermann's) M42.0
- Kienböck's (juvenile) M92.2
- – of adults M93.1
- Köhler's
- – patellar M92.4
- – tarsal navicular M92.6
- Legg-Perthes (-Calvé) (-Waldenström) M91.1
- limb
- – lower NEC (juvenile) M92.8
- – upper NEC (juvenile) M92.3
- lunate bone (carpal) (juvenile) M92.2
- – adult M93.1
- Mauclaire's M92.2
- metacarpal (head) (juvenile) M92.2
- metatarsus (fifth) (head) (juvenile) (second) M92.7
- navicular (juvenile) M92.6
- os
- – calcis (juvenile) M92.6
- – tibiale externum (juvenile) M92.6
- Osgood-Schlatter M92.5

Osteochondrosis—*continued*
- Panner's M92.0
- patellar center (juvenile) (primary) (secondary) M92.4
- pelvis (juvenile) M91.0
- Pierson's M91.0
- radius (head) (juvenile) M92.1
- Scheuermann's M42.0
- Sever's M92.6
- Sinding-Larsen M92.4
- spine M42.9
- – adult M42.1
- – juvenile M42.0
- symphysis pubis (juvenile) M91.0
- talus (juvenile) M92.6
- tarsus (navicular) (juvenile) M92.6
- tibia (proximal) (tubercle) (juvenile) M92.5
- tuberculous – *see* Tuberculosis, bone
- ulna (lower) (juvenile) M92.1
- van Neck's M91.0
- vertebral (*see also* Osteochondrosis, spine) M42.9
Osteoclastoma (M9250/1) D48.0
- malignant (M9250/3) – *see* Neoplasm, bone, malignant
Osteodynia M89.8
Osteodystrophy Q78.9
- azotemic N25.0
- congenital Q78.9
- parathyroid, secondary E21.1
- renal N25.0
Osteofibroma (M9262/0) – *see* Neoplasm, bone, benign
Osteofibrosarcoma (M9182/3) – *see* Neoplasm, bone, malignant
Osteogenesis imperfecta Q78.0
Osteogenic – *see* condition
Osteolysis M89.5
Osteoma (M9180/0) – *see also* Neoplasm, bone, benign
- osteoid (M9191/0)
- – giant (M9200/0) D16.9
Osteomalacia M83.9
- adult M83.9
- – drug-induced NEC M83.5
- – due to
- – – malabsorption (postsurgical) M83.2
- – – malnutrition M83.3
- – specified NEC M83.8
- aluminum-induced M83.4
- infantile (*see also* Rickets) E55.0
- juvenile (*see also* Rickets) E55.0
- pelvis M83.8

Osteomalacia—*continued*
- puerperal M83.0
- senile M83.1
- vitamin-D-resistant E83.3† M90.8*
Osteomyelitis (infective) (septic) (suppurative) M86.9
- acute M86.1
- - hematogenous M86.0
- chronic (or old) M86.6
- - with draining sinus M86.4
- - hematogenous NEC M86.5
- - multifocal M86.3
- echinococcal B67.2† M90.2*
- Garré's M86.8
- gonococcal A54.4† M90.2*
- jaw (acute) (chronic) (lower) (neonatal) (suppurative) (upper) K10.2
- nonsuppurating M86.8
- orbit H05.0
- petrous bone H70.2
- Salmonella (arizonae) (cholerae-suis) (enteritidis) (typhimurium) A02.2† M90.2*
- sclerosing, nonsuppurative M86.8
- specified NEC M86.8
- subacute M86.2
- syphilitic A52.7† M90.2*
- - congenital (early) A50.0† M90.2*
- tuberculous – *see* Tuberculosis, bone
- typhoid A01.0† M90.2*
- vertebra M46.2
Osteomyelofibrosis D47.4
Osteomyelosclerosis D47.4
Osteonecrosis M87.9
- in (due to)
- - caisson disease T70.3† M90.3*
- - drugs M87.1
- - hemoglobinopathy NEC D58.2† M90.4*
- - trauma (previous) M87.2
- jaw (drug-induced) (radiation-induced) K10.2
- secondary NEC M87.3
- specified NEC M87.8
Osteopathia condensans disseminata Q78.8
Osteopathy
- after poliomyelitis M89.6
- in (due to) renal osteodystrophy N25.0† M90.8*
Osteoperiostitis (*see also* Osteomyelitis) M86.8
Osteopetrosis (familial) Q78.2
Osteophyte M25.7

Osteopoikilosis Q78.8
Osteoporosis M81.9
- with pathological fracture M80.9
- disuse M81.2
- - with pathological fracture M80.2
- drug-induced M81.4
- - with pathological fracture M80.4
- idiopathic M81.5
- - with pathological fracture M80.5
- in (due to)
- - endocrine disease NEC E34.9† M82.1*
- - multiple myelomatosis C90.0† M82.0*
- localized (Lequesne) M81.6
- postmenopausal M81.0
- - with pathological fracture M80.0
- postoophorectomy M81.1
- - with pathological fracture M80.1
- postsurgical malabsorption M81.3
- - with pathological fracture M80.3
- post-traumatic M81.8
- - with pathological fracture M80.8
- senile M81.8
- - with pathological fracture M80.8
- specified NEC M81.8
- - with pathological fracture M80.8
Osteopsathyrosis (idiopathica) Q78.0
Osteoradionecrosis, jaw (acute) (chronic) (lower) (suppurative) (upper) K10.2
Osteosarcoma (M9180/3) – *see also* Neoplasm, bone, malignant
- chondroblastic (M9181/3) C41.9
- fibroblastic (M9182/3) C41.9
- in Paget's disease of bone (M9184/3) C41.9
- juxtacortical (M9190/3) C41.9
- parosteal (M9190/3) C41.9
- small cell (M9185/3) C41.9
- telangiectatic (M9183/3) C41.9
Osteosclerosis Q78.2
- acquired M85.8
- congenita Q77.4
- fragilitas (generalisata) Q78.2
- myelofibrosis D47.4
Osteosclerotic anemia D64.8
Osteosis cutis L94.2
Osterreicher-Turner syndrome Q87.2
Ostium
- atrioventriculare commune Q21.2
- primum (arteriosum) (defect) (persistent) Q21.2
- secundum (arteriosum) (defect) (patent) (persistent) Q21.1
Ostrum-Furst syndrome Q75.8
Otalgia H92.0

Othematoma, pinna (nontraumatic)
  H61.1
Otitis H66.9
– adhesive H74.1
– externa H60.9
– – acute H60.5
– – – actinic H60.5
– – – chemical H60.5
– – – contact H60.5
– – – eczematoid H60.5
– – – reactive H60.5
– – chronic H60.8
– – diffuse H60.3
– – hemorrhagic H60.3
– – in (due to)
– – – aspergillosis B44.8† H62.2*
– – – candidiasis B37.2† H62.2*
– – – erysipelas A46† H62.0*
– – – herpes (simplex) virus infection
      B00.1† H62.1*
– – – – zoster B02.8† H62.1*
– – – impetigo L01.0† H62.4*
– – – infectious disease NEC B99†
      H62.3*
– – – mycosis NEC B36.9† H62.2*
– – – parasitic disease NEC B89† H62.3*
– – – viral disease NEC B34.9† H62.1*
– – – zoster B02.8† H62.1*
– – infective NEC H60.3
– – malignant H60.2
– – mycotic B36.9† H62.2*
– – necrotizing H60.2
– – Pseudomonas aeruginosa H60.2
– – specified NEC H60.8
– interna H83.0
– media H66.9
– – with effusion (nonpurulent) H65.9
– – acute or subacute H66.9
– – – with effusion H65.1
– – – allergic H65.1
– – – exudative H65.1
– – – mucoid H65.1
– – – necrotizing (in) H66.0
– – – – measles B05.3† H67.1*
– – – – scarlet fever A38† H67.0*
– – – nonsuppurative NEC H65.1
– – – purulent H66.0
– – – sanguinous H65.1
– – – secretory H65.0
– – – seromucinous H65.1
– – – serous H65.0
– – – suppurative H66.0
– – allergic H65.9
– – catarrhal H65.9

Otitis—*continued*
– media—*continued*
– – chronic H66.9
– – – with effusion (nonpurulent) H65.4
– – – allergic H65.4
– – – catarrhal H65.2
– – – exudative H65.4
– – – mucinous H65.3
– – – mucoid H65.3
– – – nonsuppurative NEC H65.4
– – – purulent H66.3
– – – secretory H65.3
– – – seromucinous H65.4
– – – serous H65.2
– – – suppurative H66.3
– – – – atticoantral H66.2
– – – – benign H66.1
– – – – specified NEC H66.3
– – – – tubotympanic H66.1
– – – transudative H65.3
– – exudative H65.9
– – in (due to)
– – – influenza (specific virus not
      identified) J11.8† H67.1*
– – – – avian virus identified J09† H67.1*
– – – – other virus identified J10.8†
        H67.1*
– – – measles B05.3† H67.1*
– – – scarlet fever A38† H67.0*
– – – tuberculosis A18.6† H67.0*
– – – viral disease NEC B34.9† H67.1*
– – mucoid H65.9
– – nonsuppurative H65.9
– – postmeasles B05.3† H67.1*
– – purulent H66.4
– – secretory H65.9
– – seromucinous H65.9
– – serous H65.9
– – suppurative H66.4
– – transudative H65.9
– – tuberculous A18.6† H67.0*
Otocephaly Q18.2
Otolith syndrome H81.8
Otomycosis (diffuse) (in) B36.9† H62.2*
– aspergillosis B44.8† H62.2*
– candidiasis B37.8† H62.2*
– moniliasis B37.8† H62.2*
Otorrhagia (nontraumatic) H92.2
– traumatic – *see* Injury, by type
Otorrhea H92.1
– cerebrospinal G96.0
Otosclerosis H80.9
– cochlear H80.2

Otosclerosis—*continued*
– involving
– – otic capsule H80.2
– – oval window
– – – nonobliterative H80.0
– – – obliterative H80.1
– – round window H80.2
– nonobliterative H80.0
– obliterative H80.1
– specified NEC H80.8
Otospongiosis (*see also* Otosclerosis)
H80.9
Otto's disease or pelvis M24.7
Outcome of delivery Z37.9
– multiple (births) Z37.9
– – all liveborn Z37.5
– – all stillborn Z37.7
– – some liveborn Z37.6
– single Z37.9
– – liveborn Z37.0
– – stillborn Z37.1
– twins Z37.9
– – both liveborn Z37.2
– – both stillborn Z37.4
– – one liveborn, one stillborn Z37.3
Outlet – *see also condition*
– double, right ventricle (congenital) Q20.1
Outstanding ears (bilateral) Q17.5
Ovalocytosis (congenital)
(hereditary) (*see also* Elliptocytosis)
D58.1
Ovariocele N83.4
Ovaritis (cystic) (*see also* Salpingo-
oophoritis) N70.9
Ovary, ovarian – *see also condition*
– resistant syndrome E28.3
Overactive
– adrenal cortex NEC E27.0
– bladder N32.8
– disorder, associated with mental
retardation and stereotyped movements
F84.4
– hypothalmus E23.3
– thyroid (*see also* Hyperthyroidism) E05.9
Overactivity R46.3
Overbite (deep) (excessive) (horizontal)
(vertical) K07.2
Overbreathing (*see also* Hyperventilation)
R06.4
Overdevelopment – *see* Hypertrophy
Overdistension – *see* Distension
Overdose, overdosage (drug) T50.9
– specified drug or substance – *see* Table of
drugs and chemicals

Overeating R63.2
– nonorganic origin F50.4
– psychogenic F50.4
Overexertion (effects) (exhaustion) T73.3
Overexposure (effects) T73.9
– exhaustion T73.2
Overfeeding R63.2
– newborn P92.4
Overgrowth, bone NEC M89.3
Overheated (places) – *see* Heat
Overjet K07.2
Overlapping toe (acquired) M20.5
– congenital (fifth toe) Q66.8
Overload
– fluid E87.7
– potassium (K) E87.5
– sodium (Na) E87.0
Overnutrition (*see also* Hyperalimentation)
R63.2
Overproduction – *see also* Hypersecretion
– catecholamine E27.5
– growth hormone E22.0
Overprotection, child by parent Z62.1
Overriding
– aorta Q25.4
– finger (acquired) M20.0
– – congenital Q68.1
– toe (acquired) M20.5
– – congenital Q66.8
Oversize fetus P08.1
– affecting management of pregnancy
O36.6
– causing disproportion O33.5
– – with obstructed labor O66.2
– – affecting fetus or newborn P03.1
– exceptionally large (more than 4500 g)
P08.0
Overweight (*see also* Obesity) E66.9
Oviduct – *see condition*
Ovotestis Q56.0
Ovulation (cycle)
– failure or lack of N97.0
– pain N94.0
Ovum – *see condition*
Owren's disease D68.2
Ox heart – *see* Hypertrophy, cardiac
Oxalosis E74.8
Oxaluria E74.8
Oxycephaly Q75.0
– syphilitic, congenital A50.0
Oxyuriasis B80
Oxyuris vermicularis (infection)
(infestation) B80
Ozena J31.0

P

Pachyderma, pachydermia L85.9
– larynx (verrucosa) J38.7
Pachydermatocele (congenital) Q82.8
Pachydermoperiostosis M89.4
– clubbed nail M89.4† L62.0*
Pachygyria Q04.3
**Pachymeningitis (adhesive) (basal)
(cerebral) (spinal)** (*see also* Meningitis)
G03.9
Pachyonychia (congenital) Q84.5
Pacinian tumor (M9507/0) – *see* Neoplasm,
skin, benign
Pad, knuckle or Garrod's M72.1
Paget's disease
– with infiltrating duct carcinoma
(M8541/3) – *see* Neoplasm, breast,
malignant
– bone M88.9
– – osteosarcoma in (M9184/3) – *see*
Neoplasm, bone, malignant
– – skull M88.0
– – specified NEC M88.8
– breast (M8540/3) C50.0
– extramammary (M8542/3) – *see also*
Neoplasm, skin, malignant
– – anus (M8542/3) C21.0
– – – margin (M8542/3) C44.5
– – – skin (M8542/3) C44.5
– intraductal carcinoma (M8543/3) – *see*
Neoplasm, breast, malignant
– malignant (M8540/3)
– – breast C50.0
– – specified site NEC (M8542/3) – *see*
Neoplasm, skin, malignant
– – unspecified site C50.0
– mammary (M8540/3) C50.0
– nipple (M8540/3) C50.0
– osteitis deformans M88.9
Pain(s) R52.9
– abdominal R10.4
– – lower abdomen R10.3
– – – pelvic or perineal R10.2
– – severe R10.0
– – upper abdomen R10.1
– acute NEC R52.0
– anus K62.8
– arm M79.6
– back (postural) M54.9
– – low M54.5

Pain(s)—*continued*
– back—*continued*
– – psychogenic F45.4
– – specified NEC M54.8
– bladder R39.8
– bone M89.8
– breast N64.4
– – psychogenic F45.4
– cecum R10.3
– chest R07.4
– – anterior wall R07.3
– – ischemic I20.9
– – on breathing R07.1
– chronic NEC R52.2   – Pain control.
– – intractable R52.1
– – specified NEC R52.2
– coccyx M53.3
– colon R10.4
– coronary – *see* Angina
– due to device, implant or graft (*see also*
Complications, by site and type) T85.8
– – arterial graft NEC T82.8
– – breast (implant) T85.8
– – catheter NEC T85.8
– – – dialysis (renal) T82.8
– – – – intraperitoneal T85.8
– – – infusion NEC T82.8
– – – – spinal (epidural) (subdural) T85.8
– – – urinary (indwelling) T83.8
– – electronic (electrode) (pulse generator)
(stimulator)
– – – bone T84.8
– – – cardiac T82.8
– – – nervous system (brain) (peripheral
nerve) (spinal) T85.8
– – – urinary T83.8
– – fixation, internal (orthopedic) NEC
T84.8
– – gastrointestinal (bile duct) (esophagus)
T85.8
– – genital NEC T83.8
– – heart NEC T82.8
– – infusion NEC T85.8
– – joint prosthesis T84.8
– – ocular (corneal graft) (orbital implant)
NEC T85.8
– – orthopedic NEC T84.8
– – specified NEC T85.8
– – urinary NEC T83.8

Pain(s)—*continued*
- due to device, implant or graft—*continued*
- – vascular NEC T82.8
- – ventricular intracranial shunt T85.8
- ear H92.0
- epigastric, epigastrium R10.1
- eye H57.1
- face, facial R51
- – atypical G50.1
- false (labor) – *see* Labor, false
- female genital organs NEC N94.8
- finger M79.6
- flank R10.4
- foot M79.6
- gas (intestinal) R14
- gastric R10.1
- generalized R52.9
- genital organ
- – female N94.8
- – male N50.8
- – psychogenic F45.4
- groin R10.3
- hand M79.6
- head (*see also* Headache) R51
- heart (*see also* Pain, precordial) R07.2
- infra-orbital (*see also* Neuralgia, trigeminal) G50.0
- intermenstrual N94.0
- jaw K10.8
- joint M25.5
- – psychogenic F45.4
- kidney N23
- labor, false or spurious – *see* Labor, false
- leg M79.6
- limb (lower) (upper) M79.6
- loin M54.5
- low back M54.5
- lower abdomen R10.3
- – pelvic or perineal R10.2
- lumbar region M54.5
- mastoid H92.0
- maxilla K10.8
- metacarpophalangeal (joint) M25.5
- metatarsophalangeal (joint) M25.5
- mouth K13.7
- muscle M79.1
- nasal J34.8
- nasopharynx J39.2
- neck NEC M54.2
- – psychogenic F45.4
- nerve NEC M79.2
- neuromuscular M79.2
- nose J34.8
- ocular H57.1

Pain(s)—*continued*
- ophthalmic H57.1
- orbital region H57.1
- ovary N94.8
- over heart (*see also* Pain, precordial) R07.2
- ovulation N94.0
- pelvic R10.2
- penis N48.8
- – psychogenic F45.4
- pericardial (*see also* Pain, precordial) R07.2
- perineal R10.2
- pharynx J39.2
- pleura, pleural, pleuritic R07.3
- precordial (region) R07.2
- – psychogenic F45.4
- psychogenic (any site) (persistent) F45.4
- radicular (spinal) (*see also* Radiculitis) M54.1
- rectum K62.8
- respiration R07.1
- rheumatoid, muscular M79.1
- rib R07.3
- root (spinal) (*see also* Radiculitis) M54.1
- sciatic M54.3
- scrotum N50.8
- – psychogenic F45.4
- seminal vesicle N50.8
- shoulder M25.5
- spermatic cord N50.8
- spinal root (*see also* Radiculitis) M54.1
- stomach R10.1
- – psychogenic F45.4
- testis N50.8
- – psychogenic F45.4
- thoracic spine M54.6
- – with radicular and visceral pain M54.1
- throat R07.0
- tibia M89.8
- toe M79.6
- tongue K14.6
- tooth K08.8
- trigeminal (*see also* Neuralgia, trigeminal) G50.0
- ureter N23
- uterus NEC N94.8
- – psychogenic F45.4
- vertebrogenic (syndrome) M54.8
- vesical R39.8

Painful – *see also* Pain
- coitus
- – female N94.1
- – male N48.8

Progressive
Supranuclear
Palsy
G23.1

– – psychogenic F45.8
– micturition R30.9
– respiration R07.1
Painter's colic T56.0
Palate – *see condition*
Palatoplegia K13.7
Palatoschisis (*see also* Cleft, palate) Q35.9
Palilalia R48.8
Palliative care Z51.5
Pallor R23.1
– optic disk, temporal H47.2
Palmar – *see also condition*
– fascia – *see condition*
Palpable
– cecum K63.8
– kidney N28.8
– ovary N83.8
– spleen (*see also* Splenomegaly) R16.1
Palpitations (heart) R00.2
– psychogenic F45.3
Palsy (*see also* Paralysis) G83.9
– atrophic diffuse (progressive) G12.2
– Bell's (*see also* Palsy, facial) G51.0
– brachial plexus NEC G54.0
– – fetus or newborn (birth injury) P14.3
– brain – *see* Palsy, cerebral
– bulbar (chronic) (progressive) G12.2
– – of childhood (Fazio-Londe) G12.1
– – pseudo- NEC G12.2
– – supranuclear NEC G12.2
– cerebral (congenital) G80.9
– – ataxic G80.4
– – athetoid G80.3
– – choreathetoid G80.3
– – diplegic G80.8
– – – spastic G80.1
– – dyskinetic G80.3
– – – athetoid G80.3
– – – choreathetoid G80.3
– – – dystonic G80.3
– – – dystonic G80.3
– – hemiplegic G80.8
– – – spastic G80.2
– – mixed G80.8
– – monoplegic G80.8
– – – spastic G80.1

Palsy—*continued*
– cerebral—*continued*
– – not congenital acute I64
– – paraplegic G80.8
– – – spastic G80.1
– – quadriplegic G80.8
– – – spastic G80.0
– – spastic G80.1
– – – diplegic G80.1
– – – hemiplegic G80.2
– – – monoplegic G80.1
– – – quadriplegic G80.0
– – – specified NEC G80.1
– – – tetraplegic G80.0
– – specified NEC G80.8
– – syphilitic A52.1
– – – congenital A50.4
– – tetraplegic G80.8
– – – spastic G80.0
– cranial nerve – *see also* Disorder, nerve, cranial
– – multiple (in) G52.7
– – – infectious disease NEC B99† G53.1*
– – – neoplastic disease NEC (M8000/1) (*see also* Neoplasm) D48.9† G53.3*
– – – parasitic disease NEC B89† G53.1*
– – – sarcoidosis D86.8† G53.2*
– creeping G12.2
– diver's T70.3
– Erb's P14.0
– facial G51.0
– – newborn (birth injury) P11.3
– glossopharyngeal G52.1
– Klumpke(-Déjerine) P14.1
– lead T56.0
– median nerve (tardy) G56.1
– nerve G58.9
– – specified NEC G58.8
– peroneal nerve (acute) (tardy) G57.3
– pseudobulbar NEC G12.2
– radial nerve (acute) G56.3
– seventh nerve (*see also* Palsy, facial) G51.0
– shaking (*see also* Parkinsonism) G20
– ulnar nerve (tardy) G56.2
– wasting G12.2
Paludism – *see* Malaria
Panangiitis M30.0
Panaris, panaritium (with lymphangitis) L03.0
Panarteritis nodosa M30.0
– brain or cerebral I67.7

Pancarditis (acute) (chronic) I51.8
– rheumatic I09.8
– – active or acute I01.8
Pancolitis, ulcerative (chronic) K51.0
Pancoast's syndrome or tumor (M8010/3)
C34.1
Pancreas, pancreatic – see condition
Pancreatitis K85.9
– acute (edematous) (hemorrhagic)
(recurrent) K85.-
– – alcohol-induced K85.2
– – biliary K85.1
– – drug-induced K85.3
– – gallstone K85.1
– – idiopathic K85.0
– – specified NEC K85.8
– annular (acute) K85.-
– chronic (infectious) K86.1
– – alcohol-induced K86.0
– – recurrent K86.1
– – relapsing K86.1
– cystic (chronic) K86.1
– cytomegaloviral B25.2† K87.1*
– edematous (acute) K85.-
– fibrous (chronic) K86.1
– gangrenous K85.-
– hemorrhagic (acute) K85.-
– interstitial (chronic) K86.1
– – acute K85.-
– malignant K85.-
– mumps B26.3† K87.1*
– recurrent (chronic) K86.1
– relapsing, chronic K86.1
– subacute K85.-
– suppurative K85.-
– syphilitic A52.7† K87.1*
Pancreatoblastoma (M8971/3) – see
Neoplasm, pancreas, malignant
Pancreolithiasis K86.8
Pancytolysis D75.8
Pancytopenia (acquired) D61.9
– with malformations D61.0
– congenital D61.0
Panencephalitis, subacute, sclerosing
A81.1
Panhematopenia D61.9
– constitutional D61.0
– splenic, primary D73.1
Panhemocytopenia D61.9
– constitutional D61.0
Panhypopituitarism E23.0
– prepubertal E23.0

Panic (attack) (state) F41.0
– reaction to exceptional stress (transient)
F43.0
Panmyelophthisis D61.9
Panmyelosis (acute) C94.4
– with myelofibrosis, acute C94.4
Panner's disease M92.0
Panneuritis endemica E51.1† G63.4*
Panniculitis M79.3
– back M54.0
– febrile nodular nonsuppurative (Weber-
Christian) M35.6
– lupus L93.2
– neck M54.0
– nodular, nonsuppurative M35.6
– relapsing (febrile nodular
nonsuppurative)(Weber-Christian) M35.6
– sacral M54.0
Panniculus adiposus (abdominal) E65
Pannus (cornea) H16.4
– allergic H16.4
– degenerativus H16.4
– keratic H16.4
– trachomatosus, trachomatous (active)
A71.1
Panophthalmitis H44.0
Pansinusitis (chronic) (hyperplastic)
(nonpurulent) (purulent) J32.4
– acute J01.4
– tuberculous A16.8
– – with bacteriological and histological
confirmation A15.8
Panuveitis (sympathetic) H44.1
Panvalvular disease (unspecified origin)
I08.9
– specified NEC (unspecified origin) I08.8
Papanicolaou smear, cervix Z12.4
– as part of routine gynecological
examination Z01.4
– for suspected neoplasm Z12.4
– – no disease found Z03.1
– routine Z01.4
Papilledema (choked disk) H47.1
Papillitis H46
– anus K62.8
– optic H46
– rectum K62.8
– tongue K14.0
Papilloma (M8050/0) – see also Neoplasm,
benign

Note: Except where otherwise indicated, the
morphological varieties of papilloma in the
list below should be coded by site as for
"Neoplasm, benign".

Papilloma—*continued*

- acuminatum (anogenital) (female) (male) A63.0
- bladder (urinary) (transitional cell) (M8120/1) D41.4
- – benign (M8120/0) D30.3
- choroid plexus (lateral ventricle) (third ventricle) (M9390/0) D33.0
- – anaplastic (M9390/3) C71.5
- – fourth ventricle D33.1
- – malignant (M9390/3) C71.5
- ductal (M8503/0)
- dyskeratotic (M8052/0)
- epidermoid (M8052/0)
- hyperkeratotic (M8052/0)
- intracystic (M8504/0)
- intraductal (M8503/0)
- inverted (M8053/0)
- keratotic (M8052/0)
- parakeratotic (M8052/0)
- renal pelvis (transitional cell) (M8120/1) D41.1
- – benign (M8120/0) D30.1
- Schneiderian (M8121/0)
- – specified site – *see* Neoplasm, benign
- – unspecified site D14.0
- serous surface (M8461/0)
- – borderline malignancy (M8461/1)
- – – specified site – *see* Neoplasm, uncertain behavior
- – – unspecified site D39.1
- – specified site – *see* Neoplasm, benign
- – unspecified site D27
- squamous (cell) (M8052/0)
- transitional (cell) (M8120/0)
- – bladder (urinary) (M8120/1) D41.4
- – inverted type (M8121/1) – *see* Neoplasm, uncertain behavior
- – renal pelvis (M8120/1) D41.1
- – ureter (M8120/1) D41.2
- ureter (transitional cell) (M8120/1) D41.2
- – benign (M8120/0) D30.2
- urothelial (M8120/1) – *see* Neoplasm, uncertain behavior
- verrucous (M8051/0)
- villous (M8261/1) – *see* Neoplasm, uncertain behavior
- – adenocarcinoma in (M8261/3) – *see* Neoplasm, malignant
- – – in situ (M8261/2) – *see* Neoplasm, in situ
- yaws, plantar or palmar A66.1

Papillomata, multiple, of yaws A66.1

Papillomatosis (M8060/0) – *see also* Neoplasm, benign
- confluent and reticulated L83
- cystic, breast N60.1
- intraductal (diffuse) (M8505/0) – *see* Neoplasm, benign
- subareolar duct (M8506/0) D24

Papillomavirus, as cause of disease classified elsewhere B97.7

Papillon-Leage and Psaume syndrome Q87.0

Papule(s) R23.8
- carate (primary) A67.0
- fibrous, of nose (M8724/0) D22.3
- Gottron's L94.4
- pinta (primary) A67.0

Papulosis, lymphomatoid C86.6 — *parapsoriasis* L41.2

Papyraceous fetus P95
- complicating pregnancy O31.0

Para-albuminemia E88.0

Paracephalus Q89.7

Paracoccidioidomycosis B41.9
- disseminated B41.7
- generalized B41.7
- mucocutaneous-lymphangitic B41.8
- pulmonary B41.0† J17.2*
- specified NEC B41.8
- visceral B41.8

Paradentosis K05.4

Paraffinoma T88.8

Paraganglioma (M8680/1)
- adrenal (M8700/0) D35.0
- aortic body (M8691/1) D44.7
- – malignant (M8691/3) C75.5
- carotid body (M8692/1) D44.6
- chromaffin (M8700/0) – *see also* Neoplasm, benign
- – malignant (M8700/3) – *see* Neoplasm, malignant
- extra-adrenal (M8693/1)
- – malignant (M8693/3)
- – – specified site – *see* Neoplasm, malignant
- – – unspecified site C75.5
- – specified site – *see* Neoplasm, uncertain behavior
- – unspecified site D44.7
- gangliocytic (M8683/0)
- – specified site – *see* Neoplasm, benign
- – unspecified site D13.2
- glomus jugulare (M8690/1) D44.7
- jugular (M8690/1) D44.7
- malignant (M8680/3)

Paraganglioma—*continued*
– malignant—*continued*
– – specified site – *see* Neoplasm,
   malignant
– – unspecified site C75.5
– nonchromaffin (M8693/1)
– – malignant (M8693/3)
– – – specified site – *see* Neoplasm,
      malignant
– – – unspecified site C75.5
– – specified site – *see* Neoplasm, uncertain
   behavior
– – unspecified site D44.7
– parasympathetic (M8682/1)
– – specified site – *see* Neoplasm, uncertain
   behavior
– – unspecified site D44.7
– specified site – *see* Neoplasm, uncertain
   behavior
– sympathetic (M8681/1)
– – specified site – *see* Neoplasm, uncertain
   behavior
– – unspecified site D44.7
– unspecified site D44.7
Parageusia R43.2
– psychogenic F45.8
Paragonimiasis B66.4
Paragranuloma
– Hodgkin C81.0
– nodular C81.0
Parahemophilia D68.2
Parakeratosis R23.4
– variegata L41.5
Paralysis, paralytic (complete)
   (incomplete) (*see also* Paresis) G83.9
– with syphilis A52.1
– abducent (nerve) H49.2
– accommodation H52.5
– – hysterical F44.8
– agitans (*see also* Parkinsonism) G20
– – arteriosclerotic G21.4
– alternating G83.8
– – oculomotor G83.8
– amyotrophic G12.2
– anus (sphincter) K62.8
– arm G83.2
– – both G83.0
– – hysterical F44.4
– – psychogenic F44.4
– – transient R29.8
– – – traumatic NEC (*see also* Injury,
      nerve, upper limb) T11.3
– ascending (spinal), acute G61.0
– association G12.2

Paralysis, paralytic—*continued*
– ataxic (hereditary) G11.9
– – general (syphilitic) A52.1
– atrophic G58.9
– – infantile, acute (*see also* Poliomyelitis,
      paralytic) A80.3
– – progressive G12.2
– – spinal (acute) (*see also* Poliomyelitis,
      paralytic) A80.3
– axillary G54.0
– Bell's G51.0
– Benedikt's I67.9† G46.3*
– birth injury P14.9
– bladder (neurogenic) (sphincter) N31.2
– – puerperal, postpartum O90.8
– bowel, colon or intestine (*see also* Ileus)
   K56.0
– brachial plexus NEC G54.0
– – birth injury P14.3
– – newborn P14.3
– bronchial J98.0
– Brown-Séquard G83.8
– bulbar (chronic) (progressive) G12.2
– – infantile (*see also* Poliomyelitis,
      paralytic) A80.3
– – poliomyelitic (*see also* Poliomyelitis,
      paralytic) A80.3
– – pseudo- G12.2
– – supranuclear G12.2
– cardiac I46.9
– cervical sympathetic G90.2
– Cestan-Chenais I63.0† G46.3*
– Charcot-Marie-Tooth type G60.0
– colon NEC K56.0
– compressed air T70.3
– congenital (cerebral) – *see* Palsy, cerebral
– conjugate movement (gaze) (of eye)
   H51.0
– – cortical (nuclear) (supranuclear) H51.0
– convergence H51.1
– cordis (*see also* Failure, heart) I50.9
– creeping G12.2
– deglutition R13
– – hysterical F44.4
– dementia A52.1
– descending (spinal) NEC G12.2
– diaphragm (flaccid) J98.6
– – due to accidental section of phrenic
      nerve during procedure T81.2
– diplegic – *see* Diplegia
– divergence (nuclear) H51.8
– diver's T70.3
– Duchenne's
– – birth injury P14.0

Paralysis, paralytic—*continued*
- Duchenne's—*continued*
- – – due to or associated with
- – – – motor neuron disease G12.2
- – – – muscular dystrophy G71.0
- – due to intracranial or spinal birth injury –
  see Palsy, cerebral
- embolic (current episode) I63.4
- Erb(-Duchenne) (birth) (newborn) P14.0
- Erb's syphilitic spastic spinal A52.1
- esophagus K22.8
- eye muscle (extrinsic) H49.9
- – intrinsic H52.5
- facial (nerve) G51.0
- – birth injury P11.3
- – newborn P11.3
- familial (periodic) (recurrent) G72.3
- – spastic G11.4
- fauces J39.2
- gait R26.1
- gaze, conjugate H51.0
- general (progressive) (syphilitic) A52.1
- – juvenile A50.4
- glottis J38.0
- gluteal G54.1
- Gubler-Millard I67.9† G46.3∗
- hand G83.2
- – hysterical F44.4
- – psychogenic F44.4
- hemiplegic – *see* Hemiplegia
- hysterical F44.4
- ileus (*see also* Ileus) K56.0
- infantile (*see also* Poliomyelitis, paralytic)
  A80.3
- – bulbar (*see also* Poliomyelitis,
  paralytic) A80.3
- – cerebral – *see* Palsy, cerebral
- – spastic – *see* Palsy, cerebral, spastic
- infective (*see also* Poliomyelitis,
  paralytic) A80.3
- internuclear H51.2
- intestine NEC K56.0
- iris H57.0
- – due to diphtheria (toxin) A36.8†
  H22.8∗
- ischemic, Volkmann's (complicating
  trauma) T79.6
- jake T62.2
- Jamaica ginger G62.2
- juvenile general A50.4
- Klumpke(-Déjerine) (birth injury)
  (newborn) P14.1
- labioglossal (laryngeal) (pharyngeal)
  G12.2

Paralysis, paralytic—*continued*
- Landry's G61.0
- laryngeal nerve (bilateral) (recurrent)
  (superior) (unilateral) J38.0
- larynx J38.0
- – due to diphtheria (toxin) A36.2
- lateral G12.2
- lead T56.0
- left side – *see* Hemiplegia
- leg G83.1
- – both (*see also* Paraplegia) G82.2
- – hysterical F44.4
- – psychogenic F44.4
- – transient or transitory R29.8
- levator palpebrae superioris H02.4
- limb NEC G83.3
- – all four (*see also* Tetraplegia) G82.5
- – transient (cause unknown) R29.8
- lip K13.0
- Lissauer's A52.1
- lower limb G83.1
- – both (*see also* Paraplegia) G82.2
- medullary (tegmental) G83.8
- mesencephalic NEC G83.8
- – tegmental G83.8
- middle alternating G83.8
- Millard-Gubler-Foville I67.9† G46.3∗
- monoplegic – *see* Monoplegia
- motor NEC G83.9
- muscle, muscular NEC G72.8
- – due to nerve lesion NEC G58.9
- – eye (extrinsic) H49.9
- – – intrinsic H52.5
- – – oblique H49.1
- – ischemic (cmplicating trauma)
  (Volksmann's) T79.6
- – progressive G12.2
- – pseudohypertrophic G71.0
- nerve – *see also* Disorder, nerve
- – birth injury P14.9
- – facial G51.0
- – – birth injury P11.3
- – – newborn P11.3
- – fourth or trochlear H49.1
- – newborn (birth injury) P14.9
- – phrenic (birth injury) P14.2
- – radial G56.3
- – – birth injury P14.3
- – – newborn P14.3
- – seventh or facial G51.0
- – – newborn (birth injury) P11.3
- – sixth or abducent H49.2
- – syphilitic A52.1† G59.8∗
- – third or oculomotor H49.0

Paralysis, paralytic—*continued*
- ocular NEC H49.9
- oculofacial, congenital (Moebius) Q87.0
- oculomotor (nerve) H49.0
- – external bilateral H49.0
- palate (soft) K13.7
- periodic (familial) (hyperkalemic) (hypokalemic) (myotonic) (normokalemic) G72.3
- peripheral autonomic nervous system – *see* Neuropathy, peripheral, autonomic
- peroneal (nerve) G57.3
- pharynx J39.2
- poliomyelitis (current) (*see also* Poliomyelitis, paralytic) A80.3
- progressive (atrophic) (bulbar) (spinal) G12.2
- – general A52.1
- – infantile acute (*see also* Poliomyelitis, paralytic) A80.3
- pseudobulbar G12.2
- pseudohypertrophic (muscle) G71.0
- psychogenic F44.4
- quadriplegic (*see also* Tetraplegia) G82.5
- radial nerve G56.3
- – birth injury P14.3
- rectus muscle (eye) H49.9
- respiratory (muscle) R06.8
- – center NEC G93.8
- right side – *see* Hemiplegia
- saturnine T56.0
- senile NEC G83.9
- shaking (*see also* Parkinsonism) G20
- spastic G83.9
- – cerebral – *see* Palsy, cerebral, spastic
- – congenital (cerebral) – *see* Palsy, cerebral, spastic
- – familial G11.4
- – hereditary G11.4
- – not infantile or congenital (cerebral) G83.9
- – syphilitic (spinal) A52.1
- sphincter, bladder (*see also* Paralysis, bladder) N31.2
- spinal (cord) G83.8
- – acute (*see also* Poliomyelitis, paralytic) A80.3
- – ascending acute G61.0
- – atrophic (acute) (*see also* Poliomyelitis, paralytic) A80.3
- – – spastic, syphilitic A52.1
- – congenital NEC – *see* Palsy, cerebral
- – infantile (*see also* Poliomyelitis, paralytic) A80.3

Paralysis, paralytic—*continued*
- spinal—*continued*
- – progressive G12.2
- – spastic NEC – *see* Palsy, cerebral, spastic
- sternomastoid G52.8
- stomach K31.8
- stroke (current episode) I64
- supranuclear G12.2
- sympathetic G90.8
- – cervical G90.2
- – nervous system – *see* Neuropathy, peripheral, autonomic
- syndrome G83.9
- – specified NEC G83.8
- syphilitic spastic spinal (Erb's) A52.1
- throat J39.2
- – diphtheritic A36.0† G99.8*
- – muscle J39.2
- tick T63.4
- Todd's G83.8
- tongue K14.8
- transient
- – arm or leg NEC R29.8
- – traumatic NEC (*see also* Injury, nerve) T14.4
- trapezius G52.8
- traumatic, transient NEC (*see also* Injury, nerve) T14.4
- trembling (*see also* Parkinsonism) G20
- trochlear (nerve) H49.1
- upper limb G83.2
- – both (*see also* Diplegia) G83.0
- uremic N18.5† G99.8*
- uveoparotitic D86.8
- uvula K13.7
- – postdiphtheritic A36.0
- vasomotor NEC G90.8
- velum palatinum K13.7
- vesical (*see also* Paralysis, bladder) N31.2
- vocal cords J38.0
- Volkmann's (complicating trauma) T79.6
- wasting G12.2
- Weber's I67.8† G46.3*

Paramedial urethrovesical orifice Q64.7
Paramenia N92.6
Parametritis (*see also* Disease, pelvis, inflammatory) N73.2
Parametrium, parametric – *see condition*
Paramnesia (*see also* Amnesia) R41.3
Paramolar K00.1
- causing crowding K07.3
Paramyloidosis E85.8

Paramyoclonus multiplex G25.3
Paramyotonia (congenita) G71.1
Parangi (*see also* Yaws) A66.9
Paranoia F22.0
– alcoholic F10.5
– drug-induced – *code to* F11-F19 with
  fourth character .5
– querulans F22.8
– senile F03
Paranoid
– dementia (senile) F03
– – praecox (*see also* Schizophrenia) F20.9
– personality F60.0
– psychosis F22.0
– – alcoholic F10.5
– – climacteric F22.8
– – involutional F22.8
– – menopausal F22.8
– – psychogenic (acute) F23.3
– – senile F03
– reaction (acute) F23.3
– – chronic F22.0
– schizophrenia F20.0
– state F22.0
– – climacteric F22.8
– – induced by drug – *see* F11-F19 with
  fourth character .5
– – involution F22.8
– – menopausal F22.8
– – senile F03
– – simple F22.0
– – specified NEC F22.8
– tendencies F61
– traits F61
Paraparesis (*see also* Paraplegia) G82.2
Paraphasia R47.0
Paraphilia F65.9
Paraphimosis (congenital) N47
– chancroidal A57
Paraphrenia, paraphrenic (late) F22.0
– schizophrenia F20.0
Paraplegia (lower) G82.2
– ataxic – *see* Degeneration, combined,
  spinal cord
– congenital (cerebral) G80.8
– – spastic G80.1
– flaccid G82.0
– functional (hysterical) F44.4
– hereditary, spastic G11.4
– hysterical F44.4
– Pott's A18.0† M49.0*
– psychogenic F44.4
– spastic G82.1
– – Erb's spinal, syphilitic A52.1

Paraplegia—*continued*
– spastic—*continued*
– – hereditary G11.4
– – tropical G04.1
– syphilitic (spastic) A52.1
– traumatic (spinal cord), current episode
  T09.3
– tropical spastic G04.1
Paraproteinemia D89.2
– benign (familial) D89.2
– monoclonal D47.2
– secondary to malignant disease D47.2
Parapsoriasis L41.9
– guttata L41.1
– large plaque L41.4
– retiform, retiformis L41.5
– small plaque L41.3
– specified NEC L41.8
– varioliformis (acuta) L41.0
Parasitic – *see also* condition
– twin Q89.4
Parasitism B89
– intestinal NEC B82.9
– skin NEC B88.9
– specified – *see* Infestation
Parasitophobia F40.2
Parasomnia G47.8
– nonorganic origin F51.9
Paraspadias Q54.9
Paraspasmus facialis G51.8
Parasuicide
– history of (personal) Z91.5
– – in family Z81.8
– observation following alleged Z03.8
Parathyroid gland – *see* condition
Parathyroid tetany E20.9
Paratrachoma A74.0† H13.1*
Paratyphoid (fever) – *see* Fever,
  paratyphoid
Paratyphus – *see* Fever, paratyphoid
Paraurethral duct Q64.7
Paraurethritis (*see also* Urethritis) N34.2
– gonococcal (acute) (chronic) (with
  abscess) A54.1
Paravaccinia B08.0
Paravaginitis (*see also* Vaginitis) N76.0
Parencephalitis (*see also* Encephalitis)
  G04.9
Paresis (*see also* Paralysis) G83.9
– Bernhardt's G57.1
– bladder (sphincter) (*see also* Paralysis,
  bladder) N31.2
– – tabetic A52.1

Paresis—*continued*
- bowel, colon or intestine (*see also* Ileus) K56.0
- extrinsic muscle, eye H49.9
- general (progressive) (syphilitic) A52.1
- – juvenile A50.4
- heart (*see also* Failure, heart) I50.9
- insane (syphilitic) A52.1
- juvenile (general) A50.4
- peripheral progressive (idiopathic) G60.3
- pseudohypertrophic G71.0
- syphilitic (general) A52.1
- – congenital A50.4
- vesical NEC N31.2

Paretic – *see condition*

Parinaud's
- conjunctivitis H10.8
- oculoglandular syndrome H10.8
- ophthalmoplegia H49.8
- syndrome (ophthalmoplegia) H49.8

Parkinsonism (idiopathic) (primary) G20
- with neurogenic orthostatic hypotension (symptomatic) G90.3
- arteriosclerotic G21.4
- dementia in G20† F02.3*
- due to drugs G21.1
- – neuroleptic G21.0
- postencephalitic G21.3
- secondary G21.9
- – due to
- – – arteriosclerosis G21.4
- – – drugs NEC G21.1
- – – – neuroleptic G21.0
- – – encephalitis G21.3
- – – external agents NEC G21.2
- – – syphilis A52.1† G22*
- – – specified NEC G21.8
- syphilitic A52.1† G22*
- treatment-induced NEC G21.1
- vascular G21.4

Parkinson's disease, syndrome or tremor (*see also* Parkinsonism) G20

Parodontitis (*see also* Periodontitis) K05.3

Parodontosis K05.4

Paronychia (with lymphangitis) L03.0
- candidal B37.2
- tuberculous (primary) A18.4

Parorexia NEC F50.8
- psychogenic F50.8

Parosmia R43.1
- psychogenic F45.8

Parotid gland – *see condition*

Parotitis, parotiditis (acute) (chronic) (nonepidemic) (nonspecific toxic) (not

mumps) (purulent) (septic) (suppurative) K11.2
- epidemic (*see also* Mumps) B26.9
- infectious (*see also* Mumps) B26.9
- postoperative K91.8
- surgical K91.8

Parrot fever A70

Parrot's disease (early congenital syphilitic pseudoparalysis) A50.0

Parry-Romberg syndrome G51.8

Parry's disease E05.0

Pars planitis H30.2

Parsonage-Aldren-Turner syndrome G54.5

Particolored infant Q82.8

Parturition – *see* Delivery

Parulis K04.7
- with sinus K04.6

Parvovirus, as cause of disease classified elsewhere B97.6

Pasini and Pierini's atrophoderma L90.3

Passage
- false, urethra N36.0
- of sounds or bougies – *see* Attention, artificial opening

Passive – *see condition*

Pasteurellosis (*see also* Infection, Pasteurella) A28.0

Patau's syndrome (*see also* Trisomy, 13) Q91.7

Patches
- mucous (syphilitic) A51.3
- – congenital A50.0
- smokers' (mouth) K13.2

Patellar – *see condition*

Patent – *see also* Imperfect, closure
- canal of Nuck Q52.4
- cervix N88.3
- – complicating pregnancy O34.3
- – – affecting fetus or newborn P01.0
- ductus arteriosus or botalli Q25.0
- foramen
- – botalli Q21.1
- – ovale Q21.1
- interauricular septum Q21.1
- omphalomesenteric duct Q43.0
- os (uteri) – *see* Patent, cervix
- ostium secundum Q21.1
- urachus Q64.4
- vitelline duct Q43.0

Paterson(-Brown)-Kelly syndrome D50.1
- fire-setting F63.1
- gambling F63.0
- ovum O02.0

Paterson(-Brown)-Kelly syndrome—
continued
- stealing F63.2
Pattern, sleep-wake, irregular G47.2
Patulous – *see also* Patent
- eustachian tube H69.0
Paxton's disease B36.8
Pearl(s)
- enamel K00.2
- Epstein's K09.8
Pearl-worker's disease M86.8
Pectenosis K62.4
Pectoral – *see condition*
Pectus
- carinatum (congenital) Q67.7
- - acquired M95.4
- - rachitic (late effect) E64.3
- excavatum (congenital) Q67.6
- - acquired M95.4
- - rachitic (late effect) E64.3
Pederosis F65.4
Pediculosis B85.2
- capitis (head-louse) (any site) B85.0
- corporis (body-louse) (any site) B85.1
- mixed (classifiable to more than one of
  the subcategories B85.0-B85.3) B85.4
- pubis (pubic-louse) (any site) B85.3
- vestimenti B85.1
- vulvae B85.3
Pediculus (infestation) – *see* Pediculosis
Pedophilia F65.4
Peg-shaped teeth K00.2
Pelade (*see also* Alopecia, areata) L63.9
Pelger-Huet anomaly or syndrome D72.0
Peliosis (rheumatica) D69.0
- hepatis K76.4
- - with toxic liver disease K71.8
Pelizaeus-Merzbacher disease E75.2
Pellagra (alcoholic) E52
Pellegrini-Stieda disease or syndrome
  M76.4
Pellizzi's syndrome E34.8
Pel's crisis A52.1
Pelvic – *see also condition*
- examination (periodic) (routine) Z01.4
- kidney, congenital Q63.2
Pelviolithiasis (*see also* Calculus, kidney)
  N20.0
Pelviperitonitis – *see also* Peritonitis, pelvic
- gonococcal A54.2
- puerperal O85
Pelvis – *see condition*
Pemphigoid L12.9
- benign, mucous membrane L12.1

Pemphigoid—*continued*
- bullous L12.0
- cicatricial L12.1
- juvenile L12.2
- ocular L12.1† H13.3*
- specified NEC L12.8
Pemphigus L10.9
- benign familial (chronic) Q82.8
- Brazilian L10.3
- conjunctiva L12.1† H13.3*
- drug-induced L10.5
- erythematosus L10.4
- foliaceous L10.2
- gangrenous (*see also* Gangrene) R02
- neonatorum L00
- ocular L12.1† H13.3*
- specified NEC L10.8
- syphilitic (congenital) A50.0
- vegetans L10.1
- vulgaris L10.0
- wildfire L10.3
Pendred's syndrome E07.1
Pendulous
- abdomen, in pregnancy or childbirth
  O34.8
- - affecting fetus or newborn P03.8
- breast N64.8
Penetrating wound – *see also* Wound, open
- with internal injury – *see* Injury, by site
- eyeball S05.6
- - with foreign body S05.5
- orbit (with or without foreign body)
  S05.4
Penicillosis B48.4
Penis – *see condition*
Penitis N48.2
Pentalogy of Fallot Q21.8
Pentasomy X syndrome Q97.1
Pentosuria (essential) E74.8
Peregrinating patient F68.1
Perforation, perforated (nontraumatic)
- accidental during procedure (blood vessel)
  (nerve) (organ) T81.2
- appendix
- - with
- - - peritonitis, generalized K35.2
- - - peritonitis, localized K35.3
- bile duct (common) (hepatic) K83.2
- bladder (urinary)
- - obstetric trauma O71.5
- - traumatic S37.2
- bowel K63.1
- - fetus or newborn P78.0
- - obstetric trauma O71.5

Perforation, perforated—*continued*
- bowel—*continued*
- – traumatic S36.9
- broad ligament N83.8
- – obstetric trauma O71.6
- by
- – device, implant or graft (*see also*
  Complications, by site and type) T85.6
- – – arterial graft NEC T82.3
- – – – coronary (bypass) T82.2
- – – – breast (implant) T85.4
- – – – catheter NEC T85.6
- – – – dialysis (renal) T82.4
- – – – – intraperitoneal T85.6
- – – – infusion NEC T82.5
- – – – – spinal (epidural) (subdural)
        T85.6
- – – – urinary (indwelling) T83.0
- – – electronic (electrode) (pulse
      generator) (stimulator)
- – – – bone T84.3
- – – – cardiac T82.1
- – – – nervous system (brain) (peripheral
        nerve) (spinal) T85.1
- – – – urinary T83.1
- – – fixation, internal (orthopedic) NEC
      T84.2
- – – – bones of limb T84.1
- ⇥ – – gastrointestinal (bile duct)
      (esophagus) T85.5
- – – genital NEC T83.4
- – – – intrauterine contraceptive device
        T83.3
- – – heart NEC T82.5
- – – – valve (prosthesis) T82.0
- – – – – graft T82.2
- – – joint prosthesis T84.0
- – – ocular (canal graft) (orbital implant)
      NEC T85.3
- – – – intraocular lens T85.2
- – – orthopedic NEC T84.4
- – – – bone graft T84.3
- – – specified NEC T85.6
- – – urinary NEC T83.1
- – – – graft T83.2
- – – vascular NEC T82.5
- – – ventricular intracranial shunt T85.0
- – foreign body (external site) – *see also*
    Wound, open, by site
- – – internal site – *see* Foreign body
- – – left accidentally in operation wound
      T81.5
- – instrument (any) during a procedure,
    accidental T81.2

Perforation, perforated—*continued*
- cervix (uteri) N88.8
- – obstetric trauma O71.3
- colon K63.1
- – fetus or newborn P78.0
- – obstetric trauma O71.5
- – traumatic S36.5
- common duct (bile) K83.2
- cornea (due to ulceration) H16.0
- cystic duct K82.2
- diverticulum (intestine) (*see also*
  Diverticula) K57.8
- ear drum – *see* Perforation, tympanum
- esophagus K22.3
- eye, traumatic (*see also* Penetrating
  wound, eyeball) S05.6
- gallbladder K82.2
- heart valve – *see* Endocarditis
- ileum K63.1
- – fetus or newborn P78.0
- – obstetric trauma O71.5
- – traumatic S36.4
- instrumental, surgical (blood vessel)
  (nerve) (organ) T81.2
- intestine NEC K63.1
- – obstetric trauma O71.5
- – traumatic S36.9
- – ulcerative NEC K63.1
- – – fetus or newborn P78.0
- jejunum, jejunal K63.1
- – fetus or newborn P78.0
- – obstetric trauma O71.5
- – traumatic S36.4
- – ulcer – *see* Ulcer, gastrojejunal, with
    perforation
- mastoid (antrum) (cell) H70.8
- membrana tympani – *see* Perforation,
  tympanum
- nasal
- – septum J34.8
- – – congenital Q30.3
- – – syphilitic A52.7† J99.8*
- – sinus J34.8
- – – congenital Q30.8
- palate (*see also* Cleft, palate) Q35.9
- – soft (*see also* Cleft, palate, soft) Q35.3
- – – syphilitic A52.7† K93.8*
- – syphilitic A52.7† K93.8*
- palatine vault (*see also* Cleft, palate, hard)
  Q35.1
- – syphilitic A52.7† K93.8*
- – – congenital A50.5
- pars flaccida (ear drum) H72.1

Perforation, perforated—*continued*
- pelvic
- – floor S31.0
- – – obstetric trauma O70.1
- – organ NEC S37.8
- – – with abortion (subsequent episode) O08.6
- – – – current episode – *see* Abortion
- – – obstetric trauma O71.5
- perineum – *see* Laceration, perineum
- pharynx J39.2
- rectum K63.1
- – fetus or newborn P78.0
- – obstetric trauma O71.5
- – traumatic S36.6
- sigmoid K63.1
- – fetus or newborn P78.0
- – obstetric trauma O71.5
- – traumatic S36.5
- sinus (accessory) (chronic) (nasal) J34.8
- surgical (accidental) (blood vessel) (by instrument) (nerve) (organ) T81.2
- traumatic
- – external – *see* Wound, open
- – internal organ – *see* Injury, by site
- tympanum (membrane) (persistent post-traumatic) (postinflammatory) H72.9
- – attic H72.1
- – central H72.0
- – marginal NEC H72.2
- – pars flaccida H72.1
- – specified NEC H72.8
- – traumatic S09.2
- typhoid, gastrointestinal A01.0
- ulcer – *see* Ulcer, by site, with perforation
- ureter N28.8
- urethra N36.8
- – obstetric trauma O71.5
- uterus
- – by intrauterine contraceptive device T83.3
- – obstetric trauma O71.1
- – traumatic S37.6
- uvula K13.7
- – syphilitic A52.7† K93.8*
- vagina – *see* Laceration, vagina

Periadenitis mucosa necrotica recurrens K12.0

Periappendicitis (*see also* Appendicitis) K37

Periarteritis nodosa (disseminated) (infectious) (necrotizing) M30.0

Periarthritis (joint) M77.9
- Duplay's M75.0

Periarthritis—*continued*
- gonococcal A54.4† M73.8*
- humeroscapularis M75.0
- scapulohumeral M75.0
- shoulder M75.0
- wrist M77.2

Periarthrosis (angioneural) – *see* Periarthritis

Pericapsulitis, adhesive (shoulder) M75.0

Pericarditis (with decompensation) (with effusion) I31.9
- with rheumatic fever (conditions in I00) I01.0
- – active (*see also* Pericarditis, rheumatic) I01.0
- – inactive or quiescent I09.2
- acute (nonrheumatic) I30.9
- – with chorea (acute) (rheumatic) (Sydenham's) I02.0
- – benign I30.8
- – nonspecific I30.0
- – rheumatic I01.0
- adhesive or adherent (chronic) I31.0
- – acute – *see* Pericarditis, acute
- – rheumatic I09.2
- bacterial (acute) (subacute) (with serous or seropurulent effusion) I30.1
- calcareous I31.1
- chronic (nonrheumatic) I31.9
- constrictive (chronic) I31.1
- coxsackie(virus) B33.2† I32.1*
- fibrinocaseous (tuberculous) A18.8† I32.0*
- fibrinopurulent I30.1
- fibrinous I30.8
- fibrous I31.0
- gonococcal A54.8† I32.0*
- idiopathic I30.0
- in systemic lupus erythematosus M32.1† I32.8*
- infective I30.1
- meningococcal A39.5† I32.0*
- pneumococcal I30.1
- purulent I30.1
- rheumatic (active) (acute) (with effusion) (with pneumonia) I01.0
- – with chorea (acute) (rheumatic) (Sydenham's) I02.0
- – chronic or inactive (with chorea) I09.2
- septic I30.1
- serofibrinous I30.8
- staphylococcal I30.1
- streptococcal I30.1
- suppurative I30.1

Pericarditis—*continued*
- syphilitic A52.0† I32.0*
- tuberculous A18.8† I32.0*
- uremic N18.5† I32.8*
- viral I30.1

Pericardium, pericardial – *see condition*

Pericellulitis – *see* Cellulitis

Pericementitis (*see also* Periodontitis) K05.3

Perichondritis
- auricle H61.0
  bronchus J98.0
- ear (external) H61.0
- external auditory canal H61.0
- larynx J38.7
- - syphilitic A52.7† J99.8*
- nose J34.8
- pinna H61.0
- trachea J39.8

Pericoronitis (chronic) K05.3
- acute K05.2

Peridiverticulitis (intestine) (*see also* Diverticula) K57.9

Periendocarditis (*see also* Endocarditis) I38

Periepididymitis (*see also* Epididymitis) N45.9

Perifolliculitis L08.8
- capitis abscedens (et suffodiens) L66.3
- superficial pustular L01.0

Perihepatitis K65.8
- chlamydial A74.8† K67.0*
- gonococcal A54.8† K67.1*

Perilabyrinthitis (acute) H83.0

Perimeningitis – *see* Meningitis

Perimetritis (*see also* Endometritis) N71.9

Perimetrosalpingitis (*see also* Salpingo-oophoritis) N70.9

Perinephric, perinephritic – *see condition*

Perinephritis (*see also* Infection, kidney) N15.9
- purulent (*see also* Abscess, kidney) N15.1

Perineum, perineal – *see condition*

Perineuritis NEC M79.2

Periodic – *see condition*

Periodontitis (chronic) (complex) (simplex) K05.3
- acute K05.2
- apical K04.5
- - acute (pulpal origin) K04.4

Periodontosis (juvenile) K05.4

Periods – *see also* Menstruation
- heavy N92.0

Periods—*continued*
- irregular N92.6
- shortened intervals (irregular) N92.1

Perionychia (with lymphangitis) L03.0

Perioophoritis (*see also* Salpingo-oophoritis) N70.9

Periorchitis (*see also* Orchitis) N45.9

Periosteum, periosteal – *see condition*

Periostitis (circumscribed) (diffuse) (infective) M86.9
- with osteomyelitis M86.8
- - acute M86.1
- - chronic NEC M86.6
- - subacute M86.2
- alveolar K10.3
- alveolodental K10.3
- gonorrheal A54.4† M90.1*
- jaw (lower) (upper) K10.2
- monomelic M86.9
- orbital H05.0
- syphilitic A52.7† M90.1*
- - congenital (early) A50.0† M90.1*
- - secondary A51.4† M90.1*
- tuberculous (*see also* Tuberculosis, bone) A18.0† M90.0*
- yaws (early) (hypertrophic) (late) A66.6† M90.1*

Periostosis M89.8
- with osteomyelitis M86.8
- hyperplastic M89.8

Periphlebitis (*see also* Phlebitis) I80.9
- retina H35.0

Periproctitis K62.8

Periprostatitis (*see also* Prostatitis) N41.9

Perirectal – *see condition*

Perirenal – *see condition*

Perisalpingitis (*see also* Salpingo-oophoritis) N70.9

Perisplenitis (infectional) D73.8

Peristalsis, visible or reversed R19.2

Peritendinitis (*see also* Tenosynovitis) M77.9
- adhesive (shoulder) M75.0

Peritoneum, peritoneal – *see condition*

Peritonitis (adhesive) (fibrinous) (with effusion) K65.9
- with or following
- - abscess K65.0
- - appendicitis K35.3
- - - generalized K35.2
- - - - with mention of perforation or rupture K35.2
- - - localized K35.3

Peritonitis—*continued*
- with or following—*continued*
- − appendicitis—*continued*
- − − localized—*continued*
- − − − with mention of perforation or rupture K35.3
- − diverticular disease (intestine) K57.8
- acute K65.0
- aseptic T81.6
- bile, biliary K65.8
- chemical T81.6
- chlamydial A74.8† K67.0∗
- congenital NEC P78.1
- diaphragmatic K65.0
- diffuse NEC K65.0
- diphtheritic A36.8† K67.8∗
- disseminated NEC K65.0
- due to foreign substance accidentally left during a procedure (chemical) (powder) (talc) T81.6
- fibrocaseous (tuberculous) A18.3† K67.3∗
- fibropurulent K65.0
- following
- − abortion (subsequent episode) O08.0
- − − current episode – *see* Abortion
- − ectopic or molar pregnancy O08.0
- general(ized) K65.0
- gonococcal A54.8† K67.1∗
- meconium (newborn) P78.0
- neonatal P78.1
- − meconium P78.0
- pancreatic K65.0
- paroxysmal, familial E85.0
- − benign E85.0
- pelvic
- − female N73.5
- − − acute N73.3
- − − chronic NEC N73.4
- − − − with adhesions N73.6
- − male K65.0
- periodic, familial E85.0
- proliferative, chronic K65.8
- puerperal, postpartum, childbirth O85
- purulent K65.0
- septic K65.0
- subdiaphragmatic K65.0
- subphrenic K65.0
- suppurative K65.0
- syphilitic A52.7† K67.2∗
- − congenital (early) A50.0† K67.2∗
- tuberculous A18.3† K67.3∗
- urine K65.8

Peritonsillar – *see condition*

Peritonsillitis J36
Periureteritis N28.8
Periurethral – *see condition*
Periurethritis (gangrenous) (*see also* Urethritis) N34.2
Periuterine – *see condition*
Perivaginitis (*see also* Vaginitis) N76.0
Perivasculitis, retinal H35.0
Perivasitis (chronic) N49.1
Perivesiculitis (seminal) (*see also* Vesiculitis) N49.0
Perlèche NEC (due to) K13.0
- candidiasis B37.8
- moniliasis B37.8
- vitamin B$_2$ (riboflavin) deficiency E53.0† K93.8∗
Pernicious – *see condition*
Pernio T69.1
Persecution
- delusion (of) F22.0
- social Z60.5
Perseveration (tonic) R48.8
Persistence, persistent (congenital)
- anal membrane Q42.3
- − with fistula Q42.2
- arteria stapedia Q16.3
- atrioventricular canal Q21.2
- branchial cleft Q18.0
- bulbus cordis in left ventricle Q21.8
- canal of Cloquet Q14.0
- capsule (opaque) Q12.8
- cilioretinal artery or vein Q14.8
- cloaca Q43.7
- communication – *see* Fistula, congenital
- convolutions
- − aortic arch Q25.4
- − fallopian tube Q50.6
- − oviduct Q50.6
- − uterine tube Q50.6
- double aortic arch Q25.4
- ductus arteriosus (botalli) Q25.0
- fetal
- − circulation P29.3
- − form of cervix (uteri) Q51.8
- − hemoglobin, hereditary (HPFH) D56.4
- foramen
- − botalli Q21.1
- − ovale Q21.1
- Gartner's duct Q50.6
- hemoglobin, fetal (hereditary) (HPFH) D56.4
- hyaloid
- − artery (generally incomplete) Q14.0
- − system Q14.8

509

Persistence, persistent—*continued*
- hymen, in pregnancy or childbirth O34.7
- lanugo Q84.2
- left
- − − posterior cardinal vein Q26.8
- − − root with right arch of aorta Q25.4
- − − superior vena cava Q26.1
- − Meckel's diverticulum Q43.0
- nail(s), anomalous Q84.6
- occipitoposterior (position) O32.8
- − − affecting fetus or newborn P03.1
- − causing obstructed labor O64.0
- occipitotransverse (position) O64.0
- − − affecting fetur or newborn P03.1
- omphalomesenteric duct Q43.0
- ostium
- − − atrioventriculare commune Q21.2
- − − primum Q21.2
- − − secundum Q21.1
- ovarian rests in fallopian tube Q50.6
- pancreatic tissue in intestinal tract Q43.8
- primary (deciduous)
- − − teeth K00.6
- − − vitreous hyperplasia Q14.0
- pupillary membrane Q13.8
- right aortic arch Q25.4
- sinus
- − − urogenitalis
- − − − female Q52.8
- − − − male Q55.8
- − − venosus with imperfect incorporation in right auricle Q26.8
- thymus (gland) (hyperplasia) E32.0
- thyroglossal duct Q89.2
- truncus arteriosus or communis Q20.0
- tunica vasculosa lentis Q12.2
- urachus Q64.4
- vitelline duct Q43.0

Personality (disorder) F60.9
- accentuation of traits (type A pattern) Z73.1
- affective F34.0
- aggressive F60.3
- amoral F60.2
- anankastic F60.5
- antisocial F60.2
- anxious F60.6
- asocial F60.2
- asthenic F60.7
- avoidant F60.6
- borderline F60.3
- change (enduring) (after) (due to) F62.9
- − − catastrophic experience F62.0
- − − chronic pain F62.8

Personality—*continued*
- change—*continued*
- − − concentration camp experience F62.0
- − − disaster F62.0
- − − prolonged exposure to terrorism F62.0
- − − psychiatric illness F62.1
- − − secondary (nonspecific) F61
- − − specified NEC F62.8
- − − torture F62.0
- − − troublesome F61
- compulsive F60.5
- cycloid F34.0
- cyclothymic F34.0
- dependent F60.7
- depressive F34.1
- dissocial F60.2
- dual F44.8
- eccentric F60.8
- emotionally unstable F60.3
- expansive paranoid F60.0
- explosive F60.3
- fanatic F60.0
- haltlose type F60.8
- histrionic F60.4
- hyperthymic F34.0
- hypothymic F34.1
- hysterical F60.4
- immature F60.8
- inadequate F60.7
- labile (emotional) F60.3
- mixed (nonspecific) F61
- morally defective F60.2
- multiple F44.8
- narcissistic F60.8
- obsessional F60.5
- obsessive(-compulsive) F60.5
- organic F07.0
- paranoid F60.0
- passive(-dependent) F60.7
- passive-aggressive F60.8
- pathologic NEC F60.9
- pattern defect or disturbance F60.9
- pseudopsychopathic (organic) F07.0
- pseudoretarded (organic) F07.0
- psychoinfantile F60.4
- psychoneurotic NEC F60.8
- psychopathic F60.2
- querulant F60.0
- sadistic F60.8
- schizoid F60.1
- self-defeating F60.7
- sensitive paranoid F60.0
- sociopathic (amoral) (antisocial) (asocial) (dissocial) F60.2

Personality—*continued*
- specified NEC F60.8
- type A Z73.1
- unstable (emotional) F60.3
Perthes' disease M91.1
Pertussis (*see also* Whooping cough) A37.9
Perversion, perverted
- appetite F50.8
- - psychogenic F50.8
- sense of smell and taste R43.8
- - psychogenic F45.8
- sexual (*see also* Deviation, sexual) F65.9
Pervious, congenital – *see also* Imperfect, closure
- ductus arteriosus Q25.0
Pes, deformity (congenital) (*see also* Talipes) Q66.8
- acquired NEC M21.6
- adductus Q66.8
Pest, pestis (*see also* Plague) A20.9
- bubonica A20.0
- fulminans A20.0
- minor A20.8
- pneumonica A20.2
Petechia, petechiae R23.3
- fetus or newborn P54.5
Peter's anomaly Q13.4
Petit mal G40.7
- with grand mal seizures G40.6
- epilepsy (childhood) (idiopathic) (juvenile) G40.3
- impulsive G40.3
- status (epilepticus) G41.1
Petit's hernia – *see* Hernia, abdomen, specified site NEC
Petriellidosis B48.2
Petrositis H70.2
Peutz-Jeghers disease or syndrome Q85.8
Peyronie's disease N48.6
Pfeiffer's disease B27.0
Phagedena (dry) (moist) (*see also* Gangrene) R02
- geometric L88
- penis N48.2
- tropical (*see also* Ulcer, skin) L98.4
- vulva N76.6
Phagedenic – *see condition*
Phakoma H35.8
Phakomatosis (*see also* specific eponymous syndromes) Q85.9
- Bourneville's Q85.1
- specified NEC Q85.8

Phantom limb syndrome (without pain) G54.7
- with pain G54.6
Pharyngeal pouch syndrome D82.1
Pharyngitis (acute) (catarrhal) (gangrenous) (infective) (subacute) (suppurative) (ulcerative) J02.9
- with influenza, flu or grippe (*see also* Influenza, with, respiratory manifestations) J11.1
- aphthous B08.5
- atrophic J31.2
- chlamydial A56.4
- chronic (atrophic) (granular) (hypertrophic) J31.2
- coxsackievirus B08.5
- diphtheritic A36.0
- enteroviral vesicular B08.5
- follicular (chronic) J31.2
- fusospirochetal A69.1
- gonococcal A54.5
- granular (chronic) J31.2
- herpesviral B00.2
- hypertrophic J31.2
- influenzal (*see also* Influenza, with, respiratory manifestations) J11.1
- lymphonodular, acute (enteroviral) B08.8
- pneumococcal J02.8
- purulent J02.9
- putrid J02.9
- septic J02.0
- sicca J31.2
- specified organism NEC J02.8
- staphylococcal J02.8
- streptococcal J02.0
- syphilitic, congenital (early) A50.0
- tuberculous A16.8
- - with bacteriological and histological confirmation A15.8
- vesicular, enteroviral B08.5
- viral NEC J02.8
Pharyngoconjunctivitis, viral B30.2†
H13.1*
Pharyngolaryngitis (acute) J06.0
- chronic J37.0
Pharyngoplegia J39.2
Pharyngotonsillitis J06.8
- herpesviral B00.2
Pharyngotracheitis (acute) J06.8
- chronic J42
Pharynx, pharyngeal – *see condition*
Phenomenon
- Arthus' – *see* Arthus' phenomenon
- jaw-winking Q07.8

Phenomenon—*continued*
- lupus erythematosus (L.E.) cell M32.9
- Raynaud's (secondary) I73.0
- vasomotor R55
- vasospastic I73.9
- vasovagal R55
- Wenckebach's I44.1

Phenylketonuria E70.1
- classical E70.0
- maternal E70.1

Pheochromoblastoma (M8700/3)
- specified site – *see* Neoplasm, malignant
- unspecified site C74.1

Pheochromocytoma (M8700/0)
- malignant (M8700/3)
- – specified site – *see* Neoplasm, malignant
- – unspecified site C74.1
- specified site – *see* Neoplasm, benign
- unspecified site D35.0

Pheohyphomycosis (*see also* Chromomycosis) B43.9

Pheomycosis – *see* Chromomycosis

Phimosis (congenital) (due to infection) N47
- chancroidal A57

Phlebectasia (*see also* Varicose, vein) I83.9
- congenital Q27.4

Phlebitis (infective) (pyemic) (septic) (suppurative) I80.9
- breast, superficial I80.8
- cavernous (venous) sinus – *see* Phlebitis, intracranial (venous) sinus
- cerebral (venous) sinus – *see* Phlebitis, intracranial (venous) sinus
- chest wall, superficial I80.8
- complicating pregnancy O22.9
- – deep O22.8
- – superficial O22.2
- cranial (venous) sinus – *see* Phlebitis, intracranial (venous) sinus
- due to implanted device – *see* Complications, by site and type
- during or resulting from a procedure T81.7
- femoral (superficial) I80.1
- following infusion, therapeutic injection or transfusion T80.1
- hepatic veins I80.8
- iliofemoral I80.1
- intracranial (venous) sinus (any) G08
- – nonpyogenic I67.6
- intraspinal venous sinuses and veins G08
- – nonpyogenic G95.1

Phlebitis—*continued*
- lateral (venous) sinus – *see* Phlebitis, intracranial (venous) sinus
- longitudinal sinus – *see* Phlebitis, intracranial (venous) sinus
- lower limb I80.3
- – deep (vessels) NEC I80.2
- – superficial (vessels) I80.0
- migrans, migrating (superficial) I82.1
- pelvic
- – following
- – – abortion (subsequent episode) O08.0
- – – – current episode – *see* Abortion
- – – ectopic or molar pregnancy O08.0
- – puerperal, postpartum O87.1
- portal K75.1
- postoperative T81.7
- pregnancy O22.9
- – deep O22.8
- – superficial O22.2
- puerperal, postpartum, childbirth O87.9
- – deep O87.1
- – pelvic O87.1
- – superficial O87.0
- retina H35.0
- saphenous I80.0
- sinus (meninges) – *see* Phlebitis, intracranial (venous) sinus
- specified site NEC I80.8
- syphilitic A52.0† I98.8*
- ulcerative I80.9
- – leg I80.3
- – – deep (vessels) NEC I80.2
- – – superficial (vessels) I80.0
- umbilicus I80.8
- uterus (septic) (*see also* Endometritis) N71.9
- varicose (leg) (lower limb) I83.1
- – – with ulcer I83.2

Phleboliths I87.8

Phlebosclerosis I87.8

Phlebothrombosis (*see also* Thrombosis) I82.9
- antepartum, deep O22.3
- pregnancy, deep O22.3
- puerperal, deep O87.1

Phlegmasia
- alba dolens (puerperal) O87.1
- – complicating pregnancy O22.3
- – nonobstetric I80.1
- cerulea dolens I80.2

Phlegmon – *see* Abscess

Phlegmonous – *see condition*

Phlyctenulosis (allergic) (keratoconjunctivitis) (nontuberculous) H16.2
- cornea H16.2
- tuberculous A18.5† H19.2*
Phobia, phobic F40.9
- animal F40.2
- examination F40.2
- reaction F40.9
- simple F40.2
- social F40.1
- specific (isolated) F40.2
- specified NEC F40.8
- state F40.9
Phocas' disease N60.1
Phocomelia Q73.1
- lower limb Q72.1
- upper limb Q71.1
Phoria H50.5
Phosphate-losing tubular disorder N25.0
Phosphatemia E83.3
Phosphaturia E83.3
Photodermatitis (sun) L56.8
- chronic L57.8
- due to drug L56.8
- light other than sun L59.8
Photokeratitis H16.1
Photophobia H53.1
Photophthalmia H16.1
Photopsia H53.1
Photoretinitis H31.0
Photosensitivity, photosensitization of skin (sun) L56.8
- light other than sun L59.8
Phrenitis – *see* Encephalitis
Phrynoderma (vitamin A deficiency) E50.8† L86*
Phthiriasis (pubis) B85.3
- with any infestation classifiable to B85.0-B85.2 B85.4
- eyelid B85.3† H03.0*
Phthirus infestation – *see* Phthiriasis
Phthisis (*see also* Tuberculosis) A16.9
- bulbi (infectional) H44.5
- eyeball (due to infection) H44.5
Phycomycosis – *see* Zygomycosis
Physalopteriasis B81.8
Physical therapy NEC Z50.1
Phytobezoar T18.9
- intestine T18.3
- stomach T18.2
Pian (*see also* Yaws) A66.9
Pianoma A66.1

Pica F50.8
- in adults F50.8
- infant or child F98.3
Picking, nose F98.8
Pick-Niemann disease E75.2
Pick's
- disease or syndrome (brain) G31.0
- – dementia in G31.0† F02.0*
- tubular adenoma (M8640/0)
- – specified site – *see* Neoplasm, benign
- – unspecified site
- – – female D27
- – – male D29.2
Pickwickian syndrome E66.2
Piebaldism E70.3
Piedra B36.8
- black B36.3
- white B36.2
Pierre Robin deformity or syndrome Q87.0
Pierson's disease or osteochondrosis M91.0
Pig-bel A05.2
Pigeon
- breast or chest (acquired) M95.4
- – congenital Q67.7
- – rachitic (late effect) E64.3
- breeder's disease or lung J67.2
- fancier's disease or lung J67.2
- toe M20.5
Pigmentation (abnormal) L81.9
- conjunctiva H11.1
- cornea H18.0
- diminished melanin formation NEC L81.6
- iron L81.8
- lids, congenital Q82.8
- limbus corneae H18.0
- metals L81.8
- optic papilla, congenital Q14.2
- retina, congenital (grouped) (nevoid) Q14.1
- scrotum, congenital Q82.8
- tattoo L81.8
Piles – *see* Hemorrhoids
Pili
- annulati or torti (congenital) Q84.1
- incarnati L73.1
Pill-roller hand (intrinsic) (*see also* Parkinsonism) G20
Pilomatrixoma (M8110/0) – *see* Neoplasm, skin, benign
- malignant (M8110/3) – *see* Neoplasm, skin, malignant

Pilonidal – *see condition*
Pimple R23.8
Pinched nerve – *see* Neuropathy,
  entrapment
Pindborg tumor (M9340/0) D16.5
– upper jaw (bone) (M9340/0) D16.4
Pineal body or gland – *see condition*
Pinealoblastoma (M9362/3) C75.3
Pinealoma (M9360/1) D44.5
Pineoblastoma (M9362/3) C75.3
Pineocytoma (M9361/1) D44.5
Pinguecula H11.1
Pinhole meatus (*see also* Stricture, urethra)
  N35.9
Pink
– disease T56.1
– eye H10.0
Pinkus' disease (lichen nitidus) L44.1
Pinpoint
– meatus (*see also* Stricture, urethra) N35.9
– os (uteri) (*see also* Stricture, cervix)
  N88.2
Pins and needles R20.2
Pinta A67.9
– cardiovascular lesions A67.2† I98.1*
– chancre (primary) A67.0
– erythematous plaques A67.1
– hyperchromic lesions A67.1
– hyperkeratosis A67.1
– lesions A67.9
– – cardiovascular A67.2† I98.1*
– – hyperchromic A67.1
– – intermediate A67.1
– – late A67.2
– – mixed A67.3
– – primary A67.0
– – skin (achromic) (cicatricial)
  (dyschromic) A67.2
– – – hyperchromic A67.1
– – – mixed (achromic and hyperchromic)
    A67.3
– papule (primary) A67.0
– skin lesions (achromic) (cicatricial)
  (dyschromic) A67.2
– – hyperchromic A67.1
– – mixed (achromic and hyperchromic)
  A67.3
– vitiligo A67.2
Pintids A67.1
Pinworm (disease) (infection) (infestation)
  B80
Piroplasmosis B60.0
Pistol wound – *see* Gunshot wound

Pithecoid pelvis Q74.2
– with disproportion (fetopelvic) O33.0
– – affecting fetus or newborn P03.1
– – causing obstructed labor O65.0
Pithiatism F48.8
Pitted – *see* Edema
Pitting (*see also* Edema) R60.9
– lip R60.0
– nail L60.8
Pituitary gland – *see condition*
Pituitary-snuff-taker's disease J67.8
Pityriasis (capitis) L21.0
– alba L30.5
– circinata L42
– furfuracea L21.0
– Hebra's L26
– lichenoides L41.0
– – chronica L41.1
– – et varioliformis (acuta) L41.0
– maculata L30.5
– nigra B36.1
– rosea L42
– rotunda L44.8
– rubra pilaris L44.0
– simplex L30.5
– versicolor B36.0
Placenta, placental – *see also condition*
– ablatio (*see also* Abruptio placentae)
  O45.9
– – affecting fetus or newborn P02.1
– abnormal, abnormality NEC O43.1
– – with hemorrhage O46.8
– – – affecting fetus or newborn P02.1
– – – antepartum NEC O46.8
– – – intrapartum O67.8
– – affecting fetus or newborn P02.2
– abruptio (*see also* Abruptio placentae)
  O45.9
– – affecting fetus or newborn P02.1
– accreta O43.2
– adherent (morbidly) O43.2
– battledore O43.1
– bipartita O43.1
– circumvallata O43.1
– cyst (amniotic) O43.1
– deficiency – *see* Placenta, insufficiency
– detachment (partial) (premature) (with
  hemorrhage) (*see also* Abruptio placentae)
  O45.9
– dimidiata O43.1
– disease NEC O43.9
– – affecting fetus or newborn P02.2
– duplex O43.1
– dysfunction O43.8

Placenta, placental—*continued*
- fenestrata O43.1
- fibrosis O43.8
- hematoma O43.8
- hemorrhage O46.8
- – abruptio placentae (*see also* Abruptio placentae) O45.9
- – placenta previa O44.1
- hyperplasia O43.8
- increta O43.2
- infarction O43.8
- – affecting fetus or newborn P02.2
- insertion, vicious (*see also* Placenta, previa) O44.1
- insufficiency
- – affecting fetus or newborn P02.2
- – affecting management of pregnancy O36.5
- lateral (*see also* Placenta, previa) O44.1
- low implantation or insertion (with hemorrhage) O44.1
- low-lying (*see also* Placenta, previa) O44.1
- malformation O43.1
- malposition (*see also* Placenta, previa) O44.1
- marginal (hemorrhage) (rupture) O44.1
- – affecting fetus or newborn P02.0
- membranacea O43.1
- morbidly adherentt O43.2
- multilobed O43.1
- multipartita O43.1
- necrosis O43.8
- percreta O43.2
- polyp O90.8
- previa (central) (complete) (marginal) (partial) (total) (with hemorrhage) O44.1
- – affecting fetus or newborn P02.0
- – without hemorrhage O44.0
- retention (with postpartum hemorrhage) O72.0
- – fragments, complicating puerperium (delayed hemorrhage) O72.2
- – – without hemorrhage O73.1
- – without hemorrhage O73.0
- separation (normally implanted) (partial) (premature) (with hemorrhage) (*see also* Abruptio placentae) O45.9
- septuplex O43.1
- small – *see* Placenta, insufficiency
- softening (premature) O43.8
- spuria O43.1
- succenturiata O43.1
- syphilitic O98.1

Placenta, placental—*continued*
- transmission of chemical substance – *see* Absorption, chemical, through placenta
- trapped (with postpartum hemorrhage) O72.0
- – without hemorrhage O73.0
- tripartita, triplex O43.1
- varicose vessels O43.8

Placentitis
- affecting fetus or newborn P02.7
- complicating pregnancy O41.1

Plagiocephaly Q67.3

Plague A20.9
- abortive A20.8
- ambulatory A20.8
- asymptomatic A20.8
- bubonic A20.0
- cellulocutaneous A20.1
- cutaneobubonic A20.1
- meningitis A20.3† G01*
- pharyngeal A20.8
- pneumonic (primary) (secondary) A20.2
- pulmonary, pulmonic A20.2
- septicemic A20.7
- tonsillar A20.8

Plaque(s)
- artery, arterial – *see* Arteriosclerosis
- calcareous – *see* Calcification
- epicardial I31.8
- erythematous, of pinta A67.1
- Hollenhorst's H34.2
- pleural (without asbestos) J92.9
- – with asbestos J92.0
- tongue K13.2

Plasmacytoma NEC C90.3
- extramedullary C90.2
- medullary C90.0
- solitary C90.3

Plasmacytosis D72.8

Plaster ulcer L89.-
- stage
- – I L89.0
- – II L89.1
- – III L89.2
- – IV L89.3

Platybasia Q75.8

Platyonychia (congenital) Q84.6
- acquired L60.8

Platypelloid pelvis M95.5
- with disproportion (fetopelvic) O33.0
- – affecting fetus or newborn P03.1
- – causing obstructed labor O65.0
- congenital Q74.2

Platyspondylisis Q76.4

Plaut(-Vincent) infection – *see* Vincent's, infection
Pleura, pleural – *see condition*
Pleuralgia R07.3
Pleurisy (acute) (adhesive) (chronic) (double) (dry) (fibrinous) (subacute) R09.1
– with
– – effusion J90
– – – chylous, chyliform J94.0
– – – influenzal (*see also* Influenza, with, respiratory manifestations) J11.1
– – – tuberculous NEC (non-primary) A16.5
– – – – with bacteriological and histological confirmation A15.6
– – – – primary (progressive) A16.7
– – – – – with bacteriological and histological confirmation A15.7
– – influenza, flu, or grippe (*see also* Influenza, with, respiratory manifestations) J11.1
– – tuberculosis – *see* Pleurisy, tuberculous (non-primary)
– encysted (*see also* Pleurisy, with effusion) J90
– exudative (*see also* Pleurisy, with effusion) J90
– fibrinopurulent, fibropurulent (*see also* Pyothorax) J86.9
– hemorrhagic – *see* Hemothorax
– influenzal (*see also* Influenza, with, respiratory manifestations) J11.1
– pneumococcal J90
– purulent (*see also* Pyothorax) J86.9
– septic J86.9
– serofibrinous (*see also* Pleurisy, with effusion) J90
– seropurulent (*see also* Pyothorax) J86.9
– serous (*see also* Pleurisy, with effusion) J90
– staphylococcal J90
– streptococcal J90
– suppurative (*see also* Pyothorax) J86.9
– traumatic (current) (post) S27.6
– tuberculous (with effusion) (non-primary) A16.5
– – with bacteriological and histological confirmation A15.6
– – primary (progressive) A16.7
– – – with bacteriological and histological confirmation A15.7
Pleuritis sicca – *see* Pleurisy

Pleurodynia R07.3
– epidemic B33.0
Pleuropericarditis (*see also* Pericarditis) I31.9
Pleuropneumonia (acute) (bilateral) (double) (septic) (*see also* Pneumonia) J18.8
– chronic (*see also* Fibrosis, lung) J84.1
Pleuro-pneumonia-like-organism (PPLO), as cause of disease classified elsewhere B96.0
Pleurorrhea (*see also* Pleurisy, with, effusion) J90
Plica, tonsil J35.8
Plicated tongue K14.5
Plug
– bronchus NEC J98.0
– meconium (newborn), syndrome P76.0
– mucus (*see also* Asphyxia, mucus) T17.9
Plumbism T56.0
Plummer's disease E05.2
Plummer-Vinson syndrome D50.1
Pluricarential syndrome of infancy E40
Plus (and minus) hand (intrinsic) M21.8
Pneumathemia – *see* Air, embolism, by type
Pneumatic hammer (drill) syndrome T75.2
Pneumatocele J98.4
– intracranial G93.8
Pneumatosis
– cystoides intestinalis K63.8
– intestinalis K63.8
– peritonei K66.8
Pneumaturia R39.8
Pneumoblastoma (M8972/3) – *see* Neoplasm, lung, malignant
Pneumocephalus G93.8
Pneumococcus, pneumococcal – *see condition*
Pneumoconiosis NEC (due to) (inhalation of) J64
– with tuberculosis (any type in A15-A16) J65
– aluminum J63.0
– asbestos J61
– bagasse, bagassosis J67.1
– bauxite J63.1
– beryllium J63.2
– coalworker's (simple) J60
– collier's J60
– cotton dust J66.0
– diatomite (diatomaceous earth) J62.8

Pneumoconiosis NEC—*continued*
- dust
- – inorganic NEC J63.8
- – lime J62.8
- – marble J62.8
- – organic NEC J66.8
- graphite J63.3
- grinder's J62.8
- kaolin J62.8
- mica J62.8
- millstone maker's J62.8
- mineral fibers NEC J61
- miner's J60
- moldy hay J67.0
- potter's J62.8
- rheumatoid M05.1† J99.0∗
- sandblaster's J62.8
- silica, silicate NEC J62.8
- – with carbon J60
- stonemason's J62.8
- talc (dust) J62.0

Pneumocystosis B59† J17.3∗
- resulting from HIV disease B20.6

Pneumohemopericardium I31.2

Pneumohemothorax – *see also* Hemothorax
- traumatic S27.2

Pneumohydropericardium (*see also* Pericarditis) I31.9

Pneumohydrothorax (*see also* Hydrothorax) J94.8

Pneumomediastinum J98.2
- congenital or perinatal P25.2

Pneumomycosis NEC B49† J99.8∗

Pneumonia (acute) (double) (migratory) (purulent) (septic) (unresolved) J18.9
- with
- – influenza, flu, or grippe (specific virus not identified) J11.0
- – – avian influenza virus identified J09
- – – other influenza virus identified J10.0
- – lung abscess J85.1
- – – due to specified organism – *see* Pneumonia, in (due to)
- adenoviral J12.0
- adynamic J18.2
- alba (early congenital syphilitic) A50.0† J17.0∗
- allergic (eosinophilic) J82
- anthrax A22.1† J17.0∗
- apex, apical – *see* Pneumonia, lobar
- Ascaris B77.8† J17.3∗
- aspiration J69.0

Pneumonia—*continued*
- aspiration—*continued*
- – due to
- – – food (regurgitated), milk, vomit J69.0
- – – gastric secretions J69.0
- – – oils, essences J69.1
- – – solids, liquids NEC J69.8
- – newborn P24.9
- – – meconium P24.0
- atypical NEC J18.9
- bacillus J15.9
- – specified NEC J15.8
- bacterial J15.9
- – specified NEC J15.8
- basal, basic, basilar – *see* Pneumonia, lobar
- broncho, bronchial (confluent) (croupous) (diffuse) (disseminated) (involving lobes) (lobar) J18.0
- – with influenza (*see also* Pneumonia, with, influenza) J11.0
- – allergic (eosinophilic) J82
- – aspiration (*see also* Pneumonia, aspiration) J69.0
- – bacterial J15.9
- – – specified NEC J15.8
- – chronic (*see also* Fibrosis, lung) J84.1
- – Eaton's agent J15.7
- – Escherichia coli (E. coli) J15.5
- – Friedländer's bacillus J15.0
- – Haemophilus influenzae J14
- – hypostatic J18.2
- – influenzal (*see also* Pneumonia, with, influenza) J11.0
- – inhalation (*see also* Pneumonia, aspiration) J69.0
- – – due to fumes or vapors (chemical) J68.0
- – – of oils or essences J69.1
- – Klebsiella (pneumoniae) J15.0
- – lipid, lipoid J69.1
- – – endogenous J84.8
- – Mycoplasma (pneumoniae) J15.7
- – pleuro-pneumonia-like-organisms (PPLO) J15.7
- – pneumococcal J13
- – Proteus J15.6
- – Pseudomonas J15.1
- – specified organism NEC J16.8
- – staphylococcal J15.2
- – streptococcal NEC J15.4
- – viral, virus (*see also* Pneumonia, viral) J12.9

Pneumonia—*continued*
- Candida B37.1† J17.2*
- caseous (*see also* Tuberculosis, pulmonary) A16.2
- catarrhal (*see also* Pneumonia, broncho) J18.0
- chlamydial J16.0
- – congenital P23.1
- cholesterol J84.8
- chronic J98.4
- cirrhotic (chronic) (*see also* Fibrosis, lung) J84.1
- confluent – *see* Pneumonia, broncho
- congenital (infective) P23.9
- – due to
- – – bacterium NEC P23.6
- – – Chlamydia P23.1
- – – Escherichia coli P23.4
- – – Haemophilus influenzae P23.6
- – – infective organism NEC P23.8
- – – Klebsiella pneumoniae P23.6
- – – Mycoplasma P23.6
- – – Pseudomonas P23.5
- – – staphylococcus P23.2
- – – streptococcus (except group B) P23.6
- – – – group B P23.3
- – – viral agent P23.0
- – specified NEC P23.8
- cytomegaloviral B25.0† J17.1*
- deglutition (*see also* Pneumonia, aspiration) J69.0
- diffuse – *see* Pneumonia, broncho
- disseminated (focal) – *see* Pneumonia, broncho
- Eaton's agent J15.7
- embolic, embolism (*see also* Embolism, pulmonary) I26.9
- Enterobacter J15.6
- eosinophilic J82
- Escherichia coli (E. coli) J15.5
- fibroid, fibrous (chronic) (*see also* Fibrosis, lung) J84.1
- Friedländer's bacillus J15.0
- gangrenous J85.0
- giant cell (measles) B05.2† J17.1*
- gonococcal A54.8† J17.0*
- grippal (*see also* Pneumonia, with, influenza) J11.0
- Haemophilus influenzae (broncho) (lobar) J14
- hypostatic (broncho) (lobar) J18.2
- in (due to)
- – actinomycosis A42.0† J17.0*

Pneumonia—*continued*
- in—*continued*
- – adenovirus J12.0
- – anthrax A22.1† J17.0*
- – ascariasis B77.8† J17.3*
- – aspergillosis B44.-† J17.2*
- – Bacillus anthracis A22.1† J17.0*
- – candidiasis B37.1† J17.2*
- – chickenpox B01.2† J17.1*
- – Chlamydia J16.0
- – – neonatal P23.1
- – coccidioidomycosis B38.2† J17.2*
- – – acute B38.0† J17.2*
- – – chronic B38.1† J17.2*
- – cytomegalovirus disease B25.0† J17.1*
- – Eaton's agent J15.7
- – Enterobacter J15.6
- – Escherichia coli (E. coli) J15.5
- – Friedländer's bacillus J15.0
- – fumes and vapors (chemical) (inhalation) J68.0
- – gonorrhea A54.8† J17.0*
- – Haemophilus influenzae (H. influenzae) J14
- – histoplasmosis B39.2† J17.2*
- – – acute B39.0† J17.2*
- – – chronic B39.1† J17.2*
- – human metapneumovirus J12.3
- – influenza (*see also* Pneumonia, with, influenza) J11.0
- – Klebsiella (pneumoniae) J15.0
- – measles B05.2† J17.1*
- – Mycoplasma (pneumoniae) J15.7
- – nocardiosis, nocardiasis A43.0† J17.0*
- – ornithosis A70† J17.8*
- – parainfluenza virus J12.2
- – pleuro-pneumonia-like-organism (PPLO) J15.7
- – pneumococcus J13
- – pneumocystosis (Pneumocystis carinii) (Pneumocystis jirovecii) B59† J17.3*
- – – resulting from HIV disease B20.6
- – Proteus J15.6
- – Pseudomonas NEC J15.1
- – – pseudomallei A24.1
- – psittacosis A70† J17.8*
- – Q fever A78† J17.8*
- – respiratory syncytial virus J12.1
- – rheumatic fever I00† J17.8*
- – rubella B06.8† J17.1*
- – Salmonella (infection) A02.2† J17.0*
- – – typhi A01.0† J17.0*
- – schistosomiasis B65.-† J17.3*
- – sepsis A41.-† J17.0*

Pneumonia—*continued*
- in—*continued*
-   – Serratia marcescens J15.6
-   – specified
-    – bacterium NEC J15.8
-    – organism NEC J16.8
-   – Spirochaeta NEC A69.8† J17.8*
-   – staphylococcus J15.2
-   – Streptococcus J15.4
-    – group B J15.3
-    – pneumoniae J13
-    – specified NEC J15.4
-   – toxoplasmosis B58.3† J17.3*
-   – tularemia A21.2† J17.0*
-   – typhoid fever A01.0† J17.0*
-   – varicella B01.2† J17.1*
-   – virus (*see also* Pneumonia, viral) J12.9
-   – whooping cough A37.-† J17.0*
-   – Yersinia pestis A20.2
- influenzal (*see also* Pneumonia, with, influenza) J11.0
- inhalation of food or vomit (*see also* Pneumonia, aspiration) J69.0
- interstitial J84.9
-   – plasma cell B59† J17.3*
-   – usual J84.1
- Klebsiella (pneumoniae) J15.0
- lipid, lipoid (exogenous) J69.1
- lobar (disseminated) (interstitial) J18.1
-   – with influenza (*see also* Pneumonia, with, influenza) J11.0
-   – bacterial J15.9
-    – specified NEC J15.8
-   – chronic (*see also* Fibrosis, lung) J84.1
-   – Escherichia coli (E. coli) J15.5
-   – Friedländer's bacillus J15.0
-   – Haemophilus influenzae J14
-   – influenzal (*see also* Pneumonia, with, influenza) J11.0
-   – Klebsiella (pneumoniae) J15.0
-   – pneumococcal J13
-   – Proteus J15.6
-   – Pseudomonas J15.1
-   – specified organism NEC J16.8
-   – staphylococcal J15.2
-   – streptococcal NEC J15.4
-   – Streptococcus pneumoniae J13
-   – viral, virus (*see also* Pneumonia, viral) J12.9
- lobular – *see* Pneumonia, broncho
- Löffler's J82
- massive – *see* Pneumonia, lobar
- meconium P24.0
- Mycoplasma (pneumoniae) J15.7

Pneumonia—*continued*
- necrotic J85.0
- neonatal P23.9
-   – aspiration P24.9
- parainfluenza virus J12.2
- parenchymatous (*see also* Fibrosis, lung) J84.1
- patchy – *see* Pneumonia, broncho
- plasma cell (of infants) B59† J17.3*
- pleurolobar – *see* Pneumonia, lobar
- pleuro-pneumonia-like-organism (PPLO) J15.7
- pneumococcal (broncho) (lobar) J13
- Pneumocystis (carinii) (jirovecii) B59† J17.3*
-   – resulting from HIV disease B20.6
- postinfectional NEC B99† J17.8*
- postmeasles B05.2† J17.1*
- Proteus J15.6
- Pseudomonas J15.1
- psittacosis A70† J17.8*
- radiation J70.0
- respiratory syncytial virus J12.1
- resulting from a procedure J95.8
- rheumatic I00† J17.8*
- Salmonella (arizonae) (cholerae-suis) (enteritidis) (typhimurium) A02.2† J17.0*
-   – typhi A01.0† J17.0*
- Serratia marcescens J15.6
- specified NEC J18.8
-   – bacterium NEC J15.8
-   – organism NEC J16.8
-   – virus NEC J12.8
- spirochetal NEC A69.8† J17.8*
- staphylococcal (broncho) (lobar) J15.2
- static, stasis J18.2
- streptococcal NEC (broncho) (lobar) J15.4
-   – group B J15.3
- Streptococcus pneumoniae J13
- syphilitic, congenital (early) A50.0† J17.0*
- traumatic (complication) (early) (secondary) T79.8
- tuberculous (any) (*see also* Tuberculosis, pulmonary) A16.2
- tularemic A21.2† J17.0*
- viral, virus (broncho) (interstitial) (lobar) J12.9
-   – with influenza, flu, or grippe (*see also* Pneumonia, with, influenza) J11.0
-   – adenoviral J12.0
-   – congenital P23.0

Pneumonia—*continued*
- viral, virus—*continued*
- – parainfluenza J12.2
- – respiratory syncytial J12.1
- – specified NEC J12.8
- white (congenital) A50.0† J17.0∗
Pneumonic – *see condition*
Pneumonitis (acute) (primary) (*see also*
 Pneumonia) J18.9
- air-conditioner J67.7
- allergic (due to) J67.9
- – organic dust NEC J67.8
- – red cedar dust J67.8
- – sequoiosis J67.8
- – wood dust J67.8
- aspiration J69.0
- – due to anesthesia J95.4
- – – during
- – – – labor and delivery O74.0
- – – – pregnancy O29.0
- – – – puerperium O89.0
- chemical, due to gases, fumes or vapors
 (inhalation) J68.0
- cholesterol J84.8
- due to
- – beryllium J68.0
- – cadmium J68.0
- – detergent J69.8
- – fluorocarbon-polymer J68.0
- – food, vomit (aspiration) J69.0
- – gases, fumes or vapors (inhalation)
 J68.0
- – inhalation
- – – blood J69.8
- – – essences J69.1
- – – food (regurgitated), milk, vomit
 J69.0
- – – oils, essences J69.1
- – – solids, liquids NEC J69.8
- – manganese J68.0
- – nitrogen dioxide J68.0
- – oils, essences J69.1
- – solids, liquids NEC J69.8
- – toxoplasmosis (acquired) B58.3†
 J17.3∗
- – – congenital P37.1† J17.3∗
- – vanadium J68.0
- eosinophilic J82
- hypersensitivity (*see also* Pneumonitis,
 allergic) J67.9
- lymphoid, interstitial, resulting from HIV
 disease B22.1
- meconium P24.0
- neonatal aspiration P24.9

Pneumonitis—*continued*
- postanesthetic
- – correct substance properly administered
 J95.8
- – in labor and delivery O74.0
- – in pregnancy O29.0
- – overdose or wrong substance given
 T41.2
- – – specified anesthetic – *see* Table of
 drugs and chemicals
- – postpartum, puerperal O89.0
- postoperative J95.8
- radiation J70.0
- rubella, congenital P35.0
- ventilation (air-conditioning) J67.7
Pneumonoconiosis – *see* Pneumoconiosis
Pneumopathy NEC J98.4
- alveolar J84.0
- due to organic dust NEC J66.8
- parietoalveolar J84.0
Pneumopericarditis (*see also* Pericarditis)
 I31.9
Pneumopericardium (*see also* Pericarditis)
 I31.9
- congenital P25.3
- fetus or newborn P25.3
- traumatic (post) S26.8
Pneumophagia (psychogenic) F45.3
Pneumopleurisy,
 pneumopleuritis (*see also* Pneumonia)
 J18.8
Pneumopyopericardium I30.1
Pneumopyothorax (*see also*
 Pyopneumothorax) J86.9
Pneumorrhagia (*see also* Hemorrhage,
 lung) R04.8
- tuberculous (*see also* Tuberculosis,
 pulmonary) A16.2
Pneumothorax J93.9
- acute J93.8
- chronic J93.8
- congenital P25.1
- due to operative injury of chest wall or
 lung J95.8
- – accidental puncture or laceration T81.2
- perinatal period P25.1
- specified NEC J93.8
- spontaneous NEC J93.1
- – fetus or newborn P25.1
- – tension J93.0
- tension (spontaneous) J93.0
- traumatic S27.0
- – with hemothorax S27.2

Pneumothorax—*continued*
- tuberculous NEC (*see also* Tuberculosis, pulmonary) A16.2
Podagra M10.9
Podencephalus Q01.9
Poikilocytosis R71
Poikiloderma L81.6
- Civatte's L57.3
- congenital Q82.8
- vasculare atrophicans L94.5
Poikilodermatomyositis M33.1
Pointed ear (congenital) Q17.3
Poison ivy, oak, sumac or other plant dermatitis (allergic) (contact) L23.7
Poisoning (acute) (*see also* Table of drugs and chemicals) T65.9
- bacterial toxins NEC A05.9
- berries, noxious T62.1
- botulism A05.1
- ciguatera fish T61.0
- Clostridium botulinum A05.1
- drug – *see* Table of drugs and chemicals
- epidemic, fish (noxious) (*see also* Poisoning, ichthyotoxism) T61.9
- – bacterial A05.9
- fava bean D55.0
- fish (noxious) (*see also* Poisoning, ichthyotoxism) T61.2
- – bacterial (*see also* Intoxication, foodborne, by agent) A05.9
- food (acute) (diseased) (infected) (noxious) NEC T62.9
- – bacterial (*see also* Intoxication, foodborne, by agent) A05.9
- – noxious or naturally toxic T62.9
- – – berries T62.1
- – – fish NEC T61.2
- – – – ciguatera T61.0
- – – – scombroid T61.1
- – – mushrooms T62.0
- – – plants NEC T62.2
- – – seafood T61.9
- – – – specified NEC T61.8
- – – specified NEC T62.8
- ichthyotoxism T61.9
- – due to
- – – ciguatera T61.0
- – – fish NEC T61.2
- – – scombroid T61.1
- – – seafood T61.9
- – – – specified NEC T61.8
- – – shellfish NEC T61.2
- mushroom (noxious) T62.0
- mussels (noxious) T61.2

Poisoning—*continued*
- mussels—*continued*
- – bacterial (*see also* Intoxication, foodborne, by agent) A05.9
- noxious foodstuffs T62.9
- – specified NEC T62.8
- plants, noxious T62.2
- ptomaine – *see* Poisoning, food
- Salmonella (arizonae) (cholerae-suis) (enteritidis) (typhimurium) A02.9
- scombroid fish T61.1
- seafood (noxious) T61.9
- – bacterial (*see also* Intoxication, foodborne, by agent) A05.9
- – specified NEC T61.8
- shellfish (noxious) T61.2
- – bacterial (*see also* Intoxication, foodborne, by agent) A05.9
- staphylococcus, food A05.0
Poker spine M45
Poland's syndrome Q79.8
Polioencephalitis (acute) (bulbar) A80.9
- inferior G12.2
- influenzal (specific virus not identified) J11.8† G05.1∗
- – avian influenza virus identified J09† G05.1∗
- – other influenza virus identified J10.8† G05.1∗
- superior hemorrhagic (acute) (Wernicke's) E51.2† G32.8∗
- Wernicke's E51.2† G32.8∗
Polioencephalomyelitis (acute) (anterior) A80.9
- with beriberi E51.2† G32.8∗
Poliomeningoencephalitis – *see* Meningoencephalitis
Poliomyelitis (acute) (anterior) (epidemic) A80.9
- with paralysis (bulbar) (*see also* Poliomyelitis, paralytic) A80.3
- abortive A80.4
- ascending (progressive) (*see also* Poliomyelitis, paralytic) A80.3
- bulbar (paralytic) (*see also* Poliomyelitis, paralytic) A80.3
- congenital P35.8
- nonepidemic A80.9
- nonparalytic A80.4
- paralytic A80.3
- – vaccine-associated A80.0
- – wild virus
- – – imported A80.1
- – – indigenous A80.2

Poliomyelitis—*continued*
- spinal, acute A80.9

Poliosis (eyebrow) (eyelashes) L67.1
- circumscripta, acquired L67.1

Pollakiuria R35
- psychogenic F45.3

Pollinosis J30.1

Polyadenitis (*see also* Adenitis) I88.9
- malignant A20.0

Polyangiitis M30.0
- microscopic M31.7
- overlap syndrome M30.8

Polyarteritis
- microscopic M31.7
- nodosa
- - with lung involvement M30.1
- - juvenile M30.2
- - related condition NEC M30.8

Polyarthralgia M25.5
- psychogenic F45.4

Polyarthritis, polyarthropathy (*see also* Arthritis) M13.0
- due to or associated with other specified conditions – *see* Arthritis
- epidemic (Australian) (with exanthema) B33.1
- infective – *see* Arthritis, infectious
- inflammatory M06.4
- juvenile (chronic) (seronegative) M08.3
- migratory – *see* Fever, rheumatic
- rheumatic, acute – *see* Fever, rheumatic

Polyarthrosis M15.9
- post-traumatic M15.3
- primary M15.0
- specified NEC M15.8

Polycarential syndrome of infancy E40

Polychondritis (atrophic) (chronic) M94.8
- relapsing M94.1

Polycoria Q13.2

Polycystic (disease)
- degeneration, kidney Q61.3
- - autosomal dominant (adult type) Q61.2
- - autosomal recessive (infantile type) Q61.1
- kidney Q61.3
- - autosomal dominant (adult type) Q61.2
- - autosomal recessive (infantile type) Q61.1
- liver Q44.6
- lung J98.4
- - congenital Q33.0
- ovary, ovaries E28.2

Polycythemia (acquired) (secondary) NEC D75.1
- benign (familial) D75.0
- due to
- - erythropoietin D75.1
- - fall in plasma volume D75.1
- - high altitude D75.1
- - stress D75.1
- emotional D75.1
- familial (benign) D75.0
- hypertonica D75.1
- hypoxemic D75.1
- neonatorum P61.1
- nephrogenous D75.1
- primary D45
- relative D75.1
- rubra vera D45
- vera D45

Polydactylism, polydactyly Q69.9

Polydipsia R63.1

Polydystrophy, pseudo-Hurler E77.0

Polyembryoma (M9072/3) – *see* Neoplasm, malignant

Polyglandular
- deficiency E31.0
- dyscrasia E31.9
- dysfunction E31.9

Polyhydramnios O40
- affecting fetus or newborn P01.3

Polymastia Q83.1

Polymenorrhea N92.0

Polymyalgia M35.3
- arteritica, giant cell M31.5
- rheumatica M35.3
- - with giant cell arteritis M31.5

Polymyositis (acute) (chronic) (hemorrhagic) M33.2
- with involvement of
- - lung M33.2† J99.1*
- - skin M33.9
- ossificans (generalisata) (progressiva) M61.1

Polyneuritis, polyneuritic (*see also* Polyneuropathy) G62.9
- acute (post-)infective G61.0
- cranialis G52.7
- diabetic (*see also* E10-E14 with fourth character .4) E14.4† G63.2*
- diphtheritic A36.8† G63.0*
- due to lack of vitamin NEC E56.9† G63.4*
- endemic E51.1† G63.4*
- erythredema T56.1
- febrile, acute G61.0

Polyneuritis, polyneuritic—*continued*
- infective (acute) G61.0
- nutritional E63.9† G63.4*
- postinfective (acute) G61.0
- specified NEC G62.8

Polyneuropathy (peripheral) G62.9
- alcoholic G62.1
- amyloid (Portuguese) E85.1† G63.3*
- arsenical G62.2
- diabetic (*see also* E10-E14 with fourth
  character .4) E14.4† G63.2*
- drug-induced G62.0
- hereditary G60.9
- – specified NEC G60.8
- idiopathic progressive G60.3
- in (due to)
- – alcohol G62.1
- – amyloidosis, familial (Portuguese)
  E85.1† G63.3*
- – antitetanus serum G61.1
- – arsenic G62.2
- – avitaminosis NEC E56.9† G63.4*
- – beriberi E51.1† G63.4*
- – collagen vascular disease NEC M35.9†
  G63.5*
- – deficiency of B vitamins E53.9†
  G63.4*
- – diabetes (*see also* E10-E14 with fourth
  character .4) E14.4† G63.2*
- – diphtheria A36.8† G63.0*
- – drug or medicament G62.0
- – – overdose or wrong substance given
  or taken T50.9
- – – – specified drug – *see* Table of drugs
  and chemicals
- – endocrine disease NEC E34.9† G63.3*
- – herpes zoster B02.2† G63.0*
- – hypoglycemia E16.2† G63.3*
- – infectious
- – – disease NEC B99† G63.0*
- – – mononucleosis B27.-† G63.0*
- – lack of vitamin NEC E56.9† G63.4*
- – lead G62.2
- – leprosy A30.-† G63.0*
- – Lyme disease A69.2† G63.0*
- – malignant neoplasm NEC
  (M8000/3) (*see also* Neoplasm,
  malignant) C80.-† G63.1*
- – metabolic disease NEC E88.9† G63.3*
- – microscopic polyangiitis M31.7†
  G63.5*
- – mumps B26.8† G63.0*

Polyneuropathy—*continued*
- in—*continued*
- – neoplastic disease NEC
  (M8000/1) (*see also* Neoplasm)
  D48.9† G63.1*
- – nutritional deficiency NEC E63.9†
  G63.4*
- – organophosphate compounds G62.2
- – parasitic disease NEC B89† G63.0*
- – pellagra E52† G63.4*
- – polyarteritis nodosa M30.0† G63.5*
- – porphyria E80.2† G63.3*
- – radiation G62.8
- – rheumatoid arthritis M05.3† G63.6*
- – sarcoidosis D86.8† G63.8*
- – serum G61.1
- – syphilis (late) A52.1† G63.0*
- – – congenital A50.4† G63.0*
- – systemic
- – – connective tissue disorder M35.9†
  G63.5*
- – – lupus erythematosus M32.1† G63.5*
- – toxic agent NEC G62.2
- – triorthocresyl phosphate G62.2
- – tuberculosis A17.8† G63.0*
- – uremia N18.5† G63.8*
- – vitamin B₁₂ deficiency E53.8† G63.4*
- – – with anemia (pernicious) D51.0†
  G63.4*
- – – – due to dietary deficiency D51.3†
  G63.4*
- – zoster B02.2† G63.0*
- inflammatory G61.9
- – specified NEC G61.8
- nutritional E63.9† G63.4*
- postherpetic (zoster) B02.2† G63.0*
- radiation-induced G62.8
- sensory (hereditary) (idiopathic) G60.8
- specified NEC G62.8
- syphilitic (late) A52.1† G63.0*
- – congenital A50.4† G63.0*

Polyopia H53.8
Polyorchism, polyorchidism Q55.2
Polyostotic fibrous dysplasia Q78.1
Polyotia Q17.0
Polyp, polypus

Note: Polyps of organs or sites that do not
appear in the list below should be coded to
the residual category for diseases of the
organ or site concerned.

- accessory sinus J33.8
- adenocarcinoma in (M8210/3) – *see*
  Neoplasm, malignant

Polyp, polypus—*continued*
- adenocarcinoma in situ in (M8210/2) –
  see Neoplasm, in situ
- adenoid tissue J33.0
- adenomatous (M8210/0) – *see also*
  Neoplasm, benign
- – adenocarcinoma in (M8210/3) – *see*
  Neoplasm, malignant
- – adenocarcinoma in situ in (M8210/2) –
  see Neoplasm, in situ
- – carcinoma in (M8210/3) – *see*
  Neoplasm, malignant
- – carcinoma in situ in (M8210/2) – *see*
  Neoplasm, in situ
- – multiple (M8221/0) – *see* Neoplasm,
  benign
- – – adenocarcinoma in (M8221/3) – *see*
  Neoplasm, malignant
- – – adenocarcinoma in situ in
  (M8221/2) – *see* Neoplasm, in situ
- antrum J33.8
- anus, anal (canal) K62.0
- bladder (M8120/1) D41.4
- carcinoma in (M8210/3) – *see* Neoplasm,
  malignant
- carcinoma in situ in (M8210/2) – *see*
  Neoplasm, in situ
- cervix (uteri) N84.1
- – in pregnancy or childbirth O34.4
- – – affecting fetus or newborn P03.8
- – – causing obstructed labor O65.5
- – mucous N84.1
- choanal J33.0
- colon K63.5
- – adenomatous (M8210/0) – *see* Polyp,
  adenomatous
- – inflammatory K51.4
- corpus uteri N84.0
- dental K04.0
- duodenum K31.7
- ear (middle) H74.4
- endometrium N84.0
- ethmoidal (sinus) J33.8
- fallopian tube N84.8
- female genital tract N84.9
- – specified NEC N84.8
- frontal (sinus) J33.8
- gingiva, gum K06.8
- labium (majus) (minus) N84.3
- larynx (mucous) J38.1
- malignant (M8000/3) – *see* Neoplasm,
  malignant
- maxillary (sinus) J33.8
- middle ear H74.4

Polyp, polypus—*continued*
- nasal (mucous) J33.9
- – cavity J33.0
- nasopharyngeal J33.0
- nose (mucous) J33.9
- oviduct N84.8
- pharynx J39.2
  placenta O90.8
- pudendum N84.3
- pulpal (dental) K04.0
- rectum (nonadenomatous) K62.1
- – adenomatous – *see* Polyp, adenomatous
- septum (nasal) J33.0
- sinus (accessory) (ethmoidal) (frontal)
  (maxillary) (sphenoidal) J33.8
- sphenoidal (sinus) J33.8
- stomach K31.7
- – adenomatous (M8210/0) – *see* Polyp,
  adenomatous
- tube, fallopian N84.8
- turbinate, mucous membrane J33.8
- umbilical, newborn P83.6
- ureter N28.8
- urethra N36.2
- uterus (body) (corpus) (mucous) N84.0
- – cervix N84.1
- – in pregnancy or childbirth O34.1
- – – affecting fetus or newborn P03.8
- – – causing obstructed labor O65.5
- vagina N84.2
- vocal cord (mucous) J38.1
- vulva N84.3

Polyphagia R63.2
Polyploidy Q92.7
Polypoid – *see condition*
Polyposis – *see also* Polyp
- colon (adenomatous) (M8220/0) D12.6
- – adenocarcinoma in (M8220/3) C18.9
- – carcinoma in (M8220/3) C18.9
- familial (M8220/0) D12.6
- intestinal (adenomatous) (M8220/0)
  D12.6
- – lymphomatous, malignant C83.9
- multiple, adenomatous
  (M8221/0) (*see also* Neoplasm, benign)
  D36.9
Polyradiculitis (*see also* Polyneuropathy)
  G62.9
**Polyradiculoneuropathy (acute)
  (postinfective)** G61.0
Polyserositis
- periodic, familial E85.0
- tuberculous A19.9
- – acute A19.1

Polyserositis—*continued*
- tuberculous—*continued*
- – chronic A19.8
Polysyndactyly Q70.4
Polytrichia L68.3
Polyunguia Q84.6
Polyuria (nocturnal) R35
- psychogenic F45.3
Pompe's disease (glycogen storage) E74.0
Pompholyx L30.1
Poncet's disease (tuberculous arthritis) A18.0† M01.1*
Pond fracture S02.9
Ponos B55.0
Pons, pontine – *see condition*
Poor
- contractions, labor O62.2
- – affecting fetus or newborn P03.6
- fetal growth NEC P05.9
- – affecting management of pregnancy O36.5
- personal hygiene R46.0
- prenatal care, affecting management of pregnancy Z35.3
- urinary stream R39.1
- vision NEC H54.9
Poradenitis, nostras inguinalis or venerea A55
Porencephaly (congenital) (developmental) Q04.6
- acquired G93.0
- nondevelopmental G93.0
Porocephaliasis B88.8
Porokeratosis Q82.8
Poroma, eccrine (M8402/0) – *see* Neoplasm, skin, benign
Porphyria (South African) (Swedish) E80.2
- acquired E80.2
- acute intermittent (hepatic) E80.2
- cutanea tarda (hereditary) (symptomatic) E80.1
- due to drugs
- – correct substance properly administered E80.2
- – overdose or wrong substance given or taken T50.9
- – – specified drug – *see* Table of drugs and chemicals
- erythropoietic (congenital) (hereditary) E80.0
- hepatocutaneous type E80.1
- secondary E80.2
- toxic NEC E80.2

Porphyria—*continued*
- variegata E80.2
Porphyrinuria, porphyruria – *see* Porphyria
Portal – *see condition*
Posada-Wernicke disease B38.7
Position
- fetus, abnormal (*see also* Presentation, fetal) O32.9
- teeth, faulty K07.3
Positive
- culture (nonspecific)
- – nose R84.5
- – sputum R84.5
- – throat R84.5
- – wound R89.5
- serology for syphilis A53.0
- – false R76.2
- – with signs or symptoms – *code as* Syphilis, by site and stage
- test, human immunodeficiency virus (HIV) R75
- VDRL A53.0
- – with signs or symptoms – *code as* Syphilis, by site and stage
- – false R76.2
Postcardiotomy syndrome I97.0
Postcaval ureter Q62.6
Postcholecystectomy syndrome K91.5
Postcommissurotomy syndrome I97.0
Postconcussional syndrome F07.2
Postcontusional syndrome F07.2
Postcricoid region – *see condition*
Post-dates (pregnancy) (mother) O48
Postencephalitic syndrome F07.1
Posterolateral sclerosis (spinal cord) – *see* Degeneration, combined
Postexanthematous – *see condition*
Postfebrile – *see condition*
Postgastrectomy dumping syndrome K91.1
Postherpetic neuralgia (zoster) (trigeminal) B02.2† G53.0*
Posthitis N48.1
Postimmunization complication or reaction – *see* Complications, vaccination
Postinfectious – *see condition*
Postlaminectomy syndrome NEC M96.1
Postleukotomy syndrome F07.0
Postmastectomy lymphedema (syndrome) I97.2
Postmaturity, postmature (fetus or newborn) P08.2
- affecting management of pregnancy O48

Postmeasles complication NEC (*see also condition*) B05.8
Postmenopausal
- endometrium (atrophic) N95.8
- - suppurative (*see also* Endometritis) N71.9
- osteoporosis M81.0
- - with pathological fracture M80.0
Postnatal – *see condition*
Postoperative – *see condition*
Postpartum – *see condition*
Postpolio syndrome G14
Postpoliomyelitic – *see also condition*
- osteopathy M89.6
- syndrom G14
Postschizophrenic depression F20.4
Postsurgery status NEC (*see also* Status (post)) Z98.8
Post-term (pregnancy) (mother) O48
- infant P08.2
Post-traumatic brain syndrome, nonpsychotic F07.2
Postures, hysterical F44.2
Postvaccinal reaction or complication – *see* Complications, vaccination
Postvalvulotomy syndrome I97.0
Potter's
- asthma J62.8
- facies Q60.6
- lung J62.8
- syndrome (with renal agenesis) Q60.6
Pott's
- curvature (spinal) A18.0† M49.0∗
- disease or paraplegia A18.0† M49.0∗
- spinal curvature A18.0† M49.0∗
- tumor, puffy (*see also* Osteomyelitis) M86.8
Pouch
- bronchus Q32.4
- Douglas' – *see condition*
- esophagus, esophageal, congenital Q39.6
- - acquired K22.5
- gastric K31.4
- pharynx Q38.7
Poultryman's itch B88.0
Poverty NEC Z59.6
- extreme Z59.5
Prader-Willi syndrome Q87.1
Preauricular appendage or tag Q17.0
Prebetalipoproteinemia (familial) E78.1
Precipitate labor or delivery O62.3
- affecting fetus or newborn P03.5
Precocious
- menarche E30.1

Precocious—*continued*
- menstruation E30.1
- puberty E30.1
- - central E22.8
- thelarche E30.8
Precocity, sexual (female) (male) (constitutional) (cryptogenic) (idiopathic) NEC E30.1
with adrenal hyperplasia E25.9
- - congenital E25.0
Precordial pain R07.2
- psychogenic F45.4
Prediabetes, prediabetic R73.0
- complicating pregnancy, childbirth or puerperium O99.8
Predislocation status of hip at birth Q65.6
Pre-eclampsia O14.9
- with pre-existing hypertension O11
- affecting fetus or newborn P00.0
- mild O13
- moderate O14.0
- severe O14.1
- superimposed O11
Pre-excitation atrioventricular conduction I45.6
Pregnancy (single) (uterine)
- abdominal (ectopic) O00.0
- - affecting fetus or newborn P01.4
- - viable fetus O36.7
- abnormal NEC O26.9
- ampullar O00.1
- broad ligament O00.8
- cervical O00.8
- complicated by (*see also* Pregnancy, management, affected by)
- - abnormal, abnormality
- - - cervix O34.4
- - - cord (umbilical) O69.9
- - - glucose tolerance NEC O99.8
- - - pelvic organs or tissues O34.9
- - - - affecting fetus or newborn P03.8
- - - - causing obstructed labour O65.5
- - - - - affecting fetus or newborn P03.1
- - - - specified NEC O34.8
- - - pelvis (bony) (major) NEC O33.0
- - - perineum or vulva O34.7
- - - placenta, placental (vessel) O43.1
- - - - accreta O43.2
- - - - increta O43.2
- - - - morbidly adherent O43.2
- - - - percreta O43.2
- - - position
- - - - placenta O44.1

Pregnancy—*continued*
- complicated by—*continued*
-   – abnormal, abnormality—*continued*
-    – position—*continued*
-     – placenta—*continued*
-      – without hemorrhage O44.0
-     – uterus O34.5
-    – uterus (congenital) O34.0
-   – abscess or cellulitis
-    – bladder O23.1
-    – genital organ or tract O23.5
-   – adverse effect of anesthesia O29.9
-   – albuminuria O12.1
-    – with
-     – edema O12.2
-     – hypertension (*see also* Pre-eclampsia) O14.9
-   – alcohol dependence (F10.2) O99.3
-   – amnionitis O41.1
-   – anaphylactoid syndrome of pregnancy O88.1
-   – anemia (conditions in D50-D64) O99.0
-   – atrophy (acute) (subacute) (yellow), liver O26.6
-   – bicornis or bicornuate uterus O34.0
-   – bone and joint disorders of back, pelvis and lower limbs O99.8
-   – breech presentation O32.1
-   – cardiovascular diseases (conditions in I00-I09, I20-I52, I70-I99) O99.4
-   – cerebrovascular disorders (conditions in I60-I69) O99.4
-   – cervicitis O23.5
-   – chloasma (gravidarum) O26.8
-   – cholestasis (intrahepatic) O26.6
-   – compound presentation O32.6
-   – conditions in
-    – A00-A07, O98.8
-    – A08, O98.5
-    – A09, O98.8
-    – A15-A19, O98.0
-    – A24-A49, O98.8
-    – A50-A53, O98.1
-    – A54.-, O98.2
-    – A55-A64, O98.3
-    – A65-A79, O98.8
-    – A80-B09, O98.5
-    – B15-Bl9, O98.4
-    – B20-B24 O98.7
-    – B25-B34, O98.5
-    – B35-B49, O98.8
-    – B50-B64, O98.6
-    – B65-B88, O98.8
-    – B89, O98.2

Pregnancy—*continued*
- complicated by—*continued*
-   – conditions in—*continued*
-    – B90-B94, O98.8
-    – C00-D48, O99.8
-    – D50-D64, O99.0
-    – D65-D89, O99.1
-    – E00-E07, O99.2
-    – E10-E14, O24.-
-    – E15-E34, O99.2
-    – E40-E46, O25
-    – E50-E89, O99.2
-    – F00-F52, O99.3
-    – F54-F99, O99.3
-    – G00-G99, O99.3
-    – H00-H95, O99.8
-    – I00-I09, O99.4
-    – I10, pre-existing O10.0
-    – I11.-, pre-existing O10.1
-    – I12.-, pre-existing O10.2
-    – I13.-, pre-existing O10.3
-    – I15.-, pre-existing O10.4
-    – I20-I99, O99.4
-    – J00-J99, O99.5
-    – K00-K66, O99.6
-    – K70-K77, O26.6
-    – K80-K93, O99.6
-    – L00-L99, O99.7
-    – M00-M82, O99.8
-    – M83.2-M99, O99.8
-    – N00-N07, O26.8
-    – N10-N12, O23.0
-    – N13.0-N13.5, O26.8
-    – N13.6, O23.3
-    – N13.7-N13.9, O26.8
-    – N14-N15.0, O99.8
-    – N15.1, O23.0
-    – N15.8-N15.9, O99.8
-    – N17-N19, O26.8
-    – N20-N39, O99.8
-    – N60-N64, O99.8
-    – N80-N90, O99.8
-    – N99.0, O75.4
-    – N99.8, O75.4
-    – N99.9, O75.4
-    – Q00-Q99, NEC O99.8
-    – R73.0, O99.8
-   – congenital malformations, deformations and chromosomal abnormalities NEC O99.8
-   – contracted pelvis (general) O33.1
-    – inlet O33.2
-    – outlet O33.3

Pregnancy—*continued*
- complicated by—*continued*
- - convulsions (eclamptic)
  (uremic) (*see also* Eclampsia) O15.0
- - cystitis O23.1
- - cystocele O34.8
- - death of fetus (near term) O36.4
- - - early pregnancy O02.1
- - deciduitis O41.1
- - diabetes (mellitus) O24.9
- - diseases of
- - - blood NEC (conditions in D65-D77)
  O99.1
- - - cardiovascular system NEC
  (conditions in I00-I09, I20-I99)
  O99.4
- - - digestive system NEC (conditions in
  K00-K93) O99.6
- - - ear and mastoid process (conditions
  in H60-H95) O99.8
- - - eye and adnexa (conditions in H00-
  H59) O99.8
- - - genitourinary system NEC
  (conditions in N00-N99) O99.8
- - - musculoskeletal system and
  connective tissue (conditions in M00-
  M99) O99.8
- - - nervous system (conditions in G00-
  G99) O99.3
- - - respiratory system (conditions in J00-
  J99) O99.5
- - - skin and subcutaneous tissue NEC
  (conditions in L00-L99) O99.7
- - disorders of liver O26.6
- - displacement, uterus NEC O34.5
- - disproportion – *see* Disproportion
- - drug dependence (conditions in F11-
  F19, fourth character .2) O99.3
- - early delivery (with spontaneous labor)
  NEC O60.1
- - - without spontaneous labor (cesarean
  section) (induction) O60.3
- - eclampsia, eclamptic (coma)
  (convulsions) (delirium) (nephritis)
  (uremia) O15.0
- - - with pre-existing hypertension
  O15.0
- - edema O12.0
- - - with gestational hypertension,
  mild (*see also* Pre-eclampsia) O13
- - effusion, amniotic fluid O41.8
- - - delayed delivery following O75.6
- - embolism O88.2
- - - air O88.0

Pregnancy—*continued*
- complicated by—*continued*
- - embolism—*continued*
- - - amniotic fluid O88.1
- - - blood-clot O88.2
- - - pulmonary NEC O88.2
- - - pyemic O88.3
- - - septic O88.3
- - endocrine diseases NEC O99.2
- - endometritis O23.5
- - - decidual O41.1
- - excessive weight gain NEC O26.0
- - exhaustion O26.8
- - face presentation O32.3
- - failure, fetal head, to enter pelvic brim
  O32.4
- - false labor (pains) (*see also* Labor,
  false) O47.9
- - fatigue O26.8
- - fatty metamorphosis of liver O26.6
- - fetal
- - - disproportion due to deformity (fetal)
  O33.7
- - - problem O36.9
- - - - specified NEC O36.8
- - fibroid (tumor) (uterus) O34.1
- - genital infection O23.5
- - glomerular diseases (conditions in N00-
  N07) O26.8
- - - with hypertension, pre-existing
  O10.2
- - gonococcal infection O98.2
- - hemorrhage NEC
- - - antepartum (*see also* Hemorrhage,
  antepartum) O46.9
- - - before 22 completed weeks' gestation
  O20.9
- - - - specified NEC O20.8
- - - due to premature separation, placenta
  O45.9
- - - early O20.9
- - - - specified NEC O20.8
- - - threatened abortion O20.0
- - hemorrhoids O22.4
- - herniation of uterus O34.5
- - high head at term O32.4
- - human immunodeficiency virus (HIV)
  disease O98.7
- - hydatidiform mole (M9100/0) (*see also*
  Mole, hydatidiform) O01.9
- - hydramnios O40
- - hydrocephalic fetus (disproportion)
  O33.6

Vaginal Thrush in pregnancy
O23.5 + B37.3 D + N77.1 A

Pregnancy—*continued*
– complicated by—*continued*
– – hydrops
– – – amnii O40
– – – fetalis NEC O36.2
– – hydrorrhea O42.9
– – hyperemesis (gravidarum) – *see* Hyperemesis, gravidarum
– – hypertension (*see also* Hypertension, complicating pregnancy) O16
– – hypertensive
– – – heart and renal disease, pre-existing O10.3
– – – heart disease, pre-existing O10.1
– – – renal disease, pre-existing O10.2
– – immune disorders NEC (conditions in D80-D89) O99.1
– – incarceration, uterus O34.5
– – incompetent cervix O34.3
– – infection(s)
– – – amniotic fluid or sac O41.1
– – – bladder O23.1
– – – genital organ or tract O23.5
– – – genitourinary tract NEC O23.9
– – – kidney O23.0
– – – – with a predominantly sexual mode of transmission NEC O98.3
– – – specified NEC O98.8
– – – urethra O23.2
– – – urinary (tract) O23.4
– – – – specified part NEC O23.3
– – infectious or parasitic disease NEC O98.9
– – insufficient weight gain O26.1
– – malaria O98.6
– – malformation
– – – placenta, placental (vessel) O43.1
– – – uterus (congenital) O34.0
– – malnutrition (conditions in E40-E46) O25
– – malposition
– – – fetus – *see* Presentation, fetal
– – – uterus O34.5
– – malpresentation of fetus (*see also* Presentation, fetal) O32.9
– – – in multiple gestation O32.5
– – – specified NEC O32.8
– – mental disorders (conditions in F00-F99) O99.3
– – mentum presentation O32.3
– – metabolic disorders O99.2
– – missed
– – – abortion O02.1
– – – delivery O36.4

Pregnancy—*continued*
– complicated by—*continued*
– – morbidly adherent placenta O43.2
– – necrosis, liver (conditions in K72.-) O26.6
– – neoplasms NEC O99.8
– – nephropathy NEC O26.8
– – nutritional diseases NEC O99.2
– – oblique lie or presentation O32.2
– – oligohydramnios NEC O41.0
– – onset of contractions before 37 weeks' gestation – *see* Labor, early onset
– – – with
– – – – pre-term delivery O60.1
– – – – term delivery O60.2
– – – without delivery O60.0
– – oophoritis O23.5
– – oversize fetus O33.5
– – papyraceous fetus O31.0
– – peripheral neuritis O26.8
– – phlebothrombosis (superficial) O22.2
– – – deep O22.3
– – placenta, placental
– – – abnormality O43.1
– – – abruptio or ablatio (*see also* Abruptio placentae) O45.9
– – – accreta O43.2
– – – detachment (*see also* Abruptio placentae) O45.9
– – – disease O43.9
– – – dysfunction O43.8
– – – increta O43.2
– – – infarction O43.8
– – – low implantation (with hemorrhage) O44.1
– – – – without hemorrhage O44.0
– – – malformation O43.1
– – – malposition (with hemorrhage) O44.1
– – – – without hemorrhage O44.0
– – – morbidly adherent O43.2
– – – percreta O43.2
– – – previa (with hemorrhage) O44.1
– – – – without hemorrhage O44.0
– – – separation, premature (*see also* Abruptio placentae) O45.9
– – – transfusion syndrome O43.0
– – placentitis O41.1
– – polyhydramnios O40
– – postmaturity O48
– – pre-eclampsia O14.9
– – – mild O13
– – – moderate O14.0
– – – severe O14.1

Pregnancy—*continued*
- complicated by—*continued*
- - premature rupture of membranes – *see*
  Rupture, membranes, premature
- - previous
- - - nonobstetric condition Z35.8
- - - poor obstetric history Z35.2
- - - premature delivery Z35.2
- - - trophoblastic disease (conditions in
  O01.-) Z35.1
- - primigravida
- - - elderly (supervision only) Z35.5
- - - very young (supervision only) Z35.6
- - prolapse, uterus O34.5
- - proteinuria O12.1
- - - with
- - - - edema O12.2
- - - - hypertension (*see also* Pre-
  eclampsia) O14.9
- - protozoal diseases O98.6
- - pruritus (neurogenic) O26.8
- - psychosis or psychoneurosis O99.3
- - ptyalism O26.8
- - pyelitis O23.0
- - renal disease or failure NEC O26.8
- - - with secondary hypertension, pre-
  existing O10.4
- - - hypertensive, pre-existing O10.2
- - retention, retained
- - - dead ovum O02.0
- - - intrauterine contraceptive device
  O26.3
- - retroversion, uterus O34.5
- - Rh immunization, incompatibility or
  sensitization O36.0
- - rupture
- - - amnion (premature) – *see* Rupture,
  membranes, premature
- - - membranes (premature) – *see*
  Rupture, membranes, premature
- - - uterus (during labor) O71.1
- - - - before onset of labor O71.0
- - salivation (excessive) O26.8
- - salpingitis O23.5
- - salpingo-oophoritis O23.5
- - sepsis (conditions in A40.-, A41.-)
  O98.8
- - signs of fetal hypoxia (unrelated to
  labor or delivery) O36.3
- - social problem Z35.7
- - spurious labor pains (*see also* Labor,
  false) O47.9
- - superfecundation O30.8
- - superfetation O30.8

Pregnancy—*continued*
- complicated by—*continued*
- - syndrome
- - - anaphylactoid of pregnancy O88.1
- - syphilis (conditions in A50-A53)
  O98.1
- - threatened
- - - abortion O20.0
- - - delivery O47.9
- - - - at or after 37 completed weeks of
  gestation O47.1
- - - - before 37 completed weeks of
  gestation O47.0
- - thrombophlebitis (superficial) O22.2
- - thrombosis O22.9
- - - venous (superficial) O22.9
- - - - deep O22.3
- - torsion of uterus O34.5
- - toxemia (*see also* Pre-eclampsia)
  O14.9
- - transverse lie or presentation O32.2
- - tuberculosis (conditions in A15-A19)
  O98.0
- - tumor
- - - ovary O34.8
- - - pelvic organs or tissues NEC O34.8
- - - uterus (body) O34.1
- - - - cervix O34.4
- - unstable lie O32.0
- - urethritis O23.2
- - vaginitis or vulvitis O23.5
- - varicose
- - - placental vessels O43.8
- - - veins (legs) O22.0
- - - - labia or vulva O22.1
- - venereal disease NEC (conditions in
  A64) O98.3
- - viral diseases (conditions in A80-B09,
  B25-B34) O98.5
- - vomiting (*see also* Hyperemesis,
  gravidarum) O21.9
- - - due to diseases classified elsewhere
  O21.8
- complications NEC O26.9
- concealed Z35.3
- confirmed Z32.1
- continuing after
- - abortion of one fetus or more O31.1
- - intrauterine death of one fetus or more
  O31.2
- cornual O00.8
- - fetus or newborn P01.4
- death from NEC O95
- delivered – *see* Delivery

Pregnancy—*continued*
- ectopic (ruptured) O00.9
- − − affecting fetus or newborn P01.4
- − − specified NEC O00.8
- extrauterine (*see also* Pregnancy, by site) O00.9
- fallopian O00.1
- false F45.8
- hidden Z35.3
- illegitimate (unwanted) Z64.0
- − − supervision of high-risk pregnancy Z35.7
- in double uterus O34.0
- incidental finding Z33
- interstitial O00.8
- intraligamentous O00.8
- intramural O00.8
- intraperitoneal O00.0
- isthmian O00.1
- management affected by
- − − abnormal, abnormality
- − − − fetus (suspected) O35.9
- − − − − specified NEC O35.8
- − − − placenta O43.1
- − − antibodies (maternal)
- − − − anti-D O36.0
- − − − blood group (ABO) O36.1
- − − − − Rh(esus) O36.0
- − − diseases of the nervous system (conditions in G00-G99) O99.3
- − − elderly primigravida (supervision only) Z35.5
- − − fetal (suspected)
- − − − abnormality or damage O35.9
- − − − − acid-base balance O36.3
- − − − − heart rate or rhythm O36.3
- − − − − specified NEC O35.8
- − − − acidemia O36.3
- − − − anencephaly O35.0
- − − − bradycardia O36.3
- − − − central nervous system malformation O35.0
- − − − chromosal abnormality (conditions in Q90-Q99) O35.1
- − − − damage from
- − − − − amniocentesis O35.7
- − − − − biopsy procedures O35.7
- − − − − drug addiction O35.5
- − − − − hematological investigation O35.7
- − − − − intrauterine contraceptive device O35.7
- − − − − intrauterine surgery O35.7
- − − − − maternal
- − − − − − alcohol addiction O35.4

Pregnancy—*continued*
- − management affected by—*continued*
- − − fetal—*continued*
- − − − damage from—*continued*
- − − − − maternal—*continued*
- − − − − − cytomegalovirus infection O35.3
- − − − − − disease NEC O35.8
- − − − − − drug addiction O35.5
- − − − − − listeriosis O35.8
- − − − − − rubella O35.3
- − − − − − toxoplasmosis O35.8
- − − − − − viral infection O35.3
- − − − − medical procedure NEC O35.7
- − − − − radiation O35.6
- − − − distress O36.3
- − − − excessive growth O36.6
- − − − growth retardation O36.5
- − − − hereditary disease O35.2
- − − − hydrocephalus O35.0
- − − − intrauterine death O36.4
- − − − poor growth O36.5
- − − − spina bifida O35.0
- − − fetomaternal hemorrhage O43.0
- − − hereditary disease in family, (possibly) affecting fetus O35.2
- − − high-risk pregnancy NEC − *see* Pregnancy, supervision
- − − incompatibility, blood groups (ABO) O36.1
- − − − Rh(esus) O36.0
- − − insufficient prenatal care (supervision only) Z35.3
- − − intrauterine death (late) O36.4
- − − isoimmunization (ABO) O36.1
- − − − Rh(esus) O36.0
- − − large-for-dates fetus O36.6
- − − light-for-dates fetus O36.5
- − − meconium in liquor O36.3
- − − mental disorder (conditions in F00-F99) O99.3
- − − multiparity (grand) (supervision only) Z35.4
- − − poor obstetric history (conditions in O10-O92) Z35.2
- − − postmaturity O48
- − − previous
- − − − abortion Z35.1
- − − − − habitual O26.2
- − − − cesarean section O34.2
- − − − difficult delivery Z35.2
- − − − forceps delivery Z35.2
- − − − hemorrage, antepartum or postpartum Z35.2

Pregnancy—*continued*
- management affected by—*continued*
- – previous—*continued*
- – – hydatidiform mole Z35.1
- – – infertility Z35.0
- – – malignancy NEC Z35.8
- – – nonobstetrical condition Z35.8
- – – premature delivery Z35.2
- – – trophoblastic disease (conditions in O01.-) Z35.1
- – – vesicular mole Z35.1
- – prolonged pregnancy O48
- – small-for-dates fetus O36.5
- – social problem Z35.7
- – very young primigravida (supervision only) Z35.6
- mesometric (mural) O00.8
- molar NEC O02.0
- – hydatidiform (M9100/0) (*see also* Mole, hydatidiform) O01.9
- multiple NEC O30.9
- – affecting fetus or newborn P01.5
- – complicated NEC O31.8
- mural O00.8
- – fetus or newborn P01.4
- ovarian O00.2
- – fetus or newborn P01.4
- postmature O48
- post-term O48
- prolonged O48
- quadruplet O30.2
- – affecting fetus or newborn P01.5
- quintuplet O30.8
- – affecting fetus or newborn P01.5
- sextuplet O30.8
- – affecting fetus or newborn P01.5
- spurious F45.8
- supervision (of) (for) (*see also* Pregnancy, management affected by)
- – high-risk Z35.9
- – – specified NEC Z35.8
- – multiparity Z35.4
- – normal NEC Z34.9
- – – first Z34.0
- – – specified NEC Z34.8
- – previous
- – – infertility Z35.0
- – – neonatal death Z35.2
- – – stillbirth Z35.2
- – specified problem NEC Z35.8
- triplet O30.1
- – affecting fetus or newborn P01.5
- tubal (with abortion) (with rupture) O00.1
- – affecting fetus or newborn P01.4

Pregnancy—*continued*
- twin O30.0
- – affecting fetus or newborn P01.5
- unwanted Z64.0

Preiser's disease M87.2

Preleukemia (related to alkylating agent) (related to Epipodophyllotoxin) (related to therapy) (syndrome) D46.9

Preluxation, hip, congenital Q65.6

Premature – *see also* condition
- adrenarche E27.0
- aging E34.8
- beats I49.4
- – atrial I49.1
- birth NEC P07.3
- closure, foramen ovale Q21.8
- contraction
- – atrial I49.1
- – atrioventricular I49.2
- – heart (extrasystole) I49.4
- – junctional I49.2
- – ventricular I49.3
- delivery (with spontaneous labor) O60.1
- – without spontaneous labor (cesarean section) (induction) O60.3
- ejaculation F52.4
- infant NEC P07.3
- – light-for-dates P05.0
- lungs P28.0
- menopause E28.3
- newborn – *see* Prematurity
- puberty E30.1
- rupture, membranes or amnion (*see also* Rupture, membranes, premature) O42.9
- – affecting fetus or newborn P01.1
- senility E34.8
- separation, placenta (partial) (*see also* Abruptio placentae) O45.9
- thelarche E30.8
- ventricular systole I49.3

Prematurity NEC (less than 37 completed weeks) P07.3
- extreme (less than 28 completed weeks) P07.2

Premenstrual tension (syndrome) N94.3

Premolarization, cuspids K00.2

Prenatal
- care, normal pregnancy Z34.9
- – first Z34.0
- – specified NEC Z34.8
- death, cause unknown – *see* Death, fetus
- screening – *see* Antenatal, screening

Presbyeosophagus - a term that has traditionally been used to describe the manifestations of degenerating motor function in the aging oesophagus

Preparatory care for subsequent treatment NEC Z51.4
- for dialysis Z49.0
Prepartum – *see condition*
Prepuce – *see condition*
Presbycardia R54
Presbycusis, presbyacusia H91.1
Presbyophrenia F03
Presbyopia H52.4
Prescription of contraceptives (initial) Z30.0
- repeat Z30.4
Presence (of)
- aortocoronary (bypass) graft Z95.1
- arteriovenous shunt for dialysis Z99.2
- artificial
- - eye (globe) Z97.0
- - heart (mechanical) Z95.8
- - - valve Z95.2
- - larynx Z96.3
- - lens (intraocular) Z96.1
- - limb (complete) (partial) Z97.1
- audiological implant (functional) Z96.2
- bladder implant (functional) Z96.0
- bone
- - conduction hearing device Z96.2
- - implant (functional) NEC Z96.7
- - joint (prosthesis) Z96.6
- cardiac
- - defibrillator (functional) Z95.0
- - implant or graft NEC Z95.9
- - - specified type NEC Z95.8
- - pacemaker Z95.0
- cerebrospinal fluid drainage device Z98.2
- cochlear implant (functional) Z96.2
- contact lens(es) Z97.3
- coronary artery graft or prosthesis Z95.5
- dental prosthetic device Z97.2
- device (external) NEC Z97.8
- - implanted (functional) Z96.9
- - - specified NEC Z96.8
- - prosthetic Z97.8
- endocrine implant (functional) Z96.4
- eustachian tube stent or device (functional) Z96.2
- external hearing-aid or device Z97.4
- finger-joint implant (functional) (prosthetic) Z96.6
- functional implant Z96.9
- - specified NEC Z96.8
- hearing-aid or device (external) Z97.4
- - implant (bone) (cochlear) (functional) Z96.2

Presence—*continued*
- heart valve implant (functional) NEC Z95.4
- - prosthetic Z95.2
- - specified type NEC Z95.4
- - xenogenic Z95.3
- hip-joint implant (functional) (prosthesis) Z96.6
- implanted device (artificial) (functional) (prosthetic) Z96.9
- - specified NEC Z96.8
- insulin pump (functional) Z96.4
- intestinal bypass or anastomosis Z98.0
- intraocular lens (functional) Z96.1
- intrauterine contraceptive device (IUD) Z97.5
- intravascular implant (functional) (prosthetic) NEC Z95.8
- - coronary artery Z95.5
- - peripheral vessel Z95.8
- joint implant (prosthetic) (any) Z96.6
- knee-joint implant (prosthetic) Z96.6
- laryngeal implant (functional) Z96.3
- mandibular implant (dental) Z96.5
- myringotomy tube(s) Z96.2
- orthopedic-joint implant (prosthetic) (any) Z96.6
- otological implant (functional) Z96.2
- skull-plate implant Z96.7
- spectacles Z97.3
- stapes implant (functional) Z96.2
- systemic lupus erythematosus inhibitor D68.6
- tendon implant (functional) (graft) Z96.7
- tooth root(s) implant Z96.5
- ureteral stent Z96.0
- urethral stent Z96.0
- urogenital implant (functional) Z96.0
- vascular implant or device Z95.9
- - access port device Z95.8
- - specified type NEC Z95.8
Presenile – *see also condition*
- dementia F03
- premature aging E34.8
Presentation, fetal
- abnormal O32.9
- - before labor, affecting fetus or newborn P01.7
- - causing obstructed labor O64.9
- - - affecting fetus or newborn (any, except breech) P03.1
- - - - breech P03.0
- - - specified NEC O64.8

Presentation, fetal—*continued*
- abnormal—*continued*
- – in multiple gestation (one or more) O32.5
- – specified NEC O32.8
- arm (mother) O32.2
- – causing obstructed labor O64.4
- breech (mother) O32.1
- – with external version before labor, affecting fetus or newborn P01.7
- – before labor, affecting fetus or newborn P01.7
- – causing obstructed labor O64.1
- – – fetus or newborn P03.0
- brow (mother) O32.3
- – causing obstructed labor O64.3
- chin (mother) O32.3
- – causing obstructed labor O64.2
- compound O32.6
- – causing obstructed labor O64.5
- cord O69.0
- extended head (mother) O32.3
- – causing obstructed labor O64.3
- face (mother) O32.3
- – causing obstructed labor O64.2
- – to pubes O32.8
- – – causing obstructed labor O64.0
- hand (mother) O32.2
- – causing obstructed labor O64.4
- leg or foot, NEC (mother) O32.1
- – causing obstructed labor O64.1
- mentum (mother) O32.3
- – causing obstructed labor O64.2
- oblique (mother) O32.2
- – causing obstructed labor O64.4
- occipitoposterior (mother) O32.8
- – causing obstructed labor O64.0
- shoulder (mother) O32.2
- – causing obstructed labor O64.4
- transverse (mother) O32.2
- – causing obstructed labor O64.8
- unstable O32.0

Prespondylolisthesis (congenital) Q76.2

Pressure
- area, skin ulcer L89.-
- – stage
- – – I L89.0
- – – II L89.1
- – – III L89.2
- – – IV L89.3
- birth, fetus or newborn, NEC P15.9
- brachial plexus G54.0
- brain G93.5
- – injury at birth NEC P11.1

Pressure—*continued*
- cone, tentorial G93.5
- hyposystolic (*see also* Hypotension) I95.9
- – incidental reading, without diagnosis of hypotension R03.1
- increased
- – intracranial (benign) G93.2
- – – injury at birth P11.0
- – intraocular H40.0
- lumbosacral plexus G54.1
- mediastinum J98.5
- necrosis (chronic) (skin) L89.2
- – stage
- – – III L89.2
- – – IV L89.3
- sore (chronic) L89.-
- – stage
- – – I L89.0
- – – II L89.1
- – – III L89.2
- – – IV L89.3
- spinal cord G95.2
- ulcer (chronic) L89.-
- – stage
- – – I L89.0
- – – II L89.1
- – – III L89.2
- – – IV L89.3
- venous, increased I87.8

Presyncope R42

Preterm infant, newborn NEC P07.3

Previa
- placenta (with hemorrhage) (*see also* Placenta, previa) O44.1
- – affecting fetus or newborn P02.0
- vasa O69.4
- – affecting fetus or newborn P02.6

Priapism N48.3

Prickling sensation (skin) R20.2

Prickly heat L74.0

Primary – *see condition*

Primigravida
- elderly, affecting management of pregnancy, labor and delivery (supervision only) Z35.5
- very young, affecting management of pregnancy, labor and delivery (supervision only) Z35.6

Primipara
- elderly, affecting management of pregnancy, labor and delivery (supervision only) Z35.5

Primipara—*continued*
- very young, affecting management of
  pregnancy, labor and delivery
  (supervision only) Z35.6
Primus varus (bilateral) Q66.3
Pringle's disease Q85.1
Prinzmetal angina I20.1
Prizefighter ear M95.1
Problem (related to) (with)
- academic Z55.8
- acculturation Z60.3
- adjustment (to)
- - change of job Z56.1
- - life-cycle transition Z60.0
- - pension Z60.0
- - retirement Z60.0
- adopted child Z63.8
- aged
- - in-law Z63.1
- - parent Z63.1
- - person NEC Z63.8
- alcoholism in family Z63.7
- atypical parenting situation Z60.1
- bankruptcy Z59.8
- behavioral (adult) F69
- birth of sibling affecting child Z61.2
- care (of)
- - provider dependency Z74.9
- - - specified NEC Z74.8
- - sick or handicapped person in family or
    household Z63.6
- career choice Z56.7
- child
- - abuse (affecting the child) Z61.6
- - custody or support proceedings Z65.3
- - child-rearing NEC Z62.9
- - specified NEC Z62.8
- communication (developmental) F80.9
- conflict or discord (with)
- - boss Z56.4
- - classmates Z55.4
- - counsellor Z64.4
- - employer Z56.4
- - family Z63.9
- - - specified NEC Z63.8
- - probation officer Z64.4
- - social worker Z64.4
- - teachers Z55.4
- - workmates Z56.4
- conviction in legal proceedings Z65.0
- - with imprisonment Z65.1
- counsellor Z64.4
- creditors Z59.8
- digestive K92.9

Problem—*continued*
- ear H93.9
- economic Z59.9
- - specified NEC Z59.8
- education Z55.9
- - specified NEC Z55.8
- eye H57.9
- failed examinations (school) Z55.2
- family Z63.9
- - specified NEC Z63.8
- feeding R63.3
- - newborn P92.9
- - - breast P92.5
- - - overfeeding P92.4
- - - slow P92.2
- - - specified NEC P92.8
- - - underfeeding P92.3
- - nonorganic F50.8
- fetal, affecting management of pregnancy
  O36.9
- finance Z59.9
- - specified NEC Z59.8
- foreclosure on loan Z59.8
- foster child Z63.8
- frightening experience(s) in childhood
  Z61.7
- genital NEC
- - female N94.9
- - male N50.9
- health care Z75.9
- - specified NEC Z75.8
- hearing H91.9
- homelessness Z59.0
- housing Z59.9
- - inadequate Z59.1
- - isolated Z59.8
- - specified NEC Z59.8
- identity (of childhood) F93.8
- illiteracy Z55.0
- impaired mobility Z74.0
- - due to prolonged bedrest R26.3
- - requiring care provider Z74.0
- imprisonment or incarceration Z65.1
- inadequate teaching, affecting education
  Z55.8
- inappropriate parental pressure Z62.6
- influencing health status NEC Z91.8
- in-law Z63.1
- institutionalization, affecting child Z62.2
- intrafamilial communication Z63.8
- landlord Z59.2
- language (developmental) F80.9
- learning (developmental) F81.9
- legal Z65.3

Problem—*continued*
- life-management Z73.9
- – specified NEC Z73.8
- lifestyle Z72.9
- – alcohol use Z72.1
- – drug use Z72.2
- – gambling Z72.6
- – high-risk sexual behavior Z72.5
- – inappropriate eating habits Z72.4
- – self-damaging behavior NEC Z72.8
- – specified NEC Z72.8
- – tobacco use Z72.0
- literacy Z55.9
- – low level Z55.0
- – specified NEC Z55.8
- living alone Z60.2
- lodgers Z59.2
- loss of love relationship in childhood Z61.0
- marital Z63.0
- – involving
- – – divorce Z63.5
- – – gender identity F66.2
- mastication K08.8
- medical
- – care, within family Z63.6
- – facilities Z75.9
- – – specified NEC Z75.8
- mental F48.9
- multiparity Z64.1
- negative life events in childhood Z61.9
- – altered pattern of family relationships Z61.2
- – frightening experience Z61.7
- – loss of
- – – love relationship Z61.0
- – – self-esteem Z61.3
- – physical abuse (alleged) Z61.6
- – removal from home Z61.1
- – sexual abuse (alleged) (by)
- – – family member Z61.4
- – – person outside family Z61.5
- – specified event NEC Z61.8
- neighbor Z59.2
- neurological NEC R29.8
- new step-parent, affecting child Z61.2
- none (feared complaint unfounded) Z71.1
- occupational NEC Z56.7
- parent Z63.1
- parent-child Z61.9
- personal hygiene Z91.2
- personality F69
- phase-of-life transition, adjustment Z60.0
- physical environment Z58.9

Problem—*continued*
- physical environment—*continued*
- – occupational Z57.9
- – – specified NEC Z57.8
- – specified NEC Z58.8
- presence of sick or handicapped person in family or household Z63.7
- – needing care Z63.6
- primary support group (family) Z63.9
- – specified NEC Z63.8
- probation officer Z64.4
- psychiatric F99
- psychosexual (development) F66.9
- psychosocial Z65.9
- – specified NEC Z65.8
- relationship, childhood F93.8
- release from prison Z65.2
- removal from home, affecting child Z61.1
- seeking and accepting known hazardous and harmful
- – behavioral or psychological interventions Z64.3
- – chemical, nutritional or physical interventions Z64.2
- sexual function (nonorganic) F52.9
- sight H54.9
- smell R43.8
- social
- – environment Z60.9
- – – specified NEC Z60.8
- – exclusion and rejection Z60.4
- – worker Z64.4
- speech NEC R47.8
- – developmental F80.9
- swallowing R13
- taste R43.8
- underachievement in school Z55.3
- unemployment Z56.0
- – threatened Z56.2
- unwanted pregnancy Z64.0
- upbringing Z62.9
- – specified NEC Z62.8
- urinary N39.9
- voice production R47.8
- work schedule (stressful) Z56.3

Procedure (surgical)
- elective (*see also* Surgery, elective) Z41.9
- – ear piercing Z41.3
- – specified NEC Z41.8
- for purpose other than remedying health state Z41.9
- – specified NEC Z41.8
- maternal (unrelated to current delivery), affecting fetus or newborn P00.6

Procedure—*continued*
– maternal—*continued*
– – nonsurgical (medical) P00.7
– not done Z53.9
– – because of
– – – administrative reasons Z53.8
– – – contraindication Z53.0
– – – patient's decision NEC Z53.2
– – – – for reasons of belief or group
    pressure Z53.1
– – – specified reason NEC Z53.8
Procidentia (uteri) (*see also* Prolapse,
  uterus) N81.3
Proctalgia K62.8
– fugax K59.4
– spasmodic K59.4
– – psychogenic F45.4
Proctitis K62.8
– amebic (acute) A06.8
– chlamydial A56.3
– gonococcal A54.6
– herpetic A60.1† K93.8∗
– radiation K62.7
– tuberculous A18.3† K93.0∗
– ulcerative (chronic) K51.2
Proctocele
– female N81.6
– male K62.3
Proctocolitis, mucosal K51.3
Proctoptosis K62.3
Proctorrhagia K62.5
Proctosigmoiditis K63.8
– ulcerative (chronic) K51.3
Proctospasm K59.4
– psychogenic F45.3
Profichet's disease M79.8
Progeria E34.8
Prognathism (mandibular) (maxillary)
  K07.1
Progonoma (melanotic) (M9363/0) – *see*
  Neoplasm, benign
Progressive – *see* condition
Prolactinoma (M8271/0)
– specified site – *see* Neoplasm, benign
– unspecified site D35.2
Prolapse, prolapsed
– anus, anal (canal) (sphincter) K62.2
– arm or hand O32.2
– – causing obstructed labor O64.4
– – in fetus or newborn P03.1
– bladder (mucosa) (sphincter) (acquired)
– – congenital (female) (male) Q64.7
– – female N81.1
– – male N32.8

Prolapse, prolapsed—*continued*
– cecostomy K91.4
– cecum K63.4
– cervix, cervical (stump) (hypertrophied)
  N81.2
– – anterior lip, obstructing labor O65.5
– – congenital Q51.8
– – postpartal, old N81.2
– ciliary body (traumatic) S05.2
– colon (pedunculated) K63.4
– colostomy K91.4
– disk (intervertebral) – *see* Displacement,
  intervertebral disk
– eye implant T85.3
– fallopian tube N83.4
– fetal limb NEC O32.8
– – in fetus or newborn P03.1
– gastric (mucosa) K31.8
– genital, female N81.9
– – specified NEC N81.8
– globe, nontraumatic H44.8
– ileostomy bud K91.4
– intervertebral disk – *see* Displacement,
  intervertebral disk
– intestine (small) K63.4
– iris (traumatic) S05.2
– – nontraumatic H21.8
– kidney N28.8
– – congenital Q63.2
– laryngeal muscles or ventricle J38.7
– leg O32.1
– – causing obstructed labor O64.1
– – in fetus or newborn P03.1
– liver K76.8
– meatus urinarius N36.3
– mitral (valve) I34.1
– organ or site, congenital NEC – *see*
  Malposition, congenital
– ovary N83.4
– pelvic floor, female N81.8
– perineum, female N81.8
– rectum (mucosa) K62.3
– spleen D73.8
– stomach K31.8
– umbilical cord
– – affecting fetus or newborn P02.4
– – complicating delivery O69.0
– urachus, congenital Q64.4
– ureter N28.8
– – with obstruction N13.5
– – – with infection N13.6
– ureterovesical orifice N28.8
– urethra (acquired) (infected) (mucosa)
  N36.3

Prolapse, prolapsed—*continued*
- urethra—*continued*
- – congenital Q64.7
- urinary meatus N36.3
- – congenital Q64.7
- uterovaginal N81.4
- – complete N81.3
- – incomplete N81.2
- uterus (with prolapse of vagina) N81.4
- – complete N81.3
- – congenital Q51.8
- – first degree N81.2
- – in pregnancy or childbirth O34.5
- – incomplete N81.2
- – postpartal (old) N81.4
- – pregnant, affecting fetus or newborn P03.8
- – second degree N81.2
- – third degree N81.3
- uveal (traumatic) S05.2
- vagina (anterior) (wall) N81.1
- – with prolapse of uterus N81.4
- – – complete N81.3
- – – incomplete N81.2
- – posterior wall N81.6
- – posthysterectomy N99.3
- vitreous (humor) H43.0
- – in wound S05.2
- womb – *see* Prolapse, uterus

Prolapsus, female (*see also* Prolapse, uterus) N81.9
- specified NEC N81.8

Proliferation of primary cutaneous CD30-positive T-cells C86.6

Proliferative – *see condition*

Prolongation of bleeding, coagulation or prothrombin time (*see also* Defect, coagulation) D68.9

Prolonged
- labor O63.9
- – affecting fetus or newborn P03.8
- – first stage O63.0
- – second stage O63.1
- QT interval R94.3
- uterine contractions in labor O62.4
- – affecting fetus or newborn P03.6

Prominence of auricle (congenital) (ear) Q17.5

Prominent ischial spine or sacral promontory
- with disproportion (fetopelvic) O33.0
- – affecting fetus or newborn P03.1
- – causing obstructed labor O65.0

Pronation
- ankle M21.6
- foot M21.6
- – congenital Q74.2

Prophylactic
- administration of
- – antibiotics Z29.2
- – immune sera (immunoglobulin) Z29.1
- chemotherapy Z29.2
- immunotherapy Z29.1
- measure Z29.9
- – specified NEC Z29.8
- organ removal (for neoplasia management) Z40.0
- sterilization Z30.2
- surgery Z40.9
- – for risk factors related to malignant neoplasm Z40.0
- – specified NEC Z40.8

Propionic acidemia E71.1

Proptosis (ocular) H05.2

Prosecution, anxiety concerning Z65.3

Prostate, prostatic – *see condition*

Prostatism N40

Prostatitis (congestive) (suppurative) N41.9
- with cystitis N41.3
- acute N41.0
- chronic N41.1
- due to Trichomonas (vaginalis) A59.0† N51.0*
- fibrous N41.1
- gonococcal (acute) (chronic) A54.2† N51.0*
- granulomatous N41.1
- hypertrophic N41.1
- specified type NEC N41.8
- subacute N41.1
- trichomonal A59.0† N51.0*
- tuberculous A18.1† N51.0*

Prostatocystitis N41.3

Prostatorrhea N42.8

Prostration R53
- heat (*see also* Heat, exhaustion) T67.5
- nervous F48.0
- senile R54

Protanomaly (anomalous trichromat) H53.5

Protanopia(complete) (incomplete) H53.5

Protein
- deficiency NEC (*see also* Malnutrition) E46
- malnutrition (*see also* Malnutrition) E46

Protein—*continued*
– sickness (prophylactic) (therapeutic)
T80.6
Proteinemia R77.9
Proteinosis
– alveolar (pulmonary) J84.0
– lipid or lipoid (of Urbach) E78.8
Proteinuria R80
– Bence Jones NEC R80
– complicating pregnancy, childbirth or
puerperium O12.1
– – significant, with gestational
hypertension (*see also* Pre-eclampsia)
O14.9
– – superimposed on pre-existing
hypertensive disorder O11
– gestational O12.1
– – with edema O12.2
– isolated R80
– – with glomerular lesion N06.9
– – – focal and segmental hyalinosis or
sclerosis N06.1
– – – membranous (diffuse) N06.2
– – – mesangial proliferative (diffuse)
N06.3
– – – minimal change N06.0
– – – specified pathology NEC N06.8
– orthostatic N39.2
– – with glomerular lesion – *see*
Proteinuria, isolated, with glomerular
lesion
– persistent N39.1
– – with glomerular lesion – *see*
Proteinuria, isolated, with glomerular
lesion
– postural N39.2
– pre-eclamptic (*see also* Pre-eclampsia)
O14.9
– – affecting fetus or newborn P00.0
**Proteus (mirabilis) (morganii), as cause of
disease classified elsewhere** B96.4
Protoporphyria, erythropoietic E80.0
Protozoal – *see also* condition
– disease B64
– – specified NEC B60.8
Protrusion, protrusio
– acetabulum (into pelvis) M24.7
– device, implant or graft (*see also*
Complications, by site and type,
mechanical) T85.6
– – arterial graft NEC T82.3
– – – coronary (bypass) T82.2
– – breast (implant) T85.4
– – catheter NEC T85.6

Protrusion, protrusio—*continued*
– device, implant or graft—*continued*
– – catheter NEC—*continued*
– – – dialysis (renal) T82.4
– – – – intraperitoneal T85.6
– – – infusion NEC T82.5
– – – – spinal (epidural) (subdural) T85.6
– – – urinary (indwelling) T83.0
– – electronic (electrode) (pulse generator)
(stimulator)
– – – bone T84.3
– – – nervous system (brain) (peripheral
nerve) (spinal) T85.1
– – fixation, internal (orthopedic) NEC
T84.2
– – – bones of limb T84.1
– – gastrointestinal (bile duct) (esophagus)
T85.5
– – genital NEC T83.4
– – – intrauterine contraceptive device
T83.3
– – heart NEC T82.5
– – – valve (prosthesis) T82.0
– – – – graft T82.2
– – joint prosthesis T84.0
– – ocular (corneal graft) (orbital implant)
NEC T85.3
– – – intraocular lens T85.2
– – orthopedic NEC T84.4
– – – bone graft T84.3
– – specified NEC T85.6
– – urinary NEC T83.1
– – – graft T83.2
– – vascular NEC T82.5
– – ventricular intracranial shunt T85.0
– intervertebral disk – *see* Displacement,
intervertebral disk
– nucleus pulposus – *see* Displacement,
intervertebral disk
Prune belly (syndrome) Q79.4
Prurigo L28.2
– Besnier's L20.0
– estivalis L56.4
– Hebra's L28.2
– mitis L28.2
– nodularis L28.1
– psychogenic F45.8
Pruritus, pruritic L29.9
– ani, anus L29.0
– – psychogenic F45.8
– anogenital L29.3
– – psychogenic F45.8
– gravidarum O26.8
– neurogenic (any site) F45.8

Pruritus, pruritic—*continued*
- psychogenic (any site) F45.8
- scroti, scrotum L29.1
- - psychogenic F45.8
- senile L29.8
- specified NEC L29.8
- - psychogenic F45.8
- Trichomonas A59.9
- vulva, vulvae L29.2
- - psychogenic F45.8

Pseudarthrosis, pseudoarthrosis (bone) M84.1
- clavicle, congenital Q74.0
- joint, following fusion or arthrodesis M96.0

Pseudoaneurysm – *see* Aneurysm
Pseudoangina (pectoris) – *see* Angina
Pseudoarthrosis – *see* Pseudarthrosis
Pseudochromhidrosis L67.8
Pseudocirrhosis, liver, pericardial I31.1
Pseudocowpox B08.0
Pseudocoxalgia M91.3
Pseudocroup J38.5
Pseudo-Cushing's syndrome, alcohol-induced E24.4
Pseudocyesis F45.8
Pseudocyst
- lung J98.4
- pancreas K86.3
- retina H33.1
Pseudoexfoliation, capsule (lens) H26.8
Pseudofolliculitis barbae L73.1
Pseudoglioma H44.8
Pseudohemophilia (Bernuth's) (hereditary) (type B) D68.0
- type A D69.8
- vascular D69.8
Pseudohermaphroditism Q56.3
- adrenal E25.8
- female Q56.2
- - with adrenocortical disorder E25.8
- - adrenal, congenital E25.0
- - without adrenocortical disorder Q56.2
- male Q56.1
- - with
- - - adrenocortical disorder E25.8
- - - androgen resistance E34.5
- - - cleft scrotum Q56.1
- - - feminizing testis E34.5
- - - 5-alpha-reductase deficiency E29.1
- - adrenal E25.8
- - without gonadal disorder Q56.1
Pseudo-Hurler's polydystrophy E77.0
Pseudohypoparathyroidism E20.1

Pseudomembranous – *see condition*
Pseudomeningocele (postprocedural) (spinal) G97.8
- post-traumatic G96.1
Pseudomenses (newborn) P54.6
Pseudomenstruation (newborn) P54.6
Pseudomonas
- aeruginosa, as cause of disease classified elsewhere B96.5
- mallei infection – *see* Infection, Burkholderia, mallei
- - as cause of disease classified elsewhere B96.8
- pseudomallei, as cause of disease classified elsewhere B96.8
Pseudomyotonia G71.1
Pseudomyxoma peritonei (M8480/6) C78.6
Pseudoneuritis, optic (disk) (nerve), congenital Q14.2
Pseudopapilledema H47.3
- congenital Q14.2
Pseudoparalysis
- arm or leg R29.8
- atonic, congenital P94.2
Pseudopelade L66.0
Pseudophakia Z96.1
Pseudopolycythemia D75.1
Pseudopolyposis of colon K51.4
Pseudopseudohypoparathyroidism E20.1
Pseudopterygium H11.8
Pseudopuberty, precocious
- female heterosexual E25.8
- male isosexual E25.8
Pseudorickets (renal) N25.0
Pseudorubella B08.2
Pseudosclerema, newborn P83.8
Pseudosclerosis (brain)
- of Westphal E83.0† G99.8*
- spastic, with dementia A81.0† F02.1*
Pseudotetanus (*see also* Convulsions) R56.8
Pseudotetany R29.0
- hysterical F44.5
Pseudotrichinosis M33.1
Pseudotruncus arteriosus Q25.4
Pseudotuberculosis (extra-intestinal) A28.2
- enterocolitis A04.8
Pseudotumor
- cerebri G93.2
- orbital H05.1
Pseudoxanthoma elasticum Q82.8
Psilosis K90.1

Psittacosis A70
– with pneumonia A70† J17.8∗
Psoitis M60.8
Psoriasis L40.9
– arthropathic L40.5† M07.3∗
– flexural L40.8
– guttate L40.4
– nummular L40.0
– plaque L40.0
– pustular (generalized) L40.1
– – palmaris et plantaris L40.3
– specified NEC L40.8
– vulgaris L40.0
Psychalgia F45.4
Psychasthenia F48.8
Psychiatric disorder or problem NEC F99
Psychoanalysis (therapy) Z50.4
Psychogenic – *see also* condition
– factors associated with physical conditions F54
Psychological and behavioral factors affecting medical condition F59
Psychoneurosis, psychoneurotic (*see also* Neurosis) F48.9
– anxiety (state) F41.1
– hysteria F44.9
– personality NEC F60.8
Psychopathy, psychopathic
– affectionless F94.2
– autistic F84.5
– personality (*see also* Disorder, personality) F60.9
– sexual (*see also* Deviation, sexual) F65.9
– state F60.2
Psychosexual identity disorder of childhood F64.2
Psychosis, psychotic F29
– acute (transient) F23.9
– – hysterical F44.9
– – specified NEC F23.8
– affecting management of pregnancy, childbirth or puerperium O99.3
– affective (*see also* Disorder, affective) F39
– – senile NEC F03
– – specified type NEC F38.8
– alcoholic F10.5
– – with
– – – delirium tremens F10.4
– – – dementia F10.7
– – – hallucinosis F10.5
– – – jealousy F10.5
– – – paranoia F10.5
– – amnestic confabulatory F10.6

Psychosis, psychotic—*continued*
– alcoholic—*continued*
– – Korsakov's F10.6
– – late-onset F10.7
– – paranoid type F10.5
– – polyneuritic F10.6
– – specified NEC F10.5
– arteriosclerotic F01.9
– childhood F84.0
– – atypical F84.1
– climacteric (*see also* Psychosis, involutional) F28
– confusional F29
– – acute or subacute F05.9
– – reactive F23.0
– cycloid (without symptoms of schizophrenia) F23.0
– – with symptoms of schizophrenia F23.1
– depressive (single episode) F32.3
– – psychogenic F32.3
– – – recurrent F33.3
– – reactive (from emotional stress, psychological trauma) F32.3
– – – recurrent F33.3
– disintegrative (childhood) F84.3
– drug-induced – *code to* F11-F19 with fourth character .5
– – late onset – *code to* F11-F19 with fourth character .7
– – paranoid and hallucinatory states – *code to* F11-F19 with fourth character .5
– due to or associated with
– – addiction, drug – *see* Psychosis, drug-induced
– – dependence
– – – alcohol (*see also* Psychosis, alcoholic) F10.5
– – – drug – *code to* F11-F19 with fourth character .5
– – epilepsy F06.8
– – Huntington's chorea F06.8
– – ischemia, cerebrovascular (generalized) F06.8
– – multiple sclerosis F06.8
– – physical disease F06.8
– – presenile dementia F03
– – senile dementia F03
– – vascular disease (arteriosclerotic) (cerebral) F01.9
– epileptic F06.8
– episode F23.9
– – due to or associated with physical condition F06.8

541

Psychosis, psychotic—*continued*
- exhaustive F43.0
- hallucinatory, chronic F28
- hypomanic F30.0
- hysterical (acute) F44.9
- induced F24
- infantile F84.0
- - atypical F84.1
- infective F05.9
- - acute F05.9
- - subacute (*see also* Delirium) F05.8
- involutional F28
- - paranoid (state) F22.8
- Korsakov's (alcoholic) F10.6
- - induced by other psychoactive
  substance – *code to* F11-F19 with
  fourth character .6
- late-onset (after alcohol or drug use) –
  code to F10-F19 with fourth character .7
- mania, manic (single episode) F30.2
- - recurrent type F31.8
- manic-depressive (*see also* Disorder,
  bipolar, affective) F31.9
- - depressed type (without psychotic
  symptoms) F33.2
- - - with psychotic symptoms F33.3
- menopausal (*see also* Psychosis,
  involutional) F28
- mixed schizophrenic and affective F25.2
- nonorganic F29
- - specified NEC F28
- organic F09
- - due to or associated with
- - - childbirth – *see* Psychosis, puerperal
- - - Creutzfeldt-Jakob disease or
    syndrome A81.0† F02.1*
- - - disease
- - - - cerebrovascular F01.9
- - - - Creutzfeldt-Jakob A81.0† F02.1*
- - - - endocrine or metabolic F06.8
- - - - - acute or subacute F05.8
- - - - liver, alcoholic (*see also*
    Psychosis, alcoholic) F10.5
- - - epilepsy, transient (acute) F05.8
- - - infection
- - - - brain (intracranial) F06.8
- - - - - acute or subacute F05.8
- - - intoxication
- - - - alcoholic (acute) F10.5
- - - - drug – *see* Psychosis, drug-
    induced
- - - puerperium – *see* Psychosis,
    puerperal

Psychosis, psychotic—*continued*
- organic—*continued*
- - due to or associated with—*continued*
- - - trauma, brain (birth) (from electric
    current) (surgical) F06.8
- - - - acute or subacute F05.8
- - infective F06.8
- - - acute or subacute F05.9
- - post-traumatic F06.8
- - - acute or subacute F05.9
- paranoiac F22.0
- paranoid F22.0
- - alcoholic F10.5
- - climacteric F22.8
- - involutional F22.8
- - menopausal F22.8
- - psychogenic (acute) F23.3
- - schizophrenic F20.0
- - senile F03
- polyneuritic, alcoholic F10.6
- postpartum F53.1
- presbyophrenic (type) F03
- presenile F03
- psychogenic F23.9
- - depressive F32.3
- - paranoid (acute) F23.3
- puerperal F53.1
- - specified type – *see* Psychosis, by type
- reactive (brief) (transient) (emotional
  stress) (psychological trauma) F23.9
- - brief with schizophrenia-like features
  F23.2
- - confusion F23.0
- - depressive F32.3
- - - recurrent F33.3
- - excitative type F30.8
- residual (after alcohol or drug use) – *code
  to* F10-F19 with fourth character .7
- schizoaffective F25.9
- - depressive type F25.1
- - manic type F25.0
- schizophrenia, schizophrenic (*see also*
  Schizophrenia) F20.9
- schizophrenia-like, in epilepsy F06.2
- schizophreniform F20.8
- - affective type F25.9
- - brief F23.2
- - confusional type F23.1
- - depressive type F25.1
- - manic type F25.0
- - mixed type F25.2
- senile NEC F03
- - depressed or paranoid type F03
- - simple deterioration F03

Psychosis, psychotic—*continued*
- senile NEC—*continued*
- – specified type – *see* Psychosis, by type
- situational (reactive) F23.9
- symbiotic (childhood) F84.3
- symptomatic F09
Psychosomatic – *see* Disorder,
  psychosomatic
Psychosyndrome, organic F07.9
Psychotherapy Z50.4
**Psychotic episode due to or associated
  with physical condition** F06.9
Pterygium (eye) H11.0
- colli Q18.3
Ptilosis (eyelid) H02.7
Ptomaine (poisoning) T62.9
Ptosis H02.4
- adiposa (false) H02.4
- cecum K63.4
- colon K63.4
- congenital (eyelid) Q10.0
- – specified site NEC – *see* Anomaly, by
  site
- eyelid (paralytic) H02.4
- – congenital Q10.0
- gastric K31.8
- intestine K63.4
- kidney N28.8
- liver K76.8
- renal N28.8
- splanchnic K63.4
- spleen D73.8
- stomach K31.8
- viscera K63.4
Ptyalism (periodic) K11.7
- hysterical F45.3
- pregnancy O26.8
- psychogenic F45.3
Pubertas praecox E30.1
Puberty (development state) Z00.3
- bleeding (excessive) N92.2
- delayed E30.0
- precocious E30.1
- – central E22.8
- premature E30.1
- – due to
- – – adrenal cortical hyperfunction E25.8
- – – pineal tumor E34.8
- – – pituitary (anterior) hyperfunction
  E22.8
Puckering, macula H35.3
Pudenda, pudendum – *see condition*

Puerperal, puerperium
- abscess
- – areola O91.0
- – Bartholin's gland O86.1
- – breast O91.1
- – cervix (uteri) O86.1
- – genital organ O86.1
- – kidney O86.2
- – mammary O91.1
- – nipple O91.0
- – peritoneum O85
- – subareolar O91.1
- – urinary tract NEC O86.2
- – uterus O86.1
- – vagina (wall) O86.1
- – vaginorectal O86.1
- – vulvovaginal gland O86.1
- adnexitis O86.1
- afibrinogenemia, or other coagulation
  defect O72.3
- albuminuria (acute) (subacute) O12.1
- – with edema O12.2
- anemia O99.0
- anesthetic death O89.8
- apoplexy O99.4
- blood dyscrasia O72.3
- cardiomyopathy O90.3
- cerebrovascular disorder (conditions in
  I60-I69) O99.4
- cervicitis O86.1
- coagulopathy (any) O72.3
- complications O90.9
- – specified NEC O90.8
- cystitis O86.2
- cystopyelitis O86.2
- death (sudden) (cause unknown) O95
- delirium NEC F05.8
- disease O90.9
- – breast NEC O92.2
- – cerebrovascular (acute) O99.4
- – nonobstetric NEC (*see also* Pregnancy,
  complicated by, conditions in) O99.8
- – renal NEC O90.8
- – tubo-ovarian O86.1
- – Valsuani's O99.0
- disorder O90.9
- – lactation O92.7
- – nonobstetric NEC (*see also* Pregnancy,
  complicated by, conditions in) O99.8
- disruption
- – cesarean wound O90.0
- – episiotomy wound O90.1
- – perineal laceration wound O90.1

Puerperal, puerperium—*continued*
- eclampsia (with pre-existing hypertension) O15.2
- embolism (pulmonary) (blood clot) O88.2
- – air O88.0
  amniotic fluid O88.1
- – fat O88.8
- – pyemic O88.3
- – septic O88.3
- endophlebitis – *see* Puerperal, phlebitis
- endotrachelitis O86.1
- failure
- – lactation (complete) O92.3
- – – partial O92.4
- – renal, acute O90.4
- fever (sepsis) O85
- – pyrexia (of unknown origin) O86.4
- fissure, nipple O92.1
- fistula
- – breast (due to mastitis) O91.1
- – nipple O91.0
- galactophoritis O91.2
- galactorrhea O92.6
- glomerular diseases (conditions in N00-N07) O90.8
- – with hypertension, pre-existing O10.2
- hematoma, subdural O99.4
- hemiplegia, cerebral O99.3
- – due to cerebral vascular disorder O99.4
- hemorrhage (*see also* Hemorrhage, postpartum) O72.1
- – brain O99.4
- – bulbar O99.4
- – cerebellar O99.4
- – cerebral O99.4
- – cortical O99.4
- – delayed (uterine) O72.2
- – extradural O99.4
- – internal capsule O99.4
- – intracranial O99.4
- – intrapontine O99.4
- – meningeal O99.4
- – pontine O99.4
- – subarachnoid O99.4
- – subcortical O99.4
- – subdural O99.4
- – uterine, delayed O72.2
- – ventricular O99.4
- hemorrhoids O87.2
- hepatorenal syndrome O90.4
- hypertrophy, breast O92.2
- induration breast (fibrous) O92.2
- infection O86.4
- – cervix O86.1

Puerperal, puerperium—*continued*
- infection—*continued*
- – generalized O85
- – genital tract NEC O86.1
- – – minor or localized NEC O86.1
- – – obstetric surgical wound O86.0
- – kidney (Bacillus coli) O86.2
- – nipple O91.0
- – peritoneum O85
- – renal O86.2
- – specified NEC O86.8
- – urinary (tract) NEC O86.2
- – – asymptomatic O86.2
- – vagina O86.1
- – vein – *see* Puerperal, phlebitis
- ischemia, cerebral O99.4
- lymphangitis O86.8
- – breast O91.2
- mammillitis O91.0
- mammitis O91.2
- mania F30.8
- mastitis O91.2
- – purulent O91.1
- metroperitonitis O85
- metrorrhagia (*see also* Hemorrhage, postpartum) O72.1
- – delayed (secondary) O72.2
- metrosalpingitis O85
- metrovaginitis O85
- milk leg O87.1
- necrosis, liver (acute) (subacute) (conditions in category K72.0) O90.8
- – with renal failure O90.4
- paralysis, bladder (sphincter) O90.8
- parametritis O85
- paravaginitis O86.1
- pelviperitonitis O85
- perimetritis O86.1
- perimetrosalpingitis O85
- perinephritis O86.2
- periphlebitis – *see* Puerperal, phlebitis
- peritoneal infection O85
- peritonitis (pelvic) O85
- perivaginitis O86.1
- phlebitis O87.9
- – deep O87.1
- – pelvic O87.1
- – superficial O87.0
- phlebothrombosis, deep O87.1
- phlegmasia alba dolens O87.1
- placental polyp O90.8
- pneumonia, embolic – *see* Puerperal, embolism

Puerperal, puerperium—*continued*
- pre-eclampsia (*see also* Pre-eclampsia) O14.9
- – with pre-existing hypertension O11
- – severe O14.1
- psychosis F53.1
- pyelitis O86.2
- pyelocystitis O86.2
- pyelonephritis O86.2
- pyelonephrosis O86.2
- pyemia O85
- pyocystitis O86.2
- pyohemia O85
- pyometra O85
- pyonephritis O86.2
- pyosalpingitis O85
- pyrexia (of unknown origin) O86.4
- renal
- – disease NEC O90.8
- – failure O90.4
- retention
- – decidua – *see* Retention, decidua
- – placenta – *see* Retention, placenta
- – secundines – *see* Retention, secundines
- salpingo-ovaritis O86.1
- salpingoperitonitis O85
- secondary perineal tear O90.1
- sepsis (pelvic) O85
- septicemia O85
- stroke O99.4
- subinvolution (uterus) O90.8
- suppuration – *see* Puerperal, abscess
- tetanus A34
- thelitis O91.0
- thrombocytopenia O72.3
- thrombophlebitis (superficial) O87.0
- – deep O87.1
- – pelvic O87.1
- thrombosis (venous) – *see* Thrombosis, puerperal
- thyroiditis O90.5
- uremia (due to renal failure) O90.4
- vaginitis O86.1
- varicose veins (legs) O87.8
- – vulva or perineum O87.8
- vulvitis O86.1
- vulvovaginitis O86.1
- white leg O87.1
Pulmolithiasis J98.4
Pulmonary – *see condition*
Pulpitis (acute) (chronic) (hyperplastic) (irreversible) (reversible) (suppurative) (ulcerative) K04.0
Pulpless tooth K04.9

Pulse
- alternating R00.8
- bigeminal R00.8
- feeble, rapid, due to shock following injury T79.4
- weak R09.8
Pulsus alternans or trigeminus R00.8
Punch drunk F07.2
Punctum lacrimale occlusion H04.5
Puncture (*see also* Wound, open) T14.1
- accidental, complicating surgery T81.2
- by
- – device, implant or graft – *see* Complications, by site and type, mechanical
- – foreign body left accidentally in operation wound T81.5
- – instrument (any) during a procedure, accidental T81.2
- internal organs – *see* Injury, by site
- multiple T01.9
- traumatic, heart S26.8
- – with hemopericardium S26.0
PUO (pyrexia of unknown origin) R50.9
Pupillary membrane (persistent) Q13.8
Pupillotonia H57.0
Purpura D69.2
- abdominal D69.0
- allergic D69.0
- anaphylactoid D69.0
- annularis telangiectodes L81.7
- arthritic D69.0
- bacterial D69.0
- capillary fragility, idiopathic D69.8
- cryoglobulinemic D89.1
- fibrinolytic (*see also* Fibrinolysis) D65
- fulminans, fulminous D65
- gangrenous D65
- hemorrhagic, hemorrhagica D69.3
- – not due to thrombocytopenia D69.0
- Henoch(-Schönlein) D69.0
- hypergammaglobulinemic (benign) (Waldenström's) D89.0
- idiopathic (thrombocytopenic) D69.3
- – nonthrombocytopenic D69.0
- infectious D69.0
- malignant D69.0
- nervosa D69.0
- nonthrombocytopenic D69.2
- – hemorrhagic D69.0
- – idiopathic D69.0
- nonthrombopenic D69.2
- rheumatica D69.0
- Schönlein(-Henoch) D69.0

Purpura—*continued*
- scorbutic E54† D77*
- senile D69.2
- simplex D69.2
- symptomatica D69.0
- thrombocytopenic (congenital) (hereditary) (*see also* Thrombocytopenia) D69.4
- idiopathic D69.3
- − neonatal, transitory P61.0
- − thrombotic M31.1
- thrombolytic (*see also* Fibrinolysis) D65
- thrombopenic (congenital) (hereditary) (*see also* Thrombocytopenia) D69.4
- thrombotic, thrombocytopenic M31.1
- toxic D69.0
- vascular D69.0
- visceral symptoms D69.0

Purulent – *see condition*
Pus (in)
- stool R19.5
- urine N39.0

Pustular rash L08.0
Pustule (nonmalignant) L08.9
- malignant A22.0

Pustulosis palmaris et plantaris L40.3
Putnam(-Dana) disease or syndrome – *see* Degeneration, combined
Putrescent pulp (dental) K04.1
Pyarthritis, pyarthrosis M00.9
- tuberculous – *see* Tuberculosis, joint
Pyelectasis N13.3
Pyelitis (congenital) (uremic) (*see also* Pyelonephritis) N12
- with
- − calculus N20.9
- − − with hydronephrosis N13.2
- − − contracted kidney N11.9
- acute N10
- − with calculus (impacted)(recurrent) N20.9
- chronic N11.9
- − with calculus N20.9
- − − with hydronephrosis N13.2
- complicating pregnancy O23.0
- − − affecting fetus or newborn P00.1
- cystica N28.8
- puerperal (postpartum) O86.2
- tuberculous A18.1† N29.1*
Pyelocystitis (*see also* Pyelonephritis) N12
- with calculus (impacted)(recurrent) N20.9

Pyelonephritis (*see also* Nephritis, tubulo-interstitial) N12
- with
- − calculus N20.9
    with hydronephrosis N13.2
- − contracted kidney N11.9
- acute N10 ·
- calculous NEC N20.9
- − with hydronephrosis N13.2
- chronic N11.9
- − with calculus N20.9
- − − with hydronephrosis N13.2
- − nonobstructive N11.8
- − − with reflux (vesicoureteral) N11.0
- − obstructive N11.1
- − specified NEC N11.8
- complicating pregnancy O23.0
- − affecting fetus or newborn P00.1
- in (due to)
- − brucellosis A23.-† N16.0*
- − cryoglobulinemia (mixed) D89.1† N16.2*
- − cystinosis E72.0† N16.3*
- − diphtheria A36.8† N16.0*
- − glycogen storage disease E74.0† N16.3*
- − leukemia NEC C95.9† N16.1*
- − lymphoma NEC C85.9† N16.1*
- − multiple myeloma C90.0† N16.1*
- − obstruction N11.1
- − salmonella infection A02.2† N16.0*
- − sarcoidosis D86.8† N16.2*
- − sepsis NEC A41.-† N16.0*
- − Sjögren's disease M35.0† N16.4*
- − toxoplasmosis B58.8† N16.0*
- − transplant rejection T86.-† N16.5*
- − Wilson's disease E83.0† N16.3*
- nonobstructive N12
- − with reflux (vesicoureteral) N11.0
- − chronic N11.8
- syphilitic A52.7† N16.0*
Pyelonephrosis (obstructive) N11.1
- chronic N11.9
Pyelophlebitis I80.8
Pyeloureteritis cystica N28.8
Pyemia, pyemic (purulent) (*see also* Sepsis) A41.9
- joint M00.9
- postvaccinal T88.0
- tuberculous – *see* Tuberculosis, miliary
Pygopagus Q89.4
Pyknoepilepsy, pyknolepsy (idiopathic) G40.3
Pylephlebitis K75.1

Pyle's syndrome Q78.5
Pylethrombophlebitis K75.1
Pyloritis K29.9
Pylorospasm (reflex) NEC K31.3
– congenital or infantile Q40.0
– neurotic F45.3
– psychogenic F45.3
Pylorus, pyloric – *see condition*
Pyoarthrosis M00.9
Pyocele
– mastoid H70.0
– sinus (accessory) (*see also* Sinusitis) J32.9
– turbinate (bone) (*see also* Sinusitis) J32.9
– urethra N34.0
Pyocolpos (*see also* Vaginitis) N76.0
Pyocystitis (*see also* Cystitis) N30.8
Pyoderma, pyodermia NEC L08.0
– gangrenosum L88
– newborn P39.4
– phagedenic L88
– vegetans L08.8
Pyodermatitis L08.0
– vegetans L08.8
Pyogenic – *see condition*
Pyohydronephrosis N13.6
Pyometra, pyometrium, pyometritis (*see also* Endometritis) N71.9
Pyomyositis (tropical) M60.0
Pyonephritis N12
Pyonephrosis N13.6
– tuberculous A18.1† N29.1∗
Pyo-oophoritis (*see also* Salpingo-oophoritis) N70.9

Pyo-ovarium (*see also* Salpingo-oophoritis) N70.9
Pyopericarditis, pyopericardium I30.1
Pyophlebitis – *see* Phlebitis
Pyopneumopericardium I30.1
Pyopneumothorax (infective) J86.9
– with fistula J86.0
– tuberculous NEC A16.5
Pyorrhea K05.3
Pyosalpinx, pyosalpingitis (*see also* Salpingo-oophoritis) N70.9
– acute N70.0
– chronic N70.1
Pyosepticemia – *see* Sepsis
Pyosis of Corlett or Manson L00
Pyothorax J86.9
– with fistula J86.0
– tuberculous NEC A16.5
– – with bacteriological and histological confirmation A15.6
Pyoureter N28.8
– tuberculous A18.1† N29.1∗
Pyrexia (of unknown origin) R50.9
– atmospheric T67.0
– during labor NEC O75.2
– heat T67.0
– newborn, environmentally-induced P81.0
– persistent R50.8
– puerperal O86.4
Pyroglobulinemia NEC E88.0
Pyromania F63.1
Pyrosis R12
Pyuria (bacterial) N39.0

Q

Q fever A78
– with pneumonia A78† J17.8*
Quadricuspid aortic valve Q23.8
Quadriplegia G82.5
– congenital (cerebral) G80.8
– – spastic G80.0
– embolic (current episode) I63.4
– flaccid G82.3
– – congenital (cerebral) G80.8
– – – spastic G80.0
– newborn NEC P11.9
– spastic G82.4
– – congenital (cerebral) G80.0
– spinal G82.4
– thrombotic (current episode) I63.3
– traumatic T91.3
– – current episode S14.1

Quadruplet, affecting fetus or newborn
P01.5
– pregnancy O30.2
Quarrelsomeness F60.3
Queensland fever A77.3
Quervain's disease M65.4
Queyrat's erythroplasia (M8080/2)
– penis D07.4
– specified site – *see* Neoplasm, skin, in situ
– unspecified site D07.4
Quincke's disease or edema T78.3
– hereditary D84.1
Quinsy (gangrenous) J36
Quintan fever A79.0
Quintuplet, affecting fetus or newborn
P01.5
– pregnancy O30.8

R

Rabies A82.9
– inoculation reaction – *see* Complications, vaccination
– sylvatic A82.0
– urban A82.1
Rachischisis (*see also* Spina bifida) Q05.9
– with hydrocephalus (*see also* Spina bifida, with hydrocephalus) Q05.4
Rachitic – *see also* condition
– deformities of spine (late effect) E64.3
– pelvis (late effect) E64.3
– – with disproportion (fetopelvic) O33.0
– – – affecting fetus or newborn P03.1
– – – causing obstructed labor O65.0
Rachitis, rachitism (*see also* Rickets) E55.0
– sequelae E64.3
Radial nerve – *see* condition
Radiation
– effects or sickness NEC T66
– exposure NEC Z58.4
– – occupational Z57.1
Radiculitis (pressure) (vertebrogenic) M54.1
– brachial NEC M54.1
– cervical NEC M54.1
– due to displacement of intervertebral disk – *see* Neuritis, due to displacement, intervertebral disk
– lumbar, lumbosacral NEC M54.1
– syphilitic A52.1† G99.8*
– thoracic (with visceral pain) NEC M54.1
Radiculomyelitis (*see also* Encephalitis) G04.9
– toxic due to Corynebacterium diphtheriae A36.8† G05.0*
Radiculopathy (*see also* Radiculitis) M54.1
Radioactive substances, adverse effects NEC T66
Radiodermal burns (acute, chronic, or occupational) – *see* Burn
Radiodermatitis L58.9
– acute L58.0
– chronic L58.1
Radiology, maternal, affecting fetus or newborn P00.7
Radionecrosis NEC T66
Radiotherapy session Z51.0

Radium, adverse effect NEC T66
Rage, meaning rabies – *see* Rabies
Raillietiniasis B71.8
Railroad neurosis F48.8
Railway spine F48.8
Raised – *see also* Elevated
– antibody titre R76.0
Rales R09.8
Ramifying renal pelvis Q63.8
Ramsay-Hunt disease or syndrome (*see also* Hunt's disease) B02.2† G53.0*
– meaning dyssynergia cerebellaris myoclonica G11.1
Ranula K11.6
– congenital Q38.4
Rape T74.2
Rapid
– feeble pulse, due to shock, following injury T79.4
– heart(beat) R00.0
– – psychogenic F45.3
– second stage (delivery) O62.3
– – affecting fetus or newborn P03.5
Rarefaction, bone M85.8
Rash R21
– canker A38
– diaper L22
– drug (internal use) L27.0
– – contact (*see also* Dermatitis, due to, drugs, external) L25.1
– following immunization T88.1
– food (*see also* Dermatitis, due to, food) L27.2
– heat L74.0
– napkin (psoriasiform) L22
– nettle (*see also* Urticaria) L50.9
– pustular L08.0
– scarlet A38
– serum (prophylactic) (therapeutic) T80.6
– wandering, tongue K14.1
Rasmussen's aneurysm (*see also* Tuberculosis, pulmonary) A16.2
Rathke's pouch tumor (M9350/1) D44.3
Raynaud's disease, gangrene, phenomenon or syndrome I73.0
R.D.S. (newborn) (*see also* Syndrome, respiratory distress) P22.0

Reaction – *see also* Disorder
- adaption (*see also* Reaction, adjustment) F43.2
- adjustment (anxiety) (conduct disorder) (depressiveness) (distress) (emotional disturbance) F43.2
- – with mutism, elective (adolescent) (child) F94.0
- affective (*see also* Disorder, affective) F39
- allergic (*see also* Allergy) T78.4
- – drug, medicament or biological – *see* Allergy, drug
- – food (any) (ingested) NEC T78.1
- – – dermatitis L27.2
- – serum T80.6
- anaphylactic – *see* Shock, anaphylactic
- anesthesia – *see* Anesthesia, complication
- antitoxin (prophylactic) (therapeutic) – *see* Complications, vaccination
- anxiety F41.1
- Arthus – *see* Arthus' phenomenon
- asthenic F48.0
- compulsive F42.1
- conversion F44.9
- crisis, acute F43.0
- depressive (single episode) F32.9
- – psychotic F32.3
- – recurrent   *see* Disorder, depressive, recurrent
- dissociative F44.9
- drug NEC T88.7
- – addictive – *code to* F11-F19 with fourth character .9
- – – transmitted via placenta or breast milk – *see* Absorption, drug, addictive, through placenta
- – allergic – *see* Allergy, drug
- – correct substance properly administered T88.7
- – lichenoid L43.2
- – newborn P93
- – overdose or poisoning T50.9
- – – specified drug – *see* Table of drugs and chemicals
- – photoallergic L56.1
- – phototoxic L56.0
- – withdrawal – *code to* F11-F19 with fourth character .3
- – – infant of dependent mother P96.1
- – – newborn P96.1
- – wrong substance given or taken in error T50.9

Reaction—*continued*
- drug NEC—*continued*
- – wrong substance given or taken in error—*continued*
- – – specified drug – *see* Table of drugs and chemicals
- fear F40.9
- – child (abnormal) F93.1
- fluid loss, cerebrospinal G97.1
- foreign
- – body NEC M60.2
- – substance accidentally left during a procedure (chemical) (powder) (talc) T81.6
- grief F43.2
- Herxheimer's T78.2
- hyperkinetic – *see* Hyperkinesia
- hypochondriacal F45.2
- hypoglycemic, due to insulin E16.0
- – with coma (diabetic) – *code to* E10-E14 with fourth character .0
- – – nondiabetic E15
- – therapeutic misadventure T38.3
- hypomanic F30.0
- hysterical F44.9
- immunization – *see* Complications, vaccination
- incompatibility
- – blood group (ABO) (infusion) (transfusion) T80.3
- – Rh (factor) (infusion) (transfusion) T80.4
- inflammatory – *see* Infection
- infusion – *see* Complications, infusion
- inoculation (immune serum) – *see* Complications, vaccination
- insulin T78.4
- leukemoid (lymphocytic) (monocytic) (myelocytic) D72.8
- LSD (acute) F16.0
- lumbar puncture G97.1
- manic-depressive – *see* Disorder, bipolar, affective
- neurasthenic F48.0
- neurogenic (*see also* Neurosis) F48.9
- neurotic F48.9
- nitritoid – *see* Crisis, nitritoid
- obsessive-compulsive F42.9
- organic, acute or subacute (*see also* Delirium) F05.9
- paranoid (acute) F23.3
- – chronic F22.0
- – senile F03
- phobic F40.9

Reaction—*continued*
- postradiation NEC T66
- post-traumatic stress, uncomplicated
  Z73.3
- psychogenic F99
- psychoneurotic (*see also* Neurosis) F48.9
- – compulsive F42.1
- – obsessive F42.0
- psychophysiological (*see also* Disorder,
  somatoform) F45.9
- psychotic F23.9
- – due to or associated with physical
  condition F06.8
- radiation NEC T66
- scarlet fever toxin – *see* Complications,
  vaccination
- schizophrenic F23.2
- – acute (brief) (undifferentiated) F23.2
- – latent F21
- – undifferentiated (acute) (brief) F23.2
- serological for syphilis – *see* Serology for
  syphilis
- serum (prophylactic) (therapeutic) T80.6
- – immediate T80.5
- situational (*see also* Reaction, adjustment)
  F43.2
- – acute F43.0
- – maladjustment F43.2
- somatization (*see also* Disorder,
  somatoform) F45.9
- spinal puncture G97.1
- stress (severe) F43.9
- – acute (agitation) ("daze")
  (disorientation) (disturbance of
  consciousness) (flight reaction) (fugue)
  F43.0
- – specified NEC F43.8
- surgical procedure – *see* Complications,
  surgical procedure
- tetanus antitoxin – *see* Complications,
  vaccination
- toxic, to local anesthesia T81.8
- – in labor and delivery O74.4
- – in pregnancy O29.3
- – postpartum, puerperal O89.3
- toxin-antitoxin – *see* Complications,
  vaccination
- transfusion (allergic) (blood) (bone
  marrow) (lymphocytes) – *see*
  Complications, transfusion)
- tuberculin skin test, abnormal R76.1
- ultraviolet NEC T66
- vaccination (any) – *see* Complications,
  vaccination

Reaction—*continued*
- withdrawing, child or adolescent F93.2
- X-ray NEC T66
Reactive depression – *see* Reaction,
  depressive
Rearrangement, chromosomal
- balanced (in) Q95.9
- – abnormal individual (autosomal) Q95.2
- – – non-sex (autosomal) chromosomes
  Q95.2
- – – sex/non-sex chromosomes Q95.3
- – specified NEC Q95.8
Recanalization, thrombus – *see*
  Thrombosis
Recession
- chamber angle (eye) H21.5
- gingival (generalized) (localized)
  (postinfective) (postoperative) K06.0
Recklinghausen's disease (M9540/1)
  Q85.0
- bones E21.0
Reclus' disease (cystic) N60.1
Recruitment, auditory H93.2
Rectalgia K62.8
Rectitis K62.8
Rectocele
- female N81.6
- in pregnancy or childbirth O34.8
- – causing obstructed labor O65.5
- – – affecting fetus or newborn P03.1
- male K62.3
Rectosigmoid junction – *see condition*
Rectosigmoiditis K63.8
- ulcerative (chronic) K51.3
Rectourethral – *see condition*
Rectovaginal – *see condition*
Rectovesical – *see condition*
Rectum, rectal – *see condition*
Recurrent – *see condition*
Red-cedar lung or pneumonitis J67.8
Reduced ventilatory or vital capacity
  R94.2
Redundant, redundancy
- anus (congenital) Q43.8
- clitoris N90.8
- colon (congenital) Q43.8
- foreskin (congenital) N47
- intestine (congenital) Q43.8
- labia N90.6
- organ or site, congenital NEC – *see*
  Accessory
- panniculus (abdominal) E65
- prepuce (congenital) N47
- pylorus K31.8

Redundant, redundancy—*continued*
- rectum (congenital) Q43.8
- scrotum N50.8
- sigmoid (congenital) Q43.8
- skin (of face) L57.4
- – eyelids H02.3
- stomach K31.8
Reduplication – *see* Duplex, duplication
Reflex – *see also condition*
- hyperactive gag J39.2
- pupillary, abnormal H57.0
- vasovagal R55
Reflux
- esophageal K21.9
- – with esophagitis K21.0
- – neonatal P78.8
- gastroesophageal K21.9
- – with esophagitis K21.0
- – in newborn P78.8
- mitral – *see* Insufficiency, mitral
- ureteral N13.7
- – with pyelonephritis (chronic) N11.0
- – – with calculus (impacted) (recurrent)
  N20.9
- vesicoureteral NEC (with scarring) N13.7
- – with pyelonephritis (chronic) N11.0
- – congenital Q62.7
Reforming, artificial openings – *see*
  Attention to, artificial, opening
Refractive error H52.7
Refsum's disease or syndrome G60.1
Refusal of
- food, psychogenic F50.8
- immunization or vaccination because of
- – patient's decision NEC Z28.2
- – reasons of belief or group pressure
  Z28.1
- treatment (because of) Z53.2
- – patient's decision NEC Z53.2
- – reasons of belief or group pressure
  Z53.1
Regulation
- feeding (elderly) (infant) R63.3
- menstrual Z30.3
Regurgitation
- aortic (valve) (*see also* Insufficiency,
  aortic) I35.1
- – syphilitic A52.0† I39.1∗
- food (*see also* Vomiting) R11
- – with reswallowing – *see* Rumination
- – newborn P92.1
- gastric contents (*see also* Vomiting) R11
- heart – *see* Endocarditis
- mitral (valve) – *see* Insufficiency, mitral

Regurgitation—*continued*
- mitral—*continued*
- – congenital Q23.3
- myocardial – *see* Endocarditis
- pulmonary (heart) (valve) I37.1
- – congenital Q22.2
- – syphilitic A52.0† I39.3∗
- tricuspid (*see also* Insufficiency,
  tricuspid) I07.1
- – nonrheumatic (*see also* Insufficiency,
  tricuspid, nonrheumatic) I36.1
- valve, valvular – *see* Endocarditis
- vesicoureteral N13.7
- – with pyelonephritis (chronic) N11.0
Rehabilitation Z50.9
- alcohol Z50.2
- cardiac Z50.0
- drug Z50.3
- occupational (therapy) Z50.7
- personal history of Z92.5
- specified NEC Z50.8
- substance abuse NEC Z50.8
- – alcohol Z50.2
- – drug Z50.3
- tobacco use Z50.8
- vocational Z50.7
Reifenstein's syndrome E34.5
Reinsertion, contraceptive device Z30.5
Reiter's disease, syndrome or urethritis
  M02.3
Rejection
- food, psychogenic F50.8
- transplant T86.9
- – bone T86.8
- – – marrow T86.0
- – heart T86.2
- – – with lung(s) T86.3
- – intestine T86.8
- – kidney T86.1
- – liver T86.4
- – lung(s) T86.8
- – – with heart T86.3
- – organ (immune or nonimmune cause)
  T86.9
- – pancreas T86.8
- – skin (allograft) (autograft) T86.8
- – specified NEC T86.8
Relaxation
- anus (sphincter) K62.8
- – psychogenic F45.8
- arch (foot) M21.4
- – congenital Q66.5
- back ligaments M53.2
- bladder (sphincter) N31.2

Relaxation—*continued*
- cardioesophageal K21.9
- diaphragm J98.6
- joint (capsule) (paralytic) M25.2
- – congenital NEC Q74.8
- lumbosacral (joint) M53.2
- pelvic floor N81.8
- perineum N81.8
- posture R29.3
- rectum (sphincter) K62.8
- sacroiliac (joint) M53.2
- scrotum N50.8
- urethra (sphincter) N36.8
- vesical N31.2

Release from prison, anxiety concerning
Z65.2

Remains
- canal of Cloquet Q14.0
- capsule (opaque) Q14.8

Remission in
- bipolar affective disorder F31.7
- recurrent depressive disorder F33.4

Remnant
- fingernail L60.8
- – congenital Q84.6
- meniscus, knee M23.3
- thyroglossal duct Q89.2
- tonsil J35.8
- – infected (chronic) J35.0
- urachus Q64.4

Removal (from) (of)
- cardiac pulse generator (battery) (end-of-life) Z45.0
- catheter (indwelling) (urinary) Z46.6
- – from artificial opening – *see* Attention to, artificial, opening
- – vascular NEC Z45.2
- device
- – contraceptive Z30.5
- – fixation (internal) Z47.0
- – – external Z47.8
- – traction Z47.8
- dressing Z48.0
- home in childhood (to foster home or institution) Z61.1
- Kirschner wire Z47.0
- myringotomy device (stent) (tube) Z45.8
- organ, prophylactic (for neoplasm management) Z40.0
- pin Z47.0
- plaster cast Z47.8
- plate (fracture) Z47.0
- rod Z47.0
- screw Z47.0

Removal—*continued*
- splint, external Z47.8
- suture Z48.0
- traction device, external Z47.8
- vascular access device or catheter Z45.2

Ren
- arcuatus Q63.1
- mobile, mobilis N28.8
- – congenital Q63.8
- unguliformis Q63.1

Renal – *see condition*

Rendu-Osler-Weber disease or syndrome
I78.0

Reninoma (M8361/1) D41.0

Renon-Delille syndrome E23.3

Reovirus, as cause of disease classified elsewhere B97.5

Repair
- pelvic floor, previous, in pregnancy or childbirth O34.8
- scarred tissue Z42.9
  - breast Z42.1
- – head and neck Z42.0
- – lower extremity Z42.4
- – specified NEC Z42.8
- – trunk Z42.2
- – upper extremity Z42.3

Repeated falls NEC R29.6

Replaced chromosome by ring or dicentric Q93.2

Replacement by artificial or mechanical device or prosthesis of
- bladder Z96.0
- blood vessel NEC Z95.8
- bone NEC Z96.7
- cochlea Z96.2
- coronary artery Z95.5
- eustachian tube Z96.2
- eye globe Z97.0
- heart Z95.8
- – valve NEC Z95.4
- intestine Z96.8
- joint Z96.6
- larynx Z96.3
- lens Z96.1
- limb(s) Z97.1
- mandible NEC (for tooth root implant(s)) Z96.5
- organ NEC Z96.8
- peripheral vessel NEC Z95.8
- stapes Z96.2
- teeth Z97.2
- tendon Z96.7
- tissue NEC Z96.8

Replacement by artificial or mechanical device or prosthesis of—*continued*
- tooth root(s) Z96.5
- vessel NEC Z95.8
- – coronary (artery) Z95.5
Request for expert evidence Z04.8
Reserve, decreased or low
- cardiac – *see* Disease, heart
- kidney N28.8
Residual – *see also condition*
- affective disorder (due to alcohol or drug use) – *code to* F10-F19 with fourth character .7
- disorder of personality and behavior (due to alcohol or drug use) – *code to* F10-F19 with fourth character .7
- ovary syndrome N99.8
- state, schizophrenic F20.5
- urine R39.1
Resistance, resistant (to)
- activated protein C (factor V Leiden mutation) D68.5
- antibiotic(s), by bacterial agent
- – methicillin U80.1
- – multiple U88
- – penicillin U80.0
- – penicillin-related U80.8
- – specified (single) NEC U89.8
- – – multiple U88
- – vancomycin U81.0
- – vancomycin-related U81.8
Resorption
- dental (roots) K03.3
- – alveoli K08.8
- teeth (external) (internal) (pathological) (roots) K03.3
Respiration
- Cheyne-Stokes R06.3
- decreased due to shock, following injury T79.4
- disorder of, psychogenic F45.3
- insufficient, or poor R06.8
- – newborn NEC P28.5
- sighing, psychogenic F45.3
Respiratory – *see also condition*
- syncytial virus, as cause of disease classified elsewhere B97.4
Respite care Z75.5
Response, drug
- photoallergic L56.1
- phototoxic L56.0
Restless legs (syndrome) G25.8
Restlessness R45.1
Restriction of housing space Z59.1

Rests, ovarian, in fallopian tube Q50.6
Restzustand (schizophrenic) F20.5
Retained – *see* Retention
Retardation
- development, developmental, specific (*see also* Disorder, developmental) F89
- – arithmetical skills F81.2
- – learning F81.9
- – – language (skills) (expressive) F80.1
- – motor function F82
- – reading F81.0
- – spelling (without reading disorder) F81.1
- endochondral bone growth M89.2
- growth (*see also* Retardation, physical) R62.8
- – fetus P05.9
- – – affecting management of pregnancy O36.5
- intrauterine growth P05.9
- – affecting management of pregnancy O36.5
- mental F79.-
- – with
- – – autistic features F84.1
- – – overactivity and stereotyped movements F84.4
- – mild (IQ 50-69) F70.-
- – moderate (IQ 35-49) F71.-
- – profound (IQ under 20) F73.-
- – severe (IQ 20-34) F72.-
- – specified NEC F78.-
- motor function, specific F82
- physical (child) R62.8
- – due to malnutrition E45
- – fetus P05.9
- reading (specific) F81.0
- spelling (specific) (without reading disorder) F81.1
Retching (*see also* Vomiting) R11
Retention, retained
- cyst – *see* Cyst
- dead
- – fetus (at or near term) (mother) O36.4
- – – early fetal death O02.1
- – ovum O02.0
- decidua (following delivery) (fragments) (with hemorrhage) O72.2
- – with abortion – *see* Abortion, by type
- – without hemorrhage O73.1
- deciduous tooth K00.6
- dental root K08.3
- fecal (*see also* Constipation) K59.0

Retention, retained—*continued*
- fetus, dead O36.4
- – early O02.1
- fluid R60.9
- foreign body – *see also* Foreign body, retained
- – current trauma – *code as* Foreign body, by site or type
- intrauterine contraceptive device, in pregnancy O26.3
- membranes (complicating delivery) (with hemorrhage) O72.2
- – with abortion – *see* Abortion, by type
- – without hemorrhage O73.1
- meniscus (*see also* Derangement, meniscus) M23.3
- menses N94.8
- milk (puerperal, postpartum) O92.7
- nitrogen, extrarenal R39.2
- ovary syndrome N99.8
- placenta (total) (with hemorrhage) O72.0
- – portions or fragments (with hemorrhage) O72.2
- – – without hemorrhage O73.1
- – without hemorrhage O73.0
- products of conception
- – early pregnancy (dead fetus) O02.1
- – following
- – – abortion – *see* Abortion, by type
- – – delivery (with hemorrhage) O72.2
- – – – without hemorrhage O73.1
- secundines (following delivery) (with hemorrhage) O72.0
- – with abortion – *see* Abortion, by type
- – complicating puerperium (delayed hemorrhage) O72.2
- – partial O72.2
- – – – without hemorrhage O73.1
- – – without hemorrhage O73.0
- smegma, clitoris N90.8
- urine R33
- – psychogenic F45.3
- water (in tissues) (*see also* Edema) R60.9
Reticulation, dust – *see* Pneumoconiosis
Reticuloendotheliosis
- acute infantile C96.0
- leukemic C91.4
- malignant C96.9
- nonlipid C96.0
Reticulohistiocytoma (giant-cell) D76.3
Reticuloid, actinic L57.1
Reticulolymphosarcoma (diffuse) C85.9
- follicular C82.9
- nodular C82.9

Reticulosarcoma (diffuse) C83.3
Reticulosis (skin)
- acute, of infancy C96.0
- hemophagocytic, familial D76.1
- histiocytic medullary C96.9
- lipomelanotic I89.8
- malignant (midline) C86.0
- nonlipid C96.0
- polymorphic C83.8
- Sézary C84.1
Retina, retinal – *see condition*
Retinitis (*see also* Chorioretinitis) H30.9
- albuminurica N18.5† H32.8∗
- arteriosclerotic I70.8† H36.8∗
- diabetic (*see also* E10-E14 with fourth character .3) E14.3† H36.0∗
- disciformis H35.3
- focal H30.0
- gravidarum O26.8
- juxtapapillaris H30.0
- luetic – *see* Retinitis, syphilitic
- pigmentosa H35.5
- punctata albescens H35.5
- renal N18.5† H32.8∗
- syphilitic (early) (secondary) A51.4† H32.0∗
- – central, recurrent A52.7† H32.0∗
- – congenital (early) A50.0† H32.0∗
- – late A52.7† H32.0∗
- tuberculous A18.5† H32.0∗
Retinoblastoma (M9510/3) C69.2
- differentiated (M9511/3) C69.2
- undifferentiated (M9512/3) C69.2
Retinochoroiditis (*see also* Chorioretinitis) H30.9
- disseminated H30.1
- – syphilitic A52.7† H32.0∗
- focal H30.0
- juxtapapillaris H30.0
Retinopathy (background) (Coats) (exudative) (hypertensive) H35.0
- arteriosclerotic I70.8† H36.8∗
- atherosclerotic I70.8† H36.8∗
- central serous H35.7
- circinate H35.0
- diabetic (*see also* E10-E14 with fourth character .3) E14.3† H36.0∗
- in (due to)
- – atherosclerosis I70.8† H36.8∗
- – diabetes (*see also* E10-E14 with fourth character .3) E14.3† H36.0∗
- – sickle-cell disorders D57.-† H36.8∗
- of prematurity H35.1
- pigmentary, congenital H35.5

Retinopathy—*continued*
- proliferative NEC H35.2
- - sickle-cell D57.-† H36.8∗
- solar H31.0
Retinoschisis H33.1
- congenital Q14.1
Retractile testis Q55.2
Retraction
- cervix (*see also* Retroversion, uterus) N85.4
- drum (membrane) H73.8
- finger M20.0
- lid H02.5
- lung J98.4
- mediastinum J98.5
- nipple N64.5
- - congenital Q83.8
- - gestational O92.0
- - puerperal, postpartum O92.0
- palmar fascia M72.0
- pleura (*see also* Pleurisy) R09.1
- ring, uterus (Bandl's) (pathological) O62.4
- - affecting fetus or newborn P03.6
- sternum (congenital) Q76.7
- - acquired M95.4
- syndrome H50.8
- uterus (*see also* Retroversion, uterus) N85.4
- valve (heart) – *see* Endocarditis
Retraining
- activities of daily living NEC Z50.8
- cardiac Z50.0
Retrobulbar – *see condition*
Retrocecal – *see condition*
Retrocession – *see* Retroversion
Retrodisplacement – *see* Retroversion
Retroflection, retroflexion – *see* Retroversion
Retrognathia, retrognathism (mandibular) (maxillary) K07.1
Retrograde menstruation N92.5
Retroperineal – *see condition*
Retroperitoneal – *see condition*
Retroperitonitis (*see also* Peritonitis) K65.9
Retropharyngeal – *see condition*
Retroplacental – *see condition*
Retroposition – *see* Retroversion
Retrosternal thyroid Q89.2
Retroversion, retroverted
- cervix (*see also* Retroversion, uterus) N85.4

Retroversion, retroverted—*continued*
- female NEC (*see also* Retroversion, uterus) N85.4
- iris H21.5
- testis (congenital) Q55.2
- uterus, uterine N85.4
- - congenital Q51.8
- - in pregnancy or childbirth O34.5
- - - causing obstructed labor O65.5
- - - - affecting fetus or newborn P03.1
Retrovirus, as cause of disease classified elsewhere B97.3
Rett's disease or syndrome F84.2
Reverse peristalsis R19.2
Reye's syndrome G93.7
Rh (factor)
- hemolytic disease (fetus or newborn) P55.0
- incompatibility, immunization or sensitization
- - affecting management of pregnancy O36.0
- - fetus or newborn P55.0
- - transfusion reaction T80.4
- negative mother affecting fetus or newborn P55.0
- transfusion reaction T80.4
Rhabdomyolysis (idiopathic) NEC M62.8
- traumatic T79.6
Rhabdomyoma (M8900/0) – *see also* Neoplasm, connective tissue, benign
- adult (M8904/0) D21.9
- fetal (M8903/0) D21.9
- glycogenic (M8904/0) D21.9
Rhabdomyosarcoma (M8900/3) – *see also* Neoplasm, connective tissue, malignant
- alveolar (M8920/3) C49.9
- embryonal (M8910/3) C49.9
- mixed type (M8902/3) C49.9
- pleomorphic (M8901/3) C49.9
Rhabdosarcoma (M8900/3) – *see* Rhabdomyosarcoma
Rhesus (factor) incompatibility – *see* Rh, incompatibility
Rheumatic (acute) (chronic) (subacute)
- chorea – *see* Chorea, rheumatic
- fever (acute) – *see* Fever, rheumatic
- heart (*see also* Disease, heart, rheumatic) I09.9
- - specified NEC I09.8
- pneumonia I00† J17.8∗
Rheumatism (articular) (neuralgic) (nonarticular) M79.0
- palindromic (any site) M12.3

∗ See Standards Manual XIII-15

Rheumatoid – *see also* condition
- arthritis M06.9
- – with involvement of organs NEC M05.3
- – seronegative M06.0
- – seropositive M05.9
- – – specified NEC M05.8
- lung (disease) M05.1† J99.0∗
- myocarditis M05.3† I41.8∗
- pericarditis M05.3† I32.8∗
- polyarthritis M06.9
- vasculitis M05.2

Rhinitis (catarrhal) (fibrinous) (membranous) J31.0
- with sore throat – *see* Nasopharyngitis
- acute J00
- allergic J30.4
- – with asthma J45.0
- – due to pollen J30.1
- – nonseasonal J30.3
- – perennial J30.3
- – seasonal NEC J30.2
- – specified NEC J30.3
- atrophic (chronic) J31.0
- chronic J31.0
- granulomatous (chronic) J31.0
- hypertrophic (chronic) J31.0
- infective J00
- obstructive (chronic) J31.0
- pneumococcal J00
- purulent (chronic) J31.0
- syphilitic A52.7† J99.8∗
- – congenital A50.0† J99.8∗
- tuberculous A16.8
- – with bacteriological and histological confirmation A15.8
- ulcerative (chronic) J31.0
- vasomotor J30.0

Rhinoantritis (chronic) (*see also* Sinusitis, maxillary) J32.0
Rhinodacryolith H04.5
Rhinolith (nasal sinus) J34.8
Rhinomegaly J34.8
Rhinopharyngitis (acute) (subacute) (*see also* Nasopharyngitis) J00
- chronic J31.1
- destructive ulcerating A66.5† J99.8∗
- mutilans A66.5† J99.8∗
Rhinophyma L71.1
Rhinorrhea J34.8
- cerebrospinal (fluid) G96.0
- paroxysmal (*see also* Rhinitis, allergic) J30.3

Rhinorrhea—*continued*
- spasmodic (*see also* Rhinitis, allergic) J30.3
Rhinosalpingitis H68.0
Rhinoscleroma A48.8
Rhinosporidiosis B48.1
Rhinovirus infection NEC B34.8
Rhythm
- atrioventricular nodal I49.8
- disorder I49.9
- – coronary sinus I49.8
- – ectopic I49.8
- – nodal I49.8
- escape I49.9
- heart, abnormal I49.9
- idioventricular I44.2
- nodal I49.8
- sleep, inversion G47.2
Rhytidosis facialis L98.8
Rib – *see also* condition
- cervical Q76.5
Riboflavin deficiency E53.0
Rice bodies M24.0
- knee M23.4
Richter's hernia – *see* Hernia, abdomen, with obstruction
Richter syndrome C91.1
Ricinism T62.2
Rickets (active) (acute) (adolescent) (chest wall) (congenital) (current) (infantile) (intestinal) E55.0
- adult – *see* Osteomalacia
- celiac K90.0
- inactive E64.3
- kidney N25.0
- renal N25.0
- sequelae, any E64.3
- vitamin-D-resistant E83.3† M90.8∗
Rickettsial disease NEC A79.9
- specified type NEC A79.8
Rickettsialpox (Rickettsia akari) A79.1
Rickettsiosis NEC A79.9
- due to
- – Ehrlichia sennetsu A79.8
- – Rickettsia akari (rickettsialpox) A79.1
- specified type NEC A79.8
- tick-borne A77.9
- vesicular A79.1
Rider's bone M61.5
Ridge, alveolus – *see also* condition
- flabby K06.8
Ridged ear, congenital Q17.3
Riedel's
- lobe, liver Q44.7

Riedel's—*continued*
- struma, thyroiditis or disease E06.5
Rieger's anomaly or syndrome Q13.8
Riehl's melanosis L81.4
Rietti-Greppi-Micheli anemia D56.9
Rieux's hernia – *see* Hernia, abdomen,
  specified site NEC
Riga-Fede disease K14.0
Riggs' disease K05.3
Rigid, rigidity – *see also condition*
- abdominal R19.3
- - with severe abdominal pain R10.0
- articular, multiple, congenital Q68.8
- cervix (uteri)
- - in pregnancy or childbirth O34.4
- - - affecting fetus or newborn P03.8
- - - causing obstructed labor O65.5
- - - - affecting fetus or newborn P03.1
- hymen (acquired) (congenital) N89.6
- pelvic floor
- - in pregnancy or childbirth O34.8
- - - affecting fetus or newborn P03.8
- - - causing obstructed labor O65.5
- - - - affecting fetus or newborn P03.1
- perineum or vulva
- - in pregnancy or childbirth O34.7
- - - causing obstructed labor O65.5
- - - - affecting fetus or newborn P03.1
- spine M53.8
- vagina
- - in pregnancy or childbirth O34.6
- - - causing obstructed labor O65.5
- - - - affecting fetus or newborn P03.8
Rigors R68.8
- with fever R50.8
Riley-Day syndrome G90.1
Ring(s)
- aorta (vascular) Q25.4
- Bandl's O62.4
- - fetus or newborn P03.6
- contraction, complicating delivery O62.4
- - affecting fetus or newborn P03.6
- esophageal, lower (muscular) K22.2
- Fleischer's (cornea) H18.0
- hymenal, tight N89.6
- Kayser-Fleischer (cornea) H18.0
- retraction, uterus, pathological O62.4
- - affecting fetus or newborn P03.6
- Schatzki's (esophagus) (lower) K22.2
- - congenital Q39.3
- Soemmerring's H26.4
- vascular (congenital) Q25.8
- - aorta Q25.4
Ringed hair (congenital) Q84.1

Ringworm B35.9
- beard B35.0
- black dot B35.0
- body B35.4
- Burmese B35.5
- corporeal B35.4
- foot B35.3
- groin B35.6
- hand B35.2
- honeycomb B35.0
- nails B35.1
- perianal (area) B35.6
- scalp B35.0
- specified NEC B35.8
- Tokelau B35.5
Rise, venous pressure I87.8
Risk, suicidal R45.8
- constituting part of a mental disorder – *see condition*
Ritter's disease L00
Rivalry, sibling F93.3
River blindness B73† H45.1*
Robert's pelvis Q74.2
- with disproportion (fetopelvic) O33.0
- - causing obstructed labor O65.0
Robin(-Pierre) syndrome Q87.0
Robinow-Silvermann-Smith syndrome Q87.1
Robinson's (hidrotic) ectodermal dysplasia or syndrome Q82.4
Robles' disease B73
Rocky Mountain fever (spotted) A77.0
Roentgen ray, adverse effect NEC T66
Roeteln (*see also* Rubella) B06.9
Roger's disease Q21.0
Rokitansky-Aschoff sinuses (gallbladder) K82.8
Romano-Ward syndrome I45.8
Romberg's disease or syndrome G51.8
Roof, mouth – *see condition*
Rosacea L71.9
- acne L71.9
- keratitis L71.8† H19.3*
- specified NEC L71.8
Rosenbach's erysipeloid A26.0
Rosenthal's disease or syndrome D68.1
Roseola B09
- infantum B08.2
Ross River disease or fever B33.1
Rossbach's disease K31.8
- psychogenic F45.3
Rostan's asthma (*see also* Failure, ventricular, left) I50.1
Rot, Barcoo (*see also* Ulcer, skin) L98.4

Rotation
- anomalous, incomplete or insufficient, intestine Q43.3
- manual, affecting fetus or newborn P03.8
- spine, incomplete or insufficient M43.8
- tooth, teeth K07.3
- vertebra, incomplete or insufficient M43.8

Rotes Quérol disease or syndrome M48.1
Roth(-Bernhardt) disease or syndrome (meralgia paraesthetica) G57.1
Rothmund(-Thomson) syndrome Q82.8
Rotor's disease or syndrome E80.6
Round
- back (with wedging of vertebrae) M40.2
- - late effect of rickets E64.3
- worms (large) (infestation) NEC B82.0
- - ascariasis B77.-

Roussy-Lévy syndrome G60.0
Rubella B06.9
- complicating pregnancy, childbirth or puerperium O98.5
- complication NEC B06.8
- - neurological B06.0† G99.8*
- congenital P35.0
- maternal
- - affecting fetus or newborn P00.2
- - - manifest rubella in infant P35.0
- - care for (suspected) damage to fetus O35.3
- - suspected damage to fetus affecting management of pregnancy O35.3
- specified complications NEC B06.8

Rubeola (meaning measles) (*see also* Measles) B05.9
- meaning rubella (*see also* Rubella) B06.9
Rubeosis, iris H21.1
Rubinstein-Taybi syndrome Q87.2
Rudimentary (congenital) – *see also* Agenesis
- arm Q71.9
- cervix uteri Q51.8
- eye Q11.2
- lobule of ear Q17.3
- patella Q74.1
- tracheal bronchus Q32.4
- uterus Q51.8
- - in male Q56.1
- vagina Q52.0

Ruled out condition (*see also* Observation, suspected) Z03.9
Rumination R11
- disorder of infancy F98.2
- neurotic F42.0

Rumination—*continued*
- newborn P92.1
- obsessional F42.0
- psychogenic F42.0
Rupia (syphilitic) A51.3
- congenital A50.0
- tertiary A52.7† L99.8*
Rupture, ruptured
- abscess (spontaneous) – *code as* Abscess, by site
- aneurysm – *see* Aneurysm
- anus (sphincter) – *see* Laceration, anus
- aorta, aortic (*see also* Aneurysm, aorta) I71.8
- - abdominal I71.3
- - arch I71.1
- - ascending I71.1
- - descending I71.8
- - - abdominal I71.3
- - - thoracic I71.1
- - syphilitic A52.0† I79.0*
- - thorax, thoracic I71.1
- - transverse I71.1
- - traumatic (thoracic) S25.0
- - - abdominal S35.0
- - valve or cusp (*see also* Endocarditis, aortic) I35.8
- appendix
- - with
- - - peritonitis, generalized K35.2
- - - peritonitis, localized K35.3
- arteriovenous fistula, brain I60.8
- artery I77.2
- - brain (*see also* Hemorrhage, intracerebral) I61.9
- - coronary (*see also* Infarct, myocardium) I21.9
- - heart (*see also* Infarct, myocardium) I21.9
- - pulmonary I28.8
- - traumatic (complication) (*see also* Injury, blood vessel) T14.5
- bile duct (common) (hepatic) K83.2
- bladder (nontraumatic) (sphincter) (spontaneous) N32.4
- - following abortion O08.6
- - obstetrical trauma O71.5
- - traumatic S37.2
- blood vessel (*see also* Hemorrhage) R58
- - brain (*see also* Hemorrhage, intracerebral) I61.9
- - heart (*see also* Infarct, myocardium) I21.9

Rupture, ruptured—*continued*
- blood vessel—*continued*
- – traumatic (complication) (*see also* Injury, blood vessel) T14.5
- bone – *see* Fracture
- bowel (nontraumatic) K63.1
- – fetus or newborn P78.0
- – obstetric trauma O71.5
- – traumatic S36.9
- brain
- – aneurysm (congenital) (*see also* Hemorrhage, subarachnoid) I60.9
- – – syphilitic A52.0† I68.8*
- – hemorrhagic (*see also* Hemorrhage, intracerebral) I61.9
- capillaries I78.8
- cardiac (wall) I21.9
- – concurrent with acute myocardial infarction – *see* Infarct, myocardium
- – following acute myocardial infarction (current complication) I23.3
- – – with hemopericardium I23.0
- cartilage (articular) (current) (*see also* Sprain) T14.3
- – knee S83.3
- – semilunar – *see* Tear, meniscus
- cecum (with peritonitis) K65.0
- cerebral aneurysm (congenital) – *see* Hemorrhage, subarachnoid
- cervix (uteri)
- – obstetrical trauma O71.3
- – traumatic S37.6
- chordae tendineae NEC I51.1
- – concurrent with acute myocardial infarction – *see* Infarct, myocardium
- – following acute myocardial infarction (current complication) I23.4
- choroid (direct) (indirect) (traumatic) H31.3
- circle of Willis I60.6
- colon (nontraumatic) K63.1
- – fetus or newborn P78.0
- – obstetric trauma O71.5
- – traumatic S36.5
- cornea (traumatic) – *see* Rupture, eye
- coronary (artery) (thrombotic) (*see also* Infarct, myocardium) I21.9
- corpus luteum (infected) (ovary) N83.1
- cyst – *see* Cyst
- cystic duct K82.2
- Descemet's membrane H18.3
- – traumatic – *see* Rupture, eye
- diaphragm, traumatic S27.8

Rupture, ruptured—*continued*
- diverticulum (intestine) (*see also* Diverticula) K57.8
- duodenal stump K31.8
- ear drum (nontraumatic) (*see also* Perforation, tympanic membrane) H72.9
- – with otitis media – *see* Otitis media
- – traumatic, current episode S09.2
- esophagus K22.3
- eye (without prolapse or loss of intraocular tissue) S05.3
- – with prolapse or loss of intraocular tissue S05.2
- fallopian tube NEC (nonobstetric) (nontraumatic) N83.8
- – due to pregnancy O00.1
- fontanel P13.1
- gallbladder K82.2
- gastric (*see also* Rupture, stomach) K31.8
- – vessel K92.2
- globe (eye) (traumatic) – *see* Rupture, eye
- graafian follicle (hematoma) N83.0
- heart – *see* Rupture, cardiac
- – traumatic S26.8
- hymen (nonintentional) (nontraumatic) N89.8
- ileum (nontraumatic) K63.1
- – fetus or newborn P78.0
- – obstetric trauma O71.5
- – traumatic S36.4
- internal organ, traumatic – *see* Injury, by site
- intervertebral disk – *see* Displacement, intervertebral disk
- intestine NEC (nontraumatic) K63.1
- – fetus or newborn P78.0
- – obstetric trauma O71.5
- – traumatic S36.9
- iris H21.5
- – traumatic – *see* Rupture, eye
- jejunum, jejunal (nontraumatic) K63.1
- – fetus or newborn P78.0
- – obstetric trauma O71.5
- – traumatic S36.4
- joint capsule – *see* Sprain
- kidney S37.0
- – birth injury P15.8
- – nontraumatic N28.8
- lacrimal duct (traumatic) S05.8
- lens (cataract) (traumatic) H26.1
- ligament – *see* Sprain
- liver S36.1
- – birth injury P15.0
- lymphatic vessel I89.8

Rupture, ruptured—*continued*
- marginal sinus (placental) (with hemorrhage) O46.8
- − − with placenta previa O44.1
- − − − affecting fetus or newborn P02.0
- − − affecting fetus or newborn P02.1
- membrana tympani (nontraumatic) (*see also* Perforation, tympanic membrane) H72.9
- membranes (spontaneous)
- − − artificial
- − − − delayed delivery following O75.5
- − − − − affecting fetus or newborn P01.1
- − − delayed delivery following O75.6
- − − − affecting fetus or newborn P01.1
- − − premature O42.9
- − − − affecting fetus or newborn P01.1
- − − − labor delayed by therapy O42.2
- − − − onset of labor
- − − − − after 24 hours O42.1
- − − − − delayed by therapy O42.2
- − − − − within 24 hours O42.0
- meningeal artery I60.8
- meniscus (knee) (*see also* Tear, meniscus) S83.2
- − − old (*see also* Derangement, meniscus) M23.2
- − − site other than knee – *code as* Sprain
- mesentery (nontraumatic) K66.8
- mitral (valve) I34.8
- muscle (traumatic) NEC – *see* Injury, muscle
- − − nontraumatic M62.1
- musculotendinous junction NEC, nontraumatic M66.5
- mycotic aneurysm causing cerebral hemorrhage (*see also* Hemorrhage, subarachnoid) I60.9
- myocardium, myocardial (*see also* Infarct, myocardium) I21.9
- − − traumatic S26.8
- operation wound T81.3
- ovary, ovarian N83.8
- − − corpus luteum cyst N83.1
- − − follicle (graafian) N83.0
- oviduct (nonobstetric) (nontraumatic) N83.8
- − − due to pregnancy O00.1
- pancreas (nontraumatic) K86.8
- − − traumatic S36.2
- papillary muscle NEC I51.2
- − − following acute myocardial infarction (current complication) I23.5

Rupture, ruptured—*continued*
- pelvic
- − − floor, complicating delivery O70.1
- − − organ NEC, obstetrical trauma O71.5
- perineum (nonobstetric) (nontraumatic) N90.8
- − − complicating delivery O70.9
- − − − first degree O70.0
- − − − fourth degree O70.3
- − − − second degree O70.1
- − − − third degree O70.2
- postoperative wound T81.3
- prostate (traumatic) S37.8
- pulmonary
- − − artery I28.8
- − − valve (heart) I37.8
- − − vessel I28.8
- pyosalpinx (*see also* Salpingo-oophoritis) N70.9
- rectum (nontraumatic) K63.1
- − − fetus or newborn P78.0
- − − obstetric trauma O71.5
- − − traumatic S36.6
- retina, retinal (traumatic) (without detachment) H33.3
- − − with detachment H33.0
- rotator cuff (complete) (incomplete) (nontraumatic) M75.1
- sclera S05.3
- semilunar cartilage, knee S83.2
- sigmoid (nontraumatic) K63.1
- − − fetus or newborn P78.0
- − − obstetric trauma O71.5
- − − traumatic S36.5
- spinal cord (*see also* Injury, spinal cord, by region) T09.3
- − − fetus or newborn (birth injury) P11.5
- spleen (traumatic) S36.0
- − − birth injury P15.1
- − − congenital (birth injury) P15.1
- − − due to Plasmodium vivax malaria B51.0† D77*
- − − nontraumatic D73.5
- − − spontaneous D73.5
- splenic vein R58
- stomach (nontraumatic) (spontaneous) K31.8
- − − traumatic S36.3
- supraspinatus (complete) (incomplete) (nontraumatic) M75.1
- symphysis pubis
- − − obstetric O71.6
- − − traumatic S33.4
- synovium (cyst) M66.1

Rupture, ruptured—*continued*
- tendon (traumatic) – *see also* Injury, muscle
- – – nontraumatic M66.5
- – spontaneous M66.5
- – – extensor M66.2
- – – flexor M66.3
- – – specified NEC M66.4
- thoracic duct I89.8
- tonsil J35.8
- traumatic
- – ankle ligament S93.2
- – aorta (thoracic) S25.0
- – – abdominal S35.0
- – diaphragm S27.8
- – external site – *see* Wound, open, by site
- – eye (*see also* Rupture, eye) S05.3
- – internal organ – *see* Injury, by site
- – intervertebral disk T09.2
- – – cervical S13.0
- – – lumbar S33.0
- – – thoracic S23.0
- – kidney S37.0
- – ligament (*see also* Sprain) T14.3
- – – carpus (radiocarpal) (ulnocarpal) S63.3
- – – collateral (hand) S63.4
- – – – wrist S63.3
- – – finger at metacarpo- and interphalangeal joint(s) (collateral) (palmar) (volar plate) S63.4
- – – foot S93.2
- – – palmar S63.4
- – – radial collateral S53.2
- – – radiocarpal S63.3
- – – ulnar collateral S53.3
- – – ulnocarpal S63.3
- – – wrist (collateral) S63.3
- – liver S36.1
- – membrana tympani S09.2
- – muscle or tendon – *see* Injury, muscle
- – pancreas S36.2
- – rectum S36.6
- – sigmoid S36.5
- – spleen S36.0
- – stomach S36.3
- – symphysis pubis S33.4
- – tympanum, tympanic (membrane) S09.2

Rupture, ruptured—*continued*
- traumatic—*continued*
- – – ureter S37.1
- – – uterus S37.6
- – – vagina S31.4
- tricuspid (heart) (valve) I07.8
- tube, tubal (nonobstetric) (nontraumatic) N83.8
- – abscess (*see also* Salpingo-oophoritis) N70.9
- – due to pregnancy O00.1
- tympanum, tympanic (membrane) (nontraumatic) (*see also* Perforation, tympanic membrane) H72.9
- – multiple H72.8
- – total H72.8
- – traumatic S09.2
- umbilical cord, complicating delivery O69.8
- – affecting fetus or newborn P50.1
- ureter (traumatic) S37.1
- – nontraumatic N28.8
- urethra (nontraumatic) N36.8
- – following abortion O08.6
- – obstetrical trauma O71.5
- – traumatic S37.3
- uterosacral ligament (nonobstetric) (nontraumatic) N83.8
- uterus (traumatic) S37.6
- – during or after labor O71.1
- – – affecting fetus or newborn P03.8
- – nonpuerperal, nontraumatic N85.8
- – pregnant (during labor) O71.1
- – – before labor O71.0
- vagina S31.4
- – complicating delivery (*see also* Laceration, vagina, complicating delivery) O71.4
- valve, valvular (heart) – *see* Endocarditis
- varicose vein – *see* Varicose vein
- varix – *see* Varix
- vena cava R58
- vessel R58
- – pulmonary I28.8
- viscus R19.8
- vulva, complicating delivery O70.0

Russell-Silver syndrome Q87.1
Rust's disease (tuberculous cervical spondylitis) A18.0† M49.0∗

S

Saber, sabre tibia (syphilitic) A50.5†
M90.2∗
Sac, lacrimal – *see condition*
Saccharopinuria E72.3
Saccular – *see condition*
Sacculation
– aorta (nonsyphilitic) (*see also* Aneurysm,
aorta) I71.9
– – ruptured I71.8
– – syphilitic A52.0† I79.0∗
– bladder N32.3
– intralaryngeal (congenital) (ventricular)
Q31.3
– larynx (congenital) (ventricular) Q31.3
– organ or site, congenital – *see* Distortion
– pregnant uterus O34.5
– ureter N28.8
– urethra N36.1
**Sachs' amaurotic familial idiocy or
disease** E75.0
Sachs-Tay disease E75.0
Sacks-Libman disease M32.1† I39.8∗
Sacralgia M53.3
Sacralization Q76.4
Sacrodynia M53.3
Sacroiliac joint – *see condition*
Sacroiliitis NEC M46.1
Sacrum – *see condition*
Saddle
– back M40.5
– embolus, aorta I74.0
– nose M95.0
– – due to syphilis A50.5
Sadism (sexual) F65.5
Sadomasochism F65.5
Saemisch's ulcer (cornea) H16.0
Sahib disease B55.0
Sailor's skin L57.8
Saint
– Anthony's fire (*see also* Erysipelas) A46
– Vitus' dance – *see* Chorea, Sydenham's
Saint's triad (*see also* Hernia, diaphragm)
K44.9
Salaam
– attack(s) G40.4
– tic R25.8
Salicylism
– abuse F55

Salicylism—*continued*
– overdose or wrong substance given or
taken T39.0
Salivary duct or gland – *see condition*
Salivation, excessive K11.7
Salmonella – *see* Infection, Salmonella
Salmonellosis A02.0
Salpingitis (fallopian tube) (*see also*
Salpingo-oophoritis) N70.9
– acute N70.0
– chlamydial A56.1† N74.4∗
– chronic N70.1
– ear H68.0
– eustachian (tube) H68.0
– gonococcal (acute) (chronic) A54.2†
N74.3∗
– specific (acute) (chronic) (gonococcal)
A54.2† N74.3∗
– tuberculous (acute) (chronic) A18.1†
N74.1∗
– venereal (acute) (chronic) (gonococcal)
A54.2† N74.3∗
Salpingocele N83.4
**Salpingo-oophoritis (purulent) (ruptured)
(septic) (suppurative)** N70.9
– acute N70.0
– – following
– – – abortion (subsequent episode) O08.0
– – – – current episode – *see* Abortion
– – – ectopic or molar pregnancy O08.0
– – gonococcal A54.2† N74.3∗
– chronic (*see also* Salpingo-oophoritis, by
type, chronic) N70.1
– complicating pregnancy O23.5
– – affecting fetus or newborn P00.8
– following
– – abortion (subsequent episode) O08.0
– – – current episode – *see* Abortion
– – ectopic or molar pregnancy O08.0
– gonococcal (acute) (chronic) A54.2†
N74.3∗
– puerperal O86.1
– specific A54.2† N74.3∗
– tuberculous (acute) (chronic) A18.1†
N74.1∗
– venereal A54.2† N74.3∗
Salpingo-ovaritis (*see also* Salpingo-
oophoritis) N70.9

Salpingoperitonitis (*see also* Salpingo-
oophoritis) N70.9
Salzmann's nodular dystrophy H18.4
Sampson's cyst or tumor N80.1
San Joaquin (Valley) fever B38.0† J99.8∗
**Sandblaster's asthma, lung or
pneumoconiosis** J62.8
Sander's disease (paranoia) F22.0
Sandhoff's disease E75.0
**Sanfilippo (type B) (type C) (type D)
syndrome** E76.2
Sanger-Brown ataxia G11.2
Sao Paulo fever or typhus A77.0
Saponification, mesenteric K65.8
Sarcocele (benign)
– syphilitic (late) A52.7† N51.1∗
– – congenital A50.5† N51.1∗
Sarcocystosis A07.8
Sarcoepiplomphalocele Q79.2
Sarcoid (*see also* Sarcoidosis) D86.9
– arthropathy D86.8† M14.8∗
– Boeck's D86.9
– Darier-Roussy D86.3
– myocarditis D86.8† I41.8∗
– myositis D86.8† M63.3∗
Sarcoidosis D86.9
– combined sites NEC D86.8
– lung D86.0
– – and lymph nodes D86.2
– lymph nodes D86.1
– – and lung D86.2
– skin D86.3
– specified type NEC D86.8
Sarcoma – *see also* Neoplasm, connective
tissue, malignant
– alveolar soft part (M9581/3) C49.9
– ameloblastic (M9330/3) C41.1
– – upper jaw (bone) C41.0
– botryoid, botryoides (M8910/3) C49.9
– cerebellar (M9480/3) C71.6
– – circumscribed (arachnoidal) (M9471/3)
C71.6
– circumscribed (arachnoidal) cerebellar
(M9471/3) C71.6
– clear cell (M9044/3)
– – kidney (M8964/3) C64
– dendritic cells (accessory cells) (follicular)
(interdigitating) C96.4
– embryonal (M8991/3) C49.9
– endometrial (stromal) (M8930/3) C54.1
– – isthmus C54.0
– epithelioid (cell) (M8804/3) C49.9
– Ewing's (M9260/3) – *see* Neoplasm, bone,
malignant

Sarcoma—*continued*
– giant cell (except of bone) (M8802/3)
– – bone (M9250/3) – *see* Neoplasm, bone,
malignant
– glomoid (M8710/3) C49.9
– granulocytic C92.3
– hemangioendothelial (M9130/3) C49.9
– histiocytic C96.8
– Hodgkin C81.3
– immunoblastic (diffuse) C83.3
– Kaposi's (M9140/3)
– – connective tissue C46.1
– – lymph node(s) C46.3
– – multiple organs C46.8
– – palate (hard) (soft) C46.2
– – resulting from HIV disease B21.0
– – skin C46.0
– – specified site NEC C46.7
– – unspecified site C46.9
– Kupffer cell (M9124/3) C22.3
– Langerhans-cell C96.4
– leptomeningeal (M9530/3) – *see*
Neoplasm, meninges, malignant
– lymphangioendothelial (M9170/3) C49.9
– lymphoblastic C83.5
– lymphocytic C85.9
– mast cell C96.2
– melanotic (M8720/3) – *see* Melanoma
– meningeal (M9530/3) – *see* Neoplasm,
meninges, malignant
– meningothelial (M9530/3) – *see*
Neoplasm, meninges, malignant
– mesenchymal (M8800/3)
– – mixed (M8990/3) C49.9
– mesothelial (M9050/3) – *see*
Mesothelioma
– monstrocellular (M9481/3)
– – specified site – *see* Neoplasm,
malignant
– – unspecified site C71.9
– myeloid C92.3
– neurogenic (M9540/3) – *see* Neoplasm,
nerve, malignant
– odontogenic (M9270/3) C41.1
– – upper jaw (bone) C41.0
– osteoblastic (M9180/3) – *see* Neoplasm,
bone, malignant
– osteogenic (M9180/3) – *see also*
Neoplasm, bone, malignant
– – juxtacortical (M9190/3) – *see*
Neoplasm, bone, malignant
– – periosteal (M9190/3) – *see* Neoplasm,
bone, malignant

Sarcoma—*continued*
- periosteal (M8812/3) – *see also*
  Neoplasm, bone, malignant
- – osteogenic (M9190/3) – *see* Neoplasm,
  bone, malignant
- plasma cell C90.3
- pleomorphic cell (M8802/3)
- reticulum cell (diffuse) C83.3
- – nodular C96.9
- – pleomorphic cell type C83.3
- rhabdoid (M8963/3) – *see* Neoplasm,
  malignant
- round cell (M8803/3) C49.9
- small cell (M8803/3) C49.9
- soft tissue (M8800/3) C49.9
- spindle cell (M8801/3) C49.9
- stromal (endometrial) (M8930/3) C54.1
- – isthmus (M8930/3) C54.0
- synovial (M9040/3)
- – biphasic (M9043/3) C49.9
- – epithelioid cell (M9042/3) C49.9
- – spindle cell (M9041/3) C49.9
Sarcomatosis
- meningeal (M9539/3) – *see* Neoplasm,
  meninges, malignant
- specified site NEC (M8800/3) – *see*
  Neoplasm, connective tissue, malignant
- unspecified site (M8800/6) C79.9
- – ~~primary site not indicated C80.9~~
- – ~~primary site unknown, so stated C80.0~~
Sarcosinemia E72.5
Sarcosporidiosis (intestinal) A07.8
**SARS (Severe acute respiratory
  syndrome)** U04.9
Saturnine – *see condition*
Saturnism T56.0
Satyriasis F52.7
Sauriasis – *see* Ichthyosis
Scabies (any site) B86
Scald – *see* Burn
Scaling, skin R23.4
Scalp – *see condition*
Scapegoating, affecting child Z62.3
Scaphocephaly Q75.0
Scapulalgia M89.8
Scar, scarring (*see also* Cicatrix) L90.5
- adherent L90.5
- atrophic L90.5
- cervix
- – in pregnancy or childbirth O34.4
- – – affecting fetus or newborn P03.8
- – – causing obstructed labor O65.5
- chorioretinal H31.0
- – postsurgical H59.8

Scar, scarring—*continued*
- choroid H31.0
- conjunctiva H11.2
- cornea H17.9
- – xerophthalmic H17.8
- – – vitamin A deficiency E50.6† H19.8*
- due to
- – previous cesarean section, complicating
  pregnancy or childbirth O34.2
- – – affecting fetus or newborn P03.8
- duodenum, obstructive K31.5
- hypertrophic L91.0
- keloid L91.0
- labia N90.8
- lung (base) J98.4
- macula H31.0
- muscle M62.8
- myocardium, myocardial I25.2
- painful L90.5
- posterior pole (eye) H31.0
- psychic Z91.4
- retina H31.0
- trachea J39.8
- uterus N85.8
- – in pregnancy or childbirth O34.2
- – – affecting fetus or newborn P03.8
- vagina N89.8
- – postoperative N99.2
- vulva N90.8
Scarabiasis B88.2
Scarlatina A38
- myocarditis (acute) A38† I41.0*
- – old (*see also* Myocarditis) I51.4
**Schamberg's disease (progressive
  pigmentary dermatosis)** L81.7
**Schatzki's ring (acquired) (esophagus)
  (lower)** K22.2
- congenital Q39.3
Schaumann's
- benign lymphogranulomatosis D86.1
- disease or syndrome (*see also*
  Sarcoidosis) D86.9
Scheie's syndrome E76.0
Schenck's disease B42.1
Scheuermann's disease or osteochondrosis
  M42.0
Schilder(-Flatau) disease G37.0
Schilder-Addison complex E71.3
Schilling-type monocytic leukemia C93.0
**Schimmelbusch's disease, cystic mastitis
  or hyperplasia** N60.1
Schistosoma infestation – *see*
  Schistosomiasis

Schistosomiasis B65.9
– Asiatic B65.2
– bladder B65.0
– colon B65.1
– cutaneous B65.3
– Eastern B65.2
– genitourinary tract B65.0
– intestinal B65.1
– lung NEC B65.-† J99.8∗
– – pneumonia B65.-† J17.3∗
– Manson's (intestinal) B65.1
– oriental B65.2
– pulmonary NEC B65.-† J99.8∗
– – pneumonia B65.-† J17.3∗
– Schistosoma
– – haematobium B65.0
– – japonicum B65.2
– – mansoni B65.1
– specified type NEC B65.8
– urinary B65.0
– vesical B65.0
Schizencephaly Q04.6
Schizoaffective psychosis F25.9
Schizodontia K00.2
Schizoid personality F60.1
Schizophrenia, schizophrenic F20.9
– acute (brief) (undifferentiated) F23.2
– atypical (form) F20.3
– borderline F21
– catalepsy F20.2
– catatonic (type) (excited) (withdrawn) F20.2
– cenesthopathic, cenesthesiopathic F20.8
– childhood type F84.5
– chronic undifferentiated F20.5
– cyclic F25.2
– disorganized (type) F20.1
– flexibilitas cerea F20.2
– hebephrenic (type) F20.1
– incipient F21
– latent F21
– negative type F20.5
– paranoid (type) F20.0
– paraphrenic F20.0
– postpsychotic depression F20.4
– prepsychotic F21
– prodromal F21
– pseudoneurotic F21
– pseudopsychopathic F21
– reaction F23.2
– residual (state) (type) F20.5
– Restzustand F20.5
– schizoaffective (type) – see Psychosis, schizoaffective

Schizophrenia, schizophrenic—*continued*
– simple (type) F20.6
– simplex F20.6
– specified type NEC F20.8
– stupor F20.2
– syndrome of childhood NEC F84.5
– undifferentiated (type) F20.3
– – chronic F20.5
Schizothymia (persistent) F60.1
Schlatter-Osgood disease or osteochondrosis M92.5
Schlatter's tibia M92.5
Schmidt's syndrome (polyglandular, autoimmune) E31.0
Schmincke's carcinoma or tumor (M8082/3) – *see* Neoplasm, nasopharynx, malignant
Schmitz(-Stutzer) dysentery A03.0
Schmorl's disease or nodes M51.4
Schneiderian
– carcinoma (M8121/3)
– – specified site – *see* Neoplasm, malignant
– – unspecified site C30.0
– papilloma (M8121/0)
– – specified site – *see* Neoplasm, benign
– – unspecified site D14.0
Scholz(-Bielchowsky-Henneberg) disease or syndrome E75.2
Schönlein(-Henoch) disease or purpura (primary) (rheumatic) D69.0
Schüller-Christian disease or syndrome C96.5
Schultze's type acroparesthesia, simple I73.8
Schultz's disease or syndrome D70
Schwalbe-Ziehen-Oppenheim disease G24.1
Schwannoma (M9560/0) – *see also* Neoplasm, nerve, benign
– malignant (M9560/3) – *see also* Neoplasm, nerve, malignant
– – with rhabdomyoblastic differentiation (M9561/3) – *see* Neoplasm, nerve, malignant
– melanocytic (M9560/0) – *see* Neoplasm, nerve, benign
– pigmented (M9560/0) – *see* Neoplasm, nerve, benign
Schwartz(-Jampel) syndrome Q78.8
Schweninger-Buzzi anetoderma L90.1
Sciatic – *see condition*
Sciatica (infective) M54.3
– with lumbago M54.4

Sciatica—*continued*
- with lumbago—*continued*
- - - due to intervertebral disk disorder
  M51.1† G55.1*
- due to displacement of intervertebral disk
  (with lumbago) M51.1† G55.1*

Scimitar syndrome Q26.8

Sclera – *see condition*

Sclerectasia H15.8

Scleredema
- adultorum M34.8
- Buschke's M34.8
- newborn P83.0

Sclerema
- adiposum (newborn) P83.0
- adultorum M34.8
- edematosum (newborn) P83.0
- newborn P83.0

Scleriasis – *see* Scleroderma

Scleritis (annular) (anterior)
  (granulomatous) (posterior)
  (suppurative) H15.0
- in (due to) zoster B02.3† H19.0*
- syphilitic A52.7† H19.0*
- tuberculous (nodular) A18.5† H19.0*

Sclerochoroiditis H31.8

Scleroconjunctivitis H15.0

Sclerocystic ovary syndrome E28.2

Sclerodactyly, sclerodactylia L94.3

Scleroderma, sclerodermia (diffuse)
  (generalized) M34.9
- circumscribed L94.0
- linear L94.1
- localized L94.0
- newborn P83.8
- pulmonary M34.8† J99.1*

Sclerokeratitis H16.8
- tuberculous A18.5† H19.2*

Scleroma nasi A48.8

Scleromalacia (perforans) H15.8

Scleromyxedema L98.5

Sclérose en plaques G35

Sclerosis, sclerotic
- adrenal (gland) E27.8
- Alzheimer's G30.9
- - dementia in G30.9† F00.9*
- amyotrophic (lateral) G12.2
- aorta, aortic I70.0
- - valve (*see also* Endocarditis, aortic)
  I35.8
- artery, arterial, arteriolar, arteriovascular –
  see Arteriosclerosis
- ascending multiple G35
- brain G37.9

Sclerosis, sclerotic—*continued*
- brain—*continued*
- - artery, arterial I67.2
- - atrophic lobar G31.0
- - - dementia in G31.0† F02.0*
- - diffuse G37.0
- - - familial (chronic) (infantile) E75.2
- - - infantile (chronic) (familial) E75.2
- - - Pelizaeus-Merzbacher type E75.2
- - disseminated G35
- - infantile (degenerative) (diffuse)
    (familial) E75.2
- - insular G35
- - Krabbe's E75.2
- - miliary G35
- - multiple G35
- - Pelizaeus-Merzbacher E75.2
- - presenile (Alzheimer's) G30.0
- - - dementia in G30.0† F00.0*
- - progressive familial E75.2
- - senile (arteriosclerotic) I67.2
- - stem, multiple G35
- - tuberous Q85.1
- bulbar, multiple G35
- bundle of His I44.3
- cardiac I25.1
- cardiorenal (*see also* Hypertension,
  cardiorenal) I13.9
- cardiovascular (*see also* Disease,
  cardiovascular) I51.6
- - renal (*see also* Hypertension,
  cardiorenal) I13.9
- centrolobar, familial E75.2
- cerebellar – *see* Sclerosis, brain
- cerebral – *see* Sclerosis, brain
- cerebrospinal (disseminated) (multiple)
  G35
- cerebrovascular I67.2
- choroid H31.1
- combined (spinal cord) – *see also*
  Degeneration, combined
- - multiple G35
- concentric (Balo) G37.5
- cornea H17.8
- coronary (artery) I25.1
- corpus cavernosum
- - female N90.8
- - male N48.6
- diffuse (brain) (spinal cord) G37.0
- disseminated G35
- dorsolateral (spinal cord) – *see*
  Degeneration, combined
- extrapyramidal G25.9

Sclerosis, sclerotic—*continued*
- focal and segmental (glomerular) – *code to* N00-N07 with fourth character .1
- Friedreich's (spinal cord) G11.1
- funicular (spermatic cord) N50.8
- general (vascular) – *see* Arteriosclerosis
- gland (lymphatic) I89.8
- globoid body, diffuse E75.2
- hepatic K74.1
- – alcoholic K70.2
- hereditary
- – cerebellar G11.9
- – – spinal (Friedreich's ataxia) G11.1
- insular G35
- kidney – *see* Sclerosis, renal
- larynx J38.7
- lateral (amyotrophic) (descending) (primary) (spinal) G12.2
- lens, senile nuclear H25.1
- liver K74.1
- – with fibrosis K74.2
- – – alcoholic K70.2
- – alcoholic K70.2
- – cardiac K76.1
- lobar, atrophic (of brain) G31.0
- – dementia in G31.0† F02.0*
- lung (*see also* Fibrosis, lung) J84.1
- mitral I05.8
- Mönckeberg's I70.2
- multiple (brain stem) (cerebral) (generalized) (spinal cord) G35
- myocardium, myocardial I25.1
- ovary N83.8
- pancreas K86.8
- penis N48.6
- peripheral arteries I70.2
- plaques G35
- pluriglandular E31.8
- polyglandular E31.8
- posterolateral (spinal cord) – *see* Degeneration, combined
- presenile (Alzheimer's) G30.0
- – dementia in G30.0† F00.0*
- primary, lateral G12.2
- progressive, systemic M34.0
- pulmonary (*see also* Fibrosis, lung) J84.1
- – artery I27.0
- – valve (heart) (*see also* Endocarditis, pulmonary) I37.8
- renal N26
- – with
- – – cystine storage disease E72.0† N29.8*

Sclerosis, sclerotic—*continued*
- renal—*continued*
- – with—*continued*
- – – hypertension (*see also* Hypertension, kidney) I12.9
- – – hypertensive heart disease (conditions in I11.-) (*see also* Hypertension, cardiorenal) I13.9
- – arteriolar (hyaline) (hyperplastic) (*see also* Hypertension, kidney) I12.9
- retina (senile) (vascular) H35.0
- senile (vascular) – *see* Arteriosclerosis
- spinal (cord) (progressive) G95.8
- – combined – *see also* Degeneration, combined
- – – multiple G35
- – – syphilitic A52.1† G32.0*
- – disseminated G35
- – dorsolateral – *see* Degeneration, combined
- – hereditary (Friedreich's) (mixed form) G11.1
- – lateral (amyotrophic) G12.2
- – multiple G35
- – posterior (syphilitic) A52.1† G32.8*
- stomach K31.8
- subendocardial, congenital I42.4
- systemic M34.9
- – with
- – – lung involvement M34.8† J99.1*
- – – myopathy M34.8† G73.7*
- – drug-induced M34.2
- – due to chemicals NEC M34.2
- – progressive M34.0
- – specified NEC M34.8
- tricuspid (heart) (valve) I07.8
- tuberous (brain) Q85.1
- tympanic membrane H73.8
- valve, valvular (heart) – *see* Endocarditis
- vascular – *see* Arteriosclerosis
- vein I87.8

Sclerotenonitis H15.0
Scoliosis (acquired) (postural) M41.9
- adolescent (idiopathic) M41.1
- congenital Q67.5
- – due to bony malformation Q76.3
- – failure of segmentation (hemivertebra) Q76.3
- – hemivertebra fusion Q76.3
- – postural Q67.5
- idiopathic NEC M41.2
- – infantile M41.0
- – juvenile M41.1

Scoliosis—*continued*
- neuromuscular M41.4
- paralytic M41.4
- postradiation therapy M96.5
- rachitic (late effect or sequelae) E64.3
- secondary (to) NEC M41.5
- – cerebral palsy, Friedreich's ataxia, poliomyelitis and other neuromuscular disorders M41.4
- specified form NEC M41.8
- thoracogenic M41.3
- tuberculous A18.0† M49.0*

Scoliotic pelvis with disproportion (fetopelvic) O33.0
- affecting fetus or newborn P03.1
- causing obstructed labor O65.0

Scorbutus, scorbutic (*see also* Scurvy) E54
- anemia D53.2

Scotoma (arcuate) (Bjerrum) (central) (ring) H53.4
- scintillating H53.1

Scratch – *see* Injury, superficial

Screening (for) Z13.9
- alcoholism Z13.3
- anemia Z13.0
- anomaly, congenital Z13.7
- antenatal – *see* Antenatal, screening
- arterial hypertension Z13.6
- arthropod-borne viral disease NEC Z11.5
- bacteriuria, asymptomatic Z13.8
- behavioral disorder Z13.3
- bronchitis, chronic Z13.8
- brucellosis Z11.2
- cardiovascular disorder NEC Z13.6
- cataract Z13.5
- Chagas' disease Z11.6
- chlamydial diseases Z11.8
- cholera Z11.0
- chromosomal abnormalities Z13.7
- – athletes Z10.3
- – by amniocentesis Z36.0
- – postnatal Z13.7
- congenital
- – dislocation of hip Z13.7
- – eye disorder Z13.5
- – malformation or deformation Z13.7
- contamination NEC Z13.8
- cystic fibrosis Z13.8
- dengue fever Z11.5
- dental disorder Z13.8
- depression Z13.3
- developmental handicap Z13.3
- – in early childhood Z13.4
- diabetes mellitus Z13.1

Screening—*continued*
- diphtheria Z11.2
- disease or disorder Z13.9
- – bacterial NEC Z11.2
- – blood or blood-forming organ Z13.0
- – cardiovascular NEC Z13.6
- – Chagas' Z11.6
- – chlamydial Z11.8
- – dental Z13.8
- – developmental NEC Z13.3
- – – in early childhood Z13.4
- – ear NEC Z13.5
- – endocrine NEC Z13.8
- – eye NEC Z13.5
- – gastrointestinal NEC Z13.8
- – genitourinary NEC Z13.8
- – heart NEC Z13.6
- – human immunodeficiency virus (HIV) infection Z11.4
- – immunity NEC Z13.0
- – infectious Z11.9
- – mental Z13.3
- – metabolic NEC Z13.8
- – neurological Z13.8
- – nutritional NEC Z13.2
- – protozoal Z11.6
- – – intestinal Z11.0
- – respiratory NEC Z13.8
- – rheumatic NEC Z13.8
- – rickettsial Z11.8
- – sexually transmitted NEC Z11.3
- – – human immunodeficiency virus (HIV) Z11.4
- – sickle-cell (trait) Z13.0
- – skin Z13.8
- – specified NEC Z13.8
- – spirochetal Z11.8
- – thyroid Z13.8
- – vascular NEC Z13.6
- – venereal Z11.3
- – viral NEC Z11.5
- – – human immunodeficiency virus (HIV) Z11.4
- – – intestinal Z11.0
- drugs Z04.0
- emphysema Z13.8
- encephalitis, viral (mosquito- or tick-borne) Z11.5
- fever
- – dengue Z11.5
- – hemorrhagic Z11.5
- – yellow Z11.5
- filariasis Z11.6
- galactosemia Z13.8

Screening—*continued*
- gastrointestinal condition NEC Z13.8
- genitourinary condition NEC Z13.8
- glaucoma Z13.5
- gout Z13.8
- helminthiasis (intestinal) Z11.6
- hematopoietic malignancy Z12.8
- hemoglobinopathies NEC Z13.0
- – antenatal Z36.8
- hemorrhagic fever Z11.5
- Hodgkin's disease Z12.8
- hormones Z04.0
- human immunodeficiency virus (HIV)
  Z11.4
- hypertension Z13.6
- immunity disorders Z13.0
- infection
- – intestinal (disease) Z11.0
- – – helminthiasis Z11.6
- – – specified NEC Z11.0
- – mycotic Z11.8
- – parasitic NEC Z11.8
- ingestion of radioactive substance Z13.8
- leishmaniasis Z11.6
- leprosy Z11.2
- leptospirosis Z11.8
- leukemia Z12.8
- lymphoma Z12.8
- malaria Z11.6
- malnutrition Z13.2
- measles Z11.5
- mental disorder or retardation Z13.3
- metabolic errors, inborn Z13.8
- multiphasic Z13.9
- mycoses Z11.8
- neoplasm (of) Z12.9
- – bladder Z12.6
- – blood Z12.8
- – breast Z12.3
- – cervix Z12.4
- – hematopoietic system Z12.8
- – intestinal tract NEC Z12.1
- – lymph (glands) Z12.8
- – prostate Z12.5
- – respiratory organs Z12.2
- – specified site NEC Z12.8
- – stomach Z12.0
- nephropathy Z13.8
- neurological condition Z13.8
- obesity Z13.8
- parasitic infestation Z11.9
- – specified NEC Z11.8
- phenylketonuria Z13.8
- plague Z11.2

Screening—*continued*
- poisoning (chemical) (heavy metal) Z13.8
- poliomyelitis Z11.5
- postnatal, chromosomal abnormalities
  Z13.7
- prenatal *see* Antenatal, screening
- protozoal disease Z11.6
- – intestinal Z11.0
- radiation exposure Z13.8
- respiratory condition NEC Z13.8
- – tuberculous Z11.1
- rheumatoid arthritis Z13.8
- rubella Z11.5
- schistosomiasis Z11.6
- sexually-transmitted disease NEC Z11.3
- – human immunodeficiency virus (HIV)
  Z11.4
- sickle-cell disease or trait Z13.0
- skin condition Z13.8
- sleeping sickness Z11.6
- special Z13.9
- – specified NEC Z13.8
- stimulants Z04.0
- tetanus Z11.2
- trachoma Z11.8
- trypanosomiasis Z11.6
- tuberculosis, respiratory Z11.1
- venereal disease Z11.3
- viral encephalitis (mosquito- or tick-
  borne) Z11.5
- whooping cough Z11.2
- worms, intestinal Z11.6
- yaws Z11.8
- yellow fever Z11.5

**Scrofula, scrofulosis (tuberculosis of
  cervical lymph glands)** A18.2
Scrofulide (primary) (tuberculous) A18.4
**Scrofuloderma, scrofulodermia (any site)
  (primary)** A18.4
**Scrofulosus lichen (primary)
  (tuberculous)** A18.4
Scrofulous – *see condition*
Scrotal tongue K14.5
Scrotum – *see condition*
Scurvy, scorbutic E54
- anemia D53.2
- gum E54† K93.8∗
- infantile E54
- rickets E54† M90.8∗
Seasickness T75.3
Seatworm (infection) (infestation) B80
Sebaceous – *see also condition*
- cyst (*see also* Cyst, sebaceous) L72.1

Seborrhea, seborrheic R23.8
– capitis L21.0
– dermatitis L21.9
– – infantile L21.1
– eczema L21.9
– – infantile L21.1
– keratosis L82
– sicca L21.0
Seckel's syndrome Q87.1
Seclusion, pupil H21.4
Secondary
– dentin (in pulp) K04.3
– neoplasm (M8000/6) – *see* Table of
neoplasms, secondary
Secretion
– catecholamine, by pheochromocytoma
E27.5
– hormone
– – antidiuretic, inappropriate (syndrome)
E22.2
– – by
– – – carcinoid tumor E34.0
– – – pheochromocytoma E27.5
– – ectopic NEC E34.2
– urinary
– – excessive R35
– – suppression R34
Section
– cesarean (*see also* Delivery, cesarean)
O82.9
– – affecting fetus or newborn P03.4
– – postmortem, affecting fetus or newborn
P01.6
– – previous, in pregnancy or childbirth
O34.2
– – – affecting fetus or newborn P03.8
– nerve, traumatic – *see* Injury, nerve
Seeking and accepting known hazardous
and harmful
– behavioral or psychological interventions
Z64.3
– chemical, nutritional or physical
interventions Z64.2
Segmentation, incomplete (congenital) –
see also Fusion
– bone NEC Q78.8
– lumbosacral (joint) (vertebra) Q76.4
Seizure(s) (*see also* Convulsions) R56.8
– akinetic G40.3
– apoplexy, apoplectic I64
– atonic G40.3
– autonomic (hysterical) F44.5
– brain or cerebral I64
– convulsive (*see also* Convulsions) R56.8

Seizure(s)—*continued*
– cortical (focal) (motor) G40.1
– epileptic (*see also* Epilepsy) G40.9
– – complex partial G40.2
– – localized onset G40.0
– – nonspecific (atonic) (clonic)
(myoclonic) (tonic) (tonic-clonic)
G40.3
– – simple partial G40.1
– epileptiform, epileptoid R56.8
– – focal G40.1
– febrile R56.0
– heart – *see* Disease, heart
– hysterical F44.5
– jacksonian (focal) (motor type) (sensory
type) G40.1
– newborn P90
– paralysis I64
– uncinate G40.2
Selenium deficiency, dietary E59
Self-damaging behavior (lifestyle) Z72.8
Self-harm (attempted)
– history (personal) Z91.5
– – in family Z81.8
– observation following (alleged) attempt
Z03.8
Self-mutilation
– history (personal) Z91.5
– – in family Z81.8
– observation following (alleged) attempt
Z03.8
Self neglect R46.8
– causing insufficient intake of food and
water R63.6
Self-poisoning
– history (personal) Z91.5
– – in family Z81.8
– observation following (alleged) attempt
Z03.6
Semicoma R40.1
Seminoma (M9061/3)
– anaplastic (M9062/3)
– – specified site – *see* Neoplasm,
malignant
– – unspecified site C62.9
– specified site – *see* Neoplasm, malignant
– spermatocytic (M9063/3)
– – specified site – *see* Neoplasm,
malignant
– – unspecified site C62.9
– unspecified site C62.9
Senear-Usher disease or syndrome L10.4
Senectus R54

Enterococcus faecalis
-Strep Group D

Senescence (without mention of psychosis) R54
Senile, senility (*see also condition*) R54
– with
– – acute confusional state F05.1
– – mental changes NEC F03
– – psychosis NEC (*see also* Psychosis, senile) F03
– asthenia R54
– cervix (atrophic) N88.8
– debility R54
– endometrium (atrophic) N85.8
– fallopian tube (atrophic) N83.3
– ovary (atrophic) N83.3
– premature E34.8
– wart (*see also* Keratosis, seborrheic) L82
Sensation
– burning (skin) R20.8
– loss of R20.8
– prickling (skin) R20.2
– tingling (skin) R20.2
Sense loss
– smell R43.1
– taste R43.2
– – and smell mixed R43.8
– touch R20.8
Sensibility disturbance of skin (deep) (vibratory) R20.8
Sensitive, sensitivity (*see also* Allergy) T78.4
– carotid sinus G90.0
– cold, autoimmune D59.1
– dentin K03.8
– methemoglobin D74.8
Sensitiver Beziehungswahn F22.0
Sensitization, auto-erythrocytic D69.2
Separation
– anxiety, abnormal (of childhood) F93.0
– apophysis, traumatic – *code as* Fracture, by site
– choroid H31.4
– epiphysis, epiphyseal, traumatic – *code as* Fracture, by site
– fracture – *see* Fracture
– joint (traumatic) (current) – *code as* Dislocation, by site
– placenta (normally implanted) (premature) (*see also* Abruptio placentae) O45.9
– pubic bone, obstetrical trauma O71.6
– retina, retinal – *see* Detachment, retina
– symphysis pubis, obstetrical trauma O71.6

Separation—*continued*
– tracheal ring, incomplete, congenital Q32.1
Sepsis (generalized) (*see also* Infection) A41.9
– actinomycotic A42.7
– adrenal haemorrhage syndrome (meningococcal) A39.1† E35.1*
– anaerobic A41.4
– Bacillus anthracis A22.7
– bacterial, newborn P36.9
– – due to
– – – anaerobes NEC P36.5
– – – Escherichia coli P36.4
– – – Staphylococcus NEC P36.3
– – – – aureus P36.2
– – – streptococcus NEC P36.1
– – – – group B P36.0
– – specified type NEC P36.8
– Brucella (*see also* Brucellosis) A23.9
– candidal B37.7
– cryptogenic A41.9
– due to device, implant or graft (*see also* Complications, by site and type, infection or inflammation) T85.7
– – arterial graft NEC T82.7
– – breast (implant) T85.7
– – catheter NEC T85.7
– – – dialysis (renal) T82.7
– – – – intraperitoneal T85.7
– – – infusion NEC T82.7
– – – – spinal (epidural) (subdural) T85.7
– – – urinary (indwelling) T83.5
– – electronic (electrode) (pulse generator) (stimulator)
– – – bone T84.7
– – – cardiac T82.7
– – – nervous system (brain) (peripheral nerve) (spinal) T85.7
– – – urinary T83.5
– – fixation, internal (orthopedic) NEC T84.6
– – – orthopedic NEC T84.7
– – gastrointestinal (bile duct) (esophagus) T85.7
– – genital NEC T83.6
– – heart NEC T82.7
– – – valve (prosthesis) T82.6
– – – – graft T82.7
– – joint prosthesis T84.5
– – ocular (corneal graft) (orbital implant) NEC T85.7
– – orthopedic NEC T84.7
– – specified NEC T85.7

Neutropenic Sepsis A41.- +D70.X [handwritten]

Sepsis—*continued*
- due to device, implant or graft—*continued*
- – urinary NEC T83.5
- – vascular NEC T82.7
- – ventricular intracranial shunt T85.7
- during labour O75.3
- Erysipelothrix (erysipeloid) (rhusiopathiae) A26.7
- Escherichia coli A41.5 [underlined]
- extraintestinal yersiniosis A28.2
- following
- – abortion (subsequent episode) O08.0
- – – current episode – *see* Abortion
- – ectopic or molar pregnancy O08.0
- – immunization T88.0
- – infusion, therapeutic injection or transfusion T80.2
- gangrenous A41.9
- gonococcal A54.8
- Gram-negative (organism) A41.5
- – anaerobic A41.4
- Haemophilus influenzae A41.3
- herpesviral B00.7
- intraocular H44.0
- Listeria monocytogenes A32.7
- localized, in operation wound T81.4
- meliodosis A24.1
- meningeal – *see* Meningitis
- meningococcal A39.4
- – acute A39.2
- – chronic A39.3
- newborn NEC P36.9
- – due to
- – – anaerobes NEC P36.5
- – – Escherichia coli P36.4
- – – Staphylococcus NEC P36.3
- – – – aureus P36.2
- – – streptococcus NEC P36.1
- – – – group B P36.0
- – specified NEC P36.8
- Pasteurella multocida A28.0
- pelvic, puerperal, postpartum, childbirth O85
- pneumococcal A40.3
- puerperal, postpartum, childbirth (pelvic) O85
- Salmonella (arizonae) (cholerae-suis) (enteritidis) (typhimurium) A02.1
- severe, as a result of disease classified elsewhere R65.1
- Shigella (*see also* Dysentery, bacillary) A03.9
- specified organism NEC A41.8
- Staphylococcus, staphylococcal A41.2

Sepsis—*continued*
- Staphylococcus, staphylococcal— *continued*
- – aureus A41.0
- – coagulase-negative A41.1
- – specified NEC A41.1
- Streptococcus, streptococcal A40.9
- – agalactiae A40.1
- – group
- – – A A40.0
- – – B A40.1
- – – D A40.2
- – neonatal P36.1
- – pneumoniae A40.3
- – pyogenes A40.0
- – specified NEC A40.8
- tracheostomy stoma J95.0
- tularemic A21.7
- umbilical (newborn) (organism unspecified) P36.-
- – tetanus A33
- urinary N39.0
- Yersinia pestis A20.7

Septate – *see* Septum
Septic – *see also* condition
- arm (with lymphangitis) L03.1
- embolus – *see* Embolism
- finger (with lymphangitis) L03.0
- foot (with lymphangitis), except toe(s) L03.1
- gallbladder (acute) K81.0
- hand (with lymphangitis) L03.1
- joint M00.9
- leg (with lymphangitis), except toe(s) L03.1
- nail L03.0
- sore (*see also* Abscess) L02.9
- – throat J02.0
- – – streptococcal J02.0
- spleen (acute) D73.8
- throat (*see also* Pharyngitis) J02.0
- thrombus – *see* Thrombosis
- toe (with lymphangitis) L03.0
- tonsils, chronic J35.0
- umbilical cord P38
- uterus (*see also* Endometritis) N71.9

Septicemia, septicemic (generalized) (suppurative) – *see* Sepsis
Septum, septate (congenital) – *see also* Anomaly, by site
- anal Q42.3
- – with fistula Q42.2
- aqueduct of Sylvius Q03.0

Septum, septate—*continued*
- aqueduct of Sylvius—*continued*
- – – with spina bifida (*see also* Spina bifida,
  with hydrocephalus) Q05.4
- uterus (*see also* Double uterus) Q51.2
- vagina Q52.1
- – in pregnancy or childbirth O34.6
- – – causing obstructed labor O65.5

Sequelae (of) – *see also condition*
- abscess, intracranial or intraspinal
  (conditions in G06.-) G09
- amputation
- – postoperative NEC (late) T98.3
- – traumatic T94.1
- – – face T90.8
- – – head (parts) T90.8
- – – limb
- – – – lower T93.6
- – – – upper T92.6
- – – multiple body regions T94.0
- – – trunk T91.8
- burn and corrosion T95.9
- – classified according to extent of body
  surface involved T95.4
- – eye T95.8
- – face, head and neck T95.0
- – limb
- – – lower T95.3
- – – upper T95.2
- – multiple body regions T95.8
- – specified site NEC T95.8
- – trunk T95.1
- calcium deficiency E64.8
- cerebrovascular disease NEC I69.8
- childbirth complication O94
- – resulting in death (one year or more
  after delivery) O97.-
- – – between 42 days and one year after
  delivery O96.-
- complication(s) of
- – childbirth (delivery), pregnancy or
  puerperium O94
- – – resulting in death (one year or more
  after delivery) O97.-
- – – – between 42 days and one year after
  delivery O96.-
- – surgical and medical care T98.3
- – trauma (conditions in T79.-) T98.2
- contusion T94.1
- – face T90.0
- – head T90.0
- – limb
- – – lower T93.8
- – – upper T92.8

Sequelae—*continued*
- contusion—*continued*
- – – multiple body regions T94.0
- – – neck T91.0
- – – trunk T91.0
- corrosion – *see* Sequelae, burn and
  corrosion
- crushing injury T94.1
- – face T90.8
- – head T90.8
- – limb
- – – lower T93.6
- – – upper T92.6
- – multiple body regions T94.0
- – neck T91.8
- – trunk T91.8
- delivery complication O94
- – resulting in death (one year or more
  after delivery) O97.-
- – – between 42 days and one year after
  delivery O96.-
- dislocation T94.1
- – jaw T90.8
- – limb
- – – lower T93.3
- – – upper T92.3
- – lower back T91.8
- – multiple body regions T94.0
- – neck T91.8
- – pelvis T91.8
- – thorax T91.8
- – trunk T91.8
- effect of external cause NEC T98.1
- encephalitis or encephalomyelitis
  (conditions in G04.-) G09
- – in infectious disease NEC B94.8
- – viral B94.1
- external cause NEC T98.1
- foreign body entering natural orifice
  T98.0
- fracture T94.1
- – facial bones T90.2
- – femur T93.1
- – finger and thumb T92.2
- – limb
- – – lower NEC T93.2
- – – – femur T93.1
- – – upper NEC T92.1
- – – – finger and thumb T92.2
- – – – wrist and hand T92.2
- – multiple body regions T94.0
- – pelvis T91.2
- – shoulder (girdle) T92.1
- – skull T90.2

Sequelae—*continued*
- fracture—*continued*
- − − spine T91.1
- − − thorax, thoracic T91.2
- − − − spine T91.1
- − − wrist and hand T92.2
- − frostbite T95.9
- − − eye T95.8
- − − face, head and neck T95.0
- − − limb
- − − − lower T95.3
- − − − upper T95.2
- − − multiple body regions T95.8
- − − specified site NEC T95.8
- − − trunk T95.1
- − Hansen's disease B92
- − hemorrhage
- − − intracerebral I69.1
- − − intracranial, nontraumatic NEC I69.2
- − − subarachnoid I69.0
- − hepatitis, viral B94.2
- − hyperalimentation E68
- − infarction, cerebral I69.3
- − infection, pyogenic, intracranial or intraspinal G09
- − infectious disease B94.9
- − − specified NEC B94.8
- − injury NEC T94.1
- − − blood vessel T94.1
- − − − abdomen and pelvis T91.8
- − − − head T90.8
- − − − − intracranial T90.5
- − − − − − with skull fracture T90.2
- − − − limb
- − − − − lower T93.8
- − − − − upper T92.8
- − − − neck T91.8
- − − − thorax T91.8
- − − brain T90.5
- − − eye and orbit T90.4
- − − head T90.9
- − − − specified NEC T90.8
- − − internal organ T91.9
- − − − abdomen T91.5
- − − − specified NEC T91.8
- − − − thorax T91.4
- − − intra-abdominal (organs) T91.5
- − − intracranial (organs) T90.5
- − − − with skull fracture T90.2
- − − intrathoracic (organs) T91.4
- − − limb
- − − − lower T93.9
- − − − − specified NEC T93.8
- − − − upper T92.9

Sequelae—*continued*
- − injury NEC—*continued*
- − − limb—*continued*
- − − − upper—*continued*
- − − − − specified NEC T92.8
- − − multiple body regions T94.0
- − − muscle T94.1
- − − − limb
- − − − − lower T93.5
- − − − − upper T92.5
- − − − multiple body regions T94.0
- − − − neck T91.8
- − − − trunk T91.8
- − − neck T91.9
- − − − specified NEC T91.8
- − − nerve NEC T94.1
- − − − cranial T90.3
- − − − multiple body regions T94.0
- − − − neck T91.8
- − − − peripheral NEC T94.1
- − − − − lower limb and pelvic girdle T93.4
- − − − − upper limb and shoulder girdle T92.4
- − − − roots and plexus(es), spinal T91.8
- − − − trunk T91.8
- − − spine, spinal T91.8
- − − − cord T91.3
- − − − nerve root(s) and plexus(es) T91.8
- − − superficial T94.1
- − − − face T90.0
- − − − head T90.0
- − − − limb
- − − − − lower T93.8
- − − − − upper T92.8
- − − − multiple body regions T94.0
- − − − neck T91.0
- − − − trunk T91.0
- − − tendon T94.1
- − − − face and head T90.8
- − − − limb
- − − − − lower T93.5
- − − − − upper T92.5
- − − − multiple body regions T94.0
- − − − neck T91.8
- − − − trunk T91.8
- − − trunk T91.9
- − − − specified NEC T91.8
- − leprosy B92
- − meningitis
- − − bacterial (conditions in G00.-) G09
- − − other or unspecified cause (conditions in G03.-) G09
- − muscle (and tendon) injury T94.1

Sequelae—*continued*
- muscle—*continued*
- - face T90.8
- - head T90.8
- - limb
- - - lower T93.5
- - - upper T92.5
- - multiple body regions T94.0
- - neck T91.8
- - trunk T91.8
- myelitis (*see also* Sequelae, encephalitis) G09
- niacin deficiency E64.8
- nutritional deficiency E64.9
- - specified NEC E64.8
- obstetric cause O94
- - resulting in death (one year or more after delivery) O97.-
- - - between 42 days and one year after delivery O96.-
- parasitic disease B94.9
- phlebitis or thrombophlebitis of intracranial or intraspinal venous sinuses and veins (conditions in G08) G09
- poisoning due to
- - drug, medicament or biological substance T96
- - nonmedicinal substance T97
- poliomyelitis (acute) B91
- pregnancy complication(s) O94
- - resulting in death (one year or more after delivery) O97.-
- - - between 42 days and one year after delivery O96.-
- protein-energy malnutrition E64.0
- puerperium complication(s) O94
- - resulting in death (one year or more after delivery) O97.-
- - - between 42 days and one year after delivery O96.-
- radiation T98.1
- rickets E64.3
- selenium deficiency E64.8
- sprain and strain T94.1
- - jaw T90.8
- - limb
- - - lower T93.3
- - - upper T92.3
- - multiple body regions T94.0
- - neck T91.8
- - trunk T91.8
- stroke NEC I69.4
- tendon and muscle injury – *see* Sequelae, muscle injury

Sequelae—*continued*
- thiamine deficiency E64.8
- toxic effect of
- - drug, medicament or biological substance T96
- - nonmedicinal substance T97
  trachoma B94.0
- tuberculosis B90.9
- - bones and joints B90.2
- - central nervous system B90.0
- - genitourinary B90.1
- - pulmonary (respiratory) B90.9
- - specified organs NEC B90.8
- viral
- - encephalitis B94.1
- - hepatitis B94.2
- vitamin deficiency NEC E64.8
- - A E64.1
- - B E64.8
- - C E64.2
- wound, open T94.1
- - eye and orbit T90.4
- - face T90.1
- - head T90.1
- - limb
- - - lower T93.0
- - - upper T92.0
- - multiple body regions T94.0
- - neck T91.0
- - trunk T91.0

Sequestration – *see also* Sequestrum
- lung, congenital Q33.2

Sequestrum
- bone M86.6
- dental K10.2
- jaw bone K10.2
- orbit H05.1
- sinus (accessory) (nasal) (*see also* Sinusitis) J32.9

Sequoiosis, lung, or pneumonitis J67.8

Serology for syphilis
- doubtful
- - with signs or symptoms – *code as* Syphilis, by site and stage
- - follow-up of latent syphilis – *see* Syphilis, latent
- false-positive R76.2
- positive A53.0
- - with signs or symptoms – *code as* Syphilis, by site and stage
- - false R76.2
- reactivated A53.0

Seroma – *see* Hematoma

Seropurulent – *see condition*

Serositis, multiple K65.8
− peritoneal K65.8
Serous − *see condition*
Sertoli cell
− adenoma (M8640/0)
− − specified site − *see* Neoplasm, benign
− − unspecified site
− − − female D27
− − − male D29.2
− carcinoma (M8640/3)
− − specified site − *see* Neoplasm,
  malignant
− − unspecified site C62.9
− − − female C56
− − − male C62.9
− tumor (M8640/0)
− − with lipid storage (M8641/0)
− − − specified site − *see* Neoplasm, benign
− − − unspecified site
− − − − female D27
− − − − male D29.2
− − specified site − *see* Neoplasm, benign
− − unspecified site
− − − female D27
− − − male D29.2
Sertoli-Leydig cell tumor (M8631/0)
− specified site − *see* Neoplasm, benign
− unspecified site
− − female D27
− − male D29.2
Serum
− allergy, allergic reaction T80.6
− − shock T80.5
− complication or reaction NEC T80.6
− disease NEC T80.6
− hepatitis (*see also* Hepatitis, viral, type B)
  B16.9
− intoxication T80.6
− neuropathy G61.1
− poisoning NEC T80.6
− rash NEC T80.6
− sickness NEC T80.6
− urticaria T80.6
Sesamoiditis M86.8
Sever's disease or osteochondrosis M92.6
Sex
− chromosome mosaics Q97.8
− − lines with various numbers of X
  chromosomes Q97.2
− education Z70.8
Sextuplet, affecting fetus or newborn
  P01.5
− pregnancy O30.8

Sexuality, pathologic (*see also* Deviation,
  sexual) F65.9
Sézary disease, reticulosis or syndrome
  C84.1
Shadow, lung R91
Shaking palsy or paralysis (*see also*
  Parkinsonism) G20
Shallowness, acetabulum M24.8
Shaver's disease J63.1
Sheath (tendon) − *see condition*
Sheathing, retinal vessels H35.0
Shedding
− nail L60.8
− premature, primary (deciduous) teeth
  K00.6
Sheehan's disease or syndrome E23.0
Shelf, rectal K62.8
Shell teeth K00.5
Shellshock (current) F43.0
− lasting state F43.1
Shield kidney Q63.1
Shift
− auditory threshold (temporary) H93.2
− mediastinal R93.8
Shiga(-Kruse) dysentery A03.0
Shigella (dysentery), shigellosis (*see also*
  Dysentery, bacillary) A03.9
Shin splints T79.6
Shingles − *see* Herpes, zoster
Shipyard disease or eye B30.0† H19.2∗
Shirodkar suture, in pregnancy O34.3
Shock R57.9
− adrenal (cortical) (Addisonian) E27.2
− adverse food reaction (anaphylactic)
  T78.0
− allergic − *see* Shock, anaphylactic
− anaphylactic T78.2
− − chemical − *see* Table of drugs and
  chemicals
− − correct medicinal substance properly
  administered T88.6
− − drug or medicinal substance
− − − correct substance properly
  administered T88.6
− − − overdose or wrong substance given
  or taken T50.9
− − − − specified drug − *see* Table of drugs
  and chemicals
− − following sting(s) T63.9
− − − arthropod NEC T63.4
− − − bee T63.4
− − − hornet T63.4
− − − insect NEC T63.4
− − − jelly-fish T63.6

Shock—*continued*
- anaphylactic—*continued*
- – following sting(s)—*continued*
- – – marine animal NEC T63.6
- – – scorpion T63.2
- – – sea-anemone T63.6
- – – shellfish T63.6
- – – starfish T63.6
- – – wasp T63.4
- – food T78.0
- – – marine animal NEC T63.6
- – immunization T80.5
- – serum T80.5
- anaphylactoid – *see* Shock, anaphylactic
- anesthetic
- – correct substance properly administered T88.2
- – overdose or wrong substance given T41.1
- – – specified anesthetic – *see* Table of drugs and chemicals
- birth, fetus or newborn NEC P96.8
- cardiogenic R57.0
- chemical substance – *see* Table of drugs and chemicals
- culture F43.2
- drug T78.2
- – correct substance properly administered T88.6
- – overdose or wrong drug given or taken T50.9
- – – specified drug – *see* Table of drugs and chemicals
- during or after labor and delivery O75.1
- electric T75.4
- endotoxic R57.8
- – due to surgical procedure T81.1
- – during or following procedure T81.1
- following
- – abortion (subsequent episode) O08.3
- – – current episode – *see* Abortion
- – ectopic or molar pregnancy O08.3
- – injury (delayed) (immediate) T79.4
- – labor and delivery O75.1
- food (anaphylactic) T78.0
- hypovolemic R57.1
- – surgical T81.1
- – traumatic T79.4
- lightning T75.0
- lung J80
- obstetric O75.1
- – following abortion (subsequent episode) O08.3
- – – current episode – *see* Abortion

Shock—*continued*
- postoperative T81.1
- psychic F43.0
- septic R57.2
- – due to
- – – infusion, therapeutic injection or transfusion T80.2
- – – surgical procedure T81.1
- – following
- – – abortion (subsequent episode) O08.0
- – – – current episode – *see* Abortion
- – – ectopic or molar pregnancy O08.0
- specified NEC R57.8
- spinal (*see also* Injury, spinal cord, by region) T09.3
- surgical T81.1
- therapeutic misadventure NEC (*see also* Complications) T81.1
- toxic, syndrome A48.3
- transfusion – *see* Complications, transfusion
- traumatic (delayed) (immediate) T79.4

Shoemaker's chest M95.4
Shoplifting, without manifest psychiatric disorder Z03.2
Short, shortening, shortness
- arm (acquired) M21.7
- – congenital Q71.8
- breath R06.0
- common bile duct, congenital Q44.5
- cord (umbilical), complicating delivery O69.3
- – affecting fetus or newborn P02.6
- cystic duct, congenital Q44.5
- esophagus (congenital) Q39.8
- femur (acquired) M21.7
- – congenital Q72.4
- frenum, frenulum, linguae (congenital) Q38.1
- hip (acquired) M21.7
- – congenital Q65.8
- leg (acquired) M21.7
- – congenital Q72.8
- limbed stature, with immunodeficiency D82.2
- metatarsus (congenital) Q66.8
- – acquired M21.8
- organ or site, congenital NEC – *see* Distortion
- palate, congenital Q38.5
- radius (acquired) M21.7
- – congenital Q71.4
- rib syndrome Q77.2
- stature NEC (*see also* Dwarfism) E34.3

Short, shortening—*continued*
- stature NEC—*continued*
- – constitutional E34.3
- – hypochondroplastic Q77.4
- – hypophyseal E23.0
- – Laron-type E34.3
- – Lorain-Levi E23.0
- – nutritional E45
- – pituitary E23.0
- – psychosocial E34.3
- – renal N25.0
- – thanatophoric Q77.1
- tendon M67.1
- – with contracture of joint M24.5
- – Achilles (acquired) M67.0
- – – congenital Q66.8
- – congenital Q79.8
- thigh (acquired) M21.7
- – congenital Q72.4
- tibialis anterior (tendon) M67.1
- umbilical cord
- – complicating delivery O69.3
- – – affecting fetus or newborn P02.6
- urethra N36.8
- uvula, congenital Q38.5
- vagina (congenital) Q52.4

Shortsightedness H52.1
Shoulder – *see condition*
Shovel-shaped incisors K00.2
Shower, thromboembolic – *see* Embolism
Shunt
- arteriovenous (dialysis) Z99.2
- – pulmonary (acquired) NEC I28.0
- – – congenital Q25.7
- cerebral ventricle (communicating) in situ Z98.2
- surgical, prosthetic, with complications – *see* Complications, graft, arterial

Shutdown, renal (*see also* Failure, kidney) N19
- following
- – abortion (subsequent episode) O08.4
- – – current episode – *see* Abortion
- – ectopic or molar pregnancy O08.4

Shy-Drager syndrome G90.3
Sialadenitis, sialitis, sialoadenitis (any gland) (chronic) (suppurative) K11.2
Sialectasia K11.8
Sialidosis E77.1
Sialoadenopathy K11.9
Sialodochitis (fibrinosa) K11.2
Sialodocholithiasis K11.5
Sialolithiasis K11.5
Sialometaplasia, necrotizing K11.8

Sialorrhea (*see also* Ptyalism) K11.7
Sialosis K11.7
Siamese twin Q89.4
Sibling rivalry, affecting child Z61.2
Sicard's syndrome G52.7
Sicca syndrome M35.0
- with
- – keratoconjunctivits M35.0† H19.3*
- – lung involvement M35.0† J99.1*
- – myopathy M35.0† G73.7*
- – renal tubulo-interstitial disorders M35.0† N16.4*

Sick R69
- or handicapped person in family Z63.7
- – needing care at home Z63.6
- sinus (syndrome) I49.5

Sick-euthyroid syndrome E07.8
Sickle-cell anemia (*see also* Disease, sickle-cell) D57.1
- with crisis D57.0

Sicklemia (*see also* Disease, sickle-cell) D57.1
Sickness
- air (travel) T75.3
- alpine T70.2
- altitude T70.2
- aviator's T70.2
- balloon T70.2
- car T75.3
- catheter NEC T85.8
- compressed air T70.3
- decompression T70.3
- motion T75.3
- mountain T70.2
- protein T80.6
- radiation NEC T66
- roundabout (motion) T75.3
- sea T75.3
- serum NEC T80.6
- sleeping (African) (*see also* Trypanosomiasis, African) B56.9
- swing (motion) T75.3
- train (railway) (travel) T75.3
- travel (any vehicle) T75.3

Siderosilicosis J62.8
Siderosis (lung) J63.4
- eye (globe) H44.3
Siemens' syndrome Q82.8
Sighing R06.8
- psychogenic F45.3
Sigmoid – *see also condition*
- flexure – *see condition*
- kidney Q63.1

Sigmoiditis (*see also* Enteritis) A09.9
- infectious A09.0
- noninfectious K52.9
Silicosiderosis J62.8
Silicosis, silicotic (complicated) (simple) J62.8
- with tuberculosis J65
Silicotuberculosis J65
Silo-filler's disease J68.8
Silver's syndrome Q87.1
Simian malaria B53.1
Simmonds' cachexia or disease E23.0
Simons' disease or syndrome E88.1
Simple, simplex – *see condition*
Simulation, conscious (of illness) Z76.5
Sin Nombre virus disease (Hantavirus (cardio-)pulmonary syndrome B33.4† J17.1*
Sinding-Larsen disease or osteochondrosis M92.4
Singer's node or nodule J38.2
Single
- atrium Q21.2
- umbilical artery Q27.0
- ventricle Q20.4
Singultus R06.6
- epidemicus B33.0
Sinus – *see also* Fistula
- arrest I45.5
- arrhythmia I49.8
- bradycardia R00.1
- branchial cleft (external) (internal) Q18.0
- coccygeal L05.9
- – with abscess L05.0
- dental K04.6
- dermal (congenital) L05.9
- – with abscess L05.0
- – coccygeal, pilonidal – *see* Sinus, coccygeal
- infected, skin NEC L08.8
- marginal, ruptured or bleeding O46.8
- – with placenta previa O44.1
- – – affecting fetus or newborn P02.0
- – affecting fetus or newborn P02.1
- medial, face and neck Q18.8
- pause I45.5
- pericranii Q01.9
- pilonidal (infected) (rectum) L05.9
- – with abscess L05.0
- pretragal Q18.1
- preauricular Q18.1
- rectovaginal N82.3
- Rokitansky-Aschoff (gallbladder) K82.8
- tachycardia R00.0

Sinus—*continued*
- tachycardia—*continued*
- – paroxysmal I47.1
- testis N50.8
- tract (postinfective) – *see* Fistula
Sinusitis (accessory) (chronic) (hyperplastic) (nasal) (nonpurulent) (purulent) J32.9
- acute J01.9
- – ethmoidal J01.2
- – frontal J01.1
- – involving more than one sinus but not pansinusitis J01.8
- – maxillary J01.0
- – specified NEC J01.8
- – sphenoidal J01.3
- allergic (*see also* Rhinitis, allergic) J30.4
- due to high altitude T70.1
- ethmoidal J32.2
- – acute J01.2
- frontal J32.1
- – acute J01.1
- influenzal (*see also* Influenza, with, respiratory manifestations) J11.1
- involving more than one sinus but not pansinusitis J32.8
- maxillary J32.0
- – acute J01.0
- sphenoidal J32.3
- – acute J01.3
- tuberculous, any sinus A16.8
- – with bacteriological and histological confirmation A15.8
Sinusitis-bronchiectasis-situs inversus (syndrome) (triad) Q89.3
Sirenomelia (syndrome) Q87.2
Siriasis T67.0
Siti A65
Situational
- disturbance (transient) (*see also* Reaction, adjustment) F43.2
- – acute F43.0
- maladjustment (*see also* Reaction, adjustment) F43.2
- reaction (*see also* Reaction, adjustment) F43.2
- – acute F43.0
Situs inversus or transversus (abdominalis) (thoracis) Q89.3
Sixth disease B08.2
Sjögren-Larsson syndrome Q87.1
Sjögren's syndrome or disease (*see also* Sicca syndrome) M35.0
Skeletal – *see condition*

Skene's gland – *see condition*
Skenitis (*see also* Urethritis) N34.2
Skerljevo A65
Skevas-Zerfus disease T63.6
Skin – *see also condition*
– clammy R23.1
Slate-dresser's or slate-miner's lung J62.8
Sleep
– apnea G47.3
– – newborn P28.3
– disorder or disturbance G47.9
– – nonorganic origin F51.9
– – specified NEC G47.8
– disturbance G47.9
– rhythm inversion G47.2
– – nonorganic origin F51.2
– terrors F51.4
– walking F51.3
– – hysterical F44.8
Sleeping sickness NEC (*see also* Sickness, sleeping) B56.9
Sleeplessness G47.0
– psychogenic F51.0
Sleep-wake schedule disorder G47.2
Slim disease (in HIV infection) B22.2
Slipped, slipping
– epiphysis M93.9
– – traumatic (old) M93.9
– – – current – *code as* Fracture, by site
– – upper femoral (nontraumatic) M93.0
– intervertebral disk – *see* Displacement, intervertebral disk
– ligature, umbilical P51.8
– patella M22.3
– rib M89.8
– sacroiliac joint M53.2
– ulnar nerve, nontraumatic G56.2
– vertebra NEC (*see also* Spondylolisthesis) M43.1
Sloughing (multiple) (phagedena) (skin) (*see also* Gangrene) R02
– abscess (*see also* Abscess) L02.9
– appendix K38.8
– fascia M79.8
– scrotum N50.8
– ulcer (*see also* Ulcer, skin) L98.4
Slow
– feeding, newborn P92.2
– fetal growth NEC P05.9
– – affecting management of pregnancy O36.5
– heart(beat) R00.1
– rebound (transient) following surgery Z48.8

Slowing, urinary stream R39.1
Sluder's neuralgia (syndrome) G44.8
Slurring, slurred speech R47.8
Small(ness)
– fetus or newborn for gestational age P05.1
– introitus, vagina N89.6
– kidney (unknown cause) N27.9
– – bilateral N27.1
– – unilateral N27.0
– ovary (congenital) Q50.3
– pelvis
– – with disproportion (fetopelvic) O33.1
– – – affecting fetus or newborn P03.1
– – – causing obstructed labor O65.1
– uterus N85.8
Small-and-light-for-dates (infant) P05.1
– affecting management of pregnancy O36.5
Small-for-dates (infant) P05.1
– affecting management of pregnancy O36.5
Smallpox B03
Smith-Lemli-Opitz syndrome Q87.1
Smith's fracture (separation) S52.5
Smoker's
– palate K13.2
– throat J31.2
Smoking, passive Z58.7
Smothering spells R06.8
Snapping
– finger M65.3
– hip M24.8
– – involving iliotibial band M76.3
– knee M23.8
– – involving iliotibial band M76.3
Sneddon-Wilkinson disease or syndrome L13.1
Sneezing (intractable) R06.7
Sniffing
– cocaine (habitual) F14.2
– gasoline F18.-
– – addiction F18.2
– glue (airplane) F18.-
– – addiction F18.2
– petrol F18.-
– – addiction F18.2
Snoring R06.5
Snow blindness H16.1
Snuffles (non-syphilitic) R06.5
– newborn P28.8
– syphilitic (infant) A50.0† J99.8*
Social
– exclusion Z60.4

Social—*continued*
- exclusion—*continued*
- – due to discrimination or persecution (perceived) Z60.5
- migrant Z59.0
- – acculturation difficulty Z60.3
- rejection Z60.4
- – due to discrimination or persecution Z60.5
- role conflict NEC Z73.5
- skills inadequacy NEC Z73.4
- transplantation Z60.3

Sodoku A25.0
Soemmerring's ring H26.4
Soft – *see also* condition
- nails L60.3

Softening
- bone – *see* Osteomalacia
- brain (necrotic) (progressive) G93.8
- – arteriosclerotic I63.8
- – congenital Q04.8
- – embolic I63.4
- – hemorrhagic (*see also* Hemorrhage, intracerebral) I61.9
- – occlusive I63.5
- – thrombotic I63.3
- cartilage M94.8
- cerebellar – *see* Softening, brain
- cerebral – *see* Softening, brain
- cerebrospinal – *see* Softening, brain
- spinal cord G95.8
- stomach K31.8

Soldier's heart F45.3
Solitary kidney, congenital Q60.0
Solvent abuse F18.1
Somatization reaction, somatic reaction – *see* Disorder, somatoform
Somnambulism F51.3
- hysterical F44.8

Somnolence R40.0
- nonorganic origin F51.1
- periodic G47.8

Sonne dysentery A03.3
Sore
- chiclero B55.1
- Delhi B55.1
- desert (*see also* Ulcer, skin) L98.4
- eye H57.1
- Lahore B55.1
- mouth K13.7
- muscle M79.1
- Naga (*see also* Ulcer, skin) L98.4
- oriental B55.1
- pressure L89.-

Sore—*continued*
- pressure—*continued*
- – stage
- – – I L89.0
- – – II L89.1
- – – III L89.2
- – – IV L89.3
- skin NEC L98.-
- soft A57
- throat (acute) (*see also* Pharyngitis) J02.9
- – with influenza, flu, or grippe (*see also* Influenza, with, respiratory manifestations) J11.1
- – chronic J31.2
- – coxsackie (virus) B08.5
- – diphtheritic A36.0
- – herpesviral B00.2
- – influenzal (*see also* Influenza, with, respiratory manifestations) J11.1
- – septic J02.0
- – streptococcal (ulcerative) J02.0
- – viral NEC J02.8
- – – coxsackie B08.5
- tropical (*see also* Ulcer, skin) L98.4
- veldt (*see also* Ulcer, skin) L98.4

Soto's syndrome Q87.3
Spacing, abnormal, tooth, teeth K07.3
Spade-like hand (congenital) Q68.1
Spading nail L60.8
- congenital Q84.6

Sparganosis B70.1
Spasm(s), spastic, spasticity (*see also* condition) R25.2
- accommodation H52.5
- ampulla of Vater K83.4
- anus, ani (sphincter) (reflex) K59.4
- – psychogenic F45.3
- artery NEC I73.9
- – cerebral G45.9
- Bell's G51.3
- bladder (sphincter, external or internal) N32.8
- – psychogenic F45.3
- bronchus, bronchiole J98.0
- cardia K22.0
- cardiac I20.1
- carpopedal (*see also* Tetany) R29.0
- cerebral (arteries) (vascular) G45.9
- cervix, complicating delivery O62.4
- – affecting fetus or newborn P03.6
- ciliary body (of accommodation) H52.5
- colon K58.9
- – with diarrhea K58.0
- – psychogenic F45.3

Spasm(s), spastic—*continued*
- common duct K83.8
- compulsive (*see also* Tic) F95.9
- conjugate H51.8
- coronary (artery) I20.1
- diaphragm (reflex) R06.6
- – epidemic B33.0
- – psychogenic F45.3
- duodenum K59.8
- epidemic diaphragmatic (transient) B33.0
- esophagus (diffuse) K22.4
- – psychogenic F45.3
- facial G51.3
- fallopian tube N83.8
- gastrointestinal (tract), psychogenic F45.3
- glottis J38.5
- – hysterical F44.4
- – psychogenic F45.3
- – – conversion reaction F44.4
- habit (*see also* Tic) F95.9
- heart I20.1
- hemifacial (clonic) G51.3
- hourglass – *see* Contraction, hourglass
- hysterical F44.4
- infantile G40.4
- inferior oblique, eye H51.8
- intestinal (*see also* Syndrome, irritable bowel) K58.9
- – psychogenic F45.3
- larynx, laryngeal J38.5
- – hysterical F44.4
- – psychogenic F45.3
- – – conversion reaction F44.4
- levator palpebrae superioris H02.5
- lightning G40.4
- nervous F45.8
- nodding F98.4
- occupational F48.8
- oculogyric H51.8
- – psychogenic F45.8
- ophthalmic artery H34.2
- perineal, female N94.8
- pharynx (reflex) J39.2
- – hysterical F45.3
- – psychogenic F45.3
- psychogenic F45.8
- pylorus NEC K31.3
- – congenital or infantile Q40.0
- – psychogenic F45.3
- rectum (sphincter) K59.4
- – psychogenic F45.3
- retinal (artery) H34.2
- sigmoid (*see also* Syndrome, irritable bowel) K58.9

Spasm(s), spastic—*continued*
- sigmoid—*continued*
- – psychogenic F45.3
- sphincter of Oddi K83.4
- stomach K31.8
- – neurotic F45.3
- throat J39.2
- – hysterical F45.3
- – psychogenic F45.3
- tic F95.9
- tongue K14.8
- torsion (progressive) G24.1
- trigeminal nerve (*see also* Neuralgia, trigeminal) G50.0
- ureter N13.5
- urethra (sphincter) N35.9
- uterus N85.8
- – complicating labor O62.4
- – – affecting fetus or newborn P03.6
- vagina N94.2
- – psychogenic F52.5
- vascular NEC I73.9
- vasomotor NEC I73.9
- vein NEC I87.8
- viscera R10.4
Spasmodic – *see condition*
Spasmus nutans F98.4
Spastic, spasticity – *see also* Spasm
- child (cerebral) (congenital) (paralysis) G80.1
Speaker's throat R49.8
Specific, specified – *see condition*
Speech defect, disorder, disturbance, impediment NEC R47.8
- psychogenic, in childhood and adolescence F98.8
Spencer's disease A08.1
Sperm counts Z31.4
- postvasectomy Z30.8
Spermatic cord – *see condition*
Spermatocele N43.4
- congenital Q55.4
Spermatocystitis N49.0
Spermatocytoma (M9063/3)
- specified site – *see* Neoplasm, malignant
- unspecified site C62.9
Spermatorrhea N50.8
Sphacelus (*see also* Gangrene) R02
Sphenoidal – *see condition*
Sphenoiditis (chronic) (*see also* Sinusitis, sphenoidal) J32.3
Sphericity, increased, lens (congenital) Q12.4

**Spherocytosis (congenital) (familial)
(hereditary)** D58.0
- hemoglobin disease D58.0
- sickle-cell (disease) D57.8
Spherophakia Q12.4
Sphincter – *see condition*
Sphincteritis, sphincter of Oddi (*see also*
Cholangitis) K83.0
Sphingolipidosis E75.3
- specified NEC E75.2
Sphingomyelinosis E75.3
Spider
- fingers Q87.4
- nevus I78.1
- toes Q87.4
- vascular I78.1
Spiegler-Fendt benign lymphocytoma
L98.8
Spielmeyer-Vogt disease E75.4
Spina bifida (aperta) Q05.9
- with hydrocephalus NEC Q05.4
- cervical Q05.5
- – with hydrocephalus Q05.0
- dorsal Q05.6
- – with hydrocephalus Q05.1
- fetus (suspected), affecting management
of pregnancy O35.0
- lumbar Q05.7
- – with hydrocephalus Q05.2
- lumbosacral Q05.7
- – with hydrocephalus Q05.2
- occulta Q76.0
- sacral Q05.8
- – with hydrocephalus Q05.3
- thoracic Q05.6
- – with hydrocephalus Q05.1
- thoracolumbar Q05.6
- – with hydrocephalus Q05.1
Spindle, Krukenberg's H18.0
Spine, spinal – *see condition*
Spiradenoma (eccrine) (M8403/0) – *see*
Neoplasm, skin, benign
Spirillosis A25.0
Spirochetal – *see condition*
Spirochetosis A69.9
- icterohemorrhagic A27.0
Spirometrosis B70.1
Spitting blood (*see also* Hemoptysis) R04.2
Splanchnoptosis K63.4
Spleen, splenic – *see condition*
**Splenitis (interstitial) (malignant)
(nonspecific)** D73.8
- tuberculous A18.8† D77*
Splenocele D73.8

Splenomegaly, splenomegalia R16.1
- with hepatomegaly R16.2
- congenital Q89.0
- congestive, chronic D73.2
- Egyptian B65.1† D77*
- Gaucher's E75.2
- idiopathic R16.1
- malarial (*see also* Malaria) B54† D77*
- neutropenic D70
- Niemann-Pick E75.2
- syphilitic A52.7† D77*
- – congenital (early) A50.0† D77*
Splenopathy D73.9
Splenoptosis D73.8
Splenosis D73.8
Splinter – *code as* Injury, superficial, by site
Split, splitting
- foot Q72.7
- heart sounds R01.2
- lip, congenital (*see also* Cleft, lip) Q36.9
- nails L60.3
- urinary stream R39.1
Spondylarthrosis M47.9
Spondylitis M46.9
- ankylopoietica M45
- ankylosing (chronic) M45
- – with lung involvement M45† J99.8*
- atrophic (ligamentous) M45
- chronic M46.9
- deformans (chronic) M47.9
- gonococcal A54.4† M49.3*
- gouty M10.0
- in (due to)
- – brucellosis A23.-† M49.1*
- – enterobacteria A04.9† M49.2*
- – tuberculosis A18.0† M49.0*
- infectious NEC M46.5
- juvenile ankylosing (chronic) M08.1
- Kümmell's M48.3
- Marie-Strümpell M45
- muscularis M48.8
- psoriatic L40.5† M07.2*
- rheumatoid M45
- rhizomelica M45
- sacroiliac NEC M46.1
- senescent, senile M47.9
- traumatic (chronic) or post-traumatic
M48.3
- tuberculous A18.0† M49.0*
- typhosa A01.0† M49.2*
Spondyloarthrosis M47.9
Spondylolisthesis (acquired) M43.1
- with disproportion (fetopelvic) O33.0
- – affecting fetus or newborn P03.1

Spondylolisthesis—*continued*
- with disproportion—*continued*
- - causing obstructed labor O65.0
- congenital Q76.2
- degenerative M43.1
- traumatic (old) M43.1
- - acute (lumbar) (lumbosacral) S33.1
- - - site other than lumbosacral – *code as* Fracture, vertebra, by region
Spondylolysis (acquired) M43.0
- congenital Q76.2
- lumbosacral region M43.0
- - with disproportion (fetopelvic) O33.0
- - - affecting fetus or newborn P03.1
- - - causing obstructed labor O65.8
Spondylopathy M48.9
- infective NEC M46.5
- inflammatory M46.9
- - specified NEC M46.8
- neuropathic, in
- - syringomyelia and syringobulbia G95.0† M49.4*
- - tabes dorsalis A52.1† M49.4*
- specified NEC M48.8
- traumatic M48.3
Spondylosis M47.9
- with
- - compression (of)
- - - nerve root or plexus M47.2† G55.2*
- - disproportion (fetopelvic) O33.0
- - - affecting fetus or newborn P03.1
- - - causing obstructed labor O65.0
- - myelopathy NEC M47.1† G99.2*
- - radiculopathy M47.2
- cervical M47.8
- coccyx M47.8
- lumbar M47.8
- sacral, sacrococcygeal M47.8
- specified NEC M47.8
- traumatic M48.3
Sponge
- inadvertently left in operation wound T81.5
- kidney (medullary) Q61.5
Sponge-diver's disease T63.6
Spongioblastoma (M9422/3)
- multiforme (M9440/3)
- - specified site – *see* Neoplasm, malignant
- - unspecified site C71.9
- polare (M9423/3)
- - specified site – *see* Neoplasm, malignant
- - unspecified site C71.9

Spongioblastoma—*continued*
- primitive polar (M9443/3)
- - specified site – *see* Neoplasm, malignant
- - unspecified site C71.9
- specified site – *see* Neoplasm, malignant
- unspecified site C71.9
Spongioneuroblastoma (M9504/3) – *see* Neoplasm, malignant
Spontaneous – *see also condition*
- fracture (cause unknown) M84.4
Spoon nail L60.3
- congenital Q84.6
Sporadic – *see condition*
Sporothrix schenckii infection – *see* Sporotrichosis
Sporotrichosis B42.9
- arthritis B42.8† M01.6*
- disseminated B42.7
- generalized B42.7
- lymphocutaneous (fixed) (progressive) B42.1
- pulmonary B42.0† J99.8*
- specified NEC B42.8
Spots
- Bitot's
- - in the young child E50.1† H13.8*
- - vitamin A deficiency E50.1† H13.8*
- café au lait L81.3
- Cayenne pepper I78.1
- cotton wool, retina H34.2
- de Morgan's I78.1
- liver L81.4
Spotted fever – *see* Fever, spotted
Spotting, intermenstrual NEC (regular) N92.3
- irregular N92.1
Sprain, strain (joint) (ligament) T14.3
- Achilles tendon S86.0
- acromioclavicular joint or ligament S43.5
- ankle S93.4
- anterior longitudinal, cervical S13.4
- atlas, atlanto-axial, atlanto-occipital S13.4
- back T09.2
- breast bone S23.4
- broad ligament S37.8
- calcaneofibular S93.4
- carpal S63.5
- carpometacarpal S63.7
- cartilage
- - costal S23.4
- - semilunar (knee) S83.6
- - - with current tear S83.2

Sprain, strain—*continued*
- cartilage—*continued*
- – thyroid region S13.5
- – xiphoid S23.4
- cervical, cervicodorsal, cervicothoracic S13.4
- chondrocostal, chondrosternal S23.4
- coccyx S33.7
- coracoclavicular S43.7
- coracohumeral S43.4
- costal cartilage S23.4
- cricoarytenoid articulation or ligament S13.5
- cricothyroid articulation S13.5
- cruciate, knee S83.5
- deltoid, ankle S93.4
- dorsal (spine) S23.3
- elbow S53.4
- femur, head S73.1
- fibular collateral, knee S83.4
- fibulocalcaneal S93.4
- finger(s) S63.6
- foot S93.6
- hand S63.7
- hip S73.1
- iliofemoral S73.1
- innominate
- – acetabulum S73.1
- – pubic junction S33.7
- – sacral junction S33.6
- internal collateral, ankle S93.4
- interphalangeal
- – finger S63.6
- – toe S93.5
- ischiocapsular S73.1
- ischiofemoral S73.1
- jaw (articular disk) (cartilage) S03.4
- knee NEC S83.6
- – cruciate (anterior) (posterior) S83.5
- – lateral (fibular) collateral S83.4
- – medial (tibial) collateral S83.4
- – patellar ligament S76.1
- – specified NEC S83.6
- – tibiofibular joint and ligament, superior S83.6
- lateral collateral, knee S83.4
- limb
- – lower T13.2
- – – with upper limb(s) (multiple sites) T03.4
- – – multiple sites T03.3
- – upper T11.2
- – – with lower limb(s) (multiple sites) T03.4

Sprain, strain—*continued*
- limb—*continued*
- – upper—*continued*
- – – multiple sites T03.2
- lumbar (spine) S33.5
- lumbosacral S33.5
- mandible (articular disk) S03.4
- medial collateral, knee S83.4
- meniscus
- – knee S83.6
- – – with current tear S83.2
- – – old M23.2
- metacarpal (distal) (proximal) S63.7
- metacarpophalangeal S63.6
- metatarsophalangeal S93.5
- midcarpal S63.7
- midtarsal S93.6
- multiple T03.9
- – body regions NEC T03.8
- – head with
- – – neck T03.0
- – – other body regions T03.8
- – limb
- – – lower T03.3
- – – – with
- – – – – thorax, lower back and pelvis T03.8
- – – – – upper limb(s) T03.4
- – – upper T03.2
- – – – with
- – – – – lower limb(s) T03.4
- – – – – thorax, lower back and pelvis T03.8
- – neck with
- – – head T03.0
- – – other body regions NEC T03.8
- – specified NEC T03.8
- – thorax with lower back and pelvis T03.1
- – trunk T03.1
- neck NEC S13.6
- nose S03.5
- orbicular, hip S73.1
- patella S83.6
- pelvis NEC S33.7
- phalanx
- – finger S63.6
- – toe S93.5
- pubofemoral S73.1
- radiocarpal S63.5
- radiohumeral S53.4
- rib (cage) S23.4
- rotator cuff (tendon) S46.0
- – capsule S43.4

Sprain, strain—*continued*
- round ligament S37.8
- – femur S73.1
- sacral (spine) S33.7
- sacrococcygeal S33.7
- sacroiliac (region) S33.7
- – chronic or old M53.2
- – joint S33.6
- sacrotuberous S33.7
- scaphoid (hand) S63.7
- scapula(r) S43.7
- semilunar cartilage (knee) S83.6
- – with current tear S83.2
- – old M23.2
- shoulder joint S43.4
- – blade S43.7
- – girdle NEC S43.7
- spine T09.2
- – cervical S13.4
- – coccyx S33.7
- – lumbar S33.5
- – sacral S33.7
- – thoracic S23.3
- sternoclavicular joint S43.6
- sternum S23.4
- symphysis pubis S33.7
- talofibular S93.4
- tarsal S93.6
- tarsometatarsal S93.6
- temporomandibular S03.4
- thoracic (spine) S23.3
- thorax NEC S23.5
- thumb S63.6
- thyroid cartilage or region S13.5
- tibia (proximal end) S83.6
- tibial collateral, knee S83.4
- tibiofibular
- – distal S93.4
- – superior S83.6
- toe(s) S93.5
- ulnohumeral S53.4
- vertebra (*see also* Sprain, spine) T09.2
- wrist (cuneiform) (scaphoid) (semilunar) S63.5
- xiphoid cartilage S23.4

Sprengel's deformity (congenital) Q74.0
Sprue K90.1
- nontropical K90.0
- tropical K90.1
Spur, bone M77.9
- calcaneal M77.3
- iliac crest M76.2
- nose (septum) J34.8

Sputum
- blood-stained R04.2
- excessive (cause unknown) R09.3
Squamous – *see also* condition
- epithelium in
- – cervical canal (congenital) Q51.8
- – uterine mucosa (congenital) Q51.8
Squashed nose M95.0
- congenital Q67.4
Squint (*see also* Strabismus) H50.9
- accommodative H50.0
St Hubert's disease A82.9
Stab – *see also* Wound, open
- internal organs – *see* Injury, by site
Stafne's cyst or cavity K10.0
Staggering gait R26.0
- hysterical F44.4
Staghorn calculus (*see also* Calculus, kidney) N20.0
Stähli's line (cornea) (pigment) H18.0
Stain, portwine Q82.5
Staining, tooth, teeth (hard tissues) (extrinsic) (due to) K03.6
- accretions K03.6
- deposits (betel) (black) (green) (materia alba) (orange) (soft) (tobacco) K03.6
- intrinsic NEC K00.8
- metals (copper) (silver) K03.7
- pulpal bleeding K03.7
Stammering F98.5
Standstill
- auricular I45.5
- cardiac (*see also* Arrest, cardiac) I46.9
- sinoatrial I45.5
- ventricular (*see also* Arrest, cardiac) I46.9
Stannosis J63.5
Stanton's disease (*see also* Melioidosis) A24.4
Staphylitis (acute) (catarrhal) (chronic) (gangrenous) (membranous) (suppurative) (ulcerative) K12.2
Staphylococcal scalded skin syndrome L00
Staphylococcemia A41.2
Staphylococcus, staphylococcal – *see also* condition
- as cause of disease classified elsewhere B95.8
- aureus, as cause of disease classified elsewhere B95.6
- specified NEC, as cause of disease classified elsewhere B95.7

Staphyloma (anterior) (ciliary) (equatorial) (posterior) (sclera) H15.8
- cornea H18.7
Stargardt's disease H35.5
Starvation T73.0
- edema (*see also* Malnutrition, severe) E43
Stasis
- bile (noncalculous) K83.1
- bronchus J98.0
- - with infection (*see also* Bronchitis) J40
- cardiac (*see also* Failure, heart, congestive) I50.0
- cecum or colon K59.8
- dermatitis I83.1
- duodenal K31.5
- eczema I83.1
- ileum K59.8
- intestinal K59.8
- jejunum K59.8
- liver (cirrhotic) – *see* Cirrhosis, cardiac
- lymphatic I89.8
- pulmonary (*see also* Edema, lung) J81
- ulcer I83.0
- urine R33
- venous I87.8
State (of)
- affective and paranoid, mixed, organic psychotic F06.8
- agitated R45.1
- - acute reaction to stress F43.0
- anxiety (neurotic) F41.1
- apprehension F41.1
- burn-out Z73.0
- climacteric, female N95.1
- clouded epileptic or paroxysmal G40.8
- compulsive F42.1
- - mixed with obsessional thoughts F42.2
- confusional (psychogenic) F44.8
- - acute or subacute (*see also* Delirium) F05.9
- - - with senility or dementia F05.1
- - epileptic F05.8
- - reactive (from emotional stress, psychological trauma) F44.8
- convulsive (*see also* Convulsions) R56.8
- crisis F43.0
- depressive NEC F32.9
- - neurotic F34.1
- dissociative F44.9
- emotional shock (stress) R45.7
- hallucinatory, induced by drug – *see* F11-F19 with fourth character .5
- menopausal N95.1

State—*continued*
- menopausal—*continued*
- - artificial N95.3
- neurotic NEC F48.9
- - with depersonalization F48.1
- obsessional F42.0
- - mixed with compulsive acts F42.2
- onciroid (schizophrenia-like) F23.2
- organic
- - hallucinatory (nonalcoholic) F06.0
- - paranoid(-hallucinatory) F06.2
- panic F41.0
- paranoid F22.0
- - climacteric F22.8
- - induced by drug – *code to* F10-F19 with fourth character .5
- - involutional F22.8
- - menopausal F22.8
- - organic F06.2
- - senile F03
- - simple F22.0
- phobic F40.9
- postleukotomy F07.0
- pregnant (*see also* Pregnancy) Z33
- psychogenic, twilight F44.8
- psychopathic (constitutional) F60.2
- psychotic, organic F06.8
- - mixed paranoid and affective F06.8
- - senile or presenile NEC F03
- residual schizophrenic F20.5
- restlessness R45.1
- stress (emotional) R45.7
- tension (mental) F48.9
- - specified NEC F48.8
- twilight
- - epileptic F05.8
- - psychogenic F44.8
- vital exhaustion Z73.0
- withdrawal – *see* Withdrawal, state
Status (post)
- absence, epileptic G41.1
- adrenalectomy (bilateral) (unilateral) E89.6
- anastomosis Z98.0
- angioplasty (peripheral) NEC Z95.8
- - coronary artery NEC Z95.5
- aortocoronary bypass Z95.1
- arthrodesis Z98.1
- artificial opening (of) Z93.9
- - gastrointestinal tract NEC Z93.4
- - specified NEC Z93.8
- - urinary tract NEC Z93.6
- - vagina Z93.8
- asthmaticus J46

Status—*continued*
- cholecystectomy Z90.4
- colectomy (complete) (partial) Z90.4
- colostomy Z93.3
- convulsivus idiopathicus G41.0
- coronary artery angioplasty Z95.5
- cystectomy (urinary bladder) Z90.6
- cystostomy Z93.5
- epilepticus G41.9
- – complex partial G41.2
- – focal motor G41.8
- – grand mal G41.0
- – partial G41.8
- – petit mal G41.1
- – psychomotor G41.2
- – specified NEC G41.8
- – temporal lobe G41.2
- – tonic-clonic G41.0
- gastrectomy (complete) (partial) Z90.3
- gastrostomy Z93.1
- grand mal G41.0
- human immunodeficiency virus (HIV) infection, asymptomatic Z21
- hysterectomy (complete) (partial) Z90.7
- ileostomy Z93.2
- intestinal bypass Z98.0
- laryngectomy Z90.0
- marmoratus G80.3
- mastectomy (bilateral) (unilateral) Z90.1
- medicament regimen for a long term (current) NEC Z92.2
- – anticoagulants Z92.1
- – aspirin Z92.2
- migrainosus G43.2
- nephrectomy (bilateral) (unilateral) Z90.5
- nephrostomy Z93.6
- oophorectomy (bilateral) (unilateral) Z90.7
- pacemaker
- – brain Z96.8
- – cardiac Z95.0
- – specified NEC Z96.8
- pancreatectomy Z90.4
- petit mal G41.1
- pneumonectomy (complete) (partial) Z90.2
- postcommotio cerebri F07.2
- postoperative NEC Z98.8
- postpartum NEC (routine follow-up) Z39.2
- – care immediately after delivery Z39.0
- postsurgical NEC Z98.8
- renal dialysis Z99.2

Status—*continued*
- salpingo-oophorectomy (bilateral) (unilateral) Z90.7
- shunt, cerebrospinal fluid Z98.2
- splenectomy D73.0
- thyroidectomy (hypothyroidism) E89.0
- tracheostomy Z93.0
- transplant – *see* Transplant
- ureterostomy Z93.6
- urethrostomy Z93.6
Stave fracture S62.4
Stealing
- child problem F91.8
- – in company with others F91.2
- pathological (compulsive) F63.2
Steam burn – *see* Burn
Steatocystoma multiplex L72.2
Steatohepatitis (nonalcoholic) K75.8
Steatoma L72.1
- eyelid (cystic) H01.1
- – infected H00.0
Steatorrhea (chronic) K90.4
- idiopathic (adult) (infantile) K90.0
- pancreatic K90.3
- tropical K90.1
Steatosis E88.8
- heart (*see also* Degeneration, myocardial) I51.5
- kidney N28.8
- liver NEC K76.0
Steele-Richardson-Olszewski disease or syndrome G23.1
Steinbrocker's syndrome G90.8
Steinert's disease G71.1
Stein-Leventhal syndrome E28.2
Stenocardia I20.8
Stenocephaly Q75.8
Stenosis (cicatricial) – *see also* Stricture
- anus, anal (canal) (sphincter) K62.4
- – and rectum K62.4
- – congenital Q42.3
- – – with fistula Q42.2
- aorta (ascending) (supraventricular) (congenital) Q25.3
- – arteriosclerotic I70.0
- – calcified I70.0
- aortic (valve) I35.0
- – with insufficiency I35.2
- – congenital Q23.0
- – rheumatic I06.0
- – – with
- – – – incompetence, insufficiency or regurgitation I06.2

Stenosis—*continued*
- aortic—*continued*
- – rheumatic—*continued*
- – – with—*continued*
- – – – incompetence, insufficiency or regurgitation—*continued*
- – – – – with mitral (valve) disease I08.0
- – – – – – with tricuspid (valve) disease I08.3
- – – – – mitral (valve) disease I08.0
- – – – – – with tricuspid (valve) disease I08.3
- – – – – tricuspid (valve) disease I08.2
- – – – – – with mitral (valve) disease I08.3
- – – specified cause NEC I35.0
- – – syphilitic A52.0† I39.1*
- aqueduct of Sylvius (congenital) Q03.0
- – – with spina bifida (*see also* Spina bifida, with hydrocephalus) Q05.4
- – – acquired G91.1
- artery NEC I77.1
- – – cerebral – *see* Occlusion, artery, cerebral
- – – precerebral (*see also* Occlusion, artery, precerebral) I65.9
- – – – bilateral (multiple) I65.3
- – – – basilar I65.1
- – – – carotid I65.2
- – – – vertebral I65.0
- – – – specified NEC I65.8
- – – pulmonary Q25.6
- bile duct (common) (hepatic) K83.1
- – – congenital Q44.3
- bladder-neck (acquired) N32.0
- – – congenital Q64.3
- brain G93.8
- bronchus J98.0
- – – congenital Q32.3
- – – syphilitic A52.7† J99.8*
- cardia (stomach) K22.2
- cardiovascular (*see also* Disease, cardiovascular) I51.6
- caudal M48.0
- cervix, cervical (canal) N88.2
- – – congenital Q51.8
- – – in pregnancy or childbirth O34.4
- – – – affecting fetus or newborn P03.8
- – – – causing obstructed labor O65.5
- – – – – affecting fetus or newborn P03.1
- colon (*see also* Obstruction, intestine) K56.6
- – – congenital Q42.9

Stenosis—*continued*
- colon—*continued*
- – – congenital—*continued*
- – – – specified NEC Q42.8
- colostomy K91.4
- common (bile) duct K83.1
- – – congenital Q44.3
- coronary (artery) I25.1
- cystic duct (*see also* Obstruction, gallbladder) K82.0
- due to presence of device, implant or graft (*see also* Complications, by site and type, specified NEC) T85.8
- – – arterial graft NEC T82.8
- – – breast (implant) T85.8
- – – catheter T83.8
- – – – dialysis (renal) T82.8
- – – – – intraperitoneal T85.8
- – – – infusion NEC T82.8
- – – – – spinal (epidural) (subdural) T85.8
- – – – urinary (indwelling) T83.8
- – – fixation, internal (orthopedic) NEC T84.8
- – – gastrointestinal (bile duct) (esophagus) T85.8
- – – genital NEC T83.8
- – – heart NEC T82.8
- – – joint prosthesis T84.8
- – – ocular (corneal graft) (orbital implant) NEC T85.8
- – – orthopedic NEC T84.8
- – – specified NEC T85.8
- – – urinary NEC T83.8
- – – vascular NEC T82.8
- – – ventricular intracranial shunt T85.8
- duodenum K31.5
- – – congenital Q41.0
- ejaculatory duct NEC N50.8
- endocervical os – *see* Stenosis, cervix
- enterostomy K91.4
- esophagus K22.2
- – – congenital Q39.3
- – – syphilitic A52.7† K23.8*
- – – – congenital A50.5† K23.8*
- eustachian tube H68.1
- external ear canal (acquired) H61.3
- – – congenital Q16.1
- gallbladder (*see also* Obstruction, gallbladder) K82.0
- glottis J38.6
- hymen N89.6
- ileum K56.6
- – – congenital Q41.2
- intervertebral foramina M99.8

Stenosis—*continued*
- intervertebral foramina—*continued*
- – connective tissue M99.7
- – disk M99.7
- – osseous M99.6
- – subluxation M99.6
- intestine (*see also* Obstruction, intestine) K56.6
- – congenital (small) Q41.9
- – – large Q42.9
- – – – specified NEC Q42.8
- – – specified NEC Q41.8
- jejunum K56.6
- – congenital Q41.1
- lacrimal duct, punctum or sac H04.5
- – congenital Q10.5
- lacrimonasal duct H04.5
- – congenital Q10.5
- larynx J38.6
- – congenital NEC Q31.8
     subglottic Q31.1
- – syphilitic A52.7† J99.8∗
- – – congenital A50.5† J99.8∗
- mitral (chronic) (inactive) (valve) I05.0
- – with
- – – aortic valve disease (unspecified origin) I08.0
- – – incompetence, insufficiency or regurgitation I05.2
- – – active or acute I01.1
- – – – with rheumatic or Sydenham's chorea I02.0
- – congenital Q23.2
- – specified cause, except rheumatic I34.2
- – syphilitic A52.0† I39.0∗
- myocardium, myocardial (*see also* Degeneration, myocardial) I51.5
- nares (anterior) (posterior) J34.8
- – congenital Q30.0
- nasal duct H04.5
- – congenital Q10.5
- nasolacrimal duct H04.5
- – congenital Q10.5
- neural canal M99.8
- – connective tissue M99.4
- – intervertebral disk M99.5
- – osseous M99.3
- – subluxation M99.2
- oesophagus – *see* Stenosis, esophagus
- organ or site, congenital NEC – *see* Atresia, by site
- pulmonary (artery) (congenital) (supravalvular) (subvalvular) Q25.6
- – acquired I28.8

Stenosis—*continued*
- pulmonary—*continued*
- – in tetralogy of Fallot Q21.3
- – infundibular Q24.3
- – valve I37.0
- – – with insufficiency I37.2
- – – congenital Q22.1
- – – rheumatic I09.8
- – – – with aortic, mitral or tricuspid (valve) disease (unspecified origin) I08.8
- – vessel NEC I28.8
- pylorus (acquired) (hypertrophic) K31.1
- – adult K31.1
- – congenital Q40.0
- – infantile Q40.0
- rectum (sphincter) (*see also* Stricture, rectum) K62.4
- renal artery I70.1
- – congenital Q27.1
- salivary duct (any) K11.8
- spinal M48.0
- stomach, hourglass K31.2
- subaortic (congenital) Q24.4
- – hypertrophic I42.1
- subglottic
- – congenital Q31.1
- – postprocedural J95.5
- trachea J39.8
- – congenital Q32.1
- – syphilitic A52.7† J99.8∗
- – tuberculous NEC A16.4
- tricuspid (valve) I07.0
- – with
- – – aortic (valve) disease (unspecified origin) I08.2
- – – incompetence, insufficiency or regurgitation I07.2
- – – – with aortic (valve) disease (unspecified origin) I08.2
- – – – – with mitral (valve) disease (unspecified origin) I08.3
- – – mitral (valve) disease (unspecified origin) I08.1
- – – – with aortic (valve) disease (unspecified origin) I08.3
- – congenital Q22.4
- – nonrheumatic I36.0
- – – with insufficiency I36.2
- tubal N97.1
- ureteropelvic junction, congenital Q62.1
- ureterovesical orifice, congenital Q62.1
- urethra (valve) N35.9
- – congenital Q64.3

Stenosis—*continued*
– urinary meatus, congenital Q64.3
– vagina N89.5
– – congenital Q52.4
– – in pregnancy or childbirth O34.6
– – – affecting fetus or newborn P03.8
– – – causing obstructed labor O65.5
– – – – affecting fetus or newborn P03.1
– valve (cardiac) (heart) (*see also*
  Endocarditis) I38
– – congenital Q24.8
– vena cava (inferior) (superior) I87.1
– – congenital Q26.0
– vesicourethral orifice Q64.3
– vulva N90.5
Stercolith (impaction) K56.4
– appendix K38.1
Stercoraceous, stercoral ulcer K63.3
– anus or rectum K62.6
Stereotypies NEC F98.4
Sterility
– female – *see* Infertility, female
– male N46
Sterilization, admission for Z30.2
Sternalgia (*see also* Angina) I20.9
Sternopagus Q89.4
Sternum bifidum Q76.7
Steroid
– effects (adverse) (adrenocortical)
  (iatrogenic)
– – cushingoid
– – – overdose or wrong substance given
    or taken T38.0
– – diabetes
– – – correct substance properly
    administered E13.-
– – – overdose or wrong substance given
    or taken T38.0
– – due to
– – – correct substance properly
    administered E27.3
– – – overdose or wrong substance given
    or taken T38.0
– – fever
– – – correct substance properly
    administered R50.9
– – – overdose or wrong substance given
    or taken T38.0
– – withdrawal
– – – correct substance properly
    administered E27.3
– – – overdose or wrong substance given
    or taken T38.0

Stevens-Johnson disease or syndrome
  L51.1
Stewart-Morel syndrome M85.2
Sticker's disease B08.3
Sticky eye H10.0
Stiff neck (*see also* Torticollis) M43.6
Stiff-man syndrome G25.8
Stiffness, joint M25.6
– ankle M25.6
– arthrodesis status Z98.1
– elbow M25.6
– finger M25.6
– hip M25.6
– knee M25.6
– multiple sites NEC M25.6
– sacroiliac M53.3
– shoulder M25.6
– specified NEC M25.6
– spine M53.8
– surgical fusion, status Z98.1
– wrist M25.6
Stigmata, congenital syphilis A50.5
Stillbirth NEC P95
Stilling's syndrome H50.8
Still's disease or syndrome (juvenile)
  M08.2
– adult-onset M06.1
**Sting (venomous) (with allergic or
  anaphylactic shock)** T63.9
– arthropod NEC T63.4
– fish T63.5
– insect, venomous NEC (bee) (hornet)
  (wasp) T63.4
– – nonvenomous – *see* Injury, superficial
– jellyfish (Portuguese man-of-war) T63.6
– marine animal NEC T63.6
– plant L24.7
– scorpion T63.2
– sea anemone T63.6
– shellfish T63.6
– starfish T63.6
Stippled epiphyses Q78.8
Stitch
– abscess T81.4
– burst (in operation wound) T81.3
Stokes-Adams disease or syndrome I45.9
Stokvis(-Talma) disease D74.8
Stomach – *see* condition
Stomatitis (denture) (ulcerative) K12.1
– angular K13.0
– aphthous K12.0
– candidal B37.0
– diphtheritic A36.8

Stomatitis—*continued*
- due to vitamin deficiency
- – – B group NEC E53.9† K93.8*
- – – B2 (riboflavin) E53.0† K93.8*
- epidemic B08.8
- epizootic B08.8
- gangrenous A69.0
- Geotrichum B48.3† K93.8*
- herpesviral B00.2
- herpetiformis K12.0
- membranous, acute K12.1
- monilial B37.0
- mycotic B37.0
- necrotizing ulcerative A69.0
- spirochetal A69.1
- suppurative (acute) K12.2
- ulceromembranous A69.1
- vesicular K12.1
- – with exanthem (enteroviral) B08.4
- – virus disease A93.8
- Vincent's A69.1
Stomatocytosis D58.8
Stomatomycosis B37.0
Stomatorrhagia K13.7
Stone(s) – *see also* Calculus
- bladder (diverticulum) N21.0
- kidney N20.0
- prostate N42.0
- pulpal (dental) K04.2
- renal N20.0
- salivary gland or duct (any) K11.5
- urethra (impacted) N21.1
- urinary (duct) (impacted) (passage) N20.9
- – bladder (diverticulum) N21.0
- – lower tract NEC N21.9
- – – specified NEC N21.8
- xanthine E79.8† N22.8*
Stonecutter's lung J62.8
Stonemason's asthma, disease, lung or pneumoconiosis J62.8
Stoppage
- heart (*see also* Arrest, cardiac) I46.9
- urine R33
Storm, thyroid E05.5
Strabismus (alternating) (congenital) (nonparalytic) H50.9
- concomitant NEC H50.4
- – convergent H50.0
- – divergent H50.1
- convergent H50.0
- divergent H50.1
- due to adhesions, scars H50.6
- intermittent H50.3
- latent H50.5

Strabismus—*continued*
- mechanical H50.6
- paralytic H49.9
- – specified NEC H49.8
- specified NEC H50.8
- vertical H50.2
Strain – *see also* Sprain
- eye NEC H53.1
- heart – *see* Disease, heart
- low back M54.5
- mental NEC Z73.3
- – work-related Z56.6
- muscle M62.6
- – traumatic – *see* Injury, muscle, by site
- physical NEC Z73.3
- – work-related Z56.6
- postural M70.9
- psychological NEC Z73.3
Strand, vitreous H43.3
Strangulation, strangulated T71
- appendix K38.8
- asphyxiation or suffocation by T71
- bladder-neck N32.0
- bowel or colon K56.2
- hernia (*see also* Hernia, by site, with obstruction) K46.0
- – with gangrene (*see also* Hernia, by site, with gangrene) K46.1
- intestine K56.2
- – with hernia (*see also* Hernia, by site, with obstruction) K46.0
- – – with gangrene (*see also* Hernia, by site, with gangrene) K46.1
- mesentery K56.2
- mucus (*see also* Asphyxia, mucus) T17.9
- omentum K56.2
- organ or site, congenital NEC – *see* Atresia, by site
- ovary N83.5
- stomach due to hernia (*see also* Hernia, by site, with obstruction) K46.0
- – with gangrene (*see also* Hernia, by site, with gangrene) K46.1
- umbilical cord – *see also* Compression, umbilical cord
- – fetus or newborn P02.5
- vesicourethral orifice N32.0
Strangury R30.0
Strawberry gallbladder K82.4
Streak(s)
- macula, angioid H35.3
- ovarian Q50.3
Strephosymbolia F81.0
- secondary to organic lesion R48.8

Streptobacillosis A25.1
Streptococcemia (*see also* Sepsis,
streptococcal) A40.9
Streptococcus, streptococcal – *see also*
condition
– as cause of disease classified elsewhere
B95.5
– group
– – A, as cause of disease classified
elsewhere B95.0
– – B, as cause of disease classified
elsewhere B95.1
– – D, as cause of disease classified
elsewhere B95.2
– pneumoniae, as cause of disease classified
elsewhere B95.3
– specified NEC, as cause of disease
classified elsewhere B95.4
Streptomycosis B47.1
Streptotrichosis A48.8
Stress
– fetal – *see* Distress, fetal
– mental NEC Z73.3
– – work-related Z56.6
– physical NEC Z73.3
– – work-related Z56.6
– reaction (*see also* Reaction, stress) F43.9
– work schedule Z56.3
Stretching, nerve – *see* Injury, nerve
Striae albicantes, atrophicae or distensae
(cutis) L90.6
Stricture (*see also* Stenosis) R68.8
– anus (sphincter) K62.4
– – congenital Q42.3
– – – with fistula Q42.2
– – infantile Q42.3
– – – with fistula Q42.2
– aorta (ascending) (congenital) (*see also*
Stenosis, aorta) Q25.3
– – supravalvular, congenital Q25.3
– aortic (valve) (*see also* Stenosis, aortic)
I35.0
– – congenital Q23.0
– aqueduct of Sylvius (congenital) Q03.0
– – with spina bifida (*see also* Spina bifida,
with hydrocephalus) Q05.4
– – acquired G91.1
– artery I77.1
– – basilar (*see also* Occlusion, artery,
basilar) I65.1
– – carotid (*see also* Occlusion, artery,
carotid) I65.2
– – congenital (peripheral) Q27.8
– – – cerebral Q28.3

Stricture—*continued*
– artery—*continued*
– – congenital—*continued*
– – – coronary Q24.5
– – – retinal Q14.1
– – coronary I25.1
– – precerebral (*see also* Occlusion, artery,
precerebral) I65.9
– – pulmonary (congenital) Q25.6
– – – acquired I28.8
– – vertebral (*see also* Occlusion, artery,
vertebral) I65.0
– auditory canal (external) (congenital)
Q16.1
– – acquired H61.3
– bile duct (common) (hepatic) K83.1
– – congenital Q44.3
– – postoperative K91.8
– bladder N32.8
– – neck N32.0
– bowel (*see also* Obstruction, intestine)
K56.6
– bronchus J98.0
– – congenital Q32.3
– – syphilitic A52.7† J99.8*
– cardia (stomach) K22.2
– cardiac (*see also* Disease, heart) I51.9
– – orifice (stomach) K22.2
– cecum (*see also* Obstruction, intestine)
K56.6
– cervix, cervical (canal) N88.2
– – congenital Q51.8
– – in pregnancy or childbirth O34.4
– – – causing obstructed labor O65.5
– – – – affecting fetus or newborn P03.1
– colon (*see also* Obstruction, intestine)
K56.6
– – congenital Q42.9
– – – specified NEC Q42.8
– common (bile) duct K83.1
– coronary (artery) I25.1
– – congenital Q24.5
– cystic duct (*see also* Obstruction,
gallbladder) K82.0
– duodenum K31.5
– – congenital Q41.0
– ear canal (external) (congenital) Q16.1
– – acquired H61.3
– ejaculatory duct N50.8
– esophagus K22.2
– – congenital Q39.3
– – syphilitic A52.7† K23.8*
– – – congenital A50.5† K23.8*
– eustachian tube H68.1

Stricture—*continued*
- eustachian tube—*continued*
- – congenital Q16.4
- fallopian tube N97.1
- – gonococcal A54.2† N74.3∗
- – tuberculous A18.1† N74.1∗
- gallbladder (*see also* Obstruction, gallbladder) K82.0
- glottis J38.6
- heart (*see also* Disease, heart) I51.9
- – valve (*see also* Endocarditis) I38
- hepatic duct K83.1
- hourglass, of stomach K31.2
- hymen N89.6
- hypopharynx J39.2
- ileum K56.6
- – congenital Q41.2
- intestine (*see also* Obstruction, intestine) K56.6
- – congenital (small) Q41.9
- – – large Q42.9
- – – – specified NEC Q42.8
- – – specified NEC Q41.8
- – ischemic K55.1
- jejunum K56.6
- – congenital Q41.1
- lacrimal passages H04.5
- – congenital Q10.5
- larynx J38.6
- – congenital NEC Q31.8
- – – subglottic Q31.1
- – syphilitic A52.7† J99.8∗
- – – congenital A50.5† J99.8∗
- meatus
- – ear (congenital) Q16.1
- – – acquired H61.3
- – osseous (ear) (congenital) Q16.1
- – – acquired H61.3
- – urinarius (*see also* Stricture, urethra) N35.9
- – – congenital Q64.3
- mitral (valve) (*see also* Stenosis, mitral) I05.0
- – congenital Q23.2
- nares (anterior) (posterior) J34.8
- – congenital Q30.0
- nasal duct H04.5
- – congenital Q10.5
- nasolacrimal duct H04.5
- – congenital Q10.5
- nasopharynx J39.2
- – syphilitic A52.7† J99.8∗
- nose J34.8
- nostril (anterior) (posterior) J34.8

Stricture—*continued*
- nostril—*continued*
- – syphilitic A52.7† J99.8∗
- – – congenital A50.5† J99.8∗
- oesophagus – *see* Stricture, esophagus
- organ or site, congenital NEC – *see* Atresia, by site
- os uteri (*see also* Stricture, cervix) N88.2
- osseous meatus (ear) (congenital) Q16.1
- – acquired H61.3
- oviduct – *see* Stricture, fallopian tube
- pelviureteric junction N13.5
- – with
- – – hydronephrosis N13.0
- – – – with infection N13.6
- – – pyelonephritis (chronic) N11.1
- penis, by foreign body T19.8
- pharynx J39.2
- prostate N42.8
- pulmonary
- – artery (congenital) Q25.6
- – – acquired I28.8
- – valve I37.0
- – – congenital Q22.1
- – vessel NEC I28.8
- punctum lacrimale H04.5
- – congenital Q10.5
- pylorus (hypertrophic) K31.1
- – adult K31.1
- – congenital Q40.0
- – infantile Q40.0
- rectosigmoid K56.6
- rectum (sphincter) K62.4
- – congenital Q42.1
- – – with fistula Q42.0
- – due to
- – – chlamydial lymphogranuloma A55
- – – irradiation K91.8
- – gonococcal A54.6
- – inflammatory (chlamydial) A55
- – syphilitic A52.7† K93.8∗
- – tuberculous A18.3† K93.0∗
- renal artery I70.1
- – congenital Q27.1
- salivary duct or gland (any) K11.8
- sigmoid (flexure) (*see also* Obstruction, intestine) K56.6
- spermatic cord N50.8
- stoma, following
- – colostomy K91.4
- – enterostomy K91.4
- – gastrostomy K91.8
- – tracheostomy J95.0
- stomach K31.8

Stricture—*continued*
- stomach—*continued*
- – congenital Q40.2
- – hourglass K31.2
- subglottic J38.6
- syphilitic NEC A52.7
- trachea J39.8
- – congenital Q32.1
- – syphilitic A52.7† J99.8*
- – tuberculous NEC A16.4
- tricuspid (valve) (*see also* Stenosis, tricuspid) I07.0
- – congenital Q22.4
- tunica vaginalis N50.8
- ureter (postoperative) N13.5
- – with
- – – hydronephrosis N13.1
- – – – with infection N13.6
- – – pyelonephritis (chronic) N11.1
- – congenital Q62.1
- – tuberculous A18.1† N29.1*
- ureteropelvic junction N13.5
- – with
- – – hydronephrosis N13.0
- – – – with infection N13.6
- – – pyelonephritis (chronic) N11.1
- ureterovesical orifice N13.5
- – with infection N13.6
- urethra (anterior) (meatal) (organic) (posterior) (spasmodic) N35.9
- – associated with schistosomiasis B65.0† N29.1*
- – congenital Q64.3
- – – valvular (posterior) Q64.2
- – gonococcal, gonorrheal A54.0
- – infective NEC N35.1
- – late effect of injury N35.0
- – postcatheterization N99.1
- – postinfective NEC N35.1
- – postprocedural or postoperative N99.1
- – post-traumatic N35.0
- – sequela of
- – – childbirth N35.0
- – – injury N35.0
- – specified NEC N35.8
- – syphilitic A52.7† N37.8*
- – traumatic N35.0
- – valvular (posterior), congenital Q64.2
- urinary meatus (*see also* Stricture, urethra) N35.9
- – congenital Q64.3
- uterus, uterine (synechiae) N85.6
- – os (external) (internal) – *see* Stricture, cervix

Stricture—*continued*
- vagina (outlet) (*see also* Stenosis, vagina) N89.5
- – congenital Q52.4
- valve (cardiac) (heart) (*see also* Endocarditis) I38
- vas deferens N50.8
- – congenital Q55.4
- vein I87.1
- vena cava (inferior) (superior) NEC I87.1
- – congenital Q26.0
- vesicourethral orifice N32.0
- – congenital Q64.3
- vulva (acquired) N90.5
Stridor R06.1
- congenital (larynx) NEC P28.8
Stridulous – *see condition*
Stroke (apoplectic) (brain) (paralytic) I64
- epileptic – *see* Epilepsy
- heart – *see* Disease, heart
- heat T67.0
- lightning T75.0
Stromatosis, endometrial (M8931/1) D39.0
Strongyloides stercoralis infestation (*see also* Strongyloidiasis) B78.9
Strongyloidiasis, strongyloidosis B78.9
- cutaneous B78.1† L99.8*
- disseminated B78.7
- intestinal B78.0
Struck by lightning T75.0
Struma (*see also* Goiter) E04.9
- lymphomatosa E06.3
- ovarii (M9090/0) D27
- – with carcinoid (M9091/1) D39.1
- – malignant (M9090/3) C56
- Riedel's E06.5
Strumipriva cachexia E03.4
Strümpell-Marie spine M45
Strümpell-Westphal pseudosclerosis E83.0
Stuart deficiency disease (factor X) D68.2
Stuart-Prower factor deficiency (factor X) D68.2
Student's elbow M70.2
Stunting, nutritional E45
Stupor R40.1
- catatonic F20.2
- depressive F32.8
- dissociative F44.2
- manic F30.2
- manic-depressive F31.8
- psychogenic (anergic) F44.2

Stupor—*continued*
– reaction to exceptional stress (transient) F43.0
Sturge (-Weber) (-Dimitri))(-Kalischer) disease or syndrome Q85.8
Stuttering F98.5
Sty, stye (external) (internal) (meibomian) (zeisian) H00.0
Subacidity, gastric K31.8
– psychogenic F45.3
Subacute – *see condition*
Subarachnoid – *see condition*
Subcortical – *see condition*
Subcutaneous, subcuticular – *see condition*
Subdural – *see condition*
Subendocardium – *see condition*
Subependymoma (M9383/1)
– specified site – *see* Neoplasm, uncertain behavior
– unspecified site D43.2
Suberosis J67.3
Subglossitis – *see* Glossitis
Subinvolution
– breast (postlactational) (postpuerperal) N64.8
– puerperal O90.8
– uterus (nonpuerperal) N85.3
– – puerperal O90.8
Sublingual – *see condition*
Subluxatable hip Q65.6
Subluxation – *see also* Dislocation
– atlantoaxial, recurrent M43.4
– – with myelopathy M43.3
– complex, vertebral M99.1
– congenital NEC – *see also* Malposition, congenital
– – hip Q65.5
– – – bilateral Q65.4
– – – unilateral Q65.3
– – joint (excluding hip)
– – – lower limb Q68.8
– – – shoulder Q68.8
– – – upper limb Q68.8
– lens H27.1
– patella, recurrent M22.1
– pathological M24.3
– symphysis (pubis), in pregnancy, childbirth or puerperium O26.7
– vertebral, recurrent NEC M43.5
Submaxillary – *see condition*
Submersion (fatal) (nonfatal) T75.1
Submucous – *see condition*
Subnormal accommodation (old age) H52.4

Subnormality, mental F79.-
– mild F70.-
– moderate F71.-
– profound F73.-
– severe F72.-
Subphrenic – *see condition*
Subscapular nerve – *see condition*
Subseptus uterus Q51.8
Substernal thyroid E04.9
Substitution disorder F44.9
Subtentorial – *see condition*
Subthyroidism (acquired) (*see also* Hypothyroidism) E03.9
– congenital E03.1
Succenturiate placenta O43.1
Sucking thumb, child (excessive) F98.8
Sudamen, sudamina L74.1
Sudden
– death, cause unknown R96.0
– – during childbirth O95
– – infant R95
– – obstetric O95
– – puerperal, postpartum O95
– heart failure (*see also* Failure, heart) I50.9
– infant death syndrome R95
Sudeck's atrophy, disease or syndrome M89.0
Suffocation (*see also* Asphyxia) R09.0
– by
– – bed clothes T71
– – bunny bag T71
– – cave-in T71
– – constriction T71
– – drowning T75.1
– – inhalation
– – – food or foreign body (*see also* Asphyxia, food) T17.9
– – – gases, fumes, or vapors NEC T59.9
– – – – specified agent – *see* Table of drugs and chemicals
– – – oil or gasoline (*see also* Asphyxia, food) T17.9
– – overlying T71
– – plastic bag T71
– – pressure T71
– – strangulation T71
– mechanical T71
Sugar
– blood
– – high R73.9
– – low E16.2
– in urine R81

Suicide, suicidal (attempted)
- by poisoning – *see* Table of drugs and chemicals
- history of (personal) Z91.5
- – in family Z81.8
- observation following alleged attempt Z03.8
- risk R45.8
- – constituting part of a mental disorder – *see condition*
- tendencies R45.8
- – constituting part of a mental disorder – *see condition*
- trauma NEC (*see also* Nature and site of injury) T14.9

Sulfhemoglobinemia, sulphemoglobinemia (acquired) (with methemoglobinemia) D74.8
Summer – *see condition*
Sunburn L55.9
- first degree L55.0
- second degree L55.1
- specified NEC L55.8
- third degree L55.2

Sunstroke T67.0
Superfecundation O30.8
Superfetation O30.8
Superinvolution (uterus) N85.8
Supernumerary (congenital)
- aortic cusps Q23.8
- auditory ossicles Q16.3
- bone Q79.8
- breast Q83.1
- carpal bones Q74.0
- cusps, heart valve NEC Q24.8
- – aortic Q23.8
- – pulmonary Q22.3
- digit(s) Q69.9
- ear Q17.0
- fallopian tube Q50.6
- finger Q69.0
- hymen Q52.4
- kidney Q63.0
- lacrimonasal duct Q10.6
- lobule (ear) Q17.0
- muscle Q79.8
- nipple(s) Q83.3
- organ or site not listed – *see* Accessory
- ovary Q50.3
- oviduct Q50.6
- pulmonary cusps Q22.3
- rib Q76.6
- – cervical or first (syndrome) Q76.5
- roots (of teeth) K00.2

Supernumerary—*continued*
- tarsal bones Q74.2
- teeth K00.1
- – causing crowding K07.3
- testis Q55.2
- thumb Q69.1
- toe Q69.2
- uterus Q51.2
- vagina Q52.1
- vertebra Q76.4

Supervision (of)
- contraceptive method previously prescribed Z30.5
- dietary Z71.3
- high-risk pregnancy (*see also* Pregnancy, supervision) Z35.9
- lactation Z39.1
- pregnancy – *see* Pregnancy, supervision of

Supplementary teeth K00.1
- causing crowding K07.3

Suppression
- kidney (*see also* Failure, kidney) N19
- lactation O92.5
- menstruation N94.8
- ovarian secretion E28.3
- urine, urinary secretion R34

Suppuration, suppurative – *see also condition*
- accessory sinus (chronic) (*see also* Sinusitis) J32.9
- antrum (chronic) (*see also* Sinusitis, maxillary) J32.0
- bladder (*see also* Cystitis) N30.8
- brain G06.0
- breast N61
- – puerperal, postpartum or gestational O91.1
- dental periosteum K10.3
- ear (middle) NEC H66.4
- – external NEC H60.3
- – internal H83.0
- ethmoidal (chronic) (sinus) (*see also* Sinusitis, ethmoidal) J32.2
- fallopian tube (*see also* Salpingo-oophoritis) N70.9
- frontal (chronic) (sinus) (*see also* Sinusitis, frontal) J32.1
- gallbladder (acute) K81.0
- intracranial G06.0
- joint M00.9
- labyrinthine H83.0
- lung – *see* Abscess, lung
- mammary gland N61
- – puerperal, postpartum O91.1

Suppuration, suppurative—*continued*
– maxilla, maxillary K10.2
– – sinus (chronic) (*see also* Sinusitis, maxillary) J32.0
– muscle M60.0
– nasal sinus (chronic) (*see also* Sinusitis) J32.9
– pancreas, acute K85.-
– pelvis, pelvic
– – female (*see also* Disease, pelvis, inflammatory) N73.9
– – male K65.0
– pericranial (*see also* Osteomyelitis) M86.8
– salivary duct or gland (any) K11.2
– sinus (accessory) (chronic) (nasal) (*see also* Sinusitis) J32.9
– sphenoidal sinus (chronic) (*see also* Sinusitis, sphenoidal) J32.3
– thymus (gland) E32.1
– thyroid (gland) E06.0
– tonsil (*see also* Tonsillitis) J03.9
– – chronic J35.0
– uterus (*see also* Endometritis) N71.9
Suprarenal (gland) – *see condition*
Suprascapular nerve – *see condition*
Suprasellar – *see condition*
Surfer's knots or nodules T14.0
Surgery
– elective Z41.9
– – breast augmentation or reduction (cosmetic) Z41.1
– – face-lift (cosmetic) Z41.1
– – hair transplant Z41.0
– – specified type NEC Z41.8
– not done – *see* Procedure (surgical), not done
– plastic
– – corrective, restorative – *see* Surgery, reconstructive
– – cosmetic Z41.1
– – – breast augmentation or reduction Z41.1
– – – face-lift Z41.1
– – – hair transplant Z41.0
– – following healed injury or operation – *see* Surgery, reconstructive
– – for unacceptable cosmetic appearance Z41.1
– previous, in pregnancy or childbirth
– – cervix O34.4
– – – causing obstructed labor O65.5
– – – – affecting fetus or newborn P03.1
– – pelvic soft tissues NEC O34.8

Surgery—*continued*
– previous, in pregnancy or childbirth—*continued*
– – pelvic soft tissues NEC—*continued*
– – – affecting fetus or newborn P03.8
– – – causing obstructed labor O65.5
– – – – affecting fetus or newborn P03.1
– – perineum or vulva O34.7
– – uterus O34.2
– – – causing obstructed labor O65.5
– – – – affecting fetus or newborn P03.1
– – vagina O34.6
– prophylactic Z40.9
– – for risk factors related to malignant neoplasm Z40.0
– – specified NEC Z40.8
– reconstructive (following healed injury or operation) Z42.9
– – breast Z42.1
– – head and neck Z42.0
– – lower limb Z42.4
– – specified NEC Z42.8
– – trunk Z42.2
– – – breast Z42.1
– – upper limb Z42.3
Surgical
– emphysema T81.8
– operation NEC R69
– procedures, complication or misadventure – *see* Complications, surgical procedures
– shock T81.1
Surveillance (of) (for) (*see also* Observation) Z04.9
– alcohol abuse Z71.4
– contraceptive
– – device Z30.5
– – drugs Z30.4
– dietary Z71.3
– drug abuse Z71.5
Suspected condition, ruled out (*see also* Observation, suspected) Z03.9
Suspended uterus
– in pregnancy or childbirth O34.5
– – causing obstructed labor O65.5
– – – affecting fetus or newborn P03.1
Sutton's nevus (M8723/0) D22.9
Suture
– burst (in operation wound) T81.3
– inadvertently left in operation wound T81.5
Swab inadvertently left in operation wound T81.5

Swallowed foreign body (*see also* Foreign body) T18.9
Swan-neck deformity (finger) M20.0
Swearing, compulsive F42.8
– in Gilles de la Tourette's syndrome F95.2
Sweat, sweats
– fetid L75.0
– night R61.9
Sweating, excessive R61.9
Sweet's disease or dermatosis L98.2
Swelling (of)
– abdomen, abdominal (not referable to any particular organ) R19.0
– ankle M25.4
– arm M79.8
– Calabar B74.3
– cervical gland R59.0
– chest, localized R22.2
– extremity (lower) (upper) M79.8
– finger M79.8
– foot M79.8
– glands R59.9
– – generalized R59.1
– – localized R59.0
– hand M79.8
– head (localized) R22.0
– inflammatory – *see* Inflammation
– intra-abdominal R19.0
– joint M25.4
– leg M79.8
– limb M79.8
– localized (skin) R22.9
– – chest R22.2
– – head R22.0
– – limb
– – – lower R22.4
– – – upper R22.3
– – multiple sites R22.7
– – neck R22.1
– – trunk R22.2
– neck (localized) R22.1
– pelvic R19.0
– scrotum N50.8
– testis N50.8
– toe M79.8
– tubular N28.8
– umbilical R19.0
– wandering, due to Gnathostoma (spinigerum) B83.1
– white – *see* Tuberculosis, arthritis
Swift(-Feer) disease T56.1
Swimmer's
– cramp T75.1
– ear H60.3

Swimmer's—*continued*
– itch B65.3
Swollen – *see* Swelling
Swyer's syndrome Q99.1
Sycosis L73.8
– barbae (not parasitic) L73.8
contagiosa (mycotic) B35.0
– lupoides L73.8
– mycotic B35.0
– parasitic B35.0
– vulgaris L73.8
Sydenham's chorea – *see* Chorea, Sydenham's
Symblepharon H11.2
– congenital Q10.3
Sympathetic – *see* condition
Sympatheticotonia G90.8
Sympathicoblastoma (M9500/3)
– specified site – *see* Neoplasm, malignant
– unspecified site C74.9
Sympathicogonioma (M9500/3) – *see* Sympathicoblastoma
Sympathoblastoma (M9500/3) – *see* Sympathicoblastoma
Sympathogonioma (M9500/3) – *see* Sympathicoblastoma
Symphalangy (fingers) (toes) Q70.9
Symptoms specified NEC R68.8
– factitious, self-induced F68.1
– involving
– – abdomen NEC R19.8
– – appearance NEC R46.8
– – awareness NEC R41.8
– – behavior NEC R46.8
– – cardiovascular system NEC R09.8
– – chest NEC R09.8
– – circulatory system NEC R09.8
– – cognitive functions NEC R41.8
– – development NEC R62.8
– – digestive system NEC R19.8
– – emotional state NEC R45.8
– – food and fluid intake R63.8
– – general perceptions and sensations R44.8
– – musculoskeletal system NEC R29.8
– – nervous system NEC R29.8
– – pelvis NEC R19.8
– – respiratory system NEC R09.8
– – skin and integument NEC R23.8
– – urinary system NEC R39.8
– neurotic F48.8
Sympus Q74.2
Syncephalus Q89.4

Synchondrosis
– abnormal Q78.8
– ischiopubic M91.0
Synchysis (scintillans) (senile) (vitreous body) H43.8
Syncope R55
– bradycardia R00.1
– cardiac R55
– carotid sinus G90.0
– due to spinal (lumbar) puncture G97.1
– fatal unexplained R96.0
– heart R55
– heat T67.1
– psychogenic F48.8
– tussive R05
– vasoconstriction R55
Syndactylism, syndactyly Q70.9
– complex (with synostosis) Q70.9
– – fingers Q70.0
– – toes Q70.2
– fingers (without synostosis) Q70.1
– – with synostosis Q70.0
– simple (without synostosis) Q70.9
– – fingers Q70.1
– – toes Q70.3
– toes (without synostosis) Q70.3
– – with synostosis Q70.2
Syndrome – *see also* Disease
– 5q-minus (related to alkylating agent) (related to Epipodophyllotoxin) (related to therapy) D46.6
– abdominal
– – acute R10.0
– – migraine G43.1
– – muscle deficiency Q79.4
– acquired immunodeficiency – *see* Human, immunodeficiency virus (HIV) disease
– acute abdominal R10.0
– adiposogenital E23.6
– adrenal
– – hemorrhage (meningococcal) A39.1† E35.1*
– – meningococcic A39.1† E35.1*
– adrenocortical E27.0
– – with Cushing's syndrome – *see* Cushing's
– adrenogenital E25.9
– – congenital, associated with enzyme deficiency E25.0
– afferent loop NEC K91.8
– alcohol withdrawal F10.3
– – with delirium F10.4
– alveolar hypoventilation E66.2
– alveolocapillary block J84.1

Syndrome—*continued*
– amnesic, amnestic (confabulatory) (due to) F1X.6
– – alcohol-induced F10.6
– – drug-induced – *code to* F11-F19 with fourth character .6
– – organic
– – – alcohol-induced F10.6
– – – drug-induced – *code to* F11-F19 with fourth character .6
– – sedative or hypnotic F13.6
– amyostatic (Wilson's disease) E83.0
– anaphylactoid, of pregnancy O88.1
– androgen resistance E34.5
– anginal (*see also* Angina) I20.9
– anterior
– – chest wall R07.3
– – spinal artery G95.1
– – – compression M47.0† G99.2*
– antibody deficiency D80.9
– – agammaglobulinemic D80.1
– – – hereditary D80.0
– – hypogammaglobulinemic D80.1
– – – hereditary D80.0
– anticardiolipin D68.6
– antiphospholipid (-antibody) D68.6
– aortic
– – arch M31.4
– – bifurcation I74.0
– aortomesenteric duodenum occlusion K31.5
– argentaffin E34.0
– aspiration, of newborn (massive) P24.9
– – meconium P24.0
– ataxia-telangiectasia G11.3
– autoerythrocyte sensitization (Gardner-Diamond) D69.2
– autoimmune polyglandular E31.0
– autosomal (*see also* Abnormal, autosomes NEC) Q99.9
– bare lymphocyte D81.6
– basilar artery G45.0
– battered
– – baby or child T74.1
– – spouse T74.1
– bilateral polycystic ovarian E28.2
– black widow spider bite T63.3
– blind loop K90.2
– – congenital Q43.8
– – postsurgical K91.2
– blue diaper E70.8
– brachial plexus G54.0
– brain F06.9

Syndrome—*continued*
- brain—*continued*
- − acute or subacute (*see also* Delirium) F05.9
- − − alcoholic (chronic) F10.7
- − − congenital − *see* Retardation, mental
- − − organic F06.9
- − − − post-traumatic (nonpsychotic) F07.2
- − − − − psychotic F06.8
- − − personality change F07.0
- − − post-traumatic, nonpsychotic F07.2
- − − psychotic F06.8
- − brain stem stroke I67.9† G46.3∗
- − broad ligament laceration N83.8
- − bronze baby P83.8
- − bubbly lung P27.0
- − bulbar (progressive) G12.2
- − burning feet E53.9
- − carcinoid E34.0
- − cardiopulmonary-obesity E66.2
- − cardiorenal (*see also* Hypertension, cardiorenal) I13.9
- − cardiorespiratory distress (idiopathic), newborn P22.0
- − cardiovascular renal (*see also* Hypertension, cardiorenal) I13.9
- − carotid
- − − artery (hemispheric) G45.1
- − − − internal G45.1
- − − sinus G90.0
- − carpal tunnel G56.0
- − cat-cry Q93.4
- − cauda equina G83.4
- − causalgia G56.4
- − celiac artery compression I77.4
- − cerebellar
- − − hereditary G11.9
- − − stroke I67.9† G46.4∗
- − cerebral artery
- − − anterior I66.1† G46.1∗
- − − middle I66.0† G46.0∗
- − − posterior I66.2† G46.2∗
- − cervical (root) M53.1
- − − disk M50.1† G55.1∗
- − − fusion Q76.1
- − − posterior, sympathicus M53.0
- − − rib Q76.5
- − − sympathetic paralysis G90.2
- − cervicobrachial (diffuse) M53.1
- − cervicocranial M53.0
- − cervicothoracic outlet G54.0
- − child maltreatment NEC T74.9
- − chondrocostal junction M94.0

Syndrome—*continued*
- chromosome
- − − 18 long arm deletion Q93.5
- − − 21 long arms deletion Q93.5
- − − 4 short arm deletion Q93.3
- − − 5 short arm deletion Q93.4
- − chronic pain personality F62.8
- − climacteric N95.1
- − clumsiness, clumsy child F82
- − cluster headache G44.0
- − cold injury (newborn) P80.0
- − compartment (deep) (posterior) T79.6
- − − non-traumatic M62.2
- − compression T79.5
- − − anterior spinal and vertebral artery M47.0† G99.2∗
- − − cauda equina G83.4
- − − celiac artery I77.4
- − concussion F07.2
- − congenital
- − − affecting multiple systems NEC Q87.8
- − − facial diplegia Q87.0
- − − muscular hypertrophy-cerebral Q87.8
- − − oculo-auriculovertebral Q87.0
- − − oculofacial diplegia (Moebius) Q87.0
- − − rubella (manifest) P35.0
- − congestion-fibrosis (pelvic), female N94.8
- − congestive dysmenorrhea N94.6
- − connective tissue M35.9
- − − overlap NEC M35.1
- − conus medullaris G95.8
- − coronary
- − − acute NEC I24.9   I20.0 I24.9
- − − intermediate I20.0
- − costochondral junction M94.0
- − costoclavicular G54.0
- − craniovertebral M53.0
- − cri-du-chat Q93.4
- − crush T79.5
- − cryptophthalmos Q87.0
- − defibrination (*see also* Fibrinolysis) D65
- − − with
- − − − antepartum hemorrhage O46.0
- − − − intrapartum hemorrhage O67.0
- − − − premature separation of placenta O45.0
- − − fetus or newborn P60
- − − postpartum O72.3
- − delayed sleep phase G47.2
- − demyelinating G37.9
- − dependence − *code to* F10-F19 with fourth character .2
- − depersonalization(-derealization) F48.1

DiGeorge Syndrome D82.1

Syndrome—*continued*
- distal intestinal obstruction E84.1
- dorsolateral medullary I66.3† G46.4*
- drug withdrawal, infant of dependent mother P96.1
- dry eye H04.1
- due to abnormality
- – chromosomal Q99.9
- – – sex
- – – – female phenotype Q97.9
- – – – male phenotype Q98.9
- – – specified NEC Q99.8
- dumping (postgastrectomy) K91.1
- dyspraxia, developmental F82
- ectopic ACTH E24.3
- effort (psychogenic) F45.3
- empty nest Z60.0
- entrapment – *see* Neuropathy, entrapment
- eosinophilia-myalgia M35.8
- epidemic vomiting A08.1
- epileptic (*see also* Epilepsy) G40.9
- – special G40.5
- erythrocyte fragmentation D59.4
- exhaustion F48.0
- extrapyramidal G25.9
- – specified NEC G25.8
- eye retraction H50.8
- eyelid-malar-mandible Q87.0
- facial pain, paroxysmal G50.0
- familial eczema-thrombocytopenia (Wiskott-Aldrich) D82.0
- fatigue F48.0
- – chronic G93.3
- – postviral G93.3
- fertile eunuch E23.0
- fetal
- – alcohol (dysmorphic) Q86.0
- – hydantoin Q86.1
- first arch Q87.0
- flatback M40.3
- floppy
- – baby P94.2
- – mitral valve I34.1
- fragile X Q99.2
- frontal lobe F07.0
- functional
- – bowel K59.9
- – prepuberal castrate E29.1
- ganglion (basal ganglia brain) G25.9
- gastroesophageal laceration-hemorrhage K22.6
- gastrojejunal loop obstruction K91.8
- generalized, neoplastic (malignant) C79.9
- – primary site not indicated C80.9

Syndrome—*continued*
- generalized, neoplastic – *continued*
- – primary site unknown, so stated C80.0
- genito-anorectal A55
- giant platelet (Bernard-Soulier) D69.1
- goiter-deafness E07.1
- gray (newborn) P93
- – platelet D69.1
- gustatory sweating G50.8
- Hantavirus (cardio-)pulmonary (HPS) (HCPS) B33.4† J17.1*
- hand-shoulder G90.8
- headache NEC G44.8
- HELLP (hemolysis, elevated liver enzymes and low platelet count) O14.2
- hemolytic-uremic D59.3
- hemophagocytic, infection-associated D76.2
- hepatic flexure K59.8
- hepatorenal K76.7
- – following delivery O90.4
- – postoperative or postprocedural K91.8
- – postpartum, puerperal O90.4
- histamine-like (fish poisoning) T61.1
- histiocytosis NEC D76.3
- HIV infection, acute B23.0
- hyperabduction G54.0
- hyperimmunoglobulin E (IgE) D82.4
- hyperkalemic E87.5
- hyperkinetic (*see also* Hyperkinesia) F90.9
- – heart I51.8
- hypermobility M35.7
- hypersomnia-bulimia G47.8
- hyperventilation F45.3
- hypokalemic E87.6
- hyponatremic E87.1
- hypopituitarism E23.0
- hypoplastic left-heart Q23.4
- hypopotassemia E87.6
- hypotension, maternal O26.5
- idiopathic cardiorespiratory distress, newborn P22.0
- iliotibial band M76.3
- immobility, immobilization (paraplegic) M62.3
- immunodeficiency
- – acquired – *see* Human, immunodeficiency virus (HIV) disease
- – combined D81.9
- impingement, shoulder M75.4
- inappropriate secretion of antidiuretic hormone E22.2
- infant of diabetic mother P70.1

Syndrome—*continued*
- infant of diabetic mother—*continued*
- – gestational diabetes P70.0
- infantilism (pituitary) E23.0
- inferior vena cava I87.1
- inspissated bile (newborn) P59.1
- institutional (childhood) F94.2
- intermediate coronary I20.0
- interspinous ligament M48.8
- iodine-deficiency, congenital E00.9
- – type
- – – mixed E00.2
- – – myxedematous E00.1
- – – neurological E00.0
- irritable
- – bowel K58.9
- – – with diarrhea K58.0
- – – psychogenic F45.3
- – heart (psychogenic) F45.3
- – weakness F48.0
- jaw-winking Q07.8
- jugular foramen G52.7
- labyrinthine H83.2
- lacunar NEC I67.9† G46.7*
- lateral
- – cutaneous nerve of thigh G57.1
- – medullary I66.3† G46.4*
- lenticular, progressive E83.0
- limbic epilepsy personality F07.0
- lobotomy F07.0
- long QT I45.8
- low
- – atmospheric pressure T70.2
- – back M54.5
- – – psychogenic F45.4
- lower radicular, newborn (birth injury) P14.8
- malabsorption K90.9
- – postsurgical K91.2
- malformation, congenital, due to
- – alcohol Q86.0
- – exogenous cause NEC Q86.8
- – hydantoin Q86.1
- – warfarin Q86.2
- malignant neuroleptic G21.0
- mandibulofacial dysostosis Q75.4
- manic-depressive (*see also* Disorder, bipolar, affective) F31.9
- maple-syrup-urine E71.0
- maternal hypotension O26.5
- meconium plug (newborn) P76.0
- megavitamin-B$_6$ E67.2
- menopause N95.1
- – postartificial N95.3

Syndrome—*continued*
- menstruation N94.3
- mesenteric
- – artery (superior) K55.1
- – vascular insufficiency K55.1
  micrognathia-glossoptosis Q87.0
- midbrain NEC G93.8
- middle lobe (lung) J98.1
- migraine G43.9
- milk-alkali E83.5
- Miller Fisher G61.0
- monofixation H50.4
- mucocutaneous lymph node (acute febrile) (MCLS) M30.3
- multiple operations F68.1
- myasthenic (in) G70.9
- – diabetes mellitus – *code to* E10-E14 with fourth character .4
- – endocrine disease NEC E34.9† G73.0*
- – neoplastic disease NEC (M8000/1) (*see also* Neoplasm) D48.9† G73.2*
- – thyrotoxicosis (hyperthyroidism) E05.9† G73.0*
- myelodysplastic (related to alkylating agent) (related to   Epipodophyllotoxin) (related to therapy) D46.9
- – specified NEC D46.7
- myeloproliferative (chronic) D47.1
- nail patella Q87.2
- neonatal abstinence P96.1
- nephritic (*see also* Nephritis) N05.-

Note: Where a term is indexed only at the three-character level, e.g. N03.-, reference should be made to the list of fourth-character subdivisions in Volume 1 at N00-N08.

- – with edema – *see* Nephrosis
- – acute N00.-
- – chronic N03.-
- – rapidly progressive N01.-
- nephrotic (congenital) (*see also* Nephrosis) N04.-
- oculomotor H51.9
- ophthalmoplegia-cerebellar ataxia H49.0
- oro-facial-digital Q87.0
- organic amnesic (not alcohol- or drug-induced) F04
- osteoporosis-osteomalacia M83.8
- otolith H81.8
- oto-palatal-digital Q87.0
- ovary
- – polycystic E28.2
- – residual N99.8

POEMS syndrome   D47.7

rare syndrome defined as combination of Plasma Cell proliferation disorder (typically myeloma), polyneuropathy, + effects on other organs

Syndrome—*continued*
- ovary—*continued*
- – – resistant E28.3
- – – sclerocystic E28.2
- – pain – *see* Pain
- – paralysis agitans (*see also* Parkinsonism) G20
- – paralytic G83.9
- – – specified NEC G83.8
- – parkinsonian (*see also* Parkinsonism) G20
- – paroxysmal facial pain G50.0
- – pellagroid E52
- – pelvic congestion-fibrosis, female N94.8
- – penta X Q97.1
- – peptic ulcer – *see* Ulcer, peptic
- – phantom limb (without pain) G54.7
- – – with pain G54.6
- – pharyngeal pouch D82.1
- – pigmentary pallidal degeneration (progressive) G23.0
- – pineal E34.8
- – placental
- – – dysfunction O43.8
- – – – affecting fetus or newborn P02.2
- – – insufficiency O43.8
- – – – affecting fetus or newborn P02.2
- – – transfusion (mother) O43.0
- – – – in fetus or newborn P02.3
- – pluricarential, of infancy E40
- – plurideficiency E40
- – pluriglandular (compensatory) (M8360/1) D44.8
- – – autoimmune E31.0
- – pneumatic hammer T75.2
- – polyangiitis overlap M30.8
- – polycarential, of infancy E40
- – polyglandular (M8360/1) D44.8
- – – autoimmune E31.0
- – pontine NEC G93.8
- – popliteal web Q87.8
- – post-artificial-menopause N95.3
- – postcardiotomy I97.0
- – postcholecystectomy K91.5
- – postcommissurotomy I97.0
- – postconcussional F07.2
- – postcontusional F07.2
- – postencephalitic F07.1
- – posterior cervical sympathetic M53.0
- – postgastrectomy (dumping) K91.1
- – postgastric surgery K91.1
- – postlaminectomy NEC M96.1
- – postleukotomy F07.0
- – postmastectomy lymphedema I97.2

Syndrome—*continued*
- – postmyocardial infarction I24.1
- – postoperative NEC T81.9
- – postpartum panhypopituitary (Sheehan) E23.0
- – postphlebitic I87.0
- – postpolio (postpoliomyelitic) G14
- – postthrombotic I87.0
- – postvagotomy K91.1
- – postvalvulotomy I97.0
- – postviral NEC R53
- – – fatigue G93.3
- – potassium intoxication E87.5
- – precerebral artery (bilateral) (multiple) G45.2
- – preinfarction I20.0
- – preleukemic D46.9
- – premature senility E34.8
- – premenstrual tension N94.3
- – prolonged QT I45.8
- – prune belly Q79.4
- – psycho-organic (nonpsychotic severity) F07.9
- – – acute or subacute F05.9
- – – specified NEC F07.8
- – pulmonary
- – – arteriosclerosis I27.0
- – – dysmaturity (Wilson-Mikity) P27.0
- – – renal (hemorrhagic) (Goodpasture's) M31.0
- – pure
- – – motor lacunar I67.9† G46.5*
- – – sensory lacunar I67.9† G46.6*
- – radicular NEC M54.1
- – – upper limbs, newborn (birth injury) P14.3
- – reactive airways dysfunction J68.3
- – residual ovary N99.8
- – resistant ovary E28.3
- – respiratory
- – – distress (idiopathic) (newborn) P22.0
- – – – adult J80
- – – severe acute U04.9
- – restless legs G25.8
- – retraction H50.8
- – right
- – – heart, hypoplastic Q22.6
- – – ventricular obstruction – *see* Failure, heart, congestive
- – rotator cuff, shoulder M75.1
- – salt
- – – depletion E87.1
- – – – due to heat NEC T67.8

Syndrome—*continued*
- salt—*continued*
- – depletion—*continued*
- – – due to heat NEC—*continued*
- – – – causing heat exhaustion or prostration T67.4
- – low E87.1
- salt-losing N28.8
- scalenus anticus (anterior) G54.0
- scapuloperoneal G71.0
- schizophrenic, of childhood NEC F84.5
- scimitar Q26.8
- septicemic adrenal hemorrhage A39.1† E35.1*
- severe acute respiratory (SARS) U04.9
- shock-lung J80
- shock, toxic A48.3
- short rib Q77.2
- shoulder-hand M89.0
- sicca M35.0
- sick-euthyroid E07.8
- sick sinus I49.5
- sirenomelia Q87.2
- spasmodic
- – upward movement, eyes H51.8
- – winking F95.8
- spinal cord injury (*see also* Injury, spinal cord, by region) T09.3
- splenic flexure K59.8
- staphylococcal scalded skin L00
- stiff man G25.8
- straight back, congenital Q76.4
- stroke I64
- subclavian steal G45.8
- subcoracoid-pectoralis minor G54.0
- sudden infant death R95
- superior
- – cerebellar artery I63.8
- – mesenteric artery K55.1
- – vena cava I87.1
- supine hypotensive (maternal) O26.5
- supraspinatus M75.1
- sweat retention L74.0
- sympathetic
- – cervical paralysis G90.2
- – pelvic, female N94.8
- systemic inflammatory response as a result of disease classified elsewhere R65.9
- – infectious origin
- – – with organ failure (severe sepsis) R65.1
- – – without organ failure R65.0

Syndrome—*continued*
- systemic inflammatory response as a result of disease classified elsewhere—*continued*
- – non-infectious origin
- – – with organ failure R65.3
- – – without organ failure R65.2
- – unspecified origin, as a result of disease classified elsewhere R65.9
- tachycardia-bradycardia I49.5
- TAR (thrombocytopenia with absent radius) Q87.2
- tarsal tunnel G57.5
- teething K00.7
- tegmental G93.8
- telangiectasic-pigmentation-cataract Q82.8
- temporal pyramidal apex H66.0
- temporomandibular joint-pain-dysfunction K07.6
- testicular feminization E34.5
- thalamic G93.8
- thoracic outlet (compression) G54.0
- thrombocytopenia with absent radius (TAR) Q87.2
- thyroid-adrenocortical insufficiency E31.0
- tibial
- – anterior M76.8
- – posterior M76.8
- toxic shock A48.3
- traumatic vasospastic T75.2
- triple X, female Q97.0
- trisomy NEC Q92.9
- – 13 Q91.7
- – – meiotic nondisjunction Q91.4
- – – mitotic nondisjunction Q91.5
- – – mosaicism Q91.5
- – – translocation Q91.6
- – 18 Q91.3
- – – meiotic nondisjunction Q91.0
- – – mitotic nondisjunction Q91.1
- – – mosaicism Q91.1
- – – translocation Q91.2
- – 20 (q) (p) Q92.8
- – 21 Q90.9
- – – meiotic nondisjunction Q90.0
- – – mitotic nondisjunction Q90.1
- – – mosaicism Q90.1
- – – translocation Q90.2
- – 22 Q92.8
- tumor lysis (following antineoplastic drug therapy)(spontaneous) NEC E88.3

Williams syndrome - other deletions from the autosomes - Q93.8

Syndrome—*continued*
- twin (to twin) transfusion
- – in fetus or newborn P02.3
- – mother O43.0
- upward gaze H51.8
- uremia, chronic (*see also* Disease, kidney, chronic) N18.9
- urethral N34.3
- urethro-oculo-articular M02.3
- vago-hypoglossal G52.7
- vascular NEC in cerebrovascular disease I67.9† G46.8∗
- vasomotor I73.9
- vasospastic (traumatic) T75.2
- vasovagal R55
- VATER Q87.2
- vena cava (inferior) (superior) (obstruction) I87.1
- vertebral
- – artery G45.0
- – – compression M47.0† G99.2∗
- – steal G45.0
- vertebro-basilar artery G45.0
- vertebrogenic (pain) M54.8
- vertiginous H81.9
- virus B34.9
- visceral larva migrans B83.0
- visual disorientation H53.8
- vitamin B₆ deficiency E53.1
- vitreal corneal H59.0
- vitreous (following cataract surgery) (touch) H59.0
- wasting, resulting from HIV disease B22.2
- whiplash S13.4
- whistling face Q87.0
- withdrawal – *see* Withdrawal, state
- – drug
- – – infant of dependent mother P96.1
- – – therapeutic use, newborn P96.2
- XXXX, female Q97.1
- 48,XXXX Q97.1
- XXXXX, female Q97.1
- 49,XXXXX Q97.1
- XXXXY Q98.1
- XXY Q98.0
- yellow nail L60.5
Synechia (anterior) (iris) (posterior) (pupil) H21.5
- intra-uterine N85.6
Synesthesia R20.8
Syngamiasis, syngamosis B83.3
Synodontia K00.2
Synorchidism, synorchism Q55.1

Synostosis (congenital) Q78.8
- astragalo-scaphoid Q74.2
- radioulnar Q74.0
Synovial sarcoma (M9040/3) – *see* Neoplasm, connective tissue, malignant
Synovioma (malignant) (M9040/3) – *see also* Neoplasm, connective tissue, malignant
- benign (M9040/0) – *see* Neoplasm, connective tissue, benign
Synoviosarcoma (M9040/3) – *see* Neoplasm, connective tissue, malignant
Synovitis M65.9
- chronic crepitant, hand or wrist M70.0
- gonococcal A54.4† M68.0∗
- gouty M10.0
- in (due to)
- – crystals M65.8
- – gonorrhea A54.4† M68.0∗
- – syphilis (late) A52.7† M68.0∗
- – use, overuse, pressure M70.9
- – – specified NEC M70.8
- infective NEC M65.1
- specified NEC M65.8
- syphilitic A52.7† M68.0∗
- – congenital (early) A50.0
- toxic M67.3
- transient M67.3
- traumatic, current – *see* Sprain
- tuberculous – *see* Tuberculosis, synovitis
- villonodular (pigmented) M12.2
Syphilid A51.3
- congenital A50.0
- newborn A50.0
- tubercular (late) A52.7† L99.8∗
- – congenital A50.0
Syphilis, syphilitic (acquired) A53.9
- abdomen (late) A52.7
- acoustic nerve A52.1† H94.0∗
- adenopathy (secondary) A51.4
- adrenal (gland) (with cortical hypofunction) A52.7† E35.1∗
- age under 2 years NEC (*see also* Syphilis, congenital, early) A50.2
- – acquired A51.9
- alopecia (secondary) A51.3† L99.8∗
- anemia (late) A52.7† D63.8∗
- aneurysm (aorta) (ruptured) A52.0† I79.0∗
- – central nervous system A52.0† I68.8∗
- – congenital A50.5† I79.0∗
- anus (late) A52.7† K93.8∗
- – primary A51.1
- – secondary A51.3

Syphilis, syphilitic—*continued*
- aorta (abdominal) (arch) (thoracic) A52.0† I79.1*
- – aneurysm A52.0† I79.0*
- aortic (insufficiency) (regurgitation) (stenosis) A52.0† I39.1*
- – aneurysm A52.0† I79.0*
- arachnoid (adhesive) (cerebral) (spinal) A52.1† G01*
- asymptomatic – *see* Syphilis, latent
- ataxia (locomotor) A52.1
- atrophoderma maculatum A51.3† L99.8*
- auricular fibrillation A52.0† I52.0*
- bladder (late) A52.7† N33.8*
- bone A52.7† M90.2*
- – secondary A51.4† M90.2*
- brain A52.1† G94.8*
- breast (late) A52.7
- bronchus (late) A52.7† J99.8*
- bubo (primary) A51.0
- bulbar palsy A52.1
- bursa (late) A52.7† M73.1*
- cardiac decompensation A52.0† I52.0*
- cardiovascular A52.0† I98.0*
- causing death under 2 years of age (*see also* Syphilis, congenital, early) A50.2
- – stated to be acquired A51.9
- central nervous system (late) (recurrent) (relapse) (tertiary) A52.3
- – with
- – – ataxia A52.1
- – – general paralysis A52.1
- – – – juvenile A50.4
- – – paresis (general) A52.1
- – – – juvenile A50.4
- – – tabes (dorsalis) A52.1
- – – – juvenile A50.4
- – – taboparesis A52.1
- – – – juvenile A50.4
- – aneurysm A52.0† I68.8*
- – congenital A50.4
- – juvenile A50.4
- – serology doubtful, negative, or positive A52.3
- – specified nature or site NEC A52.1
- – vascular A52.0† I68.8*
- cerebral A52.1† G94.8*
- – meningovascular A52.1† G01*
- – nerves (multiple palsies) A52.1† G53.1*
- – sclerosis A52.1† G94.8*
- – thrombosis A52.0† I68.8*
- cerebrospinal (tabetic type) A52.1

Syphilis, syphilitic—*continued*
- cerebrovascular A52.0† I68.8*
- cervix (late) A52.7† N74.2*
- chancre (multiple) A51.0
- – extragenital A51.2
- – Rollet's A51.0
- Charcot's joint A52.1† M14.6*
- chorioretinitis A51.4† H32.0*
- – late A52.7† H32.0*
- choroiditis – *see* Syphilis, chorioretinitis
- choroidoretinitis – *see* Syphilis, chorioretinitis
- ciliary body (secondary) A51.4† H22.0*
- – late A52.7† H22.0*
- colon (late) A52.7† K93.8*
- combined spinal sclerosis A52.1† G32.0*
- complicating pregnancy, childbirth or puerperium O98.1
- – affecting fetus or newborn P00.2
- condyloma (latum) A51.3
- congenital A50.9
- – with
- – – paresis (general) A50.4
- – – tabes (dorsalis) A50.4
- – – taboparesis A50.4
- – chorioretinitis, choroiditis A50.0† H32.0*
- – early, or less than 2 years after birth NEC A50.2
- – – with manifestations A50.0
- – – latent (without manifestations) A50.1
- – – – negative spinal fluid test A50.1
- – – – serology positive A50.1
- – – symptomatic A50.0
- – interstitial keratitis A50.3† H19.2*
- – juvenile neurosyphilis A50.4
- – late, or 2 years or more after birth NEC A50.7
- – – chorioretinitis, choroiditis A50.3† H32.0*
- – – interstitial keratitis A50.3† H19.2*
- – – juvenile neurosyphilis A50.4
- – – latent (without manifestations) A50.6
- – – – negative spinal fluid test A50.6
- – – – serology positive A50.6
- – – symptomatic or with manifestations NEC A50.5
- conjugal A53.9
- – tabes A52.1
- conjunctiva (late) A52.7† H13.1*
- cord bladder A52.1
- cornea, late A52.7† H19.2*

Syphilis, syphilitic—*continued*
- coronary (artery) (sclerosis) A52.0†
  I52.0*
- cranial nerve A52.1† G53.8*
- – multiple palsies A52.1† G53.1*
- cutaneous – *see* Syphilis, skin
- dacryocystitis (late) A52.7† H06.0*
- degeneration, spinal cord A52.1
- dementia paralytica A52.1
- – juvenilis A50.4
- destruction of bone A52.7† M90.2*
- dilatation, aorta A52.0† I79.0*
- due to blood transfusion A53.9
- dura mater A52.1† G01*
- ear A52.7† H94.8*
- – inner A52.7† H94.8*
- – – nerve (eighth) A52.1† H94.0*
- – – neurorecurrence A52.1† H94.0*
- early NEC A51.9
- – cardiovascular A52.0† I98.0*
- – latent (less than 2 years after infection)
  (without manifestations) A51.5
- – – negative spinal fluid test A51.5
- – – serological relapse after treatment
  A51.5
- – – serology positive A51.5
- – relapse (treated, untreated) A51.9
- – skin A51.3
- – symptomatic A51.9
- – – extragenital chancre A51.2
- – – primary, except extragenital chancre
  A51.0
- – – secondary (*see also* Syphilis,
  secondary) A51.3
- – – – relapse (treated, untreated) A51.4
- – ulcer A51.3
- eighth nerve (neuritis) A52.1† H94.0*
- endemic A65
- endocarditis A52.0† I39.8*
- – aortic A52.0† I39.1*
- – pulmonary A52.0† I39.3*
- epididymis (late) A52.7† N51.1*
- epiglottis (late) A52.7† J99.8*
- epiphysitis (congenital) (early) A50.0†
  M90.2*
- episcleritis (late) A52.7† H19.0*
- esophagus A52.7† K23.8*
- eustachian tube A52.7† J99.8*
- eye A52.7† H58.8*
- eyelid (late) (with gumma) A52.7†
  H03.1*
- fallopian tube (late) A52.7† N74.2*
- fracture A52.7† M90.2*
- gallbladder (late) A52.7† K87.0*

Syphilis, syphilitic—*continued*
- gastric (late) (polyposis) A52.7† K93.8*
- general A53.9
- – paralysis A52.1
- – – juvenile A50.4
- genital (primary) A51.0
- glaucoma A52.7† H42.8*
- gumma NEC A52.7
- – cardiovascular system A52.0† I98.0*
- – central nervous system A52.3
- – congenital A50.5
- heart (block) (decompensation) (disease)
  (failure) A52.0† I52.0*
- – valve NEC A52.0† I39.8*
- hemianesthesia A52.1
- hemianopsia A52.7† H58.1*
- hemiparesis A52.1
- hemiplegia A52.1
- hepatic artery A52.0† I79.8*
- hepatis A52.7† K77.0*
- hereditaria tarda (*see also* Syphilis,
  congenital, late) A50.7
- hereditary (*see also* Syphilis, congenital)
  A50.9
- hyalitis A52.7† H45.8*
- inactive – *see* Syphilis, latent
- infantum – *see* Syphilis, congenital
- inherited – *see* Syphilis, congenital
- internal ear A52.7† H94.8*
- intestine (late) A52.7† K93.8*
- iris, iritis (secondary) A51.4† H22.0*
- – late A52.7† H22.0*
- joint (late) A52.7† M14.8*
- keratitis (congenital) (interstitial) (late)
  A50.3† H19.2*
- kidney (late) A52.7† N29.0*
- lacrimal passages (late) A52.7† H06.0*
- larynx (late) A52.7† J99.8*
- late A52.9
- – cardiovascular A52.0† I98.0*
- – central nervous system A52.3
- – kidney A52.7† N29.0*
- – latent (2 years or more after infection)
  (without manifestations) A52.8
- – – negative spinal fluid test A52.8
- – – serology positive A52.8
- – paresis A52.1
- – specified site NEC A52.7
- – symptomatic or with manifestations
  A52.7
- – tabes A52.1
- latent A53.0
- – with signs or symptoms – *code as*
  Syphilis, by site and stage

Syphilis, syphilitic—*continued*
- latent—*continued*
- – central nervous system A52.2
- – early, or less than 2 years after infection A51.5
- – follow-up of latent syphilis A53.0
- – – date of infection unspecified A53.0
- – – late, or 2 years or more after infection A52.8
- – late, or 2 years or more after infection A52.8
- – positive serology A53.0
- – – date of infection unspecified A53.0
- – – early, or less than 2 years after infection A51.5
- – – late, or 2 years or more after infection A52.8
- lens (late) A52.7† H28.8*
- leukoderma A51.3† L99.8*
- – late A52.7† L99.8*
- lienitis A52.7† D77*
- lip A51.3
- – chancre (primary) A51.2
- – late A52.7† K93.8*
- Lissauer's paralysis A52.1
- liver A52.7† K77.0*
- locomotor ataxia A52.1
- lung A52.7† J99.8*
- lymph gland (early) (secondary) A51.4
- – late A52.7† I98.8*
- lymphadenitis (secondary) A51.4
- macular atrophy of skin A51.3† L99.8*
- – striated A52.7† L99.8*
- maternal, affecting fetus or newborn P00.2
- – manifest syphilis in infant – *see* Syphilis, congenital
- mediastinum (late) A52.7† J99.8*
- meninges (adhesive) (brain) (spinal cord) A52.1† G01*
- meningitis A52.1† G01*
- – acute (secondary) A51.4† G01*
- – congenital A50.4† G01*
- meningoencephalitis A52.1† G05.0*
- meningovascular A52.1† G01*
- – congenital A50.4† G01*
- mesarteritis A52.0† I79.8*
- – brain A52.0† I68.1*
- middle ear A52.7† H75.8*
- mitral stenosis A52.0† I39.0*
- monoplegia A52.1
- mouth (secondary) A51.3
- – late A52.7† K93.8*
- mucocutaneous (secondary) A51.3

Syphilis, syphilitic—*continued*
- mucocutaneous—*continued*
- – late A52.7
- mucous
- – membrane (secondary) A51.3
- – – late A52.7
- – patches A51.3
- – – congenital A50.0
- muscle A52.7† M63.0*
- myocardium A52.0† I41.0*
- nasal sinus (late) A52.7† J99.8*
- neonatorum – *see* Syphilis, congenital
- nephrotic syndrome (secondary) A51.4† N08.0*
- nerve palsy (any cranial nerve) A52.1† G53.8*
- – multiple A52.1† G53.1*
- nervous system, central A52.3
- neuritis A52.1† G59.8*
- – acoustic A52.1† H94.0*
- neurorecidive of retina A52.1† H36.8*
- neuroretinitis A52.1† H36.8*
- nodular superficial (late) A52.7
- nonvenereal A65
- nose (late) A52.7† J99.8*
- – saddle back deformity A50.5
- occlusive arterial disease A52.0† I79.8*
- oculopathy A52.7† H58.8*
- oesophagus (late) A52.7† K23.8*
- ophthalmic (late) A52.7† H58.8*
- optic nerve (atrophy) (neuritis) (papilla) A52.1† H48.0*
- orbit (late) A52.7† H06.3*
- organic A53.9
- osseous (late) A52.7† M90.2*
- osteochondritis (congenital) (early) A50.0† M90.2*
- osteoporosis A52.7† M90.2*
- ovary (late) A52.7† N74.2*
- oviduct (late) A52.7† N74.2*
- palate (late) A52.7† K93.8*
- pancreas (late) A52.7† K87.1*
- paralysis A52.1
- – general A52.1
- – – juvenile A50.4
- paresis (general) A52.1
- – juvenile A50.4
- paresthesia A52.1
- Parkinson's disease or syndrome A52.1† G22*
- paroxysmal tachycardia A52.0† I52.0*
- pemphigus (congenital) A50.0
- penis (chancre) A51.0
- – late A52.7† N51.8*

Syphilis, syphilitic—*continued*
- pericardium A52.0† I32.0*
- perichondritis, larynx (late) A52.7† J99.8*
- periosteum (late) A52.7† M90.1*
- – congenital (early) A50.0† M90.1*
- – early (secondary) A51.4† M90.1*
- peripheral nerve A52.7† G59.8*
- petrous bone (late) A52.7† M90.2*
- pharynx (late) A52.7† J99.8*
- – secondary A51.3
- pituitary (gland) A52.7† E35.8*
- placenta O98.1
- pleura (late) A52.7† J99.8*
- pontine lesion A52.1† G94.8*
- portal vein A52.0† I98.0*
- primary A51.0
- – anal A51.1
- – and secondary (*see also* Syphilis, secondary) A51.4
- – extragenital chancre NEC A51.2
- – fingers A51.2
- – genital A51.0
- – lip A51.2
- – specified site NEC A51.2
- – tonsils A51.2
- prostate (late) A52.7† N51.0*
- ptosis (eyelid) A52.7† H03.1*
- pulmonary (late) A52.7† J99.8*
- – artery A52.0† I98.0*
- pyelonephritis (late) A52.7† N16.0*
- recently acquired, symptomatic NEC A51.9
- rectum (late) A52.7† K93.8*
- respiratory tract (late) A52.7† J99.8*
- retina, late A52.7† H32.0*
- retrobulbar neuritis A52.1† H48.1*
- salpingitis A52.7† N74.2*
- sclera (late) A52.7† H19.0*
- sclerosis
- – cerebral A52.1† G94.8*
- – coronary A52.0† I52.0*
- – multiple A52.1† G99.8*
- scotoma (central) A52.7† H58.1*
- scrotum (late) A52.7† N51.8*
- secondary (and primary) A51.4
- – adenopathy A51.4
- – anus A51.3
- – bone A51.4† M90.2*
- – chorioretinitis, choroiditis A51.4† H32.0*
- – hepatitis A51.4† K77.0*
- – liver A51.4† K77.0*
- – lymphadenitis A51.4

Syphilis, syphilitic—*continued*
- secondary—*continued*
- – meningitis (acute) A51.4† G01*
- – mouth A51.3
- – mucous membranes A51.3
- – periosteum, periostitis A51.4† M90.1*
- – pharynx A51.3
- – relapse (treated, untreated) A51.4
- – skin A51.3
- – specified form NEC A51.4
- – tonsil A51.3
- – ulcer A51.3
- – viscera NEC A51.4
- – vulva A51.3
- seminal vesicle (late) A52.7† N51.8*
- seropositive
- – with signs or symptoms – *code as* Syphilis, by site and stage
- – follow-up of latent syphilis – *see* Syphilis, latent
- – only finding – *see* Syphilis, latent
- seventh nerve (paralysis) A52.1† G53.8*
- sinus, sinusitis (late) A52.7† J99.8*
- skeletal system A52.7† M90.2*
- skin (early) (secondary) (with ulceration) A51.3
- – late or tertiary A52.7† L99.8*
- small intestine A52.7† K93.8*
- spastic spinal paralysis A52.1
- spermatic cord (late) A52.7† N51.8*
- spinal (cord) A52.1
- spleen A52.7† D77*
- splenomegaly A52.7† D77*
- spondylitis A52.7† M49.3*
- staphyloma A52.7† H19.8*
- stigmata (congenital) A50.5
- stomach A52.7† K93.8*
- synovium A52.7† M68.0*
- tabes dorsalis (late) A52.1
- – juvenile A50.4
- tabetic type A52.1
- – juvenile A50.4
- taboparesis A52.1
- – juvenile A50.4
- tachycardia A52.0† I52.0*
- tendon (late) A52.7† M68.0*
- tertiary A52.9
- – with symptoms NEC A52.7
- – cardiovascular A52.0† I98.0*
- – central nervous system A52.3
- – multiple NEC A52.7
- – specified site NEC A52.7
- testis A52.7† N51.1*
- thorax A52.7

Syphilis, syphilitic—*continued*
- throat A52.7† J99.8∗
- thymus (gland) (late) A52.7† E35.8∗
- thyroid (late) A52.7† E35.0∗
- tongue (late) A52.7† K93.8∗
- tonsil (lingual) (late) A52.7† J99.8∗
- – primary A51.2
- – secondary A51.3
- trachea (late) A52.7† J99.8∗
- tunica vaginalis (late) A52.7† N51.8∗
- ulcer (any site) (early) (secondary) A51.3
- – late A52.7
- – – perforating A52.7
- – – – foot A52.1
- urethra (late) A52.7† N37.0∗
- urogenital (late) A52.7
- uterus (late) A52.7† N74.2∗
- uveal tract (secondary) A51.4† H22.0∗
- – late A52.7† H22.0∗
- uveitis (secondary) A51.4† H22.0∗
- – late A52.7† H22.0∗
- uvula (late) (perforated) A52.7† K93.8∗
- vagina A51.0
- – late A52.7† N77.1∗
- valvulitis NEC A52.0† I39.8∗
- vascular A52.0† I98.0∗
- – brain (cerebral) A52.0† I68.8∗
- ventriculi A52.7† K93.8∗
- vesicae urinariae (late) A52.7† N33.8∗
- viscera (abdominal) (late) A52.7
- – secondary A51.4
- vitreous (opacities) (late) A52.7† H45.8∗
- – hemorrhage A52.7† H45.0∗
- vulva A51.0

Syphilis, syphilitic—*continued*
- vulva—*continued*
- – late A52.7† N77.1∗
- – secondary A51.3

Syphiloma A52.7
- cardiovascular system A52.0† I98.0∗
- central nervous system A52.3
- circulatory system A52.0† I98.0∗
- congenital A50.5

Syphilophobia F45.2

Syringadenoma (M8400/0) – *see also* Neoplasm, skin, benign
- papillary (M8406/0) D23.9

Syringobulbia G95.0

Syringocystadenoma (M8400/0) – *see* Neoplasm, skin, benign
- papillary (M8406/0) D23.9

Syringoma (M8407/0) – *see also* Neoplasm, skin, benign
- chondroid (M8940/0) D23.9

Syringomyelia G95.0

Syringomyelitis (*see also* Encephalitis) G04.9

Syringomyelocele (*see also* Spina bifida) Q05.9
- with hydrocephalus (*see also* Spina bifida, with hydrocephalus) Q05.4

Syringopontia G95.0

System, systemic – *see also* condition
- atrophy
- – multiple (brain) (CNS) G90.3
- disease, combined – *see* Degeneration, combined
- lupus erythematosus M32.9
- – inhibitor present D68.6

T

Tabacism, tabacosis, tabagism T65.2
– meaning dependence F17.2
Tabardillo A75.9
– flea-borne A75.2
– louse-borne A75.0
Tabes, tabetic A52.1
– with
– – Charcot's joint A52.1† M14.6∗
– – cord bladder A52.1
– – crisis, viscera (any) A52.1
– – paralysis, general A52.1
– – paresis (general) A52.1
– – perforating ulcer (foot) A52.1
– arthropathy (Charcot) A52.1† M14.6∗
– bladder A52.1
– bone A52.1† M90.2∗
– cerebrospinal A52.1
– congenital A50.4
– conjugal A52.1
– dorsalis A52.1
– – juvenile A50.4
– juvenile A50.4
– latent A52.1
– mesenterica A18.3† K93.0∗
– paralysis, insane, general A52.1
– spasmodic A52.1
– syphilis (cerebrospinal) A52.1
Taboparalysis A52.1
Taboparesis (remission) A52.1
– juvenile A50.4
Tachycardia R00.0
– atrial I47.1
– auricular I47.1
– fetal – *see* Distress, fetal
– nodal I47.1
– paroxysmal I47.9
– – atrial I47.1
– – atrioventricular (AV) I47.1
– – junctional I47.1
– – nodal I47.1
– – supraventricular I47.1
– – ventricular I47.2
– psychogenic F45.3
– sick sinus I49.5
– sinoauricular R00.0
– – paroxysmal I47.1
– sinusal R00.0
– – paroxysmal I47.1
– supraventricular I47.1

Tachycardia—*continued*
– ventricular I47.2
Tachypnea R06.8
– hysterical F45.3
– psychogenic F45.3
– transitory, of newborn P22.1
Taenia infection or infestation B68.9
– mediocanellata B68.1
– saginata B68.1
– solium (intestinal form) B68.0
– – larval form (*see also* Cysticercosis)
   B69.9
Taeniasis (intestine) (*see also* Taenia)
   B68.9
Tag (hypertrophied skin) (infected) L91.8
– adenoid J35.8
– anus I84.6
– hemorrhoidal I84.6
– hymen N89.8
– perineal N90.8
– rectum I84.6
– skin L91.8
– – accessory (congenital) Q82.8
– – congenital Q82.8
– tonsil J35.8
– urethra, urethral N36.8
– vulva N90.8
Tahyna fever B33.8
Takahara's disease E80.3
Takayasu's disease or syndrome M31.4
Talcosis (pulmonary) J62.0
Talipes (congenital) Q66.8
– asymmetric Q66.8
– calcaneovalgus Q66.4
– calcaneovarus Q66.1
– calcaneus Q66.8
– cavus Q66.7
– equinovalgus Q66.6
– equinovarus Q66.0
– equinus Q66.8
– percavus Q66.7
– planovalgus Q66.6
– planus (acquired) (any degree) M21.4
– – congenital Q66.5
– – due to rickets (late effect) E64.3
– valgus Q66.6
– varus Q66.3
Tall stature, constitutional E34.4
Talma's disease M62.8

Tamponade, heart (*see also* Pericarditis)
I31.9
Tanapox (virus disease) B08.8
Tangier disease E78.6
Tantrum, child problem F91.8
Tapeworm (infection)
(infestation) (*see also* Infestation,
tapeworm) B71.9
Tapia's syndrome G52.7
TAR (thrombocytopenia with absent
radius) syndrome Q87.2
Tarsal tunnel syndrome G57.5
Tarsalgia M79.6
Tarsitis (eyelid) H01.8
– syphilitic A52.7† H03.1∗
– tuberculous A18.4† H03.1∗
Tartar (teeth) (dental calculus) K03.6
Tattoo (mark) L81.8
Tauri's disease E74.0
Taurodontism K00.2
Taussig-Bing syndrome Q20.1
Taybi's syndrome Q87.2
Tay-Sachs amaurotic familial idiocy or
disease E75.0
Teacher's node or nodule J38.2
Tear, torn (traumatic) – *see also* Wound,
open
– with abortion (subsequent episode) O08.6
– – current episode – *see* Abortion
– anus, anal (sphincter) S31.8
– – complicating delivery O70.2
– – – with mucosa O70.3
– – nontraumatic, nonpuerperal (*see also*
Fissure, anus) K60.2
– articular cartilage, old M24.1
– bladder
– – obstetrical O71.5
– – traumatic S37.2
– bowel, obstetrical trauma O71.5
– broad ligament, obstetrical trauma O71.6
– bucket handle (knee) (meniscus) S83.2
– – old M23.2
– capsule, joint – *see* Sprain
– cartilage – *see also* Sprain
– – articular, old M24.1
– – traumatic S37.6
– cervix
– – obstetrical trauma (current) O71.3
– – old N88.1
– internal organ – *see* Injury, by site
– knee cartilage
– – articular (current) S83.3
– – old M23.2
– ligament – *see* Sprain

Tear, torn—*continued*
– meniscus (knee) (current injury) S83.2
– – bucket handle S83.2
– – – old (anterior horn) (lateral) (medial)
(posterior horn) M23.2
– – old (anterior horn) (lateral) (medial)
(posterior horn) M23.2
– – site other than knee – *code as* Sprain
– muscle – *see* Injury, muscle
– pelvic
– – floor, complicating delivery O70.1
– – organ NEC, obstetric trauma O71.5
– periurethral tissue, obstetric trauma
O71.5
– rectovaginal septum – *see* Laceration,
rectovaginal septum
– retina, retinal (horseshoe) (without
detachment) H33.3
– – with detachment H33.0
– rotator cuff (complete) (incomplete)
(nontraumatic) M75.1
– – traumatic (tendon) S46.0
– – – capsule S43.4
– semilunar cartilage, knee (*see also* Tear,
meniscus) S83.2
– supraspinatus (complete) (incomplete)
(nontraumatic) M75.1
– tendon – *see* Injury, muscle
– tentorial, at birth P10.4
– umbilical cord
– – affecting fetus or newborn P50.1
– – complicating delivery O69.8
– urethra, obstetric trauma O71.5
– uterus – *see* Injury, uterus
– vagina – *see* Laceration, vagina
– vulva, complicating delivery O70.0
Tear-stone H04.5
Teeth – *see also* condition
– grinding F45.8
Teething syndrome K00.7
Telangiectasia, telangiectasis (verrucous)
I78.1
– ataxic (cerebellar) (Louis-Bar) G11.3
– hemorrhagic, hereditary (congenital)
(senile) I78.0
– spider I78.1
Telephone scatologia F65.8
Telescoped bowel or intestine (*see also*
Intussusception) K56.1
Teletherapy, adverse effect NEC T66
Temperature
– body, high (of unknown origin) R50.9
– cold, trauma from T69.9
– – newborn P80.0

Temperature—*continued*
- cold, trauma from—*continued*
- – specified effect NEC T69.8

Temple – *see condition*

Temporal – *see condition*

Temporosphenoidal – *see condition*

Tendency
- bleeding (*see also* Defect, coagulation) D68.9
- paranoid F61
- suicide R45.8
- – constituting part of a mental disorder – *see condition*
- to fall R29.6

Tenderness, abdominal R10.4

Tendinitis, tendonitis (*see also* Tenosynovitis) M77.9
- Achilles M76.6
- adhesive M65.8
- – shoulder M75.0
- bicipital M75.2
- calcific M65.2
- – shoulder M75.3
- due to use, overuse, pressure M70.9
- – specified NEC M70.8
- gluteal M76.0
- patellar M76.5
- peroneal M76.7
- psoas M76.1
- tibialis (anterior) (posterior) M76.8
- trochanteric M70.6

Tendon – *see condition*

Tendosynovitis – *see* Tenosynovitis

Tenesmus (rectal) R19.8
- vesical R30.1

Tennis elbow M77.1

Tenonitis – *see also* Tenosynovitis
- eye (capsule) H05.0

Tenontosynovitis – *see* Tenosynovitis

Tenontothecitis – *see* Tenosynovitis

Tenophyte M67.8

Tenosynovitis M65.9
- adhesive M65.8
- – shoulder M75.0
- bicipital M75.2
- gonococcal A54.4† M68.0*
- in (due to)
- – crystals M65.8
- – gonorrhea A54.4† M68.0*
- – syphilis (late) A52.7† M68.0*
- – use, overuse, pressure M70.9
- – – specified NEC M70.8
- infective NEC M65.1
- radial styloid M65.4

Tenosynovitis—*continued*
- shoulder M75.8
- – adhesive M75.0
- specified NEC M65.8
- tuberculous – *see* Tuberculosis, tenosynovitis

Tenovaginitis – *see* Tenosynovitis

Tension
- arterial, high (*see also* Hypertension) I10
- headache G44.2
- nervous R45.0
- premenstrual N94.3
- state (mental) F48.9

Tentorium – *see condition*

Teratencephalus Q89.8

Teratism Q89.7

Teratoblastoma (malignant) (M9080/3) – *see* Neoplasm, malignant

Teratocarcinoma (M9081/3) – *see also* Neoplasm, malignant
- liver C22.7

Teratoma (solid) (M9080/1) – *see also* Neoplasm, uncertain behavior
- with embryonal carcinoma, mixed (M9081/3) – *see* Neoplasm, malignant
- with malignant transformation (M9084/3) – *see* Neoplasm, malignant
- adult (cystic) (M9080/0) – *see* Neoplasm, benign
- benign (M9080/0) – *see* Neoplasm, benign
- combined with choriocarcinoma (M9101/3) – *see* Neoplasm, malignant
- cystic (adult) (M9080/0) – *see* Neoplasm, benign
- differentiated (M9080/0) – *see* Neoplasm, benign
- embryonal (M9080/3) – *see also* Neoplasm, malignant
- – liver C22.7
- immature (M9080/3) – *see* Neoplasm, malignant
- liver (M9080/3) C22.7
- – adult, benign, cystic, differentiated type or mature (M9080/0) D13.4
- malignant (M9080/3) – *see also* Neoplasm, malignant
- – anaplastic (M9082/3) – *see* Neoplasm, malignant
- – intermediate (M9083/3) – *see* Neoplasm, malignant
- – trophoblastic (M9102/3)
- – – specified site – *see* Neoplasm, malignant
- – – unspecified site C62.9

Teratoma—*continued*
- malignant—*continued*
- – undifferentiated (M9082/3) – *see*
  Neoplasm, malignant
- mature (M9080/1) – *see* Neoplasm,
  uncertain behavior
- ovary (M9080/0) D27
- – embryonal, immature or malignant
  (M9080/3) C56
- sacral, fetal, causing obstructed labor
  (mother) O66.3
- solid (M9080/1) – *see* Neoplasm,
  uncertain behavior
- testis (M9080/3) C62.9
- – adult, benign, cystic, differentiated type
  or mature (M9080/0) D29.2
- – scrotal C62.1
- – undescended C62.0
Termination
- anomalous – *see also* Malposition,
  congenital
- – right pulmonary vein Q26.3
- pregnancy – *see* Abortion
**Ternidens deminutus infection or
  infestation** B81.8
**Ternidens diminutus infection or
  infestation** B81.8
Ternidensiasis B81.8
Terror(s), night (child) F51.4
Terrorism, victim of Z65.4
Tertiary – *see condition*
Test(s)
- allergens Z01.5
- blood pressure Z01.3
- – abnormal reading – *see* Blood, pressure
- blood-alcohol Z04.0
- – positive – *see* Finding in blood
- blood-drug Z04.0
- – positive – *see* Finding in blood
- cardiac pulse generator (battery) Z45.0
- contraceptive management Z30.8
- developmental, infant or child Z00.1
- fertility Z31.4
- hearing Z01.1
- HIV (human immunodeficiency virus)
- – nonconclusive in infants R75
- – positive R75
- – – asymptomatic Z21
- intelligence NEC Z01.8
- – infant or child Z00.1
- laboratory Z01.7
- – abnormal finding – *see* Abnormal, by
  type
- – for medicolegal reason NEC Z04.8

Test(s)—*continued*
- Mantoux, abnormal result R76.1
- pregnancy (possible) (unconfirmed)
  Z32.0
- – confirmed Z32.1
- procreative Z31.4
- skin, diagnostic
- – allergy Z01.5
- – bacterial disease Z01.5
- – – special screening examination – *see*
  Screening, by name of disease
- – hypersensitivity Z01.5
- specified NEC Z01.8
- tuberculin, abnormal result R76.1
- vision Z01.0
- Wassermann Z11.3
- – positive (*see also* Serology for syphilis,
  positive) A53.0
- – – false R76.2
Testicle, testicular, testis – *see also
  condition*
- feminization syndrome E34.5
- migrans Q55.2
Tetanus, tetanic (cephalic) (convulsions)
  A35
- with abortion or ectopic gestation A34
- inoculation Z23.5
- – reaction (due to serum) – *see*
  Complications, vaccination
- neonatorum A33
- obstetric A34
- puerperal, postpartum, childbirth A34
Tetany (due to) R29.0
- alkalosis E87.3
- associated with rickets E55.0
- convulsions R29.0
- – hysterical F44.5
- functional (hysterical) F44.5
- hyperkinetic R29.0
- – hysterical F44.5
- hyperpnea R06.4
- – hysterical F45.3
- – psychogenic F45.3
- hyperventilation (*see also*
  Hyperventilation) R06.4
- – hysterical F45.3
- – psychogenic F45.3
- hysterical F44.5
- neonatal (without calcium or magnesium
  deficiency) P71.3
- parathyroid (gland) E20.9
- parathyroprival E89.2
- post-(para)thyroidectomy E89.2
- postoperative E89.2

Tetany—*continued*
- psychogenic (conversion reaction) F44.5

Tetralogy of Fallot Q21.3

Tetraplegia (*see also* Quadriplegia) G82.5

Thalassanemia – *see* Thalassemia

Thalassemia (anemia) (disease) D56.9
- with other hemoglobinopathy NEC D56.9
- alpha D56.0
- beta (severe) D56.1
- – sickle-cell D57.2
- delta-beta D56.2
- intermedia D56.1
- major D56.1
- minor D56.9
- mixed (with other hemoglobinopathy) D56.9
- sickle-cell D57.2
- specified type NEC D56.8
- trait D56.3
- variants D56.8

Thanatophoric dwarfism or short stature Q77.1

Thaysen's disease K90.0

Thecoma (M8600/0) D27
- luteinized (M8601/0) D27
- malignant (M8600/3) C56

Thelarche, premature E30.8

Thelaziasis B83.8

Thelitis N61
- puerperal, postpartum or gestational O91.0

Therapeutic – *see condition*

Therapy Z51.9
- aversive (behavior) NEC Z50.4
- – alcohol Z50.2
- – drug Z50.3
- breathing Z50.1
- detoxification
- – alcohol Z50.2
- – drug Z50.3
- intravenous (IV) without reported diagnosis Z51.8
- – following surgery Z48.8
- occupational Z50.7
- physical NEC Z50.1
- psychodynamic NEC Z50.4
- speech Z50.5
- vocational Z50.7

Thermic – *see condition*

Thermoplegia T67.0

Thesaurismosis, glycogen (*see also* Disease, glycogen storage) E74.0

Thiamin deficiency E51.9
- specified NEC E51.8

Thibierge-Weissenbach syndrome M34.8

Thickening
- bone M89.3
- breast N64.5
- epidermal L85.9
- – specified NEC L85.8
- hymen N89.6
- larynx J38.7
- nail L60.2
- – congenital Q84.5
- periosteal M89.3
- pleura J92.9
- – with asbestos J92.0
- skin R23.4
- subepiglottic J38.7
- tongue K14.8
- valve, heart – *see* Endocarditis

Thigh – *see condition*

Thinning vertebra M48.8

Thirst, excessive R63.1
- due to deprivation of water T73.1

Thomsen's disease G71.1

Thoracogastroschisis (congenital) Q79.8

Thoracopagus Q89.4

Thorax, thoracic – *see also condition*
- kidney Q63.2

Thorn's syndrome N28.8

Threadworm infection or infestation B80

Threatened
- abortion O20.0
- – with subsequent abortion O03.-
- – affecting fetus P01.8
- job loss, anxiety concerning Z56.2
- labor (*see also* Labor, false) O47.9
- – affecting fetus P01.8
- loss of job, anxiety concerning Z56.2
- miscarriage O20.0
- – affecting fetus P01.8
- premature delivery, affecting fetus P01.8
- unemployment, anxiety concerning Z56.2

Thresher's lung J67.0

Thrix annulata (congenital) Q84.1

Throat – *see condition*

Thromboangiitis obliterans (general) I73.1

Thromboarteritis – *see* Arteritis

Thromboasthenia (Glanzmann) (hemorrhagic) (hereditary) D69.1

Thrombocytasthenia (Glanzmann) D69.1

Thrombocythemia (essential) (hemorrhagic) (idiopathic) (primary) D47.3

Thrombocytopathy D69.1
- dystrophic D69.1

Thrombocytopathy—*continued*
- granulopenic D69.1

Thrombocytopenia, thrombocytopenic D69.6
- with absent radius (TAR) Q87.2
- congenital D69.4
- dilutional D69.5
- due to
- - drugs D69.5
- - extracorporeal circulation of blood D69.5
- - massive blood transfusion D69.5
- - platelet alloimmunization D69.5
- essential D69.3
- hereditary D69.4
- idiopathic D69.3
- neonatal, transitory P61.0
- - due to
- - - exchange transfusion P61.0
- - - idiopathic maternal thrombocytopenia P61.0
- - - isoimmunization P61.0
- primary NEC D69.4
- puerperal, postpartum O72.3
- secondary D69.5
- transient neonatal P61.0

Thrombocytosis, essential D47.3

Thromboembolism (*see also* Embolism) I74.9
- coronary (artery) (vein) (*see also* Infarct, myocardium) I21.9
- - not resulting in infarction I24.0
- following infusion, therapeutic injection or transfusion T80.1

Thrombopathy (Bernard-Soulier) D69.1
- constitutional D68.0
- Willebrand-Jurgens D68.0

Thrombopenia (*see also* Thrombocytopenia) D69.6

Thrombophilia
- primary D68.5

Thrombophlebitis I80.9
- antepartum (superficial) O22.2
- - affecting fetus or newborn P00.3
- - deep O22.3
- cavernous (venous) sinus G08
- - nonpyogenic I67.6
- cerebral (sinus) (vein) G08
- - nonpyogenic I67.6
- due to implanted device – *see* Complications, by site and type, specified NEC
- during or resulting from a procedure NEC T81.7

Thrombophlebitis—*continued*
- femoral (superficial) I80.1
- following infusion, therapeutic injection or transfusion T80.1
- hepatic (vein) I80.8
- idiopathic, recurrent I82.1
- iliofemoral I80.1
- intracranial venous sinus (any) G08
- - nonpyogenic I67.6
- intraspinal venous sinus and vein G08
- - nonpyogenic G95.1
- lateral (venous) sinus G08
- - nonpyogenic I67.6
- leg I80.3
- - deep (vessels) NEC I80.2
- - superficial (vessels) I80.0
- longitudinal (venous) sinus G08
- - nonpyogenic I67.6
- lower extremity I80.3
- - deep (vessels) NEC I80.2
- - superficial (vessels) I80.0
- migrans, migrating I82.1
- pelvic
- - following
- - - abortion O08.0
- - - ectopic or molar pregnancy O08.0
- - puerperal O87.1
- portal (vein) K75.1
- postoperative T81.7
- pregnancy (superficial) O22.2
- - affecting fetus or newborn P00.3
- - deep O22.3
- puerperal, postpartum, childbirth (superficial) O87.0
- - deep O87.1
- - pelvic O87.1
- sinus (intracranial) G08
- - nonpyogenic I67.6
- specified site NEC I80.8

Thrombosis, thrombotic (multiple) (progressive) (septic) (vein) (vessel) I82.9
- anal (*see also* Thrombosis, perianal) I84.3
- antepartum O22.9
- aorta, aortic I74.1
- - abdominal I74.0
- - bifurcation I74.0
- - saddle I74.0
- - thoracic I74.1
- - valve – *see* Endocarditis, aortic
- apoplexy I63.3
- appendix, septic K35.8
- artery, arteries (postinfectional) I74.9
- - auditory, internal I65.8

Thrombosis, thrombotic—*continued*
- artery, arteries—*continued*
- - basilar (*see also* Occlusion, artery,
    basilar) I65.1
- - carotid (common) (internal) (*see also*
    Occlusion, artery, carotid) I65.2
- - cerebellar (anterior inferior) (posterior
    inferior) (superior) (*see also* Occlusion,
    artery, cerebellar) I66.3
- - cerebral (*see also* Occlusion, artery,
    cerebral) I66.9
- - choroidal (anterior) I66.8
- - communicating, posterior I66.8
- - coronary (*see also* Infarct,
    myocardium) I21.9
- - - due to syphilis A52.0† I52.0*
- - - not resulting in infarction I24.0
- - hepatic I74.8
- - hypophyseal I66.8
- - iliac I74.5
- - limb I74.4
- - - lower I74.3
- - - upper I74.2
- - meningeal, anterior or posterior I66.8
- - mesenteric (with gangrene) K55.0
- - ophthalmic H34.2
- - pontine I66.8
- - precerebral (*see also* Occlusion, artery,
    precerebral) I65.9
- - pulmonary (*see also* Embolism,
    pulmonary) I26.9
- - renal N28.0
- - retinal H34.2
- - spinal, anterior or posterior G95.1
- - vertebral (*see also* Occlusion, artery,
    vertebral) I65.0
- basilar (artery) (*see also* Occlusion, artery,
  basilar) I65.1
- bland NEC I82.9
- brain (artery) (stem) (*see also* Occlusion,
  artery, cerebral) I66.9
- - due to syphilis A52.0† I68.8*
- - puerperal, postpartum, childbirth
    O99.4
- - sinus (*see also* Thrombosis, intracranial
    venous sinus) G08
- capillary I78.8
- cardiac (*see also* Infarct, myocardium)
  I21.9
- - due to syphilis A52.0† I52.0*
- - not resulting in infarction I24.0
- - valve – *see* Endocarditis

Thrombosis, thrombotic—*continued*
- carotid (artery) (common)
  (internal) (*see also* Occlusion, artery,
  carotid) I65.2
- cavernous (venous) sinus (*see also*
  Thrombosis, intracranial venous sinus)
  G08
- cerebral (artery) (*see also* Occlusion,
  artery, cerebral) I66.9
- cerebrovenous sinus (*see also*
  Thrombosis, intracranial venous sinus)
  G08
- - pregnancy O22.5
- - puerperium O87.3
- coronary (artery) (vein) (*see also* Infarct,
  myocardium) I21.9
- - due to syphilis A52.0† I52.0*
- - not resulting in infarction I24.0
- corpus cavernosum N48.8
- cortical I66.9
- deep I80.2
- due to device, implant or graft (*see also*
  Complications, by site and type, specified
  NEC) T85.8
- - arterial graft NEC T82.8
- - breast (implant) T85.8
- - catheter NEC T85.8
- - - dialysis (renal) T82.8
- - - - intraperitoneal T85.8
- - - infusion NEC T82.8
- - - - spinal (epidural) (subdural) T85.8
- - - urinary (indwelling) T83.8
- - electronic (electrode) (pulse generator)
    (stimulator)
- - - bone T84.8
- - - cardiac T82.8
- - - nervous system (brain) (peripheral
      nerve) (spinal) T85.8
- - - urinary T83.8
- - fixation, internal (orthopedic) NEC
    T84.8
- - gastrointestinal (bile duct) (esophagus)
    T85.8
- - genital NEC T83.8
- - heart T82.8
- - joint prosthesis T84.8
- - ocular (corneal graft) (orbital implant)
    NEC T85.8
- - orthopedic NEC T84.8
- - specified NEC T85.8
- - urinary NEC T83.8
- - vascular NEC T82.8
- - ventricular intracranial shunt T85.8

Thrombosis, thrombotic—*continued*
- during puerperium – *see* Thrombosis, puerperal
- endocardial (*see also* Infarct, myocardium) I21.9
- – not resulting in infarction I24.0
- eye H34.8
- femoral (superficial) I80.1
- – artery I74.3
- genital organ
- – female NEC N94.8
- – – pregnancy O22.9
- – male N50.1
- hepatic I82.0
- – artery I74.8
- iliac I80.2
- – artery I74.5
- iliofemoral I80.1
- intestine (with gangrene) K55.0
- intracardiac NEC (apical) (atrial) (auricular) (ventricular) (old) I51.3
- intracranial (arterial) I66.9
- – venous sinus (any) G08
- – – nonpyogenic origin I67.6
- – – pregnancy O22.5
- – – puerperium O87.3
- intramural (*see also* Infarct, myocardium) I21.9
- – not resulting in infarction I24.0
- intraspinal venous sinus and vein G08
- – nonpyogenic G95.1
- jugular (bulb) I82.8
- kidney (artery) N28.0
- lateral (venous) sinus – *see* Thrombosis, intracranial venous sinus
- leg I80.3
- – deep (vessels) NEC I80.2
- – superficial (vessels) I80.0
- liver I82.0
- – artery I74.8
- longitudinal (venous) sinus – *see* Thrombosis, intracranial venous sinus
- lower limb – *see* Thrombosis, leg
- lung (*see also* Embolism, pulmonary) I26.9
- meninges (brain) (arterial) I66.8
- mesenteric (artery) (with gangrene) K55.0
- mitral I34.8
- mural (*see also* Infarct, myocardium) I21.9
- – due to syphilis A52.0† I52.0*
- – not resulting in infarction I24.0
- omentum (with gangrene) K55.0

Thrombosis, thrombotic—*continued*
- ophthalmic H34.8
- parietal (*see also* Infarct, myocardium) I21.9
- – not resulting in infarction I24.0
- penis, penile N48.8
- perianal I84.3
- peripheral arteries I74.4
- portal I81
- – due to syphilis A52.0† I98.0*
- precerebral artery (*see also* Occlusion, artery, precerebral) I65.9
- pregnancy O22.9
- – cerebral venous (sinus) O22.5
- – deep-vein O22.3
- – following
- – – abortion (subsequent episode) O08.7
- – – – current episode – *see* Abortion
- – – ectopic or molar pregnancy O08.7
- puerperal, postpartum O87.9
- – brain (artery) O99.4
- – – venous (sinus) O87.3
- – cardiac O99.4
- – cerebral (artery) O99.4
- – – venous (sinus) O87.3
- – superficial O87.0
- pulmonary (artery) (vein) (*see also* Embolism, pulmonary) I26.9
- renal (artery) N28.0
- – vein I82.3
- resulting from presence of device, implant or graft (any) – *see* Complications, by site and type, specified NEC
- retina, retinal H34.8
- scrotum N50.1
- seminal vesicle N50.1
- sigmoid (venous) sinus – *see* Thrombosis, intracranial venous sinus
- silent NEC I82.9
- sinus, intracranial (any) (*see also* Thrombosis, intracranial venous sinus) G08
- specified site NEC I82.8
- spermatic cord N50.1
- spinal cord (arterial) G95.1
- – due to syphilis A52.0† I79.8*
- spleen, splenic D73.5
- – artery I74.8
- testis N50.1
- tricuspid I07.8
- tunica vaginalis N50.1
- umbilical cord (vessels), complicating delivery O69.5
- – affecting fetus or newborn P02.6

Thyroid Eye disease H06.2* (handwritten at top)

Thrombosis, thrombotic—*continued*
- vas deferens N50.1
- vena cava (inferior) (superior) I82.2
Thrombus – *see* Thrombosis
Thrush (*see also* Candidiasis) B37.9
- oral B37.0
- vaginal B37.3† N77.1*
Thumb – *see also condition*
- sucking (child problem) F98.8
Thymitis E32.8
Thymoma (benign) (M8580/0) D15.0
- malignant (M8580/3) C37
Thymus, thymic (gland) – *see condition*
Thyroglossal – *see also condition*
- cyst Q89.2
- duct, persistent Q89.2
Thyroid (body) (gland) – *see also condition*
- nodule (cystic) (nontoxic) (single) E04.1
Thyroiditis E06.9
- acute E06.0
- autoimmune E06.3
- chronic E06.5
- – with thyrotoxicosis, transient E06.2
- – fibrous E06.5
- – lymphadenoid E06.3
- de Quervain E06.1
- drug-induced E06.4
- fibrous (chronic) E06.5
- giant-cell E06.1
- granulomatous (de Quervain) (subacute) E06.1
- Hashimoto's E06.3
- iatrogenic E06.4
- ligneous E06.5
- lymphocytic (chronic) E06.3
- lymphoid E06.3
- lymphomatous E06.3
- nonsuppurative E06.1
- postpartum, puerperal O90.5
- pseudotuberculous E06.1
- pyogenic E06.0
- Riedel's E06.5
- subacute E06.1
- suppurative E06.0
- tuberculous A18.8† E35.0*
- woody E06.5
Thyrolingual duct, persistent Q89.2
Thyrotoxic
- heart disease or failure (*see also* Thyrotoxicosis) E05.9† I43.8*
- storm or crisis E05.5

Thyrotoxicosis (recurrent) E05.9
- with
- – goiter (diffuse) (*see also* Goiter, toxic) E05.0
- – – multinodular E05.2
- – – nodular E05.2
- – – uninodular E05.1
- – single thyroid nodule E05.1
- due to
- – ectopic thyroid nodule or tissue E05.3
- – ingestion of (excessive) thyroid material E05.4
- – overproduction of thyroid-stimulating hormone E05.8
- – specified cause NEC E05.8
- factitia E05.4
- heart E05.9† I43.8*
- neonatal P72.1
- transient with chronic thyroiditis E06.2
Tibia vara M92.5
Tic (disorder) F95.9
- breathing F95.8
- chronic
- – motor F95.1
- – vocal F95.1
- combined vocal and multiple motor F95.2
- de la Tourette F95.2
- degenerative (generalized) (localized) G25.6
- – facial G25.6
- douloureux (*see also* Neuralgia, trigeminal) G50.0
- – atypical G50.1
- drug-induced G25.6
- eyelid F95.8
- habit F95.9
- occupational F48.8
- orbicularis F95.8
- organic origin G25.6
- postchoreic G25.6
- salaam R25.8
- spasm F95.9
- specified NEC F95.8
- transient F95.0
Tietze's disease or syndrome M94.0
Tight fascia (lata) M62.8
Tightness
- anus K62.8
- foreskin (congenital) N47
- hymen, hymenal ring N89.6
- introitus N89.6
- rectal sphincter K62.8
- tendon (*see also* Short, tendon) M67.1
- urethral sphincter N35.9

Tilting vertebra M43.8
Tin-miner's lung J63.5
Tinea (intersecta) (tarsi) B35.9
– amiantacea L44.8
– barbae B35.0
– beard B35.0
– black dot B35.0
– blanca B36.2
– capitis B35.0
– corporis B35.4
– cruris B35.6
– flava B36.0
– foot B35.3
– imbricata (Tokelau) B35.5
– kerion B35.0
– manuum B35.2
– microsporic (*see also* Dermatophytosis)
  B35.9
– nigra B36.1
– nodosa (*see also* Piedra) B36.8
– pedis B35.3
– scalp B35.0
– specified site NEC B35.8
– sycosis B35.0
– tonsurans B35.0
– trichophytic (*see also* Dermatophytosis)
  B35.9
– unguium B35.1
– versicolor B36.0
Tingling sensation (skin) R20.2
Tinnitus (audible) (aurium) (subjective)
H93.1
Tipping pelvis M95.5
– with disproportion (fetopelvic) O33.0
– – causing obstructed labor O65.0
Tiredness R53
Tissue – *see condition*
Tobacco (nicotine)
– dependence F17.2
– harmful use F17.1
– heart T65.2
– intoxication F17.0
– maternal use, affecting fetus or newborn
  P04.2
– use NEC Z72.0
– – counseling and surveillance Z71.6
– withdrawal state F17.3
Tocopherol deficiency E56.0
Todd's
– cirrhosis K74.3
– paralysis (postepileptic) G83.8
Toe – *see condition*
Toilet, artificial opening – *see* Attention to,
  artificial, opening

Tokelau (ringworm) B35.5
Tollwut – *see* Rabies
Tommaselli's disease
– correct substance properly administered
  R31
– overdose or wrong substance given or
  taken T37.2
Tongue – *see also condition*
– tie Q38.1
Tonic pupil H57.0
Tonsil – *see condition*
**Tonsillitis (acute) (follicular) (gangrenous)
(infective) (lingual) (septic) (subacute)
(ulcerative)** J03.9   *Recurrent
                            J03.9
                          (DCS. x.1)*
– chronic J35.0
– diphtheritic A36.0
– hypertrophic J35.0
– parenchymatous J03.9
– specified organism NEC J03.8
– staphylococcal J03.8
– streptococcal J03.0
– tuberculous A16.8
– – with bacteriological and histological
    confirmation A15.8
– Vincent's A69.1
Tonsillopharyngitis J06.8
Tooth, teeth – *see condition*
Toothache K08.8
Topagnosis R20.8
Tophi (*see also* Gout) M10.-
Torn – *see* Tear
Tornwaldt's cyst or disease J39.2
Torsion
– accessory tube N83.5
– adnexa (female) N83.5
– bile duct (common) (hepatic) K83.8
– – congenital Q44.5
– bowel, colon or intestine K56.2
– cervix (*see also* Malposition, uterus)
  N85.4
– cystic duct K82.8
– dystonia – *see* Dystonia, torsion
– epididymis N44
– fallopian tube N83.5
– gallbladder K82.8
– – congenital Q44.1
– hydatid of Morgagni
– – female N83.5
– – male N44
– kidney (pedicle) (leading to infarction)
  N28.0
– Meckel's diverticulum (congenital) Q43.0
– mesentery or omentum K56.2

Torsion—*continued*
- organ or site, congenital NEC – *see* Anomaly, by site
- ovary (pedicle) N83.5
- – congenital Q50.2
- oviduct N83.5
- penis N48.8
- – congenital Q55.6
- spasm – *see* Dystonia, torsion
- spermatic cord N44
- spleen D73.5
- testis, testicle N44
- tibia M21.8
- umbilical cord in fetus or newborn P02.5
- uterus (*see also* Malposition, uterus) N85.4

Torticollis (intermittent) (spastic) M43.6
- congenital (sternomastoid) Q68.0
- due to birth injury P15.2
- hysterical F44.4
- psychogenic F45.8
- – conversion reaction F44.4
- rheumatoid M06.8
- spasmodic G24.3
- traumatic, current NEC S13.4

Tortipelvis G24.1

Tortuous
- artery I77.1
- organ or site, congenital NEC – *see* Distortion
- retinal vessel, congenital Q14.1
- urethra N36.8
- vein – *see* Varicose vein

Torture, victim of Z65.4

Torula, torular (histolytica) (infection) (*see also* Cryptococcosis) B45.9

Torulosis (*see also* Cryptococcosis) B45.9

Torus (mandibularis) (palatinus) K10.0

Tourette's syndrome F95.2

Tower skull Q75.0
- with exophthalmos Q87.0

Toxemia R68.8
- bacterial – *see* Sepsis
- burn – *see* Burn
- eclamptic (*see also* Eclampsia) O15.9
- fatigue R68.8
- kidney (*see also* Uremia) N19
- maternal (of pregnancy), affecting fetus or newborn P00.0
- myocardial – *see* Myocarditis, toxic
- of pregnancy (*see also* Pre-eclampsia) O14.9
- – affecting fetus or newborn P00.0

Toxemia—*continued*
- pre-eclamptic (*see also* Pre-eclampsia) O14.9
- septic (*see also* Sepsis) A41.9
- stasis R68.8
- uremic (*see also* Uremia) N19
- urinary (*see also* Uremia) N19

Toxic (poisoning) – *see also* condition
- from drug or nonmedicinal substance – *see* Table of drugs and chemicals
- shock syndrome A48.3
- thyroid (gland) (*see also* Thyrotoxicosis) E05.9

Toxicemia – *see* Toxemia

Toxicity T65.9
- fava bean D55.0
- from drug or nonmedicinal substance – *see* Table of drugs and chemicals

Toxicosis (*see also* Toxemia) R68.8
- capillary, hemorrhagic D69.0

Toxocariasis B83.0

Toxoplasma, toxoplasmosis (acquired) B58.9
- with
- – hepatitis B58.1† K77.0*
- – meningoencephalitis B58.2† G05.2*
- – ocular involvement B58.0† H58.8*
- – other organ invovement B58.8
- – pneumonia, pneumonitis B58.3† J17.3*
- congenital (acute) (chronic) (subacute) P37.1
- maternal, affecting fetus or newborn P00.2
- – manifest toxoplasmosis in infant or fetus (acute) (chronic) (subacute) P37.1
- resulting from HIV disease B20.8
- suspected damage to fetus affecting management of pregnancy O35.8

Trabeculation, bladder N32.8

Trachea – *see* condition

Tracheitis (acute) (catarrhal) (infantile) (membranous) (plastic) (pneumococcal) (viral) J04.1
- with
- – bronchitis (15 years of age and above) J40
- – – acute or subacute (*see also* Bronchitis, acute) J20.9
- – – chronic J42
- – – tuberculous NEC A16.4
- – – – with bacteriological and histological confirmation A15.5
- – – under 15 years of age J20.-

Tracheitis—*continued*
- with—*continued*
- – laryngitis (acute) J04.2
- – – chronic J37.1
- – – tuberculous NEC A16.4
- chronic J42
- – with
- – – bronchitis (chronic) J42
- – – laryngitis (chronic) J37.1
- diphtheritic A36.8
- due to external agent – *see* Inflammation, respiratory, upper, due to
- streptococcal J04.1
- syphilitic A52.7† J99.8*
- tuberculous A16.4
- – with bacteriological and histological confirmation A15.5

Trachelitis (nonvenereal) (*see also* Cervicitis) N72
Tracheobronchial – *see condition*
Tracheobronchitis (15 years of age and above) (*see also* Bronchitis) J40
- acute or subacute (*see also* Bronchitis, acute) J20.9
- chronic J42
- due to
- – Bordetella bronchiseptica A37.8
- – Francisella tularensis A21.8
- influenzal (*see also* Influenza, with, respiratory manifestations) J11.1
- senile (chronic) J42
- under 15 years of age J20.-

Tracheobronchopneumonitis – *see* Pneumonia, broncho
Tracheocele (external) (internal) J39.8
- congenital Q32.1
Tracheomalacia J39.8
- congenital Q32.0
Tracheopharyngitis (acute) J06.8
- chronic J42
- due to external agent – *see* Inflammation, respiratory, upper, due to
Tracheostenosis J39.8
Tracheostomy
- status Z93.0
- – attention to Z43.0
- – malfunctioning J95.0
Trachoma, trachomatous A71.9
- active (stage) A71.1
- contraction of conjunctiva A71.1
- dubium A71.0
- initial (stage) A71.0
- pannus A71.1
Train sickness T75.3

Training (in)
- activities of daily living NEC Z50.8
- orthoptic Z50.6
Trait(s)
- amoral F61
- antisocial F61
- dissocial F61
- HbAS D57.3
- Hb-S D57.3
- hemoglobin
- – abnormal NEC D58.2
- – – with thalassemia D56.3
- – C (*see also* Disease, hemoglobin C) D58.2
- – – with elliptocytosis D58.1
- – S (Hb-S) D57.3
- paranoid F61
- personality, accentuated Z73.1
- sickle-cell D57.3
- – with elliptocytosis or spherocytosis D57.3
- type A personality Z73.1
Tramp Z59.0
Trance R41.8
- hysterical F44.3
Transection, trunk (abdomen) (thorax) T05.8
Transfusion
- blood (session) Z51.3
- – reaction or complication – *see* Complications, transfusion
- – without reported diagnosis Z51.3
- fetomaternal (mother) O43.0
- maternofetal (mother) O43.0
- placental (syndrome) (mother) O43.0
- – in fetus or newborn P02.3
- reaction (adverse) – *see* Complications, transfusion
- twin-to-twin O43.0
Transient (meaning homeless) (*see also* condition) Z59.0
Translocation
- balanced
- – autosomal Q95.9
- – – in normal individual Q95.0
- – chromosomes Q95.9
- – – in normal individual Q95.0
- chromosomes NEC Q99.8
- Down's syndrome Q90.2
- trisomy
- – 13 Q91.6
- – 18 Q91.2
- – 21 Q90.2
Translucency, iris H21.2

Transmission of chemical substances through the placenta – *see* Absorption, chemical, through placenta
Transparency, lung, unilateral J43.0
Transplant(ed) (status) Z94.9
– bone Z94.6
– – marrow Z94.8
– complication NEC (*see also* Complications, graft) T86.8
– – skin NEC (infection) (rejection) T86.8
– cornea Z94.7
– hair Z41.0
– heart Z94.1
– – and lung(s) Z94.3
– – valve Z95.4
– – – prosthetic Z95.2
– – – xenogenic Z95.3
– intestine Z94.8
– kidney Z94.0
– liver Z94.4
– lung(s) Z94.2
– – and heart Z94.3
– organ Z94.9
– pancreas Z94.8
– skin Z94.5
– social Z60.3
– specified organ or tissue NEC Z94.8
– stem cells Z94.8
– tissue Z94.9
Transplants, ovarian, endometrial N80.1
Transposed – *see* Transposition
Transposition (congenital) – *see also* Malposition, congenital
– abdominal viscera Q89.3
– aorta (dextra) Q20.3
– appendix Q43.8
– colon Q43.8
– corrected Q20.5
– great vessels (complete) (partial) Q20.3
– heart Q24.0
– – with complete transposition of viscera Q89.3
– intestine (large) (small) Q43.8
– stomach Q40.2
– – with complete transposition of viscera Q89.3
– tooth, teeth K07.3
– vessels, great (complete) (partial) Q20.3
– viscera (abdominal) (thoracic) Q89.3
Transsexualism F64.0
Transverse – *see also* condition
– arrest (deep), in labor O64.0
– – affecting fetus or newborn P03.1
– lie (mother) O32.2

Transverse—*continued*
– lie—*continued*
– – before labor, affecting fetus or newborn P01.7
– – causing obstructed labor O64.8
– – – affecting fetus or newborn P03.1
Transvestism, transvestitism (dual-role) F64.1
– fetishistic F65.1
Trapped placenta (with hemorrhage) O72.0
– without hemorrhage O73.0
Trauma, traumatism (*see also* Injury) T14.9
– acoustic H83.3
– birth – *see* Birth, injury
– during delivery NEC O71.9
– maternal, during pregnancy, affecting fetus or newborn P00.5
– obstetric O71.9
– – specified NEC O71.8
– previous major, affecting management of pregnancy Z35.8
Traumatic – *see* condition
Treacher Collins syndrome Q75.4
Treitz's hernia – *see* Hernia, abdomen, specified site NEC
Trematode infestation NEC (*see also* Infestation, fluke) B66.9
Trematodiasis NEC (*see also* Infestation, fluke) B66.9
Trembles T62.8
Tremor R25.1
– drug-induced G25.1
– essential (benign) G25.0
– familial G25.0
– hereditary G25.0
– hysterical F44.4
– intention G25.2
– mercurial T56.1
– Parkinson's (*see also* Parkinsonism) G20
– psychogenic (conversion reaction) F44.4
– senilis R54
– specified type NEC G25.2
Trench
– fever A79.0
– foot T69.0
– mouth A69.1
Treponema pallidum infection (*see also* Syphilis) A53.9
Treponematosis due to
– Treponema pallidum – *see* Syphilis
– Treponema pertenue – *see* Yaws

Triad
- Hutchinson's (congenital syphilis) A50.5
- Kartagener Q89.3
- Saint's (*see also* Hernia, diaphragm) K44.9

Trichiasis (eyelid) H02.0

Trichinella spiralis infection, infestation B75

Trichinellosis, trichiniasis, trichilelliasis, trichinosis B75

Trichobezoar T18.9
- intestine T18.3
- stomach T18.2

Trichocephaliasis, trichocephalosis B79

Trichocephalus infestation B79

Trichoclasis L67.8

Trichoepithelioma (M8100/0) – *see* Neoplasm, skin, benign

Trichofolliculoma (M8101/0) – *see* Neoplasm, skin, benign

Tricholemmoma (M8102/0) – *see* Neoplasm, skin, benign

Trichomoniasis A59.9
- bladder A59.0† N33.8*
- cervix A59.0† N74.8*
- intestinal A07.8
- prostate A59.0† N51.0*
- seminal vesicles A59.0† N51.8*
- specified site NEC A59.8
- urethra A59.0† N37.0*
- urogenitalis A59.0
- vagina A59.0† N77.1*
- vulva A59.0† N77.1*

Trichomycosis
- axillaris A48.8
- nodosa, nodularis B36.8

Trichonodosis L67.8

Trichophytid, Trichophyton infection (*see also* Dermatophytosis) B35.9

Trichophytobezoar T18.9
- intestine T18.3
- stomach T18.2

Trichophytosis (*see also* Dermatophytosis) B35.9
- unguium B35.1

Trichoptilosis L67.8

Trichorrhexis (nodosa) (invaginata) L67.0

Trichosis axillaris A48.8

Trichosporosis nodosa B36.2

Trichostasis spinulosa (congenital) Q84.1

Trichostrongyliasis, trichostrongylosis (small intestine) B81.2

Trichostrongylus infection B81.2

Trichotillomania F63.3

Trichromat, trichromatopsia, anomalous (congenital) H53.5

Trichuriasis B79

Trichuris trichiura infection or infestation (any site) B79

Tricuspid (valve) – *see condition*

Trifid – *see also* Accessory
- kidney (pelvis) Q63.8
- tongue Q38.3

Trigeminy R00.8

Trigger finger (acquired) M65.3
- congenital Q74.0

Trigonitis (bladder) (pseudomembranous) N30.3

Trigonocephaly Q75.0

Trilocular heart (*see also* Cor triloculare) Q20.8

Trimethylaminuria E88.8

Tripartite placenta (*see also* Placenta, abnormal) O43.1

Triphalangeal thumb Q74.0

Triple – *see also* Accessory
- kidneys Q63.0
- uteri Q51.8
- X, female Q97.0

Triplegia G83.8
- congenital or infantile G80.8

Triplet, affecting fetus or newborn P01.5
- pregnancy O30.1

Triplication – *see* Accessory

Triploidy Q92.7

Trismus R25.2
- neonatorum A33
- newborn A33

Trisomy (syndrome) Q92.9
- autosomes NEC Q92.9
- chromosome specified NEC Q92.8
- – major (whole arm or more duplicated) Q92.2
- – minor (less than whole arm duplicated Q92.3
- – whole (nonsex chromosome)
- – – meiotic nondisjunction Q92.0
- – – mitotic nondisjunction Q92.1
- – – mosaicism Q92.1
- major partial (whole arm or more duplicated) Q92.2
- minor partial (less than whole arm duplicated) Q92.3
- partial NEC Q92.8
- – major (whole arm or more duplicated) Q92.2

Trisomy—*continued*
- partial NEC—*continued*
- – minor (less than whole arm duplicated) Q92.3
- – specified NEC Q92.8
- specified NEC Q92.8
- whole chromosome Q92.9
- – meiotic nondisjunction Q92.0
- – mitotic nondisjunction Q92.1
- – mosaicism Q92.1
- – partial Q92.9
- – specified NEC Q92.8
- 13 (partial) Q91.7
- – meiotic nondisjunction Q91.4
- – mitotic nondisjunction Q91.5
- – mosaicism Q91.5
- – translocation Q91.6
- 18 (partial) Q91.3
- – meiotic nondisjunction Q91.0
- – mitotic nondisjunction Q91.1
- – mosaicism Q91.1
- – translocation Q91.2
- 20 Q92.8
- 21 (partial) Q90.9
- – meiotic nondisjunction Q90.0
- – mitotic nondisjunction Q90.1
- – mosaicism Q90.1
- – translocation Q90.2
- 22 Q92.8
Tritanomaly, tritanopia H53.5
Trombiculosis, trombiculiasis, trombidiosis B88.0
Trophoblastic disease (M9100/0) (*see also* Mole, hydatidiform) O01.9
- previous, affecting management of pregnancy Z35.1
Trophoneurosis NEC G96.8
- disseminated M34.9
Tropical – *see condition*
Trouble – *see also* Disease
- heart – *see* Disease, heart
- kidney (*see also* Disease, renal) N28.9
- nervous R45.0
- sinus (*see also* Sinusitis) J32.9
Truancy, childhood
- socialized F91.2
- unsocialized F91.1
Truncus
- arteriosus (persistent) Q20.0
- communis Q20.0
Trunk – *see condition*
Trypanosomiasis
- African B56.9

Trypanosomiasis—*continued*
- African—*continued*
- – due to Trypanosoma brucei
- – – gambiense B56.0
- – – rhodesiense B56.1
- – East B56.1
- – West B56.0
- American (*see also* Chagas' disease) B57.2
- – with
- – – heart involvement B57.2† I41.2*
- – – other organ involvement B57.5
- Brazilian – *see* Chagas' disease
- due to Trypanosoma
- – brucei gambiense B56.0
- – brucei rhodesiense B56.1
- – cruzi – *see* Chagas' disease
- East African B56.1
- gambiensis, Gambian B56.0
- rhodesiensis, Rhodesian B56.1
- South American – *see* Chagas' disease
- West African B56.0
- where
- – African trypanosomiasis is prevalent B56.9
- – Chagas' disease is prevalent B57.2
T-shaped incisors K00.2
Tsutsugamushi (disease) (fever) A75.3
Tube, tubal, tubular – *see also condition*
- ligation, admission for Z30.2
Tubercle – *see also* Tuberculosis
- brain, solitary A17.8† G07*
- Darwin's Q17.8
- Ghon, primary infection A16.7
- – with bacteriological and histological confirmation A15.7
Tuberculid, tuberculide (indurating, subcutaneous) (lichenoid) (miliary) (papulonecrotic) (primary) (skin) A18.4
Tuberculoma – *see also* Tuberculosis
- brain A17.8† G07*
- meninges (cerebral) (spinal) A17.1† G07*
- spinal cord A17.8† G07*
Tuberculosis, tubercular, tuberculous (caseous) (degeneration) (gangrene) (necrosis) A16.9
- with pneumoconiosis (any condition in J60-J64) J65
- abdomen (lymph gland) A18.3† K93.0*
- abscess NEC (respiratory) A16.9
- – bone A18.0† M90.0*
- – – hip A18.0† M01.1*

Tuberculosis, tubercular—*continued*
– abscess NEC—*continued*
– – bone—*continued*
– – – knee A18.0† M01.1∗
– – – sacrum A18.0† M49.0∗
– – – specified site NEC A18.0† M90.0∗
– – – spine A18.0† M49.0∗
– – – vertebra A18.0† M49.0∗
– – brain A17.8† G07∗
– – breast A18.8
– – Cowper's gland A18.1† N51.8∗
– – dura (mater) (cerebral) (spinal) A17.8† G01∗
– – epidural (cerebral) (spinal) A17.8† G07∗
– – female pelvis A18.1† N74.1∗
– – frontal sinus (*see also* Tuberculosis, sinus) A16.8
– – – with bacteriological and histological confirmation A15.8
– – genital organs NEC A18.1
– – genitourinary A18.1
– – gland (lymphatic) – *see* Tuberculosis, lymph gland
– – hip A18.0† M01.1∗
– – intestine A18.3† K93.0∗
– – ischiorectal A18.3† K93.0∗
– – joint NEC A18.0† M01.1∗
– – – hip A18.0† M01.1∗
– – – knee A18.0† M01.1∗
– – – vertebral A18.0† M49.0∗
– – kidney A18.1† N29.1∗
– – knee A18.0† M01.1∗
– – lumbar (spine) A18.0† M49.0∗
– – lung (*see also* Tuberculosis, pulmonary) A16.2
– – – primary (progressive) A16.7
– – – – with bacteriological and histological confirmation A15.7
– – meninges (cerebral) (spinal) A17.0† G01∗
– – muscle A18.8† M63.0∗
– – perianal (fistula) A18.3† K93.0∗
– – perinephritic A18.1† N29.1∗
– – perirectal A18.3† K93.0∗
– – rectum A18.3† K93.0∗
– – retropharyngeal A16.8
– – – with bacteriological and histological confirmation A15.8
– – sacrum A18.0† M49.0∗
– – scrofulous A18.2
– – scrotum A18.1† N51.8∗
– – skin (primary) A18.4
– – spinal cord A17.8† G07∗

Tuberculosis, tubercular—*continued*
– abscess NEC—*continued*
– – spine or vertebra (column) A18.0† M49.0∗
– – subdiaphragmatic A18.3† K93.0∗
– – testis A18.1† N51.1∗
– – urinary A18.1
– – uterus A18.1† N74.1∗
– accessory sinus – *see* Tuberculosis, sinus
– Addison's disease A18.7† E35.1∗
– adenitis (*see also* Tuberculosis, lymph gland) A18.2
– adenoids A16.8
– – with bacteriological and histological confirmation A15.8
– adenopathy (*see also* Tuberculosis, lymph gland) A18.2
– – tracheobronchial A16.3
– – – with bacteriological and histological confirmation A15.4
– – – primary (progressive) A16.7
– – – – with bacteriological and histological confirmation A15.7
– adherent pericardium A18.8† I32.0∗
– adnexa (uteri) A18.1† N74.1∗
– adrenal (capsule) (gland) A18.7† E35.1∗
– alimentary canal A18.3† K93.0∗
– anemia A18.8† D63.8∗
– ankle (joint) A18.0† M01.1∗
– anus A18.3† K93.0∗
– apex, apical – *see* Tuberculosis, pulmonary
– appendix, appendicitis A18.3† K93.0∗
– arachnoid A17.0† G01∗
– artery, arteritis A18.8† I79.8∗
– – cerebral A18.8† I68.1∗
– arthritis (chronic) (synovial) A18.0† M01.1∗
– – spine or vertebra (column) A18.0† M49.0∗
– articular – *see* Tuberculosis, joint
– ascites A18.3
– asthma (*see also* Tuberculosis, pulmonary) A16.2
– axilla, axillary (gland) A18.2
– bilateral – *see* Tuberculosis, pulmonary
– bladder A18.1† N33.0∗
– bone A18.0† M90.0∗
– – hip A18.0† M01.1∗
– – knee A18.0† M01.1∗
– – limb NEC A18.0† M90.0∗
– – sacrum A18.0† M49.0∗
– – spine or vertebra (column) A18.0† M49.0∗

Tuberculosis, tubercular—*continued*
- bowel (miliary) A18.3† K93.0*
- brain A17.8† G07*
- breast A18.8
- broad ligament A18.1† N74.1*
- bronchi, bronchial, bronchus A16.4
- – with bacteriological and histological confirmation A15.5
- – ectasia, ectasis (bronchiectasis) – *see* Tuberculosis, pulmonary
- – fistula A16.4
- – – primary (progressive) A16.7
- – – – with bacteriological and histological confirmation A15.7
- – gland or node A16.3
- – – with bacteriological and histological confirmation A15.4
- – – primary (progressive) A16.7
- – – – with bacteriological and histological confirmation A15.7
- – lymph gland or node A16.3
- – – with bacteriological and histological confirmation A15.4
- – – primary (progressive) A16.7
- – – – with bacteriological and histological confirmation A15.7
- bronchiectasis – *see* Tuberculosis, pulmonary
- bronchitis A16.4
- – with bacteriological and histological confirmation A15.5
- bronchopleural A16.5
- bronchopneumonia, bronchopneumonic – *see* Tuberculosis, pulmonary
- bronchorrhagia A16.4
- – with bacteriological and histological confirmation A15.5
- bronchotracheal A16.4
- – with bacteriological and histological confirmation A15.5
- bronze disease A18.7† E35.1*
- buccal cavity A18.8† K93.8*
- bulbourethral gland A18.1† N51.8*
- bursa A18.0† M01.1*
- cachexia NEC A16.9
- cardiomyopathy A18.8† I43.0*
- caries (*see also* Tuberculosis, bone) A18.0† M90.0*
- cartilage A18.0† M01.1*
- – intervertebral A18.0† M49.0*
- cecum A18.3† K93.0*
- cellulitis (primary) A18.4
- cerebellum A17.8† G07*
- cerebrum, cerebral A17.8† G07*

Tuberculosis, tubercular—*continued*
- cerebrospinal A17.8† G07*
- – – meninges A17.0† G01*
- cervical (lymph gland or node) A18.2
- cervix (uteri), cervicitis A18.1† N74.0*
- chest (*see also* Tuberculosis, respiratory) A16.9
- – with bacteriological and histological confirmation A15.9
- chorioretinitis A18.5† H32.0*
- choroid, choroiditis A18.5† H32.0*
- ciliary body A18.5† H22.0*
- collier's J65
- colliquativa (primary) A18.4
- colon, colitis A18.3† K93.0*
- complex, primary A16.7
- – with bacteriological and histological confirmation A15.7
- complicating pregnancy, childbirth or puerperium O98.0
- – – affecting fetus or newborn P00.2
- congenital P37.0
- conjunctiva A18.5† II13.1*
- connective tissue (systemic) A18.8† M36.8*
- cornea (ulcer) A18.5† H19.2*
- Cowper's gland A18.1† N51.8*
- coxae A18.0† M01.1*
- coxalgia A18.0† M01.1*
- cul-de-sac of Douglas A18.1† N74.1*
- curvature, spine A18.0† M49.0*
- cutis (colliquativa) (primary) A18.4
- cyst, ovary A18.1† N74.1*
- cystitis A18.1† N33.0*
- dactylitis A18.0† M90.0*
- diarrhea A18.3† K93.0*
- diffuse (*see also* Tuberculosis, miliary) A19.9
- digestive tract A18.3† K93.0*
- disseminated (*see also* Tuberculosis, miliary) A19.9
- duodenum A18.3† K93.0*
- dura (mater) (cerebral) (spinal) A17.0† G01*
- – – abscess (cerebral) (spinal) A17.8† G07*
- dysentery A18.3† K93.0*
- ear (inner) (middle) A18.6
- – – bone A18.0† M90.0*
- – – external (primary) A18.4
- – – skin (primary) A18.4
- elbow A18.0† M01.1*
- empyema A16.5

Tuberculosis, tubercular—*continued*
- empyema—*continued*
- – with bacteriological and histological confirmation A15.6
- encephalitis A17.8† G05.0*
- endarteritis A18.8† I79.8*
- endocarditis A18.8† I39.8*
- – aortic A18.8† I39.1*
- – mitral A18.8† I39.0*
- – pulmonary A18.8† I39.3*
- – tricuspid A18.8† I39.2*
- endocrine glands NEC A18.8† E35.8*
- endometrium A18.1† N74.1*
- enteric, enterica, enteritis A18.3† K93.0*
- enterocolitis A18.3† K93.0*
- epididymis, epididymitis A18.1† N51.1*
- epidural abscess (cerebral) (spinal) A17.8† G07*
- epiglottis A16.4
- – with bacteriological and histological confirmation A15.5
- episcleritis A18.5† H19.0*
- erythema (induratum) (nodosum) (primary) A18.4
- esophagus A18.8† K23.0*
- eustachian tube A18.6† H75.0*
- exudative – *see* Tuberculosis, pulmonary
- eye A18.5
- – glaucoma A18.5† H42.8*
- eyelid (lupus) (primary) A18.4† H03.1*
- fallopian tube (acute) (chronic) A18.1† N74.1*
- fascia A18.8† M73.8*
- fauces A16.8
- – with bacteriological and histological confirmation A15.8
- female pelvic inflammatory disease A18.1† N74.1*
- first infection A16.7
- – with bacteriological and histological confirmation A15.7
- gallbladder A18.8† K87.0*
- ganglion A18.0† M68.0*
- gastritis A18.8† K93.8*
- gastrocolic fistula A18.3† K93.0*
- gastroenteritis A18.3† K93.0*
- gastrointestinal tract A18.3† K93.0*
- general, generalized (*see also* Tuberculosis, miliary) A19.9
- genital organs A18.1
- genitourinary A18.1
- genu A18.0† M01.1*
- glandula suprarenalis A18.7† E35.1*
- glandular, general A18.2

Tuberculosis, tubercular—*continued*
- glottis A16.4
- – with bacteriological and histological confirmation A15.5
- grinder's J65
- gum A18.8† K93.8*
- heart A18.8† I43.0*
- hematogenous – *see* Tuberculosis, miliary
- hemoptysis – *see* Tuberculosis, pulmonary
- hemorrhage NEC – *see* Tuberculosis, pulmonary
- hemothorax A16.5
- – with bacteriological and histological confirmation A15.6
- hepatitis A18.8† K77.0*
- hilar lymph nodes A16.3
- – with bacteriological and histological confirmation A15.4
- – primary (progressive) A16.7
- – – with bacteriological and histological confirmation A15.7
- hip (bone) (disease) (joint) A18.0† M01.1*
- hydropneumothorax A16.5
- – with bacteriological and histological confirmation A15.6
- hydrothorax A16.5
- – with bacteriological and histological confirmation A15.6
- hypoadrenalism A18.7† E35.1*
- hypopharynx A16.8
- – with bacteriological and histological confirmation A15.8
- ileocecal (hyperplastic) A18.3† K93.0*
- ileocolitis A18.3† K93.0*
- ileum A18.3† K93.0*
- iliac spine (superior) A18.0† M90.0*
- immunological findings only A16.7
- indurativa (primary) A18.4
- infantile A16.7
- – with bacteriological and histological confirmation A15.7
- infection A16.9
- – with bacteriological and histological confirmation A15.9
- – without clinical manifestations A16.7
- – – with bacteriological and histological confirmation A15.7
- infraclavicular gland A18.2
- inguinal gland A18.2
- inguinalis A18.2
- intestine (any part) A18.3† K93.0*
- iridocyclitis A18.5† H22.0*
- iris, iritis A18.5† H22.0*

Tuberculosis, tubercular—*continued*
- ischiorectal A18.3† K93.0*
- jaw A18.0† M90.0*
- jejunum A18.3† K93.0*
- joint A18.0† M01.1*
- – vertebral A18.0† M49.0*
- keratitis (interstitial) A18.5† H19.2*
- keratoconjunctivitis A18.5† H19.2*
- kidney A18.1† N29.1*
- knee (joint) A18.0† M01.1*
- kyphosis, kyphoscoliosis A18.0† M49.0*
- laryngitis A16.4
- – with bacteriological and histological
    confirmation A15.5
- larynx A16.4
- – with bacteriological and histological
    confirmation A15.5
- leptomeninges, leptomeningitis (cerebral)
    (spinal) A17.0† G01*
- lichenoides (primary) A18.4
- linguae A18.8† K93.8*
- lip A18.8† K93.8*
- liver A18.8† K77.0*
- lordosis A18.0† M49.0*
- lung – *see* Tuberculosis, pulmonary
- lupus vulgaris A18.4
- lymph gland or node (peripheral) A18.2
- – abdomen A18.3
- – bronchial A16.3
- – – with bacteriological and histological
    confirmation A15.4
- – – primary (progressive) A16.7
- – – – with bacteriological and
    histological confirmation A15.7
- – cervical A18.2
- – hilar A16.3
- – – with bacteriological and histological
    confirmation A15.4
- – – primary (progressive) A16.7
- – – – with bacteriological and
    histological confirmation A15.7
- – intrathoracic A16.3
- – – with bacteriological and histological
    confirmation A15.4
- – – primary (progressive) A16.7
- – – – with bacteriological and
    histological confirmation A15.7
- – mediastinal A16.3
- – – with bacteriological and histological
    confirmation A15.4
- – – primary (progressive) A16.7
- – – – with bacteriological and
    histological confirmation A15.7
- – mesenteric A18.3† K93.0*

Tuberculosis, tubercular—*continued*
- lymph gland or node—*continued*
- – retroperitoneal A18.3
- – tracheobronchial A16.3
- – – with bacteriological and histological
    confirmation A15.4
- – – primary (progressive) A16.7
- – – – with bacteriological and
    histological confirmation A15.7
- lymphadenitis – *see* Tuberculosis, lymph
    gland
- lymphangitis – *see* Tuberculosis, lymph
    gland
- lymphatic (gland) (vessel) – *see*
    Tuberculosis, lymph gland
- mammary gland A18.8
- marasmus NEC A16.9
- mastoiditis A18.0† H75.0*
- mediastinal lymph gland or node A16.3
- – with bacteriological and histological
    confirmation A15.4
- – primary (progressive) A16.7
- – – with bacteriological and histological
    confirmation A15.7
- mediastinum, mediastinitis A16.8
- – with bacteriological and histological
    confirmation A15.8
- – primary (progressive) A16.7
- – – with bacteriological and histological
    confirmation A15.7
- mediastinum A16.8
- – with bacteriological and histological
    confirmation A15.8
- – primary (progressive) A16.7
- – – with bacteriological and histological
    confirmation A15.7
- medulla A17.8† G07*
- melanosis, Addisonian A18.7† E35.1*
- meninges, meningitis (basilar) (cerebral)
    (cerebrospinal) (spinal) A17.0† G01*
- meningoencephalitis A17.8† G05.0*
- mesentery, mesenteric (gland or node)
    A18.3† K93.0*
- miliary A19.9
- – acute A19.2
- – – multiple sites A19.1
- – – single specified site A19.0
- – chronic A19.8
- – specified NEC A19.8
- miner's J65
- molder's J65
- mouth A18.8† K93.8*
- multiple A19.9
- – acute A19.1

Tuberculosis, tubercular—*continued*
- multiple—*continued*
- - chronic A19.8
- muscle A18.8† M63.0*
- myelitis A17.8† G05.0*
- myocardium, myocarditis A18.8† I41.0*
- nasal (passage) (sinus) A16.8
- - with bacteriological and histological
  confirmation A15.8
- nasopharynx A16.8
- - with bacteriological and histological
  confirmation A15.8
- neck gland A18.2
- nephritis A18.1† N29.1*
- nerve (mononeuropathy) A17.8† G59.8*
- nervous system NEC A17.9† G99.8*
- nose (septum) A16.8
- - with bacteriological and histological
  confirmation A15.8
- ocular A18.5
- omentum A18.3
- oophoritis (acute) (chronic) A18.1†
  N74.1*
- optic (nerve trunk) (papilla) A18.5†
  H48.8*
- orbit A18.5
- orchitis A18.1† N51.1*
- organ, specified NEC A18.8
- osseous (*see also* Tuberculosis, bone)
  A18.0† M90.0*
- osteitis (*see also* Tuberculosis, bone)
  A18.0† M90.0*
- osteomyelitis (*see also* Tuberculosis,
  bone) A18.0† M90.0*
- otitis media A18.6† H67.0*
- ovary, ovaritis (acute) (chronic) A18.1†
  N74.1*
- oviduct (acute) (chronic) A18.1† N74.1*
- pachymeningitis A17.0† G01*
- palate (soft) A18.8† K93.8*
- pancreas A18.8† K87.1*
- papulonecrotic(a) (primary) A18.4
- parathyroid glands A18.8† E35.8*
- paronychia (primary) A18.4
- parotid gland or region A18.8† K93.8*
- pelvis (bony) A18.0† M90.0*
- penis A18.1† N51.8*
- peribronchitis A16.4
- - with bacteriological and histological
  confirmation A15.5
- pericardium, pericarditis A18.8† I32.0*
- perichondritis, larynx A16.4
- - with bacteriological and histological
  confirmation A15.5

Tuberculosis, tubercular—*continued*
- periostitis (*see also* Tuberculosis, bone)
  A18.0† M90.0*
- perirectal fistula A18.3† K93.0*
- peritoneum NEC A18.3† K93.0*
- peritonitis A18.3† K67.3*
- pharynx, pharyngitis A16.8
- - with bacteriological and histological
  confirmation A15.8
- phlyctenulosis (keratoconjunctivitis)
  A18.5† H19.2*
- phthisis NEC – *see* Tuberculosis,
  pulmonary
- pituitary gland A18.8† E35.8*
- placenta O98.0
- pleura, pleural, pleurisy, pleuritis
  (fibrinous) (obliterative) (purulent)
  (simple plastic) (with effusion) A16.5
- - with bacteriological and histological
  confirmation A15.6
- - primary (progressive) A16.7
- - - with bacteriological and histological
  confirmation A15.7
- pneumonia, pneumonic – *see*
  Tuberculosis, pulmonary
- pneumothorax (spontaneous) (tense
  valvular) – *see* Tuberculosis, pulmonary
- polyneuropathy A17.8† G63.0*
- polyserositis A19.9
- - acute A19.1
- - chronic A19.8
- potter's J65
- prepuce A18.1† N51.8*
- primary (complex) A16.7
- - with bacteriological and histological
  confirmation A15.7
- proctitis A18.3† K93.0*
- prostate, prostatitis A18.1† N51.0*
- pulmonalis – *see* Tuberculosis, pulmonary
- pulmonary (cavitated) (fibrotic)
  (infiltrative) (nodular) A16.2
- - bacteriological and histological
  examination not done A16.1
- - bacteriologically and histologically
  negative A16.0
- - childhood type or first infection A16.7
- - - with bacteriological and histological
  confirmation A15.7
- - confirmed (by)
- - - culture only A15.1
- - - histologically A15.2
- - - sputum microscopy with or without
  culture A15.0
- - - unspecified means A15.3

Tuberculosis, tubercular—*continued*
- pulmonary—*continued*
- − − primary (complex) A16.7
- − − − with bacteriological and histological confirmation A15.7
- − − without mention of bacteriological or histological confirmation A16.2
- pyelitis A18.1† N29.1∗
- pyelonephritis A18.1† N29.1∗
- pyemia − *see* Tuberculosis, miliary
- pyonephrosis A18.1† N29.1∗
- pyopneumothorax A16.5
- − − with bacteriological and histological confirmation A15.6
- pyothorax A16.5
- − − with bacteriological and histological confirmation A15.6
- rectum (fistula) (with abscess) A18.3† K93.0∗
- reinfection stage − *see* Tuberculosis, pulmonary
- renal A18.1† N29.1∗
- respiratory A16.9
- − − with bacteriological and histological confirmation A15.9
- − − primary A16.7
- − − − with bacteriological and histological confirmation A15.7
- − − specified site NEC A16.8
- − − − with bacteriological and histological confirmation A15.8
- resulting from HIV disease B20.0
- retina, retinitis A18.5† H32.0∗
- retroperitoneal (lymph gland or node) A18.3
- rheumatism NEC A18.0† M01.1∗
- rhinitis A16.8
- − − with bacteriological and histological confirmation A15.8
- sacroiliac (joint) A18.0† M49.0∗
- sacrum A18.0† M49.0∗
- salivary gland A18.8† K93.8∗
- salpingitis (acute) (chronic) A18.1† N74.1∗
- sandblaster's J65
- sclera A18.5† H19.0∗
- scoliosis A18.0† M49.0∗
- scrofulous A18.2
- scrotum A18.1† N51.8∗
- seminal tract or vesicle A18.1† N51.8∗
- septic NEC (*see also* Tuberculosis, miliary) A19.9
- shoulder (joint) A18.0† M01.1∗
- − − blade A18.0† M90.0∗

Tuberculosis, tubercular—*continued*
- sigmoid A18.3† K93.0∗
- sinus (any nasal) A16.8
- − − with bacteriological and histological confirmation A15.8
- − − bone A18.0† M90.0∗
- − − epididymis A18.1† N51.1∗
- skeletal NEC A18.0† M90.0∗
- skin (any site) (primary) A18.4
- spermatic cord A18.1† N51.8∗
- spine, spinal (column) A18.0† M49.0∗
- − − cord A17.8† G07∗
- − − medulla A17.8† G07∗
- − − membrane A17.0† G01∗
- − − meninges A17.0† G01∗
- spleen, splenitis A18.8† D77∗
- spondylitis A18.0† M49.0∗
- sternoclavicular joint A18.0† M01.1∗
- stomach A18.8† K93.8∗
- stonemason's J65
- subcutaneous tissue (cellular) (primary) A18.4
- subcutis (primary) A18.4
- submaxillary (region) A18.8† K93.8∗
- supraclavicular gland A18.2
- suprarenal (capsule) (gland) A18.7† E35.1∗
- symphysis pubis A18.0† M01.1∗
- synovitis A18.0† M68.0∗
- − − articular A18.0† M01.1∗
- − − spine or vertebra A18.0† M49.0∗
- systemic − *see* Tuberculosis, miliary
- tarsitis A18.4† H03.1∗
- tendon (sheath) − *see* Tuberculosis, tenosynovitis
- tenosynovitis A18.0† M68.0∗
- − − spine or vertebra A18.0† M49.0∗
- testis A18.1† N51.1∗
- throat A16.8
- − − with bacteriological and histological confirmation A15.8
- thymus gland A18.8† E35.8∗
- thyroid gland A18.8† E35.0∗
- tongue A18.8† K93.8∗
- tonsil, tonsillitis A16.8
- − − with bacteriological and histological confirmation A15.8
- trachea, tracheal A16.4
- − − with bacteriological and histological confirmation A15.5
- − − lymph gland or node A16.3
- − − − with bacteriological and histological confirmation A15.4
- − − − primary (progressive) A16.7

Arise from cells of endocrine nervous systems ← Neuroendocrine tumour—often called carcinoid tumours. Most commonly occur in the intestine but also in pancreas, lung + rest of the body → Carcinoid (M8240/3)

INTERNATIONAL CLASSIFICATION OF DISEASES

Tuberculosis, tubercular—*continued*
- trachea, tracheal—*continued*
- – – lymph gland or node—*continued*
- – – – primary—*continued*
- – – – – with bacteriological and histological confirmation A15.7
- – tracheobronchial A16.4
- – – with bacteriological and histological confirmation A15.5
- – – lymph gland or node A16.3
- – – – with bacteriological and histological confirmation A15.4
- – – – primary (progressive) A16.7
- – – – – with bacteriological and histological confirmation A15.7
- – tubal (acute) (chronic) A18.1† N74.1*
- – tunica vaginalis A18.1† N51.8*
- – ulcer (primary) (skin) A18.4
- – – bowel or intestine A18.3† K93.0*
- – – specified NEC – *code as* Tuberculosis, by site
- – unspecified site A16.9
- – ureter A18.1† N29.1*
- – urethra, urethral (gland) A18.1† N37.0*
- – urinary organ or tract A18.1
- – uterus A18.1† N74.1*
- – uveal tract A18.5† H22.0*
- – uvula A18.8† K93.8*
- – vagina A18.1† N77.1*
- – vas deferens A18.1† N51.8*
- – verruca, verrucosa (cutis) (primary) A18.4
- – vertebra (column) A18.0† M49.0*
- – vesiculitis A18.1† N51.8*
- – vulva A18.1† N77.1*
- – – with ulceration A18.1† N77.0*
- – wrist (joint) A18.0† M01.1*

Tuberculum
- Carabelli – *see* Note at K00.2
- occlusal – *see* Note at K00.2
- paramolare K00.2

Tuberous sclerosis (brain) Q85.1

Tubo-ovarian – *see condition*

Tuboplasty, after previous sterilization Z31.0

Tubotympanitis, catarrhal (chronic) H65.2

Tularemia A21.9
- abdominal A21.3
- conjunctivitis A21.1† H13.1*
- gastrointestinal A21.3
- generalized A21.7
- ingestion A21.3
- oculoglandular A21.1

Tularemia—*continued*
- ophthalmic A21.1
- pneumonia (any), pneumonic A21.2† J17.0*
- sepsis A21.7
- specified NEC A21.8
- typhoidal A21.7
- ulceroglandular A21.0

Tumefaction – *see also* Swelling
- liver (*see also* Hypertrophy, liver) R16.0

Tumor (M8000/1) – *see also* Neoplasm, uncertain behavior
- acinar cell (M8550/1) D48.9
- acinic cell (M8550/1) D48.9
- adenocarcinoid (M8245/3) – *see* Neoplasm, malignant
- adenomatoid (M9054/0) – *see also* Neoplasm, benign
- – odontogenic (M9300/0) D16.5
- – – upper jaw (bone) D16.4
- adnexal (skin) (M8390/0) – *see* Neoplasm, skin, benign
- adrenal
- – cortical (benign) (M8370/0) D35.0
- – – malignant (M8370/3) C74.0
- – rest (M8671/0) – *see* Neoplasm, benign
- alpha-cell (M8152/0)
- – malignant (M8152/3)
- – – pancreas C25.4
- – – specified site NEC – *see* Neoplasm, malignant
- – – unspecified site C25.4
- – pancreas D13.7
- – specified site NEC – *see* Neoplasm, benign
- – unspecified site D13.7
- aneurysmal (*see also* Aneurysm) I72.9
- aortic body (M8691/1) D44.7
- Askin's (M8803/3) – *see* Neoplasm, connective tissue, malignant
- basal cell (M8090/1) – *see* Neoplasm, skin, uncertain behavior
- Bednar (M8833/3) – *see* Neoplasm, skin, malignant
- benign (unclassified) (M8000/0) – *see* Neoplasm, benign
- beta-cell (M8151/0)
- – malignant (M8151/3)
- – – pancreas C25.4
- – – specified site NEC – *see* Neoplasm, malignant
- – – unspecified site C25.4
- – pancreas D13.7

Tumor—*continued*
– beta-cell—*continued*
– – specified site NEC – *see* Neoplasm,
  benign
– – unspecified site D13.7
– Brenner (M9000/0) D27
– – borderline malignancy (M9000/1)
  D39.1
– – malignant (M9000/3) C56
– – proliferating (M9000/1) D39.1
– bronchial alveolar, intravascular
  (M9134/1) D38.1
– Brooke's (M8100/0) – *see* Neoplasm, skin,
  benign
– brown fat (M8880/0) – *see* Lipoma
– Burkitt C83.7
– calcifying epithelial odontogenic
  (M9340/0) D16.5
– – upper jaw (bone) D16.4
– carcinoid (M8240/3) – *see* Carcinoid
– carotid body (M8692/1) D44.6
– cervix, in pregnancy or childbirth O34.4
– – affecting fetus or newborn P03.8
– – causing obstructed labor O65.5
– – – affecting fetus or newborn P03.1
– chondromatous giant cell (M9230/0) – *see*
  Neoplasm, bone, benign
– chromaffin (M8700/0) – *see also*
  Neoplasm, benign
– – malignant (M8700/3) – *see* Neoplasm,
  malignant
– Cock's peculiar L72.1
– Codman's (M9230/0) – *see* Neoplasm,
  bone, benign
– dentigerous, mixed (M9282/0) D16.5
– – upper jaw (bone) D16.4
– dermoid (M9084/0) – *see* Neoplasm,
  benign
– – with malignant transformation
  (M9084/3) C56
– desmoid (extra-abdominal) (M8821/1) –
  see also Neoplasm, connective tissue,
  uncertain behavior
– – abdominal (M8822/1) D48.1
– embolus (M8000/6) – *see* Neoplasm,
  secondary
– embryonal (mixed) (M9080/1) – *see also*
  Neoplasm, uncertain behavior
– – liver (M9080/3) C22.7
– endodermal sinus (M9071/3)
– – specified site – *see* Neoplasm,
  malignant
– – unspecified site
– – – female C56

Tumor—*continued*
– endodermal sinus—*continued*
– – unspecified site—*continued*
– – – male C62.9
– endometrioid, of low malignant potential
  (M8380/1) – *see* Neoplasm, uncertain
  behavior
– epithelial
– – benign (M8010/0) – *see* Neoplasm,
  benign
– – malignant (M8010/3) – *see* Neoplasm,
  malignant
– Ewing's (M9260/3) – *see* Neoplasm, bone,
  malignant
– fatty (M8850/0) – *see* Lipoma
– fetal, causing obstructed labor (mother)
  O66.3
– fibroid (M8890/0) – *see* Leiomyoma
– G cell (M8153/1)
– – malignant (M8153/3)
– – – pancreas C25.4
– – – specified site NEC – *see* Neoplasm,
  malignant
– – – unspecified site C25.4
– – specified site – *see* Neoplasm, uncertain
  behavior
– – unspecified site D37.7
– germ cell (M9064/3) – *see also* Neoplasm,
  malignant
– – mixed (M9085/3) C80.-
– ghost cell, odontogenic (M9302/0) D16.5
– – upper jaw (bone) D16.4
– giant cell (M8003/1) – *see also* Neoplasm,
  uncertain behavior
– – bone (M9250/1) D48.0
– – – malignant (M9250/3) – *see*
  Neoplasm, bone, malignant
– – chondromatous (M9230/0) – *see*
  Neoplasm, bone, benign
– – malignant (M8003/3) – *see* Neoplasm,
  malignant
– – soft parts (M9251/1) – *see* Neoplasm,
  connective tissue, uncertain behavior
– – – malignant (M9251/3) – *see*
  Neoplasm, connective tissue,
  malignant
– glomus (M8711/0) D18.0
– – jugulare (M8690/1) D44.7
– gonadal stromal (M8590/1) – *see*
  Neoplasm, uncertain behavior
– granular cell (M9580/0) – *see also*
  Neoplasm, connective tissue, benign
– – malignant (M9580/3) – *see* Neoplasm,
  connective tissue, malignant

Tumor—*continued*
- granulosa cell (M8620/1) D39.1
- - juvenile (M8622/1) D39.1
- - malignant (M8620/3) C56
- granulosa cell-theca cell (M8621/1) D39.1
- Grawitz's (M8312/3) C64
- hemorrhoidal – *see* Hemorrhoids
- hilar cell (M8660/0) D27
- hilus cell (M8660/0) D27
- Hurthle cell (benign) (M8290/0) D34
- - malignant (M8290/3) C73
- hydatid (*see also* Echinococcus) B67.9
- hypernephroid (M8311/1) – *see* Neoplasm, uncertain bahavior
- interstitial cell (M8650/1) – *see also* Neoplasm, uncertain behavior
- - benign (M8650/0) – *see* Neoplasm, benign
- - malignant (M8650/3) – *see* Neoplasm, malignant
- intravascular bronchial alveolar (M9134/1) D38.1
- islet cell (M8150/0)
- - malignant (M8150/3)
- - - pancreas C25.4
- - - specified site NEC – *see* Neoplasm, malignant
- - - unspecified site C25.4
- - pancreas D13.7
- - specified site NEC – *see* Neoplasm, benign
- - unspecified site D13.7
- juxtaglomerular (M8361/1) D41.0
- Klatskin's (M8162/3) C22.1
- Krukenberg's (M8490/6) C79.6
- Leydig cell (M8650/1)
- - benign (M8650/0)
- - - specified site – *see* Neoplasm, benign
- - - unspecified site
- - - - female D27
- - - - male D29.2
- - malignant (M8650/3)
- - - specified site – *see* Neoplasm, malignant
- - - unspecified site
- - - - female C56
- - - - male C62.9
- - specified site – *see* Neoplasm, uncertain behavior
- - unspecified site
- - - female D39.1
- - - male D40.1
- lipid cell, ovary (M8670/0) D27

Tumor—*continued*
- lipoid cell, ovary (M8670/0) D27
- malignant (M8000/3) – *see also* Neoplasm, malignant
- - fusiform cell (type) (M8004/3) C80.-
- - giant cell (type) (M8003/3) C80.-
- - mast cell C96.2
- - mixed NEC (M8940/3) C80.-
- - plasma cell, localized NEC C90.3
- - small cell (type) (M8002/3) C80.-
- - spindle cell (type) (M8004/3) C80.-
- - unclassified (M8000/3) C80.-
- mast cell D47.0
- - malignant C96.2
- melanotic, neuroectodermal (M9363/0) – *see* Neoplasm, benign
- Merkel cell (M8247/3) – *see* Neoplasm, skin, malignant
- mesenchymal
- - malignant (M8800/3) – *see* Neoplasm, connective tissue, malignant
- - mixed (M8990/1) – *see* Neoplasm, connective tissue, uncertain behavior
- mesodermal, mixed (M8951/3) – *see also* Neoplasm, malignant
- - liver C22.4
- mesonephric (M9110/1) – *see also* Neoplasm, uncertain behavior
- - malignant (M9110/3) – *see* Neoplasm, malignant
- metastatic
- - from specified site (M8000/3) – *see* Neoplasm, malignant, by site
- - to specified site (M8000/6) – *see* Neoplasm, secondary, by site
- mixed NEC (M8940/0) – *see also* Neoplasm, benign
- - malignant (M8940/3) – *see* Neoplasm, malignant
- mucinous, of low malignant potential (M8472/3)
- - specified site – *see* Neoplasm, malignant
- - unspecified site C56
- mucocarcinoid (M8243/3)
- - specified site – *see* Neoplasm, malignant
- - unspecified site C18.1
- mucoepidermoid (M8430/1) – *see* Neoplasm, uncertain behavior
- Müllerian, mixed (M8950/3)
- - specified site – *see* Neoplasm, malignant
- - unspecified site C54.9

Tumor—*continued*
- myoepithelial (M8982/0) – *see* Neoplasm, benign
- neuroectodermal (peripheral) (M9364/3) – *see also* Neoplasm, malignant
- – primitive (M9473/3)
- – – specified site – *see* Neoplasm, malignant
- – – unspecified site C71.9
- neurogenic olfactory (M9520/3) C30.0
- nonencapsulated sclerosing (M8350/3) C73
- odontogenic (M9270/1) D48.0
- – adenomatoid (M9300/0) D16.5
- – – upper jaw (bone) D16.4
- – benign (M9270/0) D16.5
- – – upper jaw (bone) D16.4
- – calcifying epithelial (M9340/0) D16.5
- – – upper jaw (bone) D16.4
- – keratocystic (M9270/0) D16.5
- – – upper jaw (bone) D16.4
- – malignant (M9270/3) C41.1
- – – upper jaw (bone) C41.0
- – squamous (M9312/0) D16.5
- – – upper jaw (bone) D16.4
- ovarian stromal (M8590/1) D39.1
- ovary, in pregnancy or childbirth O34.8
- – affecting fetus or newborn P03.8
- – causing obstructed labor O65.5
- pacinian (M9507/0) – *see* Neoplasm, skin, benign
- Pancoast's (M8010/3) C34.1
- papillary (M8050/0) – *see also* Papilloma
- – cystic (M8452/1) D37.7
- – mucinous, of low malignant potential (M8473/3) C56
- – – specified site – *see* Neoplasm, malignant
- – – unspecified site C56
- – serous, of low malignant potential (M8462/3)
- – – specified site – *see* Neoplasm, malignant
- – – unspecified site C56
- pelvic, in pregnancy or childbirth O34.8
- – affecting fetus or newborn P03.8
- – causing obstructed labor O65.5
- – – affecting fetus or newborn P03.1
- phantom F45.8
- phyllodes (M9020/1) D48.6
- – benign (M9020/0) D24
- – malignant (M9020/3) – *see* Neoplasm, breast, malignant
- Pindborg (M9340/0) D16.5

Tumor—*continued*
- Pindborg—*continued*
- – – upper jaw (bone) D16.4
- placental site trophoblastic (M9104/1) D39.2
- plasma cell (malignant) C90.3
- polyvesicular vitelline (M9071/3)
- – specified site – *see* Neoplasm, malignant
- – unspecified site
- – – female C56
- – – male C62.9
- Pott's puffy – *see* Osteomyelitis
- Rathke's pouch (M9350/1) D44.3
- retinal anlage (M9363/0) – *see* Neoplasm, benign
- salivary gland type, mixed (M8940/0) – *see also* Neoplasm, salivary gland, benign
- – malignant (M8940/3) – *see* Neoplasm, salivary gland, malignant
- Sampson's N80.1
- Schmincke's (M8082/3) – *see* Neoplasm, nasopharynx, malignant
- sclerosing stromal (M8602/0) D27
- sebaceous (*see also* Cyst, sebaceous) L72.1
- secondary (M8000/6) – *see* Neoplasm, secondary
- serous, of low malignant potential (M8442/3)
- – specified site – *see* Neoplasm, malignant
- – unspecified site C56
- Sertoli cell (M8640/0)
- – with lipid storage (M8641/0)
- – – specified site – *see* Neoplasm, benign
- – – unspecified site
- – – – female D27
- – – – male D29.2
- – specified site – *see* Neoplasm, benign
- – unspecified site
- – – female D27
- – – male D29.2
- Sertoli-Leydig cell (M8631/0)
- – specified site – *see* Neoplasm, benign
- – unspecified site
- – – female D27
- – – male D29.2
- sex cord(-stromal) (M8590/1) – *see* Neoplasm, uncertain behavior
- – with annular tubules (M8623/1) D39.1
- skin appendage (M8390/0) – *see* Neoplasm, skin, benign

Tumor—*continued*
- smooth muscle (M8897/1) – *see* Neoplasm, connective tissue, uncertain behavior
- soft tissue
- – benign (M8800/0) – *see* Neoplasm, connective tissue, benign
- – malignant (M8800/3) – *see* Neoplasm, connective tissue, malignant
- sternomastoid (congenital) Q68.0
- stromal
- – gastrointestinal (GIST) D37.9
- – benign – *see* Neoplasm, benign
- – colon D37.4
- – esophagus D37.7
- – malignant – *see* Neoplasm, malignant
- – peritoneum D48.4
- – rectum D37.5
- – small intestine D37.2
- – specified site NEC – *see* Neoplasm, uncertain behaviour
- – stomach D37.1
- sweat gland (M8400/1) – *see also* Neoplasm, skin, uncertain behavior
- – benign (M8400/0) – *see* Neoplasm, skin, benign
- – malignant (M8400/3) – *see* Neoplasm, skin, malignant
- syphilitic, brain A52.1† G94.8*
- testicular stromal (M8590/1) D40.1
- theca cell (M8600/0) D27
- theca cell-granulosa cell (M8621/1) D39.1
- Triton, malignant (M9561/3) – *see* Neoplasm, nerve, malignant
- trophoblastic, placental site (M9104/1) D39.2
- turban (M8200/0) D23.4
- uterus (body), in pregnancy or childbirth O34.1
- – affecting fetus or newborn P03.8
- – causing obstructed labor O65.5
- – – affecting fetus or newborn P03.1
- vagina, in pregnancy or childbirth O34.6
- – affecting fetus or newborn P03.8
- – causing obstructed labor O65.5
- – – affecting fetus or newborn P03.1
- varicose (*see also* Varicose vein) I83.9
- von Recklinghausen's – *see* Neurofibromatosis
- vulva or perineum, in pregnancy or childbirth O34.7
- – affecting fetus or newborn P03.8
- – causing obstructed labor O65.5

Tumor—*continued*
- vulva or perineum, in pregnancy or childbirth—*continued*
- – causing obstructed labor—*continued*
- – – affecting fetus or newborn P03.1
- Warthin's (M8561/0) – *see* Neoplasm, salivary gland, benign
- Wilms' (M8960/3) C64
- yolk sac (M9071/3)
- – specified site – *see* Neoplasm, malignant
- – unspecified site
- – – female C56
- – – male C62.9
Tumorlet (M8040/1) – *see* Neoplasm, uncertain behavior
Tungiasis B88.1
Tunica vasculosa lentis Q12.2
Turban tumor (M8200/0) D23.4
Turner-like syndrome Q87.1
Turner's
- hypoplasia (tooth) K00.4
- syndrome Q96.9
- – specified NEC Q96.8
- tooth K00.4
Turner-Ullrich syndrome Q96.9
Tussis convulsiva (*see also* Whooping cough) A37.9
Twilight state
- epileptic F05.8
- psychogenic F44.8
Twin (pregnancy) (fetus or newborn) P01.5
- complicating pregnancy O30.0
- conjoined Q89.4
Twist, twisted
- bowel, colon or intestine K56.2
- hair (congenital) Q84.1
- mesentery or omentum K56.2
- organ or site, congenital NEC – *see* Anomaly, by site
- ovarian pedicle N83.5
- – congenital Q50.2
- umbilical cord in fetus or newborn P02.5
Twitching R25.3
Tylosis (acquired) L84
- linguae K13.2
- palmaris et plantaris (congenital) (inherited) Q82.8
- – acquired L85.1
Tympanites (abdominal) (intestinal) R14
Tympanitis H73.8
- with otitis media – *see* Otitis media
- acute H73.0

Tympanitis—*continued*
- chronic H73.1
Tympanosclerosis H74.0
Tympanum – *see condition*
Tympany
- abdomen R14
- chest R09.8
Type A behavior pattern Z73.1
Typhoenteritis A01.0
Typhoid (abortive) (ambulant) (any site) (fever) (hemorrhagic) (infection) (intermittent) (malignant) (rheumatic) A01.0
- inoculation reaction – *see* Complications, vaccination
- pneumonia A01.0† J17.0∗
Typhoperitonitis A01.0
Typhus (fever) A75.9
- abdominal, abdominalis A01.0
- African tick A77.1
- brain A75.9† G94.8∗
- cerebral A75.9† G94.8∗
- classical A75.0
- due to Rickettsia
- – prowazekii A75.0
- – – recrudescent A75.1
- – tsutsugamushi A75.3
- – typhi A75.2

Typhus—*continued*
- endemic (flea-borne) A75.2
- epidemic (louse-borne) A75.0
- exanthematic NEC A75.0
- flea-borne A75.2
- India tick A77.1
- Kenya (tick) A77.1
- louse-borne A75.0
- Mexican A75.2
- mite-borne A75.3
- murine A75.2
- North Asian tick-borne A77.2
- Queensland tick A77.3
- rat A75.2
- recrudescent A75.1
- recurrens (*see also* Fever, relapsing) A68.9
- Sao Paulo A77.0
- scrub (China) (India) (Malaysia) (New Guinea) A75.3
- shop (of Malaysia) A75.2
- Siberian tick A77.2
- tick-borne A77.9
- tropical (mite-borne) A75.3
Tyrosinemia E70.2
- newborn, transitory P74.5
Tyrosinosis E70.2
Tyrosinuria E70.2

U

Uhl's disease Q24.8
**Ulcer, ulcerated, ulcerating, ulceration,
    ulcerative** L98.4
− amebic (intestine) (*see also* Amebiasis)
    A06.1
− − skin A06.7
− anastomotic − *see* Ulcer, gastrojejunal
− anorectal K62.6
− antral − *see* Ulcer, stomach
− anus (sphincter) (solitary) K62.6
− − varicose − *see* Varicose, ulcer, anus
− aphthous (oral) (recurrent) K12.0
− − genital organ(s)
− − − female N76.6
− − − male N50.8
− artery I77.8
− atrophic NEC − *see* Ulcer, skin
− Barrett's K22.1
− bile duct (common) (hepatic) K83.8
− bladder (sphincter) (solitary) NEC N32.8
− − in schistosomiasis (bilharzial) B65.0†
    N33.8*
− − submucosal N30.1
− − tuberculous A18.1† N33.0*
− bleeding NEC K27.4
− bone M86.8
− bowel (*see also* Ulcer, intestine) K63.3
− breast N61
− bronchus J98.0
− buccal (cavity) (traumatic) K12.1
− Buruli A31.1
− cancerous (M8000/3) − *see* Neoplasm,
    malignant
− cardia K22.1
− cardioesophageal (peptic) K22.1
− cecum (*see also* Ulcer, intestine) K63.3
− cervix (uteri) (decubitus) (trophic) N86
− − with cervicitis N72
− chancroidal A57
− chiclero B55.1
− chronic (cause unknown) − *see* Ulcer, skin
− Cochin-China B55.1
− colon (*see also* Ulcer, intestine) K63.3
− conjunctiva H10.8
− cornea (annular) (catarrhal) (central)
    (infectional) (marginal) (ring) (serpent)
    (serpiginous) (with perforation) H16.0
− − dendritic (herpes simplex) B00.5†
    H19.1*

Ulcer, ulcerated—*continued*
− cornea—*continued*
− − tuberculous (phlyctenular) A18.5†
    H19.2*
− corpus cavernosum (chronic) N48.5
− crural − *see* Ulcer, lower limb
− Curling's − *see* Ulcer, peptic, acute
− Cushing's − *see* Ulcer, peptic, acute
− cystic duct K82.8
− decubitus (skin, any site) L89.-
− − cervix N86
− − stage
− − − I L89.0
− − − II L89.1
− − − III L89.2
− − − IV L89.3
− dendritic, cornea (herpes simplex) B00.5†
    H19.1*
− diabetes, diabetic (mellitus) (*see also* E10-
    E14 with fourth character .5) E14.5
− Dieulafoy's K25.0
− due to
− − infection NEC − *see* Ulcer, skin
− − radiation NEC L59.8
− − trophic disturbance (any region) − *see*
    Ulcer, skin
− − X-ray L58.1
− duodenum, duodenal (eroded) (peptic)
    K26.9
− − with
− − − hemorrhage K26.4
− − − − and perforation K26.6
− − − perforation K26.5
− − acute K26.3
− − − with
− − − − hemorrhage K26.0
− − − − − and perforation K26.2
− − − − perforation K26.1
− − chronic K26.7
− − − with
− − − − hemorrhage K26.4
− − − − − and perforation K26.6
− − − − perforation K26.5
− dysenteric NEC A09.9
− elusive N30.1
− epiglottis J38.7
− esophagus (peptic) K22.1
− − due to
− − − gastrointestinal reflux disease K21.0

Ulcer, ulcerated—*continued*
- esophagus—*continued*
- – – due to—*continued*
- – – – ingestion of chemical or medicament K22.1
- – – fungal K22.1
- – – infective K22.1
- – – varicose I85.9
- – – – bleeding I85.0
- eyelid (region) H01.8
- fauces J39.2
- fistulous NEC – *see* Ulcer, skin
- foot (indolent) (*see also* Ulcer, lower limb) L97
- – – perforating L97
- – – – leprous A30.1
- – – – syphilitic A52.1
- – – varicose (venous) I83.0
- – – – inflamed or infected I83.2
- – – venous NEC I83.0
- – – – due to venous insufficiency I87.2
- – – – inflamed or infected I83.2
- – – – postphlebitic (infected) (inflamed) (postthrombotic) I87.0
- frambesial, initial A66.0
- frenum (tongue) K14.0
- gallbladder K82.8
- gangrenous (*see also* Gangrene) R02
- gastric – *see* Ulcer, stomach
- gastrocolic – *see* Ulcer, gastrojejunal
- gastroduodenal – *see* Ulcer, peptic
- gastroesophageal – *see* Ulcer, stomach
- gastrointestinal – *see* Ulcer, gastrojejunal
- gastrojejunal (peptic) K28.9
- – – with
- – – – hemorrhage K28.4
- – – – – and perforation K28.6
- – – – perforation K28.5
- – – acute K28.3
- – – – with
- – – – – hemorrhage K28.0
- – – – – – and perforation K28.2
- – – – – perforation K28.1
- – – chronic K28.7
- – – – with
- – – – – hemorrhage K28.4
- – – – – – and perforation K28.6
- – – – – perforation K28.5
- gastrojejunocolic – *see* Ulcer, gastrojejunal
- gingiva K06.8
- gingivitis K05.1
- glottis J38.7
- gum K06.8

Ulcer, ulcerated—*continued*
- heel (*see also* Ulcer, lower limb) L97
- Hunner's N30.1
- hypopharynx J39.2
- hypopyon (chronic) (subacute) H16.0
- hypostaticum – *see* Ulcer, varicose
- ileum (*see also* Ulcer, intestine) K63.3
- intestine, intestinal K63.3
- – – amebic (*see also* Amebiasis) A06.1
- – – duodenal – *see* Ulcer, duodenum
- – – marginal (*see also* Ulcer, gastrojejunal) K28.9
- – – perforating K63.1
- – – – fetus or newborn P78.0
- – – primary, small intestine K63.3
- – – rectum K62.6
- – – stercoraceous, stercoral K63.3
- – – tuberculous A18.3† K93.0*
- – – typhoid (fever) A01.0
- – – varicose I86.8
- jejunum, jejunal – *see* Ulcer, gastrojejunal
- keratitis H16.0
- knee – *see* Ulcer, lower limb
- labium (majus) (minus) N76.6
- laryngitis (*see also* Laryngitis) J04.0
- larynx (aphthous) (contact) J38.7
- – – diphtheritic A36.2
- leg – *see* Ulcer, lower limb
- lip K13.0
- lower limb (atrophic) (chronic) (neurogenic) (perforating) (pyogenic) (trophic) (tropical) L97
- – – varicose (venous) I83.0
- – – – inflamed or infected I83.2
- – – venous NEC I83.0
- – – – due to venous insufficiency I87.2
- – – – inflamed or infected I83.2
- – – – postphlebitic (infected) (inflamed) (postthrombotic) I87.0
- luetic – *see* Ulcer, syphilitic
- lung J98.4
- – – tuberculous (*see also* Tuberculosis, pulmonary) A16.2
- malignant (M8000/3) – *see* Neoplasm, malignant
- marginal NEC – *see* Ulcer, gastrojejunal
- meatus (urinarius) N34.2
- Meckel's diverticulum Q43.0
- Meleney's (chronic undermining) L98.4
- Mooren's (cornea) H16.0
- nasopharynx J39.2
- neurogenic NEC – *see* Ulcer, skin
- nose, nasal (passage) (infective) (septum) J34.0

Ulcer, ulcerated—*continued*
- nose, nasal—*continued*
- - skin – *see* Ulcer, skin
- - varicose (bleeding) I86.8
- oesophagus – *see* Ulcer, esophagus
- oral mucosa (traumatic) K12.1
- palate (soft) K12.1
- penis (chronic) N48.5
- peptic (site unspecified) K27.9
- - with
- - - hemorrhage K27.4
- - - - and perforation K27.6
- - - perforation K27.5
- - acute K27.3
- - - with
- - - - hemorrhage K27.0
- - - - - and perforation K27.2
- - - - perforation K27.1
- - chronic K27.7
- - - with
- - - - hemorrhage K27.4
- - - - - and perforation K27.6
- - - - perforation K27.5
- - newborn P78.8
- perforating NEC K27.5
- - skin L98.4
- peritonsillar J35.8
- phagedenic (tropical) NEC – *see* Ulcer, skin
- pharynx J39.2
- phlebitis – *see* Phlebitis
- plaster L89.-
- - stage
- - - I L89.0
- - - II L89.1
- - - III L89.2
- - - IV L89.3
- popliteal space – *see* Ulcer, lower limb
- postpyloric – *see* Ulcer, duodenum
- prepuce N48.1
- prepyloric – *see* Ulcer, stomach
- pressure L89.-
- - stage
- - - I L89.0
- - - II L89.1
- - - III L89.2
- - - IV L89.3
- pyloric – *see* Ulcer, stomach
- rectosigmoid K63.3
- rectum (sphincter) (solitary) K62.6
- - stercoraceous, stercoral K62.6
- - varicose – *see* Varicose, ulcer, anus
- retina H30.0

Ulcer, ulcerated—*continued*
- rodent (M8090/3) – *see also* Neoplasm, skin, malignant
- sclera H15.0
- scrofulous (tuberculous) A18.2
- scrotum N50.8
- - tuberculous A18.1† N51.8*
- - varicose I86.1
- seminal vesicle N50.8
- sigmoid (*see also* Ulcer, intestine) K63.3
- skin (atrophic) (chronic) (neurogenic) (perforating) (pyogenic) (trophic) L98.4
- - with gangrene (*see also* Gangrene) R02
- - amebic A06.7
- - decubitus L89.-
- - - stage
- - - - I L89.0
- - - - II L89.1
- - - - III L89.2
- - - - IV L89.3
- - lower limb L97
- - tuberculous (primary) A18.4
- - varicose – *see* Ulcer, varicose
- sloughing NEC – *see* Ulcer, skin
- solitary, anus or rectum (sphincter) K62.6
- sore throat J02.9
- - streptococcal J02.0
- spermatic cord N50.8
- spine (tuberculous) A18.0† M49.0*
- stasis (venous) I83.0
- - inflamed or infected I83.2
- stercoraceous, stercoral K63.3
- - anus or rectum K62.6
- stoma, stomal – *see* Ulcer, gastrojejunal
- stomach (eroded) (peptic) (round) K25.9
- - with
- - - hemorrhage K25.4
- - - - and perforation K25.6
- - - perforation K25.5
- - acute K25.3
- - - with
- - - - hemorrhage K25.0
- - - - - and perforation K25.2
- - - - perforation K25.1
- - chronic K25.7
- - - with
- - - - hemorrhage K25.4
- - - - - and perforation K25.6
- - - - perforation K25.5
- stomatitis K12.1
- stress – *see* Ulcer, peptic
- strumous (tuberculous) A18.2
- syphilitic (any site) (early) (secondary) A51.3

Ulcer, ulcerated—*continued*
- syphilitic—*continued*
- – late A52.7
- – perforating A52.7
- – – foot A52.1
- testis N50.8
- thigh – *see* Ulcer, lower limb
- throat J39.2
- toe – *see* Ulcer, lower limb
- tongue (traumatic) K14.0
- tonsil J35.8
- trachea J39.8
- trophic – *see* Ulcer, skin
- tropical NEC L98.4
- tuberculous – *see* Tuberculosis, ulcer
- tunica vaginalis N50.8
- turbinate J34.8
- typhoid (perforating) A01.0
- urethra (meatus) (*see also* Urethritis) N34.2
- uterus N85.8
- – cervix N86
- – – with cervicitis N72
- – neck N86
- – – with cervicitis N72
- vagina N76.5
- – pessary N89.8
- valve, heart I33.0
- varicose (lower limb, any part) (venous) I83.0
- – anus – *see* Varicose, ulcer, anus
- – esophagus I85.9
- – – bleeding I85.0
- – inflamed or infected I83.2
- – nasal septum I86.8
- – rectum – *see* Varicose, ulcer, anus
- – scrotum I86.1
- – specified site NEC I86.8
- vas deferens N50.8
- venous NEC I83.0
- – due to venous insufficiency I87.2
- – inflamed or infected I83.2
- – postphlebitic (infected) (inflamed) (postthrombotic) I87.0
- vulva (acute) (infectional) N76.6
- – in (due to)
- – – Behçet's disease M35.2† N77.8*
- – – herpesviral (herpes simplex) infection A60.0† N77.0*
- – – tuberculosis A18.1† N77.0*
- X-ray L58.1
- yaws A66.4

Ulcus – *see also* Ulcer
- cutis tuberculosum A18.4

Ulcus—*continued*
- duodeni – *see* Ulcer, duodenum
- durum (syphilitic) A51.0
- – extragenital A51.2
- gastrojejunale – *see* Ulcer, gastrojejunal
- hypostaticum – *see* Ulcer, varicose
- molle (cutis) (skin) A57
- serpens corneae H16.0
- ventriculi – *see* Ulcer, stomach

Ulegyria Q04.8
Ulerythema
- ophryogenes, congenital Q84.2
- sycosiforme L73.8

Ullrich (-Bonnevie) (-Turner) syndrome Q87.1
Ullrich-Feichtiger syndrome Q87.0
Ulnar – *see* condition
Ulorrhagia, ulorrhea K06.8
Unavailability (of)
- bed at medical facility Z75.1
- health service-related agencies NEC Z75.4
- medical facilities (at) Z75.3
- – due to
- – – investigation by social service agency Z75.2
- – – lack of services at home Z75.0
- – – remoteness from facility Z75.3
- – – waiting list Z75.1
- – home Z75.0
- – outpatient clinic Z75.3
- schooling Z55.1
- social service agencies Z75.4

Uncinariasis B76.9
Uncongenial work Z56.5
Unconscious(ness) R40.2
Under observation (*see also* Observation) Z03.9
Underachievement in school Z55.3
Underdevelopment – *see also* Undeveloped
- nose Q30.1
- sexual E30.0
Underfeeding, newborn P92.3
Undernourishment (*see also* Malnutrition) E46
Undernutrition – *see* Malnutrition
Underweight R62.8
- for gestational age P05.0
Underwood's disease P83.0
Undescended – *see also* Malposition, congenital
- cecum Q43.3
- colon Q43.3
- testicle Q53.9

Undescended—*continued*
– testicle—*continued*
– – bilateral Q53.2
– – unilateral Q53.1
Undetermined cause R69
Undeveloped, undevelopment – *see also*
Hypoplasia
– brain (congenital) Q02
– cerebral (congenital) Q02
heart Q24.8
– lung Q33.6
– testis E29.1
– uterus E30.0
Undiagnosed (disease) R69
Unemployment, anxiety concerning Z56.0
– threatened Z56.2
Unequal length (acquired) (arm) (leg)
(limb) M21.7
Unextracted dental root K08.3
Unguis incarnatus L60.0
Unhappiness R45.2
Unicornate uterus Q51.4
Unilateral – *see also condition*
– development, breast N64.8
– organ or site, congenital NEC – *see*
Agenesis, by site
Unilocular heart Q20.8
Union, abnormal – *see also* Fusion
– larynx and trachea Q34.8
Universal mesentery Q43.3
Unknown cause of
– morbidity R69
– mortality R99
Unsatisfactory
– surroundings NEC Z59.1
– – physical environment Z58.9
– – – specified NEC Z58.8
– – work NEC Z56.5
Unspecified cause
– morbidity R69
– mortality R99
Unstable
– back NEC M53.2
– hip (congenital) Q65.6
– – acquired M24.8
– joint (*see also* Instability, joint) M25.3
– – secondary to removal of joint prosthesis
M96.8
– lie (mother) O32.0
– – fetus or newborn, before labor P01.7
– lumbosacral joint (congenital) Q76.4
– – acquired M53.2
– sacroiliac M53.2
– spine NEC M53.2

Unsteadiness on feet R26.8
Untruthfulness, child problem F91.8
Unverricht(-Lundborg) disease or
epilepsy G40.3
Unwanted pregnancy Z64.0
Upbringing, institutional Z62.2
Upper respiratory – *see condition*
Upset
– gastrointestinal K30
– – psychogenic F45.3
– intestinal (large) (small) K59.9
– – psychogenic F45.3
– mental F48.9
– stomach K30
– – psychogenic F45.3
Urachus – *see also condition*
– patent or persistent Q64.4
Urbach-Oppenheim disease L92.1
Urbach's lipoid proteinosis E78.8
Urbach-Wiethe disease E78.8
Urea
– blood, high (*see also* Uremia) N19
– cycle metabolism disorder E72.2
Uremia, uremic (coma) N19
– chronic (*see also* Disease, kidney,
chronic) N18.9
– complicating hypertension (*see also*
Hypertension, kidney) I12.0
– congenital P96.0
– extrarenal R39.2
– following
– – abortion (subsequent episode) O08.4
– – ectopic or molar pregnancy O08.4
– hypertensive (*see also* Hypertension,
kidney) I12.0
– maternal NEC, affecting fetus or newborn
P00.1
– newborn P96.0
– prerenal R39.2
Ureter, ureteral – *see condition*
Ureteralgia N23
Ureterectasis (*see also* Hydroureter) N13.4
Ureteritis N28.8
– cystica N28.8
– due to calculus N20.1
– – with calculus, kidney N20.2
– – – with hydronephrosis N13.2
– gonococcal (acute) (chronic) A54.2†
N29.1*
– nonspecific N28.8
Ureterocele N28.8
– congenital Q62.3
Ureterolith, ureterolithiasis (*see also*
Calculus, ureter) N20.1

Ureterostomy
– attention to Z43.6
– status Z93.6
Urethra, urethral – *see condition*
Urethralgia R39.8
Urethritis (anterior) (posterior) N34.2
– calculous N21.1
– candidal B37.4† N37.0∗
– chlamydial A56.0
– diplococcal (gonococcal) A54.0
– – with abscess (accessory gland)
    (periurethral) A54.1
– gonococcal A54.0
– – with abscess (accessory gland)
    (periurethral) A54.1
– nongonococcal N34.1
– – Reiter's M02.3
– nonspecific N34.1
– nonvenereal N34.1
– postmenopausal N34.2
– Reiter's M02.3
– specified NEC N34.2
– trichomonal or due to Trichomonas
    (vaginalis) A59.0† N37.0∗
– venereal NEC (nongonococcal) A64†
    N37.0∗
Urethrocele
– female N81.0
– – with
– – – cystocele N81.1
– – – prolapse of uterus – *see* Prolapse,
    uterus
– male N36.3
Urethrolithiasis (with colic or infection)
    N21.1
Urethrorectal – *see condition*
Urethrorrhagia N36.8
Urethrorrhea R36
Urethrostomy
– attention to Z43.6
– status Z93.6
Urethrotrigonitis N30.3
Urethrovaginal – *see condition*
Urhidrosis, uridrosis L74.8
Uric acid in blood (increased) E79.0
Uricacidemia (asymptomatic) E79.0
Uricemia (asymptomatic) E79.0
Uricosuria R82.9
Urinary – *see condition*
Urination, painful R30.9
Urine
– blood in (*see also* Hematuria) R31
– discharge, excessive R35
– extravasation R39.0

Urine—*continued*
– incontinence R32
– – nonorganic origin F98.0
– pus in N39.0
– retention or stasis R33
– – psychogenic F45.3
– secretion
– – deficient R34
– – excessive R35
Urinemia – *see* Uremia
Uroarthritis, infectious (Reiter's) M02.3
Urodialysis R34
Urolithiasis (*see also* Calculus, urinary)
    N20.9
Uronephrosis N13.3
Uropathy N39.9
– obstructive N13.9
– – specified NEC N13.8
– reflux N13.9
– – specified NEC N13.8
– vesicoureteral, reflux-associated N13.7
– – with pyelonephritis (chronic) N11.0
Urosepsis N39.0
Urticaria L50.9
– with angioneurotic edema T78.3
– – hereditary D84.1
– allergic L50.0
– cholinergic L50.5
– chronic L50.8
– contact L50.6
– dermatographic L50.3
– due to
– – cold or heat L50.2
– – food L50.0
– – plants L50.6
– factitial L50.3
– giant T78.3
– – hereditary D84.1
– idiopathic L50.1
– larynx T78.3
– – hereditary D84.1
– neonatorum P83.8
– nonallergic L50.1
– papulosa (Hebra) L28.2
– pigmentosa Q82.2
– recurrent periodic L50.8
– serum T80.6
– solar L56.3
– specified type NEC L50.8
– thermal (cold) (heat) L50.2
– vibratory L50.4
– xanthelasmoidea Q82.2

Use (of)
– anticoagulant for a long term (current) Z92.1
– aspirin for a long term (current) Z92.2
– harmful F1X.1
– – alcohol F10.1
– – drugs – *code to* F11-F19 with fourth character .1
– – inhalants F18.1
– – nonprescribed drugs, non-dependence producing F55
– – patent medicines F55
– – – maternal, affecting fetus or newborn P04.1
– – volatile solvents F18.1
– medicaments for a long term (current) NEC Z92.2
– tobacco Z72.0
Usher-Senear disease or syndrome L10.4
Uta B55.1
Uteromegaly N85.2

Uterovaginal – *see condition*
Uterovesical – *see condition*
Uveal – *see condition*
Uveitis (anterior) (*see also* Iridocyclitis) H20.9
– due to toxoplasmosis (acquired) B58.0† H22.0*
– – congenital P37.1† H22.0*
– heterochromic H20.8
– posterior – *see* Chorioretinitis
– sympathetic H44.1
– syphilitic (secondary) A51.4† H22.0*
– – congenital (early) A50.0† H22.0*
– – late A52.7† H22.0*
– tuberculous A18.5† H22.0*
Uveokeratitis (*see also* Iridocyclitis) H20.9
Uveoparotitis D86.8
Uvula – *see condition*
Uvulitis (acute) (catarrhal) (chronic) (gangrenous) (membranous) (suppurative) (ulcerative) K12.2

V

Vaccination
- complication or reaction – *see*
Complications, vaccination
- not done Z28.9
- – because of, due to
- – – contraindication Z28.0
- – – patient's decision NEC Z28.2
- – – – for reason of belief or group
pressure Z28.1
- – specified reason NEC Z28.8
- prophylactic (against) Z26.9
- – arthropod-borne viral encephalitis
Z24.1
- – cholera (alone) Z23.0
- – – with typhoid-paratyphoid (cholera +
TAB) Z27.0
- – common cold Z25.8
- – diphtheria (alone) Z23.6
- – diphtheria-tetanus-pertussis combined
(DTP) Z27.1
- – – with
- – – – poliomyelitis (DTP + polio) Z27.3
- – – – typhoid-paratyphoid (DTP + TAB)
Z27.2
- – disease (single) Z26.9
- – – bacterial NEC Z23.8
- – – combinations Z27.9
- – – – specified NEC Z27.8
- – – specified NEC Z26.8
- – – viral NEC Z25.8
- – encephalitis, viral, arthropod-borne
Z24.1
- – influenza Z25.1
- – leishmaniasis Z26.0
- – measles (alone) Z24.4
- – measles-mumps-rubella (MMR) Z27.4
- – mumps (alone) Z25.0
- – pertussis (alone) Z23.7
- – plague Z23.3
- – poliomyelitis Z24.0
- – rabies Z24.2
- – rubella (alone) Z24.5
- – smallpox Z25.8
- – tetanus toxoid (alone) Z23.5
- – tuberculosis (BCG) Z23.2
- – tularemia Z23.4
- – typhoid-paratyphoid (TAB) (alone)
Z23.1
- – viral hepatitis Z24.6

Vaccination—*continued*
- prophylactic—*continued*
- – yellow fever Z24.3
Vaccinia (generalized) (localized) B08.0
- congenital P35.8
Vacuum
- extraction (delivery) O81.4
- in sinus (accessory) (nasal) J34.8
Vagabond Z59.0
Vagabond's disease B85.1
Vagina, vaginal – *see condition*
Vaginalitis (tunica) N49.1
Vaginismus (reflex) N94.2
- nonorganic F52.5
- psychogenic F52.5
- secondary N94.2
Vaginitis (acute) N76.0
- atrophic, postmenopausal N95.2
- blennorrhagic (gonococcal) A54.0
- candidal B37.3† N77.1*
- chlamydial A56.0
- chronic N76.1
- complicating pregnancy O23.5
- – affecting fetus or newborn P00.8
- due to Trichomonas (vaginalis) A59.0†
N77.1*
- following
- – abortion (subsequent episode) O08.0
- – ectopic or molar pregnancy O08.0
- gonococcal A54.0
- – with abscess (accessory gland)
(periurethral) A54.1
- in (due to)
- – candidiasis B37.3† N77.1*
- – herpesviral (herpes simplex) infection
A60.0† N77.1*
- – pinworm infection B80† N77.1*
- monilial B37.3† N77.1*
- mycotic (candidal) B37.3† N77.1*
- postmenopausal atrophic N95.2
- puerperal (postpartum) O86.1
- senile (atrophic) N95.2
- subacute or chronic N76.1
- syphilitic (early) A51.0
- – late A52.7† N77.1*
- trichomonal A59.0† N77.1*
- tuberculous A18.1† N77.1*
- venereal NEC A64† N77.1*
Vagotonia G52.2

VAIN – *see* Neoplasia, intraepithelial, vagina
Vallecula – *see condition*
Valley fever B38.0† J99.8*
Valsuani's disease O99.0
Valve, valvular (formation) – *see also condition*
– cerebral ventricle (communicating) in situ Z98.2
– cervix, internal os Q51.8
– congenital NEC – *see* Atresia, by site
– ureter (pelvic junction) (vesical orifice) Q62.3
– urethra (congenital) (posterior) Q64.2
Valvulitis (*see also* Endocarditis) I38
– rheumatic (chronic) (inactive) (with chorea) I09.1
– – active or acute (aortic) (mitral) (pulmonary) (tricuspid) I01.1
– syphilitic A52.0† I39.8*
– – aortic A52.0† I39.1*
– – mitral A52.0† I39.0*
– – pulmonary A52.0† I39.3*
– – tricuspid A52.0† I39.2*
Valvulopathy – *see* Endocarditis
Van Bogaert's leukoencephalopathy (sclerosing) (subacute) A81.1
Van Bogaert-Scherer-Epstein disease or syndrome E75.5
Van Creveld-von Gierke disease E74.0
Van der Hoeve(-de Kleyn) syndrome Q78.0
Van der Woude's syndrome Q38.0
Van Neck's disease or osteochondrosis M91.0
Vanillism L23.6
Vapor asphyxia or suffocation NEC T59.9
– specified agent – *see* Table of drugs and chemicals
Variants, thalassemic D56.8
Variations in hair color L67.1
Varicella B01.9
– with
– – complications NEC B01.8
– – encephalitis B01.1† G05.1*
– – meningitis B01.0† G02.0*
– – pneumonia B01.2† J17.1*
– congenital P35.8
Varices – *see* Varix
Varicocele (thrombosed) (scrotum) I86.1
– ovary I86.2
– spermatic cord (ulcerated) I86.1

Varicose
– aneurysm (ruptured) I77.0
– dermatitis I83.1
– eczema I83.1
– phlebitis – *see* Varicose vein, inflamed
– placental vessel O43.8
– tumor – *see* Varicose vein
– ulcer (lower limb, any part) (venous) I83.0
– – anus I84.8
– – – external I84.4
– – – internal I84.1
– – esophagus I85.9
– – – bleeding I85.0
– – inflamed or infected I83.2
– – nasal septum I86.8
– – rectum – *see* Varicose, ulcer, anus
– – scrotum I86.1
– – specified site NEC I86.8
– vein (lower limb) (ruptured) I83.9
– – anus – *see* Hemorrhoids
– – congenital (peripheral) Q27.8
– – esophagus (ulcerated) I85.9
– – – bleeding I85.0
– – inflamed or infected I83.1
– – – with ulcer (venous) I83.2
– – pelvis I86.2
– – pregnancy (lower limb) O22.0
– – – anus or rectum O22.4
– – – genital (perineum, vagina or vulva) O22.1
– – puerperium (genital) (lower limb) O87.8
– – – anus or rectum O87.2
– – rectum – *see* Hemorrhoids, internal
– – scrotum (ulcerated) I86.1
– – specified site NEC I86.8
– – sublingual I86.0
– – ulcerated I83.0
– – – inflamed or infected I83.2
– – umbilical cord, affecting fetus or newborn P02.6
– – vulva I86.3
– vessel I83.9
– – placenta O43.8
Varicosis, varicosities, varicosity (*see also* Varix) I83.9
Variola (major) (minor) B03
Varioloid B03
Varix (lower limb) (ruptured) I83.9
– with
– – inflammation or infection I83.1
– – – with ulcer (venous) I83.2
– – stasis dermatitis I83.1

Varix—*continued*
- with—*continued*
- – stasis dermatitis—*continued*
- – – with ulcer I83.2
- – ulcer (venous) I83.0
- – – with inflammation or infection I83.2
- aneurysmal I77.0
- anus – *see* Hemorrhoids
- bladder I86.2
- broad ligament I86.2
- congenital (any site) Q27.8
- esophagus (ulcerated) I85.9
- – bleeding I85.0
- – congenital Q27.8
- – in (due to)
- – – alcoholic liver disease K70.-† I98.2*
- – – – with bleeding K70.-† I98.3*
- – – cirrhosis of liver K74.-† I98.2*
- – – – with bleeding K74.-† I98.3*
- – – schistosomiasis B65.-† I98.2*
- – – – with bleeding B65.-† I98.3*
- – – toxic liver disease K71.-† I98.2*
- – – – with bleeding K71.-† I98.3*
- gastric I86.4
- inflamed or infected I83.1
- – ulcerated I83.2
- labia (majora) I86.3
- orbit I86.8
- – congenital Q27.8
- ovary I86.2
- papillary I78.1
- pelvis I86.2
- pharynx I86.8
- placenta O43.8
- pregnancy (lower limb) O22.0
- – anus or rectum O22.4
- – genital (vagina, vulva or perineum) O22.1
- puerperium O87.8
- – genital (vagina, vulva, perineum) O87.8
- rectum – *see* Hemorrhoids, internal
- renal papilla I86.8
- retina H35.0
- scrotum (ulcerated) I86.1
- sigmoid colon I86.8
- specified site NEC I86.8
- spinal (cord) (vessels) I86.8
- spleen, splenic (vein) (with phlebolith) I86.8
- stomach I86.4
- sublingual I86.0
- ulcerated I83.0
- – inflamed or infected I83.2

Varix—*continued*
- umbilical cord, affecting fetus or newborn P02.6
- uterine ligament I86.2
- vocal cord I86.8
- vulva (in) I86.3
- – pregnancy O22.1
- – puerperium O87.8
Vas deferens – *see condition*
Vas deferentitis N49.1
Vasa previa O69.4
- affecting fetus or newborn P02.6
- hemorrhage from, affecting fetus or newborn P50.0
Vascular – *see also condition*
- loop on optic papilla Q14.2
- sheathing, retina H35.0
- spider I78.1
Vasculitis I77.6
- allergic D69.0
- cryoglobulinemic D89.1
- disseminated I77.6
- hypocomplementemic M31.8
- kidney I77.8
- livedoid L95.0
- nodular L95.8
- retina H35.0
- rheumatic – *see* Fever, rheumatic
- rheumatoid M05.2
- skin (limited to) L95.9
- – specified NEC L95.8
Vasculopathy, necrotizing M31.9
- specified NEC M31.8
Vasitis (nodosa) N49.1
- tuberculous A18.1† N51.8*
Vasodilation I73.9
Vasomotor – *see condition*
Vasoplasty, after previous sterilization Z31.0
Vasospasm I73.9
- cerebral (artery) G45.9
- peripheral NEC I73.9
- retina (artery) H34.2
Vasospastic – *see condition*
Vasovagal attack (paroxysmal) R55
- psychogenic F45.3
VATER syndrome Q87.2
Vater's ampulla – *see condition*
Vegetation, vegetative
- adenoid (nasal fossa) J35.8
- endocarditis (acute) (any valve) (subacute) I33.0
- heart (mycotic) (valve) I33.0
Veil, Jackson's Q43.3

Vein, venous – *see condition*
Veldt sore (*see also* Ulcer, skin) L98.4
Velpeau's hernia – *see* Hernia, femoral
Venofibrosis I87.8
Venom, venomous
– bite or sting (animal or insect) (with
  allergic or anaphylactic shock) T63.9
– – arthropod NEC T63.4
– – – scorpion T63.2
– – – spider T63.3
– – insect NEC T63.4
– – jellyfish T63.6
– – lizard T63.1
– – marine animal NEC T63.6
– – reptile NEC T63.1
– – sea anemone T63.6
– – sea-snake T63.0
– – shellfish T63.6
– – snake T63.0
– – starfish T63.6
– poisoning – *see* Venom, bite or sting
Venous – *see condition*
Ventilator lung, newborn P27.8
Ventouse delivery NEC O81.4
– affecting fetus or newborn P03.3
Ventral – *see condition*
Ventricle, ventricular – *see also condition*
– escape I49.3
– inversion Q20.5
Ventriculitis (cerebral) (*see also*
  Encephalitis) G04.9
Vernet's syndrome G52.7
Verneuil's disease (syphilitic bursitis)
  A52.7† M73.1*
Verruca (filiformis) (plana) (plana
  juvenilis) (plantaris) (simplex) (viral)
  (vulgaris) B07
– acuminata A63.0
– necrogenica (primary) (tuberculosa)
  A18.4
– seborrheica L82
– senile (seborrheic) L82
– tuberculosa (primary) A18.4
– venereal A63.0
Verrucosities (*see also* Verruca) B07
Verruga peruana, peruviana A44.1
Version
– with extraction O83.2
– – affecting fetus or newborn P01.7
– cervix (*see also* Malposition, uterus)
  N85.4
– uterus (postinfectional) (postpartal,
  old) (*see also* Malposition, uterus) N85.4
– – forward – *see* Anteversion, uterus

Version—*continued*
– uterus—*continued*
– – lateral – *see* Lateroversion, uterus
Vertebra, vertebral – *see condition*
Vertical talus Q66.8
Vertigo R42
– auditory H81.3
– aural H81.3
  benign paroxysmal H81.1
– central (origin) H81.4
– cerebral H81.4
– due to vibration T75.2
– epidemic A88.1† II82*
– epileptic G40.8
– hysterical F44.8
– infrasound T75.2
– labyrinthine H81.0
– Ménière's H81.0
– menopausal N95.1
– otogenic H81.3
– peripheral NEC H81.3
Very-low-density-lipoprotein-type
  (VLDL) hyperlipoproteinemia E78.1
Vesania – *see* Psychosis
Vesical – *see condition*
Vesicle
– cutaneous R23.8
– seminal – *see condition*
– skin R23.8
Vesicocolic – *see condition*
Vesicoperineal – *see condition*
Vesicorectal – *see condition*
Vesicourethrorectal – *see condition*
Vesicovaginal – *see condition*
Vesicular – *see condition*
Vesiculitis (seminal) N49.0
– amebic A06.8
– gonorrheal (acute) (chronic) A54.2†
  N51.8*
– trichomonal A59.0† N51.8*
– tuberculous A18.1† N51.8*
Vestibulitis (ear) H83.0
– nose (external) J34.8
– vulvar N76.2
Vestige, vestigial – *see also* Persistence
– branchial Q18.0
– structures in vitreous (body) (humor)
  Q14.0
Vibration
– exposure (occupational) Z57.7
– vertigo T75.2
Vibrio vulnificus, as cause of disease
  classified elsewhere B98.1

Virus–Zika – A92.8 (cc 02/16)
in pregnancy O98.5 + A92.8

Victim (of)
- crime Z65.4
- disaster Z65.5
- terrorism Z65.4
- torture NEC Z65.4
- war Z65.5

Vidal's disease L28.0
Villaret's syndrome G52.7
Villous – *see condition*
VIN – *see* Neoplasia, intraepithelial, vulva
Vincent's
- angina A69.1
- gingivitis A69.1
- stomatitis A69.0

Vinson-Plummer syndrome D50.1
Violence, physical R45.6
Viosterol deficiency (*see also* Deficiency, calciferol) E55.9
Vipoma (M8155/3) – *see* Neoplasm, malignant
Viremia B34.9
Virilism (adrenal) E25.9
- congenital E25.0
Virilization (female) E25.9
- congenital E25.0
Virus, viral NEC – *see also condition*
- as cause of disease classified elsewhere B97.8
- cytomegalovirus B25.-
- – resulting from HIV disease B20.2
- human immunodeficiency (HIV) – *see* Human, immunodeficiency virus (HIV) disease
- infection (*see also* Infection, virus) B34.9
- specified NEC B34.8
- – resulting from HIV disease B20.3
Viscera, visceral – *see condition*
Visceroptosis K63.4
Visible peristalsis R19.2
Vision, visual
- binocular, suppression H53.3
- blurred, blurring H53.8
- – hysterical F44.6
- defect, defective NEC H54.9
- disorientation (syndrome) H53.8
- disturbance H53.9
- – hysterical F44.6
- double H53.2
- examination Z01.0
- field, limitation (defect) H53.4
- hallucinations R44.1
- halos H53.1
- loss H54.9
- – both eyes H54.1

Vision, visual—*continued*
- loss—*continued*
- – complete, with or without light perception – *see* Blindness
- – one eye H54.5
- – sudden H53.1
- low (both eyes) H54.2
- – one eye (other eye normal) H54.6
- – – blindness, other eye H54.4
- perception, simultaneous without fusion H53.3
Vitality, lack of R53
- newborn P96.8
Vitamin deficiency – *see* Deficiency, vitamin
Vitelline duct, persistent Q43.0
Vitiligo L80
- eyelid H02.7
- pinta A67.2
- vulva N90.8
Vitreal corneal syndrome H59.0
Vitreoretinopathy, proliferative H35.2
- with retinal detachment H33.4
Vitreous – *see also condition*
- touch syndrome H59.0
Vocal cord – *see condition*
Vocational rehabilitation Z50.7
Vogt-Koyanagi syndrome H20.8
Vogt's disease or syndrome G80.3
Vogt-Spielmeyer amaurotic idiocy or disease E75.4
Voice
- change R49.8
- loss (*see also* Aphonia) R49.1
Volhynian fever A79.0
Volkmann's ischemic contracture or paralysis (complicating trauma) T79.6
Volvulus (bowel) (colon) (intestine) K56.2
- congenital Q43.8
- fallopian tube N83.5
- oviduct N83.5
- stomach (due to absence of gastrocolic ligament) K31.8
Vomiting (*see also* Hyperemesis) R11
- bilious (cause unknown) R11
- – following gastrointestinal surgery K91.0
- blood (*see also* Hematemesis) K92.0
- causing asphyxia, choking or suffocation (*see also* Asphyxia, food) T17.9
- cyclical R11
- – psychogenic F50.5
- epidemic A08.1

Vomiting—*continued*
- fecal matter R11
- following gastrointestinal surgery K91.0
- – psychogenic F50.5
- hysterical F50.5
- nervous F50.5
- neurotic F50.5
- newborn P92.0
- of or complicating pregnancy O21.9
- – due to
- – – diseases classified elsewhere O21.8
- – – specific cause NEC O21.8
- – early (before the end of the 22nd week of gestation) (mild) O21.0
- – – with metabolic disturbance O21.1
- – late (after 22 completed weeks' gestation) O21.2
- periodic R11
- – psychogenic F50.5
- psychogenic F50.5
- stercoral R11
- uremic – *see* Uremia
- winter (epidemic) A08.1

Vomito negro – *see* Fever, yellow
Von Bezold's abscess H70.0
Von Economo-Cruchet disease A85.8
Von Gierke's disease E74.0
Von Hippel(-Lindau) disease or syndrome Q85.8
Von Jaksch's anemia or disease D64.8
Von Recklinghausen-Applebaum disease E83.1
Von Recklinghausen's
- disease (neurofibromatosis) (M9540/1) Q85.0
- – bones E21.0

Von Willebrand (-Jurgens) (-Minot) disease or syndrome D68.0
Von Zumbusch's disease L40.1

Voyeurism F65.3
Vulva – *see condition*
Vulvitis (acute) (allergic) (aphthous) (atrophic) (gangrenous) (hypertrophic) (intertriginous) (senile) N76.2
- adhesive, congenital Q52.7
- blennorrhagic (gonococcal) A54.0
- candidal B37.3† N77.1*
- chlamydial A56.0
- complicating pregnancy O23.5
- due to Haemophilus ducreyi A57
- gonococcal A54.0
- – with abscess (accessory gland) (periurethral) A54.1
- leukoplakic N90.4
- monilial B37.3† N77.1*
- puerperal (postpartum) O86.1
- subacute or chronic N76.3
- syphilitic (early) A51.0
- – late A52.7† N77.1*
- trichomonal A59.0† N77.1*
- tuberculous A18.1† N77.1*

Vulvorectal – *see condition*
Vulvovaginitis (acute) (*see also* Vaginitis) N76.0
- amebic A06.8
- candidal B37.3† N77.1*
- chlamydial A56.0
- gonococcal (acute) (chronic) A54.0
- – with abscess (accessory gland) (periurethral) A54.1
- herpetic A60.0† N77.1*
- in (due to)
- – herpesviral (herpes simplex) infection A60.0† N77.1*
- – pinworm infection B80† N77.1*
- monilial B37.3† N77.1*
- subacute or chronic N76.1
- trichomonal A59.0† N77.1*

W

Waardenburg's syndrome (with albinism) E70.3
Waiting list, person on Z75.1
– undergoing social service agency ivestigation Z75.2
Waldenström
– hypergammaglobulinemia D89.0
– syndrome or macroglobulinemia C88.0
Walking
– difficulty R26.2
– – psychogenic F44.4
– sleep F51.3
– – hysterical F44.8
Wall, abdominal – *see condition*
Wallenberg's disease or syndrome I66.3† G46.3*
Wandering
– gallbladder, congenital Q44.1
– kidney, congenital Q63.8
– organ or site, congenital NEC – *see* Malposition, congenital, by site
– pacemaker (heart) I49.8
– spleen D73.8
War neurosis F48.8
Wart (common) (digitate) (filiform) (infectious) (juvenile) (plantar) (viral) B07
– anogenital region (venereal) A63.0
– external genital organs (venereal) A63.0
– Hassal-Henle's (of cornea) H18.4
– Peruvian A44.1
– prosector (tuberculous) A18.4
– seborrheic L82
– senile (seborrheic) L82
– tuberculous A18.4
– venereal A63.0
Warthin's tumor (M8561/0) – *see* Neoplasm, salivary gland, benign
Wasting
– disease R64
– extreme (due to malnutrition) E41
– muscle NEC M62.5
– syndrome, resulting from HIV disease B22.2
Water
– clefts (senile cataract) H25.0
– deprivation of T73.1
– intoxication E87.7
– itch B76.9

Water—*continued*
– lack of T73.1
– loading E87.7
– on
– – brain – *see* Hydrocephalus
– – chest J94.8
– pollution (exposure to) Z58.2
Waterbrash R12
Waterhouse(-Friderichsen) syndrome or disease (meningococcal) A39.1† E35.1*
Watsoniasis B66.8
Wax in ear H61.2
Weak, weakness R53
– arches (acquired) M21.4
– – congenital Q66.5
– bladder (sphincter) R32
– foot (double) – *see* Weak, arches
– heart, cardiac (*see also* Failure, heart) I50.9
– mind F70.-
– muscle M62.8
– myocardium (*see also* Failure, heart) I50.9
– newborn P96.8
– pelvic fundus N81.8
– senile R54
– valvular – *see* Endocarditis
Weaning from ventilator or respirator (mechanical) Z51.8
Wear, worn, tooth, teeth (approximal) (hard tissues) (interproximal) (occlusal) K03.0
Weather, effects (of) (on)
– cold NEC T69.9
– – specified effect NEC T69.8
– hot (*see also* Heat) T67.9
– skin L57.8
Weaver's syndrome Q87.3
Web, webbed   pharyngeal –acquired K22.2
– esophagus Q39.4
– fingers Q70.1
– larynx (glottic) (subglottic) Q31.0
– neck Q18.3
– popliteal syndrome Q87.8
– toes Q70.3
Weber-Christian disease M35.6
Weber-Cockayne syndrome (epidermolysis bullosa) Q81.8
Weber-Gubler syndrome I67.9† G46.3*

Weber-Leyden syndrome I67.9† G46.3∗
Weber-Osler syndrome I78.0 ~~I67.8†~~
Weber's paralysis or syndrome ~~I67.9†~~
  G46.3∗
Wedge-shaped or wedging vertebra NEC
  M48.5
Wegener's granulomatosis or syndrome
  M31.3
– with
– – kidney involvement M31.3† N08.5∗
– – lung involvement M31.3† J99.1∗
Weight
– gain (abnormal) (excessive) R63.5
– – in pregnancy O26.0
– – – low O26.1
– loss (abnormal) (cause unknown) R63.4
– 1000-2499 grams at birth (low) P07.1
– 999 grams or less at birth (extremely low)
  P07.0
Weightlessness (effect of) T75.8
Weil(l)-Marchesani syndrome Q87.1
Weil's disease A27.0
Weingarten's syndrome J82
Wells' disease L98.3
Wen (_see also_ Cyst, sebaceous) L72.1
Wenckebach's block or phenomenon
  I44.1
Werdnig-Hoffmann
– atrophy, muscular G12.0
– disease or syndrome G12.0
Werlhof's disease D69.3
Werner's disease or syndrome E34.8
Werner-Schultz disease D70
Wernicke-Korsakov syndrome (_see also_
  Korsakov's disease, psychosis or
  syndrome (alcoholic)) F10.6
Wernicke-Posada disease B38.7
Wernicke's
– developmental aphasia F80.2
– disease or syndrome E51.2† G32.8∗
– encephalopathy E51.2† G32.8∗
– polioencephalitis, superior E51.2†
  G32.8∗
West African fever B50.8
Westphal-Strümpell syndrome E83.0
West's syndrome G40.4
Wharton's duct – _see condition_
Wheal (_see also_ Urticaria) L50.9
Wheezing R06.2
Whiplash injury S13.4
Whipple's disease K90.8† M14.8∗
Whipworm (disease) (infection)
  (infestation) B79
Whistling face Q87.0

White – _see also condition_
– leg, puerperal, postpartum or childbirth
  O87.1
– mouth B37.0
– spot lesions, teeth K02.0
Whitehead L70.0
Whitlow (with lymphangitis) L03.0
– herpesviral B00.8† L99.8∗
Whitmore's disease or fever (_see also_
  Melioidosis) A24.4
Whooping cough A37.9
  with pneumonia A37.-† J17.0∗
– Bordetella
– – bronchiseptica A37.8
– – parapertussis A37.1
– – pertussis A37.0
Wide cranial sutures, newborn P96.3
Widening aorta (_see also_ Aneurysm, aorta)
  I71.9
– ruptured I71.8
Wilkinson-Sneddon disease or syndrome
  L13.1
Willebrand-Jurgens thrombopathy D68.0
Willige-Hunt disease or syndrome G23.1
Wilms' tumor (M8960/3) C64
Wilson-Mikity syndrome P27.0
Wilson's
– disease or syndrome E83.0
– hepatolenticular degeneration E83.0
– lichen ruber L43.9
Window – _see also_ Imperfect, closure
– aorticopulmonary Q21.4
Winter – _see condition_
Wiskott-Aldrich syndrome D82.0
Withdrawal
– state, symptoms, syndrome – _code to_ F10-
  F19 with fourth character .3
– – with delirium – _code to_ F10-F19 with
  fourth character .4
– – alcohol F10.3
– – – with delirium F10.4
– – amfetamine (or related substance)
  F15.3
– – – with delirium F15.4
– – caffeine F15.3
– – cannabinoids F12.3
– – cocaine F14.3
– – – with delirium F14.4
– – drug NEC F19.3
– – – with delirium F19.4
– – hallucinogens F16.3
– – – with delirium F16.4
– – hypnotics F13.3
– – – with delirium F13.4

Withdrawal—*continued*
- state, symptoms—*continued*
- – newborn
- – – correct therapeutic substance properly administered P96.2
- – – infant of dependent mother P96.1
- – opioids F11.3
- – – with delirium F11.4
- – phencyclidine (PCP) F19.3
- – – with delirium F19.4
- – psychoactive substances NEC F19.3
- – – with delirium F19.4
- – sedatives F13.3
- – – with delirium F13.4
- – steroid NEC (correct substance properly administered) E27.3
- – – overdose or wrong substance given or taken T38.0
- – stimulants NEC F15.3
- – – with delirium F15.4
- – tobacco F17.3
- – volatile solvents F18.3
- – – with delirium F18.4
- therapeutic substance, neonatal P96.2
Witts' anemia D50.8
Witzelsucht F07.0
Woakes' ethmoiditis or syndrome J33.1
Wolff-Hirschorn syndrome Q93.3
Wolff-Parkinson-White syndrome I45.6
Wolhynian fever A79.0
Wolman's disease E75.5
Wood lung or pneumonitis J67.8
Woolly hair (congenital) Q84.1
Word
- blindness (congenital) (developmental) F81.0
- deafness (congenital) (developmental) F80.2
Worm(s) (infection) (infestation) (*see also* Infestation) B83.9
- guinea B72
- in intestine NEC B82.0
Worm-eaten soles A66.3
Worn out (*see also* Exhaustion) R53
Worried well Z71.1
Worries R45.2
Wound, open (animal bite) (cut) (laceration) (puncture wound) (shot wound) (with penetrating foreign body) T14.1
- abdomen, abdominal S31.8
- – and lower back, pelvis, multiple S31.7
- – wall S31.1
- alveolar (process) S01.5

Wound, open—*continued*
- ankle S91.0
- – and foot, multiple S91.7
- anterior chamber, eye – *see* Wound, ocular
- anus S31.8
- arm
- – meaning upper limb – *see* Wound, open, limb, upper
- – upper S41.1
- – – and shoulder (level), multiple S41.7
- auditory canal (external) (meatus) S01.3
- auricle, ear S01.3
- axilla S41.8
- back S21.2
- – lower S31.0
- blood vessel – *see* Injury, blood vessel
- breast S21.0
- brow S01.1
- buttock S31.0
- calf S81.8
- canaliculus lacrimalis S01.1
- – with wound of eyelid S01.1
- canthus, eye S01.1
- cervical esophagus S11.2
- cheek (external) S01.4
- – internal S01.5
- chest (wall) (external) S21.9
- – back S21.2
- – front S21.1
- chin S01.8
- choroid – *see* Wound, ocular
- ciliary body (eye) – *see* Wound, ocular
- clitoris S31.4
- conjunctiva (*see also* Wound, ocular) S05.0
- cornea (*see also* Wound, ocular) S05.8
- costal region S21.9
- – back S21.2
- – front S21.1
- Descemet's membrane – *see* Wound, ocular
- digit(s)
- – foot S91.1
- – – with damage to nail (matrix) S91.2
- – hand S61.0
- – – with damage to nail (matrix) S61.1
- ear (canal) (external) S01.3
- – drum S09.2
- elbow S51.0
- epididymis S31.3
- epigastric region S31.1
- epiglottis S11.8
- esophagus (thoracic) S27.8

Wound, open—*continued*
- esophagus—*continued*
- – cervical S11.2
- eye – *see* Wound, ocular
- eyeball – *see* Wound, ocular
- eyelid S01.1
- face NEC S01.8
- finger(s) S61.0
- – with damage to nail (matrix) S61.1
- flank S31.1
- foot S91.3
- – and ankle, multiple S91.7
- forearm S51.9
- – multiple S51.7
- – specified NEC S51.8
- forehead S01.8
- genital organs (external) NEC S31.5
- globe (eye) (*see also* Wound, ocular) S05.-
- groin S31.1
- gum S01.5
- hand S61.9
- – and wrist, multiple S61.7
- – specified NEC S61.8
- head S01.9
- – multiple S01.7
- – scalp S01.0
- – specified NEC S01.8
- heel S91.3
- hip S71.0
- – and thigh, multiple S71.7
- hymen S31.4
- hypochondrium S31.1
- hypogastric region S31.1
- iliac (region) S31.1
- inguinal region S31.1
- instep S91.3
- interscapular region S21.2
- intraocular – *see* Wound, ocular
- iris – *see* Wound, ocular
- jaw S01.8
- knee S81.0
- labium (majus) (minus) S31.4
- lacrimal duct S05.8
- – with wound of eyelid S01.1
- larynx S11.0
- leg
- – lower S81.9
- – – and knee, multiple S81.7
- – – multiple S81.7
- – – specified NEC S81.8
- – meaning lower limb – *see* Wound, open, limb, lower

Wound, open—*continued*
- limb
- – lower NEC T13.1
- – – multiple sites T01.3
- – upper NEC T11.1
- – – multiple sites T01.2
- lip S01.5
- loin S31.0
- lower back S31.0
- – and abdomen, pelvis, multiple S31.7
- lumbar region S31.0
- malar region S01.8
- mammary S21.0
- mastoid region S01.8
- mouth S01.5
- multiple T01.9
- – abdomen, lower back and pelvis S31.7
- – ankle (and foot) S91.7
- – arm, upper (and shoulder) S41.7
- – calf S81.7
- – foot (and ankle) S91.7
- – forearm (and elbow) S51.7
- – hand (and wrist) S61.7
- – head S01.7
- – – with
- – – – neck T01.0
- – – – other body regions T01.8
- – hip (and thigh) S71.7
- – knee (and lower leg) S81.7
- – leg, lower (and knee) S81.7
- – limb
- – – lower T01.3
- – – – with
- – – – – abdomen, lower back and pelvis T01.8
- – – – – thorax T01.8
- – – – – upper limb(s) T01.6
- – – upper T01.2
- – – – with
- – – – – abdomen, lower back and pelvis T01.8
- – – – – lower limb(s) T01.6
- – – – – thorax T01.8
- – neck S11.7
- – – with
- – – – head T01.0
- – – – other body regions T01.8
- – shoulder (and upper arm) S41.7
- – specified sites NEC T01.8
- – thigh (and hip) S71.7
- – thorax S21.7
- – – with
- – – – abdomen, lower back and pelvis T01.1

Wound, open—*continued*
- multiple—*continued*
- - wrist (and hand) S61.7
- nail
- - finger(s) S61.1
- - thumb S61.1
- - toe(s) S91.2
- nape (neck) S11.8
- nasopharynx S01.8
- neck S11.9
- - multiple S11.7
- - specified part NEC S11.8
- nose, nasal (septum) (sinus) S01.2
- ocular S05.9
- - adnexa S05.8
- - avulsion (traumatic enucleation) S05.7
- - eyelid S01.1
- - laceration and rupture S05.3
- - - with prolapse or loss of intraocular
    tissue S05.2
- - muscle (extraocular) S05.4
- - orbit (penetrating) (with or without
    foreign body) S05.4
- - penetrating (eyeball) S05.6
- - - with foreign body S05.5
- - - orbit (with or without foreign body)
    S05.4
- - periocular area S01.1
- - specified NEC S05.8
- oral cavity S01.5
- orbit, penetrating (with or without foreign
    body) S05.4
- palate S01.5
- palm S61.8
- pelvis, pelvic (floor) S31.0
- - and abdomen, lower back, multiple
    S31.7
- - girdle NEC S71.8
- - region S31.0
- penetrating – *code as* Wound, by site
- penis S31.2
- perineum S31.0
- periocular area (with or without lacrimal
    passages) S01.1
- pharynx S11.2
- pinna S01.3
- popliteal space S81.8
- prepuce S31.2
- pubic region S31.1
- pudendum S31.4
- rectovaginal septum S31.8
- sacral region S31.0
- sacroiliac region S31.0

Wound, open—*continued*
- salivary gland S01.5
- scalp S01.0
- scalpel, fetus or newborn (birth injury)
    P15.8
- scapular region S41.8
- sclera – *see* Wound, ocular
- scrotum S31.3
- shin S81.8
- shoulder S41.0
- - and upper arm (level), multiple S41.7
- - girdle S41.8
- skin NEC T14.1
- skull S01.8
- spermatic cord (scrotal) S31.3
- - pelvic region S37.8
- sternal region S21.1
- submaxillary region S01.8
- submental region S01.8
- supraclavicular region S11.8
- temple, temporal region S01.8
- temporomandibular area S01.4
- testis S31.3
- thigh S71.1
- - and hip, multiple S71.7
- thorax, thoracic (external) (wall) S21.9
- - back S21.2
- - front S21.1
- - multiple S21.7
- - specified NEC S21.8
- throat S11.8
- thumb S61.0
- - with damage to nail (matrix) S61.1
- thyroid (gland) S11.1
- toe(s) S91.1
- - with damage to nail (matrix) S91.2
- tongue S01.5
- trachea (cervical region) S11.0
- - intrathoracic S27.5
- trunk NEC T09.1
- - multiple sites T01.1
- tunica vaginalis S31.3
- tympanum, tympanic membrane S09.2
- umbilical region S31.1
- uvula S01.5
- vagina S31.4
- vitreous (humor) – *see* Wound, ocular
- vulva S31.4
- wrist S61.9
- - and hand, multiple S61.7
- - specified NEC S61.8
Wright's syndrome G54.0
Wrist – *see condition*

657

Wrong drug (given in error) NEC T50.9
– specified drug or substance – *see* Table of
  drugs and chemicals
Wry neck – *see* Torticollis

Wuchereria (bancrofti) infestation B74.0
Wuchereriasis B74.0
Wuchernde Struma Langhans (M8332/3)
  C73

X

Xanthelasma (eyelid) (palpebrarum)
H02.6
Xanthinuria, hereditary E79.8
Xanthoastrocytoma, pleomorphic
(M9424/3)
– specified site – *see* Neoplasm, malignant
– unspecified site C71.9
Xanthofibroma (M8830/0) – *see* Neoplasm,
connective tissue, benign
Xanthogranuloma D76.3
Xanthoma(s), xanthomatosis (primary)
(familial) (hereditary) E75.5
– cerebrotendinous E75.5
– cutaneotendinous E75.5
– disseminatum (skin) E78.2
– eruptive E78.2
– hypercholesterolemic E78.0
– hyperlipidemic E78.5
– joint E75.5
– multiple (skin) E78.2
– tendon (sheath) E75.5
– tubero-eruptive E78.2
– tuberosum E78.2
– verrucous, oral mucosa K13.4
Xanthosis R23.8
Xenophobia F40.1
Xeroderma – *see also* Ichthyosis
– acquired L85.0
– – eyelid H01.1
– pigmentosum Q82.1
– vitamin A deficiency E50.8† L86*

Xerophthalmia (vitamin A deficiency)
E50.7† H19.8*
– unrelated to vitamin A deficiency H16.2
Xerosis
– conjunctiva H11.1
– – with Bitot's spots H11.1
– – – vitamin A deficiency E50.1† H13.8*
– – vitamin A deficiency E50.0† H13.8*
– cornea H18.8
– – with ulceration H16.0
– – – vitamin A deficiency E50.3† H19.8*
– – vitamin A deficiency E50.2† H19.8*
– cutis L85.3
– skin L85.3
Xerostomia K11.7
Xiphopagus Q89.4
XO syndrome Q96.9
X-ray (of)
– abnormal findings – *see* Abnormal,
diagnostic imaging
– breast (mammogram) Z12.3
– – routine Z01.6
– chest
– – for suspected tuberculosis Z03.0
– – routine Z01.6
– effects, adverse NEC T66
– routine NEC Z01.6
XXXX syndrome, female Q97.1
XXXXX syndrome, female Q97.1
XXXXY syndrome Q98.1
XXY syndrome Q98.0

Y

Yaba pox virus disease B08.8
Yawning R06.8
− psychogenic F45.3
Yaws A66.9
− bone lesions A66.6† M90.2*
− chancre A66.0
− cutaneous, less than five years after
  infection A66.2
− early (cutaneous) (macular)
  (maculopapular) (micropapular) (papular)
  A66.2
− − frambeside A66.2
− − skin lesions NEC A66.2
− eyelid A66.-† H03.1*
− ganglion A66.6
− gangosis, gangosa A66.5† J99.8*
− gumma, gummata A66.4
− − bone A66.6† M90.2*
− gummatous
− − frambeside A66.4
− − osteitis A66.6† M90.2*
− − periostitis A66.6† M90.1*
− hydrarthrosis A66.6† M14.8*
− hyperkeratosis (early) (late) A66.3
− initial lesions A66.0

Yaws—*continued*
− joint lesions A66.6† M14.8*
− juxta-articular nodules A66.7
− late nodular (ulcerated) A66.4
− latent (without clinical manifestations)
  (with positive serology) A66.8
− mother A66.0
− mucosal A66.7
− multiple papillomata A66.1
− nodular, late (ulcerated) A66.4
− osteitis A66.6† M90.2*
− papilloma, plantar or palmar A66.1
− periostitis (hypertrophic) A66.6† M90.1*
− specified NEC A66.7
− ulcers A66.4
− wet crab A66.1
Yellow
− atrophy (liver) (*see also* Failure, hepatic)
  K72.9
− fever − *see* Fever, yellow
− jack − *see* Fever, yellow
− jaundice − *see* Jaundice
− nail syndrome L60.5
Yersiniosis − *see also* Infection, Yersinia
− extraintestinal A28.2
− intestinal A04.6

Z

Zellweger's syndrome Q87.8
Zenker's diverticulum (esophagus) K22.5
Ziehen-Oppenheim disease G24.1
Zieve's syndrome K70.0
Zinc
− deficiency, dietary E60
− metabolism disorder E83.2

Zollinger-Ellison syndrome E16.4
Zona − *see* Herpes, zoster
Zoophobia F40.2
Zoster (herpes) − *see* Herpes, zoster
Zygomycosis B46.9
− specified NEC B46.8
Zymotic − *see condition*

Section II

External causes of injury

A

Abandonment (causing exposure to weather conditions) (with intent to injure or kill) NEC Y06.9
– by
– – acquaintance or friend Y06.2
– – parent Y06.1
– – specified person NEC Y06.8
– – spouse or partner Y06.0
Abuse (adult) (child) (mental) (physical) (sexual) (*see also* Maltreatment) Y07.9
Accident (to) X59.9-
– aircraft (in transit) (powered) NEC (*see also* Accident, transport) V95.9
– – due to, caused by cataclysm – *see* Cataclysm, by type
– animal-rider NEC (*see also* Accident, transport) V80.9
– animal-drawn vehicle NEC (*see also* Accident, transport) V80.9
– automobile NEC (*see also* Accident, transport) V49.9
– boat, boating NEC V94.-
– bus NEC (*see also* Accident, transport) V79.9
– car NEC (*see also* Accident, transport) V49.9
– caused by, due to
– – animal NEC W64
– – cold (excessive) (*see also* Exposure, cold) X31
– – corrosive liquid, substance – *see* Table of drugs and chemicals
– – cutting or piercing instrument (*see also* Contact, with, by type of instrument) W45
– – electric
– – – current (*see also* Exposure, electric current) W87
– – – motor (*see also* Contact, with, by type of machine) W31
– – – – current (of) W86
– – environmental factor NEC X58
– – explosive material (*see also* Explosion) W40
– – fire, flames (*see also* Exposure, fire) X09
– – firearm missile (*see also* Discharge, by type of firearm) W34
– – heat (excessive) (*see also* Heat) X30

Accident—*continued*
– caused by, due to—*continued*
– – ignition (*see also* Ignition) X09
– – lifting device (*see also* Contact, with, by type of lifting device) W24
– – lightning NEC X33
– – machine, machinery NEC (*see also* Contact, with, by type of machine) W31
– – natural factor NEC X58
– – radiation (*see also* Radiation) W91
– – steam (*see also* Burn, steam) X13
– – thunderbolt NEC X33
– – transmission device (*see also* Contact, with, by type of transmission device) W24
– coach NEC (*see also* Accident, transport) V79.9
– diving W16
– – with
– – – drowning or submersion (*see also* Drowning) W74
– – – insufficient air supply W81
– heavy transport vehicle NEC (*see also* Accident, transport) V69.9
– late effect of (*see also* Sequelae) Y86
– machine, machinery NEC (*see also* Contact, with, by type of machine) W31
– motorcycle NEC (*see also* Accident, transport) V29.9
– motor vehicle NEC (traffic) (*see also* Accident, transport) V89.2
– nonmotor vehicle NEC (nontraffic) (*see also* Accident, transport) V89.1
– – traffic NEC V89.3
– pedal cycle NEC (*see also* Accident, transport) V19.9
– pick-up truck or van (*see also* Accident, transport) V59.9
– railway vehicle (any) (in motion) NEC (*see also* Accident, transport) V81.9
– – due to cataclysm – *see* Cataclysm, by type
– sequelae of (*see also* Sequelae) Y86
– ski(ing) W02
– specified cause NEC X58
– streetcar NEC (*see also* Accident, transport) V82.9

Table of land transport accidents

Victim and mode of transport	Pedestrian or animal	Pedal cycle	Two- or three-wheeled motor vehicle	Car (automobile), pick-up truck or van	Heavy transport vehicle or bus (coach)	Other motor vehicle	Railway train or vehicle	Other nonmotor vehicle including animal-drawn vehicle	Fixed or stationary object	Noncollision transport accident	Other or unspecified transport accident
Pedestrian	(W51)	V01	V02	V03	V04	V09	V05	V06	(W22)	-	V09
Pedal cyclist	V10	V11	V12	V13	V14	V19	V15	V16	V17	V18	V19
Motorcycle rider	V20	V21	V22	V23	V24	V29	V25	V26	V27	V23	V29
Occupant of:											
– three-wheeled motor vehicle	V30	V31	V32	V33	V34	V39	V35	V36	V37	V33	V39
– car (automobile)	V40	V41	V42	V43	V44	V49	V45	V46	V47	V43	V49
– pick-up truck or van	V50	V51	V52	V53	V54	V59	V55	V56	V57	V53	V59
– heavy transport vehicle	V60	V61	V62	V63	V64	V69	V65	V66	V67	V68	V69
– bus (coach)	V70	V71	V72	V73	V74	V79	V75	V76	V77	V78	V79
– animal-drawn vehicle (or animal rider)	V80.1	V80.2	V80.3	V80.4	V80.4	V80.5	V80.6	V80.7	V80.8	V80.0	V80.9

Accident—*continued*
- transport (involving injury to) (*see also*
  Table of land transport accidents) V99
- – agricultural vehicle (nontraffic) V84.9
- – – driver V84.5
- – – passenger V84.6
- – – person on outside V84.7
- – – traffic V84.3
- – – – driver V84.0
- – – – passenger V84.1
- – – – person on outside V84.2
- – – while boarding or alighting V84.4
- – aircraft
- – – person (injured by)
- – – – falling from, in or on aircraft
  V97.0
- – – – machinery on aircraft V97.8
- – – – on ground V97.3
- – – – rotating propeller V97.3
- – – – struck by object falling from
  aircraft V97.3
- – – – sucked into jet V97.3
- – – – while boarding or alighting V97.1
- – all-terrain or off-road vehicle
  (nontraffic) V86.9
- – – driver V86.5
- – – passenger V86.6
- – – person on outside V86.7
- – – traffic V86.3
- – – – driver V86.0
- – – – passenger V86.1
- – – – person on outside V86.2
- – – while boarding or alighting V86.4
- – animal-rider or animal-drawn vehicle
  occupant (in) V80.9
- – – collision (with)
- – – – animal V80.1
- – – – – being ridden V80.7
- – – – animal-drawn vehicle V80.7
- – – – bus or heavy transport vehicle
  V80.4
- – – – car, pick-up truck or van V80.4
- – – – fixed or stationary object V80.8
- – – – nonmotor vehicle V80.7
- – – – pedal cycle V80.2
- – – – pedestrian V80.1
- – – – railway train or vehicle V80.6
- – – – specified NEC V80.5
- – – – streetcar V80.7
- – – – two- or three-wheeled motor
  vehicle V80.3
- – – noncollision V80.0
- – bus occupant (in) V79.9

Accident—*continued*
- transport—*continued*
- – bus occupant—*continued*
- – – collision (motor vehicle) (with)
  V79.6
- – – – animal V70.-
- – – – – being ridden V76.-
- – – – animal-drawn vehicle V76.-
- – – – bus or heavy transport vehicle
  V74.-
- – – – car, pick-up truck or van V73.-
- – – – fixed or stationary object V77.-
- – – – nonmotor vehicle V76.-
- – – – nontraffic V79.2
- – – – – driver V79.0
- – – – – passenger V79.1
- – – – pedal cycle V71.-
- – – – pedestrian V70.-
- – – – railway train or vehicle V75.-
- – – – streetcar V76.-
- – – – traffic V79.6
- – – – – driver V79.4
- – – – – passenger V79.5
- – – – two- or three-wheeled motor
  vehicle V72.-
- – – noncollision V78.-
- – – nontraffic V79.3
- – – overturning V78.-
- – – specified NEC V79.8
- – car occupant (in) V49.9
- – – collision (motor vehicle) (with)
  V49.6
- – – – animal V40.-
- – – – – being ridden V46.-
- – – – animal-drawn vehicle V46.-
- – – – bus or heavy transport vehicle
  V44.-
- – – – car, pick-up truck or van V43.-
- – – – fixed or stationary object V47.-
- – – – nonmotor vehicle V46.-
- – – – nontraffic V49.2
- – – – – driver V49.0
- – – – – passenger V49.1
- – – – pedal cycle V41.-
- – – – pedestrian V40.-
- – – – railway train or vehicle V45.-
- – – – streetcar V46.-
- – – – traffic V49.6
- – – – – driver V49.4
- – – – – passenger V49.5
- – – – two- or three-wheeled motor
  vehicle V42.-
- – – noncollision V48.-
- – – nontraffic V49.3

Accident—*continued*
- transport—*continued*
- - car occupant—*continued*
- - - overturning V48.-
- - - specified NEC V49.8
- - construction vehicle (nontraffic) V85.9
- - - driver V85.5
- - - passenger V85.6
- - - person on outside V85.7
- - - traffic V85.3
- - - - driver V85.0
- - - - passenger V85.1
- - - - person on outside V85.2
- - - while boarding or alighting V85.4
- - due to cataclysm – *see* Cataclysm, by type
- - heavy transport vehicle occupant (in) V69.9
- - - collision (motor vehicle) (with) V69.6
- - - - animal V60.-
- - - - - being ridden V66.-
- - - - animal-drawn vehicle V66.-
- - - - bus or heavy transport vehicle V64.-
- - - - car, pick-up truck or van V63.-
- - - - fixed or stationary object V67.-
- - - - nonmotor vehicle V66.-
- - - - nontraffic V69.2
- - - - - driver V69.0
- - - - - passenger V69.1
- - - - pedal cycle V61.-
- - - - pedestrian V60.-
- - - - railway train or vehicle V65.-
- - - - streetcar V66.-
- - - - traffic V69.6
- - - - - driver V69.4
- - - - - passenger V69.5
- - - - two- or three-wheeled motor vehicle V62.-
- - - noncollision V68.-
- - - nontraffic V69.3
- - - overturning V68.-
- - - specified NEC V69.8
- - industrial vehicle (nontraffic) V83.9
- - - driver V83.5
- - - passenger V83.6
- - - person on outside V83.7
- - - traffic V83.3
- - - - driver V83.0
- - - - passenger V83.1
- - - - person on outside V83.2
- - - while boarding or alighting V83.4
- - motorcycle rider V29.9

Accident—*continued*
- transport—*continued*
- - motorcycle rider—*continued*
- - - collision (motor vehicle) (with) V29.6
- - - - animal V20.-
- - - - - being ridden V26.-
- - - - animal-drawn vehicle V26.-
- - - - bus or heavy transport vehicle V24.-
- - - - car, pick-up truck or van V23.-
- - - - fixed or stationary object V27.-
- - - - nonmotor vehicle V26.-
- - - - nontraffic V29.2
- - - - - driver V29.0
- - - - - passenger V29.1
- - - - pedal cycle V21.-
- - - - pedestrian V20.-
- - - - railway train or vehicle V25.-
- - - - streetcar V26.-
- - - - traffic V29.6
- - - - - driver V29.4
- - - - - passenger V29.5
- - - - two- or three-wheeled motor vehicle V22.-
- - - noncollision V28.-
- - - nontraffic V29.3
- - - overturning V28.-
- - - specified NEC V29.8
- - occupant (of)
- - - aircraft (powered) V95.9
- - - - fixed wing (commercial) V95.3
- - - - - private V95.2
- - - - nonpowered V96.9
- - - - specified NEC V95.8
- - - all-terrain vehicle (ATV) (*see also* Accident, transport, all-terrain or off-road vehicle) V86.9
- - - animal-drawn vehicle V80.9
- - - automobile V49.9
- - - balloon V96.0
- - - battery-powered vehicle (airport passenger vehicle) (truck) V83.9
- - - bicycle – *see* Accident, transport, pedal cyclist
- - - - motorized – *see* Accident, transport, motorcycle rider
- - - boat NEC V94.-
- - - bulldozer (*see also* Accident, transport, construction vehicle) V85.9
- - - bus V79.9
- - - cable car (on rails) V82.9
- - - - not on rails V98

Accident—*continued*
- transport—*continued*
- − occupant—*continued*
- − − car V49.9
- − − − cable (on rails) V82.9
- − − − − not on rails V98
- − − coach V79.9
- − − coal-car (*see also* Accident, transport, industrial vehicle) V83.9
- − − earth-leveler (*see also* Accident, transport, construction vehicle) V85.9
- − − farm machinery (self-propelled) (*see also* Accident, transport, agricultural vehicle) V84.9
- − − forklift (*see also* Accident, transport, industrial vehicle) V83.9
- − − glider (unpowered) V96.2
- − − − hang V96.1
- − − − powered (microlight) (ultralight) V95.1
- − − hang-glider V96.1
- − − harvester (*see also* Accident, transport, agricultural vehicle) V84.9
- − − heavy (transport) vehicle V69.9
- − − helicopter V95.0
- − − hovercraft (open water) NEC V94.3
- − − ice-yacht V98
- − − kite (carrying person) V96.8
- − − land-yacht V98
- − − logging car (*see also* Accident, transport, industrial vehicle) V83.9
- − − mechanical shovel (*see also* Accident, transport, construction vehicle) V85.9
- − − microlight V95.1
- − − minibus V49.9
- − − moped – *see* Accident, transport, motorcycle rider
- − − motorcycle (with sidecar) – *see* Accident, transport, motorcycle rider
- − − motor scooter – *see* Accident, transport, motorcycle rider
- − − pedal cycle – *see* Accident, transport, pedal cyclist
- − − pick-up (truck) V59.9
- − − railway (train) (vehicle) (monorail) (two rail) (elevated) (subterranean) V81.9
- − − − collision (with)
- − − − − motor vehicle
- − − − − − nontraffic V81.0
- − − − − − traffic V81.1
- − − − − object NEC V81.3

Accident—*continued*
- transport—*continued*
- − occupant—*continued*
- − − railway—*continued*
- − − − collision—*continued*
- − − − − rolling stock V81.2
- − − rickshaw – *see also* Accident, transport, pedal cyclist
- − − − motorized – *see* Accident, transport, three-wheeled motor vehicle
- − − − pedal driven V19.9
- − − road-roller (*see also* Accident, transport, construction vehicle) V85.9
- − − ship NEC V94.-
- − − ski-lift (chair) (gondola) V98
- − − snowmobile (*see also* Accident, transport, all-terrain or off-road vehicle) V86.9
- − − spacecraft, spaceship V95.4
- − − streetcar (interurban) (operating on public street or highway) V82.9
- − − − collision (with)
- − − − − animal being ridden or animal-drawn vehicle V82.8
- − − − − motor vehicle
- − − − − − nontraffic V82.0
- − − − − − traffic V82.1
- − − − − object NEC V82.3
- − − − − rolling stock V82.2
- − − − hit by rolling stock V82.2
- − − − operating on own right-of-way, not open to other traffic V81.-
- − − téléférique V98
- − − three-wheeled vehicle (motorized) V39.9
- − − − nonmotorized – *see* Accident, transport, pedal cyclist
- − − tractor (farm) (and trailer) (*see also* Accident, transport, agricultural vehicle) V84.9
- − − train V81.9
- − − tram V82.9
- − − tricycle – *see* Accident, transport, pedal cyclist
- − − − motorized – *see* Accident, transport, three-wheeled motor vehicle
- − − trolley V82.9
- − − tub, in mine or quarry (*see also* Accident, transport, industrial vehicle) V83.9
- − − ultralight V95.1

Accident—*continued*
- transport—*continued*
-   occupant—*continued*
-    van (*see also* Accident, transport, pick-up truck or van occupant) V59.9
-    vehicle NEC V89.9
-     heavy transport V69.9
-     motor (traffic) NEC V89.2
-      nontraffic NEC V89.0
-    watercraft NEC V94.-
-   parachutist V97.2
-    after accident to aircraft V95.9
-   pedal cyclist (in) V19.9
-    collision (motor vehicle) (with) V19.6
-     animal V10.-
-      being ridden V16.-
-     animal-drawn vehicle V16.-
-     bus or heavy transport vehicle V14.-
-     car, pick-up truck or van V13.-
-     fixed or stationary object V17.-
-     nonmotor vehicle NEC V16.-
-     nontraffic V19.2
-      driver V19.0
-      passenger V19.1
-     pedal cycle V11.-
-     pedestrian V10.-
-     railway train or vehicle V15.-
-     streetcar V16.-
-     traffic V19.6
-      driver V19.4
-      passenger V19.5
-     two- or three-wheeled motor vehicle V12.-
-    noncollision V18.-
-    nontraffic V19.3
-    specified NEC V19.8
-   pedestrian (in) V09.9
-    collision (with)
-     animal being ridden or animal-drawn vehicle V06.-
-     bus or heavy transport vehicle V04.-
-     car V03.-
-     pedal cycle V01.-
-     pick-up truck or van V03.-
-     railway train or vehicle V05.-
-     streetcar V06.-
-     two- or three-wheeled motor vehicle V02.-
-     vehicle V09.9
-      animal-drawn V06.-

Accident—*continued*
- transport—*continued*
-   pedestrian—*continued*
-    collision—*continued*
-     vehicle—*continued*
-      motor
-       nontraffic V09.0
-        traffic V09.2
-      nonmotor V06.-
-     nontraffic V09.1
-     involving motor vehicle NEC V09.0
-    traffic V09.3
-     involving motor vehicle NEC V09.2
-   person NEC (unknown means of transportation) (in) V99
-    collision (between)
-     bus and heavy transport vehicle (traffic) V87.5
-      nontraffic V88.5
-     car (with)
-      bus (traffic) V87.3
-       nontraffic V88.3
-      heavy transport vehicle (traffic) V87.4
-       nontraffic V88.4
-      pick-up truck or van (traffic) V87.2
-       nontraffic V88.2
-      railway train or vehicle (traffic) V87.6
-       nontraffic V88.6
-      two- or three-wheeled motor vehicle (traffic) V87.0
-       nontraffic V88.0
-     motor vehicle (traffic) NEC V87.7
-      nontraffic V88.7
-     two- or three-wheeled motor vehicle (traffic) (with)
-      motor vehicle NEC V87.1
-       nontraffic V88.1
-    nonmotor vehicle (collision) (noncollision) (traffic) V87.9
-     nontraffic V88.9
-   pick-up truck or van occupant V59.9
-    collision (motor vehicle) (with) V59.6
-     animal V50.-
-      being ridden V56.-
-     animal-drawn vehicle V56.-
-     bus or heavy transport vehicle V54.-
-     car, pick-up truck or van V53.-

Accident—*continued*
- transport—*continued*
- – pick-up truck or van occupant—
    continued
- – – collision—*continued*
- – – – fixed or stationary object V57.-
- – – – nonmotor vehicle V56.-
- – – – nontraffic V59.2
- – – – – driver V59.0
- – – – – passenger V59.1
- – – – pedal cycle V51.-
- – – – pedestrian V50.-
- – – – railway train or vehicle V55.-
- – – – streetcar V56.-
- – – – traffic V59.6
- – – – – driver V59.4
- – – – – passenger V59.5
- – – – two- or three-wheeled motor
    vehicle V52.-
- – – noncollision V58.-
- – – nontraffic V59.3
- – – overturning V58.-
- – – specified NEC V59.8
- – specified NEC V98
- – three-wheeled motor vehicle (in) V39.9
- – – collision (motor vehicle) (with)
    V39.6
- – – – animal V30.-
- – – – – being ridden V36.-
- – – – animal-drawn vehicle V36.-
- – – – bus or heavy transport vehicle
    V34.-
- – – – car, pick-up truck or van V33.-
- – – – fixed or stationary object V37.-
- – – – nonmotor vehicle V36.-
- – – – nontraffic V39.2
- – – – – driver V39.0
- – – – – passenger V39.1
- – – – pedal cycle V31.-
- – – – pedestrian V30.-
- – – – railway train or vehicle V35.-
- – – – streetcar V36.-
- – – – traffic V39.6
- – – – – driver V39.4
- – – – – passenger V39.5
- – – – two- or three-wheeled motor
    vehicle V32.-
- – – noncollision V38.-
- – – nontraffic V39.3
- –   – – specified NEC V39.8
- vehicle NEC V89.9
- – animal-drawn NEC (*see also* Accident,
    transport, animal rider or animal-drawn
    vehicle occupant) V80.9

Accident—*continued*
- vehicle—*continued*
- – special
- – – agricultural NEC (*see also* Accident,
    transport, agricultural vehicle) V84.9
- – – construction NEC (*see also* Accident,
    transport, construction vehicle)
    V85.9
- – – industrial NEC (*see also* Accident,
    transport, industrial vehicle) V83.9
- – three-wheeled NEC
    (motorized) (*see also* Accident,
    transport, three-wheeled motor vehicle)
    V39.9
- watercraft NEC V94.-
- – due to, caused by cataclysm – *see*
    Cataclysm, by type
Acid throwing (assault) X86
Aerosinusitis W94
After-effect, late (*see also* Sequelae) Y89.9
Air
- blast in war operations Y36.2
- sickness X51
Alpine sickness W94
Altitude sickness W94
Anaphylactic shock, anaphylaxis (*see also*
    Table of drugs and chemicals) Y57.9
Andes disease W94
Arachnidism, arachnoidism X21
Arson (with intent to injure or kill) X97
Asphyxia, asphyxiation
- by
- – any object, except food or vomitus
    W80
- – chemical in war operations Y36.7
- – food (bone) (seed) W79
- – fumes in war operations (chemical
    weapons) Y36.7
- – gas (*see also* Table of drugs and
    chemicals) X47
- – – in war operations (chemical
    weapons) Y36.7
- – – legal
- – – – execution Y35.5
- – – – intervention Y35.2
- – mechanical means (*see also*
    Suffocation) W84
- – vomitus W78
- from
- – fire (*see also* Exposure, fire) X09
- – – in war operations Y36.3
- – ignition (see also Ignition) X09

Aspiration W84
- food (any type) (into respiratory tract) (with asphyxia, obstruction respiratory tract, suffocation) W79
- foreign body (*see also* Foreign body, object or material, aspiration) W44
- mucus, not of newborn (with asphyxia, obstruction respiratory tract, suffocation) W80
- phlegm, not of newborn (with asphyxia, obstruction respiratory tract, suffocation) W80
- vomitus (with asphyxia, obstruction respiratory tract, suffocation) W78

Assassination (attempt) (*see also* Assault) Y09

Assault (homicidal) (by) (in) Y09
- acid (swallowed) X86
- bite (of human being) Y08
- bodily force (hand) (fists) (foot) Y04
- − sexual Y05
- bomb (antipersonnel) (letter) (petrol) X96
- brawl (hand) (fists) (foot) (unarmed) Y04
- burning, burns (by fire) NEC X97
- − acid (swallowed) X86
- − caustic, corrosive substance (swallowed) X86
- − − gas X88
- − chemical (from swallowing caustic, corrosive substance) X86
- − cigarette(s) X97
- − hot liquid, object or vapor X98
- − scalding X98
- − steam X98
- − vitriol (swallowed) X86
- caustic, corrosive substance (swallowed) X86
- − gas X88
- chemical X90
- − specified NEC X89
- collision, transport (vehicle(s)) Y03
- crashing of motor vehicle Y03
- cut, any part of body X99
- dagger X99
- drowning X92
- drugs or biological substances X85
- dynamite X96
- explosive(s) (material) X96
- fertilizer X89
- fight (hand) (fists) (foot) (unarmed) Y04
- − with weapon NEC Y09
- − − blunt Y00
- − − cutting or piercing X99

- − − firearm (*see also* Discharge, by type of firearm, homicide) X95
- fire X97
- firearm(s) (*see also* Discharge, by type of firearm, homicide) X95
- garrotting X91
- gases and vapors (corrosive), except drugs and biological substances X88
- gunshot (wound) NEC (*see also* Discharge, by type of firearm, homicide) X95
- hanging X91
- incendiary device X97
- injury NEC Y09
- − to child due to criminal abortion attempt NEC Y08
- knife X99
- late effect of Y87.1
- ligature X91
- noxious substance X90
- pesticides X87
- placing before moving object, train, vehicle Y02
- plant food X89
- poisoning X90
- − chemical(s) X90
- − − specified NEC X89
- − drugs or biological substances X85
- − gases and vapors (corrosive), except drugs and biological substances X88
- − noxious substances NEC X90
- − − specified NEC X89
- puncture, any part of body X99
- pushing
- − before moving object, train, vehicle Y02
- − from high place Y01
- rape Y05
- scalding X98
- sequelae of Y87.1
- sexual (by bodily force) Y05
- shooting (*see also* Discharge, by type of firearm, homicide) X95
- specified means NEC Y08
- stab, any part of body X99
- steam X98
- strangulation X91
- submersion X92
- suffocation X91
- violence NEC Y09
- vitriol (swallowed) X86
- weapon NEC Y09
- − blunt Y00
- − cutting or piercing X99

Assault—*continued*
– weapon—*continued*
– – firearm (*see also* Discharge, by type of firearm, homicide) X95
– wood preservatives X87
– wound Y09
– – cutting X99
– – gunshot (*see also* Discharge, by type of firearm, homicide) X95
– – knife X99
– – piercing X99

Assault—*continued*
– weapon—*continued*
– – puncture X99
– – stab X99
Attack by mammal NEC W55
Avalanche X36
– falling on or hitting
– – railway train or vehicle (in motion) X36
– – transport (motor) vehicle (in motion) X36
Aviator's disease W94

B

Barotitis, barodontalgia, barosinusitis, barotrauma (otitic) (sinus) W94
Battered (baby) (child) (person) (syndrome) (*see also* Maltreatment) Y07.9
Bayonet wound W26
- in
- - legal intervention Y35.4
- - war operations Y36.4
Bean in nose W79
Bed set on fire NEC X08
Beheading (by guillotine)
- homicide X99
- legal execution Y35.5
Bending, injury in X50
Bends W94
Bite, bitten by
- alligator W58
- arthropod (nonvenomous) NEC W57
- - venomous (*see also* Contact, with, by type of arthropod) X25
- black widow spider X21
- cat W55
- centipede X24
- cobra X20
- crocodile W58
- dog W54
- fer de lance X20
- Gila monster X20
- human being (accidental) W50
- - intentional Y08
- insect (nonvenomous) W57
- - venomous (*see also* Contact, with, by type of insect) X25
- krait X20
- lizard (nonvenomous) W59
- - venomous X20
- mammal NEC W55
- - marine W56
- - venomous X29
- - - specified NEC X27
- marine animal (nonvenomous) W56
- - venomous X26
- - - snake X20
- millipede W57
- - venomous (tropical) X24
- moray eel W56
- person(s) (accidental) W50
- - intentional Y08

Bite, bitten by—*continued*
- rat W53
- rattlesnake X20
- reptile NEC W59
- rodent, except rat W55
- serpent (*see also* Bite, snake) X20
- shark W56
- snake (venomous) X20
- - nonvenomous W59
- - sea X20
- spider (venomous) X21
- - nonvenomous W57
- tarantula X21
- venomous (*see also* Contact, with, by type of bite) X25
- viper X20
Blast (air) in war operations Y36.2
- from nuclear explosion Y36.5
- underwater Y36.0
Blizzard X37
Blow X59.9
- by law-enforcement agent, police (on duty) Y35.6
- - blunt object Y35.3
Blowing up (*see also* Explosion) W40
Brawl (hand) (fists) (foot) Y04
Breakage (accidental) (part of)
- ladder (causing fall) W11
- scaffolding (causing fall) W12
Broken
- glass, contact with (*see also* Contact, with, glass) W25
- power line (causing electric shock) W85
Bumping against, into (accidentally)
- object (stationary) NEC W22
- - with fall W18
- - caused by crowd or human stampede (with fall) W52
- - sports equipment W21
- person(s) W51
- - with fall W03
- - caused by crowd or human stampede (with fall) W52
- sports equipment W21
Burn, burned, burning (accidental) (by) (from) (on) X09
- acid NEC (*see also* Table of drugs and chemicals) X49
- bedlinen X08

Burn, burned—*continued*
- blowtorch (*see also* Exposure, fire) X08
- bonfire, campfire (controlled) X03
- – uncontrolled X01
- candle (*see also* Exposure, fire) X08
- caustic liquid, substance (external) (internal) NEC (*see also* Table of drugs and chemicals) X49
- chemical (external) (internal) X49
- – in war operations (chemical weapons) Y36.7
- cigar or cigarette (*see also* Exposure, fire) X08
- clothes, clothing NEC (from controlled fire) X06
- – with conflagration X00
- – – not in building or structure X01
- cooker (hot) X15
- electric blanket X16
- engine (hot) X17
- fire, flames (*see also* Exposure, fire) X09
- flare, Very pistol (*see also* Discharge, firearm) W34
- heat
- – from appliance (electrical) (household) NEC X15
- – – heating X16
- – in local application or packing during medical or surgical procedure Y63.5
- heating appliance, radiator or pipe X16
- homicide (attempt) (*see also* Assault, burning) X97
- hot
- – air X14
- – cooker X15
- – drink X10
- – engine X17
- – fat X10
- – fluid NEC X12
- – food X10
- – gases X14
- – heating appliance X16
- – household appliance NEC X15
- – kettle X15
- – liquid NEC X12
- – machinery X17
- – metal (liquid) (molten) NEC X18
- – object (not producing fire or flames) NEC X19
- – oil (cooking) X10
- – pipe X16
- – plate X15
- – radiator X16
- – saucepan (glass) (metal) X15

Burn, burned—*continued*
- hot—*continued*
- – stove (kitchen) X15
- – substance NEC X19
- – – caustic or corrosive NEC – *see* Table of drugs and chemicals
- – toaster X15
- – tool X17
- – vapor X13
- – water (bath) (bucket) (from hose) (tap) (tub) X11
- – – heated on stove X12
- hotplate X15
- ignition (*see also* Ignition) X09
- – highly flammable material (benzine) (fat) (gasoline) (kerosene) (paraffin) (petrol) X04
- – nightwear (gown, nightclothes, nightdress, pajamas, robe) X05
- in war operations (from fire-producing device or conventional weapon) NEC (*see also* War operations) Y36.3
- – nuclear explosion Y36.5
- – petrol bomb Y36.3
- inflicted by other person
- – stated as
- – – intentional, homicide (attempt) X97
- – – – by hot objects, hot vapor, or steam X98
- – – undetermined whether accidental or intentional Y26
- – – – by hot objects, hot vapor, or steam Y27
- internal, from swallowed caustic, corrosive liquid, substance X49
- iron (hot) X15
- kettle (hot) X15
- lamp (flame) (*see also* Exposure, fire) X08
- lighter (cigar) (cigarette) (*see also* Exposure, fire) X08
- lightning X33
- liquid (boiling) (hot) NEC X12
- local application of externally applied substance in medical or surgical care Y63.5
- machinery (hot) X17
- matches (*see also* Exposure, fire) X08
- mattress X08
- medicament, externally applied Y63.5
- metal (hot) (liquid) (molten) NEC X18
- nightwear (gown, nightclothes, nightdress, pajamas, robe) X05
- object (hot) NEC X19

Burn, burned—*continued*
- pipe (hot) X16
- – smoking (*see also* Exposure, fire) X08
- radiator (hot) X16
- saucepan (hot) (glass) (metal) X15
- self-inflicted (unspecified whether accidental or intentional) Y26
- – by hot object, hot vapor, or steam Y27
- – caustic or corrosive substance NEC Y33
- – stated as intentional, purposeful, suicide (attempt) X76
- – – caustic or corrosive substance NEC X83
- stated as undetermined whether accidentally or purposely inflicted Y26
- – by hot objects, hot vapor, or steam Y27
- – caustic or corrosive substance NEC Y33
- steam X13
- – pipe X16
- stove (hot) (kitchen) X15

Burn, burned—*continued*
- substance (hot) NEC X19
- – boiling X12
- – molten (metal) X18
- suicide (attempt) NEC X76
- – caustic substance X83
- therapeutic misadventure
- – heat in local application or packing during medical or surgical procedure Y63.5
- – overdose of radiation Y63.2
- toaster (hot) X15
- tool (hot) X17
- torch, welding (*see also* Exposure, fire) X08
- trash fire (controlled) (*see also* Burn, bonfire) X03
- vapor (hot) X13
- Very pistol (*see also* Discharge, firearm) W34
- vitriol X49

Butted by animal NEC W55

C

Caisson disease W94
Campfire (exposure to) (controlled) X03
– uncontrolled X01
Capital punishment (any means) Y35.5
Car sickness X51
Casualty (not due to war) NEC X59.9
– war (*see also* War operations) Y36.9
Cat bite or scratch W55
Cataclysm, cataclysmic (any injury) NEC
X39
– avalanche X36
– earth surface movement NEC X36
– earthquake X34.-
– flood X38
– landslide X36
– storm X37
– volcanic eruption X35
Catching fire (*see also* Exposure, fire) X09
Caught
– between
– – folding object W23
– – objects (moving) (stationary and
moving) W23
– – – and machinery (*see also* Contact,
with, by type of machine) W31
– – sliding door and door frame W23
– by, in
– – machinery (moving parts of) (*see also*
Contact, with, by type of machine)
W31
– – object NEC W23
– – washing-machine wringer W23
– under packing crate (due to losing grip)
W23
**Cave-in (causing asphyxia, suffocation (by
pressure))** W77
– caused by cataclysmic earth surface
movement or eruption X36
– without asphyxia or suffocation W20
Change(s) in air pressure W94
– sudden, in aircraft (ascent) (descent) W94
**Choked, choking (on) (any object except
food or vomitus)** W80
– food (bone) (seed) W79
– mucus or phlegm, not of newborn W80
– vomitus W78
Civil insurrection (*see also* War operations)
Y36.9
Cloudburst (any injury) X37

**Cold, exposure to (accidental) (excessive)
(extreme) (natural) (place)**
NEC (*see also* Exposure, cold) X31
Collapse
– building W20
– – burning (uncontrolled fire) X00
– dam or man-made structure (causing earth
movement) X36
– machinery (*see also* Contact, with, by type
of machine) W31
– structure W20
– – burning (uncontrolled fire) X00
Collision (accidental) NEC (*see also*
Accident, transport) V89.9
– pedestrian (conveyance) W51
– – with fall W03
– – and
– – – crowd or human stampede (with fall)
W52
– – – object (stationary) W22
– – – – with fall W18
– person(s) (using pedestrian
conveyance) (*see also* Collision,
pedestrian) W51
– transport vehicle NEC V89.9
– – and
– – – avalanche, fallen or not moving – *see*
Accident, transport
– – – – falling or moving X36
– – – landslide, fallen or not moving – *see*
Accident, transport
– – – – falling or moving X36
– – due to cataclysm – *see* Cataclysm, by
type
– – intentional, purposeful, suicide
(attempt) X82
Combustion, spontaneous (*see also*
Ignition) X09
**Complication (delayed) (of or following)
(medical or surgical procedure)** Y84.9
– with misadventure (*see also*
Misadventure) Y69
– amputation of limb(s) Y83.5
– anastomosis (arteriovenous) (blood
vessel) (gastrojejunal) (skin) (tendon)
(natural, artificial material, tissue) Y83.2
– aspiration (of fluid) Y84.4
– – tissue Y84.8
– biopsy Y84.8

675

Complication—*continued*
- blood
- – sampling Y84.7
- – transfusion
- – – procedure Y84.8
- bypass Y83.2
- catheterization (urinary) Y84.6
- – cardiac Y84.0
- colostomy Y83.3
- cystostomy Y83.3
- dialysis (kidney) Y84.1
- drug NEC (*see also* Table of drugs and chemicals) Y57.9
- due to misadventure (*see also* Misadventure) Y69
- duodenostomy Y83.3
- electroshock therapy Y84.3
- external stoma, creation of Y83.3
- gastrostomy Y83.3
- graft Y83.2
- hypothermia (medically induced) Y84.8
- implant, implantation (of)
- – artificial
- – – internal device (cardiac pacemaker) (electrodes in brain) (heart valve prosthesis) (orthopedic) Y83.1
- – – material or tissue (for anastomosis or bypass) Y83.2
- – – – with creation of external stoma Y83.3
- – natural tissues (for anastomosis or bypass) Y83.2
- – – with creation of external stoma Y83.3
- infusion
- – procedure Y84.8
- injection – *see* Table of drugs and chemicals
- – procedure Y84.8
- insertion of gastric or duodenal sound Y84.5
- insulin-shock therapy Y84.3
- paracentesis (abdominal) (thoracic) (aspirative) Y84.4
- procedures other than surgical operation NEC (*see also* Complication, by type of procedure) Y84.9
- – specified NEC Y84.8
- radiological procedure or therapy Y84.2
- removal of organ (partial) (total) NEC Y83.6
- sampling
- – blood Y84.7
- – fluid NEC Y84.4

Complication—*continued*
- sampling—*continued*
- – tissue Y84.8
- shock therapy Y84.3
- surgical operation NEC (*see also* Complication, by type of operation) Y83.9
- – reconstructive NEC Y83.4
- – – with
- – – – anastomosis, bypass or graft Y83.2
- – – – formation of external stoma Y83.3
- – specified NEC Y83.8
- transfusion
- – procedure Y84.8
- transplant, transplantation (heart) (kidney) (liver) (whole organ, any) Y83.0
- – partial organ Y83.4
- ureterostomy Y83.3
- vaccination – *see* Table of drugs and chemicals
- – procedure Y84.8

Compression
- diver's squeeze W94
- trachea by
- – food (lodged in esophagus) W79
- – foreign body, except food or vomitus W80
- – vomitus (lodged in esophagus) W78

Confined in low-oxygen environment W81

Conflagration – *see* Exposure, fire

Contact (accidental)
- with
- – abrasive wheel (metalworking) W31
- – animal (nonvenomous) NEC W64
- – – marine W56
- – – – venomous X26
- – – venomous X29
- – – – specified NEC X27
- – ants X25
- – arrow W21
- – – not thrown, projected or falling W45
- – arthropods NEC
- – – nonvenomous W57
- – – venomous X25
- – axe W27
- – band-saw (industrial) W31
- – bayonet (*see also* Bayonet wound) W26
- – bee(s) X23
- – bench-saw (industrial) W31
- – black widow spider X21
- – blender W29

Contact—*continued*
− with—*continued*
− − bore, earth-drilling or mining (land)
   (seabed) W31
− − can
− − − lid W45
− − − opener W27
− − − − powered W29
− − caterpillar (venomous) X25
− − centipede (venomous) X24
− − chain
− − − hoist W24
− − − − agricultural operations W30
− − − saw W29
− − chisel W27
− − circular saw W31
− − cobra X20
− − combine (harvester) W30
− − conveyer belt W24
− − cooker (hot) X15
− − coral X26
− − cotton gin W31
− − crane W24
− − − agricultural operations W30
− − dagger W26
− − dairy equipment W31
− − dart W21
− − − not thrown, projected or falling W45
− − derrick W24
− − − agricultural operations W30
− − drier (spin) (clothes) (powered) W29
− − drill (powered) W29
− − − earth (land) (seabed) W31
− − − nonpowered W27
− − drive belt W24
− − − agricultural operations W30
− − dry ice W93
− − earth(-)
− − − drilling machine (industrial) W31
− − − scraping machine (in stationary use)
   W31
− − edge of stiff paper W45
− − electric
− − − beater W29
− − − blanket X16
− − − fan W29
− − − knife W29
− − − mixer W29
− − elevator (building) W24
− − − agricultural operations W30
− − − grain W30
− − engine, hot NEC X17
− − excavating machine (in stationary use)
   W31

Contact—*continued*
− with—*continued*
− − farm machine W30
− − fer de lance X20
− − forging (metalworking) machine W31
− − fork W27
− − forklift (truck) W24
− − − agricultural operations W30
− − garden
− − − cultivator (powered) W29
− − − − riding W30
− − − fork W27
− − gas turbine W31
− − Gila monster X20
− − glass (broken) (sharp) W25
− − − due to
− − − − explosion (*see also* Explosion, by
    type) W40
− − − − fall (*see also* Fall, by type) W19
− − − − firearm discharge (*see also*
    Discharge, by type of firearm)
    W34
− − hand
− − − saw W27
− − − − powered W29
− − − tool (not powered) NEC W27
− − − − powered W29
− − harvester W30
− − hay-derrick, -mover or -rake W30
− − heat NEC X19
− − − from appliance (electrical)
   (household) X15
− − − − heating X16
− − heating
− − − appliance (hot) X16
− − − pad (electric) X16
− − hedge-trimmer (powered) W29
− − hoe W27
− − hoist (chain) (shaft) NEC W24
− − − agricultural W30
− − hornet(s) X23
− − hot
− − − air X14
− − − cooker X15
− − − drink X10
− − − engine X17
− − − fat X10
− − − food X10
− − − gases X14
− − − heating appliance X16
− − − household appliance NEC X15
− − − kettle X15
− − − liquid NEC (*see also* Burn) X12
− − − machinery X17

Contact—*continued*
- with—*continued*
- - hot—*continued*
- - - metal (liquid) (molten) NEC X18
- - - object (not producing fire or flames) NEC X19
- - - oil (cooking) X10
- - - pipe X16
- - - plate X15
- - - radiator X16
- - - saucepan (glass) (metal) X15
- - - stove (kitchen) X15
- - - substance NEC X19
- - - tapwater (from hose or tap) (in bath, bucket or tub) X11
- - - - heated on stove X12
- - - toaster X15
- - - tool X17
- - - vapor X13
- - - water (tap) in bath, bucket or tub (from hose) X11
- - - - heated on stove X12
- - hotplate X15
- - ice-pick W27
- - insect (nonvenomous) NEC W57
- - jellyfish X26
- - kettle (hot) X15
- - knife W26
- - - electric W29
- - krait X20
- - lathe (metalworking) (woodworking) W31
- - - turnings W45
- - lawnmower (powered) (ridden) W28
- - - causing electrocution W86
- - - unpowered W27
- - lift, lifting (devices) (shaft) W24
- - - agricultural operations W30
- - liquefied gas W93
- - liquid air, hydrogen, nitrogen W93
- - lizard (nonvenomous) W59
- - - venomous X20
- - machine, machinery NEC (*see also* Contact, with, by type of machine) W31
- - - agricultural, including animal-powered W30
- - - drilling, metal (industrial) W31
- - - earth-drilling W31
- - - earthmoving or scraping (in stationary use) W31
- - - excavating (in stationary use) W31
- - - hot X17
- - - lifting (devices) W24

Contact—*continued*
- with—*continued*
- - machine, machinery NEC—*continued*
- - - metalworking (industrial) W31
- - - milling, metal W31
- - - mining W31
- - - molding W31
- - - power press, metal W31
- - - prime mover W31
- - - printing W31
- - - recreational W31
- - - rolling mill, metal W31
- - - specified NEC W31
- - - spinning W31
- - - transmission W24
- - - weaving W31
- - - woodworking or forming (industrial) W31
- - marine
- - - animal W56
- - - plant, venomous X26
- - meat
- - - grinder (domestic) W29
- - - - industrial W31
- - - slicer (domestic) W29
- - - - industrial W31
- - metal, hot (liquid) (molten) NEC X18
- - millipede W57
- - - venomous (tropical) X24
- - nail W45
- - needle W27
- - - hypodermic W46
- - nematocysts X26
- - object (blunt) NEC
- - - hot NEC X19
- - - legal intervention Y35.3
- - - sharp NEC W49
- - - - inflicted by other person NEC W49
- - - - - stated as
- - - - - - intentional, homicide (attempt) X99
- - - - - - undetermined whether accidental or intentional Y28
- - - - legal intervention Y35.4
- - - - self-inflicted (unspecified whether accidental or intentional) Y28
- - - - - intentional, purposeful, suicide (attempt) X78
- - - - stated as undetermined whether accidentally or purposely inflicted Y28

Contact—*continued*
– with—*continued*
– – object—*continued*
– – – stated as undetermined whether
   accidentally or purposely inflicted
   Y29
– – overhead plane W31
– – paper (as sharp object) W45
– – paper-cutter W27
– – pipe, hot X16
– – pitchfork W27
– – plane (metal) (wood) W27
– – – overhead W31
– – plant thorns, spines, or sharp leaves
   W60
– – – toxic reaction X28
– – powered
– – – garden cultivator W29
– – – household appliance, implement, or
   machine W29
– – – saw (industrial) W31
– – – – hand W29
– – printing machine W31
– – pulley (block) (transmission) W24
– – – agricultural operations W30
– – radial-saw (industrial) W31
– – radiator (hot) X16
– – rake W27
– – rattlesnake X20
– – reaper W30
– – reptile NEC W59
– – rivet gun (powered) W29
– – road scraper – *see* Accident, transport,
   construction vehicle
– – roller coaster W31
– – rope (lifting or transmission device)
   NEC W24
– – – agricultural operations W30
– – sander W29
– – – industrial W31
– – saucepan (hot) (glass) (metal) X15
– – saw W27
– – – band (industrial) W31
– – – bench (industrial) W31
– – – chain W29
– – – hand W27
– – – – powered W29
– – sawing machine, metal W31
– – scissors W27
– – scorpion X22
– – screwdriver W27
– – – powered W29
– – sea anemone, cucumber or urchin
   (spine) X26

Contact—*continued*
– with—*continued*
– – serpent (*see also* Contact, with, snake,
   by type) X20
– – sewing-machine (electric) (powered)
   W29
– – – not powered W27
– – shaft (hoist) (lift) (transmission) NEC
   W24
– – – agricultural W30
– – shears (hand) W27
– – – powered (industrial) W31
– – – domestic W29
– – shovel W27
– – – steam (in stationary use) W31
– – snake (venomous) X20
– – – nonvenomous W59
– – – sea X20
– – spade W27
– – spider (venomous) X21
– – spin-drier W29
– – spinning machine W31
– – splinter W45
– – sports equipment W21
– – staple gun (powered) W29
– – steam X13
– – – engine W31
– – – pipe X16
– – – shovel (in stationary use) W31
– – stove (hot) (kitchen) X15
– – substance, hot NEC X19
– – – molten (metal) X18
– – sword W26
– – tarantula X21
– – thresher W30
– – tin can lid W45
– – toaster (hot) X15
– – tool NEC W27
– – – hot X17
– – – powered NEC W29
– – transmission device (belt, cable, chain,
   gear, pinion, pulley, shaft) W24
– – – agricultural operations W30
– – turbine (gas) (water-driven) W31
– – under-cutter W31
– – vehicle
– – – agricultural use (transport) – *see*
   Accident, transport, agricultural
   vehicle
– – – – in stationary use or maintenance
   W30
– – – industrial use (transport) – *see*
   Accident, transport, industrial vehicle

Contact—*continued*
− with—*continued*
− − vehicle—*continued*
− − − industrial use—*continued*
− − − − in stationary use or maintenance
  W31
− − − off-road use (transport) – *see*
  Accident, transport, all-terrain or off-
  road vehicle
− − − − in stationary use or maintenance
  W31
− − − special construction use (transport –
  see Accident, transport, construction
  vehicle
− − − − in stationary use or maintenance
  W31
− − venomous
− − − animal X29
− − − − specified NEC X27
− − − arthropod X25
− − − lizard X20
− − − marine animal NEC X26
− − − marine plant NEC X26
− − − millipede (tropical) X24
− − − plant X29
− − − − specified NEC X28
− − − snake X20
− − − spider X21
− − viper X20
− − washing-machine (powered) W29
− − wasp(s) X23
− − weaving-machine W31
− − winch W24
− − − agricultural operations W30
− − wire (for lifting and transmission
  devices) NEC W24
− − − agricultural operations W30
− − wood slivers W45
− − yellow jacket X23
Coup de soleil X32
Crash
− aircraft (powered) V95.-
− − in war operations Y36.1
− − stated as
− − − homicide (attempt) Y03
− − − suicide (attempt) X83
− − − undetermined whether accidental or
  intentional Y33
− transport vehicle NEC (*see also* Accident,
  transport) V89.9
− − homicide (attempt) Y03
− − motor NEC (traffic) V89.2
− − − homicide (attempt) Y03
− − − suicide (attempt) X82

Crash—*continued*
− transport vehicle NEC—*continued*
− − motor NEC—*continued*
− − − undetermined whether accidental or
  intentional Y32
− − suicide (attempt) X83
− − undetermined whether accidental or
  intentional Y33
**Cruelty (mental) (physical)
(sexual)** (*see also* Maltreatment) Y07.9
Crushed (accidentally) X59.9
− between objects (moving) (stationary and
  moving) (*see also* Caught) W23
− by, in
− − avalanche NEC X36
− − cave-in (with asphyxia or
  suffocation) (*see also* Suffocation, due
  to, cave-in) W77
− − − without asphyxia or suffocation
  W20
− − crowd or human stampede W52
− − door (building) W23
− − falling
− − − aircraft V95.9
− − − − in war operations Y36.1
− − − earth, material (with asphyxia or
  suffocation) (*see also* Suffocation,
  due to, cave-in) W77
− − − − without asphyxia or suffocation
  W20
− − − object NEC W20
− − landslide NEC X36
− − lizard (nonvenomous) W59
− − machinery NEC (*see also* Contact,
  with, by type of machine) W31
− − reptile NEC W59
− − snake (nonvenomous) W59
− − − venomous X20
**Cut, cutting (any part of body)
(accidental) (by)** (*see also* Contact, with,
by object or machine) W49
− during medical or surgical treatment as
  misadventure (*see also* Misadventure, cut,
  by type of procedure) Y60.9
− homicide (attempt) X99
− inflicted by other person
− − stated as
− − − intentional, homicide (attempt) X99
− − − undetermined whether accidental or
  intentional Y28
− legal
− − execution Y35.5
− − intervention Y35.4

Cut, cutting—*continued*
- machine NEC (*see also* Contact, with, by type of machine) W31
- self-inflicted (unspecified whether accidental or intentional) Y28
- – stated as intentional, purposeful, suicide (attempt) X78

Cut, cutting—*continued*
- stated as undetermined whether accidentally or purposely inflicted Y28
- suicide (attempt) X78
- war operations Y36.4

Cyclone (any injury) X37

D

**Death due to injury occurring one year or
more previously** (*see also* Sequelae)
Y89.9
**Decapitation (accidental circumstances)
NEC** X59.9
– homicide X99
– legal execution (by guillotine) Y35.5
Dehydration from lack of water (*see also*
Lack of, water) X54
Deprivation (*see also* Privation) X57
– homicidal intent (*see also* Abandonment)
Y06.9
Derailment (accidental)
– railway train or vehicle (rolling stock)
(without antecedent collision) NEC
V81.7
– – with antecedent collision NEC V81.3
– streetcar (without antecedent collision)
NEC V82.7
– – with antecedent collision NEC V82.3
**Descent parachute (voluntary) (without
accident to aircraft)** V97.2
– due to accident to aircraft V95.9
**Desertion (with intent to injure or
kill)** (*see also* Abandonment) Y06.9
Destitution (*see also* Privation) X57
**Disability, late effect or sequela of
injury** (*see also* Sequelae) Y89.9
Discharge (accidental)
– airgun (*see also* Discharge, firearm) W34
– BB gun (*see also* Discharge, firearm)
W34
– firearm NEC W34
– – homicide (attempt) X95
– – larger W33
– – – homicide (attempt) X94
– – – legal intervention Y35.0
– – – self-inflicted (unspecified whether
accidental or intentional) Y23
– – – stated as undetermined whether
accidentally or purposely inflicted
Y23
– – – suicide (attempt) X73
– – legal intervention Y35.0
– – self-inflicted (unspecified whether
accidental or intentional) Y24
– – stated as undetermined whether
accidentally or purposely inflicted Y24
– – suicide (attempt) X74

Discharge *continued*
– firework(s) W39
– gun NEC (*see also* Discharge, firearm)
W34
– – air (*see also* Discharge, firearm) W34
– – BB (*see also* Discharge, firearm) W34
– – for single hand use (*see also* Discharge,
handgun) W32
– – hand (*see also* Discharge, handgun)
W32
– – machine (*see also* Discharge, firearm,
larger) W33
– – other specified (*see also* Discharge,
firearm) W34
– – pellet (*see also* Discharge, firearm)
W34
– handgun W32
– – homicide (attempt) X93
– – legal intervention Y35.0
– – self-inflicted (unspecified whether
accidental or intentional) Y22
– – stated as undetermined whether
accidentally or purposely inflicted Y22
– – suicide (attempt) X72
– machine gun (*see also* Discharge, firearm,
larger) W33
– pistol (*see also* Discharge, handgun) W32
– – flare (*see also* Discharge, firearm)
W34
– – pellet (*see also* Discharge, firearm)
W34
– – Very (*see also* Discharge, firearm)
W34
– revolver (*see also* Discharge, handgun)
W32
– rifle (army) (hunting) (*see also* Discharge,
firearm, larger) W33
– shotgun (*see also* Discharge, firearm,
larger) W33
Disease
– Andes W94
– aviator's W94
– range W94
Diver's disease, palsy, paralysis, squeeze
W94
Diving (into water) (*see also* Accident,
diving) W16
Dog bite W54

Dragged by transport vehicle
  NEC (*see also* Accident, transport) V09.9
Drinking poison (accidental) (*see also*
  Table of drugs and chemicals) X49
**Dropped (accidentally) while being
  carried or supported by other person**
  W04
Drowning (accidental) W74
– by other person
– – intentional, homicide (attempt) X92
– – stated as undetermined whether
    accidentally or purposely inflicted Y21
– due to
– – accident
– – – machinery NEC (*see also* Contact,
      with, by type of machine) W31
– – – transport – *see* Accident, transport
– – avalanche X36
– – cataclysmic
– – – earth surface movement NEC X36
– – – storm X37
– – cloudburst X37
– – cyclone X37
– – fall overboard NEC V92.-
– – – resulting from accident to boat, ship,
      watercraft V90.-
– – hurricane X37
– – jumping into water from boat, ship,
    watercraft (burning) (crushed)
    (involved in accident) V90.-
– – – without accident to watercraft V92.-
– – tidal wave NEC X39
– – – caused by storm X37
– – torrential rain X37

Drowning—*continued*
– following fall
– – into
– – – bathtub W66
– – – quarry W70
– – – swimming-pool W68
– – – water NEC W74
– – – – natural (lake) (open sea) (river)
        (stream) W70
– – overboard NEC V92.-
– – – resulting from accident to boat, ship,
      watercraft V90.-
– homicide (attempt) X92
– in
– – bathtub W65
– – – following fall W66
– – natural water (lake) (open sea) (river)
    (stream) W69
– – – following fall W70
– – quarry W69
– – – following fall W70
– – quenching tank W73
– – reservoir W73
– – specified place NEC W73
– – swimming-pool W67
– – – following fall W68
– – war operations Y36.4
– self-inflicted (unspecified whether
  accidental or intentional) Y21
– – stated as intentional, purposeful, suicide
    (attempt) X71
– stated as undetermined whether
  accidentally or purposely inflicted Y21
– suicide (attempt) X71
Dust in eye W44

E

Earth (surface) movement NEC X36
Earth falling (on) (with asphyxia or suffocation (by pressure)) (*see also* Suffocation, due to, cave-in) W77
– without asphyxia or suffocation W20
Earthquake (any injury) X34.-
– cataclysmic earth movements X34.0
– specified effect NEC X34.8
– tsunami X34.1
Effect(s) (adverse) of
– air pressure (any) W94
– cold, excessive (exposure to) (*see also* Exposure, cold) X31
– heat (excessive) (*see also* Heat) X30
– hot
– – place (*see also* Heat) X30
– – weather X30
– insolation X30
– late – *see* Sequelae
– motion X51
– nuclear explosion or weapon in war operations (blast) (direct) (fireball) (heat) (radiation) (secondary) Y36.5
– radiation – *see* Radiation
– travel X51
Electric shock (accidental) (by) (in) (*see also* Exposure, electric current) W87
Electrocution (accidental) (*see also* Exposure, electric current) W87
Endotracheal tube wrongly placed during anesthetic procedure Y65.3
Entanglement in
– bed linen, causing suffocation W75
– wheel of pedal cycle V19.8
Entry of foreign body or material – *see* Foreign body, object or material
Execution, legal (any method) Y35.5
Exhaustion
– cold (*see also* Exposure, cold) X31
– due to excessive exertion X50
– heat (*see also* Heat) X30
Explosion (accidental) (in) (of) (on) (with secondary fire) W40
– acetylene W40
– aerosol can W36
– air tank (compressed) (in machinery) W36
– aircraft (in transit) (powered) NEC V95.9

Explosion—*continued*
– anesthetic gas in operating theatre W40
– blasting (cap) (material) W40
– boiler (machinery), not on transport vehicle W35
– butane W40
– caused by other person stated as
– – intentional, homicide (attempt) X96
– – undetermined whether accidental or intentional Y25
– coal gas W40
– detonator W40
– dump (munitions) W40
– dynamite W40
– explosive (gas) (material) NEC W40
– factory (munitions) W40
– fire-damp W40
– fireworks W39
– gas W40
– – cylinder or pressure tank (in machinery) W36
– gasoline (fumes) (tank) not in moving motor vehicle W40
– grain store W40
– grenade NEC W40
– homicide (attempt) X96
– hot water heater, tank (in machinery) W35
– in mine (of explosive gases) NEC W40
– machinery (*see also* Contact, with, by type of machine) W31
– – pressure vessel (*see also* Explosion, by type of vessel) W38
– methane W40
– mine W40
– missile NEC W40
– munitions (dump) (factory) W40
– pressure, pressurized
– – cooker W38
– – gas tank (in machinery) W36
– – hose W37
– – pipe W37
– – tire W37
– – vessel (in machinery) W38
– propane W40
– self-inflicted (unspecified whether accidental or intentional) Y25
– – stated as intentional, purposeful, suicide (attempt) X75

Explosion—*continued*
- shell (artillery) NEC W40
- stated as undetermined whether accidentally or purposely inflicted Y25
- steam or water lines (in machinery) W37
- stove W40
- suicide (attempt) X75
- vehicle tire NEC W37
- war operations (*see also* War operations, explosion) Y36.2

Exposure (to)
- cold (accidental) (excessive) (extreme) (natural) (place) X31
- – due to
- – – man-made conditions W93
- – – weather (conditions) X31
- – self-inflicted (undetermined whether accidental or intentional) Y33
- – – suicide (attempt) X83
- due to abandonment or neglect (*see also* Abandonment) Y06.9
- electric (current) W87
- – appliance (faulty) W86
- – caused by other person
- – – stated as
- – – – intentional, homicide (attempt) Y08
- – – – undetermined whether accidentally or purposely inflicted Y33
- – conductor (faulty) W86
- – control apparatus (faulty) W86
- – electric power generating plant, distribution station W86
- – high-voltage cable W85
- – homicide (attempt) Y08
- – legal execution Y35.5
- – lightning X33
- – live rail W86
- – misadventure in medical or surgical procedure in electroshock therapy Y63.4
- – motor (faulty) W86
- – self-inflicted (undetermined whether accidental or intentional) Y33
- – – stated as intentional, purposeful, suicide (attempt) X83
- – specified NEC W86
- – stated as undetermined whether accidentally or purposely inflicted Y33
- – suicide (attempt) X83
- – third rail W86
- – transformer (faulty) W86
- – transmission lines W85

Exposure—*continued*
- excessive
- – cold (*see also* Exposure, cold) X31
- – heat (natural) NEC X30
- – – man-made W92
- factor(s) X59.9
- – environmental NEC X58
- – – man-made NEC W99
- – – natural NEC X39
- – specified NEC X58
- fire (accidental) (with exposure to smoke or fumes or causing burns, or secondary explosion) X09
- – campfire X03
- – controlled (in)
- – – with ignition (of) clothing (*see also* Ignition, clothes) X06
- – – – nightwear X05
- – – bonfire X03
- – – brazier (in building or structure) X02
- – – – not in building or structure X03
- – – building or structure X02
- – – fireplace, furnace or stove (charcoal) (coal) (coke) (electric) (gas) (wood) X02
- – – not in building or structure X03
- – – trash X03
- – fireplace X02
- – fittings or furniture (in building or structure) (uncontrolled) X00
- – forest (uncontrolled) X01
- – grass (uncontrolled) X01
- – hay (uncontrolled) X01
- – homicide (attempt) X97
- – ignition of highly flammable material X04
- – in, of, on, starting in
- – – machinery (*see also* Contact, with, by type of machine) W31
- – – motor vehicle (in motion) (*see also* Accident, transport, occupant, by type of vehicle) V87.8
- – – railway train or vehicle V81.8
- – – street car (in motion) V82.8
- – – transport vehicle NEC (*see also* Accident, transport, occupant, by type of vehicle) V87.8
- – – war operations (by fire-producing device or conventional weapon) Y36.3
- – – – from nuclear explosion Y36.5
- – – watercraft (in transit) (not in transit) V91.-
- – – – localized V93.-

Exposure—*continued*
- fire—*continued*
- – lumber (uncontrolled) X01
- – mine (uncontrolled) X01
- – prairie (uncontrolled) X01
- – resulting from
- – – explosion (*see also* Explosion) W40
- – – lightning NEC X09
- – self-inflicted (unspecified whether accidental or intentional) Y26
- – – stated as intentional, purposeful, suicide (attempt) X76
- – specified NEC X08
- – started by other person
- – – stated as
- – – – intentional, homicide (attempt) X97
- – – – undetermined whether or not with intent to injure or kill Y26
- – stove X02
- – suicide (attempt) X76
- – tunnel (uncontrolled) X01
- – uncontrolled
- – – in building or structure X00
- – – not in building or structure (any) X01
- flames (*see also* Exposure, fire) X09
- forces of nature NEC X39
- G-forces (abnormal) W49
- gravitational forces (abnormal) W49

Exposure—*continued*
- heat (natural) NEC (*see also* Heat) X30
- high-pressure jet (hydraulic) (pneumatic) W41
- hydraulic jet W41
- jet, high-pressure (hydraulic) (pneumatic) W41
- lightning X33
- mechanical forces NEC W49
- – animate NEC W64
- – inanimate NEC W49
- noise W42
- noxious substance (*see also* Table of drugs and chemicals) X49
- pneumatic jet W41
- prolonged in deep-freeze unit or refrigerator W93
- radiation (*see also* Radiation) W91
- smoke (*see also* Exposure, fire) X09
- specified factors NEC X58
- sunlight NEC X32
- transmission line(s), electric W85
- vibration W43
- waves
- – infrasound W43
- – sound W42
- – supersonic W42
- weather NEC X39
- – with homicidal intent (*see also* Abandonment) Y06.9

F

Factors, supplemental
- alcohol
- – blood level
- – – under 20mg/100ml Y90.0
- – – 20-39mg/100ml Y90.1
- – – 40-59mg/100ml Y90.2
- – – 60-79mg/100ml Y90.3
- – – 80-99mg/100ml Y90.4
- – – 100-119mg/100ml Y90.5
- – – 120-199mg/100ml Y90.6
- – – 200-239mg/100ml Y90.7
- – – 240mg/100ml or more Y90.8
- – intoxication Y91.9
- – – mild Y91.0
- – – moderate Y91.1
- – – severe Y91.2
- – – – very Y91.3
- – involvement, unspecified Y91.9
- – presence in blood, but level not specified Y90.9
- environmental-pollution-related condition Y97
- lifestyle-related condition Y98
- nosocomial condition Y95
- work-related condition Y96

Failure
- in suture or ligature during surgical procedure Y65.2
- mechanical, of instrument or apparatus (any) (during any medical or surgical procedure) Y65.8
- mechanical, of instrument or apparatus (any) (during any medical or surgical procedure) Y65.8
- sterile precautions (during medical and surgical care) (*see also* Misadventure, failure, sterile precautions, by type of procedure) Y62.9
- to
- – introduce tube or instrument (except endotracheal tube during anesthesia) Y65.4
- – make curve (transport vehicle) NEC (*see also* Accident, transport) V89.9
- – remove tube or instrument (except endotracheal tube during anesthesia) Y65.4

Fall, falling (accidental) W19
- before train, vehicle or other moving object
- – stated as
- – – intentional, purposeful, suicide (attempt) X81
- – – undetermined whether accidental or intentional Y31
- building W20
- – burning (uncontrolled fire) X00
- down
- – escalator W10
- – ladder W11
- – ramp (involving ice or snow) W10
- – stairs, steps (involving ice or snow) W10
- earth (with asphyxia or suffocation (by pressure)) (*see also* Earth falling) W77
- from, off
- – aircraft NEC (with accident to aircraft NEC) V97.0
- – – while boarding or alighting V97.1
- – balcony W13
- – bed W06
- – boat, ship, watercraft NEC (with drowning or submersion) V92.-
- – – with accident to watercraft V90.-
- – bridge W13
- – building W13
- – – burning (uncontrolled fire) X00
- – chair W07
- – cliff W15
- – dock W17
- – embankment W17
- – escalator W10
- – flagpole W13
- – furniture NEC W08
- – haystack W17
- – high place NEC W17
- – – stated as undetermined whether accidentally or purposely inflicted Y30
- – incline (involving ice or snow) W10
- – ladder W11
- – machine, machinery (*see also* Contact, with, by type of machine) W31
- – – not in operation W17
- – one level to another NEC W17

Fall, falling—*continued*
- from, off—*continued*
- – one level to another NEC—*continued*
- – – intentional, purposeful, suicide (attempt) X80
- – – stated as undetermined whether accidentally or purposely inflicted Y30
- – playground equipment W09
- – railing W13
- – ramp (involving ice or snow) W10
- – roof W13
- – scaffolding W12
- – stairs, steps (involving ice or snow) W10
- – stepladder W11
- – streetcar NEC V82.6
- – – with antecedent collision NEC V82.3
- – – while boarding or alighting V82.4
- – structure NEC W13
- – – burning (uncontrolled fire) X00
- – table W08
- – toilet W18
- – tower W13
- – train NEC V81.6
- – – during derailment (without antecedent collision) V81.7
- – – – with antecedent collision V81.3
- – – while boarding or alighting V81.4
- – transport vehicle after collision – *see* Accident, transport, by type of vehicle, collision
- – tree W14
- – turret W13
- – vehicle (in motion) NEC (*see also* Accident, transport) V89.9
- – – motor NEC (*see also* Accident, transport, occupant, by type of vehicle) V87.8
- – – stationary, except while alighting, boarding, entering, leaving W17
- – viaduct W13
- – wall W13
- – wheelchair W05
- – window W13
- in, on
- – aircraft NEC V97.0
- – – with accident to aircraft V97.0
- – – while boarding or alighting V97.1
- – bath(tub) W18
- – escalator W10
- – incline W10
- – ladder W11

Fall, falling—*continued*
- in, on—*continued*
- – machine, machinery (*see also* Contact, with, by type of machine) W31
- – object, edged, pointed or sharp (with cut) (*see also* Fall, by type) W19
- – ramp (involving ice or snow) W10
- – scaffolding W12
- – staircase, stairs, steps (involving ice or snow) W10
- – streetcar (without antecedent collision) V82.5
- – – with antecedent collision V82.3
- – – while boarding or alighting V82.4
- – train (without antecedent collision) V81.5
- – – with antecedent collision V81.3
- – – during derailment (without antecedent collision) V81.7
- – – – with antecedent collision V81.3
- – – while boarding or alighting V81.4
- – transport vehicle after collision – *see* Accident, transport, by type of vehicle, collision
- – tub W18
- into
- – cavity W17
- – fire – *see* Exposure, fire, by type
- – hole W17
- – manhole W17
- – moving part of machinery (*see also* Contact, with, by type of machine) W31
- – opening in surface NEC W17
- – pit W17
- – quarry W17
- – shaft W17
- – storm drain W17
- – tank W17
- – water (with drowning or submersion) (*see also* Drowning) W74
- – well W17
- involving
- – bed W06
- – chair W07
- – furniture NEC W08
- – glass – *see* Fall, by type
- – playground equipment W09
- – skateboard(s) W02
- – skates (ice) (roller) W02
- – skis W02
- – table W08
- – wheelchair W05

Fall, falling—*continued*
- object (*see also* Struck by, object, falling)
  W20
- over
- – animal W01
- – cliff W15
- – embankment W17
- – small object W01
- rock W20
- same level NEC W18
- – from
- – – being crushed, pushed, or stepped on
  by a crowd or human stampede W52
- – – collision, pushing, shoving, by or
  with other person W03
- – – slipping, stumbling, tripping W01
- – involving ice or snow W00
- – – involving skates (ice) (roller),
  skateboard, skis W02
- snowslide (avalanche) X36
- stone W20
- structure W20
- – burning (uncontrolled fire) X00
- through floor, roof or window W13
- timber W20
- tree (caused by lightning) W20
- while being carried or supported by other
  person(s) W04

Fallen on by
- animal (not being ridden) NEC W55
- – being ridden (*see also* Accident,
  transport) V06.-

Felo-de-se – *see* Suicide

Fight (hand) (fists) (foot) (*see also* Assault,
fight) Y04

Fire (accidental) (*see also* Exposure, fire)
X09

**Fireball effects from nuclear explosion in
war operations** Y36.5

Fireworks (explosion) W39

Flash burns from explosion (*see also*
Explosion) W40

Flood (any injury) X38

Food (any type) in
- air passage (with asphyxia, obstruction, or
  suffocation) W79
- alimentary tract causing asphyxia (due to
  compression of trachea) W79

**Foreign body, object or material
(entrance into (accidental))**
- air passage (causing injury) W44
- – with asphyxia, obstruction, suffocation
  W80
- – – food W79

Foreign body, object or material—
continued
- air passage—*continued*
- – with asphyxia, obstruction—*continued*
- – – vomitus W78
- – nose (without asphyxia, obstruction,
  suffocation) W44
- – – with asphyxia, obstruction,
  suffocation W80
- – – – food W79
- – – – vomitus W78
- – – causing other injury W44
- alimentary canal (causing injury) (with
  obstruction) W44
- – with asphyxia, compression of
  respiratory passage, suffocation W80
- – – vomitus W78
- – mouth W44
- – – with asphyxia, obstruction,
  suffocation W80
- – – – vomitus W78
- – pharynx W44
- – – with asphyxia, obstruction,
  suffocation W80
- – – – vomitus W78
- aspiration (without asphyxia, obstruction
  of respiratory passage, suffocation) W44
- – with asphyxia, obstruction of
  respiratory passage, suffocation W80
- – – food W79
- – – vomitus W78
- – causing injury W44
- – mucus, not of newborn W80
- – phlegm, not of newborn W80
- – vomitus W78
- bladder (causing injury or obstruction)
  W44
- bronchus, bronchi (*see also* Foreign body,
  air passage) W44
- conjunctival sac W44
- digestive system (*see also* Foreign body,
  alimentary canal) W44
- ear (causing injury or obstruction) W44
- esophagus (causing injury or obstruction)
  W44
- – causing compression of trachea with
  interruption or obstruction of
  respiration W80
- eye (any part) W44
- ingestion W44
- inhalation (*see also* Foreign body,
  aspiration) W80
- larynx (*see also* Foreign body, air
  passage) W44

Foreign body, object or material—
continued
- mouth (*see also* Foreign body, alimentary canal, mouth) W44
- nasal passage (*see also* Foreign body, air passage, nose) W44
- nose (*see also* Foreign body, air passage, nose) W44
- oesophagus (causing injury or obstruction) W44
- – causing compression of trachea with interruption or obstruction of respiration W80
- operation wound (left in) (*see also* Misadventure, foreign object, by specified type of procedure) Y61.9
- pharynx (*see also* Foreign body, alimentary canal, pharynx) W44
- rectum (causing injury or obstruction) W44
- skin (*see also* Contact, with, by type of object) W45
- stomach (hairball) (causing injury or obstruction) W44

Foreign body, object or material—
continued
- tear ducts or glands W44
- trachea W44
- – causing suffocation NEC W80
- – – food W79
- – – vomitus W78
- urethra (causing injury or obstruction) W44
- vagina (causing injury or obstruction) W44

Forest fire (exposure to) X01
Found injured (dead) X59.9
- from exposure (to) – *see* Exposure
- on
- – highway, road(way), street V89.9
- – railway right of way V81.9

Fracture (circumstances unknown or unspecified) X59.0
- due to specified cause NEC X58

Freezing (*see also* Exposure, cold) X31
Frostbite X31
- due to man-made conditions W93

Frozen (*see also* Exposure, cold) X31

G

Garrotting, homicidal (attempted) X91
Gored W55

Gunshot wound (*see also* Discharge, by
type of firearm) W34

H

Hailstones, injured by X39
Hairball (stomach) (with obstruction)
W44
Hanged herself or himself (*see also*
Hanging, self-inflicted) Y20
Hanging (accidental) W76
– caused by other person
– – in accidental circumstances W76
– – stated as
– – – intentional, homicide (attempt) X91
– – – undetermined whether accidental or
intentional Y20
– homicide (attempt) X91
– in bed or cradle W75
– legal execution Y35.5
– self-inflicted (unspecified whether
accidental or intentional) Y20
– – in accidental circumstances W76
– – stated as intentional, purposeful, suicide
(attempt) X70
– stated as undetermined whether
accidentally or purposely inflicted Y20
– suicide (attempt) X70
Heat (effects of) (excessive) X30
– due to
– – man-made conditions, except on boat,
ship, or watercraft W92
– – weather (conditions) X30
– from
– – electric heating apparatus causing
burning X16

Heat *continued*
– from—*continued*
– – nuclear explosion in war operations
Y36.5
– inappropriate, in local application or
packing in medical or surgical procedure
Y63.5
Hemorrhage
– delayed following medical or surgical
treatment without mention of
misadventure (*see also* Complication, by
type of proce dure) Y84.9
– during medical or surgical treatment as
misadventure (*see also* Misadventure, cut,
by type of procedure) Y60.9
High
– altitude (effects) W94
– level of radioactivity, effects – *see*
Radiation
– pressure (effects) W94
– temperature, effects (*see also* Heat) X30
Hit, hitting (accidental) by – *see* Struck by
Hitting against – *see* Striking against
Homicide (attempt) (*see also* Assault) Y09
Hot
– place, effects (*see also* Heat) X30
– weather, effects X30
House fire (uncontrolled) X00
Humidity, causing problem X39
Hunger (*see also* Lack of, food) X53
– resulting from abandonment or
neglect (*see also* Abandonment) Y06.9
Hurricane (any injury) X37
Hypobarism, hypobaropathy W94

I

Ictus
- caloris (*see also* Heat) X30
- solaris X30

Ignition (accidental) (*see also* Exposure, fire) X09
- anesthetic gas in operating theatre W40
- apparel NEC X06
- - from highly flammable material X04
- bedlinen (mattress) (pillows) (sheets) (spreads) X08
- benzine X04
- clothes, clothing NEC (from controlled fire) X06
- - from
- - - highly flammable material X04
- - - uncontrolled fire (in building or structure) X00
- - - - not in building or structure X01
- explosive material (*see also* Explosion) W40
- gasoline X04
- jewelry (plastic) X06
- kerosene X04
- material
- - explosive (*see also* Explosion) W40
- - highly flammable (with secondary explosion) X04
- nightwear X05
- paraffin X04
- petrol X04

Immersion (accidental) (*see also* Drowning) W74
- hand or foot due to cold (excessive) X31

Implantation of quills of porcupine W55

Inanition (from) (hunger) (*see also* Lack of, food) X53
- resulting from homicidal intent (*see also* Abandonment) Y06.9
- thirst (*see also* Lack of, water) X54

Inappropriate operation performed Y65.5

Inattention at or after birth (homicidal intent) (infanticidal intent) (*see also* Abandonment) Y06.9

Incident, adverse
- device
- - anesthesiology Y70.-
- - cardiovascular Y71.-
- - gastroenterology Y73.-

Incident, adverse—*continued*
- device—*continued*
- - general hospital Y74.-
- - general surgical Y81.-
- - gynecological Y76.-
- - medical (specified) NEC Y82.-
- - neurological Y75.-
- - obstetric Y76.-
- - ophthalmic Y77.-
- - orthopedic Y79.-
- - otorhinolaryngological Y72.-
- - personal use Y74.-
- - physical medicine Y80.-
- - plastic surgical Y81.-
- - radiological Y78.-
- - urology Y73.-

Incineration (accidental) (*see also* Exposure, fire) X09

Infanticide (*see also* Assault) Y09

Infrasound waves (causing injury) W43

Ingestion
- foreign body (causing injury) (with obstruction) (*see also* Foreign body, alimentary canal) W44
- poisonous
- - plant(s) X49
- - substance NEC (*see also* Table of drugs and chemicals) X49

Inhalation
- excessively cold substance, man-made W93
- food (any type) (into respiratory tract) (with asphyxia, obstruction respiratory tract, suffocation) W79
- foreign body (*see also* Foreign body, aspiration) W80
- gastric contents (with asphyxia, obstruction respiratory passage, suffocation) W78
- hot air or gases X14
- liquid air, hydrogen, nitrogen W93
- mucus, not of newborn (with asphyxia, obstruction respiratory passage, suffocation) W80
- phlegm, not of newborn (with asphyxia, obstruction respiratory passage, suffocation) W80
- toxic gas – *see* Table of drugs and chemicals

Inhalation—*continued*
- vomitus (with asphyxia, obstruction respiratory passage, suffocation) W78

Injury, injured (accidental(ly)) NEC X59.~~9~~
- by, caused by, from
- - assault (*see also* Assault) Y09
- - law-enforcement agent, police, in course of legal intervention (*see also* Legal intervention) Y35.7
- - suicide (attempt) (*see also* Suicide) X84
- due to, in
- - civil insurrection – *see* War operations
- - engine in watercraft (without transport accident) V93.-
- - fight (*see also* Assault, fight) Y04
- - war operations – *see* War operations
- homicide (*see also* Assault) Y09
- inflicted (by)
- - in course of arrest (attempted), suppression of disturbance, maintenance of order, by law-enforcement agents (*see also* Legal intervention) Y35.7
- - other person
- - - stated as
- - - - accidental X59.~~9~~
- - - - intentional, homicide (attempt) (*see also* Assault) Y09
- - - - undetermined whether accidental or intentional (*see also* Injury, stated as, undetermined) Y34
- purposely (inflicted) by other person(s) (*see also* Assault) Y09
- self-inflicted (unspecified whether accidental or intentional) Y34
- - stated as
- - - accidental X59.~~9~~

Injury, injured—*continued*
- self-inflicted—*continued*
- - stated as—*continued*
- - - intentional, purposeful, suicide (attempt) X84
- specified cause NEC X58
- stated as
- - undetermined whether accidentally or purposely inflicted (by) Y34
- - - cut (any part of body) Y28
- - - cutting or piercing instrument Y28
- - - drowning Y21
- - - explosive(s) (missile) Y25
- - - falling from high place Y30
- - - hanging Y20
- - - knife Y28
- - - object (blunt) NEC Y29
- - - - sharp (any) Y28
- - - puncture (any part of body) Y28
- - - shooting (*see also* Discharge, by type of firearm, stated as undetermined whether accidentally or purposely inflicted) Y24
- - - specified means NEC Y33
- - - stab (any part of body) Y28
- - - strangulation Y20
- - - submersion Y21
- - - suffocation Y20

Insolation, effects X30
Insufficient nourishment (*see also* Lack of, food) X53
- homicidal intent (*see also* Abandonment) Y06.9

Interruption of respiration (by)
- food (lodged in esophagus) W79
- foreign body, except food or vomitus (lodged in esophagus) W80
- vomitus (lodged in esophagus) W78

Intervention, legal (*see also* Legal intervention) Y35.7

Intoxication
- drug – *see* Table of drugs and chemicals
- poison – *see* Table of drugs and chemicals

J

Jammed (accidentally)
– between objects (moving) (stationary and moving) (*see also* Caught) W23
– in object NEC W23
Jogging, excessive X50
Jumped, jumping
– before train, vehicle or other moving object (unspecified whether accidental or intentional) Y31
– – stated as intentional, purposeful, suicide (attempt) X81
– from
– – boat (into water) voluntarily, without accident (to boat), with injury (other than drowning or submersion) W16
– – – with drowning or submersion W69
– – building (*see also* Jumped, from, high place) W13

Jumped, jumping—*continued*
– from—*continued*
– – building—*continued*
– – – burning (uncontrolled fire) X00
– – high place NEC W17
– – – stated as
– – – – in undetermined circumstances Y30
– – – – intentional, purposeful, suicide (attempt) X80
– – structure (*see also* Jumped, from, high place) W13
– – – burning (uncontrolled fire) X00
– into water
– – with injury (other than drowning or submersion) W16
– – – drowning or submersion (*see also* Drowning) W74
– – from, off watercraft – *see* Jumped, from, boat

K

Kicked by
– animal NEC W55
– person(s) (accidentally) W50
– – with intent to injure or kill Y04
– – as, or caused by, a crowd or human
    stampede (with fall) W52
– – in fight Y04
Kicking against
– object (stationary) W22
– – sports equipment W21
– person (*see also* Striking against, person)
    W51
– sports equipment W21
Killed, killing (accidentally) NEC (*see also*
    Injury) X59.9
– in
– – action (*see also* War operations) Y36.9
– – brawl, fight (hand) (fists) (foot) Y04
– – – by weapon (*see also* Assault) Y09
– – – – cutting, piercing X99

Killed, killing—*continued*
– in—*continued*
– – brawl, fight—*continued*
– – – by weapon—*continued*
– – – – firearm (*see also* Discharge, by
        type of firearm, homicide) X95
– self
– – stated as
– – – accident NEC X59.9
– – – suicide (*see also* Suicide) X84
– – – undetermined whether accidental or
        intentional Y34
Knocked down (accidentally) (by) NEC
    X59.9
– animal (not being ridden) NEC (*see also*
    Struck by, by type of animal) W55
– – being ridden V06.-
– crowd or human stampede W52
– person W51
– – in brawl, fight Y04
– transport vehicle NEC (*see also* Accident,
    transport) V09.9

L

Laceration NEC (*see also* Injury) X59.9
Lack of
- air (refrigerator or closed place),
  suffocation by W81
- care (helpless person) (infant)
  (newborn) (*see also* Abandonment)
  Y06.9
- food (except as result of abandonment or
  neglect) X53
- - due to abandonment or neglect (*see also*
  Abandonment) Y06.9
- water except as result of transport accident
  X54
- - helpless person, infant,
  newborn (*see also* Abandonment)
  Y06.9
Landslide X36
- falling on, hitting
- - railway train or vehicle X36
- - transport (motor) vehicle (any) X36
Late effect – *see* Sequelae
Legal
- execution, any method Y35.5
- intervention (by) (injury from) Y35.7
- - baton Y35.3
- - bayonet Y35.4
- - blow NEC Y35.6
- - blunt object Y35.3
- - bomb (any) Y35.1
- - cutting or piercing instrument Y35.4
- - dynamite Y35.1
- - execution, any method Y35.5
- - explosive(s) (shell) Y35.1
- - firearm(s) (discharge) (any) Y35.0

Legal—*continued*
- intervention—*continued*
- - gas (asphyxiation) (poisoning) (tear)
  Y35.2
- - grenade Y35.1
- - late effect (of) Y89.0
- - manhandling Y35.6
- - sequelae (of) Y89.0
- - sharp object Y35.4
- - specified means NEC Y35.6
- - stabbing Y35.4
- - stave Y35.3
- - tear gas Y35.2
- - truncheon Y35.3
Lifting (heavy objects) (weights), excessive
  X50
Lightning (shock) (stroke) (struck by)
  X33
- causing fire (*see also* Exposure, fire) X09
Liquid (noncorrosive) in eye W44
- corrosive X49
Loss of control (transport vehicle)
  NEC (*see also* Accident, transport) V89.9
Lost at sea NEC V92.-
- in war operations Y36.4
Low
- pressure (effects) W94
- temperature (effects) (*see also* Exposure,
  cold) X31
Lying before train, vehicle or other
  moving object (unspecified whether
  accidental or intentional) Y31
- stated as intentional, purposeful, suicide
  (attempt) X81
Lynching (*see also* Assault) Y09

M

Maltreatment (syndrome) NEC Y07.9
- by
- – acquaintance or friend Y07.2
- – official authorities Y07.3
- – parent Y07.1
- – specified person(s) NEC Y07.8
- – spouse or partner Y07.0
Mangled (accidentally) NEC X59.9
Manhandling (in brawl, fight) Y04
- legal intervention Y35.6
Manslaughter (nonaccidental) (*see also* Assault) Y09
Mauled by animal NEC W55
Mauled by animal NEC W55
Medical procedure, complication of (delayed or as an abnormal reaction without mention of misadventure) (*see also* Complication, by type of procedure) Y84.9
- due to or as a result of misadventure (*see also* Misadventure) Y69
Melting (due to fire) (*see also* Exposure, fire) X09
- apparel NEC X06
- clothes, clothing NEC X06
- – nightwear X05
- fittings or furniture (burning building) (uncontrolled fire) X00
- jewelry, plastic X06
- nightwear X05
Mental cruelty (*see also* Maltreatment) Y07.9
Minamata disease X49
Misadventure(s) to patient(s) during surgical or medical care Y69
- contaminated medical or biological substance (blood, drug, fluid) Y64.9
- – administered (by)
- – – immunization Y64.1
- – – infusion Y64.0
- – – injection Y64.1
- – – specified means NEC Y64.8
- – – transfusion Y64.0
- – – vaccination Y64.1
- cut, cutting, puncture, perforation or hemorrhage (accidental) (inadvertent) (unintentional) (during) Y60.9

Misadventure(s) to patient(s) during surgical or medical care—*continued*
cut, cutting—*continued*
- – aspiration of fluid or tissue (by puncture or catheterization, except heart) Y60.6
- – biopsy (except by needle aspiration) Y60.8
- – – needle (aspirating) Y60.6
- – blood sampling Y60.6
- – catheterization Y60.6
- – – heart Y60.5
- – dialysis (kidney) Y60.2
- – endoscopic examination Y60.4
- – enema Y60.7
- – immunization Y60.3
- – infusion Y60.1
- – injection Y60.3
- – needle biopsy Y60.6
- – paracentesis (abdominal) (thoracic) Y60.6
- – perfusion Y60.2
- – puncture (lumbar) Y60.6
- – specified procedure NEC Y60.8
- – surgical operation Y60.0
- – transfusion Y60.1
- – vaccination Y60.3
- excessive amount of blood or other fluid during transfusion or infusion Y63.0
- failure
- – in dosage Y63.9
- – – electroshock therapy Y63.4
- – – infusion
- – – – excessive amount of fluid Y63.0
- – – – incorrect dilution of fluid Y63.1
- – – insulin-shock therapy Y63.4
- – – overdose – *see* Table of drugs and chemicals
- – – – radiation, in therapy Y63.2
- – – specified procedure NEC Y63.8
- – – transfusion of excessive amount of blood Y63.0
- – mechanical, of instrument or apparatus (any) (during any procedure) Y65.8
- – sterile precautions (during procedure) Y62.9
- – – aspiration of fluid or tissue (by puncture or catheterization, except heart) Y62.6

Misadventure(s) to patient(s) during surgical or medical care—*continued*
- failure—*continued*
- − − sterile precautions—*continued*
- − − − biopsy (except needle aspiration) Y62.8
- − − − − needle (aspirating) Y62.6
- − − − blood sampling Y62.6
- − − − catheterization (except heart) Y62.6
- − − − − heart Y62.5
- − − − dialysis (kidney) Y62.2
- − − − endoscopic examination Y62.4
- − − − enema Y62.8
- − − − immunization Y62.3
- − − − infusion Y62.1
- − − − injection Y62.3
- − − − needle biopsy Y62.6
- − − − paracentesis (abdominal) (thoracic) Y62.6
- − − − perfusion Y62.2
- − − − puncture (lumbar) Y62.6
- − − − removal of catheter or packing Y62.8
- − − − specified procedure NEC Y62.8
- − − − surgical operation Y62.0
- − − − transfusion Y62.1
- − − − vaccination Y62.3
- − − suture or ligature during surgical procedure Y65.2
- − − to introduce or to remove tube or instrument (except endotracheal tube during anesthesia) Y65.4
- foreign object left in body (during procedure) Y61.9
- − − aspiration of fluid or tissue (by puncture or catheterization, except heart) Y61.6
- − − biopsy (except by needle aspiration) Y61.8
- − − − needle (aspirating) Y61.6
- − − blood sampling Y61.6
- − − catheterization (except heart) Y61.6
- − − − heart Y61.5
- − − dialysis (kidney) Y61.2
- − − endoscopic examination Y61.4
- − − enema Y61.8
- − − immunization Y61.3
- − − infusion Y61.1
- − − injection Y61.3
- − − needle biopsy Y61.6
- − − paracentesis (abdominal) (thoracic) Y61.6
- − − perfusion Y61.2
- − − puncture (lumbar) Y61.6

Misadventure(s) to patient(s) during surgical or medical care—*continued*
- foreign object left in body—*continued*
- − − removal of catheter or packing Y61.7
- − − specified procedure NEC Y61.8
- − − surgical operation Y61.0
- − transfusion Y61.1
- − vaccination Y61.3
- hemorrhage (*see also* Misadventure, cut, by type of procedure) Y60.9
- inadvertent exposure of patient to radiation Y63.3
- inappropriate
- − − operation performed Y65.5
- − − temperature (too hot or too cold) in local application or packing Y63.5
- infusion (*see also* Misadventure, by type, infusion) Y69
- − − excessive amount of fluid Y63.0
- − − incorrect dilution of fluid Y63.1
- − − wrong fluid Y65.1
- late effect (of) Y88.1
- mismatched blood in transfusion Y65.0
- nonadministration of necessary drug or biological substance Y63.6
- overdose – *see* Table of drugs and chemicals
- − − radiation (in therapy) Y63.2
- perforation (*see also* Misadventure, cut, by type of procedure) Y60.9
- performance of inappropriate operation Y65.5
- puncture (*see also* Misadventure, cut, by type of procedure) Y60.9
- sequelae (of) Y88.1
- specified type NEC Y65.8
- transfusion (*see also* Misadventure, by type, transfusion) Y69
- − − excessive amount of blood Y63.0
- − − mismatched blood Y65.0
- wrong
- − − drug given in error – *see* Table of drugs and chemicals
- − − fluid in infusion Y65.1
- − − placement of endotracheal tube during anesthetic procedure Y65.3

Mismatched blood in transfusion Y65.0
Motion (effects) (sickness) X51
Mountain sickness W94
Mucus aspiration or inhalation, not of newborn (with asphyxia, obstruction respiratory passage, suffocation) W80
Mudslide (of cataclysmic nature) X36
Murder (attempt) (*see also* Assault) Y09

699

N

Nail, contact with W45
Neglect (criminal) (homicidal
intent) *(see also* Abandonment) Y06.9
Noise (causing injury) (pollution) W42

Nonadministration (of)
– drug or biological substance (necessary)
Y63.6
– surgical and medical care Y66

O

Object
- falling from, in, on, hitting, machinery (*see also* Contact, with, by type of machine) W31
- set in motion by
- – accidental explosion or rupture of pressure vessel NEC W38
- – firearm (*see also* Discharge, by type of firearm) W34
- – machine(ry) (*see also* Contact, with, by type of machine) W31

Obstruction
- air passages, larynx, respiratory passages
- – by
- – – food, any type W79
- – – material or object except food or vomitus W80
- – – mucus W80
- – – phlegm W80
- – – vomitus W78
- digestive tract, except mouth or pharynx
- – by
- – – food, any type W44
- – – foreign body (any) W44
- – – vomitus W44
- esophagus
- – by
- – – food, any type W44
- – – – with asphyxia, obstruction of respiratory passage, suffocation (due to air passage compression) W79
- – – foreign body, except food or vomitus W44
- – – vomitus W44
- – – – with asphyxia, obstruction of respiratory passage, suffocation W78

Obstruction—*continued*
- pharynx
- – by
- – – food, any type W79
- – – material or object except food or vomitus W80
- – – vomitus W78
- respiration
- – by
- – – food (lodged in esophagus) W79
- – – foreign body, except food or vomitus (lodged in esophagus) W80
- – – vomitus (lodged in esophagus) (compression of trachea) W78

Overdose (drug) – *see* Table of drugs and chemicals
- radiation Y63.2

Overexertion (lifting) (pulling) (pushing) X50

Overexposure (accidental) (to)
- cold (*see also* Exposure, cold) X31
- – due to man-made conditions W93
- heat (*see also* Heat) X30
- radiation – *see* Radiation
- radioactivity W88
- sun (sunburn) X32
- weather NEC X39
- wind NEC X39

Overheated (*see also* Heat) X30

Overlaid W75

Overturning (accidental)
- boat, ship, watercraft (causing drowning, submersion) V90.-
- – causing injury except drowning or submersion V91.-
- machinery (*see also* Contact, with, by type of machine) W31
- transport vehicle NEC (*see also* Accident, transport) V89.9

P

Parachute descent (voluntary) (without accident to aircraft) V97.2
– due to accident to aircraft V95.9
Pecked by bird W64
Perforation during medical or surgical treatment as misadventure (*see also* Misadventure, cut, by type of procedure) Y60.9
Phlegm aspiration or inhalation, not of newborn (with asphyxia, obstruction respiratory passage, suffocation) W80
Piercing (*see also* Contact, with, by type of object or machine) W49
Pinched between objects (moving) (stationary and moving) (*see also* Caught) W23
Pinned under machine(ry) (*see also* Contact, with, by type of machine) W31
Plumbism – *see* Table of drugs and chemicals, Lead
Poisoning (accidental) (by) (*see also* Table of drugs and chemicals) X49
– carbon monoxide
– – generated by
– – – motor vehicle – *see* Note 6, Volume 1, Classification and coding instructions for transport accidents before V01.-
– – – watercraft (in transit) (not in transit) V93.-
– exhaust gas
– – generated by
– – – motor vehicle – *see* Note 6, Volume 1, Classification and coding instructions for transport accidents before V01.-
– – – watercraft (in transit) (not in transit) V93.-
– fumes or smoke due to
– – explosion (*see also* Explosion) W40
– – fire (*see also* Exposure, fire) X09
– – ignition (*see also* Ignition) X09
– gas
– – in legal intervention Y35.2
– – legal execution Y35.5
– in war operations (chemical weapons) Y36.7
– legal
– – execution Y35.5

Poisoning—*continued*
  legal *continued*
  – intervention by gas Y35.2
– plant, thorns, spines, or sharp leaves (*see also* Table of drugs and chemicals) X28
– – marine or sea plants (venomous) X26
Premature cessation of surgical and medical care Y66
Pressure, external, causing asphyxia, suffocation (*see also* Suffocation) W84
Privation X57
– due to abandonment or neglect (*see also* Abandonment) Y06.9
– food (*see also* Lack of, food) X53
– water (*see also* Lack of, water) X54
Prolonged stay in
– high altitude as cause of anoxia, barodontalgia, barotitis or hypoxia W94
– weightless environment X52
Pulling, excessive X50
Puncture, puncturing (*see also* Contact, with, by type of object or machine) W49
– by
– – plant thorns, spines, sharp leaves or other mechanisms NEC W60
– – sea-urchin spine X26
– during medical or surgical treatment as misadventure (*see also* Misadventure, cut, by type of procedure) Y60.9
Pushed, pushing (accidental) (injury in) (overexertion) X50
– by other person(s) (accidental) W51
– – with fall W03
– – as, or caused by, a crowd or human stampede (with fall) W52
– – before moving object, train, vehicle
– – – stated as
– – – – intentional, homicide (attempt) Y02
– – – – undetermined whether accidentally or purposely inflicted Y33
– – from
– – – high place NEC
– – – – in accidental circumstances W17
– – – – stated as
– – – – – intentional, homicide (attempt) Y01

Pushed, pushing—*continued*
– by other person(s)—*continued*
– – from—*continued*
– – – high place NEC—*continued*
– – – – stated as—*continued*
– – – – – undetermined whether
     accidentally or purposely
     inflicted Y30

Pushed, pushing—*continued*
– by other person(s)—*continued*
– – from—*continued*
– – – transport vehicle NEC (*see also*
    Accident, transport) V89.9
– – – – stated as
– – – – – intentional, homicide (attempt)
     Y08
– – – – – undetermined whether
     accidentally or purposely
     inflicted Y33

R

Radiation (exposure to) W91
- arc lamps W89
- atomic power plant (malfunction) NEC W88
- complication of or abnormal reaction to medical radiotherapy Y84.2
- electromagnetic, ionizing W88
- gamma rays W88
- in
- – war operations (from or following nuclear explosion) (direct) (secondary) Y36.5
- – – laser(s) Y36.7
- inadvertent exposure of patient (receiving test or therapy) Y63.3
- infrared (heaters and lamps) W90
- – excessive heat from W92
- ionized, ionizing (particles, artificially accelerated) W88
- isotopes, radioactive (*see also* Radiation, radioactive isotopes) W88
- laser(s) W90
- – in war operations Y36.7
- – misadventure in medical care Y63.2
- light sources (man-made visible and ultraviolet) W89
- – natural X32
- man-made visible light W89
- microwave W90
- misadventure in medical or surgical procedure Y63.2
- natural NEC X39
- overdose (in medical or surgical procedure) Y63.2
- radar W90
- radioactive isotopes (any) W88
- – atomic power plant malfunction W88
- – misadventure in medical or surgical treatment Y63.2
- radiofrequency W90
- radium NEC W88
- sun X32
- ultraviolet (light) (man-made) W89
- – natural X32
- welding arc, torch, or light W89
- – excessive heat from W92
- X-rays (hard) (soft) W88
Range disease W94
Rape (attempted) Y05

Rat bite W53
Reaction, abnormal to medical procedure (*see also* Complication, by type of procedure) Y84.9
- with misadventure (*see also* Misadventure) Y69
- biologicals – *see* Table of drugs and chemicals
- drugs – *see* Table of drugs and chemicals
- vaccine – *see* Table of drugs and chemicals
Reduction in
- atmospheric pressure W94
- – while surfacing from
- – – deep water diving (causing caisson or diver's disease, palsy or paralysis) W94
- – – underground W94
Repetitive movements, excessive X50
Residual (effect) (*see also* Sequelae) Y89.9
Rock falling on or hitting (accidentally) person W20
Rowing, excessive X50
Run over (accidentally) (by)
- animal (not being ridden) NEC W55
- – being ridden V06.-
- machinery (*see also* Contact, with, by type of machine) W31
- transport vehicle NEC (*see also* Accident, transport) V09.9
- – intentional, homicide (attempt) Y03
- – motor NEC V09.2
- – – intentional, homicide (attempt) Y03
- – – undetermined whether accidental or intentional Y33
- – undetermined whether accidental or intentional Y33
Running
- before train, vehicle or other moving object (unspecified whether accidental or intentional) Y31
- – stated as intentional, purposeful, suicide (attempt) X81
- excessive X50
Running off, away
- animal (being ridden) (*see also* Accident, transport) V80.9
- – not being ridden W55

Running off, away—*continued*
- animal-drawn vehicle NEC (*see also*
  Accident, transport) V80.9

Running off, away—*continued*
- highway, road(way), street
- – transport vehicle NEC (*see also*
  Accident, transport) V89.9
Rupture of pressurized device (*see also*
  Explosion, by type of device) W38

S

Saturnism – *see* Table of drugs and chemicals, Lead
Scald, scalding (accidental) (by) (from) (in) X19
– air (hot) X14
– gases (hot) X14
– homicide (attempt) X98
– inflicted by other person
– – stated as
– – – intentional, homicide (attempt) X98
– – – undetermined whether accidental or intentional Y27
– liquid (boiling) (hot) NEC X12
– local application of externally applied substance in medical or surgical care Y63.5
– metal (hot) (liquid) (molten) NEC X18
– self-inflicted (unspecified whether accidental or intentional) Y27
– – stated as intentional, purposeful, suicide (attempt) X77
– stated as undetermined whether accidental or intentional Y27
– steam X13
– suicide (attempt) X77
– vapor (hot) X13
Scratched by
– cat W55
– person(s) (accidentally) W50
Seasickness X51
Self-harm NEC (*see also* external cause by type, undetermined whether accidental or intentional) Y34
– intentional (*see also* Suicide) X84
Self-inflicted (injury) NEC (*see also* external cause by type, undetermined whether accidental or intentional) Y34
– intentional (*see also* Suicide) X84
– poisoning NEC (*see also* Table of drugs and chemicals) X49
Sequelae (of) Y89.9
– accident NEC (classifiable to W00-X59) Y86
– adverse incident associated with medical device in diagnostic or therapeutic use (classifiable to Y70-Y82) Y88.2
– assault (homicidal) (any means) (classifiable to X85-Y09) Y87.1

Sequelae—*continued*
– drugs and biologicals causing adverse effects in therapeutic use (classifiable to Y40-Y59) Y88.0
– event of undetermined intent (classifiable to Y10-Y34) Y87.2
– homicide, attempt (any means) (classifiable to X85-Y09) Y87.1
– injury undetermined whether accidentally or purposely inflicted (classifiable to Y10-Y34) Y87.2
– intentional self-harm (classifiable to X60-X84) Y87.0
– legal intervention Y89.0
– medical or surgical procedure, resulting from misadventure Y88.1
– misadventure to patient during medical or surgical procedure (classifiable to Y60-Y69) Y88.1
– motor vehicle accident Y85.0
– suicide (attempt) (any means) (classifiable to X60-X84) Y87.0
– surgical and medical procedures as cause of abnormal reaction or later complication (classifiable to Y83-Y84) Y88.3
– transport accident, except motor vehicles Y85.9
– war operations Y89.1
Shock
– electric (*see also* Exposure, electric current) W87
– from electric appliance (any) (faulty) W86
Shooting, shot (accidental(ly)) (*see also* Discharge, by type of firearm) W34
– herself or himself (*see also* Discharge, by type of firearm, self-inflicted) Y24
– homicide (attempt) (*see also* Discharge, firearm, by type, homicide) X95
– in war operations Y36.4
– inflicted by other person
– – stated as
– – – intentional, homicide (attempt) (*see also* Discharge, by type of firearm) X95
– – – undetermined whether accidental or intentional (*see also* Discharge, by type of firearm, stated as undetermined intent) Y24

Shooting, shot—*continued*
- legal
- – execution Y35.5
- – intervention Y35.0
- self-inflicted (unspecified whether accidental or intentional) (*see also* Discharge, by type of firearm, self-inflicted) Y24
- – stated as
- – – intentional, purposeful, suicide (attempt) (*see also* Discharge, by type of firearm, suicide) X74
- suicide (attempt) (*see also* Discharge, by type of firearm, suicide) X74

Shoving (accidentally) by other person (*see also* Pushed, by other person) W51

Shut in (accidentally) (*see also* Suffocation)
- airtight space, except plastic bag W81
- plastic bag (*see also* Suffocation, in, plastic bag) W83
- refrigerator W81

Sickness
- air X51
- alpine W94
- car X51
- motion X51
- mountain W94
- sea X51
- travel X51

Sinking (accidental)
- boat, ship, watercraft (causing drowning or submersion) V90.-
- – causing injury except drowning or submersion V91.-

Siriasis X32

Slashed wrists (*see also* Cut, self-inflicted) Y28

Slipping (accidental) (on same level) (with fall) W01
- on
- – ice W00
- – – with skates W02
- – mud W01
- – oil W01
- – snow W00
- – – with skis W02
- – surface (slippery) (wet) NEC W01

Sliver, wood, contact with W45

Smothering, smothered (*see also* Suffocation) W84

Smouldering (due to fire) (*see also* Exposure, fire) X09

Sodomy (attempted) by force Y05
Sound waves (causing injury) W42
Splinter, contact with W45
Stab, stabbing X99
- accidental (*see also* Contact, with, by object) W49
Starvation X53
- due to abandonment or neglect (*see also* Abandonment) Y06.9
Stepped on
- by
- – animal (not being ridden) NEC W55
- – – being ridden V06.-
- – crowd or human stampede W52
- – person W50
Stepping on
- object (stationary) W22
- – with fall W18
- – sports equipment W21
- sports equipment W21
Sting (venomous) (*see also* Contact, with, by type of sting) X29
- ant X25
- arthropod NEC X25
- – nonvenomous W57
- bee X23
- caterpillar X25
- centipede X24
- coral X26
- hornet X23
- insect NEC X25
- – nonvenomous W57
- jelly fish X26
- marine animal or plant X26
- millipede, venomous X24
- nematocysts X26
- scorpion X22
- sea anemone, cucumber, or urchin (spine) X26
- wasp X23
- yellow jacket X23
Storm (cataclysmic) X37
- causing flood X38
Straining, excessive X50
Strangling – *see* Strangulation
Strangulation (accidental) W76
- by, due to, in
- – baby carriage W75
- – bed, bed linen W75
- – bib W76
- – blanket W75
- – cot, cradle W75
- – other person NEC W76
- – – in bed W75

707

Strangulation—*continued*
- by, due to—*continued*
- – other person NEC—*continued*
- – – stated as undetermined whether
  accidentally or purposely inflicted
  Y20
- – perambulator W75
- – pillow W75
- – sheet (plastic) W75
- homicide (attempt) X91
- self-inflicted (unspecified whether
  accidental or intentional) Y20
- – accidental W76
- – stated as intentional, purposeful, suicide
  (attempt) X70
- stated as undetermined whether
  accidentally or purposely inflicted Y20
- suicide (attempt) X70

**Strenuous movements (in recreational or
other activities)** X50

Striking against
- bottom (when jumping or diving into
  water) W16
- diving board (swimming-pool) (when
  jumping or diving into water) W16
- object (stationary) W22
- – with
- – – drowning or submersion (*see also*
  Drowning) W74
- – – fall W18
- – caused by crowd or human stampede
  (with fall) W52
- – moving, projected W20
- – sports equipment W21
- person(s) W51
- – with fall W03
- – as, or caused by, a crowd or human
  stampede (with fall) W52
- sports equipment W21
- wall of swimming-pool (when jumping or
  diving into water) W16
- water surface (with injury other than
  drowning or submersion) W16

Struck (accidentally) by
- alligator W58
- animal (not being ridden) NEC W55
- – being ridden V06.-
- avalanche X36
- ball (hit) (thrown) W21
- bullet (*see also* Discharge, by type of
  firearm) W34
- – in war operations Y36.4
- crocodile W58
- dog W54

Struck—*continued*
- flare, Very pistol (*see also* Discharge,
  firearm) W34
- hailstones X39
- hockey stick or puck W21
- landslide X36
- law enforcement agent (on duty) Y35.6
- – with blunt object (baton) (stave)
  (truncheon) Y35.3
- lightning X33
- machine (*see also* Contact, with, by type
  of machine) W31
- mammal NEC W55
- – marine W56
- marine animal W56
- missile
- – firearm (*see also* Discharge, by type of
  firearm) W34
- – in war operations – *see* War operations,
  missile
- object NEC W22
- – falling W20
- – – from, in, on
- – – – building W20
- – – – – burning (uncontrolled fire) X00
- – – – cataclysmic
- – – – – earth surface movement NEC
  X36
- – – – – storm X37
- – – – cave-in W20
- – – – – with asphyxiation or
  suffocation (*see also*
  Suffocation, due to, cave-in)
  W77
- – – – earthquake X34.‡
- – – – machine (in operation) (*see also*
  Contact, with, by type of machine)
  W31
- – – – structure W20
- – – – – burning X00
- – – – transport vehicle (in motion)
  NEC (*see also* Accident, transport)
  V89.9
- – – – – stationary W20
- – moving NEC W20
- – projected NEC W20
- – set in motion by explosion (*see also*
  Explosion) W40
- – thrown NEC W20
- other person(s) W50
- – with blunt object W22
- – – intentional, homicide (attempt) Y00
- – – sports equipment W21

Struck—*continued*
- other person(s)—*continued*
- – as, or caused by, a crowd or human stampede (with fall) W52
- – sports equipment W21
- police (on duty) Y35.6
- – with blunt object (baton) (stave) (truncheon) Y35.3
- sports equipment W21
- thunderbolt X33
- transport vehicle NEC (*see also* Accident, transport) V09.9
- – intentional, homicide (attempt) Y03
- – motor NEC (*see also* Accident, transport) V09.2
- – – intentional, homicide (attempt) Y03
- – – undetermined whether accidental or intentional Y33
- – undetermined whether accidental or intentional Y33
- vehicle (transport) NEC (*see also* Accident, transport) V09.9
- – stationary (falling from jack, hydraulic lift, ramp) W20

Stumbling
- over
- – animal NEC W64
- – – with fall W01
- – carpet, curb, kerb, rug or (small) object (*see also* Striking against, object) W22
- – – with fall W01
- – person W51
- – – with fall W03

Submersion (accidental) (*see also* Drowning) W74

Suffocation (accidental) (by external means) (by pressure) (mechanical) W84
- caused by other person
- – in accidental circumstances W84
- – stated as
- – – intentional, homicide (attempt) X91
- – – undetermined whether accidentally or purposely inflicted Y20
- due to, by
- – another person in bed W75
- – avalanche X36
- – bed, bed linen W75
- – bib W76
- – blanket W75
- – cave-in W77
- – – caused by cataclysmic earth surface movement X36

Suffocation—*continued*
- due to, by—*continued*
- – explosion (*see also* Explosion) W40
- – falling earth or other substance W77
- – fire (*see also* Exposure, fire) X09
- – food, any type (aspiration) (ingestion) (inhalation) W79
- – foreign body, except food or vomitus W80
- – ignition (*see also* Ignition) X09
- – landslide X36
- – machine(ry) (*see also* Contact, with, by type of machine) W31
- – material or object except food or vomitus W80
- – mucus (aspiration) (inhalation), not of newborn W80
- – phlegm (aspiration) (inhalation), not of newborn W80
- – pillow W75
- – plastic bag (*see also* Suffocation, in, plastic bag) W83
- – sheet (plastic) W75
- – specified means NEC W83
- – vomitus (aspiration) (inhalation) W78
- homicide (attempt) X91
- in
- – airtight place W81
- – baby carriage W75
- – bed W75
- – burning building X00
- – closed place W81
- – cot, cradle W75
- – perambulator W75
- – plastic bag (in accidental circumstances) W83
- – – homicide (attempt) X91
- – – self-inflicted (unspecified whether accidental or intentional) Y20
- – – – in accidental circumstances W83
- – – – stated as intentional, purposeful, suicide (attempt) X70
- – – stated as undetermined whether accidentally or purposely inflicted Y20
- – – suicide (attempt) X70
- – refrigerator W81
- infant while asleep W75
- self-inflicted Y20
- – in accidental circumstances W84
- – stated as intentional, purposeful, suicide (attempt) X70
- stated as undetermined whether accidentally or purposely inflicted Y20

Suffocation—*continued*
– suicide (attempt) X70
Suicide, suicidal (attempted) (by) X84
– blunt object X79
– burning, burns X76
– – hot object, steam or vapor X77
– caustic substance X83
– – poisoning – *see* Table of drugs and
   chemicals
– – swallowed – *see* Table of drugs and
   chemicals
– cold, extreme X83
– collision (of)
– – motor vehicle X82
– – streetcar, train or tram X82
– – transport vehicle NEC X82
– crashing of
– – aircraft X83
– – streetcar, train or tram X82
– – transport vehicle NEC X82
– cut (any part of body) X78
– cutting or piercing instrument X78
– drowning X71
– electrocution X83
– explosive(s) (material) X75
– fire, flames X76
– firearm (*see also* Discharge, by type of
   firearm, suicide) X74
– hanging X70
– hot object X77
– jumping
– – before moving object, train, vehicle
   X81
– – from high place X80
– late effect of attempt Y87.0
– lying before moving object, train, vehicle
   X81

Suicide, suicidal—*continued*
– poisoning – *see* Table of drugs and
   chemicals
– puncture (any part of body) X78
– scald X77
– sequelae of attempt Y87.0
– sharp object (any) X78
– shooting (*see also* Discharge, by type of
   firearm, suicide) X74
– specified means NEC X83
– stab (any part of body) X78
– steam, hot vapor X77
– strangulation X70
– submersion X71
– suffocation X70
– wound NEC X84
Sunstroke X32
Supersonic waves (causing injury) W42
**Surgical procedure, complication of
   (delayed or as an abnormal reaction
   without mention of
   misadventure)** (*see also* Complication,
   by type of procedure) Y83.9
– due to or as a result of
   misadventure (*see also* Misadventure)
   Y69
Swallowed, swallowing
– foreign body (*see also* Foreign body,
   alimentary canal) W44
– poison – *see* Table of drugs and chemicals
– substance
– – caustic or corrosive X49
– – poisonous – *see* Table of drugs and
   chemicals
Syndrome
– battered – *see* Maltreatment
– maltreatment – *see* Maltreatment

T

Tackle in sport W03
Thirst (*see also* Lack of, water) X54
Threat to breathing W84
– due to cave-in, falling earth or other
substance NEC W77
– specified NEC W83
Thrown (accidentally)
– against part (any) of or object in transport
vehicle (in motion) NEC – *see* Accident,
transport
– from, off
– – high place, intentional, homicide
(attempt) Y01
– – machinery (*see also* Contact, with, by
type of machine) W31
– – transport vehicle NEC (*see also*
Accident, transport) V89.9
Thunderbolt NEC X33
Tidal wave (any injury) NEC X39
– caused by storm X37
Took
– overdose (drug) – *see* Table of drugs and
chemicals
– poison – *see* Table of drugs and chemicals
Tornado (any injury) X37
Torrential rain (any injury) X37
Torture – *see* Maltreatment
Trampled by animal NEC W55
– being ridden V06.-

Trapped (accidentally)
– between
– – buildings (collapsing) in earthquake
X34.0̶
– – objects (moving) (stationary and
moving) (*see also* Caught) W23
– by part (any) of
– – motorcycle V29.8
– – pedal cycle V19.8
– – transport vehicle NEC (*see also*
Accident, transport) V89.9
– in low-oxygen environment W81
Travel (effects) (sickness) X51
**Tree falling on or hitting (accidentally)
(person)** W20
Tripping
– over
– – animal W64
– – – with fall W01
– – carpet, curb, kerb, rug or (small)
object (*see also* Striking against, object)
W22
– – – with fall W01
– – person W51
– – – with fall W03
Tsunami (any injury) NEC X34.1̶
Twisted by person(s) (accidentally) W50
Twisting, excessive X50

V

Vibration (causing injury) W43
Victim (of)
− avalanche X36
− earth movement NEC X36
− earthquake X34.9
− − cataclysmic earth movements X34.0
− − specified effect NEC X34.8
− − tsunami X34.1
− flood X38
− landslide X36

Victim—*continued*
− lightning X33
− storm (cataclysmic) NEC X37
− − causing flood X38
− volcanic eruption X35
Volcanic eruption (any injury) X35
**Vomitus, gastric contents, regurgitated
  food in air passages (with asphyxia,
  obstruction or suffocation)** (*see also*
  Foreign body, air passage) W78

W

Walked into stationary object (any) W22
War operations (during hostilities)
(injury) (by) (in) Y36.9
– after cessation of hostilities, injury due to
Y36.8
– air blast Y36.2
– aircraft burned, destroyed, exploded, shot
down Y36.1
– asphyxia from
– – chemical (weapons) Y36.7
– – fire, conflagration (caused by fire-
producing device or conventional
weapon) Y36.3
– – – from nuclear explosion Y36.5
– – gas or fumes Y36.7
– battle wound NEC Y36.9
– bayonet Y36.4
– biological warfare agents Y36.6
– blast (air) (effects) Y36.2
– – from nuclear explosion Y36.5
– – underwater Y36.0
– bomb (antipersonnel) (mortar) (explosion)
(fragments) Y36.2
– – after cessation of hostilities Y36.8
– bullet(s) (from carbine, machine gun,
pistol, rifle, shotgun) Y36.4
– burn from
– – chemical Y36.7
– – fire, conflagration (caused by fire-
producing device or conventional
weapon) Y36.3
– – – from nuclear explosion Y36.5
– – gas Y36.7
– burning aircraft Y36.1
– chemical Y36.7
– conventional warfare, specified form NEC
Y36.4
– crushed by falling aircraft Y36.1
– depth-charge Y36.0
– destruction of aircraft Y36.1
– disability as sequela one year or more
after injury Y89.1
– drowning Y36.4
– effect (direct) (secondary) of nuclear
weapon Y36.5
– explosion (artillery shell) (breech-block)
(cannon block) Y36.2
– – after cessation of hostilities of bomb,
mine placed in war Y36.8

War operations—*continued*
– explosion—*continued*
– – aircraft Y36.1
– – bomb (antipersonnel) (mortar) Y36.2
– – – nuclear (atom) (hydrogen) Y36.5
– – depth-charge Y36.0
– – grenade Y36.2
– – injury by fragments from Y36.2
– – land-mine Y36.2
– – marine weapon Y36.0
– – mine (land) Y36.2
– – – at sea or in harbor Y36.0
– – – marine Y36.0
– – missile (explosive) NEC (*see also* War
operations, missile) Y36.2
– – munitions (accidental) (being used in
war) (dump) (factory) Y36.2
– – nuclear (weapon) Y36.5
– – own weapons (accidental) Y36.2
– – sea-based artillery shell Y36.0
– – torpedo Y36.0
– exposure to ionizing radiation from
nuclear explosion Y36.5
– falling aircraft Y36.1
– fire or fire-producing device Y36.3
– fireball effects from nuclear explosion
Y36.5
– fragments from artillery shell, bomb NEC,
grenade, guided missile, land-mine,
rocket, shell, shrapnel Y36.2
– gas or fumes Y36.7
– grenade (explosion) (fragments) Y36.2
– guided missile (explosion) (fragments)
Y36.2
– – nuclear Y36.5
– heat from nuclear explosion Y36.5
– injury due to, but occurring after cessation
of hostilities Y36.8
– land-mine (explosion) (fragments) Y36.2
– – after cessation of hostilities Y36.8
– laser(s) Y36.7
– late effect of Y89.1
– lewisite Y36.7
– lung irritant (chemical) (fumes) (gas)
Y36.7
– marine mine Y36.0
– mine Y36.2
– – after cessation of hostilities Y36.8
– – at sea Y36.0

War operations—*continued*
– mine—*continued*
– – in harbor Y36.0
– – land (explosion) (fragments) Y36.2
– – marine Y36.0
– missile (guided) (explosion) (fragments)
  Y36.2
– – marine Y36.0
– – nuclear Y36.5
– mortar bomb (explosion) (fragments)
  Y36.2
– mustard gas Y36.7
– nerve gas Y36.7
– phosgene Y36.7
– poisoning (chemical) (fumes) (gas) Y36.7
– radiation, ionizing from nuclear explosion
  Y36.5
– rocket (explosion) (fragments) Y36.2
– saber, sabre Y36.4
– screening smoke Y36.7
– shell (aircraft) (artillery) (cannon) (land-
  based) (explosion) (fragments) Y36.2
– – sea-based Y36.0
– shooting Y36.4
– – after cessation of hostilities Y36.8
– – bullet(s) Y36.4
– – pellet(s) (rifle) (shotgun) Y36.4
– shrapnel Y36.2

War operations—*continued*
– submersion Y36.4
– torpedo Y36.0
– unconventional warfare NEC Y36.7
– – biological (warfare) Y36.6
– – gas, fumes, chemicals Y36.7
    laser(s) Y36.7
– – nuclear weapon Y36.5
– – specified NEC Y36.7
– underwater blast Y36.0
– vesicant (chemical) (fumes) (gas) Y36.7
– weapon burst Y36.2
Washed
– away by flood X38
– off road by storm (transport vehicle) X37
Weather exposure NEC (*see also*
  Exposure) X39
**Weightlessness (causing injury) (effects
  of) (in spacecraft, real or simulated)**
  X52
Wound (accidental) NEC (*see also* Injury)
  X59.9
– battle (*see also* War operations) Y36.9
– gunshot (*see also* Discharge, by type of
  firearm) W34
Wreck transport vehicle NEC (*see also*
  Accident, transport) V89.9
Wrong fluid in infusion Y65.1

Section III

Table of drugs and chemicals

A

Substance	Chapter XIX	Poisoning			Adverse effect in therapeutic use
		Accidental	Intentional self-harm	Undetermined intent	
Abrine	T62.2	X49	X69	Y19	
Absinthe	T51.0	X45	X65	Y15	
Acebutolol	T44.7	X43	X63	Y13	Y51.7
Acecarbromal	T42.6	X41	X61	Y11	Y47.4
Aceclidine	T44.1	X43	X63	Y13	Y51.1
Acedapsone	T37.0	X44	X64	Y14	Y41.0
Acefylline piperazine	T48.6	X44	X64	Y14	Y55.6
Acemetacin	T39.3	X40	X60	Y10	Y45.3
Acemorphan	T40.2	X42	X62	Y12	Y45.0
Acenocoumarin	T45.5	X44	X64	Y14	Y44.2
Acenocoumarol	T45.5	X44	X64	Y14	Y44.2
Acepifylline	T48.6	X44	X64	Y14	Y55.6
Acepromazine	T43.3	X41	X61	Y11	Y49.3
Acesulfamethoxypyridazine	T37.0	X44	X64	Y14	Y41.0
Acetal	T52.8	X46	X66	Y16	
Acetaldehyde (vapor)	T52.8	X46	X66	Y16	
– liquid	T65.8	X49	X69	Y19	
p-Acetamidophenol	T39.1	X40	X60	Y10	Y45.5
Acetaminophen	T39.1	X40	X60	Y10	Y45.5
Acetanilide	T39.1	X40	X60	Y10	Y45.5
Acetarsol	T37.3	X44	X64	Y14	Y41.3
Acetazolamide	T50.2	X44	X64	Y14	Y54.2
Acetiamine	T45.2	X44	X64	Y14	Y57.7
Acetic					
– acid	T54.2	X49	X69	Y19	
– – ester (solvent) (vapor)	T52.8	X46	X66	Y16	
– – medicinal (lotion)	T49.2	X44	X64	Y14	Y56.2
– anhydride	T65.8	X49	X69	Y19	
– ether (vapor)	T52.8	X46	X66	Y16	
Acetohexamide	T38.3	X44	X64	Y14	Y42.3
Acetohydroxamic acid	T50.9	X44	X64	Y14	Y43.5
Acetomenaphthone	T45.7	X44	X64	Y14	Y44.3
Acetone (oils)	T52.4	X46	X66	Y16	
– chlorinated	T52.4	X46	X66	Y16	
– vapor	T52.4	X46	X66	Y16	
Acetonitrile	T52.8	X46	X66	Y16	
Acetophenazine	T43.3	X41	X61	Y11	Y49.3
Acetophenetedin	T39.1	X40	X60	Y10	Y45.5
Acetophenone	T52.4	X46	X66	Y16	
Acetrizoic acid	T50.8	X44	X64	Y14	Y57.5
Acetyl					
– bromide	T53.6	X46	X66	Y16	
– chloride	T53.6	X46	X66	Y16	

Substance	Chapter XIX	Poisoning Accidental	Poisoning Intentional self-harm	Poisoning Undetermined intent	Adverse effect in therapeutic use
Acetylcholine					
– chloride	T44.1	X43	X63	Y13	Y51.1
– derivative	T44.1	X43	X63	Y13	Y51.1
Acetylcysteine	T48.4	X44	X64	Y14	Y55.4
Acetyldigitoxin	T46.0	X44	X64	Y14	Y52.0
Acetyldigoxin	T46.0	X44	X64	Y14	Y52.0
Acetylene (gas)	T59.8	X47	X67	Y17	
– dichloride	T53.6	X46	X66	Y16	
– industrial	T59.8	X47	X67	Y17	
– tetrachloride	T53.6	X46	X66	Y16	
– – vapor	T53.6	X46	X66	Y16	
Acetylpheneturide	T42.6	X41	X61	Y11	Y46.6
Acetylsalicylic acid (salts)	T39.0	X40	X60	Y10	Y45.1
– enteric coated	T39.0	X40	X60	Y10	Y45.1
Acetylsulfamethoxypyridazine	T37.0	X44	X64	Y14	Y41.0
Aciclovir	T37.5	X44	X64	Y14	Y41.5
Acid (corrosive) NEC	T54.2	X49	X69	Y19	
Acidifying agent NEC	T50.9	X44	X64	Y14	Y43.5
Acipimox	T46.6	X44	X64	Y14	Y52.6
Acitretin	T50.9	X44	X64	Y14	Y57.8
Aclarubicin	T45.1	X44	X64	Y14	Y43.3
Aclatonium napadisilate	T48.1	X44	X64	Y14	Y55.1
Aconitine	T46.9	X44	X64	Y14	Y52.9
Acridine	T65.6	X49	X69	Y19	
– vapor	T59.8	X47	X67	Y17	
Acriflavinium chloride	T49.0	X44	X64	Y14	Y56.0
Acrinol	T49.0	X44	X64	Y14	Y56.0
Acrivastine	T45.0	X44	X64	Y14	Y43.0
Acrolein (gas)	T59.8	X47	X67	Y17	
– liquid	T54.1	X49	X69	Y19	
Acrylamide	T65.8	X49	X69	Y19	
Acrylic resin	T49.3	X44	X64	Y14	Y56.3
Acrylonitrile	T65.8	X49	X69	Y19	
ACTH	T38.8	X44	X64	Y14	Y42.8
Actinomycin C	T45.1	X44	X64	Y14	Y43.3
Actinomycin D	T45.1	X44	X64	Y14	Y43.3
Activated charcoal	T47.6	X44	X64	Y14	Y53.6
Acyclovir	T37.5	X44	X64	Y14	Y41.5
Adenine	T45.2	X44	X64	Y14	Y57.7
– arabinoside	T37.5	X44	X64	Y14	Y41.5
Adhesive NEC	T65.8	X49	X69	Y19	
Adicillin	T36.0	X44	X64	Y14	Y40.0
Adiphenine	T44.3	X43	X63	Y13	Y51.3
Adipiodone	T50.8	X44	X64	Y14	Y57.5
Adrenaline	T44.5	X43	X63	Y13	Y51.5
Adrenergic NEC	T44.9	X43	X63	Y13	Y51.9
– blocking agent NEC	T44.8	X43	X63	Y13	Y51.8
– – beta, heart	T44.7	X43	X63	Y13	Y51.7
– specified NEC	T44.9	X43	X63	Y13	Y51.9

Substance	Chapter XIX	Accidental	Poisoning Intentional self-harm	Undetermined intent	Adverse effect in therapeutic use
Adrenochrome					
– (mono) semicarbazone	T46.9	X44	X64	Y14	Y52.9
– derivative	T46.9	X44	X64	Y14	Y52.9
Adrenocorticotrophic hormone	T38.8	X44	X64	Y14	Y42.8
Adrenocorticotrophin	T38.8	X44	X64	Y14	Y42.8
– long-acting	T38.8	X44	X64	Y14	Y42.8
Adriamycin	T45.1	X44	X64	Y14	Y43.3
Aerosol spray NEC	T65.9	X49	X69	Y19	
Aflatoxin	T64	X49	X69	Y19	
Afloqualone	T42.8	X41	X61	Y11	Y46.8
Agar	T47.4	X44	X64	Y14	Y53.4
Agonist					
– predominantly					
– – Alpha-adrenoreceptor	T44.4	X43	X63	Y13	Y51.4
– – Beta-adrenoreceptor	T44.5	X43	X63	Y13	Y51.5
AHLG	T50.9	X44	X64	Y14	Y59.3
Air contaminant(s), source or type not specified	T65.9	X49	X69	Y19	
Ajmaline	T46.2	X44	X64	Y14	Y52.2
Akritoin	T37.8	X44	X64	Y14	Y41.8
Alacepril	T46.4	X44	X64	Y14	Y52.4
Albendazole	T37.4	X44	X64	Y14	
Albumin					
– bovine	T45.8	X44	X64	Y14	Y44.6
– human serum	T45.8	X44	X64	Y14	Y44.6
– – salt-poor	T45.8	X44	X64	Y14	Y44.6
– normal human serum	T45.8	X44	X64	Y14	Y44.6
Albuterol	T48.6	X44	X64	Y14	Y55.6
Albutoin	T42.0	X41	X61	Y11	Y46.2
Alclofenac	T39.3	X40	X60	Y10	Y45.3
Alclometasone	T49.0	X44	X64	Y14	Y56.0
Alcohol	T51.9	X45	X65	Y15	
– absolute	T51.0	X45	X65	Y15	
– allyl	T51.8	X45	X65	Y15	
– amyl	T51.3	X45	X65	Y15	
– beverage	T51.0	X45	X65	Y15	
– butyl	T51.3	X45	X65	Y15	
– dehydrated	T51.0	X45	X65	Y15	
– denatured	T51.0	X45	X65	Y15	
– deterrent NEC	T50.6	X44	X64	Y14	Y57.3
– ethyl	T51.0	X45	X65	Y15	
– grain	T51.0	X45	X65	Y15	
– industrial	T51.0	X45	X65	Y15	
– isopropyl	T51.2	X45	X65	Y15	
– methyl	T51.1	X45	X65	Y15	
– propyl	T51.3	X45	X65	Y15	
– rubbing	T51.2	X45	X65	Y15	
– surgical	T51.0	X45	X65	Y15	
– vapor (from any type of alcohol)	T59.8	X47	X67	Y17	
– wood	T51.1	X45	X65	Y15	
Alcuronium (chloride)	T48.1	X44	X64	Y14	Y55.1

Substance	Chapter XIX	Poisoning Accidental	Intentional self-harm	Undetermined intent	Adverse effect in therapeutic use
Aldesulfone sodium	T37.1	X44	X64	Y14	Y41.1
Aldicarb	T60.0	X48	X68	Y18	
Aldosterone	T50.0	X44	X64	Y14	Y54.0
Aldrin (dust)	T60.1	X48	X68	Y18	
Alexitol sodium	T47.1	X44	X64	Y14	Y53.1
Alfacalcidol	T45.2	X44	X64	Y14	Y54.7
Alfadolone	T41.1	X44	X64	Y14	Y48.1
Alfaxalone	T41.1	X44	X64	Y14	Y48.1
Alfentanil	T40.4	X42	X62	Y12	Y45.0
Alfuzosin (hydrochloride)	T44.8	X43	X63	Y13	Y51.8
Algeldrate	T47.1	X44	X64	Y14	Y53.1
Algin	T47.8	X44	X64	Y14	Y53.8
Alglucerase	T45.3	X44	X64	Y14	Y43.6
Alimemazine	T43.3	X41	X61	Y11	Y49.3
Alizapride	T45.0	X44	X64	Y14	Y43.0
Alkali (caustic)	T54.3	X49	X69	Y19	
Alkalizing agent NEC	T50.9	X44	X64	Y14	Y43.5
Alkonium (bromide)	T49.0	X44	X64	Y14	Y56.0
Alkylating drug NEC	T45.1	X44	X64	Y14	Y43.3
− antimyeloproliferative	T45.1	X44	X64	Y14	Y43.3
− lymphatic	T45.1	X44	X64	Y14	Y43.3
Alkylisocyanate	T65.0	X49	X69	Y19	
Allantoin	T49.4	X44	X64	Y14	Y56.4
Allethrin	T49.0	X48	X68	Y18	Y56.0
Allobarbital	T42.3	X41	X61	Y11	Y47.0
Allopurinol	T50.4	X44	X64	Y14	Y54.8
Allyl					
− alcohol	T51.8	X45	X65	Y15	
− disulfide	T46.6	X44	X64	Y14	Y52.6
Allylestrenol	T38.5	X44	X64	Y14	Y42.5
Allylthiourea	T49.3	X44	X64	Y14	Y56.3
Allypropymal	T42.3	X41	X61	Y11	Y47.0
Almagate	T47.1	X44	X64	Y14	Y53.1
Almasilate	T47.1	X44	X64	Y14	Y53.1
Alminoprofen	T39.3	X40	X60	Y10	Y45.2
Almitrine	T50.7	X44	X64	Y14	Y50.0
Aloes	T47.2	X44	X64	Y14	Y53.2
Aloglutamol	T47.1	X44	X64	Y14	Y53.1
Aloin	T47.2	X44	X64	Y14	Y53.2
Aloxiprin	T39.0	X40	X60	Y10	Y45.1
Alpha					
− acetyldigoxin	T46.0	X44	X64	Y14	Y52.0
− amylase	T45.3	X44	X64	Y14	Y43.6
− tocoferol(acetate)	T45.2	X44	X64	Y14	Y57.7
Alpha-adrenergic blocking drug	T44.6	X43	X63	Y13	Y51.6
Alphadolone	T41.1	X44	X64	Y14	Y48.1
Alphaprodine	T40.4	X42	X62	Y12	Y45.0
Alphaxalone	T41.1	X44	X64	Y14	Y48.1
Alprazolam	T42.4	X41	X61	Y11	Y47.1
Alprenolol	T44.7	X43	X63	Y13	Y51.7
Alprostadil	T46.7	X44	X64	Y14	Y52.7

Substance		Poisoning			Adverse effect in therapeutic use
	Chapter XIX	Accidental	Intentional self-harm	Undetermined intent	
Alsactide	T38.8	X44	X64	Y14	Y42.8
Alseroxylon	T46.5	X44	X64	Y14	Y52.5
Alteplase	T45.6	X44	X64	Y14	Y44.5
Altizide	T50.2	X44	X64	Y14	Y54.3
Altretamine	T45.1	X44	X64	Y14	Y43.3
Alum (medicinal)	T49.4	X44	X64	Y14	Y56.4
– nonmedicinal (ammonium) (potassium)	T56.8	X49	X69	Y19	
Alumin(i)um					
– acetate	T49.2	X44	X64	Y14	Y56.2
– – solution	T49.0	X44	X64	Y14	Y56.0
– bis (acetylsalicylate)	T39.0	X40	X60	Y10	Y45.1
– carbonate (gel, basic)	T47.1	X44	X64	Y14	Y53.1
– chlorhydroxide-complex	T47.1	X44	X64	Y14	Y53.1
– chloride	T49.2	X44	X64	Y14	Y56.2
– clofibrate	T46.6	X44	X64	Y14	Y52.6
– diacetate	T49.2	X44	X64	Y14	Y56.2
– glycinate	T47.1	X44	X64	Y14	Y53.1
– hydroxide (gel)	T47.1	X44	X64	Y14	Y53.1
– hydroxide-magnesium carb. gel	T47.1	X44	X64	Y14	Y53.1
– magnesium silicate	T47.1	X44	X64	Y14	Y53.1
– nicotinate	T46.7	X44	X64	Y14	Y52.7
– phosphate	T47.1	X44	X64	Y14	Y53.1
– salicylate	T39.0	X40	X60	Y10	Y45.1
– silicate	T47.1	X44	X64	Y14	Y53.1
– sodium silicate	T47.1	X44	X64	Y14	Y53.1
– sulfate	T49.0	X44	X64	Y14	Y56.0
– tannate	T47.6	X44	X64	Y14	Y53.6
Alverine	T44.3	X43	X63	Y13	Y51.3
Amanitine	T62.0	X49	X69	Y19	
Amantadine	T42.8	X41	X61	Y11	Y46.7
Ambazone	T49.6	X44	X64	Y14	Y56.6
Ambenonium (chloride)	T44.0	X43	X63	Y13	Y51.0
Ambroxol	T48.4	X44	X64	Y14	Y55.4
Ambuphylline	T48.6	X44	X64	Y14	Y55.6
Amcinonide	T49.0	X44	X64	Y14	Y56.0
Amdinocilline	T36.0	X44	X64	Y14	Y40.0
Ametazole	T50.8	X44	X64	Y14	Y57.6
Amethocaine	T41.3	X44	X64	Y14	Y48.3
– regional	T41.3	X44	X64	Y14	Y48.3
– spinal	T41.3	X44	X64	Y14	Y48.3
Amezinium metilsulfate	T44.9	X43	X63	Y13	Y51.9
Amfebutamone	T43.2	X41	X61	Y11	Y49.2
Amfenac	T39.3	X40	X60	Y10	Y45.3
Amfepramone	T50.5	X44	X64	Y14	Y57.0
Amfetamine	T43.6	X41	X61	Y11	Y49.7
Amfetaminil	T43.6	X41	X61	Y11	Y49.7
Amfomycin	T36.8	X44	X64	Y14	Y40.8
Amidefrine mesilate	T48.5	X44	X64	Y14	Y55.5
Amidone	T40.3	X42	X62	Y12	Y45.0
Amidopyrine	T39.2	X40	X60	Y10	Y45.8

721

Substance	Chapter XIX	Poisoning			Adverse effect in therapeutic use
		Accidental	Intentional self-harm	Undetermined intent	
Amidotrizoate	T50.8	X44	X64	Y14	Y57.5
Amiflamine	T43.1	X41	X61	Y11	Y49.1
Amikacin	T36.5	X44	X64	Y14	Y40.5
Amikhelline	T46.3	X44	X64	Y14	Y52.3
Amiloride	T50.2	X44	X64	Y14	Y54.5
Aminaphtone	T45.5	X44	X64	Y14	Y44.2
Amineptine	T43.0	X41	X61	Y11	Y49.0
Aminoacetic acid (derivatives)	T50.3	X44	X64	Y14	Y54.6
Aminoacridine	T49.0	X44	X64	Y14	Y56.0
Aminobenzoic acid (-p)	T49.3	X44	X64	Y14	Y56.3
4-Aminobutyric acid	T43.8	X41	X61	Y11	Y49.8
Aminocaproic acid	T45.6	X44	X64	Y14	Y44.3
Aminofenazone	T39.2	X40	X60	Y10	Y45.8
Aminoglutethimide	T45.1	X44	X64	Y14	Y43.3
Aminoglycoside	T36.5	X44	X64	Y14	Y40.5
Aminohippuric acid	T50.8	X44	X64	Y14	Y57.6
Aminomethylbenzoic acid	T45.6	X44	X64	Y14	Y44.3
Aminometradine	T50.2	X44	X64	Y14	Y54.5
Aminophenazone	T39.2	X40	X60	Y10	Y45.8
Aminophenol	T54.0	X49	X69	Y19	
4-Aminophenol derivatives	T39.1	X40	X60	Y10	Y45.5
Aminophylline	T48.6	X44	X64	Y14	Y55.6
Aminopterin sodium	T45.1	X44	X64	Y14	Y43.1
Aminopyrine	T39.2	X40	X60	Y10	Y45.8
8-Aminoquinoline drugs	T37.2	X44	X64	Y14	Y41.2
Aminorex	T50.5	X44	X64	Y14	Y57.0
Aminosalicylic acid	T37.1	X44	X64	Y14	Y41.1
Aminosalylum	T37.1	X44	X64	Y14	Y41.1
Amiodarone	T46.2	X44	X64	Y14	Y52.2
Amiphenazole	T50.7	X44	X64	Y14	Y50.0
Amisulpride	T43.5	X41	X61	Y11	Y49.5
Amitriptyline	T43.0	X41	X61	Y11	Y49.0
Amitriptylinoxide	T43.0	X41	X61	Y11	Y49.0
Amlexanox	T48.6	X44	X64	Y14	Y55.6
Ammonia (fumes) (gas) (vapor)	T59.8	X47	X67	Y17	
– aromatic spirit	T48.7	X44	X64	Y14	Y55.7
– liquid (household)	T54.3	X49	X69	Y19	
Ammoniated mercury	T49.0	X44	X64	Y14	Y56.0
Ammonium					
– acid tartrate	T49.5	X44	X64	Y14	Y56.5
– bromide	T42.6	X41	X61	Y11	Y47.4
– chloride	T50.9	X44	X64	Y14	Y43.5
– compounds (household) NEC	T54.3	X49	X69	Y19	
– – fumes (any usage)	T59.8	X47	X67	Y17	
– – industrial	T54.3	X49	X69	Y19	
– sulfamate	T60.3	X48	X68	Y18	
– sulfonate resin	T47.8	X44	X64	Y14	Y53.8
Amobarbital (sodium)	T42.3	X41	X61	Y11	Y47.0
Amodiaquine	T37.2	X44	X64	Y14	Y41.2
Amoxapine	T43.0	X41	X61	Y11	Y49.0
Amoxicillin	T36.0	X44	X64	Y14	Y40.0

Substance	Chapter XIX	Poisoning			Adverse effect in therapeutic use
		Accidental	Intentional self-harm	Undetermined intent	
Amperozide	T43.5	X41	X61	Y11	Y49.5
Amphetamine NEC	T43.6	X41	X61	Y11	Y49.7
Amphotalide	T37.4	X44	X64	Y14	Y41.4
Amphotericin B	T36.7	X44	X64	Y14	Y40.7
Ampicillin	T36.0	X44	X64	Y14	Y40.0
Amsacrine	T45.1	X44	X64	Y14	Y43.3
Amygdaline	T62.2	X49	X69	Y19	
Amyl					
– acetate	T52.8	X46	X66	Y16	
– – vapor	T59.8	X47	X67	Y17	
– alcohol	T51.3	X45	X65	Y15	
– chloride	T53.6	X46	X66	Y16	
– formate	T52.8	X46	X66	Y16	
– nitrite	T46.3	X44	X64	Y14	Y52.3
– propionate	T65.8	X49	X69	Y19	
Amylase	T47.5	X44	X64	Y14	Y53.5
Amyleine, regional	T41.3	X44	X64	Y14	Y48.3
Amylene					
– dichloride	T53.6	X46	X66	Y16	
– hydrate	T51.3	X45	X65	Y15	
Amylmetacresol	T49.6	X44	X64	Y14	Y56.6
Amylobarbitone	T42.3	X41	X61	Y11	Y47.0
Amylocaine, regional	T41.3	X44	X64	Y14	Y48.3
Amylopectin	T47.6	X44	X64	Y14	Y53.6
Anabolic steroid	T38.7	X44	X64	Y14	Y42.7
Analeptic NEC	T50.7	X44	X64	Y14	Y50.0
Analgesic NEC	T39.8	X40	X60	Y10	Y45.8
– anti-inflammatory NEC	T39.9	X40	X60	Y10	Y45.9
– – propionic acid derivative	T39.3	X40	X60	Y10	Y45.2
– antirheumatic NEC	T39.9	X40	X60	Y10	Y45.9
– aromatic NEC	T39.1	X40	X60	Y10	Y45.5
– narcotic NEC	T40.6	X42	X62	Y12	Y45.0
– – combination	T40.6	X42	X62	Y12	Y45.0
– – obstetric	T40.6	X42	X62	Y12	Y45.0
– non-narcotic NEC	T39.9	X40	X60	Y10	Y45.9
– – combination	T39.9	X40	X60	Y10	Y45.9
– nonopioid	T39.9	X40	X60	Y10	Y45.9
– pyrazole	T39.2	X40	X60	Y10	Y45.8
Analgin	T39.2	X40	X60	Y10	Y45.8
Ancrod	T45.6	X44	X64	Y14	Y44.9
Androgen	T38.7	X44	X64	Y14	Y42.7
Androgen-estrogen mixture	T38.7	X44	X64	Y14	Y42.7
Androstanolone	T38.7	X44	X64	Y14	Y42.7
Anesthesia					
– caudal	T41.3	X44	X64	Y14	Y48.3
– endotracheal	T41.0	X44	X64	Y14	Y48.0
– epidural	T41.3	X44	X64	Y14	Y48.3
– inhalation	T41.0	X44	X64	Y14	Y48.0
– local	T41.3	X44	X64	Y14	Y48.3
– mucosal	T41.3	X44	X64	Y14	Y48.3
– muscle relaxation	T48.1	X44	X64	Y14	Y55.1

Substance	Chapter XIX	Poisoning Accidental	Poisoning Intentional self-harm	Poisoning Undetermined intent	Adverse effect in therapeutic use
Anesthesia					
– nerve blocking	T41.3	X44	X64	Y14	Y48.3
– plexus blocking	T41.3	X44	X64	Y14	Y48.3
– potentiated	T41.2	X44	X64	Y14	Y48.2
– rectal	T41.2	X44	X64	Y14	Y48.2
– regional	T41.3	X44	X64	Y14	Y48.3
– surface	T41.3	X44	X64	Y14	Y48.3
Anesthetic NEC (see also Anesthesia)	T41.4	X44	X64	Y14	Y48.4
– with muscle relaxant	T41.2	X44	X64	Y14	Y48.2
– gaseous NEC	T41.0	X44	X64	Y14	Y48.0
– general NEC	T41.2	X44	X64	Y14	Y48.2
– infiltration NEC	T41.3	X44	X64	Y14	Y48.3
– inhaled	T41.0	X44	X64	Y14	Y48.0
– intravenous NEC	T41.1	X44	X64	Y14	Y48.1
– local NEC	T41.3	X44	X64	Y14	Y48.3
– rectal	T41.2	X44	X64	Y14	Y48.2
– regional NEC	T41.3	X44	X64	Y14	Y48.3
– spinal NEC	T41.3	X44	X64	Y14	Y48.3
– thiobarbiturate	T41.1	X44	X64	Y14	Y48.1
Aneurine	T45.2	X44	X64	Y14	Y57.7
Angiotensinamide	T44.9	X43	X63	Y13	Y51.9
Anileridine	T40.4	X42	X62	Y12	Y45.0
Aniline (dye) (liquid)	T65.3	X49	X69	Y19	
Anise oil	T47.5	X44	X64	Y14	Y53.5
Anisidine	T65.3	X49	X69	Y19	
Anisindione	T45.5	X44	X64	Y14	Y44.2
Anisotropine methylbromide	T44.3	X43	X63	Y13	Y51.3
Anistreplase	T45.6	X44	X64	Y14	Y44.5
Anorexiant (central)	T50.5	X44	X64	Y14	Y57.0
Ansamycin	T36.6	X44	X64	Y14	Y40.6
Ant poison – see Insecticide					
Antacid NEC	T47.1	X44	X64	Y14	Y53.1
Antagonist					
– Alpha-adrenoreceptor NEC	T44.6	X43	X63	Y13	Y51.6
– Beta-adrenoreceptor NEC	T44.7	X43	X63	Y13	Y51.7
– aldosterone	T50.0	X44	X64	Y14	Y54.1
– anticoagulant	T45.7	X44	X64	Y14	Y44.3
– extrapyramidal NEC	T44.3	X43	X63	Y13	Y51.3
– folic acid	T45.1	X44	X64	Y14	Y43.1
– heavy metal	T45.8	X44	X64	Y14	Y43.8
– H₂ receptor	T47.0	X44	X64	Y14	Y53.1
– narcotic analgesic	T50.7	X44	X64	Y14	Y50.1
– opiate	T50.7	X44	X64	Y14	Y50.1
– pyrimidine	T45.1	X44	X64	Y14	Y43.1
– serotonin	T46.5	X44	X64	Y14	Y52.5
Antazolin(e)	T45.0	X44	X64	Y14	Y43.0
Anterior pituitary hormone NEC	T38.8	X44	X64	Y14	Y42.8
Anthelminthic NEC	T37.4	X44	X64	Y14	Y41.4
Anthiolimine	T37.4	X44	X64	Y14	Y41.4
Anthralin	T49.4	X44	X64	Y14	Y56.4

| Substance | Chapter XIX | Poisoning | | | Adverse effect in therapeutic use |
		Accidental	Intentional self-harm	Undetermined intent	
Antiadrenergic NEC	T44.8	X43	X63	Y13	Y51.8
Antiandrogen NEC	T38.6	X44	X64	Y14	Y42.6
Antiallergic NEC	T45.0	X44	X64	Y14	Y43.0
Anti-anemic (drug) (preparation)	T45.8	X44	X64	Y14	Y44.9
Antianxiety drug NEC	T43.5	X41	X61	Y11	Y47.9
Antiarteriosclerotic drug	T46.6	X44	X64	Y14	Y52.6
Antiasthmatic drug NEC	T48.6	X44	X64	Y14	Y55.6
Antibiotic NEC	T36.9	X44	X64	Y14	Y40.9
– aminoglycoside	T36.5	X44	X64	Y14	Y40.5
– anticancer	T45.1	X44	X64	Y14	Y43.3
– antifungal	T36.7	X44	X64	Y14	Y40.7
– antineoplastic	T45.1	X44	X64	Y14	Y43.3
– ENT	T49.6	X44	X64	Y14	Y56.6
– eye	T49.5	X44	X64	Y14	Y56.5
– fungicidal (local)	T49.0	X44	X64	Y14	Y56.0
– intestinal	T36.8	X44	X64	Y14	Y40.8
– Beta-lactam NEC	T36.1	X44	X64	Y14	Y40.1
– local	T49.0	X44	X64	Y14	Y56.0
– polypeptide	T36.8	X44	X64	Y14	Y40.8
– specified NEC	T36.8	X44	X64	Y14	Y40.8
– throat	T49.6	X44	X64	Y14	Y56.6
Anticholesterolemic drug NEC	T46.6	X44	X64	Y14	Y52.6
Anticholinergic NEC	T44.3	X43	X63	Y13	Y51.3
Anticholinesterase	T44.0	X43	X63	Y13	Y51.0
– organophosphorus	T44.0	X43	X63	Y13	Y51.0
Anticoagulant NEC	T45.5	X44	X64	Y14	Y44.2
– antagonist	T45.7	X44	X64	Y14	Y44.3
Anti-common-cold drug NEC	T48.5	X44	X64	Y14	Y55.5
Anticonvulsant NEC	T42.6	X41	X61	Y11	Y46.6
– barbiturate	T42.3	X41	X61	Y11	Y47.0
– combination (with barbiturate)	T42.3	X41	X61	Y11	Y47.0
– deoxybarbiturates	T42.3	X41	X61	Y11	Y46.3
– hydantoin	T42.0	X41	X61	Y11	Y46.2
– hypnotic NEC	T42.6	X41	X61	Y11	Y47.8
– oxazolidinedione	T42.2	X41	X61	Y11	Y46.1
– pyrimidinedione	T42.6	X41	X61	Y11	Y46.6
– succinimide	T42.2	X41	X61	Y11	Y46.0
Anti-D immunoglobulin (human)	T50.9	X44	X64	Y14	Y59.3
Antidepressant NEC	T43.2	X41	X61	Y11	Y49.2
– monoamine-oxidase-inhibitor	T43.1	X41	X61	Y11	Y49.1
– triazolpyridine	T43.2	X41	X61	Y11	Y49.2
– tricyclic or tetracyclic	T43.0	X41	X61	Y11	Y49.0
Antidiabetic NEC	T38.3	X44	X64	Y14	Y42.3
– biguanide	T38.3	X44	X64	Y14	Y42.3
– – and sulfonyl combined	T38.3	X44	X64	Y14	Y42.3
– combined	T38.3	X44	X64	Y14	Y42.3
– sulfonylurea	T38.3	X44	X64	Y14	Y42.3
Antidiarrheal drug NEC	T47.6	X44	X64	Y14	Y53.6
– absorbent	T47.6	X44	X64	Y14	Y53.6
Antidiphtheria serum	T50.9	X44	X64	Y14	Y59.3
Antidiuretic hormone	T38.8	X44	X64	Y14	Y42.8

Substance	Chapter XIX	Poisoning Accidental	Intentional self-harm	Undetermined intent	Adverse effect in therapeutic use
Antidote NEC	T50.6	X44	X64	Y14	Y57.2
– heavy metal	T45.8	X44	X64	Y14	Y43.8
Antidysrhythmic NEC	T46.2	X44	X64	Y14	Y52.2
Antiemetic drug	T45.0	X44	X64	Y14	Y43.0
Antiepiletic	T42.7	X41	X61	Y11	Y46.6
– mixed NEC	T42.5	X41	X61	Y11	Y46.6
– specified NEC	T42.6	X41	X61	Y11	Y46.6
Antiestrogen NEC	T38.6	X44	X64	Y14	Y42.6
Antifertility pill	T38.4	X44	X64	Y14	Y42.4
Antifibrinolytic drug	T45.6	X44	X64	Y14	Y44.3
Antifilarial drug	T37.4	X44	X64	Y14	Y41.4
Antiflatulent	T47.5	X44	X64	Y14	Y53.5
Antifreeze	T65.9	X49	X69	Y19	
– ethylene glycol	T51.8	X45	X65	Y15	
Antifungal					
– antibiotic (systemic)	T36.7	X44	X64	Y14	Y40.7
– anti-infective NEC	T37.9	X44	X64	Y14	Y41.9
– disinfectant, local	T49.0	X44	X64	Y14	Y56.0
– nonmedicinal (spray)	T60.3	X48	X68	Y18	
Anti-gastric-secretion drug NEC	T47.1	X44	X64	Y14	Y53.1
Antigonadotrophin NEC	T38.6	X44	X64	Y14	Y42.6
Antihallucinogen	T43.5	X41	X61	Y11	Y49.5
Antihemophilic					
– factor	T45.8	X44	X64	Y14	Y44.6
– fraction	T45.8	X44	X64	Y14	Y44.6
– globulin concentrate	T45.7	X44	X64	Y14	Y44.3
– human plasma	T45.8	X44	X64	Y14	Y44.6
– plasma, dried	T45.7	X44	X64	Y14	Y44.3
Antihemorrhoidal preparation	T49.2	X44	X64	Y14	Y56.2
Antiheparin drug	T45.7	X44	X64	Y14	Y44.3
Antihookworm drug	T37.4	X44	X64	Y14	Y41.4
Anti-human lymphocytic globulin	T50.9	X44	X64	Y14	Y59.3
Antihyperlipidemic drug	T46.6	X44	X64	Y14	Y52.6
Antihypertensive drug NEC	T46.5	X44	X64	Y14	Y52.5
Anti-infective NEC	T37.9	X44	X64	Y14	Y41.9
– bismuth, local	T49.0	X44	X64	Y14	Y56.0
– ENT	T49.6	X44	X64	Y14	Y56.6
– eye NEC	T49.5	X44	X64	Y14	Y56.5
– local NEC	T49.0	X44	X64	Y14	Y56.0
– – specified NEC	T49.0	X44	X64	Y14	Y56.0
– mixed	T37.9	X44	X64	Y14	Y41.9
Anti-inflammatory drug, NEC	T39.3	X40	X60	Y10	Y45.9
– local	T49.0	X44	X64	Y14	Y56.0
– nonsteroidal NEC	T39.3	X40	X60	Y10	Y45.3
– specified NEC	T39.3	X40	X60	Y10	Y45.8
Antikaluretic	T50.3	X44	X64	Y14	Y54.6
Antiknock (tetraethyl lead)	T56.0	X49	X69	Y19	
Antilipemic drug NEC	T46.6	X44	X64	Y14	Y52.6

| Substance | Chapter XIX | Poisoning | | | Adverse effect in therapeutic use |
		Accidental	Intentional self-harm	Undetermined intent	
Antimalarial	T37.2	X44	X64	Y14	Y41.2
– prophylactic NEC	T37.2	X44	X64	Y14	Y41.2
– pyrimidine derivative	T37.2	X44	X64	Y14	Y41.2
Antimetabolite	T45.1	X44	X64	Y14	Y43.1
Antimitotic agent	T45.1	X44	X64	Y14	Y43.3
Antimony (compounds) (vapor) NEC	T56.8	X49	X69	Y19	
– dimercaptosuccinate	T37.3	X44	X64	Y14	Y41.3
– hydride	T56.8	X49	X69	Y19	
– pesticide (vapor)	T60.8	X48	X68	Y18	
– potassium (sodium) tartrate	T37.8	X44	X64	Y14	Y41.8
– sodium dimercaptosuccinate	T37.3	X44	X64	Y14	Y41.3
Antimuscarinic NEC	T44.3	X43	X63	Y13	Y51.3
Antimycobacterial drug NEC	T37.1	X44	X64	Y14	Y41.1
– combination	T37.1	X44	X64	Y14	Y41.1
Antinausea drug	T45.0	X44	X64	Y14	Y43.0
Antinematode drug	T37.4	X44	X64	Y14	Y41.4
Antineoplastic NEC	T45.1	X44	X64	Y14	Y43.3
– alkaloidal	T45.1	X44	X64	Y14	Y43.2
– combination	T45.1	X44	X64	Y14	Y43.3
– – estrogen	T38.5	X44	X64	Y14	Y42.5
– steroid	T38.7	X44	X64	Y14	Y42.7
Antiparasitic drug (systemic)	T37.9	X44	X64	Y14	Y41.9
– local	T49.0	X44	X64	Y14	Y56.0
– specified NEC	T37.8	X44	X64	Y14	Y41.8
Antiparkinsonism drug NEC	T42.8	X41	X61	Y11	Y46.7
Antiperspirant NEC	T49.2	X44	X64	Y14	Y56.2
Antiphlogistic NEC	T39.4	X40	X60	Y10	Y45.4
Antiplatyhelminthic drug	T37.4	X44	X64	Y14	Y41.4
Antiprotozoal drug NEC	T37.3	X44	X64	Y14	Y41.3
– local	T49.0	X44	X64	Y14	Y56.0
Antipruritic drug NEC	T49.1	X44	X64	Y14	Y56.1
Antipsychotic drug NEC	T43.5	X41	X61	Y11	Y49.5
– phenothiazine	T43.3	X41	X61	Y11	Y49.3
Antipyretic NEC	T39.8	X40	X60	Y10	Y45.8
Antipyrine	T39.2	X40	X60	Y10	Y45.8
Antirabies hyperimmune serum	T50.9	X44	X64	Y14	Y59.3
Antirheumatic NEC	T39.4	X40	X60	Y10	Y45.4
Antirigidity drug NEC	T42.8	X41	X61	Y11	Y46.8
Antischistosomal drug	T37.4	X44	X64	Y14	Y41.4
Antiscorpion sera	T50.9	X44	X64	Y14	Y59.3
Antitapeworm drug	T37.4	X44	X64	Y14	Y41.4
Antitetanus immunoglobulin	T50.9	X44	X64	Y14	Y59.3
Antithyroid drug NEC	T38.2	X44	X64	Y14	Y42.2
Antitoxin					
– diphtheria	T50.9	X44	X64	Y14	Y59.3
– gas gangrene	T50.9	X44	X64	Y14	Y59.3
– tetanus	T50.9	X44	X64	Y14	Y59.3
Antitrichomonal drug	T37.3	X44	X64	Y14	Y41.3

Substance	Chapter XIX	Poisoning			Adverse effect in therapeutic use
		Accidental	Intentional self-harm	Undetermined intent	
Antitussive NEC	T48.3	X44	X64	Y14	Y55.3
– codeine mixture	T40.2	X42	X62	Y12	Y45.0
– opiate	T40.2	X42	X62	Y12	Y45.0
Antivaricose drug	T46.8	X44	X64	Y14	Y52.8
Antivenin, antivenom (sera)	T50.9	X44	X64	Y14	Y59.3
– crotaline	T50.9	X44	X64	Y14	Y59.3
– spider bite	T50.9	X44	X64	Y14	Y59.3
Antivertigo drug	T45.0	X44	X64	Y14	Y43.0
Antiviral drug NEC	T37.5	X44	X64	Y14	Y41.5
– eye	T49.5	X44	X64	Y14	Y56.5
Antiwhipworm drug	T37.4	X44	X64	Y14	Y41.4
Antrafenine	T39.3	X40	X60	Y10	Y45.3
ANTU (alpha naphthylthiourea)	T60.4	X48	X68	Y18	
Apalcillin	T36.0	X44	X64	Y14	Y40.0
APC	T48.5	X44	X64	Y14	Y55.5
Aplonidine	T44.4	X43	X63	Y13	Y51.4
Apomorphine	T47.7	X44	X64	Y14	Y53.7
Apraclonidine (hydrochloride)	T44.4	X43	X63	Y13	Y51.4
Aprindine	T46.2	X44	X64	Y14	Y52.2
Aprobarbital	T42.3	X41	X61	Y11	Y47.0
Aprotinin	T45.6	X44	X64	Y14	Y44.3
Aptocaine	T41.3	X44	X64	Y14	Y48.3
Aqua fortis	T54.2	X49	X69	Y19	
Ara-A	T37.5	X44	X64	Y14	Y41.5
Ara-C	T45.1	X44	X64	Y14	Y43.1
Arachis oil	T49.3	X44	X64	Y14	Y56.3
Arecoline	T44.1	X43	X63	Y13	Y51.1
Arginine	T50.9	X44	X64	Y14	Y57.1
– glutamate	T50.9	X44	X64	Y14	Y57.1
Arsenate of lead	T57.0	X48	X68	Y18	
Arsenic, arsenicals (compounds) (dust) (vapor) NEC	T57.0	X48	X68	Y18	
Arsine (gas)	T57.0	X49	X69	Y19	
Arsthinol	T37.3	X44	X64	Y14	Y41.3
Articaine	T41.3	X44	X64	Y14	Y48.3
Asbestos	T57.8	X49	X69	Y19	
Ascaridole	T37.4	X44	X64	Y14	Y41.4
Ascorbic acid	T45.2	X44	X64	Y14	Y57.7
Asparaginase	T45.1	X44	X64	Y14	Y43.3
Aspirin (aluminum) (soluble)	T39.0	X40	X60	Y10	Y45.1
Aspoxicillin	T36.0	X44	X64	Y14	Y40.0
Astemizole	T45.0	X44	X64	Y14	Y43.0
Astringent (local)	T49.2	X44	X64	Y14	Y56.2
– specified NEC	T49.2	X44	X64	Y14	Y56.2
Astromicin	T36.5	X44	X64	Y14	Y40.5
Ataractic drug NEC	T43.5	X41	X61	Y11	Y49.5
Atenolol	T44.7	X43	X63	Y13	Y51.7
Atracurium besilate	T48.1	X44	X64	Y14	Y55.1
Atropine	T44.3	X43	X63	Y13	Y51.3
– derivative	T44.3	X43	X63	Y13	Y51.3
– methonitrate	T44.3	X43	X63	Y13	Y51.3

Amoxyclav
Amoxycillin + Augmentin
Augmentin — Clavulanic Acid

Substance	Poisoning				Adverse effect in therapeutic use
	Chapter XIX	Accidental	Intentional self-harm	Undetermined intent	
Attapulgite	T47.6	X44	X64	Y14	Y53.6
Auramine	T65.8	X49	X69	Y19	
Auranofin	T39.4	X40	X60	Y10	Y45.4
Aurantiin	T46.9	X44	X64	Y14	Y52.9
Aurothioglucose	T39.4	X40	X60	Y10	Y45.4
Aurothioglycanide	T39.4	X40	X60	Y10	Y45.4
Aurothiomalate sodium	T39.4	X40	X60	Y10	Y45.4
Aurotioprol	T39.4	X40	X60	Y10	Y45.4
Autonomic nervous system agent NEC	T44.9	X43	X63	Y13	Y51.9
Axerophthol	T45.2	X44	X64	Y14	Y57.7
Azacitidine	T45.1	X44	X64	Y14	Y43.1
Azacyclonol	T43.5	X41	X61	Y11	Y49.5
Azadirachta	T60.2	X48	X68	Y18	
Azanidazole	T37.3	X44	X64	Y14	Y41.3
Azapetine	T46.7	X44	X64	Y14	Y52.7
Azapropazone	T39.2	X40	X60	Y10	Y45.3
Azaribine	T45.1	X44	X64	Y14	Y43.1
Azatadine	T45.0	X44	X64	Y14	Y43.0
Azatepa	T45.1	X44	X64	Y14	Y43.3
Azathioprine	T45.1	X44	X64	Y14	Y43.4
Azelaic acid	T49.0	X44	X64	Y14	Y56.0
Azelastine	T45.0	X44	X64	Y14	Y43.0
Azidocillin	T36.0	X44	X64	Y14	Y40.0
Azidothymidine	T37.5	X44	X64	Y14	Y41.5
Azinphos (ethyl) (methyl)	T60.0	X48	X68	Y18	
Aziridine (chelating)	T54.1	X49	X69	Y19	
Azithromycin	T36.3	X44	X64	Y14	Y40.3
Azlocillin	T36.0	X44	X64	Y14	Y40.0
Azobenzene smoke	T65.8	X48	X68	Y18	
AZT	T37.5	X44	X64	Y14	Y41.5
Aztreonam	T36.1	X44	X64	Y14	Y40.1
Azuresin	T50.8	X44	X64	Y14	Y57.6

B

Substance		Poisoning			Adverse effect in therapeutic use
	Chapter XIX	Accidental	Intentional self-harm	Undetermined intent	
Bacampicillin	T36.0	X44	X64	Y14	Y40.0
Bacillus					
− lactobacillus	T47.8	X44	X64	Y14	Y53.8
− subtilis	T47.6	X44	X64	Y14	Y53.6
Bacitracin zinc	T49.0	X44	X64	Y14	Y56.0
− with neomycin	T49.0	X44	X64	Y14	Y56.0
Baclofen	T42.8	X41	X61	Y11	Y46.8
BAL	T45.8	X44	X64	Y14	Y43.8
Bambuterol	T48.6	X44	X64	Y14	Y55.6
Bamethan (sulfate)	T46.7	X44	X64	Y14	Y52.7
Bamifylline	T48.6	X44	X64	Y14	Y55.6
Bamipine	T45.0	X44	X64	Y14	Y43.0
Barbexaclone	T42.6	X41	X61	Y11	Y46.6
Barbital	T42.3	X41	X61	Y11	Y47.0
− sodium	T42.3	X41	X61	Y11	Y47.0
Barbitone	T42.3	X41	X61	Y11	Y47.0
Barbiturate NEC	T42.3	X41	X61	Y11	Y47.0
− with tranquillizer	T42.3	X41	X61	Y11	Y47.0
Barium (carbonate) (chloride) (sulfite)	T57.8	X49	X69	Y19	
− pesticide	T60.4	X48	X68	Y18	
− sulfate (medicinal)	T50.8	X44	X64	Y14	Y57.5
Barrier cream	T49.3	X44	X64	Y14	Y56.3
Basic fuchsin	T49.0	X44	X64	Y14	Y56.0
Battery acid or fluid	T54.2	X49	X69	Y19	
Bay rum	T51.8	X45	X65	Y15	
BCG (vaccine)	T50.9	X44	X64	Y14	Y58.0
BCNU	T45.1	X44	X64	Y14	Y43.3
Beclamide	T42.6	X41	X61	Y11	Y46.6
Beclometasone	T44.5	X43	X63	Y13	Y51.5
Befunolol	T49.5	X44	X64	Y14	Y56.5
Bekanamycin	T36.5	X44	X64	Y14	Y40.5
Belladonna					
− alkaloids	T44.3	X43	X63	Y13	Y51.3
− extract	T44.3	X43	X63	Y13	Y51.3
− herb	T44.3	X43	X63	Y13	Y51.3
Bemegride	T50.7	X44	X64	Y14	Y50.0
Benactyzine	T44.3	X43	X63	Y13	Y51.3
Benaprizine	T44.3	X43	X63	Y13	Y51.3
Benazepril	T46.4	X44	X64	Y14	Y52.4
Bencyclane	T46.7	X44	X64	Y14	Y52.7
Bendazac	T39.3	X40	X60	Y10	Y45.3
Bendazol	T46.3	X44	X64	Y14	Y52.3
Bendrofluazide	T50.2	X44	X64	Y14	Y54.3

| Substance | Chapter XIX | Poisoning | | | Adverse effect in therapeutic use |
		Accidental	Intentional self-harm	Undetermined intent	
Bendroflumethiazide	T50.2	X44	X64	Y14	Y54.3
Benethamine penicillin	T36.0	X44	X64	Y14	Y40.0
Benexate	T47.1	X44	X64	Y14	Y53.1
Benfluorex	T46.6	X44	X64	Y14	Y52.6
Benfotiamine	T45.2	X44	X64	Y14	Y57.7
Benomyl	T60.0	X48	X68	Y18	
Benorilate	T39.0	X40	X60	Y10	Y45.1
Benoxinate	T41.3	X44	X64	Y14	Y48.3
Benperidol	T43.4	X41	X61	Y11	Y49.4
Benproperine	T48.3	X44	X64	Y14	Y55.3
Benserazide	T42.8	X41	X61	Y11	Y46.7
Bentazepam	T42.4	X41	X61	Y11	Y47.1
Bentiromide	T50.8	X44	X64	Y14	Y57.6
Bentonite	T49.3	X44	X64	Y14	Y56.3
Benzalbutyramide	T46.6	X44	X64	Y14	Y52.6
Benzalkonium (chloride)	T49.0	X44	X64	Y14	Y56.0
Benzamine	T41.3	X44	X64	Y14	Y48.3
– lactate	T49.1	X44	X64	Y14	Y56.1
Benzamphetamine	T50.5	X44	X64	Y14	Y57.0
Benzapril hydrochloride	T46.5	X44	X64	Y14	Y52.5
Benzathine benzylpenicillin	T36.0	X44	X64	Y14	Y40.0
Benzatropine	T42.8	X41	X61	Y11	Y46.7
Benzbromarone	T50.4	X44	X64	Y14	Y54.8
Benzenamine	T65.3	X49	X69	Y19	
Benzene	T52.1	X46	X66	Y16	
– homologues (acetyl) (dimethyl) (methyl)(solvent)	T52.2	X46	X66	Y16	
Benzethonium (chloride)	T49.0	X44	X64	Y14	Y56.0
Benzfetamine	T50.5	X44	X64	Y14	Y57.0
Benzhexol	T44.3	X43	X63	Y13	Y51.3
Benzhydramine (chloride)	T45.0	X44	X64	Y14	Y43.0
Benzidine	T65.8	X49	·X69	Y19	
Benzilonium bromide	T44.3	X43	X63	Y13	Y51.3
Benzimidazole	T60.3	X48	X68	Y18	
Benzin(e) – see Ligroin					
Benziodarone	T46.3	X44	X64	Y14	Y52.3
Benznidazole	T37.3	X44	X64	Y14	Y41.3
Benzocaine	T41.3	X44	X64	Y14	Y48.3
Benzoctamine	T43.0	X41	X61	Y11	Y49.0
Benzodiazepine NEC	T42.4	X41	X61	Y11	Y47.1
Benzoic acid	T49.0	X44	X64	Y14	Y56.0
– with salicylic acid	T49.0	X44	X64	Y14	Y56.0
Benzoin (tincture)	T48.5	X44	X64	Y14	Y55.5
Benzol (benzene)	T52.1	X46	X66	Y16	
– vapor	T52.0	X46	X66	Y16	
Benzonatate	T48.3	X44	X64	Y14	Y55.3
Benzophenones	T49.3	X44	X64	Y14	Y56.3
Benzopyrone	T46.9	X44	X64	Y14	Y52.9
Benzothiadiazide	T50.2	X44	X64	Y14	Y54.3
Benzoxonium chloride	T49.0	X44	X64	Y14	Y56.0
Benzoyl peroxide	T49.0	X44	X64	Y14	Y56.0

Bisphosphonates   Y54.7

Substance	Chapter XIX	Poisoning			Adverse effect in therapeutic use
		Accidental	Intentional self-harm	Undetermined intent	
Benzoylpas calcium	T37.1	X44	X64	Y14	Y41.1
Benzperidin	T43.5	X41	X61	Y11	Y49.5
Benzphetamine	T50.5	X44	X64	Y14	Y57.0
Benzpyrinium bromide	T44.1	X43	X63	Y13	Y51.1
Benzquinamide	T45.0	X44	X64	Y14	Y43.0
Benzthiazide	T50.2	X44	X64	Y14	Y54.3
Benztropine					
– anticholinergic	T44.3	X43	X63	Y13	Y51.3
– antiparkinson	T42.8	X41	X61	Y11	Y46.7
Benzydamine	T49.0	X44	X64	Y14	Y56.0
Benzyl					
– acetate	T52.8	X46	X66	Y16	
– alcohol	T49.0	X44	X64	Y14	Y56.0
– benzoate	T49.0	X44	X64	Y14	Y56.0
– benzoic acid	T49.0	X44	X64	Y14	Y56.0
– nicotinate	T46.6	X44	X64	Y14	Y52.6
– penicillin	T36.0	X44	X64	Y14	Y40.0
Benzylhydrochlorthiazide	T50.2	X44	X64	Y14	Y54.3
Benzylpenicillin	T36.0	X44	X64	Y14	Y40.0
Benzylthiouracil	T38.2	X44	X64	Y14	Y42.2
Bephenium hydroxynaphthoate	T37.4	X44	X64	Y14	Y41.4
Bepridil	T46.1	X44	X64	Y14	Y52.1
Bergamot oil	T65.8	X49	X69	Y19	
Bergapten	T50.9	X44	X64	Y14	Y57.8
Berries, poisonous	T62.1	X49	X69	Y19	
Beryllium (compounds)	T56.7	X49	X69	Y19	
Beta-acetyldigoxin	T46.0	X44	X64	Y14	Y52.0
Beta-adrenergic blocking agent, heart	T44.7	X43	X63	Y13	Y51.7
Beta-benzalbutyramide	T46.6	X44	X64	Y14	Y52.6
Betacarotene	T45.2	X44	X64	Y14	Y57.7
Beta-eucaine	T49.1	X44	X64	Y14	Y56.1
Beta-galactosidase	T47.5	X44	X64	Y14	Y53.5
Betahistine	T46.7	X44	X64	Y14	Y52.7
Betaine	T47.5	X44	X64	Y14	Y53.5
Betamethasone	T49.0	X44	X64	Y14	Y56.0
Betamicin	T36.8	X44	X64	Y14	Y40.8
Betanidine	T46.5	X44	X64	Y14	Y52.5
Beta-sitosterol(s)	T46.6	X44	X64	Y14	Y52.6
Betaxolol	T44.7	X43	X63	Y13	Y51.7
Betazole	T50.8	X44	X64	Y14	Y57.6
Bethanechol	T44.1	X43	X63	Y13	Y51.1
– chloride	T44.1	X43	X63	Y13	Y51.1
Bethanidine	T46.5	X44	X64	Y14	Y52.5
Betoxycaine	T41.3	X44	X64	Y14	Y48.3
Bevantolol	T44.7	X43	X63	Y13	Y51.7
Bevonium metilsulfate	T44.3	X43	X63	Y13	Y51.3
Bezafibrate	T46.6	X44	X64	Y14	Y52.6
Bezitramide	T40.4	X42	X62	Y12	Y45.0
BHA	T50.9	X44	X64	Y14	Y57.4
Bhang	T40.7	X42	X62	Y12	Y49.6

Substance	Chapter XIX	Accidental	Poisoning Intentional self-harm	Undetermined intent	Adverse effect in therapeutic use
BHC (medicinal)	T49.0	X44	X64	Y14	Y56.0
– nonmedicinal (vapor)	T53.6	X46	X66	Y16	
Bialamicol	T37.3	X44	X64	Y14	Y41.3
Bibenzonium bromide	T48.3	X44	X64	Y14	Y55.3
Bibrocathol	T49.5	X44	X64	Y14	Y56.5
Bichromates (calcium) (potassium) (sodium)(crystals)	T57.8	X49	X69	Y19	
Biclotymol	T49.6	X44	X64	Y14	Y56.6
Bicucculine	T50.7	X44	X64	Y14	Y50.0
Bifemelane	T43.2	X41	X61	Y11	Y49.2
Bile salts	T47.5	X44	X64	Y14	Y53.5
Binifibrate	T46.6	X44	X64	Y14	Y52.6
Binitrobenzol	T65.3	X46	X66	Y16	
Bioflavonoid(s)	T46.9	X44	X64	Y14	Y52.9
Biological substance NEC	T50.9	X44	X64	Y14	Y59.9
Biotin	T45.2	X44	X64	Y14	Y57.7
Biperiden	T44.3	X43	X63	Y13	Y51.3
Bisacodyl	T47.2	X44	X64	Y14	Y53.2
Bisbentiamine	T45.2	X44	X64	Y14	Y57.7
Bisbutiamine	T45.2	X44	X64	Y14	Y57.7
Bisdequalinium (salts) (diacetate)	T49.6	X44	X64	Y14	Y56.6
Bishydroxycoumarin	T45.5	X44	X64	Y14	Y44.2
Bismuth salts	T47.6	X44	X64	Y14	Y53.6
– aluminate	T47.1	X44	X64	Y14	Y53.1
– formic iodide	T49.0	X44	X64	Y14	Y56.0
– glycolylarsenate	T49.0	X44	X64	Y14	Y56.0
– nonmedicinal (compounds) NEC	T65.9	X49	X69	Y19	
– subcarbonate	T47.6	X44	X64	Y14	Y53.6
– subsalicylate	T37.8	X44	X64	Y14	Y41.8
Bisoprolol	T44.7	X43	X63	Y13	Y51.7
Bisoxatin	T47.2	X44	X64	Y14	Y53.2
Bisulepin (hydrochloride)	T45.0	X44	X64	Y14	Y43.0
Bithionol	T37.8	X44	X64	Y14	Y41.8
Bitolterol	T48.6	X44	X64	Y14	Y55.6
Bitoscanate	T37.4	X44	X64	Y14	Y41.4
Bitter almond oil	T62.8	X49	X69	Y19	
Bittersweet	T62.2	X49	X69	Y19	
Blast furnace gas (carbon monoxide from)	T58	X47	X67	Y17	
Bleach	T54.9	X49	X69	Y19	
Bleaching agent (medicinal)	T49.4	X44	X64	Y14	Y56.4
Bleomycin	T45.1	X44	X64	Y14	Y43.3
Blockers, calcium-channel	T46.1	X44	X64	Y14	Y52.1
Blood	T45.8	X44	X64	Y14	Y44.6
– dried	T45.8	X44	X64	Y14	Y44.6
– drug affecting NEC	T45.9	X44	X64	Y14	Y44.9
– expander NEC	T45.8	X44	X64	Y14	Y44.7
– fraction NEC	T45.8	X44	X64	Y14	Y44.6
Bone meal	T62.8	X49	X69	Y19	
Bopindolol	T44.7	X43	X63	Y13	Y51.7
Borane complex	T57.8	X49	X69	Y19	

| Substance | Chapter XIX | Poisoning | | | Adverse effect in therapeutic use |
		Accidental	Intentional self-harm	Undetermined intent	
Borate(s)	T57.8	X49	X69	Y19	
− buffer	T50.9	X44	X64	Y14	Y57 4
− cleanser	T55	X49	X69	Y19	
− sodium	T57.8	X49	X69	Y19	
Borax (cleanser)	T55	X49	X69	Y19	
Bordeaux mixture	T60.3	X48	X68	Y18	
Boric acid	T49.0	X44	X64	Y14	Y56.0
Bornaprine	T44.3	X43	X63	Y13	Y51.3
Boron	T57.8	X49	X69	Y19	
− hydride NEC	T57.8	X49	X69	Y19	
− − fumes or gas	T57.8	X47	X67	Y17	
− trifluoride	T59.8	X47	X67	Y17	
Botulinus antitoxin (type A, B)	T50.9	X44	X64	Y14	Y59.3
Brallobarbital	T42.3	X41	X61	Y11	Y47.0
Bran (wheat)	T47.4	X44	X64	Y14	Y53.4
Brass (fumes)	T56.8	X49	X69	Y19	
Bretylium tosilate	T46.2	X44	X64	Y14	Y52.2
Brinase	T45.3	X44	X64	Y14	Y43.6
Brodifacoum	T60.4	X48	X68	Y18	
Bromazepam	T42.4	X41	X61	Y11	Y47.1
Bromazine	T45.0	X44	X64	Y14	Y43.0
Brombenzylcyanide	T59.3	X47	X67	Y17	
Bromelains	T45.3	X44	X64	Y14	Y43.6
Bromethalin	T60.4	X48	X68	Y18	
Bromhexine	T48.4	X44	X64	Y14	Y55.4
Bromide salts	T42.6	X41	X61	Y11	Y47.4
Bromindione	T45.5	X44	X64	Y14	Y44.2
Bromine					
− sedative	T42.6	X41	X61	Y11	Y47.4
− vapor	T59.8	X47	X67	Y17	
Bromisoval	T42.6	X41	X61	Y11	Y47.4
Bromobenzylcyanide	T59.3	X47	X67	Y17	
Bromochlorosalicylanilide	T49.0	X44	X64	Y14	Y56.0
Bromocriptine	T42.8	X41	X61	Y11	Y46.7
Bromodiphenhydramine	T45.0	X44	X64	Y14	Y43.0
Bromoform	T42.6	X41	X61	Y11	Y47.4
Bromopride	T47.8	X44	X64	Y14	Y53.8
Bromosalicylchloranitide	T49.0	X44	X64	Y14	Y56.0
Bromoxynil	T60.3	X48	X68	Y18	
Bromperidol	T43.4	X41	X61	Y11	Y49.4
Brompheniramine	T45.0	X44	X64	Y14	Y43.0
Bromsulfophthalein	T50.8	X44	X64	Y14	Y57.6
Bromvaletone	T42.6	X41	X61	Y11	Y47.4
Bronchodilator NEC	T48.6	X44	X64	Y14	Y55.6
Brotizolam	T42.4	X41	X61	Y11	Y47.1
Brovincamine	T46.7	X44	X64	Y14	Y52.7
Broxaterol	T48.6	X44	X64	Y14	Y55.6
Broxuridine	T45.1	X44	X64	Y14	Y43.1
Broxyquinoline	T37.8	X44	X64	Y14	Y41.8
Bruceine	T48.2	X44	X64	Y14	Y55.2
Brucine	T65.1	X49	X69	Y19	

Substance	Chapter XIX	Poisoning			Adverse effect in therapeutic use
		Accidental	Intentional self-harm	Undetermined intent	
Brunswick green – *see* Copper					
Bryonia	T47.2	X44	X64	Y14	Y53.2
Buclizine	T45.0	X44	X64	Y14	Y43.0
Buclosamide	T49.0	X44	X64	Y14	Y56.0
Bucolome	T39.3	X40	X60	Y10	Y45.3
Budesonide	T44.5	X43	X63	Y13	Y51.5
Budralazine	T46.5	X44	X64	Y14	Y52.5
Bufexamac	T39.3	X40	X60	Y10	Y45.3
Buflomedil	T46.7	X44	X64	Y14	Y52.7
Buformin	T38.3	X44	X64	Y14	Y42.3
Bufrolin	T48.6	X44	X64	Y14	Y55.6
Bufylline	T48.6	X44	X64	Y14	Y55.6
Bulk filler	T50.5	X44	X64	Y14	Y57.0
– cathartic	T47.4	X44	X64	Y14	Y53.4
Bumadizone	T39.3	X40	X60	Y10	Y45.3
Bumetanide	T50.1	X44	X64	Y14	Y54.4
Bunaftine	T46.2	X44	X64	Y14	Y52.2
Bunamiodyl	T50.8	X44	X64	Y14	Y57.5
Bunazosin	T44.6	X43	X63	Y13	Y51.6
Bunitrolol	T44.7	X43	X63	Y13	Y51.7
Buphenine	T46.7	X44	X64	Y14	Y52.7
Bupivacaine	T41.3	X44	X64	Y14	Y48.3
– spinal	T41.3	X44	X64	Y14	Y48.3
Bupranolol	T44.7	X43	X63	Y13	Y51.7
Buprenorphine	T40.4	X42	X62	Y12	Y45.0
Bupropion	T43.2	X41	X61	Y11	Y49.2
Burimamide	T47.1	X44	X64	Y14	Y53.1
Buserelin	T38.8	X44	X64	Y14	Y42.8
Buspirone	T43.5	X41	X61	Y11	Y49.5
Busulfan, busulphan	T45.1	X44	X64	Y14	Y43.3
Butacaine	T41.3	X44	X64	Y14	Y48.3
Butalamine	T46.7	X44	X64	Y14	Y52.7
Butalbital	T42.3	X41	X61	Y11	Y47.0
Butamben	T41.3	X44	X64	Y14	Y48.3
Butamirate	T48.3	X44	X64	Y14	Y55.3
Butane (distributed in mobile container)	T59.8	X47	X67	Y17	
– distributed through pipes	T59.8	X47	X67	Y17	
– incomplete combustion	T58	X47	X67	Y17	
Butanilicaine	T41.3	X44	X64	Y14	Y48.3
Butanol	T51.3	X45	X65	Y15	
Butanone, 2-butanone	T52.4	X46	X66	Y16	
Butantrone	T49.4	X44	X64	Y14	Y56.4
Butaperazine	T43.3	X41	X61	Y11	Y49.3
Butetamate	T48.6	X44	X64	Y14	Y55.6
Butethal	T42.3	X41	X61	Y11	Y47.0
Butizide	T50.2	X44	X64	Y14	Y54.3
Butobarbital	T42.3	X41	X61	Y11	Y47.0
– sodium	T42.3	X41	X61	Y11	Y47.0
Butobarbitone	T42.3	X41	X61	Y11	Y47.0
Butoconazole (nitrate)	T49.0	X44	X64	Y14	Y56.0

Substance		Poisoning			Adverse effect in therapeutic use
	Chapter XIX	Accidental	Intentional self-harm	Undetermined intent	
Butorphanol	T40.4	X42	X62	Y12	Y45.0
Butriptyline	T43.0	X41	X61	Y11	Y49.0
Butropium bromide	T44.3	X43	X63	Y13	Y51.3
Butyl					
– acetate (secondary)	T52.8	X46	X66	Y16	
– alcohol	T51.3	X45	X65	Y15	
– aminobenzoate	T41.3	X44	X64	Y14	Y48.3
– butyrate	T52.8	X46	X66	Y16	
– carbinol	T51.3	X45	X65	Y15	
– carbitol	T52.3	X46	X66	Y16	
– cellosolve	T52.3	X46	X66	Y16	
– formate	T52.8	X46	X66	Y16	
– lactate	T52.8	X46	X66	Y16	
– propionate	T52.8	X46	X66	Y16	
– scopolamine bromide	T44.3	X43	X63	Y13	Y51.3
– thiobarbital sodium	T41.1	X44	X64	Y14	Y48.1
Butylated hydroxyanisole	T50.9	X44	X64	Y14	Y57.4
Butylchloral hydrate	T42.6	X41	X61	Y11	Y47.2
Butyltoluene	T52.2	X46	X66	Y16	

C

Substance	Chapter XIX	Poisoning			Adverse effect in therapeutic use
		Accidental	Intentional self-harm	Undetermined intent	
Cabergoline	T42.8	X41	X61	Y11	Y46.7
Cacodyl, cacodylic acid	T57.0	X48	X68	Y18	
Cactinomycin	T45.1	X44	X64	Y14	Y43.3
Cadexomer iodine	T49.0	X44	X64	Y14	Y56.0
Cadmium (chloride) (fumes) (oxide)	T56.3	X49	X69	Y19	
Cadralazine	T46.5	X44	X64	Y14	Y52.5
Caffeine	T43.6	X41	X61	Y11	Y50.2
Calamine (lotion)	T49.3	X44	X64	Y14	Y56.3
Calcifediol	T45.2	X44	X64	Y14	Y54.7
Calciferol	T45.2	X44	X64	Y14	Y54.7
Calcitonin	T50.9	X44	X64	Y14	Y54.7
Calcitriol	T45.2	X44	X64	Y14	Y54.7
Calcium					
– actylsalicylate	T39.0	X40	X60	Y10	Y45.1
– benzamidosalicylate	T37.1	X44	X64	Y14	Y41.1
– bromide	T42.6	X41	X61	Y11	Y47.4
– bromolactobionate	T42.6	X41	X61	Y11	Y47.4
– carbaspirin	T39.0	X40	X60	Y10	Y45.1
– carbimide	T50.6	X44	X64	Y14	Y57.3
– carbonate	T47.1	X44	X64	Y14	Y53.1
– chloride	T50.9	X44	X64	Y14	Y54.9
– – anhydrous	T50.9	X44	X64	Y14	Y54.9
– cyanide	T57.8	X48	X68	Y18	
– disodium edetate	T45.8	X44	X64	Y14	Y43.8
– dobesilate	T46.9	X44	X64	Y14	Y52.9
– ferrous citrate	T45.4	X44	X64	Y14	Y44.0
– folinate	T45.8	X44	X64	Y14	Y44.1
– glubionate	T50.3	X44	X64	Y14	Y54.6
– gluconate	T50.3	X44	X64	Y14	Y54.6
– gluconogalactogluconate	T50.3	X44	X64	Y14	Y54.6
– hydrate, hydroxide	T54.3	X49	X69	Y19	
– hypochlorite	T37.8	X44	X64	Y14	Y41.8
– iodide	T48.4	X44	X64	Y14	Y55.4
– iopodate	T50.8	X44	X64	Y14	Y57.5
– lactate	T50.3	X44	X64	Y14	Y54.6
– leucovorin	T45.8	X44	X64	Y14	Y44.1
– oxide	T54.3	X49	X69	Y19	
– pantothenate	T45.2	X44	X64	Y14	Y57.7
– phosphate	T50.3	X44	X64	Y14	Y54.6
– salicylate	T39.0	X40	X60	Y10	Y45.1
– salts	T50.3	X44	X64	Y14	Y54.9
Calculus-dissolving drug	T50.9	X44	X64	Y14	Y57.8
Calomel	T49.0	X44	X64	Y14	Y56.0
Caloric agent	T50.3	X44	X64	Y14	Y54.6

| Substance | Chapter XIX | Poisoning | | | Adverse effect in therapeutic use |
		Accidental	Intentional self-harm	Undetermined intent	
Calusterone	T38.7	X44	X64	Y14	Y42.7
Camazepam	T42.4	X41	X61	Y11	Y47.1
Camomile	T49.0	X44	X64	Y14	Y56.0
Camphor					
− insecticide	T60.2	X48	X68	Y18	
− medicinal	T49.8	X44	X64	Y14	Y56.8
Camylofin	T44.3	X43	X63	Y13	Y51.3
Cancer chemotherapy drug regimen	T45.1	X44	X64	Y14	Y43.3
Candicidin	T49.0	X44	X64	Y14	Y56.0
Cannabinol	T40.7	X42	X62	Y12	Y49.6
Cannabis (derivatives)	T40.7	X42	X62	Y12	Y49.6
Canrenoic acid	T50.0	X44	X64	Y14	Y54.1
Canrenone	T50.0	X44	X64	Y14	Y54.1
Canthaxanthin	T50.9	X44	X64	Y14	Y57.8
Capillary-active drug NEC	T46.9	X44	X64	Y14	Y52.9
Capreomycin	T36.8	X44	X64	Y14	Y40.8
Capsicum	T49.4	X44	X64	Y14	Y56.4
Captafol	T60.3	X48	X68	Y18	
Captan	T60.3	X48	X68	Y18	
Captopril	T46.4	X44	X64	Y14	Y52.4
Caramiphen	T44.3	X43	X63	Y13	Y51.3
Carazolol	T44.7	X43	X63	Y13	Y51.7
Carbachol	T44.1	X43	X63	Y13	Y51.1
Carbacrylamine (resin)	T50.3	X44	X64	Y14	Y54.6
Carbamate (insecticide)	T60.0	X48	X68	Y18	
Carbamazepine	T42.1	X41	X61	Y11	Y46.4
Carbamide	T47.3	X44	X64	Y14	Y53.3
− peroxide	T49.0	X44	X64	Y14	Y56.0
Carbaril	T60.0	X48	X68	Y18	
Carbarsone	T37.3	X44	X64	Y14	Y41.3
Carbaryl	T60.0	X48	X68	Y18	
Carbasalate calcium	T39.0	X40	X60	Y10	Y45.1
Carbazochrome (salicylate) (sodium sulfonate)	T49.4	X44	X64	Y14	Y56.4
Carbenicillin	T36.0	X44	X64	Y14	Y40.0
Carbenoxolone	T47.1	X44	X64	Y14	Y53.1
Carbetapentane	T48.3	X44	X64	Y14	Y55.3
Carbethyl salicylate	T39.0	X40	X60	Y10	Y45.1
Carbidopa (with levodopa)	T42.8	X41	X61	Y11	Y46.7
Carbimazole	T38.2	X44	X64	Y14	Y42.2
Carbinol	T51.1	X45	X65	Y15	
Carbinoxamine	T45.0	X44	X64	Y14	Y43.0
Carbiphene	T39.8	X40	X60	Y10	Y45.8
Carbitol	T52.3	X46	X66	Y16	
Carbo medicinalis	T47.6	X44	X64	Y14	Y53.6
Carbocisteine	T48.4	X44	X64	Y14	Y55.4
Carbocromen	T46.3	X44	X64	Y14	Y52.3
Carbol fuchsin	T49.0	X44	X64	Y14	Y56.0
Carbolic acid (see also Phenol)	T54.0	X49	X69	Y19	
Carbolonium (bromide)	T48.1	X44	X64	Y14	Y55.1

Substance	Chapter XIX	Accidental	Poisoning Intentional self-harm	Undetermined intent	Adverse effect in therapeutic use
Carbon					
– bisulfide (liquid)	T65.4	X49	X69	Y19	
– – vapor	T65.4	X47	X67	Y17	
– dioxide (gas)	T59.7	X47	X67	Y17	
– – medicinal	T41.5	X44	X64	Y14	Y48.5
– – nonmedicinal	T59.7	X47	X67	Y17	
– – snow	T49.4	X44	X64	Y14	Y56.4
– disulfide (liquid)	T65.4	X49	X69	Y19	
– – vapor	T65.4	X47	X67	Y17	
– monoxide (from incomplete combustion)	T58	X47	X67	Y17	
– tetrachloride (vapor) NEC	T53.0	X46	X66	Y16	
– – liquid (cleansing agent) NEC	T53.0	X46	X66	Y16	
– – solvent	T53.0	X46	X66	Y16	
Carbonic acid gas	T59.7	X47	X67	Y17	
– anhydrase inhibitor NEC	T50.2	X44	X64	Y14	Y54.2
Carbophenothion	T60.0	X48	X68	Y18	
Carboplatin	T45.1	X44	X64	Y14	Y43.3
Carboprost	T48.0	X44	X64	Y14	Y55.0
Carboquone	T45.1	X44	X64	Y14	Y43.3
Carboxymethylcellulose	T47.4	X44	X64	Y14	Y53.4
S-Carboxymethylcysteine	T48.4	X44	X64	Y14	Y55.4
Carbromal	T42.6	X41	X61	Y11	Y47.4
Carbutamide	T38.3	X44	X64	Y14	Y42.3
Carbuterol	T48.6	X44	X64	Y14	Y55.6
Cardiac rhythm regulator NEC	T46.2	X44	X64	Y14	Y52.2
– specified NEC	T46.2	X44	X64	Y14	Y52.2
Cardiotonic (glycoside) NEC	T46.0	X44	X64	Y14	Y52.0
Cardiovascular drug NEC	T46.9	X44	X64	Y14	Y52.9
Carfecillin	T36.0	X44	X64	Y14	Y40.0
Carfenazine	T43.3	X43	X63	Y13	Y49.3
Carindacillin	T36.0	X44	X64	Y14	Y40.0
Carisoprodol	T42.8	X41	X61	Y11	Y46.8
Carmellose	T47.4	X44	X64	Y14	Y53.4
Carminative	T47.5	X44	X64	Y14	Y53.5
Carmofur	T45.1	X44	X64	Y14	Y43.1
Carmustine	T45.1	X44	X64	Y14	Y43.3
Carotene	T45.2	X44	X64	Y14	Y57.7
Carphenazine	T43.3	X41	X61	Y11	Y49.3
Carpipramine	T42.4	X41	X61	Y11	Y47.1
Carprofen	T39.3	X40	X60	Y10	Y45.3
Carpronium chloride	T44.3	X43	X63	Y13	Y51.3
Carrageenan	T47.8	X44	X64	Y14	Y53.8
Carteolol	T44.7	X43	X63	Y13	Y51.7
Cascara (sagrada)	T47.2	X44	X64	Y14	Y53.2
Castor					
– bean	T62.2	X49	X69	Y19	
– oil	T47.2	X44	X64	Y14	Y53.2
Catalase	T45.3	X44	X64	Y14	Y43.6
Catha (tea)	T43.6	X41	X61	Y11	Y49.7

Substance	Chapter XIX	Poisoning Accidental	Intentional self-harm	Undetermined intent	Adverse effect in therapeutic use
Cathartic NEC	T47.4	X44	X64	Y14	Y53.4
– anthacene derivative	T47.2	X44	X64	Y14	Y53.2
– bulk	T47.4	X44	X64	Y14	Y53.4
– emollient NEC	T47.4	X44	X64	Y14	Y53.4
– irritant NEC	T47.2	X44	X64	Y14	Y53.2
mucilage	T47.4	X44	X64	Y14	Y53.4
– vegetable	T47.2	X44	X64	Y14	Y53.2
Cathine	T50.5	X44	X64	Y14	Y57.0
Cation exchange resin	T50.3	X44	X64	Y14	Y54.6
Caustic(s) NEC	T54.9	X49	X69	Y19	
– alkali	T54.3	X49	X69	Y19	
– hydroxide	T54.3	X49	X69	Y19	
– potash	T54.3	X49	X69	Y19	
– soda	T54.3	X49	X69	Y19	
Cefacetrile	T36.1	X44	X64	Y14	Y40.1
Cefaclor	T36.1	X44	X64	Y14	Y40.1
Cefadroxil	T36.1	X44	X64	Y14	Y40.1
Cefalexin	T36.1	X44	X64	Y14	Y40.1
Cefaloglycin	T36.1	X44	X64	Y14	Y40.1
Cefaloridine	T36.1	X44	X64	Y14	Y40.1
Cefalosporins	T36.1	X44	X64	Y14	Y40.1
Cefalotin	T36.1	X44	X64	Y14	Y40.1
Cefamandole	T36.1	X44	X64	Y14	Y40.1
Cefamycin antibiotic	T36.1	X44	X64	Y14	Y40.1
Cefapirin	T36.1	X44	X64	Y14	Y40.1
Cefatrizine	T36.1	X44	X64	Y14	Y40.1
Cefazedone	T36.1	X44	X64	Y14	Y40.1
Cefazolin	T36.1	X44	X64	Y14	Y40.1
Cefbuperazone	T36.1	X44	X64	Y14	Y40.1
Cefetamet	T36.1	X44	X64	Y14	Y40.1
Cefixime	T36.1	X44	X64	Y14	Y40.1
Cefmenoxime	T36.1	X44	X64	Y14	Y40.1
Cefmetazole	T36.1	X44	X64	Y14	Y40.1
Cefminox	T36.1	X44	X64	Y14	Y40.1
Cefonicid	T36.1	X44	X64	Y14	Y40.1
Cefoperazone	T36.1	X44	X64	Y14	Y40.1
Ceforanide	T36.1	X44	X64	Y14	Y40.1
Cefotaxime	T36.1	X44	X64	Y14	Y40.1
Cefotetan	T36.1	X44	X64	Y14	Y40.1
Cefotiam	T36.1	X44	X64	Y14	Y40.1
Cefoxitin	T36.1	X44	X64	Y14	Y40.1
Cefpimizole	T36.1	X44	X64	Y14	Y40.1
Cefpiramide	T36.1	X44	X64	Y14	Y40.1
Cefradine	T36.1	X44	X64	Y14	Y40.1
Cefroxadine	T36.1	X44	X64	Y14	Y40.1
Cefsulodin	T36.1	X44	X64	Y14	Y40.1
Ceftazidime	T36.1	X44	X64	Y14	Y40.1
Cefteram	T36.1	X44	X64	Y14	Y40.1
Ceftezole	T36.1	X44	X64	Y14	Y40.1
Ceftizoxime	T36.1	X44	X64	Y14	Y40.1
Ceftriaxone	T36.1	X44	X64	Y14	Y40.1

Substance	Chapter XIX	Accidental	Poisoning Intentional self-harm	Undetermined intent	Adverse effect in therapeutic use
Cefuroxime	T36.1	X44	X64	Y14	Y40.1
Cefuzonam	T36.1	X44	X64	Y14	Y40.1
Celiprolol	T44.7	X43	X63	Y13	Y51.7
Cellulose					
– cathartic	T47.4	X44	X64	Y14	Y53.4
– hydroxyethyl	T47.4	X44	X64	Y14	Y53.4
– oxidized	T49.4	X44	X64	Y14	Y56.4
Cephaloridine	T36.1	X44	X64	Y14	Y40.1
Cephalosporins	T36.1	X44	X64	Y14	Y40.1
Cephalothin	T36.1	X44	X64	Y14	Y40.1
Cephalotin	T36.1	X44	X64	Y14	Y40.1
Cephradine	T36.1	X44	X64	Y14	Y40.1
Cerium oxalate	T45.0	X44	X64	Y14	Y43.0
Cerous oxalate	T45.0	X44	X64	Y14	Y43.0
Ceruletide	T50.8	X44	X64	Y14	Y57.6
Cetalkonium (chloride)	T49.0	X44	X64	Y14	Y56.0
Cethexonium chloride	T49.0	X44	X64	Y14	Y56.0
Cetiedil	T46.7	X44	X64	Y14	Y52.7
Cetirizine	T45.0	X44	X64	Y14	Y43.0
Cetomacrogol	T50.9	X44	X64	Y14	Y57.4
Cetotiamine	T45.2	X44	X64	Y14	Y57.7
Cetraxate	T47.1	X44	X64	Y14	Y53.1
Cetrimide	T49.0	X44	X64	Y14	Y56.0
Cetrimonium (bromide)	T49.0	X44	X64	Y14	Y56.0
Cetylpyridinium chloride	T49.0	X44	X64	Y14	Y56.0
Chamomile	T49.0	X44	X64	Y14	Y56.0
Ch'an su	T46.0	X44	X64	Y14	Y52.0
Charcoal	T47.6	X44	X64	Y14	Y53.6
– activated	T47.6	X44	X64	Y14	Y53.6
– fumes (carbon monoxide)	T58	X47	X67	Y17	
– – industrial	T58	X47	X67	Y17	
Chaulmosulfone	T37.1	X44	X64	Y14	Y41.1
Chelating agent NEC	T50.6	X44	X64	Y14	Y57.2
Chemical substance NEC	T65.9	X49	X69	Y19	
Chenodeoxycholic acid	T47.5	X44	X64	Y14	Y53.5
Chenodiol	T47.5	X44	X64	Y14	Y53.5
Chenopodium	T37.4	X44	X64	Y14	Y41.4
Chinidin(e)	T46.2	X44	X64	Y14	Y52.2
Chiniofon	T37.8	X44	X64	Y14	Y41.8
Chlophedianol	T48.3	X44	X64	Y14	Y55.3
Chloral	T42.6	X41	X61	Y11	Y47.2
– derivative	T42.6	X41	X61	Y11	Y47.2
– hydrate	T42.6	X41	X61	Y11	Y47.2
Chloralodol	T42.6	X41	X61	Y11	Y47.2
Chloralose	T60.4	X48	X68	Y18	
Chlorambucil	T45.1	X44	X64	Y14	Y43.3
Chloramine (-T)	T49.8	X44	X64	Y14	Y56.8
Chloramphenicol	T36.2	X44	X64	Y14	Y40.2
Chloramphenicolum	T36.2	X44	X64	Y14	Y40.2
Chlorate (potassium) (sodium) NEC	T60.3	X48	X68	Y18	
– herbicide	T60.3	X48	X68	Y18	

Substance	Chapter XIX	Poisoning			Adverse effect in therapeutic use
		Accidental	Intentional self-harm	Undetermined intent	
Chlorazanil	T50.2	X44	X64	Y14	Y54.5
Chlorbenzene, chlorbenzol	T53.7	X46	X66	Y16	
Chlorbenzoxamine	T44.3	X43	X63	Y13	Y51.3
Chlorbutol	T42.6	X41	X61	Y11	Y47.2
Chlorcyclizine	T45.0	X44	X64	Y14	Y43.0
Chlordan(e) (dust)	T60.1	X48	X68	Y18	
Chlordiazepoxide	T42.4	X41	X61	Y11	Y47.1
Chlordiethyl benzamide	T49.3	X44	X64	Y14	Y56.3
Chlorethyl – *see* Ethyl chloride					
Chlorfenvinphos	T60.0	X48	X68	Y18	
Chlorhexamide	T45.1	X44	X64	Y14	Y43.3
Chlorhexidine	T49.0	X44	X64	Y14	Y56.0
Chlorimipramine	T43.0	X41	X61	Y11	Y49.0
Chlorinated					
– camphene	T53.6	X48	X68	Y18	
– diphenyl	T53.7	X49	X69	Y19	
– hydrocarbons NEC	T53.9	X48	X68	Y18	
– – solvents	T53.9	X46	X66	Y16	
– lime (bleach)	T54.3	X49	X69	Y19	
– – and boric acid solution	T49.0	X44	X64	Y14	Y56.0
– naphthalene	T60.1	X48	X68	Y18	
– pesticide NEC	T60.8	X48	X68	Y18	
– soda – *see also* Sodium hypochlorite					
– – solution	T49.0	X44	X64	Y14	Y56.0
Chlorine (fumes) (gas)	T59.4	X47	X67	Y17	
– bleach	T54.3	X49	X69	Y19	
– compound gas NEC	T59.4	X47	X67	Y17	
– disinfectant	T59.4	X47	X67	Y17	
– releasing agents NEC	T59.4	X47	X67	Y17	
Chlorisondamine chloride	T46.9	X44	X64	Y14	Y52.9
Chlormadinone	T38.5	X44	X64	Y14	Y42.5
Chlormephos	T60.0	X48	X68	Y18	
Chlormerodrin	T50.2	X44	X64	Y14	Y54.5
Chlormethiazole	T42.6	X41	X61	Y11	Y47.8
Chlormethine	T45.1	X44	X64	Y14	Y43.3
Chlormezanone	T42.6	X41	X61	Y11	Y47.8
Chloroacetic acid	T60.3	X48	X68	Y18	
Chloroacetone	T59.3	X47	X67	Y17	
Chloroacetophenone	T59.3	X47	X67	Y17	
Chloroaniline	T53.7	X49	X69	Y19	
Chlorobenzene, chlorobenzol	T53.7	X46	X66	Y16	
Chlorobromomethane (fire extinguisher)	T53.6	X46	X66	Y16	
Chlorobutanol	T42.6	X41	X61	Y11	Y47.2
Chlorocresol	T49.0	X44	X64	Y14	Y56.0
Chlorodehydromethyltestosterone	T38.7	X44	X64	Y14	Y42.7
Chlorodinitrobenzene	T53.7	X46	X66	Y16	
– dust or vapor	T53.7	X47	X67	Y17	
Chlorodiphenyl	T53.7	X49	X69	Y19	
Chloroethane – *see* Ethyl chloride					

Substance	Chapter XIX	Accidental	Poisoning Intentional self-harm	Undetermined intent	Adverse effect in therapeutic use
Chloroethylene	T53.6	X46	X66	Y16	
Chlorofluorocarbons	T53.5	X46	X66	Y16	
Chloroform (fumes) (vapor)	T53.1	X46	X66	Y16	
– anesthetic	T41.0	X44	X64	Y14	Y48.0
– solvent	T53.1	X46	X66	Y16	
– water, concentrated	T41.0	X44	X64	Y14	Y48.0
Chloronitrobenzene	T53.7	X49	X69	Y19	
– dust or vapor	T53.7	X46	X66	Y16	
Chlorophacinone	T60.4	X48	X68	Y18	
Chlorophenol	T53.7	X46	X66	Y16	
Chlorophenothane	T60.1	X48	X68	Y18	
Chlorophyll	T50.9	X44	X64	Y14	Y57.4
Chloropicrin (fumes)	T53.6	X46	X66	Y16	
– pesticide	T60.8	X48	X68	Y18	
Chloroprocaine	T41.3	X44	X64	Y14	Y48.3
– spinal	T41.3	X44	X64	Y14	Y48.3
Chloropurine	T45.1	X44	X64	Y14	Y43.1
Chloropyramine	T45.0	X44	X64	Y14	Y43.0
Chloropyrifos	T60.0	X48	X68	Y18	
Chloropyrilene	T45.0	X44	X64	Y14	Y43.0
Chloroquine	T37.2	X44	X64	Y14	Y41.2
Chlorothalonil	T60.3	X48	X68	Y18	
Chlorothiazide	T50.2	X44	X64	Y14	Y54.3
Chlorothymol	T49.4	X44	X64	Y14	Y56.4
Chlorotrianisene	T38.5	X44	X64	Y14	Y42.5
Chlorovinyldichloroarsine, not in war	T57.0	X49	X69	Y19	
Chloroxine	T49.4	X44	X64	Y14	Y56.4
Chloroxylenol	T49.0	X44	X64	Y14	Y56.0
Chlorphenamine	T45.0	X44	X64	Y14	Y43.0
Chlorphenesin	T42.8	X41	X61	Y11	Y46.8
Chlorpheniramine	T45.0	X44	X64	Y14	Y43.0
Chlorphenoxamine	T45.0	X44	X64	Y14	Y43.0
Chlorphentermine	T50.5	X44	X64	Y14	Y57.0
Chlorprocaine – see Chloroprocaine					
Chlorproguanil	T37.2	X44	X64	Y14	Y41.2
Chlorpromazine	T43.3	X41	X61	Y11	Y49.3
Chlorpropamide	T38.3	X44	X64	Y14	Y42.3
Chlorprothixene	T43.4	X41	X61	Y11	Y49.4
Chlorquinaldol	T49.0	X44	X64	Y14	Y56.0
Chlorquinol	T49.0	X44	X64	Y14	Y56.0
Chlortalidone	T50.2	X44	X64	Y14	Y54.5
Chlortetracycline	T36.4	X44	X64	Y14	Y40.4
Chlorthalidone	T50.2	X44	X64	Y14	Y54.5
Chlorthion	T60.0	X48	X68	Y18	
Chlorthiophos	T60.0	X48	X68	Y18	
Chlorzoxazone	T42.8	X41	X61	Y11	Y46.8
Choke damp	T59.7	X47	X67	Y17	
Cholagogues	T47.5	X44	X64	Y14	Y53.5
Cholecalciferol	T45.2	X44	X64	Y14	Y54.7
Cholecystokinin	T50.8	X44	X64	Y14	Y57.6

743

| Substance | Chapter XIX | Poisoning | | | Adverse effect in therapeutic use |
		Accidental	Intentional self-harm	Undetermined intent	
Cholera vaccine	T50.9	X44	X64	Y14	Y58.2
Choleretic	T47.5	X44	X64	Y14	Y53.5
Cholestyramine (resin)	T46.6	X44	X64	Y14	Y52.6
Cholic acid	T47.5	X44	X64	Y14	Y53.5
Choline	T48.6	X44	X64	Y14	Y55.6
– chloride	T50.9	X44	X64	Y14	Y57.1
– dihydrogen citrate	T50.9	X44	X64	Y14	Y57.1
– salicylate	T39.0	X40	X60	Y10	Y45.1
– theophyllinate	T48.6	X44	X64	Y14	Y55.6
Cholinergic (drug) NEC	T44.1	X43	X63	Y13	Y51.1
– muscle tone enhancer	T44.1	X43	X63	Y13	Y51.1
– organophosphorus	T44.0	X43	X63	Y13	Y51.0
– trimethyl ammonium propanediol	T44.1	X43	X63	Y13	Y51.1
Cholinesterase reactivator	T50.6	X44	X64	Y14	Y57.2
Chorionic gonadotropin	T38.8	X44	X64	Y14	Y42.8
Chromate	T56.2	X49	X69	Y19	
– dust or mist	T56.2	X49	X69	Y19	
– lead (see also Lead)	T56.0	X49	X69	Y19	
Chromic					
– acid	T56.2	X49	X69	Y19	
– – dust or mist	T56.2	X49	X69	Y19	
– phosphate ^{32}P	T45.1	X44	X64	Y14	Y43.3
Chromium	T56.2	X49	X69	Y19	
– compounds – see Chromate					
– sesquioxide	T50.8	X44	X64	Y14	Y57.6
Chromomycin A₃	T45.1	X44	X64	Y14	Y43.3
Chromyl chloride	T56.2	X49	X69	Y19	
Chrysarobin	T49.4	X44	X64	Y14	Y56.4
Chymopapain	T45.3	X44	X64	Y14	Y43.6
Chymotrypsin	T45.3	X44	X64	Y14	Y43.6
Cianidanol	T50.9	X44	X64	Y14	Y57.1
Cianopramine	T43.0	X41	X61	Y11	Y49.0
Cibenzoline	T46.2	X44	X64	Y14	Y52.2
Ciclacillin	T36.0	X44	X64	Y14	Y40.0
Ciclobarbital – see Hexobarbital					
Ciclonicate	T46.7	X44	X64	Y14	Y52.7
Ciclopirox (olamine)	T49.0	X44	X64	Y14	Y56.0
Ciclosporin	T45.1	X44	X64	Y14	Y43.4
Cicutoxin	T62.2	X49	X69	Y19	
Cigarette lighter fluid	T52.0	X46	X66	Y16	
Ciguatoxin	T61.0	X49	X69	Y19	
Cilazapril	T46.4	X44	X64	Y14	Y52.4
Cimetidine	T47.0	X44	X64	Y14	Y53.0
Cimetropium bromide	T44.3	X43	X63	Y13	Y51.3
Cinchocaine	T41.3	X44	X64	Y14	Y48.3
Cinchophen	T50.4	X44	X64	Y14	Y54.8
Cinepazide	T46.7	X44	X64	Y14	Y52.7
Cinnamedrine	T48.5	X44	X64	Y14	Y55.5
Cinnarizine	T45.0	X44	X64	Y14	Y43.0
Cinoxacin	T37.8	X44	X64	Y14	Y41.8
Ciprofibrate	T46.6	X44	X64	Y14	Y52.6

Substance	Chapter XIX	Accidental	Poisoning Intentional self-harm	Undetermined intent	Adverse effect in therapeutic use
Ciprofloxacin	T36.8	X44	X64	Y14	Y40.8
Cisapride	T47.8	X44	X64	Y14	Y53.8
Cisplatin	T45.1	X44	X64	Y14	Y43.3
Citalopram	T43.2	X41	X61	Y11	Y49.2
Citric acid	T47.5	X44	X64	Y14	Y53.5
Citrovorum (factor)	T45.8	X44	X64	Y14	Y44.1
Clavulanic acid Augmentin	T36.1	X44	X64	Y14	Y40.1
Cleaner, cleansing agent NEC	T52.9	X49	X69	Y19	
− of paint or varnish	T52.9	X46	X66	Y16	
Clebopride	T47.8	X44	X64	Y14	Y53.8
Clefamide	T37.3	X44	X64	Y14	Y41.3
Clemastine	T45.0	X44	X64	Y14	Y43.0
Clemizole	T45.0	X44	X64	Y14	Y43.0
− penicillin	T36.0	X44	X64	Y14	Y40.0
Clenbuterol	T48.6	X44	X64	Y14	Y55.6
Clidanac	T39.3	X40	X60	Y10	Y45.3
Clidinium bromide	T44.3	X43	X63	Y13	Y51.3
Clindamycin	T36.8	X44	X64	Y14	Y40.8
Clinofibrate	T46.6	X44	X64	Y14	Y52.6
Clioquinol	T37.8	X44	X64	Y14	Y41.8
Clobazam	T42.4	X41	X61	Y11	Y47.1
Clobenzorex	T50.5	X44	X64	Y14	Y57.0
Clobetasol	T49.0	X44	X64	Y14	Y56.0
Clobetasone	T49.0	X44	X64	Y14	Y56.0
Clobutinol	T48.3	X44	X64	Y14	Y55.3
Clocapramine	T43.0	X41	X61	Y11	Y49.0
Clodantoin	T49.0	X44	X64	Y14	Y56.0
Clodronic acid	T50.9	X44	X64	Y14	Y54.7
Clofazimine	T37.1	X44	X64	Y14	Y41.1
Clofedanol	T48.3	X44	X64	Y14	Y55.3
Clofenamide	T50.2	X44	X64	Y14	Y54.5
Clofenotane	T49.0	X44	X64	Y14	Y56.0
Clofezone	T39.2	X40	X60	Y10	Y45.3
Clofibrate	T46.6	X44	X64	Y14	Y52.6
Clofibride	T46.6	X44	X64	Y14	Y52.6
Cloforex	T50.5	X44	X64	Y14	Y57.0
Clomacran	T43.0	X41	X61	Y11	Y49.0
Clometacin	T39.3	X40	X60	Y10	Y45.3
Clomethiazole	T42.6	X41	X61	Y11	Y47.8
Clometocillin	T36.0	X44	X64	Y14	Y40.0
Clomifene	T38.5	X44	X64	Y14	Y42.5
Clomipramine	T43.0	X41	X61	Y11	Y49.0
Clomocycline	T36.4	X44	X64	Y14	Y40.4
Clonazepam	T42.4	X41	X61	Y11	Y47.1
Clonidine	T46.5	X44	X64	Y14	Y52.5
Clonixin	T39.8	X40	X60	Y10	Y45.8
Clopamide	T50.2	X44	X64	Y14	Y54.5
Clopenthixol	T43.4	X41	X61	Y11	Y49.4
Cloperastine	T48.3	X44	X64	Y14	Y55.3
Clophedianol	T48.3	X44	X64	Y14	Y55.3
Clopirac	T39.3	X40	X60	Y10	Y45.3

| Substance | Chapter XIX | Poisoning | | | Adverse effect in therapeutic use |
		Accidental	Intentional self-harm	Undetermined intent	
Cloponone	T37.3	X44	X64	Y14	Y41.3
Cloprednol	T38.0	X44	X64	Y14	Y42.0
Cloral betaine	T42.6	X41	X61	Y11	Y47.2
Cloramfenicol	T36.2	X44	X64	Y14	Y40.2
Clorazepate (dipotassium)	T42.4	X41	X61	Y11	Y47.1
Clorexolone	T50.2	X44	X64	Y14	Y54.5
Clorfenamine	T45.0	X44	X64	Y14	Y43.0
Clorgiline	T43.1	X41	X61	Y11	Y49.1
Clorotepine	T44.3	X43	X63	Y13	Y51.3
Clorprenaline	T48.6	X44	X64	Y14	Y55.6
Clortermine	T50.5	X44	X64	Y14	Y57.0
Clotiapine	T43.5	X41	X61	Y11	Y49.5
Clotiazepam	T42.4	X41	X61	Y11	Y47.1
Clotibric acid	T46.6	X44	X64	Y14	Y52.6
Clotrimazole	T49.0	X44	X64	Y14	Y56.0
Cloxacillin	T36.0	X44	X64	Y14	Y40.0
Cloxazolam	T42.4	X41	X61	Y11	Y47.1
Cloxiquine	T49.0	X44	X64	Y14	Y56.0
Clozapine	T42.4	X41	X61	Y11	Y47.1
Coagulant NEC	T45.7	X44	X64	Y14	Y44.3
Coal (carbon monoxide from)	T58	X47	X67	Y17	
– tar	T49.1	X44	X64	Y14	Y56.1
Cobalamine	T45.2	X44	X64	Y14	Y44.1
Cobalt (nonmedicinal) (fumes) (industrial)	T56.8	X49	X69	Y19	
– medicinal (trace) (chloride)	T45.8	X44	X64	Y14	Y44.1
Cocaine	T40.5	X42	X62	Y12	Y48.3
Cocarboxylase	T45.3	X44	X64	Y14	Y43.6
Coccidioidin	T50.8	X44	X64	Y14	Y57.6
Cochineal	T65.6	X49	X69	Y19	
Codeine	T40.2	X42	X62	Y12	Y45.0
Cod-liver oil	T45.2	X44	X64	Y14	Y57.7
Coenzyme A	T50.9	X44	X64	Y14	Y57.1
Coffee	T62.8	X49	X69	Y19	
Cogalactoisomerase	T50.9	X44	X64	Y14	Y57.1
Coke fumes or gas (carbon monoxide)	T58	X47	X67	Y17	
– industrial use	T58	X47	X67	Y17	
Colaspase	T45.1	X44	X64	Y14	Y43.3
Colchicine	T50.4	X44	X64	Y14	Y54.8
Colecalciferol	T45.2	X44	X64	Y14	Y54.7
Colestipol	T46.6	X44	X64	Y14	Y52.6
Colestyramine	T46.6	X44	X64	Y14	Y52.6
Colimycin	T36.8	X44	X64	Y14	Y40.8
Colistimethate	T36.8	X44	X64	Y14	Y40.8
Colistin	T36.8	X44	X64	Y14	Y40.8
– sulfate (eye preparation)	T49.5	X44	X64	Y14	Y56.5
Collagenase	T49.4	X44	X64	Y14	Y56.4
Collodion	T49.3	X44	X64	Y14	Y56.3
Colophony adhesive	T49.3	X44	X64	Y14	Y56.3
Colorant	T50.9	X44	X64	Y14	Y57.4

Substance	Chapter XIX	Accidental	Poisoning Intentional self-harm	Undetermined intent	Adverse effect in therapeutic use
Combustion gas	T58	X47	X67	Y17	
Compound					
– 42 (warfarin)	T60.4	X48	X68	Y18	
– 269 (endrin)	T60.1	X48	X68	Y18	
– 497 (dieldrin)	T60.1	X48	X68	Y18	
– 1080 (sodium fluoroacetate)	T60.4	X48	X68	Y18	
– 3422 (parathion)	T60.0	X48	X68	Y18	
– 3911 (phorate)	T60.0	X48	X68	Y18	
– 3956 (toxaphene)	T60.1	X48	X68	Y18	
– 4069 (malathion)	T60.0	X48	X68	Y18	
– 4124 (dicapthon)	T60.0	X48	X68	Y18	
Congenor, anabolic	T38.7	X44	X64	Y14	Y42.7
Congo red	T50.8	X44	X64	Y14	Y57.6
Coniine	T62.2	X49	X69	Y19	
Conjugated estrogenic substances	T38.5	X44	X64	Y14	Y42.5
Contraceptive (oral)	T38.4	X44	X64	Y14	Y42.4
Contrast medium, radiography	T50.8	X44	X64	Y14	Y57.5
Convallaria glycosides	T46.0	X44	X64	Y14	Y52.0
Copper (dust) (fumes) (nonmedicinal) NEC	T56.4	X49	X69	Y19	
– arsenate, arsenite	T57.0	X48	X68	Y18	
– – insecticide	T60.2	X48	X68	Y18	
– gluconate	T49.0	X44	X64	Y14	Y56.0
– medicinal (trace)	T45.8	X44	X64	Y14	Y44.1
– oleate	T49.0	X44	X64	Y14	Y56.0
– sulfate	T56.4	X49	X69	Y19	
– – medicinal	T49.6	X44	X64	Y14	Y56.6
– – – eye	T49.5	X44	X64	Y14	Y56.5
Corbadrine	T49.6	X44	X64	Y14	Y56.6
Cordite	T65.8	X49	X69	Y19	
– vapor	T59.8	X47	X67	Y17	
Coronary vasodilator NEC	T46.3	X44	X64	Y14	Y52.3
Corrosive NEC	T54.9	X49	X69	Y19	
– acid NEC	T54.2	X49	X69	Y19	
– aromatics	T54.1	X49	X69	Y19	
– fumes NEC	T54.9	X47	X67	Y17	
– sublimate	T56.1	X49	X69	Y19	
Corticosteroid					
– mineral	T50.0	X44	X64	Y14	Y54.0
– ophthalmic	T49.5	X44	X64	Y14	Y56.5
Corticotrophin	T38.8	X44	X64	Y14	Y42.8
– long-acting	T38.8	X44	X64	Y14	Y42.8
– zinc hydroxide	T38.8	X44	X64	Y14	Y42.8
Cortisol	T49.0	X44	X64	Y14	Y56.0
Cortisone (acetate)	T38.0	X44	X64	Y14	Y42.0
Cortivazol	T38.0	X44	X64	Y14	Y42.0
Corynebacterium parvum	T45.1	X44	X64	Y14	Y43.3
Cosmetic preparation	T49.8	X44	X64	Y14	Y56.8
Cosmetics	T49.8	X44	X64	Y14	Y56.8
Cosyntropin	T38.8	X44	X64	Y14	Y42.8
Co-trimoxazole	T36.8	X44	X64	Y14	Y40.8

Substance	Chapter XIX	Poisoning			Adverse effect in therapeutic use
		Accidental	Intentional self-harm	Undetermined intent	
Cough mixture (syrup)	T48.4	X44	X64	Y14	Y55.4
Coumaphos	T60.0	X48	X68	Y18	
Coumarin	T45.5	X44	X64	Y14	Y44.2
Coumetarol	T45.5	X44	X64	Y14	Y44.2
Crataegus extract	T46.0	X44	X64	Y14	Y52.0
Creosol (compound)	T49.0	X44	X64	Y14	Y56.0
Creosote (coal tar) (beechwood)	T49.0	X44	X64	Y14	Y56.0
Cresol(s)	T49.0	X44	X64	Y14	Y56.0
– and soap solution	T49.0	X44	X64	Y14	Y56.0
Cresyl acetate	T49.0	X44	X64	Y14	Y56.0
Cresylic acid	T49.0	X44	X64	Y14	Y56.0
Crimidine	T60.4	X48	X68	Y18	
Croconazole	T37.8	X44	X64	Y14	Y41.8
Cromoglicic acid	T48.6	X44	X64	Y14	Y55.6
Cromolyn	T48.6	X44	X64	Y14	Y55.6
Cromonar	T46.3	X44	X64	Y14	Y52.3
Crotamiton	T49.0	X44	X64	Y14	Y56.0
Crude oil	T52.0	X46	X66	Y16	
Cryolite (vapor)	T60.1	X48	X68	Y18	
– insecticide	T60.1	X48	X68	Y18	
Cryptenamine (tannates)	T46.5	X44	X64	Y14	Y52.5
Crystal violet	T49.0	X44	X64	Y14	Y56.0
Cupric					
– acetate	T60.3	X48	X68	Y18	
– acetoarsenite	T57.0	X48	X68	Y18	
– arsenate	T57.0	X49	X69	Y19	
– gluconate	T49.0	X44	X64	Y14	Y56.0
– oleate	T49.0	X44	X64	Y14	Y56.0
– sulfate	T56.4	X49	X69	Y19	
Cyamemazine	T43.3	X41	X61	Y11	Y49.3
Cyamopsis tetragonoloba	T46.6	X44	X64	Y14	Y52.6
Cyanacetyl hydrazide	T37.1	X44	X64	Y14	Y41.1
Cyanic acid (gas)	T59.8	X47	X67	Y17	
Cyanide(s) (compounds) (potassium) (sodium) NEC	T65.0	X49	X69	Y19	
– hydrogen	T57.3	X48	X68	Y18	
Cyanoacrylate adhesive	T49.3	X44	X64	Y14	Y56.3
Cyanocobalamin	T45.8	X44	X64	Y14	Y44.1
Cyanogen (chloride) (gas) NEC	T59.8	X47	X67	Y17	
Cyclacillin	T36.0	X44	X64	Y14	Y40.0
Cyclamate	T50.9	X44	X64	Y14	Y57.4
Cyclandelate	T46.7	X44	X64	Y14	Y52.7
Cyclazocine	T50.7	X44	X64	Y14	Y50.1
Cyclizine	T45.0	X44	X64	Y14	Y43.0
Cyclobarbital	T42.3	X41	X61	Y11	Y47.0
Cyclobarbitone	T42.3	X41	X61	Y11	Y47.0
Cyclobenzaprine	T48.1	X44	X64	Y14	Y55.1
Cyclodrine	T44.3	X43	X63	Y13	Y51.3
Cycloguanil embonate	T37.2	X44	X64	Y14	Y41.2
Cycloheptadiene	T43.2	X41	X61	Y11	Y49.2
Cyclohexane	T52.8	X46	X66	Y16	

Substance	Chapter XIX	Poisoning			Adverse effect in therapeutic use
		Accidental	Intentional self-harm	Undetermined intent	
Cyclohexanol	T51.8	X45	X65	Y15	
Cyclohexanone	T52.4	X46	X66	Y16	
Cycloheximide	T60.3	X48	X68	Y18	
Cyclohexyl acetate	T52.8	X46	X66	Y16	
Cycloleucin	T45.1	X44	X64	Y14	Y43.3
Cyclomethycaine	T41.3	X44	X64	Y14	Y48.3
Cyclopenthiazide	T50.2	X44	X64	Y14	Y54.3
Cyclopentolate	T44.3	X43	X63	Y13	Y51.3
Cyclophosphamide	T45.1	X44	X64	Y14	Y43.3
Cycloplegic drug	T49.5	X44	X64	Y14	Y56.5
Cyclopropane	T41.2	X44	X64	Y14	Y48.2
Cyclopyrabital	T39.8	X40	X60	Y10	Y45.8
Cycloserine	T37.1	X44	X64	Y14	Y41.1
Cyclosporin	T45.1	X44	X64	Y14	Y43.4
Cyclothiazide	T50.2	X44	X64	Y14	Y54.3
Cycrimine	T44.3	X43	X63	Y13	Y51.3
Cyhalothrin	T60.1	X48	X68	Y18	
Cypermethrin	T60.1	X48	X68	Y18	
Cyphenothrin	T60.2	X48	X68	Y18	
Cyproheptadine	T45.0	X44	X64	Y14	Y43.0
Cyproterone	T38.6	X44	X64	Y14	Y42.6
Cysteamine	T50.6	X44	X64	Y14	Y57.2
Cytarabine	T45.1	X44	X64	Y14	Y43.1
Cytochrome C	T47.5	X44	X64	Y14	Y53.5
Cytosine arabinoside	T45.1	X44	X64	Y14	Y43.1
Cytozyme	T45.7	X44	X64	Y14	Y44.3

D

Substance	Chapter XIX	Poisoning			Adverse effect in therapeutic use
		Accidental	Intentional self-harm	Undetermined intent	
2,4-D	T60.3	X48	X68	Y18	
Dacarbazine	T45.1	X44	X64	Y14	Y43.3
Dactinomycin	T45.1	X44	X64	Y14	Y43.3
DADPS	T37.1	X44	X64	Y14	Y41.1
Dakin's solution	T49.0	X44	X64	Y14	Y56.0
Dalapon (sodium)	T60.3	X48	X68	Y18	
Danazol	T38.6	X44	X64	Y14	Y42.6
Danthron	T47.2	X44	X64	Y14	Y53.2
Dantrolene	T42.8	X41	X61	Y11	Y46.8
Dantron	T47.2	X44	X64	Y14	Y53.2
Dapsone	T37.1	X44	X64	Y14	Y41.1
Daunomycin	T45.1	X44	X64	Y14	Y43.3
Daunorubicin	T45.1	X44	X64	Y14	Y43.3
DDAVP	T38.8	X44	X64	Y14	Y42.8
DDE (bis(chlorophenyl)-dichloroethylene)	T60.2	X48	X68	Y18	
DDT (dust)	T60.1	X48	X68	Y18	
Deadly nightshade	T62.2	X49	X69	Y19	
Deamino-D-arginine vasopressin	T38.8	X44	X64	Y14	Y42.8
Deanol (aceglumate)	T50.9	X44	X64	Y14	Y50.8
Debrisoquine	T46.5	X44	X64	Y14	Y52.5
Decaborane	T57.8	X49	X69	Y19	
– fumes	T59.8	X47	X67	Y17	
Decahydronaphthalene	T52.8	X46	X66	Y16	
Decalin	T52.8	X46	X66	Y16	
Decamethonium (bromide)	T48.1	X44	X64	Y14	Y55.1
Decongestant, nasal (mucosa)	T48.5	X44	X64	Y14	Y55.5
– combination	T48.5	X44	X64	Y14	Y55.5
Deet	T60.8	X48	X68	Y18	
Deferoxamine	T45.8	X44	X64	Y14	Y43.8
Deflazacort	T38.0	X44	X64	Y14	Y42.0
Deglycyrrhizinized extract of liquorice	T48.4	X44	X64	Y14	Y55.4
Dehydrocholic acid	T47.5	X44	X64	Y14	Y53.5
Dehydroemetine	T37.3	X44	X64	Y14	Y41.3
Dekalin	T52.8	X46	X66	Y16	
Delorazepam	T42.4	X41	X61	Y11	Y47.1
Deltamethrin	T60.1	X48	X68	Y18	
Demecarium (bromide)	T49.5	X44	X64	Y14	Y56.5
Demeclocycline	T36.4	X44	X64	Y14	Y40.4
Demecolcine	T45.1	X44	X64	Y14	Y43.3
Demegestone	T38.5	X44	X64	Y14	Y42.5
Demephion -O and -S	T60.0	X48	X68	Y18	
Demethylchlortetracycline	T36.4	X44	X64	Y14	Y40.4

Substance	Chapter XIX	Accidental	Poisoning Intentional self-harm	Undetermined intent	Adverse effect in therapeutic use
Demeton -O and -S	T60.0	X48	X68	Y18	
Demulcent (external)	T49.3	X44	X64	Y14	Y56.3
– specified NEC	T49.3	X44	X64	Y14	Y56.3
Denatured alcohol	T51.0	X45	X65	Y15	
Dental drug, topical application NEC	T49.7	X44	X64	Y14	Y56.7
Dentifrice	T49.7	X44	X64	Y14	Y56.7
Deoxybarbiturates	T42.3	X41	X61	Y11	Y46.3
Deoxycortone	T50.0	X44	X64	Y14	Y54.0
2-Deoxy-5-fluorouridine	T45.1	X44	X64	Y14	Y43.1
5-Deoxy-5-fluorouridine	T45.1	X44	X64	Y14	Y43.1
Deoxyribonuclease (pancreatic)	T45.3	X44	X64	Y14	Y43.6
Depilatory	T49.4	X44	X64	Y14	Y56.4
Deprenalin	T42.8	X41	X61	Y11	Y46.7
Deprenyl	T42.8	X41	X61	Y11	Y46.7
Depressant					
– appetite	T50.5	X44	X64	Y14	Y57.0
– muscle tone, central, NEC	T42.8	X41	X61	Y11	Y46.8
Deptropine	T45.0	X44	X64	Y14	Y43.0
Dequalinium (chloride)	T49.0	X44	X64	Y14	Y56.0
Derris root	T60.2	X48	X68	Y18	
Deserpidine	T46.5	X44	X64	Y14	Y52.5
Desferrioxamine	T45.8	X44	X64	Y14	Y43.8
Desipramine	T43.0	X41	X61	Y11	Y49.0
Deslanoside	T46.0	X44	X64	Y14	Y52.0
Desloughing agent	T49.4	X44	X64	Y14	Y56.4
Desmethylimipramine	T43.0	X41	X61	Y11	Y49.0
Desmopressin	T38.8	X44	X64	Y14	Y42.8
Desogestrel	T38.5	X44	X64	Y14	Y42.5
Desonide	T49.0	X44	X64	Y14	Y56.0
Desoximetasone	T49.0	X44	X64	Y14	Y56.0
Desoxycorticosteroid	T50.0	X44	X64	Y14	Y54.0
Desoxycortone	T50.0	X44	X64	Y14	Y54.0
Desoxyephedrine	T43.6	X41	X61	Y11	Y49.7
Detaxtran	T46.6	X44	X64	Y14	Y52.6
Detergent (local) (medicinal) NEC	T49.2	X44	X64	Y14	Y56.2
– nonmedicinal	T55	X49	X69	Y19	
– specified NEC	T49.2	X44	X64	Y14	Y56.2
Detoxifying agent	T50.6	X44	X64	Y14	Y57.2
Dexamethasone	T38.0	X44	X64	Y14	Y42.0
Dexamfetamine	T43.6	X41	X61	Y11	Y49.7
Dexamphetamine	T43.6	X41	X61	Y11	Y49.7
Dexbrompheniramine	T45.0	X44	X64	Y14	Y43.0
Dexchlorpheniramine	T45.0	X44	X64	Y14	Y43.0
Dexetimide	T44.3	X43	X63	Y13	Y51.3
Dexfenfluramine	T50.5	X44	X64	Y14	Y57.0
Dexpanthenol	T45.2	X44	X64	Y14	Y57.7
Dextran (40) (70) (150)	T45.8	X44	X64	Y14	Y44.7
Dextriferron	T45.4	X44	X64	Y14	Y44.0
Dextroamphetamine	T43.6	X41	X61	Y11	Y49.7
Dextromethorphan	T48.3	X44	X64	Y14	Y55.3

Substance		Poisoning			Adverse effect in therapeutic use
	Chapter XIX	Accidental	Intentional self-harm	Undetermined intent	
Dextromoramide	T40.4	X42	X62	Y12	Y45.0
Dextropropoxyphene	T40.4	X42	X62	Y12	Y45.0
Dextrose	T50.3	X44	X64	Y14	Y54.6
– concentrated solution, intravenous	T46.8	X44	X64	Y14	Y52.8
Dextrothyroxine sodium	T38.1	X44	X64	Y14	Y42.1
DHE	T37.3	X44	X64	Y14	Y41.3
– 45	T46.5	X44	X64	Y14	Y52.5
Diacerein	T39.3	X40	X60	Y10	Y45.3
Diacetone alcohol	T52.4	X46	X66	Y16	
Diacetylmorphine	T40.1	X42	X62	Y12	Y45.0
Diachylon plaster	T49.4	X44	X64	Y14	Y56.4
Diaethylstilboestrolum	T38.5	X44	X64	Y14	Y42.5
Diagnostic agent NEC	T50.8	X44	X64	Y14	Y57.6
Dialkyl carbonate	T52.9	X46	X66	Y16	
Diallymal	T42.3	X41	X61	Y11	Y47.0
Dialysis solution (intraperitoneal)	T50.3	X44	X64	Y14	Y54.6
Diaminodiphenylsulfone	T37.1	X44	X64	Y14	Y41.1
Diamorphine	T40.1	X42	X62	Y12	Y45.0
Diamthazole	T49.0	X44	X64	Y14	Y56.0
Dianthone	T47.2	X44	X64	Y14	Y53.2
Diaphenylsulfone	T37.0	X44	X64	Y14	Y41.0
Diastase	T47.5	X44	X64	Y14	Y53.5
Diatrizoate	T50.8	X44	X64	Y14	Y57.5
Diazepam	T42.4	X41	X61	Y11	Y47.1
Diazinon	T60.0	X48	X68	Y18	
Diazomethane (gas)	T59.8	X47	X67	Y17	
Diazoxide	T46.5	X44	X64	Y14	Y52.5
Dibekacin	T36.5	X44	X64	Y14	Y40.5
Dibenzepin	T43.0	X41	X61	Y11	Y49.0
Diborane (gas)	T59.8	X47	X67	Y17	
Dibromochloropropane	T60.8	X48	X68	Y18	
Dibromodulcitol	T45.1	X44	X64	Y14	Y43.3
Dibromoethane	T53.6	X46	X66	Y16	
Dibromomannitol	T45.1	X44	X64	Y14	Y43.3
Dibromopropamidine isethionate	T49.0	X44	X64	Y14	Y56.0
Dibrompropamidine	T49.0	X44	X64	Y14	Y56.0
Dibucaine	T41.3	X44	X64	Y14	Y48.3
Dibutoline sulfate	T44.3	X43	X63	Y13	Y51.3
Dicamba	T60.3	X48	X68	Y18	
Dicapthon	T60.0	X48	X68	Y18	
Dichlobenil	T60.3	X48	X68	Y18	
Dichlone	T60.3	X48	X68	Y18	
Dichloralphenozone	T42.6	X41	X61	Y11	Y47.5
Dichlorbenzidine	T65.3	X49	X69	Y19	
Dichlorhydrin, dichlorohydrin, alpha-dichlorohydrin	T52.8	X46	X66	Y16	
Dichlorhydroxyquinoline	T37.8	X44	X64	Y14	Y41.8
Dichlorobenzene	T53.7	X46	X66	Y16	
Dichlorobenzyl alcohol	T49.6	X44	X64	Y14	Y56.6
Dichlorodifluoromethane	T53.5	X46	X66	Y16	
Dichloroethane	T52.8	X46	X66	Y16	

Substance		Poisoning			Adverse effect in therapeutic use
	Chapter XIX	Accidental	Intentional self-harm	Undetermined intent	
sym-Dichloroethyl ether	T53.6	X46	X66	Y16	
Dichloroethyl sulfide, not in war	T59.8	X47	X67	Y17	
Dichloroethylene	T53.6	X46	X66	Y16	
Dichloroformoxine, not in war	T65.8	X49	X69	Y19	
Dichloromethane (solvent)	T53.4	X46	X66	Y16	
− vapor	T53.4	X46	X66	Y16	
Dichloronaphthoquinone	T60.3	X48	X68	Y18	
Dichlorophen	T37.4	X44	X64	Y14	Y41.4
2,4-Dichlorophenoxyacetic acid	T60.3	X48	X68	Y18	
Dichloropropene	T60.3	X48	X68	Y18	
Dichloropropionic acid	T60.3	X48	X68	Y18	
Dichlorphenamide	T50.2	X44	X64	Y14	Y54.2
Dichlorvos	T60.0	X48	X68	Y18	
Diclofenac	T39.3	X40	X60	Y10	Y45.3
Diclofenamide	T50.2	X44	X64	Y14	Y54.2
Diclofensine	T43.2	X41	X61	Y11	Y49.2
Diclonixine	T39.8	X40	X60	Y10	Y45.8
Dicloxacillin	T36.0	X44	X64	Y14	Y40.0
Dicophane	T49.0	X44	X64	Y14	Y56.0
Dicoumarol, dicoumarin, dicumarol	T45.5	X44	X64	Y14	Y44.2
Dicrotophos	T60.0	X48	X68	Y18	
Dicyanogen (gas)	T65.0	X47	X67	Y17	
Dicyclomine	T44.3	X43	X63	Y13	Y51.3
Dicycloverine	T44.3	X43	X63	Y13	Y51.3
Dideoxycytidine	T37.5	X44	X64	Y14	Y41.5
Dideoxyinosine	T37.5	X44	X64	Y14	Y41.5
Dieldrin (vapor)	T60.1	X48	X68	Y18	
Diemal	T42.3	X41	X61	Y11	Y47.0
Dienestrol	T38.5	X44	X64	Y14	Y42.5
Dienoestrol	T38.5	X44	X64	Y14	Y42.5
Dietetic drug NEC	T50.9	X44	X64	Y14	Y57.8
Diethazine	T42.8	X41	X61	Y11	Y46.7
Diethyl					
− carbinol	T51.3	X45	X65	Y15	
− carbonate	T52.8	X46	X66	Y16	
− ether (vapor) (*see also* Ether)	T59.8	X47	X67	Y17	
− oxide	T52.8	X46	X66	Y16	
− toluamide (nonmedicinal)	T60.8	X48	X68	Y18	
− − medicinal	T49.8	X44	X64	Y14	Y56.8
Diethylcarbamazine	T37.4	X44	X64	Y14	Y41.4
Diethylene					
− dioxide	T52.8	X46	X66	Y16	
− glycol (monoacetate) (monobutyl ether) (monoethyl ether)	T52.3	X46	X66	Y16	
Diethylhexylphthalate	T65.8	X49	X69	Y19	
Diethylpropion	T50.5	X44	X64	Y14	Y57.0
Diethylstilbestrol	T38.5	X44	X64	Y14	Y42.5
Diethylstilboestrol	T38.5	X44	X64	Y14	Y42.5
Diethyltoluamide	T49.0	X44	X64	Y14	Y56.0
Difebarbamate	T42.3	X41	X61	Y11	Y47.0
Difenidol	T45.0	X44	X64	Y14	Y43.0

| Substance | Chapter XIX | Poisoning | | | Adverse effect in therapeutic use |
		Accidental	Intentional self-harm	Undetermined intent	
Difenoxin	T47.6	X44	X64	Y14	Y53.6
Difetarsone	T37.3	X44	X64	Y14	Y41.3
Diflorasone	149.0	X44	X64	Y14	Y56.0
Diflubenzuron	T60.1	X48	X68	Y18	
Diflucortolone	T49.0	X44	X64	Y14	Y56.0
Diflunisal	T39.0	X40	X60	Y10	Y45.1
Difluoromethyldopa	T42.8	X41	X61	Y11	Y46.7
Difluorophate	T44.0	X43	X63	Y13	Y51.0
Digestant NEC	T47.5	X44	X64	Y14	Y53.5
Digitalis (leaf) (glycoside)	T46.0	X44	X64	Y14	Y52.0
– lanata	T46.0	X44	X64	Y14	Y52.0
– purpurea	T46.0	X44	X64	Y14	Y52.0
Digitoxin	T46.0	X44	X64	Y14	Y52.0
Digitoxose	T46.0	X44	X64	Y14	Y52.0
Digoxin	T46.0	X44	X64	Y14	Y52.0
Digoxine	T46.0	X44	X64	Y14	Y52.0
Dihydralazine	T46.5	X44	X64	Y14	Y52.5
Dihydrazine	T46.5	X44	X64	Y14	Y52.5
Dihydrocodeine	T40.2	X42	X62	Y12	Y45.0
Dihydrocodeinone	T40.2	X42	X62	Y12	Y45.0
Dihydroergocornine	T46.7	X44	X64	Y14	Y52.7
Dihydroergocristine (mesilate)	T46.7	X44	X64	Y14	Y52.7
Dihydroergokryptine	T46.7	X44	X64	Y14	Y52.7
Dihydroergotamine	T46.5	X44	X64	Y14	Y52.5
Dihydroergotoxine	T46.7	X44	X64	Y14	Y52.7
– mesilate	T46.7	X44	X64	Y14	Y52.7
Dihydrohydroxycodeinone	T40.2	X42	X62	Y12	Y45.0
Dihydromorphinone	T40.2	X42	X62	Y12	Y45.0
Dihydrostreptomycin	T36.5	X44	X64	Y14	Y40.5
Dihydrotachysterol	T45.2	X44	X64	Y14	Y54.7
Dihydroxyaluminum aminoacetate	T47.1	X44	X64	Y14	Y53.1
Dihydroxyaluminum sodium carbonate	T47.1	X44	X64	Y14	Y53.1
Dihydroxyanthraquinone	T47.2	X44	X64	Y14	Y53.2
Dihydroxypropyl theophylline	T50.2	X44	X64	Y14	Y54.5
Diiodohydroxyquinoline	T37.8	X44	X64	Y14	Y41.8
Diiodotyrosine	T38.2	X44	X64	Y14	Y42.2
Diisopromine	T44.3	X43	X63	Y13	Y51.3
Diisopropylamine	T46.3	X44	X64	Y14	Y52.3
Diisopropylfluorophosphonate	T44.0	X43	X63	Y13	Y51.0
Dilazep	T46.3	X44	X64	Y14	Y52.3
Dill	T47.5	X44	X64	Y14	Y53.5
Diloxanide	T37.3	X44	X64	Y14	Y41.3
Diltiazem	T46.1	X44	X64	Y14	Y52.1
Dimazole	T49.0	X44	X64	Y14	Y56.0
Dimefline	T50.7	X44	X64	Y14	Y50.0
Dimefox	T60.0	X48	X68	Y18	
Dimemorfan	T48.3	X44	X64	Y14	Y55.3
Dimenhydrinate	T45.0	X44	X64	Y14	Y43.0
Dimercaprol (British anti-lewisite)	T45.8	X44	X64	Y14	Y43.8
Dimestrol	T38.5	X44	X64	Y14	Y42.5

	Poisoning			Adverse effect in therapeutic use
Substance	Chapter XIX	Accidental	Intentional self-harm	Undetermined intent	
Dimethicone	T47.1	X44	X64	Y14	Y53.1
Dimethindene	T45.0	X44	X64	Y14	Y43.0
Dimethisoquin	T49.1	X44	X64	Y14	Y56.1
Dimethisterone	T38.5	X44	X64	Y14	Y42.5
Dimethoate	T60.0	X48	X68	Y18	
Dimethocaine	T41.3	X44	X64	Y14	Y48.3
Dimethoxanate	T48.3	X44	X64	Y14	Y55.3
Dimethyl					
− arsine, arsinic acid	T57.0	X48	X68	Y18	
− carbinol	T51.2	X45	X65	Y15	
− carbonate	T52.8	X46	X66	Y16	
− ketone	T52.4	X46	X66	Y16	
− − vapor	T52.4	X46	X66	Y16	
− phthlate	T49.3	X44	X64	Y14	Y56.3
− sulfate (fumes)	T59.8	X47	X67	Y17	
− − liquid	T65.8	X49	X69	Y19	
− sulfoxide (nonmedicinal)	T52.8	X46	X66	Y16	
− − medicinal	T49.4	X44	X64	Y14	Y56.4
Dimethylamine sulfate	T49.4	X44	X64	Y14	Y56.4
Dimethylformamide	T52.8	X46	X66	Y16	
Dimethyltubocurarinium chloride	T48.1	X44	X64	Y14	Y55.1
Dimeticone	T47.1	X44	X64	Y14	Y53.1
Dimetilan	T60.0	X48	X68	Y18	
Dimetindene	T45.0	X44	X64	Y14	Y43.0
Dimetotiazine	T43.3	X41	X61	Y11	Y49.3
Dimorpholamine	T50.7	X44	X64	Y14	Y50.0
Dimoxyline	T46.3	X43	X63	Y13	Y52.3
Dinitrobenzene	T65.3	X46	X66	Y16	
− vapor	T59.8	X47	X67	Y17	
Dinitrobenzol	T65.3	X46	X66	Y16	
− vapor	T59.8	X47	X67	Y17	
Dinitrobutylphenol	T65.3	X46	X66	Y16	
Dinitro(-ortho-)cresol (pesticide) (spray)	T65.3	X46	X66	Y16	
Dinitrocyclohexylphenol	T65.3	X46	X66	Y16	
Dinitrophenol	T65.3	X46	X66	Y16	
Dinoprost	T48.0	X44	X64	Y14	Y55.0
Dinoprostone	T48.0	X44	X64	Y14	Y55.0
Dinoseb	T60.3	X48	X68	Y18	
Diodone	T50.8	X44	X64	Y14	Y57.5
Diosmin	T46.9	X44	X64	Y14	Y52.9
Dioxane	T52.8	X46	X66	Y16	
Dioxathion	T60.0	X48	X68	Y18	
Dioxin	T53.7	X46	X66	Y16	
Dioxopromethazine	T43.3	X41	X61	Y11	Y49.3
Dioxyline	T46.3	X44	X64	Y14	Y52.3
Dipentene	T52.8	X46	X66	Y16	
Diperodon	T41.3	X44	X64	Y14	Y48.3
Diphacinone	T60.4	X48	X68	Y18	
Diphemanil	T44.3	X43	X63	Y13	Y51.3
− metilsulfate	T44.3	X43	X63	Y13	Y51.3

Substance	Chapter XIX	Accidental	Intentional self-harm	Undetermined intent	Adverse effect in therapeutic use
		Poisoning			Adverse effect in therapeutic use
Diphenadione	T45.5	X44	X64	Y14	Y44.2
– rodenticide	T60.4	X48	X68	Y18	
Diphenhydramine	T45.0	X44	X64	Y14	Y43.0
Diphenidol	T45.0	X44	X64	Y14	Y43.0
Diphenoxylate	T47.6	X44	X64	Y14	Y53.6
Diphenylamine	T65.3	X49	X69	Y19	
Diphenylbutazone	T39.2	X40	X60	Y10	Y45.3
Diphenylchloroarsine, not in war	T57.0	X49	X69	Y19	
Diphenylhydantoin	T42.0	X41	X61	Y11	Y46.2
Diphenylmethane dye	T52.1	X46	X66	Y16	
Diphenylpyraline	T45.0	X44	X64	Y14	Y43.0
Diphtheria					
– antitoxin	T50.9	X44	X64	Y14	Y58.5
– vaccine (combination)	T50.9	X44	X64	Y14	Y58.5
Diphylline	T50.2	X44	X64	Y14	Y54.5
Dipipanone	T40.4	X42	X62	Y12	Y45.0
Dipivefrine	T49.5	X44	X64	Y14	Y56.5
Diprophylline	T50.2	X44	X64	Y14	Y54.5
Dipropyline	T48.2	X44	X64	Y14	Y55.2
Dipyridamole	T46.3	X44	X64	Y14	Y52.3
Dipyrocetyl	T39.0	X40	X60	Y10	Y45.1
Dipyrone	T39.2	X40	X60	Y10	Y45.8
Diquat (dibromide)	T60.3	X48	X68	Y18	
Disinfectant	T65.8	X49	X69	Y19	
– alkaline	T54.3	X49	X69	Y19	
– intestinal	T37.8	X44	X64	Y14	Y41.8
Disodium edetate	T50.6	X44	X64	Y14	Y57.2
Disoprofol	T41.2	X44	X64	Y14	Y48.2
Disopyramide	T46.2	X44	X64	Y14	Y52.2
Distigmine (bromide)	T44.0	X43	X63	Y13	Y51.0
Disulfamide	T50.2	X44	X64	Y14	Y54.3
Disulfiram	T50.6	X44	X64	Y14	Y57.3
Disulfoton	T60.0	X48	X68	Y18	
Ditazole	T39.3	X40	X60	Y10	Y45.3
Dithiazanine iodide	T37.4	X44	X64	Y14	Y41.4
Dithiocarbamate	T60.0	X48	X68	Y18	
Dithranol	T49.4	X44	X64	Y14	Y56.4
Diuretic NEC	T50.2	X44	X64	Y14	Y54.5
– benzothiadiazine	T50.2	X44	X64	Y14	Y54.3
– furfuryl NEC	T50.2	X44	X64	Y14	Y54.5
– loop [high-ceiling]	T50.1	X44	X64	Y14	Y54.4
– mercurial NEC	T50.2	X44	X64	Y14	Y54.5
– osmotic	T50.2	X44	X64	Y14	Y54.5
– purine NEC	T50.2	X44	X64	Y14	Y54.5
– saluretic NEC	T50.2	X44	X64	Y14	Y54.5
– sulfonamide	T50.2	X44	X64	Y14	Y54.5
– thiazide NEC	T50.2	X44	X64	Y14	Y54.3
– xanthine	T50.2	X44	X64	Y14	Y54.5
Diurgin	T50.2	X44	X64	Y14	Y54.5
Diuron	T60.3	X48	X68	Y18	
Divalproex	T42.6	X41	X61	Y11	Y46.5

| Substance | Chapter XIX | Poisoning | | | Adverse effect in therapeutic use |
		Accidental	Intentional self-harm	Undetermined intent	
Dixanthogen	T49.0	X44	X64	Y14	Y56.0
Dixyrazine	T43.3	X41	X61	Y11	Y49.3
DMSO – *see* Dimethyl sulfoxide					
DNBP	T60.3	X48	X68	Y18	
DNOC	T65.3	X46	X66	Y16	
Dobutamine	T44.5	X43	X63	Y13	Y51.5
Docusate sodium	T47.4	X44	X64	Y14	Y53.4
Dodicin	T49.0	X44	X64	Y14	Y56.0
Dofamium chloride	T49.0	X44	X64	Y14	Y56.0
Domestic gas	T58	X47	X67	Y17	
Domiodol	T48.4	X44	X64	Y14	Y55.4
Domiphen (bromide)	T49.0	X44	X64	Y14	Y56.0
Domperidone	T45.0	X44	X64	Y14	Y43.0
Dopa	T42.8	X41	X61	Y11	Y46.7
Dopamine	T44.9	X43	X63	Y13	Y51.9
Dornase	T48.4	X44	X64	Y14	Y55.4
Dosulepin	T43.0	X41	X61	Y11	Y49.0
Dothiepin	T43.0	X41	X61	Y11	Y49.0
Doxantrazole	T48.6	X44	X64	Y14	Y55.6
Doxapram	T50.7	X44	X64	Y14	Y50.0
Doxazosin	T44.6	X43	X63	Y13	Y51.6
Doxepin	T43.0	X41	X61	Y11	Y49.0
Doxifluridine	T45.1	X44	X64	Y14	Y43.1
Doxorubicin	T45.1	X44	X64	Y14	Y43.3
Doxycycline	T36.4	X44	X64	Y14	Y40.4
Doxylamine	T45.0	X44	X64	Y14	Y43.0
Dressing, live pulp	T49.7	X44	X64	Y14	Y56.7
Drocode	T40.2	X42	X62	Y12	Y45.0
Dronabinol	T40.7	X42	X62	Y12	Y49.6
Droperidol	T43.5	X41	X61	Y11	Y49.5
Dropropizine	T48.3	X44	X64	Y14	Y55.3
Drostanolone	T38.7	X44	X64	Y14	Y42.7
Drotaverine	T44.3	X43	X63	Y13	Y51.3
Drug NEC	T50.9	X44	X64	Y14	Y57.9
DTIC	T45.1	X44	X64	Y14	Y43.3
Dyclonine	T41.3	X44	X64	Y14	Y48.3
Dydrogesterone	T38.5	X44	X64	Y14	Y42.5
Dye NEC	T65.6	X49	X69	Y19	
– antiseptic	T49.0	X44	X64	Y14	Y56.0
Dyflos	T44.0	X43	X63	Y13	Y51.0
Dynamite	T65.3	X49	X69	Y19	
– fumes	T59.8	X47	X67	Y17	

757

E

| | Poisoning | | | Adverse effect in therapeutic use |
Substance	Chapter XIX	Accidental	Intentional self-harm	Undetermined intent	
Ear drug NEC	T49.6	X44	X64	Y14	Y56.6
Econazole	T49.0	X44	X64	Y14	Y56.0
Ecothiopate iodide	T49.5	X44	X64	Y14	Y56.5
Ectylurea	T42.6	X41	X61	Y11	Y47.8
Edoxudine	T49.5	X44	X64	Y14	Y56.5
Edrophonium	T44.0	X43	X63	Y13	Y51.0
– chloride	T44.0	X43	X63	Y13	Y51.0
EDTA	T50.6	X44	X64	Y14	Y57.2
Eflornithine	T37.2	X44	X64	Y14	Y41.2
Efloxate	T46.3	X44	X64	Y14	Y52.3
Elastase	T47.5	X44	X64	Y14	Y53.5
Elcatonin	T50.9	X44	X64	Y14	Y54.7
Electrolyte balance drug	T50.3	X44	X64	Y14	Y54.6
Elemental diet	T50.9	X44	X64	Y14	Y57.8
Elliptinium acetate	T45.1	X44	X64	Y14	Y43.3
Embramine	T45.0	X44	X64	Y14	Y43.0
Emepronium (salts)	T44.3	X43	X63	Y13	Y51.3
– bromide	T44.3	X43	X63	Y13	Y51.3
Emetic NEC	T47.7	X44	X64	Y14	Y53.7
Emetine	T37.3	X44	X64	Y14	Y41.3
Emollient NEC	T49.3	X44	X64	Y14	Y56.3
Emorfazone	T39.8	X40	X60	Y10	Y45.8
Emylcamate	T43.5	X41	X61	Y11	Y49.5
Enalapril	T46.4	X44	X64	Y14	Y52.4
Enalaprilat	T46.4	X44	X64	Y14	Y52.4
Encainide	T46.2	X44	X64	Y14	Y52.2
Endosulfan	T60.2	X48	X68	Y18	
Endothall	T60.3	X48	X68	Y18	
Endralazine	T46.5	X44	X64	Y14	Y52.5
Endrin	T60.1	X48	X68	Y18	
Enflurane	T41.0	X44	X64	Y14	Y48.0
Enhexymal	T42.3	X41	X61	Y11	Y47.0
Enocitabine	T45.1	X44	X64	Y14	Y43.1
Enoxacin	T36.8	X44	X64	Y14	Y40.8
Enoxaparin (sodium)	T45.5	X44	X64	Y14	Y44.2
Enpiprazole	T43.5	X41	X61	Y11	Y49.5
Enprofylline	T48.6	X44	X64	Y14	Y55.6
Enprostil	T47.1	X44	X64	Y14	Y53.1
Enterogastrone	T38.8	X44	X64	Y14	Y42.8
Enviomycin	T36.8	X44	X64	Y14	Y40.8
Enzyme NEC	T45.3	X44	X64	Y14	Y43.6
– depolymerizing	T49.8	X44	X64	Y14	Y56.8
– fibrolytic	T45.3	X44	X64	Y14	Y43.6
– gastric	T45.3	X44	X64	Y14	Y43.6

Substance	Chapter XIX	Accidental	Poisoning Intentional self-harm	Undetermined intent	Adverse effect in therapeutic use
Enzyme NEC—*continued*					
– intestinal	T47.5	X44	X64	Y14	Y53.5
– local action	T49.4	X44	X64	Y14	Y56.4
– proteolytic	T49.4	X44	X64	Y14	Y56.4
– thrombolytic	T45.3	X44	X64	Y14	Y43.6
EPAB	T41.3	X44	X64	Y14	Y48.3
Ephedra	T44.9	X43	X63	Y13	Y51.9
Ephedrine	T44.9	X43	X63	Y13	Y51.9
Epichlorhydrin, epichlorohydrin	T52.8	X46	X66	Y16	
Epicillin	T36.0	X44	X64	Y14	Y40.0
Epimestrol	T38.5	X44	X64	Y14	Y42.5
Epinephrine	T44.5	X43	X63	Y13	Y51.5
Epirizole	T39.3	X40	X60	Y10	Y45.3
Epirubicin	T45.1	X44	X64	Y14	Y43.3
Epitiostanol	T38.7	X44	X64	Y14	Y42.7
Epitizide	T50.2	X44	X64	Y14	Y54.3
EPN	T60.0	X48	X68	Y18	
EPO	T45.8	X44	X64	Y14	Y44.1
Epoetin alpha	T45.8	X44	X64	Y14	Y44.1
Epomediol	T50.9	X44	X64	Y14	Y57.1
Epoprostenol	T45.5	X44	X64	Y14	Y44.4
Epoxy resin	T65.8	X49	X69	Y19	
Eprazinone	T48.4	X44	X64	Y14	Y55.4
Epsilon aminocaproic acid	T45.6	X44	X64	Y14	Y44.3
Eptazocine	T40.4	X42	X62	Y12	Y45.0
Ergobasine	T48.0	X44	X64	Y14	Y55.0
Ergocalciferol	T45.2	X44	X64	Y14	Y54.7
Ergoloid mesylates	T46.7	X44	X64	Y14	Y52.7
Ergometrine	T48.0	X44	X64	Y14	Y55.0
Ergonovine	T48.0	X44	X64	Y14	Y55.0
Ergot NEC	T64	X49	X69	Y19	
– derivative	T48.0	X44	X64	Y14	Y55.0
– prepared	T48.0	X44	X64	Y14	Y55.0
Ergotamine	T46.5	X44	X64	Y14	Y52.5
Ergotocine	T48.0	X44	X64	Y14	Y55.0
Eritrityl tetranitrate	T46.3	X44	X64	Y14	Y52.3
Erythrityl tetranitrate	T46.3	X44	X64	Y14	Y52.3
Erythrol tetranitrate	T46.3	X44	X64	Y14	Y52.3
Erythromycin (salts)	T36.3	X44	X64	Y14	Y40.3
Erythropoietin	T45.8	X44	X64	Y14	Y44.1
– human	T45.8	X44	X64	Y14	Y44.1
Escin	T46.9	X44	X64	Y14	Y52.9
Esculin	T45.2	X44	X64	Y14	Y57.7
Esculoside	T45.2	X44	X64	Y14	Y57.7
ESDT (ether-soluble tar distillate)	T49.1	X44	X64	Y14	Y56.1
Eserine	T49.5	X44	X64	Y14	Y56.5
Esflurbiprofen	T39.3	X40	X60	Y10	Y45.2
Esmolol	T44.7	X43	X63	Y13	Y51.7
Estanozolol	T38.7	X44	X64	Y14	Y42.7
Estazolam	T42.4	X41	X61	Y11	Y47.1

Substance	Chapter XIX	Poisoning Accidental	Intentional self-harm	Undetermined intent	Adverse effect in therapeutic use
Estradiol	T38.5	X44	X64	Y14	Y42.5
– with testosterone	T38.7	X44	X64	Y14	Y42.7
– benzoate	T38.5	X44	X64	Y14	Y42.5
Estramustine	T45.1	X44	X64	Y14	Y43.3
Estriol	T38.5	X44	X64	Y14	Y42.5
Estrogen	T38.5	X44	X64	Y14	Y42.5
– with progesterone	T38.5	X44	X64	Y14	Y42.5
– conjugated	T38.5	X44	X64	Y14	Y42.5
Estrone	T38.5	X44	X64	Y14	Y42.5
Estropipate	T38.5	X44	X64	Y14	Y42.5
Etacrynate sodium	T50.1	X44	X64	Y14	Y54.4
Etacrynic acid	T50.1	X44	X64	Y14	Y54.4
Etafedrine	T48.6	X44	X64	Y14	Y55.6
Etafenone	T46.3	X44	X64	Y14	Y52.3
Etambutol	T37.1	X44	X64	Y14	Y41.1
Etamiphyllin	T48.6	X44	X64	Y14	Y55.6
Etamivan	T50.7	X44	X64	Y14	Y50.0
Etamsylate	T45.7	X44	X64	Y14	Y44.3
Etebenecid	T50.4	X44	X64	Y14	Y54.8
Etersalate	T39.0	X40	X60	Y10	Y45.1
Eterylate	T39.0	X40	X60	Y10	Y45.1
Ethacridine	T49.0	X44	X64	Y14	Y56.0
Ethacrynic acid	T50.1	X44	X64	Y14	Y54.4
Ethadione	T42.2	X41	X61	Y11	Y46.1
Ethambutol	T37.1	X44	X64	Y14	Y41.1
Ethamivan	T50.7	X44	X64	Y14	Y50.0
Ethamsylate	T45.7	X44	X64	Y14	Y44.3
Ethanol	T51.0	X45	X65	Y15	
Ethanolamine oleate	T46.8	X44	X64	Y14	Y52.8
Ethaverine	T44.3	X43	X63	Y13	Y51.3
Ethchlorvynol	T42.6	X41	X61	Y11	Y47.8
Ethenzamide	T39.0	X40	X60	Y10	Y45.1
Ether (vapor)	T41.0	X47	X67	Y17	Y48.0
– anesthetic	T41.0	X44	X64	Y14	Y48.0
– divinyl	T41.0	X44	X64	Y14	Y48.0
– ethyl (medicinal)	T41.0	X44	X64	Y14	Y48.0
– – nonmedicinal	T52.8	X46	X66	Y16	
– petroleum – see Ligroin					
– solvent	T52.8	X46	X66	Y16	
Ethiazide	T50.2	X44	X64	Y14	Y54.3
Ethidium chloride (vapor)	T59.8	X46	X66	Y16	
Ethinamate	T42.6	X41	X61	Y11	Y47.8
Ethinylestradiol, ethinyloestradiol	T38.5	X44	X64	Y14	Y42.5
– with					
– – levonorgestrel	T38.4	X44	X64	Y14	Y42.4
– – norethisterone	T38.4	X44	X64	Y14	Y42.4
Ethiodized oil (^{131}I)	T50.8	X44	X64	Y14	Y57.5
Ethion	T60.0	X48	X68	Y18	
Ethionamide	T37.1	X44	X64	Y14	Y41.1
Ethioniamide	T37.1	X44	X64	Y14	Y41.1
Ethisterone	T38.5	X44	X64	Y14	Y42.5

Substance	Chapter XIX	Accidental	Poisoning Intentional self-harm	Undetermined intent	Adverse effect in therapeutic use
Ethoheptazine	T40.4	X42	X62	Y12	Y45.0
Ethopropazine	T44.3	X43	X63	Y13	Y51.3
Ethosuximide	T42.2	X41	X61	Y11	Y46.0
Ethotoin	T42.0	X41	X61	Y11	Y46.2
Ethoxazorutoside	T46.9	X44	X64	Y14	Y52.9
2-Ethoxyethanol	T52.3	X46	X66	Y16	
Ethoxzolamide	T50.2	X44	X64	Y14	Y54.2
Ethyl					
– acetate	T52.8	X46	X66	Y16	
– alcohol	T51.0	X45	X65	Y15	
– aldehyde (vapor)	T59.8	X47	X67	Y17	
– – liquid	T52.8	X46	X66	Y16	
– aminobenzoate	T41.3	X44	X64	Y14	Y48.3
– aminophenothiazine	T43.3	X41	X61	Y11	Y49.3
– benzoate	T52.8	X46	X66	Y16	
– biscoumacetate	T45.5	X44	X64	Y14	Y44.2
– carbamate	T45.1	X44	X64	Y14	Y43.3
– carbinol	T51.3	X45	X65	Y15	
– carbonate	T52.8	X46	X66	Y16	
– chloride (anesthetic)	T41.0	X44	X64	Y14	Y48.0
– – local	T49.4	X44	X64	Y14	Y56.4
– – solvent	T53.6	X46	X66	Y16	
– dibunate	T48.3	X44	X64	Y14	Y55.3
– dichloroarsine (vapor)	T57.0	X49	X69	Y19	
– ether (see also Ether)	T52.8	X46	X66	Y16	
– formate NEC (solvent)	T52.0	X46	X66	Y16	
– fumarate	T49.4	X44	X64	Y14	Y56.4
– hydroxyisobutyrate NEC (solvent)	T52.8	X46	X66	Y16	
– iodoacetate	T59.3	X47	X67	Y17	
– lactate NEC (solvent)	T52.8	X46	X66	Y16	
– loflazepate	T42.4	X41	X61	Y11	Y47.1
– mercuric chloride	T56.1	X49	X69	Y19	
– noradrenaline	T48.6	X44	X64	Y14	Y55.6
– oxybutyrate NEC (solvent)	T52.8	X46	X66	Y16	
Ethylene (gas)	T59.8	X47	X67	Y17	
– chlorohydrin	T52.8	X46	X66	Y16	
– – vapor	T53.6	X46	X66	Y16	
– dichloride	T52.8	X46	X66	Y16	
– – vapor	T53.6	X46	X66	Y16	
– dinitrate	T52.3	X46	X66	Y16	
– glycol(s)	T52.8	X46	X66	Y16	
– – dinitrate	T52.3	X46	X66	Y16	
– – monobutyl ether	T52.3	X46	X66	Y16	
– imine	T54.1	X49	X69	Y19	
– oxide (fumigant) (nonmedicinal)	T59.8	X47	X67	Y17	
– – medicinal	T49.0	X44	X64	Y14	Y56.0
Ethylenediamine theophylline	T48.6	X44	X64	Y14	Y55.6
Ethylenediaminetetraacetic acid	T50.6	X44	X64	Y14	Y57.2
Ethylenedinitrilotetraacetate	T50.6	X44	X64	Y14	Y57.2
Ethylestrenol	T38.7	X44	X64	Y14	Y42.7

Substance	Chapter XIX	Poisoning			Adverse effect in therapeutic use
		Accidental	Intentional self-harm	Undetermined intent	
Ethylhydroxycellulose	T47.4	X44	X64	Y14	Y53.4
Ethylidene					
– chloride NEC	T53.6	X46	X66	Y16	
– diacetate	T60.3	X48	X68	Y18	
– dicoumarin	T45.5	X44	X64	Y14	Y44.2
– dicoumarol	T45.5	X44	X64	Y14	Y44.2
– diethyl ether	T52.0	X46	X66	Y16	
Ethylmorphine	T40.2	X42	X62	Y12	Y45.0
Ethylnorepinephrine	T48.6	X44	X64	Y14	Y55.6
Ethylparachlorophenoxyisobutyrate	T46.6	X44	X64	Y14	Y52.6
Ethynodiol	T38.4	X44	X64	Y14	Y42.4
– with mestranol diacetate	T38.4	X44	X64	Y14	Y42.4
Etidocaine	T41.3	X44	X64	Y14	Y48.3
Etidronate	T50.9	X44	X64	Y14	Y54.7
Etidronic acid (disodium salt)	T50.9	X44	X64	Y14	Y54.7
Etifoxine	T42.6	X41	X61	Y11	Y47.8
Etilefrine	T44.4	X43	X63	Y13	Y51.4
Etinodiol	T38.4	X44	X64	Y14	Y42.4
Etiroxate	T46.6	X44	X64	Y14	Y52.6
Etizolam	T42.4	X41	X61	Y11	Y47.1
Etodolac	T39.3	X40	X60	Y10	Y45.3
Etofamide	T37.3	X44	X64	Y14	Y41.3
Etofibrate	T46.6	X44	X64	Y14	Y52.6
Etofylline	T46.7	X44	X64	Y14	Y52.7
– clofibrate	T46.6	X44	X64	Y14	Y52.6
Etoglucid	T45.1	X44	X64	Y14	Y43.3
Etomidate	T41.1	X44	X64	Y14	Y48.1
Etomidoline	T44.3	X43	X63	Y13	Y51.3
Etoposide	T45.1	X44	X64	Y14	Y43.3
Etosalamide	T39.0	X40	X60	Y10	Y45.1
Etozolin	T50.1	X44	X64	Y14	Y54.4
Etretinate	T50.9	X44	X64	Y14	Y57.8
Etybenzatropine	T44.3	X43	X63	Y13	Y51.3
Etynodiol	T38.4	X44	X64	Y14	Y42.4
Eucaine	T41.3	X44	X64	Y14	Y48.3
Eucalyptus oil	T49.7	X44	X64	Y14	Y56.7
Eucatropine	T49.5	X44	X64	Y14	Y56.5
Evans blue	T50.8	X44	X64	Y14	Y57.6
Exalamide	T49.0	X44	X64	Y14	Y56.0
Exhaust gas	T58	X47	X67	Y17	
Expectorant NEC	T48.4	X44	X64	Y14	Y55.4
Extended insulin zinc suspension	T38.3	X44	X64	Y14	Y42.3
Extrapyramidal antagonist NEC	T44.3	X43	X63	Y13	Y51.3
Eye drug NEC	T49.5	X44	X64	Y14	Y56.5

F

Substance	Chapter XIX	Poisoning			Adverse effect in therapeutic use
		Accidental	Intentional self-harm	Undetermined intent	
FAC (fluorouracil + doxorubicin + cyclophosphamide)	T45.1	X44	X64	Y14	Y43.3
Factor					
– I (fibrinogen)	T45.8	X44	X64	Y14	Y44.6
– III (thromboplastin)	T45.8	X44	X64	Y14	Y44.6
– VIII (antihemophilic factor) (concentrate)	T45.8	X44	X64	Y14	Y44.6
– IX complex	T45.7	X44	X64	Y14	Y44.3
– – human	T45.8	X44	X64	Y14	Y44.6
Famotidine	T47.0	X44	X64	Y14	Y53.0
Fat suspension, intravenous	T50.9	X44	X64	Y14	Y57.8
Fazadinium bromide	T48.1	X44	X64	Y14	Y55.1
Febarbamate	T42.3	X41	X61	Y11	Y47.0
Fecal softener	T47.4	X44	X64	Y14	Y53.4
Fedrilate	T48.3	X44	X64	Y14	Y55.3
Felodipine	T46.1	X44	X64	Y14	Y52.1
Felypressin	T38.8	X44	X64	Y14	Y42.8
Femoxetine	T43.2	X41	X61	Y11	Y49.2
Fenalcomine	T46.3	X44	X64	Y14	Y52.3
Fenamisal	T37.1	X44	X64	Y14	Y41.1
Fenazone	T39.2	X40	X60	Y10	Y45.8
Fenbendazole	T37.4	X44	X64	Y14	Y41.4
Fenbufen	T39.3	X40	X60	Y10	Y45.2
Fenbutrazate	T50.5	X44	X64	Y14	Y57.0
Fenclofenac	T39.3	X40	X60	Y10	Y45.3
Fendiline	T46.1	X44	X64	Y14	Y52.1
Fenetylline	T43.6	X41	X61	Y11	Y49.7
Fenflumizole	T39.3	X40	X60	Y10	Y45.3
Fenfluramine	T50.5	X44	X64	Y14	Y57.0
Fenobarbital	T42.3	X41	X61	Y11	Y47.0
Fenofibrate	T46.6	X44	X64	Y14	Y52.6
Fenoprofen	T39.3	X40	X60	Y10	Y45.2
Fenoterol	T48.6	X44	X64	Y14	Y55.6
Fenoverine	T44.3	X43	X63	Y13	Y51.3
Fenoxazoline	T48.5	X44	X64	Y14	Y55.5
Fenproporex	T50.5	X44	X64	Y14	Y57.0
Fenquizone	T50.2	X44	X64	Y14	Y54.5
Fentanyl	T40.4	X42	X62	Y12	Y45.0
Fenthion	T60.0	X48	X68	Y18	
Fentiazac	T39.3	X40	X60	Y10	Y45.3
Fenticlor	T49.0	X44	X64	Y14	Y56.0
Fenylbutazone	T39.2	X40	X60	Y10	Y45.3
Feprazone	T39.2	X40	X60	Y10	Y45.8

763

| | Poisoning | | | Adverse effect |
Substance	Chapter XIX	Accidental	Intentional self-harm	Undetermined intent	in therapeutic use
Ferric *see also* Iron					
– chloride	T45.4	X44	X64	Y14	Y44.0
– citrate	T45.4	X44	X64	Y14	Y44.0
– hydroxide					
– – colloidal	T45.4	X44	X64	Y14	Y44.0
– – polymaltose	T45.4	X44	X64	Y14	Y44.0
– pyrophosphate	T45.4	X44	X64	Y14	Y44.0
Ferritin	T45.4	X44	X64	Y14	Y44.0
Ferrocholinate	T45.4	X44	X64	Y14	Y44.0
Ferrodextrane	T45.4	X44	X64	Y14	Y44.0
Ferropolimaler	T45.4	X44	X64	Y14	Y44.0
Ferrous – *see also* Iron					
– phosphate	T45.4	X44	X64	Y14	Y44.0
– salt	T45.4	X44	X64	Y14	Y44.0
– – with folic acid	T45.4	X44	X64	Y14	Y44.0
Ferrovanadium (fumes)	T59.8	X47	X67	Y17	
Ferrum – *see* Iron					
Fertilizers NEC	T65.8	X49	X69	Y19	
Fetoxilate	T47.6	X44	X64	Y14	Y53.6
Fiber, dietary	T47.4	X44	X64	Y14	Y53.4
Fibrinogen (human)	T45.8	X44	X64	Y14	Y44.6
Fibrinolysin (human)	T45.6	X44	X64	Y14	Y44.5
Fibrinolysis-affecting drug	T45.6	X44	X64	Y14	Y44.9
Fibrinolysis inhibitor NEC	T45.6	X44	X64	Y14	Y44.3
Fibrinolytic drug	T45.6	X44	X64	Y14	Y44.5
Filix mas	T37.4	X44	X64	Y14	Y41.4
Filtering cream	T49.3	X44	X64	Y14	Y56.3
Firedamp	T59.8	X47	X67	Y17	
Fish, noxious, nonbacterial	T61.2	X49	X69	Y19	
– shell	T61.2	X49	X69	Y19	
Flavine adenine dinucleotide	T45.2	X44	X64	Y14	Y57.7
Flavodic acid	T46.9	X44	X64	Y14	Y52.9
Flavoxate	T44.3	X43	X63	Y13	Y51.3
Flecainide	T46.2	X44	X64	Y14	Y52.2
Fleroxacin	T36.8	X44	X64	Y14	Y40.8
Floctafenine	T39.8	X40	X60	Y10	Y45.8
Flomoxef	T36.1	X44	X64	Y14	Y40.1
Flopropione	T44.3	X43	X63	Y13	Y51.3
Floxuridine	T45.1	X44	X64	Y14	Y43.3
Fluanisone	T43.4	X41	X61	Y11	Y49.4
Flubendazole	T37.4	X44	X64	Y14	
Fluclorolone acetonide	T49.0	X44	X64	Y14	Y56.0
Flucloxacillin	T36.0	X44	X64	Y14	Y40.0
Fluconazole	T37.8	X44	X64	Y14	Y41.8
Flucytosine	T37.8	X44	X64	Y14	Y41.8
Fludeoxyglucose (^{18}F)	T50.8	X44	X64	Y14	Y57.6
Fludiazepam	T42.4	X41	X61	Y11	Y47.1
Fludrocortisone	T50.0	X44	X64	Y14	Y54.0
Fludroxycortide	T49.0	X44	X64	Y14	Y56.0
Flufenamic acid	T39.3	X40	X60	Y10	Y45.3
Fluindione	T45.5	X44	X64	Y14	Y44.2

| Substance | Chapter XIX | Poisoning | | | Adverse effect in therapeutic use |
		Accidental	Intentional self-harm	Undetermined intent	
Flumequine	T37.8	X44	X64	Y14	Y41.8
Flumetasone	T49.0	X44	X64	Y14	Y56.0
Flunarizine	T46.7	X44	X64	Y14	Y52.7
Flunidazole	T37.8	X44	X64	Y14	Y41.8
Flunisolide	T48.6	X44	X64	Y14	Y55.6
Flunitrazepam	T42.4	X41	X61	Y11	Y47.1
Flunoxaprofen	T39.3	X40	X60	Y10	Y45.3
Fluocinolone (acetonide)	T49.0	X44	X64	Y14	Y56.0
Fluocinonide	T49.0	X44	X64	Y14	Y56.0
Fluocortin (butyl)	T49.0	X44	X64	Y14	Y56.0
Fluocortolone	T49.0	X44	X64	Y14	Y56.0
Fluopromazine	T43.3	X41	X61	Y11	Y49.3
Fluorescein	T50.8	X44	X64	Y14	Y57.6
Fluorhydrocortisone	T50.0	X44	X64	Y14	Y54.0
Fluoride (nonmedicinal) (pesticide) (sodium) NEC	T60.8	X48	X68	Y18	
– medicinal NEC	T50.9	X44	X64	Y14	Y54.9
– dental use	T49.7	X44	X64	Y14	Y56.7
Fluorine (gas)	T59.5	X47	X67	Y17	
– salt – see Fluoride(s)					
Fluormetholone	T49.0	X44	X64	Y14	Y56.0
Fluoroacetate	T60.4	X48	X68	Y18	
Fluorocarbon monomer	T53.6	X46	X66	Y16	
Fluorocytosine	T37.8	X44	X64	Y14	Y41.8
Fluorometholone	T49.0	X44	X64	Y14	Y56.0
Fluorophosphate insecticide	T60.0	X48	X68	Y18	
Fluorosol	T46.3	X44	X64	Y14	Y52.3
Fluorouracil	T45.1	X44	X64	Y14	Y43.1
Fluorphenylalanine	T49.5	X44	X64	Y14	Y56.5
Fluoxetine	T43.2	X41	X61	Y11	Y49.2
Fluoxymesterone	T38.7	X44	X64	Y14	Y42.7
Flupenthixol	T43.4	X41	X61	Y11	Y49.4
Flupentixol	T43.4	X41	X61	Y11	Y49.4
Fluphenazine	T43.3	X41	X61	Y11	Y49.3
Fluprednidene	T49.0	X44	X64	Y14	Y56.0
Fluprednisolone	T38.0	X44	X64	Y14	Y42.0
Fluradoline	T39.8	X40	X60	Y10	Y45.8
Flurandrenolone	T49.0	X44	X64	Y14	Y56.0
Flurazepam	T42.4	X41	X61	Y11	Y47.1
Flurbiprofen	T39.3	X40	X60	Y10	Y45.2
Flurotyl	T43.2	X41	X61	Y11	Y49.2
Fluroxene	T41.0	X44	X64	Y14	Y48.0
Fluspirilene	T43.5	X41	X61	Y11	Y49.5
Flutamide	T38.6	X44	X64	Y14	Y42.6
Flutazolam	T42.4	X41	X61	Y11	Y47.1
Fluticasone propionate	T49.1	X44	X64	Y14	Y56.1
Flutoprazepam	T42.4	X41	X61	Y11	Y47.1
Flutropium bromide	T48.6	X44	X64	Y14	Y55.6
Fluvoxamine	T43.2	X41	X61	Y11	Y49.2

	Poisoning			Adverse effect in therapeutic use
Substance	Chapter XIX	Accidental	Intentional self-harm	Undetermined intent	
Folic acid	T45.8	X44	X64	Y14	Y44.1
– with ferrous salt	T45.2	X44	X64	Y14	Y44.1
– antagonist	T45.1	X44	X64	Y14	Y43.1
Folinic acid	T45.8	X44	X64	Y14	Y44.1
Folium stramoniae	T48.6	X44	X64	Y14	Y55.6
Follicle-stimulating hormone, human	T38.8	X44	X64	Y14	Y42.8
Folpet	T60.3	X48	X68	Y18	
Fominoben	T48.3	X44	X64	Y14	Y55.3
Food, foodstuffs, noxious, nonbacterial, NEC	T62.9	X49	X69	Y19	
Formaldehyde (solution), gas or vapor	T59.2	X47	X67	Y17	
Formalin (vapor)	T59.2	X47	X67	Y17	Y56.0
Formic acid	T54.2	X49	X69	Y19	
– vapor	T59.8	X47	X67	Y17	
Foscarnet sodium	T37.5	X44	X64	Y14	Y41.5
Fosfestrol	T38.5	X44	X64	Y14	Y42.5
Fosfomycin	T36.8	X44	X64	Y14	Y40.8
Fosfonet sodium	T37.5	X44	X64	Y14	Y41.5
Fosfosal	T39.0	X40	X60	Y10	Y45.1
Fosinopril	T46.4	X44	X64	Y14	Y52.4
– sodium	T46.4	X44	X64	Y14	Y52.4
Foxglove	T62.2	X49	X69	Y19	
Framycetin	T36.5	X44	X64	Y14	Y40.5
Frangula	T47.2	X44	X64	Y14	Y53.2
– extract	T47.2	X44	X64	Y14	Y53.2
Frei antigen	T50.8	X44	X64	Y14	Y57.6
Freon	T53.5	X46	X66	Y16	
Fructose	T50.3	X44	X64	Y14	Y54.6
Frusemide	T50.1	X44	X64	Y14	Y54.4
FSH	T38.8	X44	X64	Y14	Y42.8
Ftorafur	T45.1	X44	X64	Y14	Y43.1
Fuel					
– automobile	T52.0	X46	X66	Y16	
– – exhaust gas, not in transit	T58	X47	X67	Y17	
– – vapor NEC	T52.0	X46	X66	Y16	
– gas (domestic use)	T58	X47	X67	Y17	
– industrial, incomplete combustion	T58	X47	X67	Y17	
Fulminate of mercury	T56.1	X49	X69	Y19	
Fumagillin	T36.8	X44	X64	Y14	Y40.8
Fumaric acid	T49.4	X44	X64	Y14	Y56.4
Fumes (from)	T59.9	X47	X67	Y17	
– carbon monoxide	T58	X47	X67	Y17	
– charcoal (domestic use)	T58	X47	X67	Y17	
– coke (in domestic stoves, fireplaces)	T58	X47	X67	Y17	
– corrosive NEC	T59.8	X47	X67	Y17	
– ether – see Ether					
– lead – see Lead					

Substance		Poisoning			Adverse effect in therapeutic use
	Chapter XIX	Accidental	Intentional self-harm	Undetermined intent	
Fumes—*continued*					
– metal – *see* Metals, or the specified metal					
– specified source NEC	T59.9	X47	X67	Y17	
Fumigant NEC	T60.9	X48	X68	Y18	
Fungi, noxious, used as food	T62.0	X49	X69	Y19	
Fungicide NEC (nonmedicinal)	T60.3	X48	X68	Y18	
Furazolidone	T37.8	X44	X64	Y14	Y41.8
Furazolium chloride	T49.0	X44	X64	Y14	Y56.0
Furfural	T52.8	X46	X66	Y16	
Furnace (coal burning) (domestic), gas from industrial	T58	X47	X67	Y17	
Furniture polish	T65.8	X49	X69	Y19	
Furosemide	T50.1	X44	X64	Y14	Y54.4
Fursultiamine	T45.2	X44	X64	Y14	Y57.7
Fusafungine	T36.8	X44	X64	Y14	Y40.8
Fusel oil (any) (amyl) (butyl) (propyl), vapor	T51.3	X45	X65	Y15	
Fusidate (ethanolamine) (sodium)	T36.8	X44	X64	Y14	Y40.8
Fusidic acid	T36.8	X44	X64	Y14	Y40.8
Fytic acid, nonasodium	T50.6	X44	X64	Y14	Y57.2

G

Constituent of daffodil

| | Poisoning | | | | Adverse effect |
Substance	Chapter XIX	Accidental	Intentional self-harm	Undetermined intent	in therapeutic use
GABA	T43.8	X41	X61	Y11	Y49.8
Gabexate	T45.6	X44	X64	Y14	Y44.3
Gadopentetic acid	T50.8	X44	X64	Y14	Y57.5
Galactose	T50.3	X44	X64	Y14	Y54.6
Beta-Galactosidase	T47.5	X44	X64	Y14	Y53.5
Galantamine	T44.0	X43	X63	Y13	Y51.0
Gallamine (triethiodide)	T48.1	X44	X64	Y14	Y55.1
Gallium citrate	T50.9	X44	X64	Y14	Y54.7
Gallopamil	T46.1	X44	X64	Y14	Y52.1
Gamma globulin NEC	T50.9	X44	X64	Y14	Y59.3
Gamma-aminobutyric acid	T43.8	X41	X61	Y11	Y49.8
Gamma-benzene hexachloride (medicinal)	T49.0	X44	X64	Y14	Y56.0
– nonmedicinal, vapor	T53.6	X46	X66	Y16	
Gamma-BHC (medicinal)	T49.0	X44	X64	Y14	Y56.0
Ganciclovir (sodium)	T37.5	X44	X64	Y14	Y41.5
Ganglionic blocking drug NEC	T44.2	X43	X63	Y13	Y51.2
– specified NEC	T44.2	X43	X63	Y13	Y51.2
Ganja	T40.7	X42	X62	Y12	Y49.6
Gas	T59.9	X47	X67	Y17	
– acetylene	T59.8	X47	X67	Y17	
– air contaminants, source or type not specified	T59.9	X47	X67	Y17	
– anesthetic	T41.0	X44	X64	Y14	Y48.0
– blast furnace	T58	X47	X67	Y17	
– butane – see Butane					
– carbon monoxide	T58	X47	X67	Y17	
– chlorine	T59.4	X47	X67	Y17	
– coal	T58	X47	X67	Y17	
– cyanide	T57.3	X47	X67	Y17	
– dicyanogen	T65.0	X47	X67	Y17	
– domestic	T58	X47	X67	Y17	
– exhaust	T58	X47	X67	Y17	
– from utility (for cooking, heating, or lighting)	T58	X47	X67	Y17	
– from wood- or coal-burning stove or fireplace	T58	X47	X67	Y17	
– fuel (domestic use)	T58	X47	X67	Y17	
– garage	T58	X47	X67	Y17	
– hydrocarbon NEC	T59.8	X47	X67	Y17	
– – liquefied – see Butane					
– hydrocyanic acid	T59.8	X47	X67	Y17	
– illuminating	T58	X47	X67	Y17	
– incomplete combustion, any	T58	X47	X67	Y17	

		Poisoning			Adverse effect in therapeutic use
Substance	Chapter XIX	Accidental	Intentional self-harm	Undetermined intent	
Gas—*continued*					
– kiln	T58	X47	X67	Y17	
– lacrimogenic	T59.3	X47	X67	Y17	
– liquefied petroleum – *see* Butane					
– marsh	T59.8	X47	X67	Y17	
– motor exhaust, not in transit	T58	X47	X67	Y17	
– mustard, not in war	T59.8	X47	X67	Y17	
– natural	T59.8	X47	X67	Y17	
– nerve, not in war	T59.9	X47	X67	Y17	
– oil	T52.0	X46	X66	Y16	
– producer	T58	X47	X67	Y17	
– propane – *see* Propane					
– refrigerant (chlorofluorocarbon)	T53.5	X47	X67	Y17	
– – not chlorofluorocarbon	T59.8	X47	X67	Y17	
– sewer	T59.9	X47	X67	Y17	
– specified source NEC	T59.9	X47	X67	Y17	
– stove	T58	X47	X67	Y17	
– therapeutic	T41.5	X44	X64	Y14	Y48.5
– water	T58	X47	X67	Y17	
Gaseous substance – *see* Gas					
Gasolene, gasoline	T52.0	X46	X66	Y16	
– vapor	T52.0	X46	X66	Y16	
Gastrointestinal drug	T47.9	X44	X64	Y14	Y53.9
– biological	T47.8	X44	X64	Y14	Y53.8
– specified NEC	T47.8	X44	X64	Y14	Y53.8
Gefarnate	T44.3	X43	X63	Y13	Y51.3
Gemeprost	T48.0	X44	X64	Y14	Y55.0
Gemfibrozil	T46.6	X44	X64	Y14	Y52.6
Gentamicin	T36.5	X44	X64	Y14	Y40.5
Gentian	T47.5	X44	X64	Y14	Y53.5
– violet	T49.0	X44	X64	Y14	Y56.0
Gepefrine	T44.4	X43	X63	Y13	Y51.4
Gestonorone caproate	T38.5	X44	X64	Y14	Y42.5
Ginger	T47.5	X44	X64	Y14	Y53.5
– jamaica	T62.2	X49	X69	Y19	
Gitalin	T46.0	X44	X64	Y14	Y52.0
– amorphous	T46.0	X44	X64	Y14	Y52.0
Gitaloxin	T46.0	X44	X64	Y14	Y52.0
Glafenine	T39.8	X40	X60	Y10	Y45.8
Glibenclamide	T38.3	X44	X64	Y14	Y42.3
Glibornuride	T38.3	X44	X64	Y14	Y42.3
Gliclazide	T38.3	X44	X64	Y14	Y42.3
Glimidine	T38.3	X44	X64	Y14	Y42.3
Glipizide	T38.3	X44	X64	Y14	Y42.3
Gliquidone	T38.3	X44	X64	Y14	Y42.3
Glisolamide	T38.3	X44	X64	Y14	Y42.3
Glisoxepide	T38.3	X44	X64	Y14	Y42.3
Globin zinc insulin	T38.3	X44	X64	Y14	Y42.3

| Substance | Chapter XIX | Poisoning | | | Adverse effect in therapeutic use |
		Accidental	Intentional self-harm	Undetermined intent	
Globulin					
– antilymphocytic	T50.9	X44	X64	Y14	Y59.3
antirhesus	T50.9	X44	X64	Y14	Y59.3
– antivenin	T50.9	X44	X64	Y14	Y59.3
– antiviral	T50.9	X44	X64	Y14	Y59.3
Glucagon	T38.3	X44	X64	Y14	Y42.3
Glucametacin	T39.3	X40	X60	Y10	Y45.3
Glucocorticoid	T38.0	X44	X64	Y14	Y42.0
Glucocorticosteroid	T38.0	X44	X64	Y14	Y42.0
Gluconic acid	T50.9	X44	X64	Y14	Y43.5
Glucosamine sulfate	T39.4	X40	X60	Y10	Y45.4
Glucose	T50.3	X44	X64	Y14	Y54.6
– with sodium chloride	T50.3	X44	X64	Y14	Y54.6
Glucurolactone	T47.8	X44	X64	Y14	Y53.8
Glue NEC	T52.8	X49	X69	Y19	
Glutamic acid	T47.5	X44	X64	Y14	Y53.5
Glutaral (medicinal)	T49.0	X44	X64	Y14	Y56.0
– nonmedicinal	T65.8	X49	X69	Y19	
Glutaraldehyde (nonmedicinal)	T65.8	X49	X69	Y19	
– medicinal	T49.0	X44	X64	Y14	Y56.0
Glutathione	T50.6	X44	X64	Y14	Y57.2
Glutethimide	T42.6	X41	X61	Y11	Y47.8
Glyburide	T38.3	X44	X64	Y14	Y42.3
Glycerin	T47.4	X44	X64	Y14	Y53.4
Glycerol	T47.4	X44	X64	Y14	Y53.4
– borax	T49.6	X44	X64	Y14	Y56.6
– intravenous	T50.3	X44	X64	Y14	Y54.6
– iodinated	T48.4	X44	X64	Y14	Y55.4
Glycerophosphate	T50.9	X44	X64	Y14	Y57.8
Glyceryl					
– guaiacolate	T48.4	X44	X64	Y14	Y55.4
– nitrate	T46.3	X44	X64	Y14	Y52.3
– trinitrate	T46.3	X44	X64	Y14	Y52.3
Glyclopyramide	T38.3	X44	X64	Y14	Y42.3
Glycobiarsol	T37.3	X44	X64	Y14	Y41.3
Glycols (ether)	T52.3	X46	X66	Y16	
Glyconiazide	T37.1	X44	X64	Y14	Y41.1
Glycopyrrolate	T44.3	X43	X63	Y13	Y51.3
Glycopyrronium	T44.3	X43	X63	Y13	Y51.3
– bromide	T44.3	X43	X63	Y13	Y51.3
Glycoside, cardiac-stimulant	T46.0	X44	X64	Y14	Y52.0
Glycyclamide	T38.3	X44	X64	Y14	Y42.3
Glycyrrhiza extract	T48.4	X44	X64	Y14	Y55.4
Glycyrrhizic acid	T48.4	X44	X64	Y14	Y55.4
Glycyrrhizinate potassium	T48.4	X44	X64	Y14	Y55.4
Glymidine sodium	T38.3	X44	X64	Y14	Y42.3
Glyphosate	T60.3	X48	X68	Y18	
Glyphylline	T48.6	X44	X64	Y14	Y55.6
Gold					
– colloidal (^{198}Au)	T45.1	X44	X64	Y14	Y43.3
– salts	T39.4	X40	X60	Y10	Y45.4

| Substance | Chapter XIX | Poisoning | | | Adverse effect in therapeutic use |
		Accidental	Intentional self-harm	Undetermined intent	
Golden sulfide of antimony	T56.8	X49	X69	Y19	
Gonadorelin	T38.8	X44	X64	Y14	Y42.8
Gonadotrophin	T38.8	X44	X64	Y14	Y42.8
– chorionic	T38.8	X44	X64	Y14	Y42.8
– serum	T38.8	X44	X64	Y14	Y42.8
Goserelin	T45.1	X44	X64	Y14	Y43.3
Grain alcohol	T51.0	X45	X65	Y15	
Gramicidin	T49.0	X44	X64	Y14	Y56.0
Granisetron	T45.0	X44	X64	Y14	Y43.0
Grease	T65.8	X49	X69	Y19	
Griseofulvin	T36.7	X44	X64	Y14	Y40.7
Guacetisal	T39.0	X40	X60	Y10	Y45.1
Guaiacol derivatives	T48.4	X44	X64	Y14	Y55.4
Guaifenesin	T48.4	X44	X64	Y14	Y55.4
Guaimesal	T48.4	X44	X64	Y14	Y55.4
Guaiphenesin	T48.4	X44	X64	Y14	Y55.4
Guamecycline	T36.4	X44	X64	Y14	Y40.4
Guanabenz	T46.5	X44	X64	Y14	Y52.5
Guanacline	T46.5	X44	X64	Y14	Y52.5
Guanadrel	T46.5	X44	X64	Y14	Y52.5
Guanethidine	T46.5	X44	X64	Y14	Y52.5
Guanfacine	T46.5	X44	X64	Y14	Y52.5
Guano	T65.8	X49	X69	Y19	
Guanochlor	T46.5	X44	X64	Y14	Y52.5
Guanoclor	T46.5	X44	X64	Y14	Y52.5
Guanoxabenz	T46.5	X44	X64	Y14	Y52.5
Guanoxan	T46.5	X44	X64	Y14	Y52.5
Guar gum (medicinal)	T46.6	X44	X64	Y14	Y52.6

H

Substance	Chapter XIX	Poisoning			Adverse effect in therapeutic use
		Accidental	Intentional self-harm	Undetermined intent	
Hachimycin	T36.7	X44	X64	Y14	Y40.7
Hair					
– dye	T49.4	X44	X64	Y14	Y56.4
– preparation NEC	T49.4	X44	X64	Y14	Y56.4
Halazepam	T42.4	X41	X61	Y11	Y47.1
Halcinolone	T49.0	X44	X64	Y14	Y56.0
Halcinonide	T49.0	X44	X64	Y14	Y56.0
Hallucinogen NEC	T40.9	X42	X62	Y12	Y49.6
Halofantrine	T37.2	X44	X64	Y14	Y41.2
Halofenate	T46.6	X44	X64	Y14	Y52.6
Halometasone	T49.0	X44	X64	Y14	Y56.0
Haloperidol	T43.4	X41	X61	Y11	Y49.4
Haloprogin	T49.0	X44	X64	Y14	Y56.0
Halothane	T41.0	X44	X64	Y14	Y48.0
Haloxazolam	T42.4	X41	X61	Y11	Y47.1
Halquinols	T49.0	X44	X64	Y14	Y56.0
Hamamelis	T49.2	X44	X64	Y14	Y56.2
Haptendextran	T45.8	X44	X64	Y14	Y44.7
Hartmann's solution	T50.3	X44	X64	Y14	Y54.6
Hashish	T40.7	X42	X62	Y12	Y49.6
HCB	T60.3	X48	X68	Y18	
HCH	T53.6	X46	X66	Y16	
– medicinal	T49.0	X44	X64	Y14	Y56.0
HCN	T57.3	X48	X68	Y18	
Heavy metal antidote	T45.8	X44	X64	Y14	Y43.8
Helium	T48.7	X44	X64	Y14	Y55.7
Hematin	T45.8	X44	X64	Y14	Y44.9
Hematinic preparation	T45.8	X44	X64	Y14	Y44.1
Hematological agent	T45.9	X44	X64	Y14	Y44.9
– specified NEC	T45.8	X44	X64	Y14	Y44.9
Hemlock	T62.2	X49	X69	Y19	
Hemostatic	T49.4	X44	X64	Y14	Y56.4
– drug, systemic	T45.7	X44	X64	Y14	Y44.3
Hemostyptic	T49.4	X44	X64	Y14	Y56.4
Heparin (sodium)	T45.5	X44	X64	Y14	Y44.2
– action reverser	T45.7	X44	X64	Y14	Y44.3
Heparin-fraction	T45.5	X44	X64	Y14	Y44.2
Heparinoid (systemic)	T45.5	X44	X64	Y14	Y44.2
Hepatic secretion stimulant	T47.8	X44	X64	Y14	Y53.8
Hepatitis B					
– immune globulin	T50.9	X44	X64	Y14	Y59.3
– vaccine	T50.9	X44	X64	Y14	Y59.0
Hepronicate	T46.7	X44	X64	Y14	Y52.7
Heptabarb	T42.3	X41	X61	Y11	Y47.0

| Substance | Chapter XIX | Poisoning | | | Adverse effect in therapeutic use |
		Accidental	Intentional self-harm	Undetermined intent	
Heptabarbitone	T42.3	X41	X61	Y11	Y47.0
Heptachlor	T60.1	X48	X68	Y18	
Heptaminol	T46.3	X44	X64	Y14	Y52.3
Herbicide NEC	T60.3	X48	X68	Y18	
Heroin	T40.1	X42	X62	Y12	Y45.0
Hesperidin	T46.9	X44	X64	Y14	Y52.9
Hetacillin	T36.0	X44	X64	Y14	Y40.0
Hetastarch	T45.8	X44	X64	Y14	Y44.7
HETP	T60.0	X48	X68	Y18	
Hexachlorobenzene (vapor)	T60.3	X48	X68	Y18	
Hexachlorocyclohexane	T53.6	X46	X66	Y16	
Hexachlorophene	T49.0	X44	X64	Y14	Y56.0
Hexadiline	T46.3	X44	X64	Y14	Y52.3
Hexadylamine	T46.3	X44	X64	Y14	Y52.3
Hexaethyl tetraphosphate	T60.0	X48	X68	Y18	
Hexafluorenium bromide	T48.1	X44	X64	Y14	Y55.1
Hexafluorodiethyl ether	T43.2	X41	X61	Y11	Y49.2
Hexafluronium (bromide)	T48.1	X44	X64	Y14	Y55.1
Hexahydrobenzol	T52.8	X46	X66	Y16	
Hexahydrocresol(s)	T51.8	X45	X65	Y15	
– arsenide	T57.0	X49	X69	Y19	
– arseniurated	T57.0	X49	X69	Y19	
– cyanide	T57.3	X49	X69	Y19	
– – gas	T59.8	X47	X67	Y17	
– fluoride (liquid)	T57.8	X49	X69	Y19	
– – vapor	T59.8	X47	X67	Y17	
– phophorated	T60.0	X48	X68	Y18	
– sulfate	T57.8	X49	X69	Y19	
– sulfide (gas)	T59.6	X47	X67	Y17	
– – arseniurated	T57.0	X49	X69	Y19	
– sulfurated	T57.8	X49	X69	Y19	
Hexahydrophenol	T51.8	X45	X65	Y15	
Hexamethonium bromide	T44.2	X43	X63	Y13	Y51.2
Hexamethylene	T52.8	X46	X66	Y16	
Hexamethylmelamine	T45.1	X44	X64	Y14	Y43.3
Hexamidine	T49.0	X44	X64	Y14	Y56.0
Hexamine (mandelate)	T37.8	X44	X64	Y14	Y41.8
Hexanone, 2-hexanone	T52.4	X46	X66	Y16	
Hexapropymate	T42.6	X41	X61	Y11	Y47.8
Hexasonium iodide	T44.3	X43	X63	Y13	Y51.3
Hexcarbacholine bromide	T48.1	X44	X64	Y14	Y55.1
Hexemal	T42.3	X41	X61	Y11	Y47.0
Hexestrol	T38.5	X44	X64	Y14	Y42.5
Hexetidine	T37.8	X44	X64	Y14	Y41.8
Hexobarbital	T42.3	X41	X61	Y11	Y47.0
– rectal	T41.2	X44	X64	Y14	Y48.2
– sodium	T41.1	X44	X64	Y14	Y48.1
Hexobendine	T46.3	X44	X64	Y14	Y52.3
Hexocyclium	T44.3	X43	X63	Y13	Y51.3
– metilsulfate	T44.3	X43	X63	Y13	Y51.3
Hexone	T52.4	X46	X66	Y16	

| Substance | Chapter XIX | Poisoning | | | Adverse effect in therapeutic use |
		Accidental	Intentional self-harm	Undetermined intent	
Hexoprenaline	T48.6	X44	X64	Y14	Y55.6
Hexylcaine	T41.3	X44	X64	Y14	Y48.3
Hexylresorcinol	T52.2	X46	X66	Y16	
HGH (human growth hormone)	T38.8	X44	X64	Y14	Y42.8
Histamine (phosphate)	T50.8	X44	X64	Y14	Y57.6
Histoplasmin	T50.8	X44	X64	Y14	Y57.6
Homatropine	T44.3	X43	X63	Y13	Y51.3
– methylbromide	T44.3	X43	X63	Y13	Y51.3
Homochlorcyclizine	T45.0	X44	X64	Y14	Y43.0
Homosalate	T49.3	X44	X64	Y14	Y56.3
Hormone NEC	T38.8	X44	X64	Y14	Y42.8
– androgenic	T38.7	X44	X64	Y14	Y42.7
– anterior pituitary NEC	T38.8	X44	X64	Y14	Y42.8
– antidiuretic	T38.8	X44	X64	Y14	Y42.8
– cancer therapy	T45.1	X44	X64	Y14	Y43.3
– luteinizing	T38.8	X44	X64	Y14	Y42.8
– ovarian	T38.5	X44	X64	Y14	Y42.5
– oxytocic	T48.0	X44	X64	Y14	Y55.0
– pituitary (posterior) NEC	T38.8	X44	X64	Y14	Y42.8
– thyroid	T38.1	X44	X64	Y14	Y42.1
Horse anti-human lymphocytic serum	T50.9	X44	X64	Y14	Y59.3
Human					
– albumin	T45.8	X44	X64	Y14	Y44.6
– growth hormone (HGH)	T38.8	X44	X64	Y14	Y42.8
– immune serum	T50.9	X44	X64	Y14	Y59.3
Hyaluronidase	T45.3	X44	X64	Y14	Y43.6
Hydantoin derivative NEC	T42.0	X41	X61	Y11	Y46.2
Hydralazine	T46.5	X44	X64	Y14	Y52.5
Hydrargaphen	T49.0	X44	X64	Y14	Y56.0
Hydrargyri aminochloridum	T49.0	X44	X64	Y14	Y56.0
Hydrastine	T48.2	X44	X64	Y14	Y55.2
Hydrazine	T54.1	X49	X69	Y19	
– monoamine oxidase inhibitors	T43.1	X41	X61	Y11	Y49.1
Hydrazoic acid, azides	T54.2	X49	X69	Y19	
Hydriodic acid	T48.4	X44	X64	Y14	Y55.4
Hydrochloric acid (liquid)	T54.2	X49	X69	Y19	
– medicinal (digestant)	T47.5	X44	X64	Y14	Y53.5
– vapor	T59.8	X47	X67	Y17	
Hydrochlorothiazide	T50.2	X44	X64	Y14	Y54.3
Hydrocodone	T40.2	X42	X62	Y12	Y45.0
Hydrocortisone (derivatives)	T49.0	X44	X64	Y14	Y56.0
– aceponate	T49.0	X44	X64	Y14	Y56.0
Hydrocyanic acid (liquid)	T57.3	X49	X69	Y19	
– gas	T65.0	X47	X67	Y17	
Hydroflumethiazide	T50.2	X44	X64	Y14	Y54.3
Hydrofluoric acid (liquid)	T54.2	X49	X69	Y19	
– vapor	T59.8	X47	X67	Y17	

Substance	Chapter XIX	Accidental	Intentional self-harm	Undetermined intent	Adverse effect in therapeutic use
Hydrogen	T59.8	X47	X67	Y17	
– chloride	T57.8	X49	X69	Y19	
– cyanide (gas)	T57.3	X48	X68	Y18	
– fluoride	T59.5	X47	X67	Y17	
– peroxide	T49.0	X44	X64	Y14	Y56.0
– sulfide	T59.6	X47	X67	Y17	
Hydromethylpyridine	T46.7	X44	X64	Y14	Y52.7
Hydromorphone	T40.2	X42	X62	Y12	Y45.0
Hydroquinidine	T46.2	X44	X64	Y14	Y52.2
Hydroquinone	T52.2	X46	X66	Y16	
– vapor	T59.8	X47	X67	Y17	
Hydrosulfuric acid (gas)	T59.8	X47	X67	Y17	
Hydrotalcite	T47.1	X44	X64	Y14	Y53.1
Hydrous wool fat	T49.3	X44	X64	Y14	Y56.3
Hydroxide, caustic	T54.3	X49	X69	Y19	
Hydroxocobalamin	T45.8	X44	X64	Y14	Y44.1
Hydroxyamfetamine	T49.5	X44	X64	Y14	Y56.5
Hydroxyamphetamine	T49.5	X44	X64	Y14	Y56.5
Hydroxycarbamide	T45.1	X44	X64	Y14	Y43.3
Hydroxychloroquine	T37.8	X44	X64	Y14	Y41.8
Hydroxyestrone	T38.5	X44	X64	Y14	Y42.5
Hydroxymethylpentanone	T52.4	X46	X66	Y16	
Hydroxyprogesterone	T38.5	X44	X64	Y14	Y42.5
– caproate	T38.5	X44	X64	Y14	Y42.5
Hydroxyquinoline (derivatives) NEC	T37.8	X44	X64	Y14	Y41.8
Hydroxystilbamidine	T37.3	X44	X64	Y14	Y41.3
Hydroxytoluene (nonmedicinal)	T54.0	X49	X69	Y19	
– medicinal	T49.0	X44	X64	Y14	Y56.0
Hydroxyurea	T45.1	X44	X64	Y14	Y43.3
Hydroxyzine	T43.5	X41	X61	Y11	Y49.5
Hyoscine	T44.3	X43	X63	Y13	Y51.3
Hyoscyamine	T44.3	X43	X63	Y13	Y51.3
Hyoscyamus	T44.3	X43	X63	Y13	Y51.3
– dry extract	T44.3	X43	X63	Y13	Y51.3
Hypnotic	T42.7	X41	X61	Y11	Y47.9
– anticonvulsant	T42.7	X41	X61	Y11	Y47.5
– specified NEC	T42.6	X41	X61	Y11	Y47.8
Hypochlorite	T49.0	X44	X64	Y14	Y56.0
Hypophysis, posterior	T38.8	X44	X64	Y14	Y42.8
Hypotensive NEC	T46.5	X44	X64	Y14	Y52.5
Hypromellose	T49.5	X44	X64	Y14	Y56.5

I

		Poisoning			Adverse effect in therapeutic use
Substance	Chapter XIX	Accidental	Intentional self-harm	Undetermined intent	
Ibacitabine	T37.5	X44	X64	Y14	Y41.5
Ibopamine	T44.9	X43	X63	Y13	Y51.9
Ibufenac	T39.3	X40	X60	Y10	Y45.3
Ibuprofen	T39.3	X40	X60	Y10	Y45.2
Ibuproxam	T39.3	X40	X60	Y10	Y45.3
Ibuterol	T48.6	X44	X64	Y14	Y55.6
Ichthammol	T49.0	X44	X64	Y14	Y56.0
Idarubicin	T45.1	X44	X64	Y14	Y43.3
Idoxuridine	T37.5	X44	X64	Y14	Y41.5
Idrocilamide	T42.8	X41	X61	Y11	Y46.8
Ifenprodil	T46.7	X44	X64	Y14	Y52.7
Ifosfamide	T45.1	X44	X64	Y14	Y43.3
Illuminating gas	T58	X47	X67	Y17	
Iloprost	T46.7	X44	X64	Y14	Y52.7
Imidazole-4-carboxamide	T45.1	X44	X64	Y14	Y43.3
Iminostilbene	T42.1	X41	X61	Y11	Y46.4
Imipenem	T36.0	X44	X64	Y14	Y40.0
Imipramine	T43.0	X41	X61	Y11	Y49.0
Imipraminoxide	T43.0	X41	X61	Y11	Y49.0
Immune					
– globulin	T50.9	X44	X64	Y14	Y59.3
– serum globulin	T50.9	X44	X64	Y14	Y59.3
Immunoglobin human (intravenous) (normal)	T50.9	X44	X64	Y14	Y59.3
– unmodified	T50.9	X44	X64	Y14	Y59.3
Immunological agent	T50.9	X44	X64	Y14	Y59.9
– specified NEC	T50.9	X44	X64	Y14	Y59.8
Immunosuppressive drug	T45.1	X44	X64	Y14	Y43.4
Indalpine	T43.2	X41	X61	Y11	Y49.2
Indanazoline	T48.5	X44	X64	Y14	Y55.5
Indapamide	T46.5	X44	X64	Y14	Y52.5
Indendione (derivatives)	T45.5	X44	X64	Y14	Y44.2
Indenolol	T44.7	X43	X63	Y13	Y51.7
Indian hemp	T40.7	X42	X62	Y12	Y49.6
Indigo carmine	T50.8	X44	X64	Y14	Y57.6
Indobufen	T45.5	X44	X64	Y14	Y44.4
Indocyanine green	T50.8	X44	X64	Y14	Y57.6
Indometacin	T39.3	X40	X60	Y10	Y45.3
Indomethacin	T39.3	X40	X60	Y10	Y45.3
– farnesil	T39.4	X40	X60	Y10	Y45.4
Indoramin	T44.6	X43	X63	Y13	Y51.6
Influenza vaccine	T50.9	X44	X64	Y14	Y59.0
Ingested substance NEC	T65.9	X49	X69	Y19	
INH	T37.1	X44	X64	Y14	Y41.1

Substance	Chapter XIX	Accidental	Poisoning Intentional self-harm	Undetermined intent	Adverse effect in therapeutic use
Inhibitor					
− angio-tensin-converting enzyme	T46.4	X44	X64	Y14	Y52.4
− carbonic-anhydrase	T50.2	X44	X64	Y14	Y54.2
− fibrinolysis	T45.6	X44	X64	Y14	Y44.3
− monoamine oxidase NEC	T43.1	X41	X61	Y11	Y49.1
− − hydrazine	T43.1	X41	X61	Y11	Y49.1
− postsynaptic	T43.8	X41	X61	Y11	Y49.8
− prothrombin synthesis	T45.5	X44	X64	Y14	Y44.2
Inosine pranobex	T37.5	X44	X64	Y14	Y41.5
Inositol	T50.9	X44	X64	Y14	Y57.1
− nicotinate	T46.7	X44	X64	Y14	Y52.7
Insect (sting), venomous	T63.4				
Insecticide NEC	T60.9	X48	X68	Y18	
− carbamate	T60.0	X48	X68	Y18	
− mixed	T60.9	X48	X68	Y18	
− organochlorine	T60.1	X48	X68	Y18	
− organophosphorus	T60.0	X48	X68	Y18	
Insulin NEC	T38.3	X44	X64	Y14	Y42.3
− defalan	T38.3	X44	X64	Y14	Y42.3
− human	T38.3	X44	X64	Y14	Y42.3
− injection, soluble	T38.3	X44	X64	Y14	Y42.3
− − biphasic	T38.3	X44	X64	Y14	Y42.3
− intermediate acting	T38.3	X44	X64	Y14	Y42.3
− protamine zinc	T38.3	X44	X64	Y14	Y42.3
− slow acting	T38.3	X44	X64	Y14	Y42.3
− zinc					
− − protamine injection	T38.3	X44	X64	Y14	Y42.3
− − suspension (amorphous) (crystalline)	T38.3	X44	X64	Y14	Y42.3
Interferon (alpha) (beta) (gamma)	T37.5	X44	X64	Y14	Y41.5
Intestinal motility control drug	T47.6	X44	X64	Y14	Y53.6
− biological	T47.8	X44	X64	Y14	Y53.8
Intravenous					
− amino acids	T50.9	X44	X64	Y14	Y57.8
− fat suspension	T50.9	X44	X64	Y14	Y57.8
Inulin	T50.8	X44	X64	Y14	Y57.6
Invert sugar	T50.3	X44	X64	Y14	Y54.6
Iobenzamic acid	T50.8	X44	X64	Y14	Y57.5
Iocarmic acid	T50.8	X44	X64	Y14	Y57.5
Iocetamic acid	T50.8	X44	X64	Y14	Y57.5
Iodamide	T50.8	X44	X64	Y14	Y57.5
Iodinated					
− contrast medium	T50.8	X44	X64	Y14	Y57.5
− glycerol	T48.4	X44	X64	Y14	Y55.4
− human serum albumin (^{131}I)	T50.8	X44	X64	Y14	Y57.6
Iodine (antiseptic, external) (tincture) NEC	T49.0	X44	X64	Y14	Y56.0
− solution	T49.0	X44	X64	Y14	Y56.0
− 125	T50.8	X44	X64	Y14	Y57.6
− 131	T50.8	X44	X64	Y14	Y57.6
Iodipamide	T50.8	X44	X64	Y14	Y57.5

		Poisoning			Adverse effect in therapeutic use
Substance	Chapter XIX	Accidental	Intentional self-harm	Undetermined intent	
Iodized (poppy seed) oil	T50.8	X44	X64	Y14	Y57.5
Iodochlorhydroxyquinoline	T37.8	X44	X64	Y14	Y41.8
Iodocholesterol (^{131}I)	T50.8	X44	X64	Y14	Y57.6
Iodoform	T49.0	X44	X64	Y14	Y56.0
Iodohippuric acid	T50.8	X44	X64	Y14	Y57.5
Iodophthalein (sodium)	T50.8	X44	X64	Y14	Y57.6
Iodopyracet	T50.8	X44	X64	Y14	Y57.6
Iodoquinol	T37.8	X44	X64	Y14	Y41.8
Iodoxamic acid	T50.8	X44	X64	Y14	Y57.5
Iofendylate	T50.8	X44	X64	Y14	Y57.5
Ioglycamic acid	T50.8	X44	X64	Y14	Y57.5
Iohexol	T50.8	X44	X64	Y14	Y57.5
Ion exchange resin					
– anion	T47.8	X44	X64	Y14	Y53.8
– cation	T50.3	X44	X64	Y14	Y54.6
– cholestyramine	T46.6	X44	X64	Y14	Y52.6
– intestinal	T47.8	X44	X64	Y14	Y53.8
Iopamidol	T50.8	X44	X64	Y14	Y57.5
Iopanoic acid	T50.8	X44	X64	Y14	Y57.5
Iophenoic acid	T50.8	X44	X64	Y14	Y57.5
Iopodate, sodium	T50.8	X44	X64	Y14	Y57.5
Iopodic acid	T50.8	X44	X64	Y14	Y57.5
Iopromide	T50.8	X44	X64	Y14	Y57.5
Iopydol	T50.8	X44	X64	Y14	Y57.5
Iotalamic acid	T50.8	X44	X64	Y14	Y57.5
Iothalamate	T50.8	X44	X64	Y14	Y57.5
Iotrol	T50.8	X44	X64	Y14	Y57.5
Iotrolan	T50.8	X44	X64	Y14	Y57.5
Iotroxate	T50.8	X44	X64	Y14	Y57.5
Iotroxic acid	T50.8	X44	X64	Y14	Y57.5
Ioversol	T50.8	X44	X64	Y14	Y57.6
Ioxaglate	T50.8	X44	X64	Y14	Y57.5
Ioxaglic acid	T50.8	X44	X64	Y14	Y57.5
Ioxitalamic acid	T50.8	X44	X64	Y14	Y57.5
Ipecacuanha, ipecac	T48.4	X44	X64	Y14	Y55.4
Ipodate, calcium	T50.8	X44	X64	Y14	Y57.5
Ipratropium (bromide)	T48.6	X44	X64	Y14	Y55.6
Ipriflavone	T46.3	X44	X64	Y14	Y52.3
Iprindole	T43.0	X41	X61	Y11	Y49.0
Iproclozide	T43.1	X41	X61	Y11	Y49.1
Iprofenin	T50.8	X44	X64	Y14	Y57.6
Iproheptine	T49.2	X44	X64	Y14	Y56.2
Iproniazid	T43.1	X41	X61	Y11	Y49.1
Iproplatin	T45.1	X44	X64	Y14	Y43.3
Iproveratril	T46.1	X44	X64	Y14	Y52.1
Iron (compounds) (medicinal) NEC	T45.4	X44	X64	Y14	Y44.0
– ammonium	T45.4	X44	X64	Y14	Y44.0
– dextran injection	T45.4	X44	X64	Y14	Y44.0
– nonmedicinal	T56.8	X49	X69	Y19	
– salts	T45.4	X44	X64	Y14	Y44.0
– sorbitex	T45.4	X44	X64	Y14	Y44.0

		Poisoning			Adverse effect in therapeutic use
Substance	Chapter XIX	Accidental	Intentional self-harm	Undetermined intent	
Iron—*continued*					
– sorbitol citric acid complex	T45.4	X44	X64	Y14	Y44.0
Irrigating fluid (vaginal)	T49.8	X44	X64	Y14	Y56.8
– eye	T49.5	X44	X64	Y14	Y56.5
Isepamicin	T36.5	X44	X64	Y14	Y40.5
Isoaminile (citrate)	T48.3	X44	X64	Y14	Y55.3
Isobenzan	T60.1	X48	X68	Y18	
Isobutyl acetate	T52.8	X46	X66	Y16	
Isocarboxazid	T43.1	X41	X61	Y11	Y49.1
Isoconazole	T49.0	X44	X64	Y14	Y56.0
Isocyanate	T65.0	X49	X69	Y19	
Isoetarine	T48.6	X44	X64	Y14	Y55.6
Isoethadione	T42.2	X41	X61	Y11	Y46.1
Isoflurane	T41.0	X44	X64	Y14	Y48.0
Isoflurophate	T44.0	X43	X63	Y13	Y51.0
Isomaltose, ferric complex	T45.4	X44	X64	Y14	Y44.0
Isometheptene	T44.3	X43	X63	Y13	Y51.3
Isoniazid	T37.1	X44	X64	Y14	Y41.1
– with					
– – rifampicin	T36.6	X44	X64	Y14	Y40.6
– – thioacetazone	T37.1	X44	X64	Y14	Y41.1
Isonicotinic acid hydrazide	T37.1	X44	X64	Y14	Y41.1
Isonipecaine	T40.4	X42	X62	Y12	Y45.0
Isonixin	T39.3	X40	X60	Y10	Y45.3
Isophorone	T65.8	X49	X69	Y19	
Isophosphamide	T45.1	X44	X64	Y14	Y43.3
Isoprenaline	T48.6	X44	X64	Y14	Y55.6
Isopromethazine	T43.3	X41	X61	Y11	Y49.3
Isopropamide	T44.3	X43	X63	Y13	Y51.3
– iodide	T44.3	X43	X63	Y13	Y51.3
Isopropanol	T51.2	X45	X65	Y15	
Isopropyl					
– acetate	T52.8	X46	X66	Y16	
– alcohol	T51.2	X45	X65	Y15	
– – medicinal	T49.4	X44	X64	Y14	Y56.4
– ether	T52.8	X46	X66	Y16	
Isopropylaminophenazone	T39.2	X40	X60	Y10	Y45.8
Isoproterenol	T48.6	X44	X64	Y14	Y55.6
Isosorbide dinitrate	T46.3	X44	X64	Y14	Y52.3
Isothipendyl	T45.0	X44	X64	Y14	Y43.0
Isotretinoin	T50.9	X44	X64	Y14	Y57.8
Isoxicam	T39.3	X40	X60	Y10	Y45.3
Isoxsuprine	T46.7	X44	X64	Y14	Y52.7
Ispagula	T47.4	X44	X64	Y14	Y53.4
– husk	T47.4	X44	X64	Y14	Y53.4
Isradipine	T46.1	X44	X64	Y14	Y52.1
Itraconazole	T37.8	X44	X64	Y14	Y41.8
Itramin tosilate	T46.3	X44	X64	Y14	Y52.3
Ivermectin	T37.4	X44	X64	Y14	Y41.4
Izoniazid	T37.1	X44	X64	Y14	Y41.1
– with thioacetazone	T37.1	X44	X64	Y14	Y41.1

J

| Substance | Chapter XIX | Poisoning | | | Adverse effect in therapeutic use |
		Accidental	Intentional self-harm	Undetermined intent	
Jalap	T47.2	X44	X64	Y14	Y53.2
Jamaica ginger	T62.2	X49	X69	Y19	
Jimson weed (stramonium)	T62.2	X49	X69	Y19	
Josamycin	T36.3	X44	X64	Y14	Y40.3
Juniper tar	T49.1	X44	X64	Y14	Y56.1

K

Substance	Chapter XIX	Accidental	Intentional self-harm	Undetermined intent	Adverse effect in therapeutic use
			Poisoning		
Kallidinogenase	T46.7	X44	X64	Y14	Y52.7
Kallikrein	T46.7	X44	X64	Y14	Y52.7
Kanamycin	T36.5	X44	X64	Y14	Y40.5
Kaolin	T47.6	X44	X64	Y14	Y53.6
– light	T47.6	X44	X64	Y14	Y53.6
Kebuzone	T39.2	X40	X60	Y10	Y45.8
Kelevan	T60.1	X48	X68	Y18	
Keratolytic drug NEC	T49.4	X44	X64	Y14	Y56.4
– anthracene	T49.4	X44	X64	Y14	Y56.4
Keratoplastic NEC	T49.4	X44	X64	Y14	Y56.4
Kerosene, kerosine (fuel) (solvent) NEC	T52.0	X46	X66	Y16	
– insecticide	T52.0	X46	X66	Y16	
– vapor	T52.0	X46	X66	Y16	
Ketamine	T41.2	X44	X64	Y14	Y48.2
Ketazolam	T42.4	X41	X61	Y11	Y47.1
Ketazon	T39.2	X40	X60	Y10	Y45.8
Ketobemidone	T40.4	X42	X62	Y12	Y45.0
Ketoconazole	T49.0	X44	X64	Y14	Y56.0
Ketols	T52.4	X46	X66	Y16	
Ketone oils	T52.4	X46	X66	Y16	
Ketoprofen	T39.3	X40	X60	Y10	Y45.2
Ketorolac	T39.8	X40	X60	Y10	Y45.8
Ketotifen	T45.0	X44	X64	Y14	Y43.0
Khat	T43.6	X41	X61	Y11	Y49.7
Khellin	T46.3	X44	X64	Y14	Y52.3
Khelloside	T46.3	X44	X64	Y14	Y52.3
Kiln gas or vapor (carbon monoxide)	T58	X47	X67	Y17	
Kitasamycin	T36.3	X44	X64	Y14	Y40.3

L

	Poisoning			Adverse effect
		Intentional	Undetermined	in therapeutic
Substance	Chapter XIX	Accidental	self-harm	intent	use
Labetalol	T44.8	X43	X63	Y13	Y51.8
Laburnum (seeds)	T62.2	X49	X69	Y19	
Lachesine	T49.5	X44	X64	Y14	Y56.5
Lacidipine	T46.5	X44	X64	Y14	Y52.5
Lacquer	T65.6	X49	X69	Y19	
Lactated potassic saline	T50.3	X44	X64	Y14	Y54.9
Lactic acid	T49.8	X44	X64	Y14	Y56.8
Lactobacillus					
– acidophilus	T47.6	X44	X64	Y14	Y53.6
– – compound	T47.6	X44	X64	Y14	Y53.6
– bifidus, lyophilized	T47.6	X44	X64	Y14	Y53.6
– bulgaricus	T47.6	X44	X64	Y14	Y53.6
– sporogenes	T47.6	X44	X64	Y14	Y53.6
Lactose (as excipient)	T50.9	X44	X64	Y14	Y57.4
Lactulose	T47.3	X44	X64	Y14	Y53.3
Laevo – see Levo-					
Lanatosides	T46.0	X44	X64	Y14	Y52.0
Lanolin	T49.3	X44	X64	Y14	Y56.3
Lassar's paste	T49.4	X44	X64	Y14	Y56.4
Latamoxef	T36.1	X44	X64	Y14	Y40.1
Laudanum	T40.0	X42	X62	Y12	Y45.0
Laughing gas	T41.0	X44	X64	Y14	Y48.0
Lauryl sulfoacetate	T49.2	X44	X64	Y14	Y56.2
Laxative NEC	T47.4	X44	X64	Y14	Y53.4
– osmotic	T47.3	X44	X64	Y14	Y53.3
– saline	T47.3	X44	X64	Y14	Y53.3
– stimulant	T47.2	X44	X64	Y14	Y53.2
Lead (dust) (fumes) (vapor) NEC	T56.0	X49	X69	Y19	
– acetate	T49.2	X44	X64	Y14	Y56.2
– alkyl (fuel additive)	T56.0	X46	X66	Y16	
– arsenate, arsenite (dust) (herbicide)(insecticide) (vapor)	T57.0	X48	X68	Y18	
– inorganic	T56.0	X49	X69	Y19	
– organic	T56.0	X49	X69	Y19	
Lefetamine	T39.8	X40	X60	Y10	Y45.8
Lenperone	T43.4	X41	X61	Y11	Y49.4
Leptazol	T50.7	X44	X64	Y14	Y50.0
Leptophos	T60.0	X48	X68	Y18	
Letosteine	T48.4	X44	X64	Y14	Y55.4
Leucinocaine	T41.3	X44	X64	Y14	Y48.3
Leucocianidol	T46.9	X44	X64	Y14	Y52.9
Leucovorin (factor)	T45.8	X44	X64	Y14	Y44.1
Leuprorelin	T38.8	X44	X64	Y14	Y42.8
Levallorphan	T50.7	X44	X64	Y14	Y50.1

Substance	Chapter XIX	Accidental	Poisoning Intentional self-harm	Poisoning Undetermined intent	Adverse effect in therapeutic use
Levamisole	T37.4	X44	X64	Y14	Y41.4
Levarterenol	T44.4	X43	X63	Y13	Y51.4
Levdropropizine	T48.3	X44	X64	Y14	Y55.3
Levobunolol	T49.5	X44	X64	Y14	Y56.5
Levocabastine (hydrochloride)	T45.0	X44	X64	Y14	Y43.0
Levocarnitine	T50.9	X44	X64	Y14	Y57.1
Levodopa	T42.8	X41	X61	Y11	Y46.7
– with carbidopa	T42.8	X41	X61	Y11	Y46.7
Levoglutamide	T50.9	X44	X64	Y14	Y57.1
Levomepromazine	T43.3	X41	X61	Y11	Y49.3
Levonordefrin	T49.6	X44	X64	Y14	Y56.6
Levonorgestrel	T38.4	X44	X64	Y14	Y42.4
– with ethinylestradiol	T38.4	X44	X64	Y14	Y42.5
Levopromazine	T43.3	X41	X61	Y11	Y49.3
Levopropoxyphene	T40.4	X42	X62	Y12	Y45.0
Levopropylhexedrine	T50.5	X44	X64	Y14	Y57.0
Levoproxyphylline	T48.6	X44	X64	Y14	Y55.6
Levorphanol	T40.4	X42	X62	Y12	Y45.0
Levothyroxine	T38.1	X44	X64	Y14	Y42.1
– sodium	T38.1	X44	X64	Y14	Y42.1
Levulose	T50.3	X44	X64	Y14	Y54.6
Lewisite (gas), not in war	T57.0	X49	X69	Y19	
Lidocaine	T41.3	X44	X64	Y14	Y48.3
– regional	T41.3	X44	X64	Y14	Y48.3
– spinal	T41.3	X44	X64	Y14	Y48.3
Lidofenin	T50.8	X44	X64	Y14	Y57.6
Lidoflazine	T46.1	X44	X64	Y14	Y52.1
Lighter fluid	T52.0	X46	X66	Y16	
Lignin hemicellulose	T47.6	X44	X64	Y14	Y53.6
Lignocaine	T41.3	X44	X64	Y14	Y48.3
– regional	T41.3	X44	X64	Y14	Y48.3
– spinal	T41.3	X44	X64	Y14	Y48.3
Ligroin(e) (solvent)	T52.0	X46	X66	Y16	
– vapor	T59.8	X47	X67	Y17	
Lime (chloride)	T54.3	X49	X69	Y19	
Limonene	T52.8	X46	X66	Y16	
Lincomycin	T36.8	X44	X64	Y14	Y40.8
Lindane (insecticide) (nonmedicinal) (vapor)	T53.6	X46	X66	Y16	
– medicinal	T49.0	X44	X64	Y14	Y56.0
Linoleic acid	T46.6	X44	X64	Y14	Y52.6
Linolenic acid	T46.6	X44	X64	Y14	Y52.6
Linseed	T47.4	X44	X64	Y14	Y53.4
Liothyronine	T38.1	X44	X64	Y14	Y42.1
Liotrix	T38.1	X44	X64	Y14	Y42.1
Lipo-alprostadil	T46.7	X44	X64	Y14	Y52.7
Lipotropic drug NEC	T50.9	X44	X64	Y14	Y57.1
Liquid					
– paraffin	T47.4	X44	X64	Y14	Y53.4
– substance NEC	T65.9	X49	X69	Y19	
Liquor creosolis compositus	T65.8	X49	X69	Y19	

783

Substance	Chapter XIX	Poisoning			Adverse effect in therapeutic use
		Accidental	Intentional self-harm	Undetermined intent	
Liquorice	T48.4	X44	X64	Y14	Y55.4
– extract	T47.8	X44	X64	Y14	Y53.8
Lisinopril	T46.4	X44	X64	Y14	Y52.4
Lisuride	T42.8	X41	X61	Y11	Y46.7
Lithium	T56.8	X49	X69	Y19	
– gluconate	T43.5	X41	X61	Y11	Y49.5
– salts (carbonate)	T43.5	X41	X61	Y11	Y49.5
Liver					
– extract	T45.8	X44	X64	Y14	Y44.1
– – for parenteral use	T45.8	X44	X64	Y14	Y44.1
– fraction 1	T45.8	X44	X64	Y14	Y44.1
– hydrolysate	T45.8	X44	X64	Y14	Y44.1
Lobeline	T50.7	X44	X64	Y14	Y50.0
Lobenzarit	T39.3	X40	X60	Y10	Y45.3
Local action drug NEC	T49.8	X44	X64	Y14	Y56.8
Lofepramine	T43.0	X41	X61	Y11	Y49.0
Lomustine	T45.1	X44	X64	Y14	Y43.3
Lonazolac	T39.3	X40	X60	Y10	Y45.3
Lonidamine	T45.1	X44	X64	Y14	Y43.3
Loperamide	T47.6	X44	X64	Y14	Y53.6
Loprazolam	T42.4	X41	X61	Y11	Y47.1
Lorajmine	T46.2	X44	X64	Y14	Y52.2
Loratidine	T45.0	X44	X64	Y14	Y43.0
Lorazepam	T42.4	X41	X61	Y11	Y47.1
Lorcainide	T46.2	X44	X64	Y14	Y52.2
Lormetazepam	T42.4	X41	X61	Y11	Y47.1
Lovastatin	T46.6	X44	X64	Y14	Y52.6
Loxapine	T43.5	X41	X61	Y11	Y49.5
Loxoprofen	T39.3	X40	X60	Y10	Y45.2
LSD	T40.8	X42	X62	Y12	Y49.6
Lubricant, eye	T49.5	X44	X64	Y14	Y56.5
Lubricating oil NEC	T52.0	X46	X66	Y16	
Lucanthone	T37.4	X44	X64	Y14	Y41.4
Lung irritant (gas) NEC	T59.8	X47	X67	Y17	
Luteinizing hormone	T38.8	X44	X64	Y14	Y42.8
Lututrin	T48.2	X44	X64	Y14	Y55.2
Lye (concentrated)	T54.3	X49	X69	Y19	
Lymecycline	T36.4	X44	X64	Y14	Y40.4
Lymphogranuloma venereum antigen	T50.8	X44	X64	Y14	Y57.6
Lynestrenol	T38.4	X44	X64	Y14	Y42.4
Lypressin	T38.8	X44	X64	Y14	Y42.8
Lysergic acid diethylamide	T40.8	X42	X62	Y12	Y49.6
Lysergide	T40.8	X42	X62	Y12	Y49.6
Lysozyme	T49.0	X44	X64	Y14	Y56.0

M

Substance	Chapter XIX	Poisoning			Adverse effect in therapeutic use
		Accidental	Intentional self-harm	Undetermined intent	
Macrogol	T50.9	X44	X64	Y14	Y57.4
Macrolide					
– anabolic drug	T38.7	X44	X64	Y14	Y42.7
– antibiotic	T36.3	X44	X64	Y14	Y40.3
Mafenide	T49.0	X44	X64	Y14	Y56.0
Magaldrate	T47.1	X44	X64	Y14	Y53.1
Magnesia magma	T47.1	X44	X64	Y14	Y53.1
Magnesium NEC	T56.8	X49	X69	Y19	
– carbonate	T47.1	X44	X64	Y14	Y53.1
– citrate	T47.4	X44	X64	Y14	Y53.4
– hydroxide	T47.1	X44	X64	Y14	Y53.1
– oxide	T47.1	X44	X64	Y14	Y53.1
– peroxide	T49.0	X44	X64	Y14	Y56.0
– salicylate	T39.0	X40	X60	Y10	Y45.1
– silicofluoride	T50.3	X44	X64	Y14	Y54.9
– sulfate	T47.4	X44	X64	Y14	Y53.4
– thiosulfate	T45.0	X44	X64	Y14	Y43.0
– trisilicate	T47.1	X44	X64	Y14	Y53.1
Malathion (medicinal)	T49.0	X44	X64	Y14	Y56.0
– insecticide	T60.0	X48	X68	Y18	
Male fern extract	T37.4	X44	X64	Y14	Y41.4
M-AMSA	T45.1	X44	X64	Y14	Y43.3
Mandelic acid	T37.8	X44	X64	Y14	Y41.8
Manganese (dioxide) (salts)	T57.2	X49	X69	Y19	
– medicinal	T50.9	X44	X64	Y14	Y54.9
Mannitol	T47.3	X44	X64	Y14	Y53.3
– hexanitrate	T46.3	X44	X64	Y14	Y52.3
Mannomustine	T45.1	X44	X64	Y14	Y43.3
Maphenide	T49.0	X44	X64	Y14	Y56.0
Maprotiline	T43.0	X41	X61	Y11	Y49.0
Marihuana	T40.7	X42	X62	Y12	Y49.6
Marijuana	T40.7	X42	X62	Y12	Y49.6
Marsh gas	T59.8	X47	X67	Y17	
Mazindol	T50.5	X44	X64	Y14	Y57.0
MCPA	T60.3	X48	X68	Y18	
Measles virus vaccine (attenuated)	T50.9	X44	X64	Y14	Y59.0
Meat, noxious	T62.8	X49	X69	Y19	
Meballymal	T42.3	X41	X61	Y11	Y47.0
Mebanazine	T43.1	X41	X61	Y11	Y49.1
Mebendazole	T37.4	X44	X64	Y14	Y41.4
Mebeverine	T44.3	X43	X63	Y13	Y51.3
Mebhydrolin	T45.0	X44	X64	Y14	Y43.0
Mebumal	T42.3	X41	X61	Y11	Y47.0
Mebutamate	T43.5	X41	X61	Y11	Y49.5

| Substance | Chapter XIX | Poisoning | | | Adverse effect in therapeutic use |
		Accidental	Intentional self-harm	Undetermined intent	
Mecamylamine	T44.2	X43	X63	Y13	Y51.2
Mechlorethamine	T45.1	X44	X64	Y14	Y43.3
Mecillinam	T36.0	X44	X64	Y14	Y40.0
Meclizine (hydrochloride)	T45.0	X44	X64	Y14	Y43.0
Meclocycline	T36.4	X44	X64	Y14	Y40.4
Meclofenamate	T39.3	X40	X60	Y10	Y45.3
Meclofenamic acid	T39.3	X40	X60	Y10	Y45.3
Meclofenoxate	T43.6	X41	X61	Y11	Y49.7
Meclozine	T45.0	X44	X64	Y14	Y43.0
Mecobalamin	T45.8	X44	X64	Y14	Y44.1
Mecoprop	T60.3	X48	X68	Y18	
Mecrilate	T49.3	X44	X64	Y14	Y56.3
Mecysteine	T48.4	X44	X64	Y14	Y55.4
Medazepam	T42.4	X41	X61	Y11	Y47.1
Medicament NEC	T50.9	X44	X64	Y14	Y57.9
Medrogestone	T38.5	X44	X64	Y14	Y42.5
Medroxalol	T44.8	X43	X63	Y13	Y51.8
Medroxyprogesterone acetate (depot)	T38.5	X44	X64	Y14	Y42.5
Medrysone	T49.0	X44	X64	Y14	Y56.0
Mefenamic acid	T39.3	X40	X60	Y10	Y45.3
Mefenorex	T50.5	X44	X64	Y14	Y57.0
Mefloquine	T37.2	X44	X64	Y14	Y41.2
Mefruside	T50.2	X44	X64	Y14	Y54.5
Megestrol	T38.5	X44	X64	Y14	Y42.5
Meglumine					
– antimoniate	T37.8	X44	X64	Y14	Y41.8
– diatrizoate	T50.8	X44	X64	Y14	Y57.5
– iodipamide	T50.8	X44	X64	Y14	Y57.5
– iotroxate	T50.8	X44	X64	Y14	Y57.5
MEK (methyl ethyl ketone)	T52.4	X46	X66	Y16	
Meladrazine	T44.3	X43	X63	Y13	Y51.3
Melaleuca alternifolia oil	T49.0	X44	X64	Y14	Y56.0
Melanocyte-stimulating hormone	T38.8	X44	X64	Y14	Y42.8
Melarsonyl potassium	T37.3	X44	X64	Y14	Y41.3
Melarsoprol	T37.3	X44	X64	Y14	Y41.3
Melitracen	T43.0	X41	X61	Y11	Y49.0
Melperone	T43.4	X41	X61	Y11	Y49.4
Melphalan	T45.1	X44	X64	Y14	Y43.3
Memantine	T42.8	X41	X61	Y11	Y46.7
Menadiol	T45.7	X44	X64	Y14	Y44.3
– sodium sulfate	T45.7	X44	X64	Y14	Y44.3
Menadione	T45.7	X44	X64	Y14	Y44.3
– sodium bisulfite	T45.7	X44	X64	Y14	Y44.3
Menaphthone	T45.7	X44	X64	Y14	Y44.3
Menaquinone	T45.7	X44	X64	Y14	Y44.3
Menatetrenone	T45.7	X44	X64	Y14	Y44.3
Meningococcal vaccine	T50.9	X44	X64	Y14	Y58.9
Menthol	T48.5	X44	X64	Y14	Y55.5
Mepacrine	T37.2	X44	X64	Y14	Y41.2
Meparfynol	T42.6	X41	X61	Y11	Y47.8

Substance	Chapter XIX	Poisoning			Adverse effect in therapeutic use
		Accidental	Intentional self-harm	Undetermined intent	
Mepartricin	T36.7	X44	X64	Y14	Y40.7
Mepenzolate	T44.3	X43	X63	Y13	Y51.3
– bromide	T44.3	X43	X63	Y13	Y51.3
Meperidine	T40.4	X42	X62	Y12	Y45.0
Mephebarbital	T42.3	X41	X61	Y11	Y47.0
Mephenesin	T42.8	X41	X61	Y11	Y46.8
Mephenhydramine	T45.0	X44	X64	Y14	Y43.0
Mephenoxalone	T42.8	X41	X61	Y11	Y46.8
Mephentermine	T44.9	X43	X63	Y13	Y51.9
Mephenytoin	T42.0	X41	X61	Y11	Y46.2
– with phenobarbital	T42.3	X41	X61	Y11	Y47.0
Mephobarbital	T42.3	X41	X61	Y11	Y47.0
Mephosfolan	T60.0	X48	X68	Y18	
Mepindolol	T44.7	X43	X63	Y13	Y51.7
Mepitiostane	T38.7	X44	X64	Y14	Y42.7
Mepivacaine	T41.3	X44	X64	Y14	Y48.3
– epidural	T41.3	X44	X64	Y14	Y48.3
Meprednisone	T38.0	X44	X64	Y14	Y42.0
Meprobamate	T43.5	X41	X61	Y11	Y49.5
Meproscillarin	T46.0	X44	X64	Y14	Y52.0
Meprylcaine	T41.3	X44	X64	Y14	Y48.3
Meptazinol	T39.8	X40	X60	Y10	Y45.8
Mepyramine	T45.0	X44	X64	Y14	Y43.0
Mequitazine	T43.3	X41	X61	Y11	Y49.3
Meralluride	T50.2	X44	X64	Y14	Y54.5
Merbromin	T49.0	X44	X64	Y14	Y56.0
Mercaptobenzothiazole salts	T49.0	X44	X64	Y14	Y56.0
Mercaptomerin	T50.2	X44	X64	Y14	Y54.5
Mercaptopurine	T45.1	X44	X64	Y14	Y43.1
Mercuramide	T50.2	X44	X64	Y14	Y54.5
Mercurochrome	T49.0	X44	X64	Y14	Y56.0
Mercurophylline	T50.2	X44	X64	Y14	Y54.5
Mercury, mercurial, mercuric, mercurous(compounds) (cyanide) (fumes)(nonmedicinal) (vapor) NEC	T56.1	X49	X69	Y19	
– anti-infective					
– – local	T49.0	X44	X64	Y14	Y56.0
– – systemic	T37.8	X44	X64	Y14	Y41.8
– chloride (ammoniated)	T49.0	X44	X64	Y14	Y56.0
– diuretic NEC	T50.2	X44	X64	Y14	Y54.5
– oxide, yellow	T49.0	X44	X64	Y14	Y56.0
Mersalyl	T50.2	X44	X64	Y14	Y54.5
Merthiolate	T49.0	X44	X64	Y14	Y56.0
Mesalazine	T47.8	X44	X64	Y14	Y53.8
Mescaline	T40.9	X42	X62	Y12	Y49.6
Mesna	T48.4	X44	X64	Y14	Y55.4
Mesoglycan	T46.6	X44	X64	Y14	Y52.6
Mesoridazine	T43.3	X41	X61	Y11	Y49.3
Mestanolone	T38.7	X44	X64	Y14	Y42.7
Mesterolone	T38.7	X44	X64	Y14	Y42.7

| | | | Poisoning | | Adverse effect in therapeutic use |
| | | | Intentional | Undetermined | |
Substance	Chapter XIX	Accidental	self-harm	intent	
Mestranol	T38.5	X44	X64	Y14	Y42.5
Mesulergine	T42.8	X41	X61	Y11	Y46.7
Mesulfen	T49.0	X44	X64	Y14	Y56.0
Mesuximide	T42.2	X41	X61	Y11	Y46.0
Metabutethamine	T41.3	X44	X64	Y14	Y48.3
Metacycline	T36.4	X44	X64	Y14	Y40.4
Metaldehyde (snail killer) NEC	T60.8	X48	X68	Y18	
Metals (heavy) (nonmedicinal)	T56.9	X49	X69	Y19	
– specified NEC	T56.8	X49	X69	Y19	
Metamfetamine	T43.6	X41	X61	Y11	Y49.7
Metamizole sodium	T39.2	X40	X60	Y10	Y45.8
Metampicillin	T36.0	X44	X64	Y14	Y40.0
Metandienone	T38.7	X44	X64	Y14	Y42.7
Metandrostenolone	T38.7	X44	X64	Y14	Y42.7
Metaphos	T60.0	X48	X68	Y18	
Metapramine	T43.0	X41	X61	Y11	Y49.0
Metaproterenol	T48.2	X44	X64	Y14	Y55.2
Metaraminol	T44.4	X43	X63	Y13	Y51.4
Metaxalone	T42.8	X41	X61	Y11	Y46.8
Metenolone	T38.7	X44	X64	Y14	Y42.7
Metergoline	T42.8	X41	X61	Y11	Y46.7
Metescufylline	T46.9	X44	X64	Y14	Y52.9
Metetoin	T42.0	X41	X61	Y11	Y46.2
Metformin	T38.3	X44	X64	Y14	Y42.3
Methacholine	T44.1	X43	X63	Y13	Y51.1
Methadone	T40.3	X42	X62	Y12	Y45.0
Methallenestril	T38.5	X44	X64	Y14	Y42.5
Methallenoestril	T38.5	X44	X64	Y14	Y42.5
Methamphetamine	T43.6	X41	X61	Y11	Y49.7
Methampyrone	T39.2	X40	X60	Y10	Y45.8
Methandienone	T38.7	X44	X64	Y14	Y42.7
Methandriol	T38.7	X44	X64	Y14	Y42.7
Methandrostenolone	T38.7	X44	X64	Y14	Y42.7
Methane	T59.8	X47	X67	Y17	
Methanethiol	T59.8	X47	X67	Y17	
Methaniazide	T37.1	X44	X64	Y14	Y41.1
Methanol (vapor)	T51.1	X45	X65	Y15	
Methantheline	T44.3	X43	X63	Y13	Y51.3
Methanthelinium bromide	T44.3	X43	X63	Y13	Y51.3
Methapyrilene	T45.0	X44	X64	Y14	Y43.0
Methaqualone (compound)	T42.6	X41	X61	Y11	Y47.8
Metharbital	T42.3	X41	X61	Y11	Y47.0
Methazolamide	T50.2	X44	X64	Y14	Y54.2
Methdilazine	T43.3	X41	X61	Y11	Y49.3
Methenamine (mandelate)	T37.8	X44	X64	Y14	Y41.8
Methenolone	T38.7	X44	X64	Y14	Y42.7
Methetoin	T42.0	X41	X61	Y11	Y46.2
Methicillin	T36.0	X44	X64	Y14	Y40.0
Methimazole	T38.2	X44	X64	Y14	Y42.2
Methiodal sodium	T50.8	X44	X64	Y14	Y57.5
Methionine	T50.9	X44	X64	Y14	Y57.1

Substance	Chapter XIX	Accidental	Poisoning Intentional self-harm	Undetermined intent	Adverse effect in therapeutic use
Methisoprinol	T37.5	X44	X64	Y14	Y41.5
Methixene	T44.3	X43	X63	Y13	Y51.3
Methocarbamol	T42.8	X41	X61	Y11	Y46.8
– skeletal muscle relaxant	T48.1	X44	X64	Y14	Y55.1
Methohexital	T41.1	X44	X64	Y14	Y48.1
Methohexitone	T41.1	X44	X64	Y14	Y48.1
Methoin	T42.0	X41	X61	Y11	Y46.2
Methopromazine	T43.3	X41	X61	Y11	Y49.3
Methoserpidine	T46.5	X44	X64	Y14	Y52.5
Methotrexate	T45.1	X44	X64	Y14	Y43.1
Methotrimeprazine	T43.3	X41	X61	Y11	Y49.3
Methoxamine	T44.4	X43	X63	Y13	Y51.4
Methoxsalen	T50.9	X44	X64	Y14	Y57.8
Methoxyaniline	T65.3	X49	X69	Y19	
Methoxychlor	T53.7	X46	X66	Y16	
Methoxy-DDT	T53.7	X46	X66	Y16	
2-Methoxyethanol	T52.3	X46	X66	Y16	
Methoxyflurane	T41.0	X44	X64	Y14	Y48.0
Methoxyphenamine	T48.6	X44	X64	Y14	Y55.6
5-Methoxypsoralen (5-MOP)	T50.9	X44	X64	Y14	Y57.8
8-Methoxypsoralen (8-MOP)	T50.9	X44	X64	Y14	Y57.8
Methscopolamine bromide	T44.3	X43	X63	Y13	Y51.3
Methsuximide	T42.2	X41	X61	Y11	Y46.0
Methyclothiazide	T50.2	X44	X64	Y14	Y54.3
Methyl					
– acetate	T52.4	X46	X66	Y16	
– acetone	T52.4	X46	X66	Y16	
– acrylate	T65.8	X49	X69	Y19	
– alcohol	T51.1	X45	X65	Y15	
– aminophenol	T65.3	X49	X69	Y19	
– benzene	T52.2	X46	X66	Y16	
– benzoate	T52.8	X46	X66	Y16	
– benzol	T52.2	X46	X66	Y16	
– bromide (gas)	T59.8	X47	X67	Y17	
– – fumigant	T60.8	X48	X68	Y18	
– butanol	T51.3	X45	X65	Y15	
– carbonate	T52.8	X46	X66	Y16	
– CCNU	T45.1	X44	X64	Y14	Y43.3
– chloride (gas)	T59.8	X47	X67	Y17	
– chloroformate	T59.3	X47	X67	Y17	
– cyclohexane	T52.8	X46	X66	Y16	
– cyclohexanol	T51.8	X45	X65	Y15	
– cyclohexanone	T52.8	X46	X66	Y16	
– cyclohexyl acetate	T52.8	X46	X66	Y16	
– demeton	T60.0	X48	X68	Y18	
– ethyl ketone	T52.4	X46	X66	Y16	
– glucamine antimonate	T37.8	X44	X64	Y14	Y41.8
– hydrazine	T65.8	X49	X69	Y19	
– iodide	T65.8	X49	X69	Y19	
– intravenous	T38.0	X44	X64	Y14	Y42.0
– isobutyl ketone	T52.4	X46	X66	Y16	

| Substance | Chapter XIX | Poisoning | | | Adverse effect in therapeutic use |
		Accidental	Intentional self-harm	Undetermined intent	
Methyl—*continued*					
– isothiocyanate	T60.3	X48	X68	Y18	
– mercaptan	T59.8	X47	X67	Y17	
– nicotinate	T49.4	X44	X64	Y14	Y56.4
– paraben	T49.0	X44	X64	Y14	Y56.0
– parathion	T60.0	X48	X68	Y18	
– propylcarbinol	T51.3	X45	X65	Y15	
– salicylate	T49.2	X44	X64	Y14	Y56.2
– sulfate (fumes)	T59.8	X47	X67	Y17	
– – liquid	T52.8	X46	X66	Y16	
Methylamphetamine	T43.6	X41	X61	Y11	Y49.7
Methylated spirit	T51.1	X45	X65	Y15	
Methylatropine nitrate	T44.3	X43	X63	Y13	Y51.3
Methylbenactyzium bromide	T44.3	X43	X63	Y13	Y51.3
Methylbenzethonium chloride	T49.0	X44	X64	Y14	Y56.0
Methylcellulose	T47.4	X44	X64	Y14	Y53.4
– laxative	T47.4	X44	X64	Y14	Y53.4
Methylchlorophenoxyacetic acid	T60.3	X48	X68	Y18	
Methyldopa	T46.5	X44	X64	Y14	Y52.5
Methyldopate	T46.5	X44	X64	Y14	Y52.5
Methylene					
– blue	T50.6	X44	X64	Y14	Y57.2
– chloride or dichloride (solvent) NEC	T53.4	X46	X66	Y16	
Methylenedioxyamphetamine	T43.6	X41	X61	Y11	Y49.7
Methylergometrine	T48.0	X44	X64	Y14	Y55.0
Methylergonovine	T48.0	X44	X64	Y14	Y55.0
Methylestrenolone	T38.5	X44	X64	Y14	Y42.5
Methylethyl cellulose	T50.9	X44	X64	Y14	Y57.4
Methylmorphine	T40.2	X42	X62	Y12	Y45.0
Methylparafynol	T42.6	X41	X61	Y11	Y47.8
Methylpentynol, methylpenthynol	T42.6	X41	X61	Y11	Y47.8
Methylphenidate	T43.6	X41	X61	Y11	Y49.7
Methylphenobarbital	T42.3	X41	X61	Y11	Y47.0
Methylpolysiloxane	T47.1	X44	X64	Y14	Y53.1
Methylprednisolone	T49.0	X44	X64	Y14	Y56.0
– intravenous	T38.0	X44	X64	Y14	Y42.0
Methylrosaniline	T49.0	X44	X64	Y14	Y56.0
Methylrosanilinium chloride	T49.0	X44	X64	Y14	Y56.0
Methyltestosterone	T38.7	X44	X64	Y14	Y42.7
Methylthionine chloride	T50.6	X44	X64	Y14	Y57.2
Methylthioninium chloride	T50.6	X44	X64	Y14	Y57.2
Methylthiouracil	T38.2	X44	X64	Y14	Y42.2
Methyprylon	T42.6	X41	X61	Y11	Y47.8
Methysergide	T46.5	X44	X64	Y14	Y52.5
Metiamide	T47.1	X44	X64	Y14	Y53.1
Metiazinic acid	T39.3	X40	X60	Y10	Y45.3
Meticillin	T36.0	X44	X64	Y14	Y40.0
Meticrane	T50.2	X44	X64	Y14	Y54.5
Metildigoxin	T46.0	X44	X64	Y14	Y52.0
Metipranolol	T49.5	X44	X64	Y14	Y56.5

Substance	Chapter XIX	Accidental	Poisoning Intentional self-harm	Undetermined intent	Adverse effect in therapeutic use
Metirosine	T46.5	X44	X64	Y14	Y52.5
Metisazone	T37.5	X44	X64	Y14	Y41.5
Metixene	T44.3	X43	X63	Y13	Y51.3
Metizoline	T48.5	X44	X64	Y14	Y55.5
Metoclopramide	T45.0	X44	X64	Y14	Y43.0
Metofenazate	T43.3	X41	X61	Y11	Y49.3
Metolazone	T50.2	X44	X64	Y14	Y54.5
Metoprine	T45.1	X44	X64	Y14	Y43.3
Metoprolol	T44.7	X43	X63	Y13	Y51.7
Metrifonate	T60.0	X48	X68	Y18	
Metrizamide	T50.8	X44	X64	Y14	Y57.5
Metrizoic acid	T50.8	X44	X64	Y14	Y57.5
Metronidazole	T37.8	X44	X64	Y14	Y41.8
Metyrapone	T50.8	X44	X64	Y14	Y57.6
Mevinphos	T60.0	X48	X68	Y18	
Mexazolam	T42.4	X41	X61	Y11	Y47.1
Mexenone	T49.3	X44	X64	Y14	Y56.3
Mexiletine	T46.2	X44	X64	Y14	Y52.2
Mezlocillin	T36.0	X44	X64	Y14	Y40.0
Mianserin	T43.0	X41	X61	Y11	Y49.0
Miconazole	T49.0	X44	X64	Y14	Y56.0
Micronomicin	T36.5	X44	X64	Y14	Y40.5
Midazolam	T42.4	X41	X61	Y11	Y47.1
Midecamycin	T36.3	X44	X64	Y14	Y40.3
Mifepristone	T38.6	X44	X64	Y14	Y42.6
Milk of magnesia	T47.1	X44	X64	Y14	Y53.1
Milverine	T44.3	X43	X63	Y13	Y51.3
Minaprine	T43.2	X41	X61	Y11	Y49.2
Minaxolone	T41.2	X44	X64	Y14	Y48.2
Mineral					
– acids	T54.2	X49	X69	Y19	
– oil (laxative) (medicinal)	T47.4	X44	X64	Y14	Y53.4
– – emulsion	T47.2	X44	X64	Y14	Y53.2
– – nonmedicinal	T52.0	X46	X66	Y16	
– salt NEC	T50.3	X44	X64	Y14	Y54.9
Mineralocorticosteroid	T50.0	X44	X64	Y14	Y54.0
Minocycline	T36.4	X44	X64	Y14	Y40.4
Minoxidil	T46.7	X44	X64	Y14	Y52.7
Miokamycin	T36.3	X44	X64	Y14	Y40.3
Miotic drug	T49.5	X44	X64	Y14	Y56.5
Mipafox	T60.0	X48	X68	Y18	
Mirex	T60.1	X48	X68	Y18	
Misonidazole	T37.3	X44	X64	Y14	Y41.3
Misoprostol	T47.1	X44	X64	Y14	Y53.1
Mithramycin	T45.1	X44	X64	Y14	Y43.3
Mitobronitol	T45.1	X44	X64	Y14	Y43.3
Mitoguazone	T45.1	X44	X64	Y14	Y43.3
Mitolactol	T45.1	X44	X64	Y14	Y43.3
Mitomycin	T45.1	X44	X64	Y14	Y43.3
Mitopodozide	T45.1	X44	X64	Y14	Y43.3
Mitotane	T45.1	X44	X64	Y14	Y43.3

Substance	Chapter XIX	Accidental	Poisoning Intentional self-harm	Undetermined intent	Adverse effect in therapeutic use
Mitoxantrone	T45.1	X44	X64	Y14	Y43.3
Mivacurium chloride	T48.1	X44	X64	Y14	Y55.1
Miyari bacteria	T47.6	X44	X64	Y14	Y53.6
Moclobemide	T43.1	X41	X61	Y11	Y49.1
Mofebutazone	T39.2	X40	X60	Y10	Y45.8
Molindone	T43.5	X41	X61	Y11	Y49.5
Molsidomine	T46.3	X44	X64	Y14	Y52.3
Mometasone	T49.0	X44	X64	Y14	Y56.0
Monoamine oxidase inhibitor NEC	T43.1	X41	X61	Y11	Y49.1
– hydrazine	T43.1	X41	X61	Y11	Y49.1
Monobenzone	T49.4	X44	X64	Y14	Y56.4
Monochloroacetic acid	T60.3	X48	X68	Y18	
Monochlorobenzene	T53.7	X46	X66	Y16	
Monoethanolamine	T46.8	X44	X64	Y14	Y52.8
– oleate	T46.8	X44	X64	Y14	Y52.8
Monooctanoin	T50.9	X44	X64	Y14	Y57.8
Monophenylbutazone	T39.2	X40	X60	Y10	Y45.8
Monosulfiram	T49.0	X44	X64	Y14	Y56.0
Monoxide, carbon	T58	X47	X67	Y17	
Monoxidine hydrochloride	T46.1	X44	X64	Y14	Y52.1
Monuron	T60.3	X48	X68	Y18	
Moperone	T43.4	X41	X61	Y11	Y49.4
Mopidamol	T45.1	X44	X64	Y14	Y43.1
MOPP (mechlorethamine + vincristine + prednisone + procarbazine)	T45.1	X44	X64	Y14	Y43.3
Morfin	T40.2	X42	X62	Y12	Y45.0
Morinamide	T37.1	X44	X64	Y14	Y41.1
Morniflumate	T39.3	X40	X60	Y10	Y45.3
Moroxydine	T37.5	X44	X64	Y14	Y41.5
Morphazinamide	T37.1	X44	X64	Y14	Y41.1
Morphine	T40.2	X42	X62	Y12	Y45.0
– antagonist	T50.7	X44	X64	Y14	Y50.1
Morsuximide	T42.2	X41	X61	Y11	Y46.0
Mosapramine	T43.5	X41	X61	Y11	Y49.5
Motor exhaust gas	T58	X47	X67	Y17	
Mouthwash (antiseptic) (zinc chloride)	T49.6	X44	X64	Y14	Y56.6
Moxastine	T45.0	X44	X64	Y14	Y43.0
Moxaverine	T44.3	X43	X63	Y13	Y51.3
Moxifensine	T43.2	X41	X61	Y11	Y49.2
Moxisylyte	T46.7	X44	X64	Y14	Y52.7
Mucilage, plant	T47.4	X44	X64	Y14	Y53.4
Mucolytic drug	T48.4	X44	X64	Y14	Y55.4
Mupirocin	T49.0	X44	X64	Y14	Y56.0
Muriatic acid – see Hydrochloric acid					
Muromonab-CD3	T45.1	X44	X64	Y14	Y43.4
Muscle relaxant – see Relaxant, muscle					
Muscle-action drug NEC	T48.2	X44	X64	Y14	Y55.2

Substance		Poisoning			Adverse effect in therapeutic use
	Chapter XIX	Accidental	Intentional self-harm	Undetermined intent	
Muscle-tone depressant, central NEC	T42.8	X41	X61	Y11	Y46.8
– specified NEC	T42.8	X41	X61	Y11	Y46.8
Mushroom, noxious	T62.0	X49	X69	Y19	
Mussel, noxious	T61.2	X49	X69	Y19	
Mustard (emetic)	T47.7	X44	X64	Y14	Y53.7
– black	T47.7	X44	X64	Y14	Y53.7
– gas, not in war	T59.9	X47	X67	Y17	
Mustine	T45.1	X44	X64	Y14	Y43.3
Mycotoxins	T64	X49	X69	Y19	
Mydriatic drug	T49.5	X44	X64	Y14	Y56.5
Myralact	T49.0	X44	X64	Y14	Y56.0
Myristicin	T65.8	X49	X69	Y19	

N

	Poisoning			Adverse effect in therapeutic use
Substance	Chapter XIX	Accidental	Intentional self-harm	Undetermined intent	
Nabilone	T40.7	X42	X62	Y12	Y49.6
Nabumetone	T39.3	X40	X60	Y10	Y45.3
Nadolol	T44.7	X43	X63	Y13	Y51.7
Nafamostat	T45.6	X44	X64	Y14	Y44.3
Nafcillin	T36.0	X44	X64	Y14	Y40.0
Nafoxidine	T38.6	X44	X64	Y14	Y42.6
Naftazone	T46.9	X44	X64	Y14	Y52.9
Naftidrofuryl (oxalate)	T46.7	X44	X64	Y14	Y52.7
Naftifine	T49.0	X44	X64	Y14	Y56.0
Nalbuphine	T40.4	X42	X62	Y12	Y45.0
Naled	T60.0	X48	X68	Y18	
Nalidixic acid	T37.8	X44	X64	Y14	Y41.8
Nalorphine	T50.7	X44	X64	Y14	Y50.1
Naloxone	T50.7	X44	X64	Y14	Y50.1
Naltrexone	T50.7	X44	X64	Y14	Y50.1
Nandrolone	T38.7	X44	X64	Y14	Y42.7
Naphazoline	T48.5	X44	X64	Y14	Y55.5
Naphtha (painters') (petroleum)	T52.0	X46	X66	Y16	
− solvent	T52.0	X46	X66	Y16	
− vapor	T52.0	X46	X66	Y16	
Naphthalene (chlorinated)	T60.1	X48	X68	Y18	
− insecticide or moth repellent	T60.1	X48	X68	Y18	
− vapor	T60.1	X48	X68	Y18	
Naphthol	T65.8	X49	X69	Y19	
Naphthylamine	T65.8	X49	X69	Y19	
Naphthylthiourea (ANTU)	T60.4	X48	X68	Y18	
Naproxen	T39.3	X40	X60	Y10	Y45.2
Narcotic NEC	T40.6	X42	X62	Y12	Y45.0
− synthetic NEC	T40.4	X42	X62	Y12	Y45.0
Nasal drug NEC	T49.6	X44	X64	Y14	Y56.6
Natamycin	T49.0	X44	X64	Y14	Y56.0
Natural gas	T59.8	X47	X67	Y17	
− incomplete combustion	T58	X47	X67	Y17	
Nealbarbital	T42.3	X41	X61	Y11	Y47.0
Nedocromil	T48.6	X44	X64	Y14	Y55.6
Nefopam	T39.8	X40	X60	Y10	Y45.8
Nemonapride	T43.5	X41	X61	Y11	Y49.5
Neoarsphenamine	T37.8	X44	X64	Y14	Y41.8
Neomycin (derivatives)	T36.5	X44	X64	Y14	Y40.5
− with					
− − bacitracin	T49.0	X44	X64	Y14	Y56.0
− − neostigmine	T44.0	X44	X64	Y14	Y51.0
Neostigmine bromide	T44.0	X43	X63	Y13	Y51.0
Nerium oleander	T62.2	X49	X69	Y19	

Substance	Chapter XIX	Poisoning			Adverse effect in therapeutic use
		Accidental	Intentional self-harm	Undetermined intent	
Nerve gas, not in war	T59.9	X47	X67	Y17	
Netilmicin	T36.5	X44	X64	Y14	Y40.5
Neuroleptic drug NEC	T43.5	X41	X61	Y11	Y49.5
– butyrophenone	T43.4	X41	X61	Y11	Y49.4
– phenothiazine	T43.3	X41	X61	Y11	Y49.3
– thioxanthene	T43.4	X41	X61	Y11	Y49.4
Neuromuscular blocking drug	T48.1	X44	X64	Y14	Y55.1
Neutral insulin injection	T38.3	X44	X64	Y14	Y42.3
Niacin	T46.7	X44	X64	Y14	Y52.7
Niacinamide	T45.2	X44	X64	Y14	Y57.7
Nialamide	T43.1	X41	X61	Y11	Y49.1
Niaprazine	T42.6	X41	X61	Y11	Y47.8
Nicametate	T46.7	X44	X64	Y14	Y52.7
Nicardipine	T46.1	X44	X64	Y14	Y52.1
Nicergoline	T46.7	X44	X64	Y14	Y52.7
Nickel (carbonyl) (tetracarbonyl) (fumes)(vapor)	T56.8	X49	X69	Y19	
Nickelocene	T56.8	X49	X69	Y19	
Niclosamide	T37.4	X44	X64	Y14	Y41.4
Nicofuranose	T46.7	X44	X64	Y14	Y52.7
Nicomorphine	T40.2	X42	X62	Y12	Y45.0
Nicorandil	T46.3	X44	X64	Y14	Y52.3
Nicotiana (plant)	T62.2	X49	X69	Y19	
Nicotinamide	T45.2	X44	X64	Y14	Y57.7
Nicotine (insecticide) (spray) (sulfate) NEC	T60.2	X48	X68	Y18	
– from tobacco	T65.2	X49	X69	Y19	
Nicotinic acid	T46.7	X44	X64	Y14	Y52.7
Nicotinyl alcohol	T46.7	X44	X64	Y14	Y52.7
Nicoumalone	T45.5	X44	X64	Y14	Y44.2
Nifedipine	T46.1	X44	X64	Y14	Y52.1
Nifenazone	T39.2	X40	X60	Y10	Y45.8
Niflumic acid	T39.3	X40	X60	Y10	Y45.3
Nifuratel	T37.8	X44	X64	Y14	Y41.8
Nifurtimox	T37.3	X44	X64	Y14	Y41.3
Nifurtoinol	T37.8	X44	X64	Y14	Y41.8
Nightshade, deadly (solanum)	T62.2	X49	X69	Y19	
Nikethamide	T50.7	X44	X64	Y14	Y50.0
Nilutamide	T38.6	X44	X64	Y14	Y42.6
Nimesulide	T39.3	X40	X60	Y10	Y45.3
Nimetazepam	T42.4	X41	X61	Y11	Y47.1
Nimodipine	T46.1	X44	X64	Y14	Y52.1
Nimorazole	T37.3	X44	X64	Y14	Y41.3
Nimustine	T45.1	X44	X64	Y14	Y43.3
Niridazole	T37.4	X44	X64	Y14	Y41.4
Nisoldipine	T46.1	X44	X64	Y14	Y52.1
Nitramine	T65.3	X49	X69	Y19	
Nitrate, organic	T46.3	X44	X64	Y14	Y52.3
Nitrazepam	T42.4	X41	X61	Y11	Y47.1
Nitrefazole	T50.6	X44	X64	Y14	Y57.3
Nitrendipine	T46.1	X44	X64	Y14	Y52.1

Substance	Chapter XIX	Poisoning Accidental	Poisoning Intentional self-harm	Poisoning Undetermined intent	Adverse effect in therapeutic use
Nitric					
– acid (liquid)	T54.2	X49	X69	Y19	
– – vapor	T59.8	X47	X67	Y17	
– oxide (gas)	T59.0	X47	X67	Y17	
Nitrimidazine	T37.3	X44	X64	Y14	Y41.3
Nitroaniline	T65.3	X49	X69	Y19	
– vapor	T59.8	X47	X67	Y17	
Nitrobenzene, nitrobenzol	T65.3	X49	X69	Y19	
– vapor	T65.3	X47	X67	Y17	
Nitrocellulose	T65.8	X49	X69	Y19	
– lacquer	T65.8	X49	X69	Y19	
Nitrodiphenyl	T65.3	X49	X69	Y19	
Nitrofural	T49.0	X44	X64	Y14	Y56.0
Nitrofurantoin	T37.8	X44	X64	Y14	Y41.8
Nitrofurazone	T49.0	X44	X64	Y14	Y56.0
Nitrogen	T59.0	X47	X67	Y17	
– mustard	T45.1	X44	X64	Y14	Y43.3
Nitroglycerin, nitroglycerol (medicinal)	T46.3	X44	X64	Y14	Y52.3
– nonmedicinal	T65.5	X49	X69	Y19	
Nitroglycol	T52.3	X46	X66	Y16	
Nitrohydrochloric acid	T54.2	X49	X69	Y19	
Nitromersol	T49.0	X44	X64	Y14	Y56.0
Nitronaphthalene	T65.8	X49	X69	Y19	
Nitrophenol	T54.0	X49	X69	Y19	
Nitropropane	T52.8	X46	X66	Y16	
Nitroprusside	T46.5	X44	X64	Y14	Y52.5
Nitrosodimethylamine	T65.3	X49	X69	Y19	
Nitrotoluene, nitrotoluol	T65.3	X49	X69	Y19	
– vapor	T65.3	X47	X67	Y17	
Nitrous					
– acid (liquid)	T54.2	X49	X69	Y19	
– – fumes	T59.8	X47	X67	Y17	
– ether spirit	T46.3	X44	X64	Y14	Y52.3
– oxide	T41.0	X44	X64	Y14	Y48.0
Nitroxoline	T37.8	X44	X64	Y14	Y41.8
Nizatidine	T47.0	X44	X64	Y14	Y53.0
Nizofenone	T43.8	X41	X61	Y11	Y49.8
Nomegestrol	T38.5	X44	X64	Y14	Y42.5
Nomifensine	T43.2	X41	X61	Y11	Y49.2
Nonoxinol	T49.8	X44	X64	Y14	Y56.8
Nonylphenoxy (polyethoxyethanol)	T49.8	X44	X64	Y14	Y56.8
Noradrenaline	T44.4	X43	X63	Y13	Y51.4
Noramidopyrine	T39.2	X40	X60	Y10	Y45.8
– methanesulfonate sodium	T39.2	X40	X60	Y10	Y45.8
Norbormide	T60.4	X48	X68	Y18	
Nordazepam	T42.4	X41	X61	Y11	Y47.1
Norepinephrine	T44.4	X43	X63	Y13	Y51.4
Norethandrolone	T38.7	X44	X64	Y14	Y42.7
Norethindrone	T38.4	X44	X64	Y14	Y42.4

Substance	Chapter XIX	Accidental	Poisoning Intentional self-harm	Undetermined intent	Adverse effect in therapeutic use
Norethisterone (acetate) (enantate)	T38.4	X44	X64	Y14	Y42.4
– with ethinylestradiol	T38.5	X44	X64	Y14	Y42.5
Noretynodrel	T38.5	X44	X64	Y14	Y42.5
Norfenefrine	T44.4	X43	X63	Y13	Y51.4
Norfloxacin	T36.8	X44	X64	Y14	Y40.8
Norgestrel	T38.4	X44	X64	Y14	Y42.4
Norgestrienone	T38.4	X44	X64	Y14	Y42.4
Normal serum albumin (human), salt-poor	T45.8	X44	X64	Y14	Y44.6
Normethandrone	T38.5	X44	X64	Y14	Y42.5
Norpseudoephedrine	T50.5	X44	X64	Y14	Y57.0
Nortestosterone (furanpropionate)	T38.7	X44	X64	Y14	Y42.7
Nortriptyline	T43.0	X41	X61	Y11	Y49.0
Noscapine	T48.3	X44	X64	Y14	Y55.3
Novobiocin	T36.5	X44	X64	Y14	Y40.5
Noxious foodstuff	T62.9	X49	X69	Y19	
– specified NEC	T62.8	X49	X69	Y19	
Noxiptiline	T43.0	X41	X61	Y11	Y49.0
Noxytiolin	T49.0	X44	X64	Y14	Y56.0
NSAID NEC	T39.3	X40	X60	Y10	Y45.3
Nutritional supplement	T50.9	X44	X64	Y14	Y57.8
Nylidrin	T46.7	X44	X64	Y14	Y52.7
Nystatin	T36.7	X44	X64	Y14	Y40.7

O

Substance	Chapter XIX	Accidental	Poisoning Intentional self-harm	Undetermined intent	Adverse effect in therapeutic use
Obidoxime chloride	T50.6	X44	X64	Y14	Y57.2
Octafonium (chloride)	T49.3	X44	X64	Y14	Y56.3
Octamethyl pyrophosphoramide	T60.0	X48	X68	Y18	
Octanoin	T50.9	X44	X64	Y14	Y57.8
Octatropine methylbromide	T44.3	X43	X63	Y13	Y51.3
Octotiamine	T45.2	X44	X64	Y14	Y57.7
Octoxinol (9)	T49.8	X44	X64	Y14	Y56.8
Octreotide	T38.9	X44	X64	Y14	Y42.9
Oestradiol	T38.5	X44	X64	Y14	Y42.5
Oestriol	T38.5	X44	X64	Y14	Y42.5
Oestrogen	T38.5	X44	X64	Y14	Y42.5
Oestrone	T38.5	X44	X64	Y14	Y42.5
Ofloxacin	T36.8	X44	X64	Y14	Y40.8
Oil (of)					
– bitter almond	T62.8	X49	X69	Y19	
– cloves	T49.7	X44	X64	Y14	Y56.7
– colors	T65.6	X49	X69	Y19	
– fumes	T59.8	X47	X67	Y17	
– lubricating	T52.0	X46	X66	Y16	
– Niobe	T52.8	X46	X66	Y16	
– vitriol (liquid)	T54.2	X49	X69	Y19	
– – fumes	T54.2	X47	X67	Y17	
Oily preparation (for skin)	T49.3	X44	X64	Y14	Y56.3
Ointment NEC	T49.3	X44	X64	Y14	Y56.3
Oleander	T62.2	X49	X69	Y19	
Oleandomycin	T36.3	X44	X64	Y14	Y40.3
Oleandrin	T46.0	X44	X64	Y14	Y52.0
Oleic acid	T46.6	X44	X64	Y14	Y52.6
Oleovitamin A	T45.2	X44	X64	Y14	Y57.7
Oleum ricini	T47.2	X44	X64	Y14	Y53.2
Olivomycin	T45.1	X44	X64	Y14	Y43.3
Olsalazine	T47.8	X44	X64	Y14	Y53.8
Omeprazole	T47.1	X44	X64	Y14	Y53.1
OMPA	T60.0	X48	X68	Y18	
Ondansetron	T45.0	X44	X64	Y14	Y43.0
Ophthalmological drug NEC	T49.5	X44	X64	Y14	Y56.5
Opiate NEC	T40.6	X42	X62	Y12	Y45.0
Opioid NEC	T40.2	X42	X62	Y12	Y45.0
Opipramol	T43.0	X41	X61	Y11	Y49.0
Opium alkaloids (total)	T40.0	X42	X62	Y12	Y45.0
– standardized powdered	T40.0	X42	X62	Y12	Y45.0
– tincture (camphorated)	T40.0	X42	X62	Y12	Y45.0
Oral rehydration salts	T50.3	X44	X64	Y14	Y54.6
Orazamide	T50.9	X44	X64	Y14	Y57.1

Substance		Poisoning			Adverse effect in therapeutic use
	Chapter XIX	Accidental	Intentional self-harm	Undetermined intent	
Orciprenaline	T48.2	X44	X64	Y14	Y55.2
Organonitrate NEC	T46.3	X44	X64	Y14	Y52.3
Organophosphates	T60.0	X48	X68	Y18	
Orgotein	T39.3	X40	X60	Y10	Y45.3
Ormeloxifene	T38.6	X44	X64	Y14	Y42.6
Ornidazole	T37.3	X44	X64	Y14	Y41.3
Ornipressin	T38.8	X44	X64	Y14	Y42.8
Ornithine aspartate	T50.9	X44	X64	Y14	Y57.1
Ornoprostil	T47.1	X44	X64	Y14	Y53.1
Orphenadrine (hydrochloride)	T42.8	X41	X61	Y11	Y46.7
Orthodichlorobenzene	T53.7	X46	X66	Y16	
Osmic acid (liquid)	T54.2	X49	X69	Y19	
− fumes	T54.2	X47	X67	Y17	
Otilonium bromide	T44.3	X43	X63	Y13	Y51.3
Otorhinolaryngological drug NEC	T49.6	X44	X64	Y14	Y56.6
Ouabain(e)	T46.0	X44	X64	Y14	Y52.0
Ovarian					
− hormone	T38.5	X44	X64	Y14	Y42.5
− stimulant	T38.5	X44	X64	Y14	Y42.5
Oxaceprol	T39.3	X40	X60	Y10	Y45.3
Oxacillin	T36.0	X44	X64	Y14	Y40.0
Oxalic acid	T54.2	X49	X69	Y19	
− ammonium salt	T50.9	X44	X64	Y14	Y57.6
Oxametacin	T39.3	X40	X60	Y10	Y45.3
Oxamniquine	T37.4	X44	X64	Y14	Y41.4
Oxandrolone	T38.7	X44	X64	Y14	Y42.7
Oxantel	T37.4	X44	X64	Y14	Y41.4
Oxapium iodide	T44.3	X43	X63	Y13	Y51.3
Oxaprotiline	T43.0	X41	X61	Y11	Y49.0
Oxaprozin	T39.3	X40	X60	Y10	Y45.2
Oxatomide	T45.0	X44	X64	Y14	Y43.0
Oxazepam	T42.4	X41	X61	Y11	Y47.1
Oxazimedrine	T50.5	X44	X64	Y14	Y57.0
Oxazolam	T42.4	X41	X61	Y11	Y47.1
Oxazolidinedione	T42.2	X41	X61	Y11	Y46.1
Ox bile extract	T47.5	X44	X64	Y14	Y53.5
Oxcarbazepine	T42.1	X41	X61	Y11	Y46.4
Oxedrine	T44.4	X43	X63	Y13	Y51.4
Oxeladin (citrate)	T48.3	X44	X64	Y14	Y55.3
Oxendolone	T38.5	X44	X64	Y14	Y42.5
Oxetacaine	T41.3	X44	X64	Y14	Y48.3
Oxethazine	T41.3	X44	X64	Y14	Y48.3
Oxetorone	T39.8	X40	X60	Y10	Y45.8
Oxiconazole	T49.0	X44	X64	Y14	Y56.0
Oxidizing agent NEC	T54.9	X49	X69	Y19	
Oxipurinol	T50.4	X44	X64	Y14	Y54.8
Oxitriptan	T43.2	X41	X61	Y11	Y49.2
Oxitropium bromide	T48.6	X44	X64	Y14	Y55.6
Oxodipine	T46.1	X44	X64	Y14	Y52.1
Oxolamine	T48.3	X44	X64	Y14	Y55.3
Oxolinic acid	T37.8	X44	X64	Y14	Y41.8

Substance	Poisoning				Adverse effect in therapeutic use
	Chapter XIX	Accidental	Intentional self-harm	Undetermined intent	
Oxomemazine	T43.3	X41	X61	Y11	Y49.3
Oxophenarsine	T37.3	X44	X64	Y14	Y41.3
Oxprenolol	T44.7	X43	X63	Y13	Y51.7
Oxtriphylline	T48.6	X44	X64	Y14	Y55.6
Oxybate sodium	T41.2	X44	X64	Y14	Y48.2
Oxybuprocaine	T41.3	X44	X64	Y14	Y48.3
Oxybutynin	T44.3	X43	X63	Y13	Y51.3
Oxychlorosene	T49.0	X44	X64	Y14	Y56.0
Oxycodone	T40.2	X42	X62	Y12	Y45.0
Oxyfedrine	T46.3	X44	X64	Y14	Y52.3
Oxygen	T41.5	X44	X64	Y14	Y48.5
Oxymesterone	T38.7	X44	X64	Y14	Y42.7
Oxymetazoline	T48.5	X44	X64	Y14	Y55.5
Oxymetholone	T38.7	X44	X64	Y14	Y42.7
Oxymorphone	T40.2	X42	X62	Y12	Y45.0
Oxypertine	T43.5	X41	X61	Y11	Y49.5
Oxyphenbutazone	T39.2	X40	X60	Y10	Y45.3
Oxyphencyclimine	T44.3	X43	X63	Y13	Y51.3
Oxyphenisatine	T47.2	X44	X64	Y14	Y53.2
Oxyphenonium bromide	T44.3	X43	X63	Y13	Y51.3
Oxypolygelatin	T45.8	X44	X64	Y14	Y44.7
Oxyquinoline (derivatives)	T37.8	X44	X64	Y14	Y41.8
Oxytetracycline	T36.4	X44	X64	Y14	Y40.4
Oxytocic drug NEC	T48.0	X44	X64	Y14	Y55.0
Oxytocin (synthetic)	T48.0	X44	X64	Y14	Y55.0
Ozone	T59.8	X47	X67	Y17	

P

| Substance | Chapter XIX | Poisoning | | | Adverse effect in therapeutic use |
		Accidental	Intentional self-harm	Undetermined intent	
Padimate	T49.3	X44	X64	Y14	Y56.3
Paint NEC	T65.6	X49	X69	Y19	
– cleaner	T52.9	X46	X66	Y16	
– fumes NEC	T59.8	X47	X67	Y17	
– lead (fumes)	T56.0	X49	X69	Y19	
– solvent NEC	T52.8	X46	X66	Y16	
– stripper	T52.8	X46	X66	Y16	
Palm kernel oil	T50.9	X44	X64	Y14	Y57.4
Pancreatic					
– digestive secretion stimulant	T47.8	X44	X64	Y14	Y53.8
– dornase	T45.3	X44	X64	Y14	Y43.6
Pancreatin	T47.5	X44	X64	Y14	Y53.5
Pancrelipase	T47.5	X44	X64	Y14	Y53.5
Pancuronium (bromide)	T48.1	X44	X64	Y14	Y55.1
Pangamic acid	T45.2	X44	X64	Y14	Y57.7
Panthenol	T45.2	X44	X64	Y14	Y57.7
Pantothenic acid	T45.2	X44	X64	Y14	Y57.7
Papain	T47.5	X44	X64	Y14	Y53.5
– digestant	T47.5	X44	X64	Y14	Y53.5
Papaveretum	T40.0	X42	X62	Y12	Y45.0
Papaverine	T44.3	X43	X63	Y13	Y51.3
Para-acetamidophenol	T39.1	X40	X60	Y10	Y45.5
Para-aminobenzoic acid	T49.3	X44	X64	Y14	Y56.3
Para-aminosalicylic acid	T37.1	X44	X64	Y14	Y41.1
Paracetaldehyde	T42.6	X41	X61	Y11	Y47.3
Paracetamol	T39.1	X40	X60	Y10	Y45.5
Parachlorophenol (camphorated)	T49.0	X44	X64	Y14	Y56.0
Paraffin(s) (wax)	T52.0	X46	X66	Y16	
– liquid (medicinal)	T47.4	X44	X64	Y14	Y53.4
– – nonmedicinal	T52.0	X46	X66	Y16	
Paraformaldehyde	T60.3	X48	X68	Y18	
Paraldehyde	T42.6	X41	X61	Y11	Y47.3
Paramethadione	T42.2	X41	X61	Y11	Y46.1
Paramethasone	T38.0	X44	X64	Y14	Y42.0
– acetate	T49.0	X44	X64	Y14	Y56.0
Paraoxon	T60.0	X48	X68	Y18	
Paraquat	T60.3	X48	X68	Y18	
Parasympatholytic NEC	T44.3	X43	X63	Y13	Y51.3
Parasympathomimetic drug NEC	T44.1	X43	X63	Y13	Y51.1
Parathion	T60.0	X48	X68	Y18	
Parathyroid extract	T50.9	X44	X64	Y14	Y54.7
Paregoric	T40.0	X42	X62	Y12	Y45.0
Pargyline	T46.5	X44	X64	Y14	Y52.5
Paris green	T57.0	X49	X69	Y19	

| Substance | Chapter XIX | Poisoning | | | Adverse effect in therapeutic use |
		Accidental	Intentional self-harm	Undetermined intent	
Paromomycin	T36.5	X44	X64	Y14	Y40.5
PAS	T37.1	X44	X64	Y14	Y41.1
Pasiniazid	T37.1	X44	X64	Y14	Y41.1
PBB (polybrominated biphenyls)	T65.8	X49	X69	Y19	
PCB	T65.8	X49	X69	Y19	
Pecazine	T43.3	X41	X61	Y11	Y49.3
Pectin	T47.6	X44	X64	Y14	Y53.6
Pefloxacin	T37.8	X44	X64	Y14	Y41.8
Pegademase, bovine	T50.9	X44	X64	Y14	Y57.8
Pelletierine tannate	T37.4	X44	X64	Y14	Y41.4
Pemirolast (potassium)	T48.6	X44	X64	Y14	Y55.6
Pemoline	T50.7	X44	X64	Y14	Y50.0
Pempidine	T44.2	X43	X63	Y13	Y51.2
Penamecillin	T36.0	X44	X64	Y14	Y40.0
Penbutolol	T44.7	X43	X63	Y13	Y51.7
Penethamate	T36.0	X44	X64	Y14	Y40.0
Penfluridol	T43.5	X41	X61	Y11	Y49.5
Penflutizide	T50.2	X44	X64	Y14	Y54.3
Pengitoxin	T46.0	X44	X64	Y14	Y52.0
Penicillamine	T50.6	X44	X64	Y14	Y57.2
Penicillin (any)	T36.0	X44	X64	Y14	Y40.0
Penicillinase	T45.3	X44	X64	Y14	Y43.6
Penicilloyl polylysine	T50.8	X44	X64	Y14	Y57.6
Penimepicycline	T36.4	X44	X64	Y14	Y40.4
Pentachloroethane	T53.6	X46	X66	Y16	
Pentachloronaphthalene	T53.7	X46	X66	Y16	
Pentachlorophenol (pesticide)	T60.3	X48	X68	Y18	
Pentaerythritol tetranitrate	T46.3	X44	X64	Y14	Y52.3
Pentaerythrityl tetranitrate	T46.3	X44	X64	Y14	Y52.3
Pentagastrin	T50.8	X44	X64	Y14	Y57.6
Pentalin	T53.6	X46	X66	Y16	
Pentamethonium bromide	T44.2	X43	X63	Y13	Y51.2
Pentamidine	T37.3	X44	X64	Y14	Y41.3
Pentanol	T51.3	X45	X65	Y15	
Pentapyrrolinium (bitartrate)	T44.2	X43	X63	Y13	Y51.2
Pentazocine	T40.4	X42	X62	Y12	Y45.0
Pentetrazole	T50.7	X44	X64	Y14	Y50.0
Penthienate bromide	T44.3	X43	X63	Y13	Y51.3
Pentifylline	T46.7	X44	X64	Y14	Y52.7
Pentobarbital	T42.3	X41	X61	Y11	Y47.0
– sodium	T42.3	X41	X61	Y11	Y47.0
Pentobarbitone	T42.3	X41	X61	Y11	Y47.0
Pentolonium tartrate	T44.2	X43	X63	Y13	Y51.2
Pentosan polysulfate (sodium)	T45.5	X44	X64	Y14	Y44.2
Pentostatin	T45.1	X44	X64	Y14	Y43.4
Pentoxifylline	T46.7	X44	X64	Y14	Y52.7
Pentoxyverine	T48.3	X44	X64	Y14	Y55.3
Pentrinat	T46.3	X44	X64	Y14	Y52.3
Pentylenetetrazole	T50.7	X44	X64	Y14	Y50.0
Pentymal	T42.3	X41	X61	Y11	Y47.0
Peplomycin	T45.1	X44	X64	Y14	Y43.3

		Poisoning			Adverse effect in therapeutic use
Substance	Chapter XIX	Accidental	Intentional self-harm	Undetermined intent	
Peppermint (oil)	T47.5	X44	X64	Y14	Y53.5
Pepsin	T47.5	X44	X64	Y14	Y53.5
– digestant	T47.5	X44	X64	Y14	Y53.5
Pepstatin	T47.1	X44	X64	Y14	Y53.1
Perazine	T43.3	X41	X61	Y11	Y49.3
Perchloroethylene	T53.3	X46	X66	Y16	
– vapor	T53.3	X46	X66	Y16	
Pergolide	T42.8	X41	X61	Y11	Y46.7
Perhexilene	T46.3	X44	X64	Y14	Y52.3
Perhexiline (maleate)	T46.3	X44	X64	Y14	Y52.3
Periciazine	T43.3	X41	X61	Y11	Y49.3
Perindopril	T46.4	X44	X64	Y14	Y52.4
Perisoxal	T39.8	X40	X60	Y10	Y45.8
Peritoneal dialysis solution	T50.3	X44	X64	Y14	Y54.6
Perlapine	T42.4	X41	X61	Y11	Y47.1
Permanganate	T65.8	X49	X69	Y19	
Permethrin	T60.1	X48	X68	Y18	
Perphenazine	T43.3	X41	X61	Y11	Y49.3
Pertussis vaccine	T50.9	X44	X64	Y14	Y58.6
Peruvian balsam	T49.0	X44	X64	Y14	Y56.0
Peruvoside	T46.0	X44	X64	Y14	Y52.0
Pesticide (dust) (fumes) (vapor) NEC	T60.9	X48	X68	Y18	
– chlorinated	T60.1	X48	X68	Y18	
Pethidine	T40.4	X42	X62	Y12	Y45.0
Petrol	T52.0	X46	X66	Y16	
– vapor	T52.0	X46	X66	Y16	
Petrolatum	T49.3	X44	X64	Y14	Y56.3
– nonmedicinal	T52.0	X46	X66	Y16	
– red veterinary	T49.3	X44	X64	Y14	Y56.3
– white	T49.3	X44	X64	Y14	Y56.3
Petroleum (products) NEC	T52.0	X46	X66	Y16	
– benzine(s) – see Ligroin					
– ether – see Ligroin					
– jelly – see Petrolatum					
– naphtha – see Ligroin					
– pesticide	T60.8	X48	X68	Y18	
– vapor	T52.0	X46	X66	Y16	
Peyote	T40.9	X42	X62	Y12	Y49.6
Phanquinone	T37.3	X44	X64	Y14	Y41.3
Phanquone	T37.3	X44	X64	Y14	Y41.3
Pharmaceutical					
– adjunct NEC	T50.9	X44	X64	Y14	Y57.4
– excipient NEC	T50.9	X44	X64	Y14	Y57.4
– sweetener	T50.9	X44	X64	Y14	Y57.4
– viscous agent	T50.9	X44	X64	Y14	Y57.4
Phemitone	T42.3	X41	X61	Y11	Y47.0
Phenacaine	T41.3	X44	X64	Y14	Y48.3
Phenacemide	T42.6	X41	X61	Y11	Y46.6
Phenacetin	T39.1	X40	X60	Y10	Y45.5
Phenaglycodol	T43.5	X41	X61	Y11	Y49.5

Substance	Chapter XIX	Poisoning			Adverse effect in therapeutic use
		Accidental	Intentional self-harm	Undetermined intent	
Phenantoin	T42.0	X41	X61	Y11	Y46.2
Phenazocine	T40.4	X42	X62	Y12	Y45.0
Phenazone	T39.2	X40	X60	Y10	Y45.8
Phenazopyridine	T39.8	X40	X60	Y10	Y45.9
Phenbutrazate	T50.5	X44	X64	Y14	Y57.0
Phencyclidine	T41.1	X40	X60	Y10	Y48.1
Phendimetrazine	T50.5	X44	X64	Y14	Y57.0
Phenelzine	T43.1	X41	X61	Y11	Y49.1
Phenemal	T42.3	X41	X61	Y11	Y47.0
Pheneticillin	T36.0	X44	X64	Y14	Y40.0
Pheneturide	T42.6	X41	X61	Y11	Y46.6
Phenformin	T38.3	X44	X64	Y14	Y42.3
Phenglutarimide	T44.3	X43	X63	Y13	Y51.3
Phenindamine	T45.0	X44	X64	Y14	Y43.0
Phenindione	T45.5	X44	X64	Y14	Y44.2
Pheniprazine	T43.1	X41	X61	Y11	Y49.1
Pheniramine	T45.0	X44	X64	Y14	Y43.0
Phenisatin	T47.2	X44	X64	Y14	Y53.2
Phenmetrazine	T50.5	X44	X64	Y14	Y57.0
Phenobarbital	T42.3	X41	X61	Y11	Y47.0
– with					
– – mephenytoin	T42.3	X41	X61	Y11	Y47.0
– – phenytoin	T42.3	X41	X61	Y11	Y47.0
– sodium	T42.3	X41	X61	Y11	Y47.0
Phenobarbitone	T42.3	X41	X61	Y11	Y47.0
Phenobutiodil	T50.8	X44	X64	Y14	Y57.5
Phenol	T49.0	X44	X64	Y14	Y56.0
– disinfectant	T54.0	X49	X69	Y19	
– in oil injection	T46.8	X44	X64	Y14	Y52.8
– medicinal	T49.1	X44	X64	Y14	Y56.1
– nonmedicinal NEC	T54.0	X49	X69	Y19	
– pesticide	T60.8	X48	X68	Y18	
– red	T50.8	X44	X64	Y14	Y57.6
Phenolic preparation	T49.1	X44	X64	Y14	Y56.1
Phenolphthalein	T47.2	X44	X64	Y14	Y53.2
Phenolsulfonphthalein	T50.8	X44	X64	Y14	Y57.6
Phenoperidine	T40.4	X42	X62	Y12	Y45.0
Phenopyrazone	T46.9	X44	X64	Y14	Y52.9
Phenoquin	T50.4	X44	X64	Y14	Y54.8
Phenothiazine (psychotropic) NEC	T43.3	X41	X61	Y11	Y49.3
– insecticide	T60.2	X48	X68	Y18	
Phenothrin	T49.0	X44	X64	Y14	Y56.0
Phenoxybenzamine	T46.7	X44	X64	Y14	Y52.7
Phenoxyethanol	T49.0	X44	X64	Y14	Y56.0
Phenoxymethylpenicillin	T36.0	X44	X64	Y14	Y40.0
Phenprobamate	T42.8	X41	X61	Y11	Y46.8
Phenprocoumon	T45.5	X44	X64	Y14	Y44.2
Phensuximide	T42.2	X41	X61	Y11	Y46.0
Phentermine	T50.5	X44	X64	Y14	Y57.0
Phenthicillin	T36.0	X44	X64	Y14	Y40.0
Phentolamine	T46.7	X44	X64	Y14	Y52.7

| Substance | Chapter XIX | Poisoning | | | Adverse effect in therapeutic use |
		Accidental	Intentional self-harm	Undetermined intent	
Phenyl					
– hydrazine	T65.3	X49	X69	Y19	
– salicylate	T49.3	X44	X64	Y14	Y56.3
Phenylalanine mustard	T45.1	X44	X64	Y14	Y43.3
Phenylbutazone	T39.2	X40	X60	Y10	Y45.3
Phenylenediamine	T65.3	X49	X69	Y19	
Phenylephrine	T44.4	X43	X63	Y13	Y51.4
Phenylmercuric					
– acetate	T49.0	X44	X64	Y14	Y56.0
– borate	T49.0	X44	X64	Y14	Y56.0
– nitrate	T49.0	X44	X64	Y14	Y56.0
Phenylmethylbarbitone	T42.3	X41	X61	Y11	Y47.0
Phenylpropanol	T47.5	X44	X64	Y14	Y53.5
Phenylpropanolamine	T44.9	X43	X63	Y13	Y51.9
Phenyltoloxamine	T45.0	X44	X64	Y14	Y43.0
Phenytoin	T42.0	X41	X61	Y11	Y46.2
– with phenobarbital	T42.3	X41	X61	Y11	Y47.0
Pholcodine	T48.3	X44	X64	Y14	Y55.3
Pholedrine	T46.9	X44	X64	Y14	Y52.9
Phorate	T60.0	X48	X68	Y18	
Phosfolan	T60.0	X48	X68	Y18	
Phosgene (gas)	T59.8	X47	X67	Y17	
Phosphamidon	T60.0	X48	X68	Y18	
Phosphate					
– laxative	T47.4	X44	X64	Y14	Y53.4
– tricresyl	T65.8	X49	X69	Y19	
Phosphine	T57.1	X49	X69	Y19	
Phosphoric acid	T54.2	X49	X69	Y19	
Phosphorus (compound) NEC	T57.1	X49	X69	Y19	
– pesticide	T60.0	X48	X68	Y18	
Phthalates	T65.8	X49	X69	Y19	
Phthalic anhydride	T65.8	X49	X69	Y19	
Phthalylsulfathiazole	T37.0	X44	X64	Y14	Y41.0
Phylloquinone	T45.7	X44	X64	Y14	Y44.3
Physostigmine	T49.5	X44	X64	Y14	Y56.5
Phytomenadione	T45.7	X44	X64	Y14	Y44.3
Picoperine	T48.3	X44	X64	Y14	Y55.3
Picosulfate (sodium)	T47.2	X44	X64	Y14	Y53.2
Picric (acid)	T54.2	X49	X69	Y19	
Picrotoxin	T50.7	X44	X64	Y14	Y50.0
Piketoprofen	T49.0	X44	X64	Y14	Y56.0
Pilocarpine	T44.1	X43	X63	Y13	Y51.1
Pilsicainide (hydrochloride)	T46.2	X44	X64	Y14	Y52.2
Pimeclone	T50.7	X44	X64	Y14	Y50.0
Pimelic ketone	T52.8	X46	X66	Y16	
Pimethixene	T45.0	X44	X64	Y14	Y43.0
Pimozide	T43.5	X41	X61	Y11	Y49.5
Pinacidil	T46.5	X44	X64	Y14	Y52.5
Pinaverium bromide	T44.3	X43	X63	Y13	Y51.3
Pinazepam	T42.4	X41	X61	Y11	Y47.1
Pindolol	T44.7	X43	X63	Y13	Y51.7

Substance	Chapter XIX	Poisoning Accidental	Intentional self-harm	Undetermined intent	Adverse effect in therapeutic use
Pindone	T60.4	X48	X68	Y18	
Pine oil (disinfectant)	T65.8	X49	X69	Y19	
Pipamazine	T45.0	X44	X64	Y14	Y43.0
Pipamperone	T43.4	X41	X61	Y11	Y49.4
Pipazetate	T48.3	X44	X64	Y14	Y55.3
Pipemidic acid	T37.8	X44	X64	Y14	Y41.8
Pipenzolate bromide	T44.3	X43	X63	Y13	Y51.3
Piperacetazine	T43.3	X41	X61	Y11	Y49.3
Piperacillin	T36.0	X44	X64	Y14	Y40.0
Piperazine	T37.4	X44	X64	Y14	Y41.4
Piperidolate	T44.3	X43	X63	Y13	Y51.3
Piperocaine	T41.3	X44	X64	Y14	Y48.3
Piperonyl butoxide	T60.8	X48	X68	Y18	
Pipethanate	T44.3	X43	X63	Y13	Y51.3
Pipobroman	T45.1	X44	X64	Y14	Y43.3
Pipofezine	T43.0	X41	X61	Y11	Y49.0
Pipotiazine	T43.3	X41	X61	Y11	Y49.3
Pipoxizine	T45.0	X44	X64	Y14	Y43.0
Pipradrol	T43.6	X41	X61	Y11	Y49.7
Piprinhydrinate	T45.0	X44	X64	Y14	Y43.0
Piproxen	T39.3	X40	X60	Y10	Y45.2
Pirarubicin	T45.1	X44	X64	Y14	Y43.3
Pirazinamide	T37.1	X44	X64	Y14	Y41.1
Pirbuterol	T48.6	X44	X64	Y14	Y55.6
Pirenzepine	T47.1	X44	X64	Y14	Y53.1
Piretanide	T50.1	X44	X64	Y14	Y54.4
Piribedil	T42.8	X41	X61	Y11	Y46.7
Piridoxilate	T46.3	X44	X64	Y14	Y52.3
Piritramide	T40.4	X42	X62	Y12	Y45.0
Pirlindole	T43.0	X41	X61	Y11	Y49.0
Piromidic acid	T37.8	X44	X64	Y14	Y41.8
Piroxicam	T39.3	X40	X60	Y10	Y45.3
− Beta-cyclodextrin complex	T39.8	X40	X60	Y10	Y45.8
Pirozadil	T46.6	X44	X64	Y14	Y52.6
Pirprofen	T39.3	X40	X60	Y10	Y45.2
Pitch	T65.8	X49	X69	Y19	
Pivampicillin	T36.0	X44	X64	Y14	Y40.0
Pivmecillinam	T36.0	X44	X64	Y14	Y40.0
Placental hormone	T38.8	X44	X64	Y14	Y42.8
Plafibride	T45.5	X44	X64	Y14	Y44.4
Plague vaccine	T50.9	X44	X64	Y14	Y58.3
Plant					
− food or fertilizer NEC	T65.8	X49	X69	Y19	
− − containing herbicide	T60.3	X48	X68	Y18	
− noxious, used as food	T62.2	X49	X69	Y19	
Plasma	T45.8	X44	X64	Y14	Y44.6
− expander NEC	T45.8	X44	X64	Y14	Y44.7
− protein fraction (human)	T45.8	X44	X64	Y14	Y44.6
Plasminogen (tissue) activator	T45.6	X44	X64	Y14	Y44.5
Plaster dressing	T49.3	X44	X64	Y14	Y56.3
Plastic dressing	T49.3	X44	X64	Y14	Y56.3

Substance	Chapter XIX	Poisoning			Adverse effect in therapeutic use
		Accidental	Intentional self-harm	Undetermined intent	
Plicamycin	T45.1	X44	X64	Y14	Y43.3
Podophyllotoxin	T49.8	X44	X64	Y14	Y56.8
Podophyllum (resin)	T49.4	X44	X64	Y14	Y56.4
Poison NEC	T65.9	X49	X69	Y19	
Pokeweed (any part)	T62.2	X49	X69	Y19	
Poldine metilsulfate	T44.3	X43	X63	Y13	Y51.3
Polidexide (sulfate)	T46.6	X44	X64	Y14	Y52.6
Polidocanol	T46.8	X44	X64	Y14	Y52.8
Poliomyelitis vaccine	T50.9	X44	X64	Y14	Y59.0
Polish (car) (floor) (furniture) (metal)(porcelain) (silver)	T65.8	X49	X69	Y19	
Poloxamer	T47.4	X44	X64	Y14	Y53.4
Polycarbophil	T47.4	X44	X64	Y14	Y53.4
Polychlorinated biphenyl	T53.7	X49	X69	Y19	
Polyester fumes	T59.8	X47	X67	Y17	
Polyestradiol phosphate	T38.5	X44	X64	Y14	Y42.5
Polyethanolamine alkyl sulfate	T49.2	X44	X64	Y14	Y56.2
Polyethylene adhesive	T49.3	X44	X64	Y14	Y56.3
Polygeline	T45.8	X44	X64	Y14	Y44.7
Polymyxin	T36.8	X44	X64	Y14	Y40.8
− B	T36.8	X44	X64	Y14	Y40.8
− E sulfate (eye preparation)	T49.5	X44	X64	Y14	Y56.5
Polynoxylin	T49.0	X44	X64	Y14	Y56.0
Polyoestradiol phosphate	T38.5	X44	X64	Y14	Y42.5
Polysilane	T47.8	X44	X64	Y14	Y53.8
Polytetrafluoroethylene (inhaled)	T59.8	X47	X67	Y17	
Polythiazide	T50.2	X44	X64	Y14	Y54.3
Polyvidone	T45.8	X44	X64	Y14	Y44.7
Polyvinylpyrrolidone	T45.8	X44	X64	Y14	Y44.7
Porfiromycin	T45.1	X44	X64	Y14	Y43.3
Posterior pituitary hormone NEC	T38.8	X44	X64	Y14	Y42.8
Potash (caustic)	T54.3	X49	X69	Y19	
Potassium (salts) NEC	T50.3	X44	X64	Y14	Y54.9
− aminobenzoate	T45.8	X44	X64	Y14	Y43.8
− aminosalicylate	T37.1	X44	X64	Y14	Y41.1
− antimony tartrate	T37.8	X44	X64	Y14	Y41.8
− bichromate	T56.2	X49	X69	Y19	
− bisulfate	T47.3	X44	X64	Y14	Y53.3
− bromide	T42.6	X41	X61	Y11	Y47.4
− canrenoate	T50.0	X44	X64	Y14	Y54.1
− carbonate	T54.3	X49	X69	Y19	
− chlorate NEC	T65.8	X49	X69	Y19	
− chloride	T50.3	X44	X64	Y14	Y54.9
− citrate	T50.9	X44	X64	Y14	Y43.5
− cyanide	T65.0	X49	X69	Y19	
− ferric hexacyanoferrate (medicinal)	T50.6	X44	X64	Y14	Y57.2
− − nonmedicinal	T65.8	X49	X69	Y19	
− fluoride	T57.8	X49	X69	Y19	
− glucaldrate	T47.1	X44	X64	Y14	Y53.1
− hydroxide	T54.3	X49	X69	Y19	

| Substance | Chapter XIX | Poisoning | | | Adverse effect in therapeutic use |
		Accidental	Intentional self-harm	Undetermined intent	
Potassium—*continued*					
– iodate	T49.0	X44	X64	Y14	Y56.0
– iodide	T48.4	X44	X64	Y14	Y55.4
– nitrate	T57.8	X49	X69	Y19	
– oxalate	T65.8	X49	X69	Y19	
– perchlorate (nonmedicinal) NEC	T65.8	X49	X69	Y19	
– – medicinal	T38.2	X44	X64	Y14	Y42.2
– permanganate (nonmedicinal)	T65.8	X49	X69	Y19	
– medicinal	T49.0	X44	X64	Y14	Y56.0
– sulfate	T47.2	X44	X64	Y14	Y53.2
Potassium-removing resin	T50.3	X44	X64	Y14	Y54.6
Potassium-retaining drug	T50.3	X44	X64	Y14	Y54.6
Povidone	T45.8	X44	X64	Y14	Y44.7
– iodine	T49.0	X44	X64	Y14	Y56.0
Practolol	T44.7	X43	X63	Y13	Y51.7
Prajmalium bitartrate	T46.2	X44	X64	Y14	Y52.2
Pralidoxime (iodide)	T50.6	X44	X64	Y14	Y57.2
– chloride	T50.6	X44	X64	Y14	Y57.2
Pramiverine	T44.3	X43	X63	Y13	Y51.3
Pramocaine	T49.1	X44	X64	Y14	Y56.1
Pramoxine	T49.1	X44	X64	Y14	Y56.1
Pranoprofen	T39.3	X40	X60	Y10	Y45.2
Prasterone	T38.7	X44	X64	Y14	Y42.7
Pravastatin	T46.6	X44	X64	Y14	Y52.6
Prazepam	T42.4	X41	X61	Y11	Y47.1
Praziquantel	T37.4	X44	X64	Y14	Y41.4
Prazitone	T43.2	X41	X61	Y11	Y49.2
Prazosin	T44.6	X43	X63	Y13	Y51.6
Prednicarbate	T49.0	X44	X64	Y14	Y56.0
Prednimustine	T45.1	X44	X64	Y14	Y43.3
Prednisolone (oral)	T38.0	X44	X64	Y14	Y42.0
– ENT agent	T49.6	X44	X64	Y14	Y56.6
– ophthalmic preparation	T49.5	X44	X64	Y14	Y56.5
– steaglate	T49.0	X44	X64	Y14	Y56.0
– topical NEC	T49.0	X44	X64	Y14	Y56.0
Prednisone	T38.0	X44	X64	Y14	Y42.0
Prednylidene	T38.0	X44	X64	Y14	Y42.0
Pregnandiol	T38.5	X44	X64	Y14	Y42.5
Premedication anesthetic	T41.2	X44	X64	Y14	Y48.2
Prenalterol	T44.5	X43	X63	Y13	Y51.5
Prenoxdiazine	T48.3	X44	X64	Y14	Y55.3
Prenylamine	T46.3	X44	X64	Y14	Y52.3
Preparation, local	T49.4	X44	X64	Y14	Y56.4
Preservative (nonmedicinal)	T65.8	X49	X69	Y19	
– medicinal	T50.9	X44	X64	Y14	Y57.4
– wood	T60.9	X48	X68	Y18	
Prethcamide	T50.7	X44	X64	Y14	Y50.0
Pridinol	T44.3	X43	X63	Y13	Y51.3
Prifinium bromide	T44.3	X43	X63	Y13	Y51.3
Prilocaine	T41.3	X44	X64	Y14	Y48.3
– regional	T41.3	X44	X64	Y14	Y48.3

Substance	Chapter XIX	Poisoning			Adverse effect in therapeutic use
		Accidental	Intentional self-harm	Undetermined intent	
Primaquine	T37.2	X44	X64	Y14	Y41.2
Primidone	T42.6	X41	X61	Y11	Y46.6
Pristinamycin	T36.3	X44	X64	Y14	Y40.3
Probenecid	T50.4	X44	X64	Y14	Y54.8
Probucol	T46.6	X44	X64	Y14	Y52.6
Procainamide	T46.2	X44	X64	Y14	Y52.2
Procaine	T41.3	X44	X64	Y14	Y48.3
– benzylpenicillin	T36.0	X44	X64	Y14	Y40.0
– regional	T41.3	X44	X64	Y14	Y48.3
– spinal	T41.3	X44	X64	Y14	Y48.3
Procarbazine	T45.1	X44	X64	Y14	Y43.3
Procaterol	T44.5	X43	X63	Y13	Y51.5
Prochlorperazine	T43.3	X41	X61	Y11	Y49.3
Procyclidine	T44.3	X43	X63	Y13	Y51.3
Producer of gas	T58	X47	X67	Y17	
Profadol	T40.4	X42	X62	Y12	Y45.0
Profenamine	T44.3	X43	X63	Y13	Y51.3
Proflavine	T49.0	X44	X64	Y14	Y56.0
Progabide	T42.6	X41	X61	Y11	Y46.6
Progesterone	T38.5	X44	X64	Y14	Y42.5
Progestogen NEC	T38.5	X44	X64	Y14	Y42.5
Proglumetacin	T39.3	X40	X60	Y10	Y45.3
Proglumide	T47.1	X44	X64	Y14	Y53.1
Proguanil	T37.2	X44	X64	Y14	Y41.2
Prolactin	T38.8	X44	X64	Y14	Y42.8
Prolactinol	T38.8	X44	X64	Y14	Y42.8
Prolintane	T43.6	X41	X61	Y11	Y49.7
Promazine	T43.3	X41	X61	Y11	Y49.3
Promegestone	T38.5	X44	X64	Y14	Y42.5
Promethazine (teoclate)	T43.3	X41	X61	Y11	Y49.3
Pronase	T45.3	X44	X64	Y14	Y43.6
Pronetalol	T44.7	X43	X63	Y13	Y51.7
Propachlor	T60.3	X48	X68	Y18	
Propafenone	T46.2	X44	X64	Y14	Y52.2
Propallylonal	T42.3	X41	X61	Y11	Y47.0
Propamidine	T49.0	X44	X64	Y14	Y56.0
Propane (distributed in mobile container)	T59.8	X47	X67	Y17	
– distributed through pipes	T59.8	X47	X67	Y17	
– incomplete combustion	T58	X47	X67	Y17	
Propanidid	T41.2	X44	X64	Y14	Y48.2
Propanil	T60.3	X48	X68	Y18	
1-Propanol	T51.3	X45	X65	Y15	
2-Propanol	T51.2	X45	X65	Y15	
Propantheline	T44.3	X43	X63	Y13	Y51.3
– bromide	T44.3	X43	X63	Y13	Y51.3
Proparacaine	T41.3	X44	X64	Y14	Y48.3
Propatylnitrate	T46.3	X44	X64	Y14	Y52.3
Propicillin	T36.0	X44	X64	Y14	Y40.0
Propiolactone	T49.0	X44	X64	Y14	Y56.0
Propiomazine	T45.0	X44	X64	Y14	Y43.0

| Substance | Chapter XIX | Poisoning | | | Adverse effect in therapeutic use |
		Accidental	Intentional self-harm	Undetermined intent	
Propionate (calcium) (sodium)	T49.0	X44	X64	Y14	Y56.0
Propofol	T41.2	X44	X64	Y14	Y48.2
Propoxur	T60.0	X48	X68	Y18	
Propoxycaine	T41.3	X44	X64	Y14	Y48.3
Propoxyphene	T40.4	X42	X62	Y12	Y45.0
Propranolol	T44.7	X43	X63	Y13	Y51.7
Propylaminophenothiazine	T43.3	X41	X61	Y11	Y49.3
Propylene	T59.8	X47	X67	Y17	
Propylhexedrine	T48.5	X44	X64	Y14	Y55.5
Propyliodone	T50.8	X44	X64	Y14	Y57.5
Propylthiouracil	T38.2	X44	X64	Y14	Y42.2
Propyphenazone	T39.2	X40	X60	Y10	Y45.8
Proquazone	T39.3	X40	X60	Y10	Y45.3
Proscillaridin	T46.0	X44	X64	Y14	Y52.0
Prostacyclin	T45.5	X44	X64	Y14	Y44.4
Prostaglandin (I_2)	T45.5	X44	X64	Y14	Y44.4
− E_1	T46.7	X44	X64	Y14	Y52.7
− E_2	T48.0	X44	X64	Y14	Y55.0
− F_2Alpha	T48.0	X44	X64	Y14	Y55.0
Prosultiamine	T45.2	X44	X64	Y14	Y57.7
Protamine sulfate	T45.7	X44	X64	Y14	Y44.3
Protease	T47.5	X44	X64	Y14	Y53.5
Protectant, skin NEC	T49.3	X44	X64	Y14	Y56.3
Protein hydrolysate	T50.9	X44	X64	Y14	Y57.8
Prothionamide	T37.1	X44	X64	Y14	Y41.1
Prothipendyl	T43.5	X41	X61	Y11	Y49.5
Prothoate	T60.0	X48	X68	Y18	
Prothrombin					
− activator	T45.7	X44	X64	Y14	Y44.3
− synthesis inhibitor	T45.5	X44	X64	Y14	Y44.2
Protionamide	T37.1	X44	X64	Y14	Y41.1
Protirelin	T38.8	X44	X64	Y14	Y42.8
Protokylol	T48.6	X44	X64	Y14	Y55.6
Protoveratrine(s) (A) (B)	T46.5	X44	X64	Y14	Y52.5
Protriptyline	T43.0	X41	X61	Y11	Y49.0
Proxibarbal	T42.3	X41	X61	Y11	Y47.0
Proxymetacaine	T41.3	X44	X64	Y14	Y48.3
Proxyphylline	T48.6	X44	X64	Y14	Y55.6
Prussian blue					
− commercial	T65.8	X49	X69	Y19	
− therapeutic	T50.6	X44	X64	Y14	Y57.2
Prussic acid	T57.3	X48	X68	Y18	
− vapor	T57.3	X48	X68	Y18	
Pseudoephedrine	T44.9	X43	X63	Y13	Y51.9
Psilocin	T40.9	X42	X62	Y12	Y49.6
Psilocybin	T40.9	X42	X62	Y12	Y49.6
Psilocybine	T40.9	X42	X62	Y12	Y49.6
Psoralene (nonmedicinal)	T65.8	X49	X69	Y19	
Psoralens (medicinal)	T50.9	X44	X64	Y14	Y57.8
Psychodysleptic drug NEC	T40.9	X42	X62	Y12	Y49.6
Psychostimulant NEC	T43.6	X41	X61	Y11	Y49.7

| | Poisoning | | | Adverse effect in therapeutic use |
Substance	Chapter XIX	Accidental	Intentional self-harm	Undetermined intent	
Psychotherapeutic drug NEC	T43.9	X41	X61	Y11	Y49.9
Psychotropic drug NEC	T43.9	X41	X61	Y11	Y49.9
– specified NEC	T43.8	X41	X61	Y11	Y49.8
Psyllium hydrophilic mucilloid	T47.4	X44	X64	Y14	Y53.4
Pteroylglutamic acid	T45.8	X44	X64	Y14	Y44.1
Pulp					
– devitalizing paste	T49.7	X44	X64	Y14	Y56.7
– dressing	T49.7	X44	X64	Y14	Y56.7
Pumpkin seed extract	T37.4	X44	X64	Y14	Y41.4
Purgative NEC (*see also* Cathartic)	T47.4	X44	X64	Y14	Y53.4
Purine analogue (antineoplastic)	T45.1	X44	X64	Y14	Y43.1
PVP	T45.8	X44	X64	Y14	Y44.7
Pyrantel	T37.4	X44	X64	Y14	Y41.4
Pyrazinamide	T37.1	X44	X64	Y14	Y41.1
Pyrazolone analgesic NEC	T39.2	X40	X60	Y10	Y45.8
Pyrethrin, pyrethrum (nonmedicinal)	T60.2	X48	X68	Y18	
Pyrethrum extract	T49.0	X44	X64	Y14	Y56.0
Pyridine	T52.8	X46	X66	Y16	
– aldoxime methiodide	T50.6	X44	X64	Y14	Y57.2
– vapor	T59.8	X47	X67	Y17	
Pyridostigmine bromide	T44.0	X43	X63	Y13	Y51.0
Pyridoxal phosphate	T45.2	X44	X64	Y14	Y57.7
Pyridoxine	T45.2	X44	X64	Y14	Y57.7
Pyrilamine	T45.0	X44	X64	Y14	Y43.0
Pyrimethamine	T37.2	X44	X64	Y14	Y41.2
– with sulfadoxine	T37.2	X44	X64	Y14	Y41.2
Pyrimidine antagonist	T45.1	X44	X64	Y14	Y43.1
Pyriminil	T60.4	X48	X68	Y18	
Pyrithione zinc	T49.4	X44	X64	Y14	Y56.4
Pyrithyldione	T42.6	X41	X61	Y11	Y47.8
Pyrogallic acid	T49.0	X44	X64	Y14	Y56.0
Pyrogallol	T49.0	X44	X64	Y14	Y56.0
Pyroxylin	T49.3	X44	X64	Y14	Y56.3
Pyrrobutamine	T45.0	X44	X64	Y14	Y43.0
Pyrrolizidine alkaloids	T62.8	X49	X69	Y19	
Pyrvinium chloride	T37.4	X44	X64	Y14	Y41.4

Q

Substance	Chapter XIX	Poisoning			Adverse effect in therapeutic use
		Accidental	Intentional self-harm	Undetermined intent	
Quarternary ammonium					
− anti-infective	T49.0	X44	X64	Y14	Y56.0
− ganglion blocking	T44.2	X43	X63	Y13	Y51.2
− parasympatholytic	T44.3	X43	X63	Y13	Y51.3
Quazepam	T42.4	X41	X61	Y11	Y47.1
Quicklime	T54.3	X49	X69	Y19	
Quillaja extract	T48.4	X44	X64	Y14	Y55.4
Quinacrine	T37.2	X44	X64	Y14	Y41.2
Quinalbarbital	T42.3	X41	X61	Y11	Y47.0
Quinalbarbitone sodium	T42.3	X41	X61	Y11	Y47.0
Quinalphos	T60.0	X48	X68	Y18	
Quinapril	T46.4	X44	X64	Y14	Y52.4
Quinestradol	T38.5	X44	X64	Y14	Y42.5
Quinestrol	T38.5	X44	X64	Y14	Y42.5
Quinethazone	T50.2	X44	X64	Y14	Y54.5
Quingestanol	T38.4	X44	X64	Y14	Y42.4
Quinidine	T46.2	X44	X64	Y14	Y52.2
Quinine	T37.2	X44	X64	Y14	Y41.2
Quinisocaine	T49.1	X44	X64	Y14	Y56.1
Quinocide	T37.2	X44	X64	Y14	Y41.2
Quinoline (derivatives) NEC	T37.8	X44	X64	Y14	Y41.8
Quinupramine	T43.0	X41	X61	Y11	Y49.0

R

Substance	Chapter XIX	Accidental	Poisoning Intentional self-harm	Undetermined intent	Adverse effect in therapeutic use
Rabies					
– immune globulin (human)	T50.9	X44	X64	Y14	Y59.3
– vaccine	T50.9	X44	X64	Y14	Y59.0
Racepinefrin	T44.5	X43	X63	Y13	Y51.5
Raclopride	T43.5	X41	X61	Y11	Y49.5
Radioactive drug NEC	T50.8	X44	X64	Y14	Y57.6
Ramifenazone	T39.2	X40	X60	Y10	Y45.8
Ramipril	T46.4	X44	X64	Y14	Y52.4
Ranitidine	T47.0	X44	X64	Y14	Y53.0
Rat poison NEC	T60.4	X48	X68	Y18	
Raubasine	T46.7	X44	X64	Y14	Y52.7
Rauwolfia (alkaloids)	T46.5	X44	X64	Y14	Y52.5
Razoxane	T45.1	X44	X64	Y14	Y43.3
Recombinant (R) – see specific protein					
Red blood cells, packed	T45.8	X44	X64	Y14	Y44.6
Red squill (scilliroside)	T60.4	X48	X68	Y18	
Reducing agent, industrial NEC	T65.8	X49	X69	Y19	
Refrigerant gas (chlorofluorocarbon)	T53.5	X46	X66	Y16	
– not chlorofluorocarbon	T59.8	X47	X67	Y17	
Rehydration salts (oral)	T50.3	X44	X64	Y14	Y54.6
Relaxant, muscle					
– anesthetic	T48.1	X44	X64	Y14	Y55.1
– skeletal NEC	T48.1	X44	X64	Y14	Y55.1
– smooth NEC	T44.3	X43	X63	Y13	Y51.3
Remoxipride	T43.5	X41	X61	Y11	Y49.5
Replacement solution	T50.3	X44	X64	Y14	Y54.6
Reproterol	T48.6	X44	X64	Y14	Y55.6
Rescinnamine	T46.5	X44	X64	Y14	Y52.5
Reserpin(e)	T46.5	X44	X64	Y14	Y52.5
Resorcin, resorcinol (nonmedicinal)	T65.8	X49	X69	Y19	
– medicinal	T49.4	X44	X64	Y14	Y56.4
Respiratory drug NEC	T48.7	X44	X64	Y14	Y55.7
– antiasthmatic NEC	T48.6	X44	X64	Y14	Y55.6
– anti-common-cold NEC	T48.5	X44	X64	Y14	Y55.5
– expectorant NEC	T48.4	X44	X64	Y14	Y55.4
– stimulant	T48.7	X44	X64	Y14	Y55.7
Retinoic acid	T49.0	X44	X64	Y14	Y56.0
Retinol	T45.2	X44	X64	Y14	Y57.7
Rhubarb					
– dry extract	T47.2	X44	X64	Y14	Y53.2
– tincture, compound	T47.2	X44	X64	Y14	Y53.2
Ribavirin	T37.5	X44	X64	Y14	Y41.5
Riboflavin	T45.2	X44	X64	Y14	Y57.7

| Substance | Chapter XIX | Poisoning | | | Adverse effect in therapeutic use |
		Accidental	Intentional self-harm	Undetermined intent	
Ribostamycin	T36.5	X44	X64	Y14	Y40.5
Ricin	T62.2	X49	X69	Y19	
Rickettsial vaccine NEC	T50.9	X44	X64	Y14	Y59.1
Rifabutin	T36.6	X44	X64	Y14	Y40.6
Rifamide	T36.6	X44	X64	Y14	Y40.6
Rifampicin	T36.6	X44	X64	Y14	Y40.6
– with isoniazid	T37.1	X44	X64	Y14	Y41.1
Rifampin	T36.6	X44	X64	Y14	Y40.6
Rifamycin	T36.6	X44	X64	Y14	Y40.6
Rifaximin	T36.6	X44	X64	Y14	Y40.6
Rimantadine	T37.5	X44	X64	Y14	Y41.5
Rimazolium metilsulfate	T39.8	X40	X60	Y10	Y45.8
Rimiterol	T48.6	X44	X64	Y14	Y55.6
Ringer (lactate) solution	T50.3	X44	X64	Y14	Y54.6
Ritodrine	T44.5	X43	X63	Y13	Y51.5
Roach killer – *see* Insecticide					
Rociverine	T44.3	X43	X63	Y13	Y51.3
Rodenticide NEC	T60.4	X48	X68	Y18	
Rokitamycin	T36.3	X44	X64	Y14	Y40.3
Rolitetracycline	T36.4	X44	X64	Y14	Y40.4
Ronifibrate	T46.6	X44	X64	Y14	Y52.6
Rosaprostol	T47.1	X44	X64	Y14	Y53.1
Rose bengal sodium (^{131}I)	T50.8	X44	X64	Y14	Y57.6
Rosoxacin	T37.8	X44	X64	Y14	Y41.8
Rotenone	T60.2	X48	X68	Y18	
Rotoxamine	T45.0	X44	X64	Y14	Y43.0
Roxatidine	T47.0	X44	X64	Y14	Y53.0
Roxithromycin	T36.3	X44	X64	Y14	Y40.3
Rt-PA	T45.6	X44	X64	Y14	Y44.5
Rubbing alcohol	T51.2	X45	X65	Y15	
Rubefacient	T49.4	X44	X64	Y14	Y56.4
Rubella vaccine	T50.9	X44	X64	Y14	Y59.0
Rubidium chloride Rb82	T50.8	X44	X64	Y14	Y57.6
Rubidomycin	T45.1	X44	X64	Y14	Y43.3
Rue	T62.2	X49	X69	Y19	
Rufocromomycin	T45.1	X44	X64	Y14	Y43.3
Russel's viper venin	T45.7	X44	X64	Y14	Y44.3
Rutinum	T46.9	X44	X64	Y14	Y52.9
Rutoside	T46.9	X44	X64	Y14	Y52.9

S

| Substance | Chapter XIX | Poisoning | | | Adverse effect in therapeutic use |
		Accidental	Intentional self-harm	Undetermined intent	
Saccharated iron oxide	T45.8	X44	X64	Y14	Y44.0
Saccharin	T50.9	X44	X64	Y14	Y57.4
Saccharomyces boulardii	T47.6	X44	X64	Y14	Y53.6
Safflower oil	T46.6	X44	X64	Y14	Y52.6
Safrazine	T43.1	X41	X61	Y11	Y49.1
Salazosulfapyridine	T37.0	X44	X64	Y14	Y41.0
Salbutamol	T48.6	X44	X64	Y14	Y55.6
Salicylamide	T39.0	X40	X60	Y10	Y45.1
Salicylate NEC	T39.0	X40	X60	Y10	Y45.1
Salicylazosulfapyridine	T37.0	X44	X64	Y14	Y41.0
Salicylic acid	T49.4	X44	X64	Y14	Y56.4
− with benzoic acid	T49.4	X44	X64	Y14	Y56.4
− derivative	T39.0	X40	X60	Y10	Y45.1
Salinazid	T37.1	X44	X64	Y14	Y41.1
Salmeterol	T48.6	X44	X64	Y14	Y55.6
Salol	T49.3	X44	X64	Y14	Y56.3
Salsalate	T39.0	X40	X60	Y10	Y45.1
Salt substitute	T50.9	X44	X64	Y14	Y57.8
Salt-replacing drug	T50.9	X44	X64	Y14	Y57.8
Salt-retaining mineralocorticoid	T50.0	X44	X64	Y14	Y54.0
Saluretic NEC	T50.2	X44	X64	Y14	Y54.5
Santonin	T37.4	X44	X64	Y14	Y41.4
Saralasin	T46.5	X44	X64	Y14	Y52.5
Sarcolysin	T45.1	X44	X64	Y14	Y43.3
Saturnine − see Lead					
Scheele's green	T57.0	X49	X69	Y19	
− insecticide	T57.0	X48	X68	Y18	
Schizontozide (blood) (tissue)	T37.2	X44	X64	Y14	Y41.2
Schradan	T60.0	X48	X68	Y18	
Schweinfurth green	T57.0	X49	X69	Y19	
− insecticide	T57.0	X48	X68	Y18	
Scilla, rat poison	T60.4	X48	X68	Y18	
Scillaren	T60.4	X48	X68	Y18	
Sclerosing agent	T46.8	X44	X64	Y14	Y52.8
Scombrotoxin	T61.1	X49	X69	Y19	
Scopolamine	T44.3	X43	X63	Y13	Y51.3
Scopolia extract	T44.3	X43	X63	Y13	Y51.3
Secbutabarbital	T42.3	X41	X61	Y11	Y47.0
Secnidazole	T37.3	X44	X64	Y14	Y41.3
Secobarbital	T42.3	X41	X61	Y11	Y47.0
Secretin	T50.8	X44	X64	Y14	Y57.6
Sedative NEC	T42.7	X41	X61	Y11	Y47.9
− mixed NEC	T42.6	X41	X61	Y11	Y47.5
Seed disinfectant or dressing	T60.8	X48	X68	Y18	

Substance	Chapter XIX	Poisoning			Adverse effect in therapeutic use
		Accidental	Intentional self-harm	Undetermined intent	
Seeds, poisonous	T62.2	X49	X69	Y19	
Selegiline	T42.8	X41	X61	Y11	Y46.7
Selenium NEC	T56.8	X49	X69	Y19	
– fumes	T59.8	X47	X67	Y17	
– sulfide	T49.4	X44	X64	Y14	Y56.4
Selenomethionine (^{75}Se)	T50.8	X44	X64	Y14	Y57.6
Semustine	T45.1	X44	X64	Y14	Y43.3
Senega syrup	T48.4	X44	X64	Y14	Y55.4
Senna	T47.2	X44	X64	Y14	Y53.2
Sennoside A+B	T47.2	X44	X64	Y14	Y53.2
Seractide	T38.8	X44	X64	Y14	Y42.8
Sermorelin	T38.8	X44	X64	Y14	Y42.8
Serrapeptase	T45.3	X44	X64	Y14	Y43.6
Serum					
– antibotulinus	T50.9	X44	X64	Y14	Y59.3
– anticytotoxic	T50.9	X44	X64	Y14	Y59.3
– antidiphtheria	T50.9	X44	X64	Y14	Y59.3
– antimeningococcus	T50.9	X44	X64	Y14	Y59.3
– anti-Rh	T50.9	X44	X64	Y14	Y59.3
– anti-snake-bite	T50.9	X44	X64	Y14	Y59.3
– antitetanic	T50.9	X44	X64	Y14	Y59.3
– antitoxic	T50.9	X44	X64	Y14	Y59.3
– complement (inhibitor)	T45.8	X44	X64	Y14	Y44.6
– convalescent	T50.9	X44	X64	Y14	Y59.3
– gonadotrophin	T38.8	X44	X64	Y14	Y42.8
– hemolytic complement	T45.8	X44	X64	Y14	Y44.6
– immune (human)	T50.9	X44	X64	Y14	Y59.3
– protective NEC	T50.9	X44	X64	Y14	Y59.3
Setastine	T45.0	X44	X64	Y14	Y43.0
Setoperone	T43.5	X41	X61	Y11	Y49.5
Sewer gas	T59.8	X47	X67	Y17	
Shampoo	T55	X49	X69	Y19	
Shellfish, noxious, nonbacterial	T61.2	X49	X69	Y19	
Sildefanil	T46.7	X44	X64	Y14	Y52.7
Silibinin	T50.9	X44	X64	Y14	Y57.1
Silicone NEC	T65.8	X49	X69	Y19	
– medicinal	T49.3	X44	X64	Y14	Y56.3
Silver	T49.0	X44	X64	Y14	Y56.0
– colloidal	T49.0	X44	X64	Y14	Y56.0
– nitrate	T49.0	X44	X64	Y14	Y56.0
– nonmedicinal (dust)	T56.8	X49	X69	Y19	
– protein	T49.5	X44	X64	Y14	Y56.5
– sulfadiazine	T49.4	X44	X64	Y14	Y56.4
Silymarin	T50.9	X44	X64	Y14	Y57.1
Simaldrate	T47.1	X44	X64	Y14	Y53.1
Simazine	T60.3	X48	X68	Y18	
Simethicone	T47.1	X44	X64	Y14	Y53.1
Simfibrate	T46.6	X44	X64	Y14	Y52.6
Simvastatin	T46.6	X44	X64	Y14	Y52.6
Sincalide	T50.8	X44	X64	Y14	Y57.6
Sisomicin	T36.5	X44	X64	Y14	Y40.5

Substance	Chapter XIX	Accidental	Poisoning Intentional self-harm	Undetermined intent	Adverse effect in therapeutic use
Sleeping draught, pill	T42.7	X41	X61	Y11	Y47.9
Smallpox vaccine	T50.9	X44	X64	Y14	Y59.0
Smelter fumes NEC	T56.9	X49	X69	Y19	
Smog	T59.1	X47	X67	Y17	
Smoke NEC	T59.8	X47	X67	Y17	
Snail killer NEC	T60.8	X48	X68	Y18	
Snake venom or bite	T63.0				
– hemocoagulase	T45.7	X44	X64	Y14	Y44.3
Snuff	T65.2	X49	X69	Y19	
Soap (powder) (product)	T55	X49	X69	Y19	
– enema	T47.4	X44	X64	Y14	Y53.4
– superfatted	T49.2	X44	X64	Y14	Y56.2
Sobrerol	T48.4	X44	X64	Y14	Y55.4
Soda (caustic)	T54.3	X49	X69	Y19	
Sodium					
– acetosulfone	T37.1	X44	X64	Y14	Y41.1
– acetrizoate	T50.8	X44	X64	Y14	Y57.5
– acid phosphate	T50.3	X44	X64	Y14	Y54.6
– alginate	T47.8	X44	X64	Y14	Y53.8
– amidotrizoate	T50.8	X44	X64	Y14	Y57.5
– aminopterin	T45.1	X44	X64	Y14	Y43.1
– amylosulfate	T47.8	X44	X64	Y14	Y53.8
– antimony gluconate	T37.3	X44	X64	Y14	Y41.3
– arsenate	T57.0	X48	X68	Y18	
– aurothiomalate	T39.4	X40	X60	Y10	Y45.4
– aurothiosulfate	T39.4	X40	X60	Y10	Y45.4
– barbiturate	T42.3	X41	X61	Y11	Y47.0
– basic phosphate	T47.4	X44	X64	Y14	Y53.4
– bicarbonate	T47.1	X44	X64	Y14	Y53.1
– bichromate	T57.8	X49	X69	Y19	
– biphosphate	T50.3	X44	X64	Y14	Y54.6
– bisulfate	T65.8	X49	X69	Y19	
– borate					
– – cleanser	T57.8	X49	X69	Y19	
– – – eye	T49.5	X44	X64	Y14	Y56.5
– – therapeutic	T49.8	X44	X64	Y14	Y56.8
– bromide	T42.6	X41	X61	Y11	Y47.4
– calcium edetate	T45.8	X44	X64	Y14	Y43.8
– carbonate NEC	T54.3	X49	X69	Y19	
– chlorate NEC	T65.8	X49	X69	Y19	
– chloride	T50.3	X44	X64	Y14	Y54.6
– – with glucose	T50.3	X44	X64	Y14	Y54.6
– chromate	T65.8	X49	X69	Y19	
– citrate	T50.9	X44	X64	Y14	Y43.5
– cromoglicate	T48.6	X44	X64	Y14	Y55.6
– cyanide	T65.0	X49	X69	Y19	
– dehydrocholate	T45.8	X44	X64	Y14	Y57.8
– dibunate	T48.4	X44	X64	Y14	Y55.4
– dioctyl sulfosuccinate	T47.4	X44	X64	Y14	Y53.4
– dipantoyl ferrate	T45.8	X44	X64	Y14	Y44.0
– etacrynate	T50.1	X44	X64	Y14	Y54.4

| Substance | Chapter XIX | Poisoning | | | Adverse effect in therapeutic use |
		Accidental	Intentional self-harm	Undetermined intent	
Sodium—*continued*					
– feredetate	T45.8	X44	X64	Y14	Y44.0
= fluoride = see Fluoride					
– fluoroacetate (dust) (pesticide)	T60.4	X48	X68	Y18	
– fusidate	T36.8	X44	X64	Y14	Y40.8
– glucaldrate	T47.1	X44	X64	Y14	Y53.1
– glucosulfone	T37.1	X44	X64	Y14	Y41.1
– glutamate	T45.8	X44	X64	Y14	Y43.5
– hydrogen carbonate	T50.3	X44	X64	Y14	Y54.6
– hydroxide	T54.3	X49	X69	Y19	
– hypochlorite (bleach) NEC	T54.3	X49	X69	Y19	
– – vapor	T54.3	X47	X67	Y17	
– indigotin disulfonate	T50.8	X44	X64	Y14	Y57.6
– iodohippurate (^{131}I)	T50.8	X44	X64	Y14	Y57.5
– iopodate	T50.8	X44	X64	Y14	Y57.5
– lactate (compound solution)	T45.8	X44	X64	Y14	Y43.5
– lauryl (sulfate)	T49.2	X44	X64	Y14	Y56.2
– magnesium citrate	T50.9	X44	X64	Y14	Y57.8
– mersalate	T50.2	X44	X64	Y14	Y54.5
– metasilicate	T65.8	X49	X69	Y19	
– metrizoate	T50.8	X44	X64	Y14	Y57.5
– monofluoroacetate (pesticide)	T60.1	X48	X68	Y18	
– morrhuate	T46.8	X44	X64	Y14	Y52.8
– nitrate (oxidizing agent)	T65.8	X49	X69	Y19	
– nitrite	T50.6	X44	X64	Y14	Y57.2
– nitroprusside	T46.5	X44	X64	Y14	Y52.5
– oxalate	T65.8	X49	X69	Y19	
– oxide/peroxide	T65.8	X49	X69	Y19	
– oxybate	T41.2	X44	X64	Y14	Y48.2
– perborate (nonmedicinal) NEC	T65.8	X49	X69	Y19	
– – medicinal	T49.0	X44	X64	Y14	Y56.0
– pertechnetate Tc99m	T50.8	X44	X64	Y14	Y57.5
– phosphate					
– – dibasic	T47.2	X44	X64	Y14	Y53.2
– – monobasic	T45.8	X44	X64	Y14	Y43.5
– phytate	T50.6	X44	X64	Y14	Y57.2
– picosulfate	T47.2	X44	X64	Y14	Y53.2
– polyhydroxyaluminium monocarbonate	T47.1	X44	X64	Y14	Y53.1
– polystyrene sulfonate	T50.3	X44	X64	Y14	Y54.6
– propyl hydroxybenzoate	T50.9	X44	X64	Y14	Y57.4
– salicylate	T39.0	X40	X60	Y10	Y45.1
– salt NEC	T50.3	X44	X64	Y14	Y54.6
– selenate	T60.2	X48	X68	Y18	
– stibogluconate	T37.3	X44	X64	Y14	Y41.3
– sulfate	T47.4	X44	X64	Y14	Y53.4
– tetradecyl sulfate	T46.8	X44	X64	Y14	Y52.8
– thiosulfate	T50.6	X44	X64	Y14	Y57.2
– tolbutamide	T38.3	X44	X64	Y14	Y42.3
– l-triiodothyronine	T38.1	X44	X64	Y14	Y42.1
– tyropanoate	T50.8	X44	X64	Y14	Y57.5

Substance	Chapter XIX	Accidental	Poisoning Intentional self-harm	Undetermined intent	Adverse effect in therapeutic use
Sodium—*continued*					
− versenate	T50.6	X44	X64	Y14	Y57.2
Sodium-free salt	T50.9	X44	X64	Y14	Y57.8
Sodium-removing resin	T50.3	X44	X64	Y14	Y54.6
Soft soap	T55	X44	X64	Y14	Y53.4
Solanine	T62.2	X49	X69	Y19	
Solapsone	T37.1	X44	X64	Y14	Y41.1
Solar lotion	T49.3	X44	X64	Y14	Y56.3
Solasulfone	T37.1	X44	X64	Y14	Y41.1
Soldering fluid	T65.8	X49	X69	Y19	
Solvent, industrial NEC	T52.9	X46	X66	Y16	
Somatorelin	T38.8	X44	X64	Y14	Y42.8
Somatostatin	T38.9	X44	X64	Y14	Y42.9
Somatotropin	T38.8	X44	X64	Y14	Y42.8
Somatrem	T38.8	X44	X64	Y14	Y42.8
Somatropin	T38.8	X44	X64	Y14	Y42.8
Soporific	T42.7	X41	X61	Y11	Y47.9
Sorbide nitrate	T46.3	X44	X64	Y14	Y52.3
Sorbitol	T47.4	X44	X64	Y14	Y53.4
Sotalol	T44.7	X43	X63	Y13	Y51.7
Soysterol	T46.6	X44	X64	Y14	Y52.6
Sparteine	T48.0	X44	X64	Y14	Y55.0
Spasmolytic					
− autonomic	T44.3	X43	X63	Y13	Y51.3
− bronchial NEC	T48.6	X44	X64	Y14	Y55.6
− quaternary ammonium	T44.3	X43	X63	Y13	Y51.3
− skeletal muscle NEC	T48.1	X44	X64	Y14	Y55.1
Spectinomycin	T36.5	X44	X64	Y14	Y40.5
Spermicide	T49.8	X44	X64	Y14	Y56.8
Spindle inactivator	T50.4	X44	X64	Y14	Y54.8
Spiperone	T43.4	X41	X61	Y11	Y49.4
Spiramycin	T36.3	X44	X64	Y14	Y40.3
Spirapril	T46.4	X44	X64	Y14	Y52.4
Spirilene	T43.5	X41	X61	Y11	Y49.5
Spirit(s) (neutral) NEC	T51.0	X45	X65	Y15	
− industrial	T51.0	X45	X65	Y15	
− of salt − *see* Hydrochloric acid					
− surgical	T51.0	X45	X65	Y15	
Spironolactone	T50.0	X44	X64	Y14	Y54.1
Spiroperidol	T43.4	X41	X61	Y11	Y49.4
Spray (aerosol)	T65.9	X49	X69	Y19	
− specified content − *see* specific substance					
Sputum viscosity-lowering drug	T48.4	X44	X64	Y14	Y55.4
Squill	T46.0	X44	X64	Y14	Y52.0
− rat poison	T60.4	X48	X68	Y18	
Stannous fluoride	T49.7	X44	X64	Y14	Y56.7
Stanolone	T38.7	X44	X64	Y14	Y42.7
Stanozolol	T38.7	X44	X64	Y14	Y42.7
Starch	T50.9	X44	X64	Y14	Y57.4
Stepronin	T48.4	X44	X64	Y14	Y55.4

Substance	Chapter XIX	Poisoning Accidental	Intentional self-harm	Undetermined intent	Adverse effect in therapeutic use
Sterculia	T47.4	X44	X64	Y14	Y53.4
Sternutator gas	T59.8	X47	X67	Y17	
Steroid					
– anabolic	T38.7	X44	X64	Y14	Y42.7
– androgenic	T38.7	X44	X64	Y14	Y42.7
– antineoplastic, hormone	T38.7	X44	X64	Y14	Y42.7
– – estrogen	T38.5	X44	X64	Y14	Y42.5
Stibine	T56.8	X49	X69	Y19	
Stibogluconate	T37.3	X44	X64	Y14	Y41.3
Stibophen	T37.4	X44	X64	Y14	Y41.4
Stilbamidine (isetionate)	T37.3	X44	X64	Y14	Y41.3
Stilbestrol	T38.5	X44	X64	Y14	Y42.5
Stilboestrol	T38.5	X44	X64	Y14	Y42.5
Stimulant					
– central nervous system	T50.9	X44	X64	Y14	Y50.9
– – specified NEC	T50.9	X44	X64	Y14	Y50.8
– respiratory	T48.7	X44	X64	Y14	Y55.7
Stone-dissolving drug	T50.9	X44	X64	Y14	Y57.8
Storage battery (cells) (acid)	T65.8	X49	X69	Y19	
Stove gas	T58	X47	X67	Y17	
Stramonium	T48.6	X44	X64	Y14	Y55.6
Streptodornase	T45.3	X44	X64	Y14	Y43.6
Streptoduocin	T36.5	X44	X64	Y14	Y40.5
Streptokinase	T45.6	X44	X64	Y14	Y44.5
Streptomycin (derivative)	T36.5	X44	X64	Y14	Y40.5
Streptonivicin	T36.5	X44	X64	Y14	Y40.5
Streptovarycin	T36.5	X44	X64	Y14	Y40.5
Streptozocin	T45.1	X44	X64	Y14	Y43.3
Streptozotocin	T45.1	X44	X64	Y14	Y43.3
Stripper (paint) (solvent)	T52.8	X46	X66	Y16	
Strobane	T60.1	X48	X68	Y18	
Strofantina	T46.0	X44	X64	Y14	Y52.0
Strophanthin (g) (k)	T46.0	X44	X64	Y14	Y52.0
Strophanthus	T46.0	X44	X64	Y14	Y52.0
Strophantin	T46.0	X44	X64	Y14	Y52.0
Strophantin-g	T46.0	X44	X64	Y14	Y52.0
Strychnine (nonmedicinal) (pesticide)(salts)	T65.1	X49	X69	Y19	
– medicinal	T48.2	X44	X64	Y14	Y55.2
Styramate	T42.8	X41	X61	Y11	Y46.8
Styrene	T65.8	X49	X69	Y19	
Succinimide, antiepileptic or anticonvulsant	T42.2	X41	X61	Y11	Y46.0
Succinylcholine	T48.1	X44	X64	Y14	Y55.1
Succinylsulfathiazole	T37.0	X44	X64	Y14	Y41.0
Sucralfate	T47.1	X44	X64	Y14	Y53.1
Sucrose	T50.3	X44	X64	Y14	Y54.6
Sufentanil	T40.4	X42	X62	Y12	Y45.0
Sulbactam	T36.0	X44	X64	Y14	Y40.0
Sulbenicillin	T36.0	X44	X64	Y14	Y40.0
Sulbentine	T49.0	X44	X64	Y14	Y56.0

Substance	Chapter XIX	Accidental	Poisoning Intentional self-harm	Undetermined intent	Adverse effect in therapeutic use
Sulfacetamide	T49.5	X44	X64	Y14	Y56.5
Sulfachlorpyridazine	T37.0	X44	X64	Y14	Y41.0
Sulfacitine	T37.0	X44	X64	Y14	Y41.0
Sulfadiasulfone sodium	T37.0	X44	X64	Y14	Y41.0
Sulfadiazine	T37.0	X44	X64	Y14	Y41.0
Sulfadimethoxine	T37.0	X44	X64	Y14	Y41.0
Sulfadimidine	T37.0	X44	X64	Y14	Y41.0
Sulfadoxine	T37.0	X44	X64	Y14	Y41.0
– with pyrimethamine	T37.2	X44	X64	Y14	Y41.2
Sulfafurazole	T37.0	X44	X64	Y14	Y41.0
Sulfaguanidine	T37.0	X44	X64	Y14	Y41.0
Sulfalene	T37.0	X44	X64	Y14	Y41.0
Sulfaloxate	T37.0	X44	X64	Y14	Y41.0
Sulfaloxic acid	T37.0	X44	X64	Y14	Y41.0
Sulfamazone	T39.2	X40	X60	Y10	Y45.8
Sulfamerazine	T37.0	X44	X64	Y14	Y41.0
Sulfameter	T37.0	X44	X64	Y14	Y41.0
Sulfamethazine	T37.0	X44	X64	Y14	Y41.0
Sulfamethizole	T37.0	X44	X64	Y14	Y41.0
Sulfamethoxazole	T37.0	X44	X64	Y14	Y41.0
– with trimethoprim	T36.8	X44	X64	Y14	Y40.8
Sulfamethoxydiazine	T37.0	X44	X64	Y14	Y41.0
Sulfamethoxypyridazine	T37.0	X44	X64	Y14	Y41.0
Sulfametoxydiazine	T37.0	X44	X64	Y14	Y41.0
Sulfamidopyrine	T39.2	X40	X60	Y10	Y45.8
Sulfamonomethoxine	T37.0	X44	X64	Y14	Y41.0
Sulfamoxole	T37.0	X44	X64	Y14	Y41.0
Sulfanilamide	T37.0	X44	X64	Y14	Y41.0
Sulfaperin	T37.0	X44	X64	Y14	Y41.0
Sulfaphenazole	T37.0	X44	X64	Y14	Y41.0
Sulfaproxyline	T37.0	X44	X64	Y14	Y41.0
Sulfapyridine	T37.0	X44	X64	Y14	Y41.0
Sulfasalazine	T37.0	X44	X64	Y14	Y41.0
Sulfasymazine	T37.0	X44	X64	Y14	Y41.0
Sulfated amylopectin	T47.8	X44	X64	Y14	Y53.8
Sulfathiazole	T37.0	X44	X64	Y14	Y41.0
Sulfatostearate	T49.2	X44	X64	Y14	Y56.2
Sulfinpyrazone	T50.4	X44	X64	Y14	Y54.8
Sulfiram	T49.0	X44	X64	Y14	Y56.0
Sulfisomidine	T37.0	X44	X64	Y14	Y41.0
Sulfisoxazole	T37.0	X44	X64	Y14	Y41.0
Sulfobromophthalein (sodium)	T50.8	X44	X64	Y14	Y57.6
Sulfobromphthalein	T50.8	X44	X64	Y14	Y57.6
Sulfogaiacol	T48.4	X44	X64	Y14	Y55.4
Sulfonamide NEC	T37.0	X44	X64	Y14	Y41.0
– eye	T49.5	X44	X64	Y14	Y56.5
Sulfonazide	T37.1	X44	X64	Y14	Y41.1
Sulforidazine	T43.3	X41	X61	Y11	Y49.3

Substance	Chapter XIX	Poisoning			Adverse effect in therapeutic use
		Accidental	Intentional self-harm	Undetermined intent	
Sulfur, sulfurated, sulfuric, sulfurous, sulfuryl (compounds NEC) (medicinal)	T49.4	X47	X67	Y17	Y56.4
– dioxide (gas)	T59.1	X47	X67	Y17	
– ointment	T49.0	X44	X64	Y14	Y56.0
Sulfuric acid	T54.2	X49	X69	Y19	
Sulglicotide	T47.1	X44	X64	Y14	Y53.1
Sulindac	T39.3	X40	X60	Y10	Y45.3
Sulisatin	T47.2	X44	X64	Y14	Y53.2
Sulisobenzone	T49.3	X44	X64	Y14	Y56.3
Sulmetozine	T44.3	X43	X63	Y13	Y51.3
Suloctidil	T46.7	X44	X64	Y14	Y52.7
Sulph- – *see also* Sulf-					
Sulphadiazine	T37.0	X44	X64	Y14	Y41.0
Sulphadimethoxine	T37.0	X44	X64	Y14	Y41.0
Sulphadimidine	T37.0	X44	X64	Y14	Y41.0
Sulphafurazole	T37.0	X44	X64	Y14	Y41.0
Sulphamethizole	T37.0	X44	X64	Y14	Y41.0
Sulphamethoxazole	T37.0	X44	X64	Y14	Y41.0
Sulphan blue	T50.8	X44	X64	Y14	Y57.6
Sulphaphenazole	T37.0	X44	X64	Y14	Y41.0
Sulphapyridine	T37.0	X44	X64	Y14	Y41.0
Sulphasalazine	T37.0	X44	X64	Y14	Y41.0
Sulphinpyrazone	T50.4	X44	X64	Y14	Y54.8
Sulpiride	T43.5	X41	X61	Y11	Y49.5
Sulprostone	T48.0	X44	X64	Y14	Y55.0
Sulpyrine	T39.2	X40	X60	Y10	Y45.8
Sultamicillin	T36.0	X44	X64	Y14	Y40.0
Sulthiame	T42.6	X41	X61	Y11	Y46.6
Sultiame	T42.6	X41	X61	Y11	Y46.6
Sultopride	T43.5	X41	X61	Y11	Y49.5
Sumatriptan	T39.8	X40	X60	Y10	Y45.8
Sunflower seed oil	T46.6	X44	X64	Y14	Y52.6
Suprofen	T39.3	X40	X60	Y10	Y45.2
Suramin (sodium)	T37.4	X44	X64	Y14	Y41.4
Sutilains	T45.3	X44	X64	Y14	Y43.6
Suxamethonium (chloride)	T48.1	X44	X64	Y14	Y55.1
Suxethonium (chloride)	T48.1	X44	X64	Y14	Y55.1
Suxibuzone	T39.2	X40	X60	Y10	Y45.8
Sweet niter spirit	T46.3	X44	X64	Y14	Y52.3
Sweetener	T50.9	X44	X64	Y14	Y57.4
Sympatholytic NEC	T44.8	X43	X63	Y13	Y51.8
– haloalkylamine	T44.8	X43	X63	Y13	Y51.8
Sympathomimetic NEC	T44.9	X43	X63	Y13	Y51.9
– anti-common-cold	T48.5	X44	X64	Y14	Y55.5
– bronchodilator	T48.6	X44	X64	Y14	Y55.6
– specified NEC	T44.9	X43	X63	Y13	Y51.9
Syrosingopine	T46.5	X44	X64	Y14	Y52.5
Systemic drug	T45.9	X44	X64	Y14	Y43.9
– specified NEC	T45.8	X44	X64	Y14	Y43.8

T

Substance		Poisoning			Adverse effect in therapeutic use
	Chapter XIX	Accidental	Intentional self-harm	Undetermined intent	
2,4,5-T	T60.3	X48	X68	Y18	
Tacrine	T44.0	X43	X63	Y13	Y51.0
Tadalafil	T46.7	X44	X64	Y14	Y52.7
Talampicillin	T36.0	X44	X64	Y14	Y40.0
Talbutal	T42.3	X41	X61	Y11	Y47.0
Talc powder	T49.3	X44	X64	Y14	Y56.3
Taleranol	T38.6	X44	X64	Y14	Y42.6
Tamoxifen	T38.6	X44	X64	Y14	Y42.6
Tannic acid	T49.2	X44	X64	Y14	Y56.2
Tar NEC	T52.0	X46	X66	Y16	
– camphor	T60.1	X48	X68	Y18	
– distillate	T49.1	X44	X64	Y14	Y56.1
– fumes	T59.8	X47	X67	Y17	
– medicinal	T49.1	X44	X64	Y14	Y56.1
– ointment	T49.1	X44	X64	Y14	Y56.1
Tartar emetic	T37.8	X44	X64	Y14	Y41.8
Tartaric acid	T65.8	X49	X69	Y19	
Tartrate, laxative	T47.4	X44	X64	Y14	Y53.4
Tauromustine	T45.1	X44	X64	Y14	Y43.3
TCA – *see* Trichloroacetic acid					
TCDD	T65.8	X49	X69	Y19	
TDI (vapor)	T65.0	X49	X69	Y19	
Tear					
– gas	T59.3	X47	X67	Y17	
– solution	T49.5	X44	X64	Y14	Y56.5
Teclothiazide	T50.2	X44	X64	Y14	Y54.3
Teclozan	T37.3	X44	X64	Y14	Y41.3
Tegafur	T45.1	X44	X64	Y14	Y43.1
Teicoplanin	T36.8	X44	X64	Y14	Y40.8
Tellurium	T56.8	X49	X69	Y19	
Temazepam	T42.4	X41	X61	Y11	Y47.1
Temocillin	T36.0	X44	X64	Y14	Y40.0
Tenamfetamine	T43.6	X41	X61	Y11	Y49.7
Teniposide	T45.1	X44	X64	Y14	Y43.3
Tenitramine	T46.3	X44	X64	Y14	Y52.3
Tenoglicin	T48.4	X44	X64	Y14	Y55.4
Tenonitrozole	T37.3	X44	X64	Y14	Y41.3
Tenoxicam	T39.3	X40	X60	Y10	Y45.3
TEPP	T60.0	X48	X68	Y18	
Teprotide	T46.5	X44	X64	Y14	Y52.5
Terazosin	T44.6	X43	X63	Y13	Y51.6
Terbufos	T60.0	X48	X68	Y18	
Terbutaline	T48.6	X44	X64	Y14	Y55.6
Terconazole	T49.0	X44	X64	Y14	Y56.0

| Substance | Chapter XIX | Poisoning | | | Adverse effect in therapeutic use |
		Accidental	Intentional self-harm	Undetermined intent	
Terfenadine	T45.0	X44	X64	Y14	Y43.0
Teriparatide (acetate)	T50.9	X44	X64	Y14	Y54.7
Terizidone	T37.1	X44	X64	Y14	Y41.1
Terlipressin	T38.8	X44	X64	Y14	Y42.8
Terodiline	T46.3	X44	X64	Y14	Y52.3
Terpin(cis) hydrate	T48.4	X44	X64	Y14	Y55.4
Tertatolol	T44.7	X43	X63	Y13	Y51.7
Testolactone	T38.7	X44	X64	Y14	Y42.7
Testosterone	T38.7	X44	X64	Y14	Y42.7
Tetanus toxoid or vaccine	T50.9	X44	X64	Y14	Y58.4
Tetrabenazine	T43.5	X41	X61	Y11	Y49.5
Tetracaine	T41.3	X44	X64	Y14	Y48.3
– regional	T41.3	X44	X64	Y14	Y48.3
– spinal	T41.3	X44	X64	Y14	Y48.3
Tetrachlorethylene – *see* Tetrachloroethylene					
2,3,7,8-Tetrachlorodibenzo-p-dioxin	T53.7	X46	X66	Y16	
Tetrachloroethane	T53.3	X46	X66	Y16	
– vapor	T53.3	X46	X66	Y16	
Tetrachloroethylene (liquid)	T53.3	X46	X66	Y16	
– medicinal	T37.4	X44	X64	Y14	Y41.4
– vapor	T53.3	X46	X66	Y16	
Tetrachloromethane – *see* Carbon tetrachloride					
Tetracosactide	T38.8	X44	X64	Y14	Y42.8
Tetracosactrin	T38.8	X44	X64	Y14	Y42.8
Tetracycline	T36.4	X44	X64	Y14	Y40.4
Tetradifon	T60.8	X48	X68	Y18	
Tetradotoxin	T61.2	X49	X69	Y19	
Tetraethyl					
– lead	T56.0	X49	X69	Y19	
– pyrophosphate	T60.0	X48	X68	Y18	
Tetrahydrocannabinol	T40.7	X42	X62	Y12	Y49.6
Tetrahydrofuran	T52.8	X46	X66	Y16	
Tetrahydronaphthalene	T52.8	X46	X66	Y16	
Tetrahydrozoline	T49.5	X44	X64	Y14	Y56.5
Tetralin	T52.8	X46	X66	Y16	
Tetramethrin	T60.2	X48	X68	Y18	
Tetramethylthiuram (disulfide) NEC	T60.3	X48	X68	Y18	
– medicinal	T49.0	X44	X64	Y14	Y56.0
Tetramisole	T37.4	X44	X64	Y14	Y41.4
Tetranicotinoyl fructose	T46.7	X44	X64	Y14	Y52.7
Tetrazepam	T42.4	X41	X61	Y11	Y47.1
Tetryl	T65.3	X49	X69	Y19	
Tetrylammonium chloride	T44.2	X43	X63	Y13	Y51.2
Tetryzoline	T49.5	X44	X64	Y14	Y56.5
Thalidomide	T45.1	X44	X64	Y14	Y43.4
Thallium (compounds) (dust) NEC	T56.8	X49	X69	Y19	
– pesticide	T60.4	X48	X68	Y18	
Thebacon	T48.3	X44	X64	Y14	Y55.3
Thenoic acid	T49.6	X44	X64	Y14	Y56.6

Substance	Chapter XIX	Accidental	Poisoning Intentional self-harm	Undetermined intent	Adverse effect in therapeutic use
Thenyldiamine	T45.0	X44	X64	Y14	Y43.0
Theobromine (calcium salicylate)	T48.6	X44	X64	Y14	Y55.6
– sodium salicylate	T48.6	X44	X64	Y14	Y55.6
Theophyllamine	T48.6	X44	X64	Y14	Y55.6
Theophylline	T48.6	X44	X64	Y14	Y55.6
– aminobenzoic acid	T48.6	X44	X64	Y14	Y55.6
– piperazine p-aminobenzoate	T48.6	X44	X64	Y14	Y55.6
Thiabendazole	T37.4	X44	X64	Y14	Y41.4
Thialbarbital	T41.1	X44	X64	Y14	Y48.1
Thiamazole	T38.2	X44	X64	Y14	Y42.2
Thiambutosine	T37.1	X44	X64	Y14	Y41.1
Thiamine	T45.2	X44	X64	Y14	Y57.7
Thiamphenicol	T36.2	X44	X64	Y14	Y40.2
Thiamylal	T41.1	X44	X64	Y14	Y48.1
– sodium	T41.1	X44	X64	Y14	Y48.1
Thiazinamium metilsulfate	T43.3	X41	X61	Y11	Y49.3
Thiethylperazine	T43.3	X41	X61	Y11	Y49.3
Thimerosal	T49.0	X44	X64	Y14	Y56.0
Thioacetazone	T37.1	X44	X64	Y14	Y41.1
– with isoniazid	T37.1	X44	X64	Y14	Y41.1
Thiobarbital sodium	T41.1	X44	X64	Y14	Y48.1
Thiobarbiturate anesthetic	T41.1	X44	X64	Y14	Y48.1
Thiobutabarbital sodium	T41.1	X44	X64	Y14	Y48.1
Thiocarbamate (insecticide)	T60.0	X48	X68	Y18	
Thiocarlide	T37.1	X44	X64	Y14	Y41.1
Thioctamide	T50.9	X44	X64	Y14	Y57.1
Thioctic acid	T50.9	X44	X64	Y14	Y57.1
Thiofos	T60.0	X48	X68	Y18	Y56.0
Thioglycolate	T49.4	X44	X64	Y14	Y56.4
Thioglycolic acid	T65.8	X49	X69	Y19	
Thioguanine	T45.1	X44	X64	Y14	Y43.1
Thiomersal	T49.0	X44	X64	Y14	Y56.0
Thionazin	T60.0	X48	X68	Y18	
Thiopental (sodium)	T41.1	X44	X64	Y14	Y48.1
Thiopentone (sodium)	T41.1	X44	X64	Y14	Y48.1
Thiopropazate	T43.3	X41	X61	Y11	Y49.3
Thioproperazine	T43.3	X41	X61	Y11	Y49.3
Thioridazine	T43.3	X41	X61	Y11	Y49.3
Thiosinamine	T49.3	X44	X64	Y14	Y56.3
Thiotepa	T45.1	X44	X64	Y14	Y43.3
Thiothixene	T43.4	X41	X61	Y11	Y49.4
Thiouracil (benzyl) (methyl) (propyl)	T38.2	X44	X64	Y14	Y42.2
Thiphenamil	T44.3	X43	X63	Y13	Y51.3
Thiram	T60.3	X48	X68	Y18	
Thonzylamine (systemic)	T45.0	X44	X64	Y14	Y43.0
– mucosal decongestant	T48.5	X44	X64	Y14	Y55.5
Thorium dioxide suspension	T50.8	X44	X64	Y14	Y57.5
Throat drug NEC	T49.6	X44	X64	Y14	Y56.6
Thromboplastin	T45.7	X44	X64	Y14	Y44.3
Thurfyl nicotinate	T46.7	X44	X64	Y14	Y52.7

Substance	Chapter XIX	Poisoning			Adverse effect in therapeutic use
		Accidental	Intentional self-harm	Undetermined intent	
Thymol	T49.0	X44	X64	Y14	Y56.0
Thymopentin	T37.5	X44	X64	Y14	Y41.5
Thymoxamine	T46.7	X44	X64	Y14	Y52.7
Thyreotrophic hormone	T38.8	X44	X64	Y14	Y42.8
Thyroglobulin	T38.1	X44	X64	Y14	Y42.1
Thyroid (hormone)	T38.1	X44	X64	Y14	Y42.1
Thyrotrophin	T38.8	X44	X64	Y14	Y42.8
Thyrotropic hormone	T38.8	X44	X64	Y14	Y42.8
Thyroxine	T38.1	X44	X64	Y14	Y42.1
Tiabendazole	T37.4	X44	X64	Y14	Y41.4
Tiamizide	T50.2	X44	X64	Y14	Y54.5
Tianeptine	T43.0	X41	X61	Y11	Y49.0
Tiapamil	T46.1	X44	X64	Y14	Y52.1
Tiapride	T43.5	X41	X61	Y11	Y49.5
Tiaprofenic acid	T39.3	X40	X60	Y10	Y45.2
Tiaramide	T39.8	X40	X60	Y10	Y45.8
Ticarcillin	T36.0	X44	X64	Y14	Y40.0
Ticlatone	T49.0	X44	X64	Y14	Y56.0
Ticlopidine	T45.5	X44	X64	Y14	Y44.2
Ticrynafen	T50.1	X44	X64	Y14	Y54.4
Tidiacic	T50.9	X44	X64	Y14	Y57.1
Tiemonium	T44.3	X43	X63	Y13	Y51.3
– iodide	T44.3	X43	X63	Y13	Y51.3
Tienilic acid	T50.1	X44	X64	Y14	Y54.4
Tifenamil	T44.3	X43	X63	Y13	Y51.3
Tigloidine	T44.3	X43	X63	Y13	Y51.3
Tilactase	T47.5	X44	X64	Y14	Y53.5
Tiletamine	T41.2	X44	X64	Y14	Y48.2
Tilidine	T40.4	X42	X62	Y12	Y45.0
Timepidium bromide	T44.3	X43	X63	Y13	Y51.3
Timiperone	T43.4	X41	X61	Y11	Y49.4
Timolol	T44.7	X43	X63	Y13	Y51.7
Tin (chloride) (dust) (oxide) NEC	T56.6	X49	X69	Y19	
Tincture, iodine – *see* Iodine					
Tinidazole	T37.3	X44	X64	Y14	Y41.3
Tinoridine	T39.8	X40	X60	Y10	Y45.8
Tiocarlide	T37.1	X44	X64	Y14	Y41.1
Tioclomarol	T45.5	X44	X64	Y14	Y44.2
Tioconazole	T49.0	X44	X64	Y14	Y56.0
Tioguanine	T45.1	X44	X64	Y14	Y43.1
Tiopronin	T50.9	X44	X64	Y14	Y57.1
Tiotixene	T43.4	X41	X61	Y11	Y49.4
Tioxolone	T49.4	X44	X64	Y14	Y56.4
Tipepidine	T48.3	X44	X64	Y14	Y55.3
Tiquizium bromide	T44.3	X43	X63	Y13	Y51.3
Tiratricol	T38.1	X44	X64	Y14	Y42.1
Tisokinase	T45.5	X44	X64	Y14	Y44.2
Tisopurine	T50.4	X44	X64	Y14	Y54.8

Substance	Chapter XIX	Accidental	Poisoning Intentional self-harm	Undetermined intent	Adverse effect in therapeutic use
Titanium (compounds) (vapor)	T56.8	X49	X69	Y19	
– dioxide	T49.3	X44	X64	Y14	Y56.3
– oxide	T49.3	X44	X64	Y14	Y56.3
– tetrachloride	T65.8	X49	X69	Y19	
Titanocene	T65.8	X49	X69	Y19	
Tizanidine	T42.8	X41	X61	Y11	Y46.8
TMTD	T60.3	X48	X68	Y18	
TNT (fumes)	T65.3	X49	X69	Y19	
Toadstool	T62.0	X49	X69	Y19	
Tobacco NEC	T65.2	X49	X69	Y19	
Tobramycin	T36.5	X44	X64	Y14	Y40.5
Tocainide	T46.2	X44	X64	Y14	Y52.2
Tocoferol	T45.2	X44	X64	Y14	Y57.7
Tocopherol	T45.2	X44	X64	Y14	Y57.7
– acetate	T45.2	X44	X64	Y14	Y57.7
Todralazine	T46.5	X44	X64	Y14	Y52.5
Tofisopam	T42.4	X41	X61	Y11	Y47.1
Toilet deodorizer	T65.8	X49	X69	Y19	
Tolamolol	T44.7	X43	X63	Y13	Y51.7
Tolazamide	T38.3	X44	X64	Y14	Y42.3
Tolazoline	T46.7	X44	X64	Y14	Y52.7
Tolbutamide (sodium)	T38.3	X44	X64	Y14	Y42.3
Tolciclate	T49.0	X44	X64	Y14	Y56.0
Tolfenamic acid	T39.3	X40	X60	Y10	Y45.3
Tolmetin	T39.3	X40	X60	Y10	Y45.3
Tolnaftate	T49.0	X44	X64	Y14	Y56.0
Tolonidine	T46.5	X44	X64	Y14	Y52.5
Toloxatone	T42.6	X41	X61	Y11	Y47.8
Tolperisone	T44.3	X43	X63	Y13	Y51.3
Toluene (liquid)	T52.2	X46	X66	Y16	
– diisocyanate	T65.0	X49	X69	Y19	
Toluidine	T65.8	X49	X69	Y19	
– vapor	T59.8	X47	X67	Y17	
Toluol (liquid)	T52.2	X46	X66	Y16	
– vapor	T52.2	X46	X66	Y16	
Toluylenediamine	T65.3	X49	X69	Y19	
Tonic NEC	T50.9	X44	X64	Y14	Y57.8
Topical action drug NEC	T49.9	X44	X64	Y14	Y56.9
– ear, nose or throat	T49.6	X44	X64	Y14	Y56.6
– eye	T49.5	X44	X64	Y14	Y56.5
– skin	T49.4	X44	X64	Y14	Y56.4
– specified NEC	T49.8	X44	X64	Y14	Y56.8
Toquizine	T44.3	X43	X63	Y13	Y51.3
Toremifene	T38.6	X44	X64	Y14	Y42.6
Tosylchloramide sodium	T49.8	X44	X64	Y14	Y56.8
Toxin, diphtheria (Schick test)	T50.8	X44	X64	Y14	Y57.6
Toxoid					
– combined	T50.9	X44	X64	Y14	Y58.9
– diphtheria	T50.9	X44	X64	Y14	Y58.5
– tetanus	T50.9	X44	X64	Y14	Y58.4
Trace element NEC	T45.8	X44	X64	Y14	Y57.8

827

Substance	Poisoning			Adverse effect in therapeutic use
	Chapter XIX	Accidental	Intentional self-harm	Undetermined intent	
Tractor fuel NEC	T52.0	X46	X66	Y16	
Tragacanth	T50.9	X44	X64	Y14	Y57.4
Tramadol	T40.4	X42	X62	Y12	Y45.0
Tramazoline	T48.5	X44	X64	Y14	Y55.5
Tranexamic acid	T45.6	X44	X64	Y14	Y44.3
Tranilast	T45.0	X44	X64	Y14	Y43.0
Tranquilizer NEC	T43.5	X41	X61	Y11	Y49.5
− with hypnotic or sedative	T42.6	X41	X61	Y11	Y47.5
− benzodiazepine NEC	T42.4	X41	X61	Y11	Y47.1
− butyrophenone NEC	T43.4	X41	X61	Y11	Y49.4
− carbamate	T43.5	X41	X61	Y11	Y49.5
− dimethylamine	T43.3	X41	X61	Y11	Y49.3
− ethylamine	T43.3	X41	X61	Y11	Y49.3
− hydroxyzine	T43.5	X41	X61	Y11	Y49.5
− major NEC	T43.5	X41	X61	Y11	Y49.5
− penothiazine NEC	T43.3	X41	X61	Y11	Y49.3
− piperazine NEC	T43.3	X41	X61	Y11	Y49.3
− piperidine	T43.3	X41	X61	Y11	Y49.3
− propylamine	T43.3	X41	X61	Y11	Y49.3
− thioxanthene NEC	T43.5	X41	X61	Y11	Y49.5
Tranylcypromine	T43.1	X41	X61	Y11	Y49.1
Trapidil	T46.3	X44	X64	Y14	Y52.3
Trazodone	T43.2	X41	X61	Y11	Y49.2
Treosulfan	T45.1	X44	X64	Y14	Y43.3
Tretamine	T45.1	X44	X64	Y14	Y43.3
Tretinoin	T49.0	X44	X64	Y14	Y56.0
Tretoquinol	T48.6	X44	X64	Y14	Y55.6
Triacetin	T49.0	X44	X64	Y14	Y56.0
Triacetoxyanthracene	T49.4	X44	X64	Y14	Y56.4
Triacetyloleandomycin	T36.3	X44	X64	Y14	Y40.3
Triamcinolone	T49.0	X44	X64	Y14	Y56.0
− hexacetonide	T49.0	X44	X64	Y14	Y56.0
Triampyzine	T44.3	X43	X63	Y13	Y51.3
Triamterene	T50.2	X44	X64	Y14	Y54.5
Triazine (herbicide)	T60.3	X48	X68	Y18	
Triaziquone	T45.1	X44	X64	Y14	Y43.3
Triazolam	T42.4	X41	X61	Y11	Y47.1
Triazole (herbicide)	T60.3	X48	X68	Y18	
Tribenoside	T46.9	X44	X64	Y14	Y52.9
Tribromoethanol, rectal	T41.2	X44	X64	Y14	Y48.2
Trichlorethylene	T53.2	X46	X66	Y16	
Trichlorfon	T60.0	X48	X68	Y18	
Trichlormethiazide	T50.2	X44	X64	Y14	Y54.3
Trichlormethine	T45.1	X44	X64	Y14	Y43.3
Trichloroacetic acid, trichloracetic acid	T54.2	X49	X69	Y19	
− medicinal	T49.4	X44	X64	Y14	Y56.4
Trichloroethane	T53.2	X46	X66	Y16	
Trichloroethylene	T53.2	X46	X66	Y16	
− vapor NEC	T41.0	X44	X64	Y14	
Trichlorofluoromethane NEC	T53.5	X46	X66	Y16	

Substance	Chapter XIX	Accidental	Intentional self-harm	Undetermined intent	Adverse effect in therapeutic use
Trichloronat(e)	T60.0	X48	X68	Y18	
2,4,5-Trichlorophenoxyacetic acid	T60.3	X48	X68	Y18	
Trichloropropane	T53.6	X46	X66	Y16	
Triclobisonium chloride	T49.0	X44	X64	Y14	Y56.0
Triclocarban	T49.0	X44	X64	Y14	Y56.0
Triclofos	T42.6	X41	X61	Y11	Y47.8
Triclosan	T49.0	X44	X64	Y14	Y56.0
Tricresyl phosphate	T65.8	X49	X69	Y19	
Tricyclamol chloride	T44.3	X43	X63	Y13	Y51.3
Tridihexethyl iodide	T44.3	X43	X63	Y13	Y51.3
Trientine	T45.8	X44	X64	Y14	Y57.2
Triethanolamine NEC	T54.3	X49	X69	Y19	
– detergent	T54.3	X49	X69	Y19	
– trinitrate (biphosphate)	T46.3	X44	X64	Y14	Y52.3
Triethanomelamine	T45.1	X44	X64	Y14	Y43.3
Triethylenemelamine	T45.1	X44	X64	Y14	Y43.3
Triethylenethiophosphoramide	T45.1	X44	X64	Y14	Y43.3
Trifluoperazine	T43.3	X41	X61	Y11	Y49.3
Trifluoroethyl vinyl ether	T41.0	X44	X64	Y14	Y48.0
Trifluperidol	T43.4	X41	X61	Y11	Y49.4
Triflupromazine	T43.3	X41	X61	Y11	Y49.3
Trifluridine	T37.5	X44	X64	Y14	Y41.5
Triflusal	T45.5	X44	X64	Y14	Y44.2
Trihexyphenidyl	T44.3	X43	X63	Y13	Y51.3
Trilostane	T38.9	X44	X64	Y14	Y42.9
Trimebutine	T44.3	X43	X63	Y13	Y51.3
Trimecaine	T41.3	X44	X64	Y14	Y48.3
Trimeprazine (tartrate)	T44.3	X43	X63	Y13	Y51.3
Trimetaphan camsilate	T44.2	X43	X63	Y13	Y51.2
Trimetazidine	T46.7	X44	X64	Y14	Y52.7
Trimethadione	T42.2	X41	X61	Y11	Y46.1
Trimethaphan	T44.2	X43	X63	Y13	Y51.2
Trimethidinium	T44.2	X43	X63	Y13	Y51.2
Trimethobenzamide	T45.0	X44	X64	Y14	Y43.0
Trimethoprim	T37.8	X44	X64	Y14	Y41.8
– with sulfamethoxazole	T36.8	X44	X64	Y14	Y40.8
Trimethylcarbinol	T51.3	X45	X65	Y15	
Trimetrexate	T45.1	X44	X64	Y14	Y43.1
Trimipramine	T43.0	X41	X61	Y11	Y49.0
Trinitrine	T46.3	X44	X64	Y14	Y52.3
Trinitrobenzol	T65.3	X49	X69	Y19	
Trinitrophenol	T65.3	X49	X69	Y19	
Trinitrotoluene (fumes)	T65.3	X49	X69	Y19	
Triorthocresyl phosphate	T65.8	X49	X69	Y19	
Trioxide of arsenic	T57.0	X48	X68	Y18	
Trioxysalen	T49.4	X44	X64	Y14	Y56.4
Tripamide	T50.2	X44	X64	Y14	Y54.5
Triparanol	T46.6	X44	X64	Y14	Y52.6
Tripelennamine	T45.0	X44	X64	Y14	Y43.0
Triperiden	T44.3	X43	X63	Y13	Y51.3
Triphenylphosphate	T65.8	X49	X69	Y19	

| | | Poisoning | | | Adverse effect in therapeutic use |
Substance	Chapter XIX	Accidental	Intentional self-harm	Undetermined intent	
Triple					
— bromides	T42.6	X41	X61	Y11	Y47.4
— carbonate	T47.1	X44	X64	Y14	Y53.1
— vaccine, including pertussis	T50.9	X44	X64	Y14	Y58.6
Triprolidine	T45.0	X44	X64	Y14	Y43.0
Trisodium hydrogen edetate	T50.6	X44	X64	Y14	Y57.2
Trisulfapyrimidines	T37.0	X44	X64	Y14	Y41.0
Trithiozine	T44.3	X43	X63	Y13	Y51.3
Tritiozine	T44.3	X43	X63	Y13	Y51.3
Tritoqualine	T45.0	X44	X64	Y14	Y43.0
Trofosfamide	T45.1	X44	X64	Y14	Y43.3
Troleandomycin	T36.3	X44	X64	Y14	Y40.3
Trolnitrate (phosphate)	T46.3	X44	X64	Y14	Y52.3
Tromantadine	T37.5	X44	X64	Y14	Y41.5
Trometamol	T50.2	X44	X64	Y14	Y54.5
Tromethamine	T50.2	X44	X64	Y14	Y54.5
Tropacine	T44.3	X43	X63	Y13	Y51.3
Tropatepine	T44.3	X43	X63	Y13	Y51.3
Tropicamide	T44.3	X43	X63	Y13	Y51.3
Trospium chloride	T44.3	X43	X63	Y13	Y51.3
Troxerutin	T46.9	X44	X64	Y14	Y52.9
Troxidone	T42.2	X41	X61	Y11	Y46.1
Tryparsamide	T37.3	X44	X64	Y14	Y41.3
Trypsin	T45.3	X44	X64	Y14	Y43.6
TSH	T38.8	X44	X64	Y14	Y42.8
Tuaminoheptane	T48.5	X44	X64	Y14	Y55.5
Tuberculin, purified protein derivative(PPD)	T50.8	X44	X64	Y14	Y57.6
Tubocurarine (chloride)	T48.1	X44	X64	Y14	Y55.1
Tulobuterol	T48.6	X44	X64	Y14	Y55.6
Turpentine (spirits of)	T52.8	X46	X66	Y16	
— vapor	T52.8	X46	X66	Y16	
Tybamate	T43.5	X41	X61	Y11	Y49.5
Tyloxapol	T48.4	X44	X64	Y14	Y55.4
Tymazoline	T48.5	X44	X64	Y14	Y55.5
Typhoid-paratyphoid vaccine	T50.9	X44	X64	Y14	Y58.1
Typhus vaccine	T50.9	X44	X64	Y14	Y59.1
Tyropanoate	T50.8	X44	X64	Y14	Y57.6
Tyrothricin	T49.6	X44	X64	Y14	Y56.6

U

| Substance | Chapter XIX | Poisoning | | | Adverse effect in therapeutic use |
		Accidental	Intentional self-harm	Undetermined intent	
Ufenamate	T39.3	X40	X60	Y10	Y45.3
Ultraviolet light protectant	T49.3	X44	X64	Y14	Y56.3
Undecenoic acid	T49.0	X44	X64	Y14	Y56.0
Undecoylium	T49.0	X44	X64	Y14	Y56.0
Undecylenic acid (derivatives)	T49.0	X44	X64	Y14	Y56.0
Unsaturated fatty acid	T46.6	X44	X64	Y14	Y52.6
Uracil mustard	T45.1	X44	X64	Y14	Y43.3
Uramustine	T45.1	X44	X64	Y14	Y43.3
Urapidil	T46.5	X44	X64	Y14	Y52.5
Urate oxidase	T50.4	X44	X64	Y14	Y54.8
Urea	T47.3	X44	X64	Y14	Y53.3
– peroxide	T49.0	X44	X64	Y14	Y56.0
– stibamine	T37.4	X44	X64	Y14	Y41.4
Urethane	T45.1	X44	X64	Y14	Y43.3
Uric acid metabolism drug NEC	T50.4	X44	X64	Y14	Y54.8
Uricosuric agent	T50.4	X44	X64	Y14	Y54.8
Urinary anti-infective	T37.8	X44	X64	Y14	Y41.8
Urofollitropin	T38.8	X44	X64	Y14	Y42.8
Urokinase	T45.6	X44	X64	Y14	Y44.5
Ursodeoxycholic acid	T50.9	X44	X64	Y14	Y57.8
Ursodiol	T50.9	X44	X64	Y14	Y57.8
Uterine relaxing factor	T44.5	X43	X63	Y13	Y51.5
Utility gas	T58	X47	X67	Y17	

V

Substance	Chapter XIX	Poisoning			Adverse effect in therapeutic use
		Accidental	Intentional self-harm	Undetermined intent	
Vaccine NEC	T50.9	X44	X64	Y14	Y59.9
– antineoplastic	T50.9	X44	X64	Y14	Y59.8
– bacterial NEC	T50.9	X44	X64	Y14	Y58.9
– – mixed NEC	T50.9	X44	X64	Y14	Y58.8
– BCG	T50.9	X44	X64	Y14	Y58.0
– cholera	T50.9	X44	X64	Y14	Y58.2
– diphtheria	T50.9	X44	X64	Y14	Y58.5
– – with tetanus	T50.9	X44	X64	Y14	Y58.8
– – – and pertussis	T50.9	X44	X64	Y14	Y58.6
– influenza	T50.9	X44	X64	Y14	Y59.0
– measles	T50.9	X44	X64	Y14	Y59.0
– – with mumps and rubella	T50.9	X44	X64	Y14	Y59.0
– mixed, viral-rickettsial	T50.9	X44	X64	Y14	Y59.8
– mumps	T50.9	X44	X64	Y14	Y59.0
– pertussis	T50.9	X44	X64	Y14	Y58.6
– – with diphtheria	T50.9	X44	X64	Y14	Y58.6
– – – and tetanus	T50.9	X44	X64	Y14	Y58.6
– plague	T50.9	X44	X64	Y14	Y58.3
– poliomyelitis	T50.9	X44	X64	Y14	Y59.0
– protozoal	T50.9	X44	X64	Y14	Y59.2
– rabies	T50.9	X44	X64	Y14	Y59.0
– rickettsial NEC	T50.9	X44	X64	Y14	Y59.1
– Rocky Mountain spotted fever	T50.9	X44	X64	Y14	Y59.1
– rubella	T50.9	X44	X64	Y14	Y59.0
– smallpox	T50.9	X44	X64	Y14	Y59.0
– TAB	T50.9	X44	X64	Y14	Y58.1
– tetanus	T50.9	X44	X64	Y14	Y58.4
– typhoid	T50.9	X44	X64	Y14	Y58.1
– typhus	T50.9	X44	X64	Y14	Y59.1
– viral NEC	T50.9	X44	X64	Y14	Y59.0
– yellow fever	T50.9	X44	X64	Y14	Y59.0
Vaccinia immune globulin	T50.9	X44	X64	Y14	Y59.3
Valerian					
– root	T42.6	X41	X61	Y11	Y47.8
– tincture	T42.6	X41	X61	Y11	Y47.8
Valethamate bromide	T44.3	X43	X63	Y13	Y51.3
Valnoctamide	T42.6	X41	X61	Y11	Y47.8
Valproate (sodium)	T42.6	X41	X61	Y11	Y46.5
Valproic acid	T42.6	X41	X61	Y11	Y46.5
Valpromide	T42.6	X41	X61	Y11	Y46.5
Vanadium	T56.8	X49	X69	Y19	
Vancomycin	T36.8	X44	X64	Y14	Y40.8

| Substance | Chapter XIX | Poisoning | | | Adverse effect in therapeutic use |
		Accidental	Intentional self-harm	Undetermined intent	
Vapor (*see also* Gas)	T59.9	X47	X67	Y17	
– kiln (carbon monoxide)	T58	X47	X67	Y17	
– lead – *see* Lead					
– specified source NEC	T59.8	X47	X67	Y17	
Vardenafil	T46.7	X44	X64	Y14	Y52.7
Varicose reduction drug	T46.8	X44	X64	Y14	Y52.8
Varnish	T65.4	X49	X69	Y19	
Vasodilator					
– coronary NEC	T46.3	X44	X64	Y14	Y52.3
– peripheral NEC	T46.7	X44	X64	Y14	Y52.7
Vasopressin	T38.8	X44	X64	Y14	Y42.8
Vecuronium bromide	T48.1	X44	X64	Y14	Y55.1
Vegetable extract, astringent	T49.2	X44	X64	Y14	Y56.2
Venom (centipede) (insect) (reptile) (snake)	T63.9				
Venous sclerosing drug NEC	T46.8	X44	X64	Y14	Y52.8
Verapamil	T46.1	X44	X64	Y14	Y52.1
Veratrum alkaloid, veratrine	T46.5	X44	X64	Y14	Y52.5
Verdigris	T60.3	X48	X68	Y18	
Versenate	T50.6	X44	X64	Y14	Y57.2
Vetrabutine	T48.0	X44	X64	Y14	Y55.0
Vidarabine	T37.5	X44	X64	Y14	Y41.5
Vienna					
– green	T57.0	X49	X69	Y19	
– – insecticide	T60.2	X48	X68	Y18	
– red	T57.0	X49	X69	Y19	
Vigabatrin	T42.6	X41	X61	Y11	Y46.6
Viloxazine	T43.2	X41	X61	Y11	Y49.2
Viminol	T39.8	X40	X60	Y10	Y45.8
Vinblastine	T45.1	X44	X64	Y14	Y43.3
Vinburnine	T46.7	X44	X64	Y14	Y52.7
Vincamine	T45.1	X44	X64	Y14	Y43.3
Vincristine	T45.1	X44	X64	Y14	Y43.3
Vindesine	T45.1	X44	X64	Y14	Y43.3
Vinorelbine tartrate	T45.1	X44	X64	Y14	Y43.3
Vinpocetine	T46.7	X44	X64	Y14	Y52.7
Vinyl					
– acetate	T65.8	X49	X69	Y19	
– bromide	T65.8	X47	X67	Y17	
– chloride	T59.8	X47	X67	Y17	
– ether	T41.0	X44	X64	Y14	Y48.0
Vinylbital	T42.3	X41	X61	Y11	Y47.0
Vinylidene chloride	T65.8	X49	X69	Y19	
Viomycin	T36.8	X44	X64	Y14	Y40.8
Viprynium	T37.4	X44	X64	Y14	Y41.4
Viquidil	T46.7	X44	X64	Y14	Y52.7
Viral vaccine NEC	T50.9	X44	X64	Y14	Y59.0
Virginiamycin	T36.8	X44	X64	Y14	Y40.8
Viscous agent	T50.9	X44	X64	Y14	Y57.4
Visnadine	T46.3	X44	X64	Y14	Y52.3

| Substance | Chapter XIX | Poisoning | | | Adverse effect in therapeutic use |
		Accidental	Intentional self-harm	Undetermined intent	
Vitamin NEC	T45.2	X44	X64	Y14	Y57.7
– A	T45.2	X44	X64	Y14	Y57.7
– B NEC	T45.2	X44	X64	Y14	Y57.7
– – nicotinic acid	T46.7	X44	X64	Y14	Y52.7
B$_1$	T45.2	X44	X64	Y14	Y57.7
– B$_2$	T45.2	X44	X64	Y14	Y57.7
– B$_6$	T45.2	X44	X64	Y14	Y57.7
– B$_{12}$	T45.2	X44	X64	Y14	Y44.1
– B$_{15}$	T45.2	X44	X64	Y14	Y57.7
– C	T45.2	X44	X64	Y14	Y57.7
– D	T45.2	X44	X64	Y14	Y54.7
– D$_2$	T45.2	X44	X64	Y14	Y54.7
– D$_3$	T45.2	X44	X64	Y14	Y54.7
– E	T45.2	X44	X64	Y14	Y57.7
– E acetate	T45.2	X44	X64	Y14	Y57.7
– K NEC	T45.7	X44	X64	Y14	Y44.3
– K$_1$	T45.7	X44	X64	Y14	Y44.3
– K$_2$	T45.7	X44	X64	Y14	Y44.3
– PP	T45.2	X44	X64	Y14	Y57.7
– ulceroprotectant	T47.1	X44	X64	Y14	Y53.1

W

Substance	Chapter XIX	Poisoning			Adverse effect in therapeutic use
		Accidental	Intentional self-harm	Undetermined intent	
Warfarin	T45.5	X44	X64	Y14	Y44.2
– rodenticide	T60.4	X48	X68	Y18	
– sodium	T60.4	X48	X68	Y18	
Water					
– balance drug	T50.3	X44	X64	Y14	Y54.6
– distilled	T50.3	X44	X64	Y14	Y54.6
– gas	T58	X47	X67	Y17	
– purified	T50.3	X44	X64	Y14	Y54.6
Wax (paraffin) (petroleum)	T52.0	X46	X66	Y16	
– automobile	T65.8	X49	X69	Y19	
White					
– arsenic	T57.0	X48	X68	Y18	
– spirit	T52.0	X46	X66	Y16	
Whitewash	T65.8	X49	X69	Y19	
Whole blood (human)	T45.8	X44	X64	Y14	Y44.6
Wisterine	T62.2	X49	X69	Y19	
Wood alcohol or spirit	T51.1	X45	X65	Y15	
Wood preservatives	T60.9	X48	X68	Y18	
Wool fat (hydrous)	T49.3	X44	X64	Y14	Y56.3

X

Substance	Chapter XIX	Poisoning			Adverse effect in therapeutic use
		Accidental	Intentional self-harm	Undetermined intent	
Xamoterol	T44.5	X43	X63	Y13	Y51.5
Xanthinol nicotinate	T46.7	X44	X64	Y14	Y52.7
Xantinol nicotinate	T46.7	X44	X64	Y14	Y52.7
Xantocillin	T36.0	X44	X64	Y14	Y40.0
Xenon (^{127}Xe) (^{133}Xe)	T50.8	X44	X64	Y14	Y57.6
Xenysalate	T49.4	X44	X64	Y14	Y56.4
Xibornol	T37.8	X44	X64	Y14	Y41.8
Xipamide	T50.2	X44	X64	Y14	Y54.5
Xylene (vapor)	T52.2	X46	X66	Y16	
Xylol (vapor)	T52.2	X46	X66	Y16	
Xylometazoline	T48.5	X44	X64	Y14	Y55.5

Y

| Substance | Chapter XIX | Poisoning | | | Adverse effect in therapeutic use |
		Accidental	Intentional self-harm	Undetermined intent	
Yeast	T45.2	X44	X64	Y14	Y57.7
– dried	T45.2	X44	X64	Y14	Y57.7
Yellow					
– fever vaccine	T50.9	X44	X64	Y14	Y59.0
– phenolphthalein	T47.2	X44	X64	Y14	Y53.2
Yew	T62.2	X49	X69	Y19	
Yohimbic acid	T40.9	X42	X62	Y12	Y49.6

Z

Substance	Poisoning				Adverse effect in therapeutic use
	Chapter XIX	Accidental	Intentional self-harm	Undetermined intent	
Zalcitabine	T37.5	X44	X64	Y14	Y41.5
Zeranol	T38.7	X44	X64	Y14	Y42.7
Zidovudine	T37.5	X44	X64	Y14	Y41.5
Zimeldine	T43.2	X41	X61	Y11	Y49.2
Zinc (compounds) (fumes) (vapor) NEC	T56.5	X49	X69	Y19	
− chloride (mouthwash)	T49.6	X44	X64	Y14	Y56.6
− chromate	T56.5	X49	X69	Y19	
− oxide	T49.3	X44	X64	Y14	Y56.3
− − plaster	T49.3	X44	X64	Y14	Y56.3
− phosphide	T60.4	X48	X68	Y18	
− pyrithionate	T49.4	X44	X64	Y14	Y56.4
− stearate	T49.3	X44	X64	Y14	Y56.3
− sulfate	T49.5	X44	X64	Y14	Y56.5
Zineb	T60.0	X48	X68	Y18	
Zinostatin	T45.1	X44	X64	Y14	Y43.3
Zipeprol	T48.3	X44	X64	Y14	Y55.3
Zofenopril	T46.4	X44	X64	Y14	Y52.4
Zolpidem	T42.6	X41	X61	Y11	Y47.8
Zomepirac	T39.3	X40	X60	Y10	Y45.3
Zopiclone	T42.6	X41	X61	Y11	Y47.8
Zorubicin	T45.1	X44	X64	Y14	Y43.3
Zotepine	T43.5	X41	X61	Y11	Y49.5
Zuclopenthixol	T43.4	X41	X61	Y11	Y49.4

Maternity Coding lead terms for Indexing

Condition - In Pregnancy
        o/ Complicating pregnancy

Pregnancy - Complicated by
        - Management affected by

Labour -

Presentation

Delivery

Laceration - (perineal tears in delivery)

Maternal Care for

Puerperium

Z37. -   Outcome of delivery